Modern Concepts and Practices in Cardiothoracic Critical Care

Adam S. Evans
Icahn School of Medicine at Mount Sinai, USA

Gregory E. Kerr
Weill Cornell Medical College, USA

Insung Chung
Icahn School of Medicine at Mount Sinai, USA

Robin Varghese
Icahn School of Medicine at Mount Sinai, USA

A volume in the Advances in Medical Technologies and Clinical Practice (AMTCP) Book Series

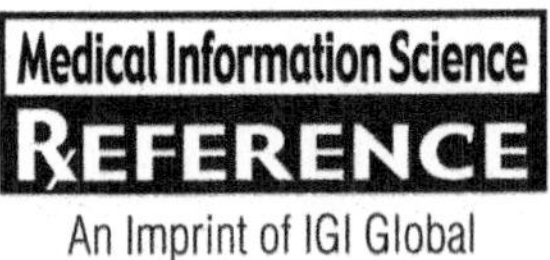

Managing Director:	Lindsay Johnston
Managing Editor:	Austin DeMarco
Director of Intellectual Property & Contracts:	Jan Travers
Acquisitions Editor:	Kayla Wolfe
Production Editor:	Christina Henning
Development Editor:	Caitlyn Martin
Typesetter:	Lisandro Gonzalez
Cover Design:	Jason Mull

Published in the United States of America by
Medical Information Science Reference (an imprint of IGI Global)
701 E. Chocolate Avenue
Hershey PA, USA 17033
Tel: 717-533-8845
Fax: 717-533-8661
E-mail: cust@igi-global.com
Web site: http://www.igi-global.com

Library of Congress Cataloging-in-Publication Data

Modern concepts and practices in cardiothoracic critical care / Adam S. Evans, Gregory E. Kerr, Insung Chiung, and Robin Varghese, editors.
pages cm
Includes bibliographical references and index.
ISBN 978-1-4666-8603-8 (hardcover) -- ISBN 978-1-4666-8604-5 (ebook) 1. Cardiac intensive care. I. Evans, Adam S., editor. II. Kerr, Gregory E., editor. III. Chiung, Insung, editor. IV. Varghese, Robin, editor.
RC684.C36M63 2015
616.1'2028--dc23

2015012069

This book is published in the IGI Global book series Advances in Medical Technologies and Clinical Practice (AMTCP) (ISSN: 2327-9354; eISSN: 2327-9370)

British Cataloguing in Publication Data
A Cataloguing in Publication record for this book is available from the British Library.

All work contributed to this book is new, previously-unpublished material. The views expressed in this book are those of the authors, but not necessarily of the publisher.

For electronic access to this publication, please contact: eresources@igi-global.com.

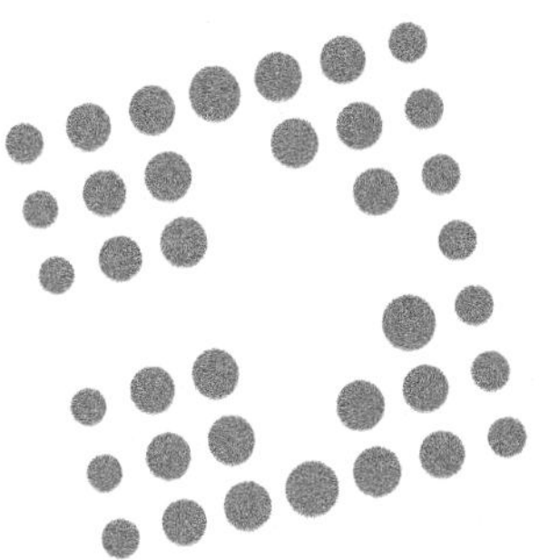

Advances in Medical Technologies and Clinical Practice (AMTCP) Book Series

Srikanta Patnaik
SOA University, India
Priti Das
S.C.B. Medical College, India

ISSN: 2327-9354
EISSN: 2327-9370

Mission

Medical technological innovation continues to provide avenues of research for faster and safer diagnosis and treatments for patients. Practitioners must stay up to date with these latest advancements to provide the best care for nursing and clinical practices.

The **Advances in Medical Technologies and Clinical Practice (AMTCP) Book Series** brings together the most recent research on the latest technology used in areas of nursing informatics, clinical technology, biomedicine, diagnostic technologies, and more. Researchers, students, and practitioners in this field will benefit from this fundamental coverage on the use of technology in clinical practices.

Coverage

- Neural Engineering
- Clinical Data Mining
- Biomedical Applications
- Telemedicine
- Medical Informatics
- Nutrition
- Nursing Informatics
- Biomechanics
- Clinical High-Performance Computing
- E-health

IGI Global is currently accepting manuscripts for publication within this series. To submit a proposal for a volume in this series, please contact our Acquisition Editors at Acquisitions@igi-global.com or visit: http://www.igi-global.com/publish/.

The Advances in Medical Technologies and Clinical Practice (AMTCP) Book Series (ISSN 2327-9354) is published by IGI Global, 701 E. Chocolate Avenue, Hershey, PA 17033-1240, USA, www.igi-global.com. This series is composed of titles available for purchase individually; each title is edited to be contextually exclusive from any other title within the series. For pricing and ordering information please visit http://www.igi-global.com/book-series/advances-medical-technologies-clinical-practice/73682. Postmaster: Send all address changes to above address.

Titles in this Series

For a list of additional titles in this series, please visit: www.igi-global.com

Recent Advances in Assistive Technologies to Support Children with Developmental Disorders
Nava R. Silton (Marymount Manhattan College, USA)
Medical Information Science Reference • copyright 2015 • 425pp • H/C (ISBN: 9781466683952) • US $210.00 (our price)

Advanced Technological Solutions for E-Health and Dementia Patient Monitoring
Fatos Xhafa (Universitat Politècnica de Catalunya, Spain) Philip Moore (School of Information Science and Engineering, Lanzhou University, China) and George Tadros (University of Warwick, UK)
Medical Information Science Reference • copyright 2015 • 389pp • H/C (ISBN: 9781466674813) • US $215.00 (our price)

Assistive Technologies for Physical and Cognitive Disabilities
Lau Bee Theng (Swinburne University of Technology, Malaysia)
Medical Information Science Reference • copyright 2015 • 321pp • H/C (ISBN: 9781466673731) • US $205.00 (our price)

Fuzzy Expert Systems for Disease Diagnosis
A.V. Senthil Kumar (Hindusthan College of Arts and Science, India)
Medical Information Science Reference • copyright 2015 • 401pp • H/C (ISBN: 9781466672406) • US $265.00 (our price)

Handbook of Research on Computerized Occlusal Analysis Technology Applications in Dental Medicine
Robert B. Kerstein, DMD (Former clinical professor at Tufts University School of Dental Medicine, USA & Private Dental Practice Limited to Prosthodontics and Computerized Occlusal Analysis, USA)
Medical Information Science Reference • copyright 2015 • 1093pp • H/C (ISBN: 9781466665873) • US $475.00 (our price)

Enhancing the Human Experience through Assistive Technologies and E-Accessibility
Christos Kouroupetroglou (Caretta-Net Technologies, Greece)
Medical Information Science Reference • copyright 2014 • 345pp • H/C (ISBN: 9781466661301) • US $265.00 (our price)

Applications, Challenges, and Advancements in Electromyography Signal Processing
Ganesh R. Naik (University of Technology Sydney (UTS), Australia)
Medical Information Science Reference • copyright 2014 • 404pp • H/C (ISBN: 9781466660908) • US $235.00 (our price)

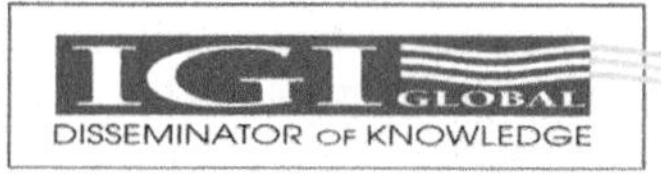

www.igi-global.com

701 E. Chocolate Ave., Hershey, PA 17033
Order online at www.igi-global.com or call 717-533-8845 x100
To place a standing order for titles released in this series, contact: cust@igi-global.com
Mon-Fri 8:00 am - 5:00 pm (est) or fax 24 hours a day 717-533-8661

To my wife Leslie, sons Jack and Max, and my parents Beth and Barry for their unwavering support. To my mentors who encouraged me to challenge the status quo-A.S.E

To my late parents for their support, inspiration and unconditional love-G.E.K.

All praise and glory to my Lord and Savior Jesus Christ. To Mina, my loving wife. To Emma, Toby and Micah who make me so proud to be their father. To my parents B.K. and Sung Ja for their unconditional love-I.C.

To my lovely wife Sarah and children Naaman, Matthew and Amelia, to my mother and late father whose love and guidance was immeasurable, and finally I thank God who is the foundation of my life-R.V.

List of Reviewers

Himani Bhatt, *Icahn School of Medicine at Mount Sinai, USA*
June Chan, *Weill Cornell Medical College, USA*
Leila Hosseinian, *Icahn School of Medicine at Mount Sinai, USA*
Koichi Nomoto, *Icahn School of Medicine at Mount Sinai, USA*
Cesar Rodriguez-Diaz, *Icahn School of Medicine at Mount Sinai, USA*
Benjamin Salter, *Icahn School of Medicine at Mount Sinai, USA*
Menachem Weiner, *Icahn School of Medicine at Mount Sinai, USA*

Table of Contents

Section 2
Preoperative Assessment and Optimization

Section 3
Pharmacology in the Cardiothoracic ICU

Section 4
A Systematic Approach to Cardiothoracic Critical Care

Section 5
Surgical Techniques and Postoperative Concerns

Section 6
Monitoring the Postoperative Cardiac Patient

Detailed Table of Contents

Section 1
Introduction to Care of the Cardiac Surgical Patient

While the timeline has been relatively abbreviated, there has been significant evolution in the field of cardiac surgery. These changes have been driven by a combination of operative innovation, changing patient demographics, and novel critical care resources, all of which have allowed today's surgeons to treat a myriad of conditions among increasingly higher risk patient cohorts. At the same time, this has forced providers to expand their clinical skill sets, embrace multidisciplinary collaboration, enhance postoperative care, and intensify the rigor by which outcomes and quality are being measured. In spite of this increasing complexity, however, mortality in cardiac surgery continues to improve. In this chapter, we highlight key historical events and describe an unprecedented trajectory and evolution in care practices that have helped shape modern cardiac surgery. We also make an appeal for additional research efforts which are needed to ensure sustained and innovative growth.

Quality improvement is a goal of all institutions but effective quality improvement programs have been difficult to create and sustain. Cardiac surgery has long been a pioneer in the quality improvement process through protocolization, large database analysis, and evidence based research. This chapter will discuss the theoretical foundation for quality improvement in medicine, and address current quality improvement strategies in the cardiothoracic ICU including care bundles, large database review, and externally promulgated quality programs such as the Surgical Care Improvement Project (SCIP) or the Physician Quality Reporting Initiative (PQRS). Controversies from national quality improvement programs including SCIP, extended staffing, and the value of quality culture will be discussed.

Education and training has been the cornerstone of medicine from the days of the Hippocratic oath. What began as an informal apprenticeship has become a standardized curriculum, with heavy influence from the education sciences, regulatory bodies and societal demands. As an area of rigorous study in its own right, physicians have a responsibility to understand education theory and their effective application in clinical practice in order to fulfill their professional obligations. This chapter will outline past and current education theory relevant to critical care practice; introduce ideas and suggestions to implement these theories, and present new and emerging paradigms that are set to change graduate medical education in the upcoming decades.

The purpose of this chapter is to emphasize and describe the team nature of critical care medicine in the Cardiothoracic Intensive Care Unit. The chapter will review the importance of various team members and discuss various staffing models (open vs closed, high intensity vs low intensity, etc.) on patient outcomes and cost. The chapter will also examine the roles of nurse practitioners and physician assistants (NP/PAs) in critical care, and will briefly review the growing role of the tele-ICU. Most studies support the concept that a multi-disciplinary ICU team, led by an intensivist, improves patient outcomes and decreases overall cost of care. The role of the tele-ICU and 24 hour in-house intensivist staffing in improving outcomes is controversial, and more research is needed in this area. Finally, a brief discussion of billing for critical care will be discussed.

Palliative care is a specialty of medicine that focuses on improving quality of life for patients with serious illness and their families. As the limitations of intensive care and the long-term sequelae of critical illness continue to be delimited, the role of palliative care for patients that are unable to achieve their original goals of care, as well as for survivors of critical illness, is changing and expanding. The purpose of this chapter is to introduce readers to the specialty of palliative care and its potential benefits for critically ill patients, and to present some of the issues related to the delivery of palliative care in surgical units.

In all areas of medicine physicians are confronted with a myriad ethical problems. It is important that intensivists are well versed on ethical issues that commonly arise in the critical care setting. This chapter will serve to provide a review of common topics, including informed consent, decision-making capacity, and surrogate decision-making. It will also highlight special circumstances related to cardiac surgical critical care, including ethical concerns associated with emerging technologies in cardiac care.

Acute coronary syndrome (ACS) is a common and sometimes lethal event, usually precipitated by sudden rupture and thrombosis of an atherosclerotic plaque. Patients presenting with ACS can be rapidly risk stratified based on signs, symptoms, electrocardiogram, and biomarkers. There is a new generation of potent and reliable antiplatelet drugs, which in concert with anticoagulation and rapid revascularization, can preserve myocardium and save lives. When choosing how to revascularize, hemodynamically stable patients with diabetes mellitus and complex coronary disease benefit more from coronary artery bypass grafting rather than percutaneous coronary intervention. Despite optimal treatment, ACS can result in deadly complications such as cardiogenic shock. Supportive care is paramount, but despite its widespread use, the utility of intraaortic balloon counterpulsation is uncertain. In the future, advanced coronary imaging may enhance preventative care, novel molecular targets will help expand treatment options, and cell-based regenerative therapies may aid myocardial recovery after acute coronary syndrome.

Valvular heart disease is a common cardiovascular disorder, with an estimated prevalence of 2.5% in the United States. The disease is particularly burdensome in adults over 75 years of age, with 13.3% having moderate to severe disease of the aortic or mitral valve. As populations grow older, diagnostic capabilities improve, and health care becomes more accessible, the number of patients with valvular heart disease undergoing both cardiac and non-cardiac surgery will continue to grow. The preoperative assessment and optimization of these patients is a complex task involving multiple specialists, including internists, cardiologists, intensivists, cardiothoracic surgeons, and anesthesiologists. As newer therapeutic options are offered to patients with numerous comorbidities, the preoperative management of these patients will require a sophisticated multimodal approach. The purpose of this chapter is to summarize the preoperative assessment and optimization of patients with valvular heart disease undergoing cardiac and non-cardiac surgery.

Advancements in the field of heart failure have significantly improved both mortality and the quality of life of millions. However, heart failure generally remains a chronic disease with an insidious progression to organ failure despite optimal medical treatment. Early consideration of advanced therapies such as mechanical circulatory support and cardiac transplantation in advanced heart failure is essential. The purpose of this chapter is to assist the reader in the identification of patients with advanced heart failure that have not yet developed irreversible end-organ dysfunction, as interventions in this narrow therapeutic window results in improved post-surgical outcomes.

Section 3
Pharmacology in the Cardiothoracic ICU

Arrhythmias, low cardiac output syndromes, and low blood pressure are commonly faced complications in the cardiothoracic surgery patient. In order to provide appropriate clinical management, one must identify underlying etiologies while recognizing and understanding available treatment options. The objective of this chapter is to review common agents utilized to manage arrhythmias and maintain hemodynamic stability following cardiac surgery. Mechanisms of action, key clinical pearls and relevant literature pertaining to each agent will be discussed.

There are multiple indications for anticoagulation in the cardiac surgery intensive care unit including cardiac valve replacement, mechanical circulatory pumps (ECMO and ventricular assist devices), deep vein thrombosis prophylaxis, treatment of heparin-induced thrombocytopenia, and treatment of other thrombotic conditions including pulmonary embolism. Anticoagulant medications broadly fall into two categories: antiplatelet drugs and inhibitors of protein clotting factors. In this chapter we will review anticoagulant medications, therapeutic drug monitoring, common indications for anticoagulation, and the risks associated with anticoagulation after cardiac surgery.

Patients in the cardiothoracic intensive care unit (CTICU) are subject to numerous physical and mental stresses. While most of these cannot be completely eliminated, intensivists have many tools in their armamentarium to alleviate patients' pain and suffering. This chapter will consider the importance of analgesia and sedation in the CTICU and the relevant consequences of over- or under-treatment. We will examine the tools available for monitoring and titrating analgesia and sedation in critically ill patients. The major classes of medications available will be reviewed, with particular attention to their clinical

This chapter addresses underlying physiology, diagnostics, and management of common cardiovascular abnormalities in the patient after cardiac surgery. The goal is to provide insights into daily management, areas of controversy, and future directions in the field. After reviewing basic physiologic principles of cardiac output and circulation; problems affecting the postoperative hemodynamic state will be addressed individually. Specific topics include the low cardiac output syndrome, right ventricular failure, myocardial ischemia, diastolic dysfunction, vasodilatory syndrome, rhythm disturbances, pericardial tamponade, and cardiac arrest. Patients with postoperative open chests, or after orthotopic heart transplantation are also discussed.

The primary goal of this chapter is to provide the reader with an overview of basic renal physiology and function and to review the identification, pathogenesis, and treatment of acute kidney injury following cardiac surgery. Particular focus will be directed toward the diagnostic criteria for acute kidney injury, short- and long-term impacts on patient outcomes, role of novel biomarkers, mechanisms of acute renal injury, general management principles, preventative strategies, and the influence of anesthetic and surgical techniques on its development. The content of this chapter will serve to underscore a particularly harmful but likely underappreciated problem affecting patients in the cardiothoracic critical care setting.

A thorough understanding of gastrointestinal issues in critical illness is necessary to optimize management of the cardiothoracic patient. Post-operatively, these patients are at increased risk of GI complications due a combination of underlying vascular disease, cardiopulmonary bypass, and low cardiac output, all of which lead to splanchnic hypoperfusion and subsequent damage to the gut mucosa. While GI complications are uncommon, they are associated with a disproportionately high rate of morbidity and mortality. Presence of unexplained fever, leukocytosis, bacteremia, hemodynamic compromise or abdominal pain or distention are concerning and require prompt assessment. Other GI management issues include delivery of adequate nutrition to counteract catabolism and promote wound healing and stress ulcer prophylaxis in patients with risk factors for upper gastrointestinal bleeding.

Infections are a major cause of mortality in intensive care unit (ICU) patients and the most common non-cardiac complications after cardiac surgery. Commonly encountered infections in the cardiothoracic ICU include pneumonia, bloodstream infections, and surgical site infections. At the beginning of this chapter, general measures of infection control and prevention are introduced. Those can help reduce infections and are best implemented in a bundled care fashion. Specifically for ICU patients, care bundles aimed at ventilator-associated pneumonia and central line-associated bloodstream infection have been successfully implemented, studied, and revised. In the next section, antibiotic treatment principles are described. Treatment with antibiotic drugs is an important part of therapy for infectious complications and is under continuous revision given the changing and diverse spectrum of microorganisms and the emergence of multidrug-resistance. In the central part of the chapter, specific infections are discussed in detail with regards to etiology, incidence, diagnosis, and therapy. Finally, the concept of systemic inflammatory response is described which is a common clinical problem after cardiac surgery, particularly with the use of cardiopulmonary bypass. Several immunologic mechanisms have been found to be associated with this and the clinical picture can be confused with sepsis.

The cardiac perioperative period presents a unique clinical scenario where the risk of life-threatening hemorrhage is balanced against the risk of thrombosis. Management practices are in a continual flux as practitioners respond to evidence showing the serious harms independently associated with anemia, bleeding and transfusion of blood (Ranucci, Aronson, et al., 2011a). Despite comprehensive transfusion guideline recommendations rates of blood transfusion range from 7.8% to 92.8% across US hospitals (Bennett-Guerrero et al., 2010). In this chapter we navigate the complex hemostasis and transfusion issues in cardiac surgery to provide clinicians a comprehensive understanding of the coagulation system in this specialized population. We emphasize a multidisciplinary team approach focused on risk stratification with preoperative optimization to minimize coagulopathy and bleeding followed by a tailored and conservative use of blood products for maximum patient benefit.

In this chapter, we review several important endocrine disorders frequently encountered in patients undergoing cardiothoracic surgery. Hyperglycemia, common in patients with and without diabetes mellitus (DM) in the perioperative period, has been linked to poor outcomes. Use of an intravenous insulin infusion early in the postoperative course, followed by transition to subcutaneous insulin, with maintenance of moderate glycemic targets (100-180 mg/dL) is currently the standard of care. Oral intake should be encouraged in the postoperative period, but if not possible, nutrition support with enteral nutrition should be considered. Critical illness related corticosteroid insufficiency (CIRCI) should be suspected in critically ill patients with refractory hypotension requiring vasopressors, especially in the setting of septic shock. Although diagnositic criteria are controversial, if suspected, empiric treatment with corticosteroids should be initiated. Nonthyroidal illness syndrome (NTIS) is common in critically ill patients and thyroid function tests should be interpreted with caution in this population.

Section 5
Surgical Techniques and Postoperative Concerns

Coronary artery bypass grafting (CABG), first introduced in 1968, is now one of the most common surgical procedures and the most common cardiac procedures worldwide. It is estimated that over 800,000 CABG surgeries are performed worldwide each year. The goals of CABG are to reduce mortality, prevent the progress of heart failure and reduce symptoms associated with coronary artery disease. This chapter deals with cardiac critical care issues that pertain to the patient undergoing CABG and potential post-operative complications.

Broadly speaking, pathology is categorized as being primarily related to valvular stenosis (AS) or regurgitation (AR), but a diseased valve may often exhibit both. The predilection of degenerative disease of the aortic valve, particularly stenosis, for the elderly has resulted in a steadily increasing prevalence as the population ages. As general life expectancy increases in the United States and other western countries, surgery to correct aortic valve disease will increase. As more elderly patients with more comorbidities present for surgery their intraoperative and perioperative care will become more complex. This chapter discusses ways for the practicing intensivist to facilitate identification and treatment in the immediate peri-operative period.

Surgery for the mitral valve has increased over the last decade, with a focus on an increasing number of valve repairs for degenerative mitral valve disease. This chapter discusses the surgical management of mitral valve disease with a focus on the pathology of mitral valve stenosis and regurgitation. With an examination into the pathophysiology of the lesions. Subsequently a discussion regarding the various surgical techniques for mitral valve surgery followed by the major and minor complications of surgery are reviewed to provide the Intensivist with an overview of possible complications. Finally a look at the future direction of the field is briefly examined.

Thoracic aortic disease most commonly presents in the form of aneurysmal dilation or dissection of the ascending or descending thoracic aorta, most commonly secondary to degenerative disease and hypertension. Several genetic connective tissue disorders are commonly associated as well. Treatment is focused on blood pressure control and surgical repair. Surgical repair of thoracic aortic disease presents unique risks, including neurologic injury involving the brain or spinal cord, and several adjuncts are available to mitigate against this risk. This chapter discusses commonly associated risk factors, preoperative testing, surgical repair, and postoperative management of thoracic aortic disease along with strategies for minimizing neurologic injury.

Orthotopic heart transplantation (OHT) has evolved as the "gold standard" therapy for end stage cardiomyopathy, Advances in the fields of immunosuppression, infection prophylaxis and treatment, surgical techniques as well as intensice care management have transformed heart transplantation from what was once considered an experimental intervention into a standard therapy. This chapter focuses on the standard care for OHT including surgical techniques, perioperative management and management of common postoperative complications.

Lung transplantation is a widely accepted surgical procedure for treatment of select patients suffering from end-stage lung disease. Recipients, however, require meticulous post-transplant care to preserve allograft lung function and to ensure optimal patient quality of life. In the post-operative period, these patients are predisposed to specific complications and pose unique considerations that clinicians caring for these patients in the intensive care setting should be familiar with managing. This chapter focuses on the early post-operative critical care management of the lung transplant recipient with specific emphasis on hemodynamic resuscitation; early lung graft dysfunction; and considerations regarding immunosuppression and infection. Non-pulmonary issues that affect the clinical care of these patients in the ICU setting are also discussed.

An increasingly important component of the therapeutic armamentarium in the treatment of cardiac and cardiopulmonary pathology, utilization of mechanical circulatory support allows clinicians to help sicker patients with more advanced disease states. A plethora of options exist, each with multiple implant techniques and management strategies. To optimize patient care in a cost-conscious environment, one must understand the advantages and disadvantages of each permutation, and have an algorithmic approach for the selection and application of available technologies. This chapter aims to provide such an understanding by reviewing surgical implant techniques and peri-operative management strategies for a number of commonly used short-term and durable devices.

Patients having major general thoracic surgery constitute an integral part of any cardiothoracic intensive care unit. Pulmonary or esophageal resection especially in a patient who has cardiopulmonary issues at baseline demands close monitoring by a critical care team postoperatively. This chapter aims to cover the important aspects of the perioperative care involved with these patients. In addition, procedures requiring an intensive care unit postoeratively such as, pneumonectomy, esophagectomy, thymectomy are dealt with in some detail where key technical aspects and care and complications specific to each are discussed.

This chapter will provide a review of modern concepts of cardiovascular monitoring with emphasis on essential hemodynamic variables in the early post cardiac surgery patient. When defining circulatory function, importance of the entire circulatory system is underscored. This includes the function and interaction of the heart, blood vessels and circulatory blood volume to deliver sufficient amount of oxygenated blood to tissue beds. In post cardiac surgery patients, the pulmonary artery catheter remains the most widely used technology to assess cardiac function. This chapter highlights the importance of validation of less invasive and noninvasive hemodynamic monitors for the management of critically ill patients and early post cardiac surgery patients. In addition, this chapter describes the evolution of monitoring of post cardiac surgery and critically ill patients, examines different monitoring technologies and address controversial questions in modern practice as well as future directions.

Bleeding in the postoperative cardiac surgical patient can be multifactorial. This chapter examines the preoperative and intraoperative risk factors for having significant postoperative bleeding. It also discuss the advantages and disadvantages of standard laboratory testing as well as point-of-care tests, such as thromboelastography (TEG) and thromboelastometry (ROTEM), in their diagnostic capabilities. Finally, we conclude with different treatment strategies in this challenging patient population along with diagnostic criteria of clinically significant postoperative bleeding and when to return to the operating room for re-exploration.

Sonography in the intensive care unit is a rapidly emerging point-of-care diagnostic tool. Literature supports the use of sonography for the evaluation of lung pathology, protocol based focused cardiac evaluation, and abdominal pathology, as well as identifying deep venous thrombosis. There is also evidence that ultrasound guided procedures such as venous access, thoracentesis, and paracentesis may decrease complications compared to a landmark based technique. However, there is ambiguity in the literature regarding definition, scope, and training in this modality as used by intensivists. The purpose of this chapter is to provide a broad overview of the role of ultrasound in the ICU and data supporting the use of point-of-care protocols. This chapter does not provide instruction on how to perform a complete transthoracic or transesophageal exam, nor does it provide a library of images of various pathologies since a reader seeking such depth would be better served by a full textbook on echocardiography.

Foreword

It is indeed a privilege to write a foreword to this comprehensive textbook on the care of the postoperative patient in the cardiothoracic intensive care unit (CTICU). Perioperative cardiac care has been a focus of my professional life for more than 40 years. In 1967, as a third year student at the University of Cape Town in South Africa, I and my classmates admired the extraordinary achievement of our Professor of Cardiac Surgery, Christiaan Barnard, in performing the world's first successful heart transplant. Ten years later, as a Fellow in Critical Care Medicine and Cardiac Anesthesiology at Stanford University, I provided anesthesia for the great Norman Shumway, a fierce competitor of Dr. Barnard's, who lost no time in telling me what he thought of my origins! Despite their differences, these two extraordinary figures had in common their pioneering spirit and ability to perform all types of cardiac surgery on adults, infants and neonates alike. What they also had in common was their strong belief that the cardiac surgeon is "Captain of the Ship" and should take sole responsibility for patient care after surgery.

Over the last three decades, the milieu of cardiothoracic surgery has dramatically altered. The quantity and intricacy of cardiac surgical procedures - as well as the technical complexity of the support provided - have increased exponentially. Patients are older, sicker, and those coming to surgery have considerably more co-morbidity than in the past. Cardiothoracic surgeons have become more subspecialized, while the number being trained is declining. Today, most cardiothoracic surgeons recognize that postoperative care is a "team sport", and that good patient outcome depends on an integrated, multidisciplinary approach. This has driven the development of the subspecialty of cardiothoracic critical care, provided by surgeons or anesthesiologists who have trained in critical care medicine, and whose knowledge and experience is reflected in this outstanding textbook.

The spectrum of cardiothoracic surgery has also increased extraordinarily. The past two decades have witnessed a drive toward minimal invasiveness, characterized by procedures such as off-pump coronary artery bypass grafting (OPCAB), robotic cardiac surgery, and transcatheter aortic valve replacement (TAVR). At the other extreme is the expanding capability for cardiovascular intervention in the patient with life-threatening acute or chronic heart failure, built upon the progression through a short-, medium- or long-term ventricular assist device (VAD) as a bridge to recovery, decision or transplant, or as destination therapy. The miniaturization of the pump oxygenator has facilitated emergent institution of extracorporeal membrane oxygenation (ECMO), and has revolutionized acute cardiovascular and pulmonary salvage and resuscitation.

As a consequence, the staff of the CTICU has to deal with a number of "tracks" of patient care. Patients without substantial comorbidity who undergo uncomplicated coronary revascularization or a single valve repair or replacement are candidates for the "fast track". This usually requires an overnight stay in the ICU only, and much of the care can be protocol driven. A middle group of patients may undergo the procedures listed above, but have substantial comorbidity, or may undergo more complex procedures such as combined valve replacement and coronary revascularization. These patients may spend several days in the ICU, or much longer if they have had perioperative complications. The third - and most challenging - group of patients undergo major, complex surgical procedures, such as mechanical circulatory support (MCS), heart or lung transplantation, or pulmonary thrombo-endarterectomy (PTE). Add to this any patient who has a catastrophic complication in the operating room requiring ECMO. Some of these patients may spend weeks in the CTICU before recovery.

The postoperative outcome of all groups of patients – but especially the latter two - is dependent on the teamwork and mutual interaction of the cardiac surgeon, cardiologist, the CTICU nursing staff, therapists (respiratory, physical and occupational), consultants in nephrology, infectious disease, gastroenterology etc., and the palliative care team. At the center of all this stands the cardiothoracic intensivist, leader of the group of physicians who not only provide 24/7 care of the patient, but also coordinate the inputs coming from so many sources.

This timely contribution to our management of the patient undergoing cardiothoracic surgery is aptly entitled "Modern Concepts and Practices", because it truly represents the multidisciplinary team approach that is essential to assuring good patient outcomes. Its contributors represent a wide constellation of specialties and subspecialties, including cardiac anesthesiologists, intensivists and cardiac surgeons from major centers throughout the United States and Canada. It address every aspect of perioperative care: the structure and function of the CTICU; preoperative assessment and optimization of cardiac surgical patient; cardiothoracic pharmacology; the multiple body systems affected by cardiac surgery; the impact of various surgical techniques; and monitoring, echocardiography and ultrasound. It is essential reading for cardiac surgeons, cardiac anesthesiologists, intensivists, CTICU nurses and therapists - and indeed, anyone involved in the perioperative management of patients undergoing cardiothoracic surgery.

Robert N. Sladen
Columbia University Medical Center, USA

Preface

Welcome to the first edition of *Modern Concepts and Practices in Cardiothoracic Critical Care.* Over the past two decades there has been a dramatic increase in patients requiring intensive care services. With cardiovascular disease ranking near the top as the etiology for admission to the intensive care unit(ICU) and the demographic trend of an aging population with multiple co-morbidities(primarily cardiac) a need for specialized cardiovascular critical care has been established. Furthermore, there will be a need for specific well-trained cardiovascular intensivists to meet the needs of this patient population. Educational resources designed to provide the latest information regarding cardiothoracic critical care are essential.

This book is intended for the medical students, residents, fellows, intensivists, anesthesiologists, cardiac surgeons, nurses, physician assistants and pharmacists who all care for patients following cardiothoracic surgery. We have tried to strike a balance between explaining the basic tenets of caring for these patients while also presenting the latest research and current controversies regarding the specialized management of these patients. We are especially grateful to the team of nationally and internationally renowned experts in cardiology, intensive care, cardiac anesthesiology, cardiac surgery, and pharmaceutical care that have each contributed chapters. This emphasizes the multidisciplinary nature of caring for patients in the cardiothoracic intensive care unit as well as their commitment and recognition of this increasingly specialized and unique field of critical care.

The book is divided into six sections. Section I involves an introduction to care of the cardiac surgical population. Here the epidemiology of the evolving cardiac surgical population is reviewed along with issues surrounding quality and safety, management of a cardiothoracic intensive care unit and training to work in this sub-specialized environment. Chapters on ethics and palliative care also round out this section helping to provide a framework for decision making in this vulnerable population. Section II focuses on the preoperative assessment and optimization of patients prior to undergoing cardiothoracic surgery. Chapters on acute coronary syndromes, valvular heart disease, and heart failure are emphasized. Section III reviews the basic pharmacology utilized in the cardiothoracic intensive care unit with an emphasis on inotropes & pressors, anticoagulation, sedation and analgesia, and vasodilating agents. Section IV involves a systems approach to cardiothoracic critical care. Over eight chapters a detailed approach of each of the current clinical areas of focus on daily rounds are reviewed. Section V emphasizes specific surgical techniques and postoperative concerns. Written specifically by surgeons, these eight chapters attempt to explain the most common procedures performed and the surgeon's viewpoint on where the postoperative team should focus their efforts. Finally, Section VI discusses physiologic monitoring of the post-operative cardiac surgical patient. Current management of bleeding via point of care technology along with methods of invasive and non-invasive monitoring and the role of ultrasound and echocardiography are reviewed.

In chapter 1, Epidemiology, the authors highlight key historical events and describe an unprecedented trajectory and evolution in care practices that have helped shape modern cardiac surgery. They also make an appeal for additional research efforts which are needed to ensure sustained and innovative growth. While the timeline has been relatively abbreviated, there has been significant evolution in the field of cardiac surgery. These changes have been driven by a combination of operative innovation, changing patient demographics, and novel critical care resources, all of which have allowed today's surgeons to treat a myriad of conditions among increasingly higher risk patient cohorts. At the same time, this has forced providers to expand their clinical skill sets, embrace multidisciplinary collaboration, enhance postoperative care, and intensify the rigor by which outcomes and quality are being measured. In spite of this increasing complexity, however, mortality in cardiac surgery continues to improve.

Quality improvement is a goal of all institutions but effective quality improvement programs have been difficult to create and sustain. Cardiac surgery has long been a pioneer in the quality improvement process through protocolization, large database analysis, and evidence based research. In Chapter 2, Quality and Safety, the authors discuss the theoretical foundation for quality improvement in medicine, and address current quality improvement strategies in the cardiothoracic ICU including care bundles, large database review, and externally promulgated quality programs such as the Surgical Care Improvement Project (SCIP) or the Physician Quality Reporting Initiative (PQRS). Controversies from national quality improvement programs including SCIP, extended staffing, and the value of quality culture will be discussed.

Education and training has been the cornerstone of medicine from the days of the Hippocratic oath. What began as an informal apprenticeship has become a standardized curriculum, with heavy influence from the education sciences, regulatory bodies and societal demands. As an area of rigorous study in its own right, Physicians have a responsibility to understand education theory and their effective application in clinical practice in order to fulfill their professional obligations. Chapter 3, Education and Training, will outline past and current education theory relevant to critical care practice; introduce ideas and suggestions to implement these theories, and present new and emerging paradigms that are set to change graduate medical education in the upcoming decades.

In chapter 4, Organization and Structure of the CTICU, the authors emphasize and describe the team nature of critical care medicine in the Cardiothoracic Intensive Care Unit. The chapter will review the importance of various team members and discuss various staffing models (open vs closed, high intensity vs low intensity, etc.) on patient outcomes and cost. The chapter will also examine the roles of nurse practitioners and physician assistants (NP/PAs) in critical care, and will briefly review the growing role of the tele-ICU. Most studies support the concept that a multi-disciplinary ICU team, led by an intensivist, improves patient outcomes and decreases overall cost of care. The role of the tele-ICU and 24 hour in-house intensivist staffing in improving outcomes is controversial, and more research is needed in this area. Finally, a brief discussion of billing for critical care will be discussed.

The purpose of chapter 5, Palliative Care, is to introduce readers to the specialty of palliative care and its potential benefits for critically ill patients, and to present some of the issues related to the delivery of palliative care in surgical units. Palliative care is a specialty of medicine that focuses on improving quality of life for patients with serious illness and their families. As the limitations of intensive care and the long-term sequelae of critical illness continue to be delimited, the role of palliative care for patients that are unable to achieve their original goals of care, as well as for survivors of critical illness, is changing and expanding.

In all areas of medicine physicians are confronted with a myriad ethical problems. It is important that intensivists are well versed on ethical issues that commonly arise in the critical care setting. Chapter 6, Ethics, will serve to provide a review of common topics, including informed consent, decision-making capacity, and surrogate decision-making. It will also highlight special circumstances related to cardiac surgical critical care, including ethical concerns associated with emerging technologies in cardiac care.

As discussed in Chapter 7, Acute coronary syndrome (ACS) is a common and sometimes lethal event, usually precipitated by sudden rupture and thrombosis of an atherosclerotic plaque. Patients presenting with ACS can be rapidly risk stratified based on signs, symptoms, electrocardiogram, and biomarkers. There is a new generation of potent and reliable antiplatelet drugs, which in concert with anticoagulation and rapid revascularization, can preserve myocardium and save lives. When choosing how to revascularize, hemodynamically stable patients with diabetes mellitus and complex coronary disease benefit more from coronary artery bypass grafting rather than percutaneous coronary intervention. Despite optimal treatment, ACS can result in deadly complications such as cardiogenic shock. Supportive care is paramount, but despite its widespread use, the utility of intraaortic balloon counterpulsation is uncertain. In the future, advanced coronary imaging may enhance preventative care, novel molecular targets will help expand treatment options, and cell-based regenerative therapies may aid myocardial recovery after acute coronary syndrome.

Valvular heart disease is a common cardiovascular disorder, with an estimated prevalence of 2.5% in the United States. The disease is particularly burdensome in adults over 75 years of age, with 13.3% having moderate to severe disease of the aortic or mitral valve. As populations grow older, diagnostic capabilities improve, and health care becomes more accessible, the number of patients with valvular heart disease undergoing both cardiac and non-cardiac surgery will continue to grow. The preoperative assessment and optimization of these patients is a complex task involving multiple specialists, including internists, cardiologists, intensivists, cardiothoracic surgeons, and anesthesiologists. As newer therapeutic options are offered to patients with numerous comorbidities, the preoperative management of these patients will require a sophisticated multimodal approach. The purpose of chapter 8, Valvular Heart Disease, is to summarize the preoperative assessment and optimization of patients with valvular heart disease undergoing cardiac and non-cardiac surgery.

Advancements in the field of heart failure have significantly improved both mortality and the quality of life of millions. However, heart failure generally remains a chronic disease with an insidious progression to organ failure despite optimal medical treatment. Early consideration of advanced therapies such as mechanical circulatory support and cardiac transplantation in advanced heart failure is essential. The purpose of chapter 9, Heart Failure, is to assist the reader in the identification of patients with advanced heart failure that have not yet developed irreversible end-organ dysfunction, as interventions in this narrow therapeutic window results in improved post-surgical outcomes.

Arrhythmias, low cardiac output syndromes, and low blood pressure are commonly faced complications in the cardiothoracic surgery patient. In order to provide appropriate clinical management, one must identify underlying etiologies while recognizing and understanding available treatment options. The objective of chapter 10, Antiarrythmics & Inotropes, is to review common agents utilized to manage arrhythmias and maintain hemodynamic stability following cardiac surgery. Mechanisms of action, key clinical pearls and relevant literature pertaining to each agent will be discussed.

There are multiple indications for anticoagulation in the cardiac surgery intensive care unit including cardiac valve replacement, mechanical circulatory pumps (ECMO and ventricular assist devices), deep vein thrombosis prophylaxis, treatment of heparin-induced thrombocytopenia, and treatment of other thrombotic conditions including pulmonary embolism. Anticoagulant medications broadly fall into two categories: antiplatelet drugs and inhibitors of protein clotting factors. In chapter 11, Anticoagulation Options, the authors review anticoagulant medications, therapeutic drug monitoring, common indications for anticoagulation, and the risks associated with anticoagulation after cardiac surgery.

Patients in the cardiothoracic intensive care unit (CTICU) are subject to numerous physical and mental stresses. While most of these cannot be completely eliminated, intensivists have many tools in their armamentarium to alleviate patients' pain and suffering. Chapter 12, Sedation and Analgesia, will consider the importance of analgesia and sedation in the CTICU and the relevant consequences of over- or under-treatment. We will examine the tools available for monitoring and titrating analgesia and sedation in critically ill patients. The major classes of medications available will be reviewed, with particular attention to their clinical effects, metabolism and excretion, and hemodynamic characteristics. Lastly, experimental evidence will be assessed regarding the best strategies for treatment of pain and agitation in the CTICU, including use of non-pharmacologic adjuvants.

Chapter 13, Vasodilating Agents, discusses the salient features of arterial and venous dilating agents commonplace in the management of the post-cardiotomy surgical patient. A keen understanding of the underlying cellular mechanism, pharmacology, indication, safety profile, and controversies of clinical utility of vasodilating agents is imperative for routine use. The evidenced-based examination of each therapeutic modality will strengthen the practitioner's fund of knowledge for management of each pathophysiological state.

Chapter 14, Neurologic Complications in the Cardiac Surgery Patient, discusses the spectrum of complications that occur in the postoperative cardiac surgery patients. It evaluates the mechanistic role of cardiopulmonary bypass and the various cardiac surgical procedures in the development of cerebral injury. Furthermore, it evaluates the role of different intraoperative monitoring in early detection of cerebral injury in these patients. Finally, it provides evidence based practice guidelines for hemodynamic management as well as treatment of complications that are diagnosed in the cardiac surgical intensive care unit.

Clinicians caring for patients with cardio-pulmonary disease invariably must manage the respiratory system. Doing so requires a basic understanding of physiology and the interaction of the heart and lung. Chapter 15, Perioperative Respiratory Care and Complications, begins with rudimentary concepts of respiratory physiology, focusing on, gas exchange, pulmonary mechanics, and cardio-pulmonary interactions. These are used to develop an approach to mechanical ventilation and routine perioperative respiratory care of the patient having undergone a cardio-pulmonary procedure. The final section of this chapter addresses specific respiratory challenges encountered in caring for the critically ill cardiothoracic patient in addition to contemporary management strategies.

Chapter 16, Cardiovascular System addresses underlying physiology, diagnostics, and management of common cardiovascular abnormalities in the patient after cardiac surgery. The goal is to provide insights into daily management, areas of controversy, and future directions in the field. After reviewing basic physiologic principles of cardiac output and circulation; problems affecting the postoperative hemodynamic state will be addressed individually. Specific topics include the low cardiac output syndrome, right ventricular failure, myocardial ischemia, diastolic dysfunction, vasodilatory syndrome, rhythm disturbances, pericardial tamponade, and cardiac arrest. Patients with postoperative open chests, or after orthotopic heart transplantation are also discussed.

The primary goal of chapter 17, Renal, is to provide the reader with an overview of basic renal physiology and function and to review the identification, pathogenesis, and treatment of acute kidney injury following cardiac surgery. Particular focus will be directed toward the diagnostic criteria for acute kidney injury, short- and long-term impacts on patient outcomes, role of novel biomarkers, mechanisms of acute renal injury, general management principles, preventative strategies, and the influence of anesthetic and surgical techniques on its development. The content of this chapter will serve to underscore a particularly harmful but likely underappreciated problem affecting patients in the cardiothoracic critical care setting.

Chapter 18 is titled Gastrointestinal. A thorough understanding of gastrointestinal (GI) issues in critical illness is necessary to optimize management of the cardiothoracic patient. Post-operatively, these patients are at increased risk of GI complications due a combination of underlying vascular disease, cardiopulmonary bypass, and low cardiac output, all of which lead to splanchnic hypoperfusion and subsequent damage to the gut mucosa. While GI complications are uncommon, they are associated with a disproportionately high rate of morbidity and mortality. Presence of unexplained fever, leukocytosis, bacteremia, hemodynamic compromise or abdominal pain or distention are concerning and require prompt assessment. Other GI management issues include delivery of adequate nutrition to counteract catabolism and promote wound healing and stress ulcer prophylaxis in patients with risk factors for upper gastrointestinal bleeding.

Infections are a major cause of mortality in intensive care unit (ICU) patients and the most common non-cardiac complications after cardiac surgery. Commonly encountered infections in the cardiothoracic ICU include pneumonia, bloodstream infections, and surgical site infections. At the beginning of this chapter, general measures of infection control and prevention are introduced. Those can help reduce infections and are best implemented in a bundled care fashion. Specifically for ICU patients, care bundles aimed at ventilator-associated pneumonia and central line-associated bloodstream infection have been successfully implemented, studied, and revised. In the next section, antibiotic treatment principles are described. Treatment with antibiotic drugs is an important part of therapy for infectious complications and is under continuous revision given the changing and diverse spectrum of microorganisms and the emergence of multidrug-resistance. In the central part of chapter 19, Infection and Immune System, specific infections are discussed in detail with regards to etiology, incidence, diagnosis, and therapy. Finally, the concept of systemic inflammatory response is described which is a common clinical problem after cardiac surgery, particularly with the use of cardiopulmonary bypass. Several immunologic mechanisms have been found to be associated with this and the clinical picture can be confused with sepsis.

The cardiac perioperative period presents a unique clinical scenario where the risk of life-threatening hemorrhage is balanced against the risk of thrombosis. In chapter 20, Hematology and Transfusion, the authors navigate the complex hemostasis and transfusion issues in cardiac surgery to provide clinicians a comprehensive understanding of the coagulation system in this specialized population. Emphasis is placed on a multidisciplinary team approach focused on risk stratification with preoperative optimization to minimize coagulopathy and bleeding followed by a tailored and conservative use of blood products for maximum patient benefit.

In chapter 21, Endocrine, the authors review several important endocrine disorders frequently encountered in patients undergoing cardiothoracic surgery. Hyperglycemia, common in patients with and without diabetes mellitus (DM) in the perioperative period, has been linked to poor outcomes. Use of an intravenous insulin infusion early in the postoperative course, followed by transition to subcutaneous insulin, with maintenance of moderate glycemic targets (100-180 mg/dL) is currently the standard of care. Oral intake should be encouraged in the postoperative period, but if not possible, nutrition support with enteral nutrition should be considered. Critical illness related corticosteroid insufficiency (CIRCI) should be suspected in critically ill patients with refractory hypotension requiring vasopressors, especially in the setting of septic shock. Although diagnositic criteria are controversial, if suspected, empiric treatment with corticosteroids should be initiated. Nonthyroidal illness syndrome (NTIS) is common in critically ill patients and thyroid function tests should be interpreted with caution in this population.

Coronary artery bypass grafting (CABG) is one of the most common surgical procedures and the most common cardiac procedures worldwide. It is estimated that over 800,000 CABG surgeries are performed worldwide each year. CABG is a procedure in which one or more stenosed (or occluded) coronary arteries are bypassed with an alternate blood vessel conduit to re-establish normal blood flow to the myocardium. The goals of CABG are to reduce mortality, prevent the progress of heart failure and reduce symptoms associated with coronary artery disease. Chapter 22, Coronary Artery Disease deals with cardiac critical care issues that pertain to the patient undergoing CABG and potential post-operative complications.

Chapter 23, Aortic Valvular Disease discusses valvular stenosis (AS) or regurgitation (AR), but a diseased valve may often exhibit both. The predilection of degenerative disease of the aortic valve, particularly stenosis, for the elderly has resulted in a steadily increasing prevalence as the population ages. As general life expectancy increases in the United States and other western countries, surgery to correct aortic valve disease will increase. As more elderly patients with more comorbidities present for surgery their intraoperative and perioperative care will become more complex. In immediate peri-operative period to facilitate identification and treatment for the practicing intensivist.

Surgery for the mitral valve has increased over the last decade, with a focus on an increasing number of valve repairs for degenerative mitral valve disease. Chapter 24, Mitral Valvular Disease discusses the surgical management of mitral valve disease with a focus on the pathology of mitral valve stenosis and regurgitation. with an examination into the pathophysiology of the lesions. Subsequently a discussion regarding the various surgical techniques for mitral valve surgery followed by the major and minor complications of surgery are reviewed to provide the Intensivist with an overview of possible complications. Finally a look at the future direction of the field is briefly examined.

Thoracic aortic disease most commonly presents in the form of aneurysmal dilation or dissection of the ascending or descending thoracic aorta, most commonly secondary to degenerative disease and hypertension. Several genetic connective tissue disorders are commonly associated as well. Treatment is focused on blood pressure control and surgical repair. Surgical repair of thoracic aortic disease presents unique risks, including neurologic injury involving the brain or spinal cord, and several adjuncts are available to mitigate against this risk. Chapter 25, Thoracic Aorta discusses commonly associated risk factors, preoperative testing, surgical repair, and postoperative management of thoracic aortic disease along with strategies for minimizing neurologic injury.

Orthotopic heart transplantation (OHT) has evolved as the "gold standard" therapy for end stage cardiomyopathy, Advances in the fields of immunosuppression, infection prophylaxis and treatment, surgical techniques as well as intensice care management have transformed heart transplantation from what was once considered an experimental intervention into a standard therapy. Chapter 26, Heart Transplantation focuses on the standard care for OHT including surgical techniques, perioperative management and management of common postoperative complications.

Lung transplantation is a widely accepted surgical procedure for treatment of select patients suffering from end-stage lung disease. Recipients, however, require meticulous post-tranplant care to preserve allograft lung function and to ensure optimal patient quality of life. In the post-operative period, these patients are predisposed to specific complications and pose unique considerations that clinicians caring for these patients in the intensive care setting should be familiar with managing. Chapter 27, Lung Transplantation focuses on the early post-operative critical care management of the lung transplant recipient with specific emphasis on hemodynamic resuscitation; early lung graft dysfunction; and considerations regarding immunosuppression and infection. Non-pulmonary issues that affect the clinical care of these patients in the ICU setting are also discussed.

An increasingly important component of the therapeutic armamentarium in the treatment of cardiac and cardiopulmonary pathology, utilization of mechanical circulatory support allows clinicians to help sicker patients with more advanced disease states. A plethora of options exist, each with multiple implant techniques and management strategies. To optimize patient care in a cost-conscious environment, one must understand the advantages and disadvantages of each permutation, and have an algorithmic approach for the selection and application of available technologies. Chapter 28, Mechanical Circulatory Support aims to provide such an understanding by reviewing surgical implant techniques and peri-operative management strategies for a number of commonly used short-term and durable devices.

Patients having major general thoracic surgery constitute an integral part of any cardiothoracic intensive care unit. Pulmonary or esophageal resection especially in a patient who has cardiopulmonary issues at baseline demands close monitoring by a critical care team postoperatively. Chapter 29, Thoracic Surgery aims to cover the important aspects of the perioperative care involved with these patients. In addition, procedures requiring an intensive care unit postoeratively such as, pneumonectomy, esophagectomy, thymectomy are dealt with in some detail where key technical aspects and care and complications specific to each are discussed.

Chapter 30, Physiologic Monitoring will provide a review of modern concepts of cardiovascular monitoring with emphasis on essential hemodynamic variables in the early post cardiac surgery patient. When defining circulatory function, importance of the entire circulatory system is underscored. This includes the function and interaction of the heart, blood vessels and circulatory blood volume to deliver sufficient amount of oxygenated blood to tissue beds. In post cardiac surgery patients, the pulmonary artery catheter remains the most widely used technology to assess cardiac function. This chapter highlights the importance of validation of less invasive and noninvasive hemodynamic monitors for the management of critically ill patients and early post cardiac surgery patients. In addition, this chapter describes the evolution of monitoring of post cardiac surgery and critically ill patients, examines different monitoring technologies and address controversial questions in modern practice as well as future directions.

Bleeding in the postoperative cardiac surgical patient can be multifactorial. Chapter 31, Coagulation Monitoring examines the preoperative and intraoperative risk factors for having significant postoperative bleeding. It also discuss the advantages and disadvantages of standard laboratory testing as well as point-of-care tests, such as thromboelastography (TEG) and thromboelastometry (ROTEM), in their diagnostic capabilities. Finally, we conclude with different treatment strategies in this challenging patient population along with diagnostic criteria of clinically significant postoperative bleeding and when to return to the operating room for reexploration.

Sonography in the intensive care unit is a rapidly emerging point-of-care diagnostic tool. Literature supports the use of sonography for the evaluation of lung pathology, protocol based focused cardiac evaluation, and abdominal pathology, as well as identifying deep venous thrombosis. There is also evidence that ultrasound guided procedures such as venous access, thoracentesis, and paracentesis may decrease complications compared to a landmark based technique. However, there is ambiguity in the literature regarding definition, scope, and training in this modality as used by intensivists. The purpose of chapter 32, Echocardiography and Ultrasound in the Intensive Care unit is to provide a broad overview of the role of ultrasound in the ICU and data supporting the use of point-of-care protocols. This chapter does not provide instruction on how to perform a complete transthoracic or transesophageal exam, nor does it provide a library of images of various pathologies since a reader seeking such depth would be better served by a full textbook on echocardiography.

This book could not have come to fruition without the administrative assistance from Natalie Benjamin in the Department of Anesthesiology at Weill Cornell Medical College as well as the team at IGI publishing.

We hope you enjoy reading!

Adam S. Evans
Icahn School of Medicine at Mount Sinai, USA

Gregory E. Kerr
Weill Cornell Medical College, USA

Insung Chung
Icahn School of Medicine at Mount Sinai, USA

Robin Varghese
Icahn School of Medicine at Mount Sinai, USA

Section 1

Introduction to Care of the Cardiac Surgical Patient

Chapter 1
Epidemiology of Cardiac Surgery and the Cardiac Surgical Patient

Jason Neil Katz
University of North Carolina, USA

Edward J. Sawey
University of North Carolina, USA

ABSTRACT

While the timeline has been relatively abbreviated, there has been significant evolution in the field of cardiac surgery. These changes have been driven by a combination of operative innovation, changing patient demographics, and novel critical care resources, all of which have allowed today's surgeons to treat a myriad of conditions among increasingly higher risk patient cohorts. At the same time, this has forced providers to expand their clinical skill sets, embrace multidisciplinary collaboration, enhance postoperative care, and intensify the rigor by which outcomes and quality are being measured. In spite of this increasing complexity, however, mortality in cardiac surgery continues to improve. In this chapter, we highlight key historical events and describe an unprecedented trajectory and evolution in care practices that have helped shape modern cardiac surgery. We also make an appeal for additional research efforts which are needed to ensure sustained and innovative growth.

INTRODUCTION

There has been remarkable growth in the field of cardiac surgery, driven largely by transformative technological advancement and changing patient characteristics. Buttressed by an evolving evidence-base focusing not only on operative outcomes but also on the provision of cost-effective care, cardiac surgery today is vastly different than ever before. Increased utilization of hybrid therapies, multidisciplinary partnerships, and interventions for the extremely high-risk patient are all now commonplace. In addition, the contemporary care of the cardiac surgical patient is no longer isolated to the operating room (OR), but rather has extended into the intensive care unit (ICU) and beyond. The burgeoning use of mechanical

DOI: 10.4018/978-1-4666-8603-8.ch001

circulatory support (MCS) in particular has, in many ways, made the ICU an extension of the OR and has forced providers to quickly expand their skill set in response to increasing critical care demands. Fortunately, despite this mounting complexity, mortality after cardiac surgery continues to decrease.

The following chapter will highlight pivotal historic and epidemiologic events that have helped to shape the face of modern cardiac surgery. Through an exploration of the current landscape and a clearer understanding of the trajectory of care, we hope to inform today's providers so that they may better anticipate the future needs of this increasingly complicated patient population. In addition, the importance of augmenting the current evidence-base through timely and collaborative investigation will be discussed throughout the text.

EVOLVING CARE FOR THE PATIENT WITH CORONARY ARTERY DISEASE

The foundations of cardiac surgery date back to the late 1800s when the treatment of angina pectoris became a focal point for operative innovation. While ligation of pain pathways and creative approaches to sympathectomy did seem to improve the symptoms of ischemia (Harken, Black, Dickson, & Wilson, 1955), these interventions did little to attenuate the other deleterious effects of progressive epicardial coronary disease (i.e. myocardial infarction, arrhythmia, and heart failure). As a result, the development of novel methods for improving collateral blood flow to the ischemic myocardium became strong motivation for evolving surgical care. In 1903, for instance, Thorel (1903) proposed a mechanism by which pericardial adhesions could improve myocardial perfusion. Through the use of either irritant therapies or mechanical intervention, other like-minded surgeons soon created and shared their unique methods for augmenting blood flow using a pericardial substrate (Moritz, Hudson, & Orgain, 1932). Shortly thereafter, muscle (Beck, 1935), omentum (O'Shaughnessy, 1936), and even intestinal grafts were employed to treat ischemia through collateralization (Key, Kergin, Martineau, & Leckey, 1954).

It wasn't until the mid-1960s, however, that vascular conduits were finally used as a means for mechanically bypassing obstructive coronary lesions. Vasilii Kolesov (Olearchyk, Vasilii, & Kolesov, 1988) was believed to have been the first to perform anastomosis of the internal mammary artery to the left anterior descending (LAD) vessel. Following closely on the heels of Kolesov's report, others described the use of saphenous vein grafts for surgical revascularization (Garrett, Dennies, & DeBakey, 1973). By many, however, Rene Favaloro is considered the "father of modern bypass surgery" – while not the first to describe this operation in detail, he was one of the first to perform the coronary artery bypass graft (CABG) procedure with consistent rigor, and one of the first to share and publish his reproducible outcomes (Favaloro, 1969).

It is, in fact, this sharing of outcomes that has been most instrumental in the widespread dissemination and ongoing evolution of CABG care. Supported by three pivotal trials espousing the benefits of surgical revascularization over medical therapy, the use of CABG for patients with coronary disease reached historical peaks in the 1980s. The Veterans Administration Cooperative Study (Detre, Murphy, & Hultgren, 1977), the European Coronary Surgery Study (European Coronary Surgery Study Group, 1979), and the National Heart, Lung, and Blood Institute (NHLBI)- sponsored Coronary Artery Surgery Study (CASS) (National Heart, Lung, and Blood Institute Coronary Artery Surgery Study, 1981), together formed the basis for contemporary surgical guidelines to treat the ischemic patient (Gibbons et al, 2003). For those with advanced disease, concomitant left ventricular contractile dysfunction, and other high-risk features, it is now acknowledged that CABG carries a demonstrable and durable survival advantage over medicines alone. This mortality benefit has since been established outside of clinical trial populations (Weintraub et al, 2012), and seems to be associated with concomitant improvements in patient quality-of-life (Graham, Norris, Galbraith, Knudtson, & Ghali, 2006; Caine, Sharples, & Wallwork, 1999). At the same time, US hospital mortality rates with CABG have steadily declined since the late 1990s, and are now threatening to drop below even 1% per patient (Agency for Healthcare Research and Quality, 2014).

The development of percutaneous coronary intervention (PCI), however, has more recently had a rather dramatic effect on the care of patients with myocardial ischemia and, as a result, has greatly influenced the evolution of cardiac surgery as a discipline. Following Andreas Grüntzig's first report on the use of transluminal balloon dilatation (or angioplasty) as an alternative means for coronary revascularization (Gruntzig, 1978), rates of PCI quickly blossomed. While little additional innovation has since bolstered surgical coronary care over the past several decades, PCI alternatively has seen marked advancements in stent technology, implantation techniques and delivery platforms, and even adjuvant pharmacotherapies – all of which have led to broadened applicability, improved outcomes, and expanded clinical indications. And while the evidence-base supporting surgical versus percutaneous methods for the treatment of symptomatic coronary artery disease (CAD) has been mixed (Mohr et al, 2013; Hlatky et al, 2009), the less invasive PCI alternative has nonetheless resulted directly in a systematic decline in CABG volumes (Figure 1A). In many cases now, CABG has become increasingly reserved for higher-risk patient profiles and for those individuals with only the most complex anatomical disease.

EVOLUTION IN NON-CORONARY CARDIAC SURGICAL CARE

Though a cornerstone of cardiac surgery, the treatment of CAD has not been the only driver for evolving operative care. The discipline, in fact, has foundations deeply rooted in our historic battlegrounds. In the 1940s, Dwight Harken, a captain in the medical corps, became instrumental in the maturation of this young field. By removing foreign bodies from in and around the heart of more than 100 injured soldiers, a precedent for cardiac manipulation was firmly established (Harken, 1946), and from there valuable surgical innovation quickly ensued. Not long afterwards, Blalock and Taussig (1945) reported on their novel operative therapy for tetralogy of Fallot, and soon other palliative treatments for a variety of congenital heart diseases followed.

Perhaps most critical to the evolution of cardiac surgery, however, was the creation and successful employment of cardiopulmonary bypass (CPB) (Gibbon Jr, 1954). Prior to the implementation of bypass, other humans – often the parents of pediatric surgical patients – would be used to control arteriovenous gas admixture through cross-circulation techniques during high-risk cardiac operations (Lillehei, 1955). With CPB, alternatively, there was now a viable means to independently support vital circulatory and ventilatory function throughout the duration of these complex surgeries. The CPB machine has now been used for decades to facilitate all forms of operative intervention on the heart and great vessels, including valve replacement and repairs, treatment of congenital defects, and the management of aortic diseases, to name a few.

The field of cardiac surgery has also been greatly influenced by the care of the heart failure patient. The first heart transplant using a cadaveric donor was performed on December 3, 1967 by Dr. Christiaan Barnard in Cape Town, South Africa, and shortly thereafter by Dr. Norman Shumway in the United States. With pivotal improvements in medical immunosuppression that soon followed, cardiac transplantation quickly saw significant growth, and has since proven to be a life-saving option for those with end-stage

Figure 1. Declining US surgical volume for coronary artery bypass graft (CABG) procedures (A), compared with increasing ventricular assist device (VAD) implantation rates (B). Adapted from the Agency for Healthcare Research and Quality (AHRQ) Healthcare Cost and Utilization (HCUP) project.

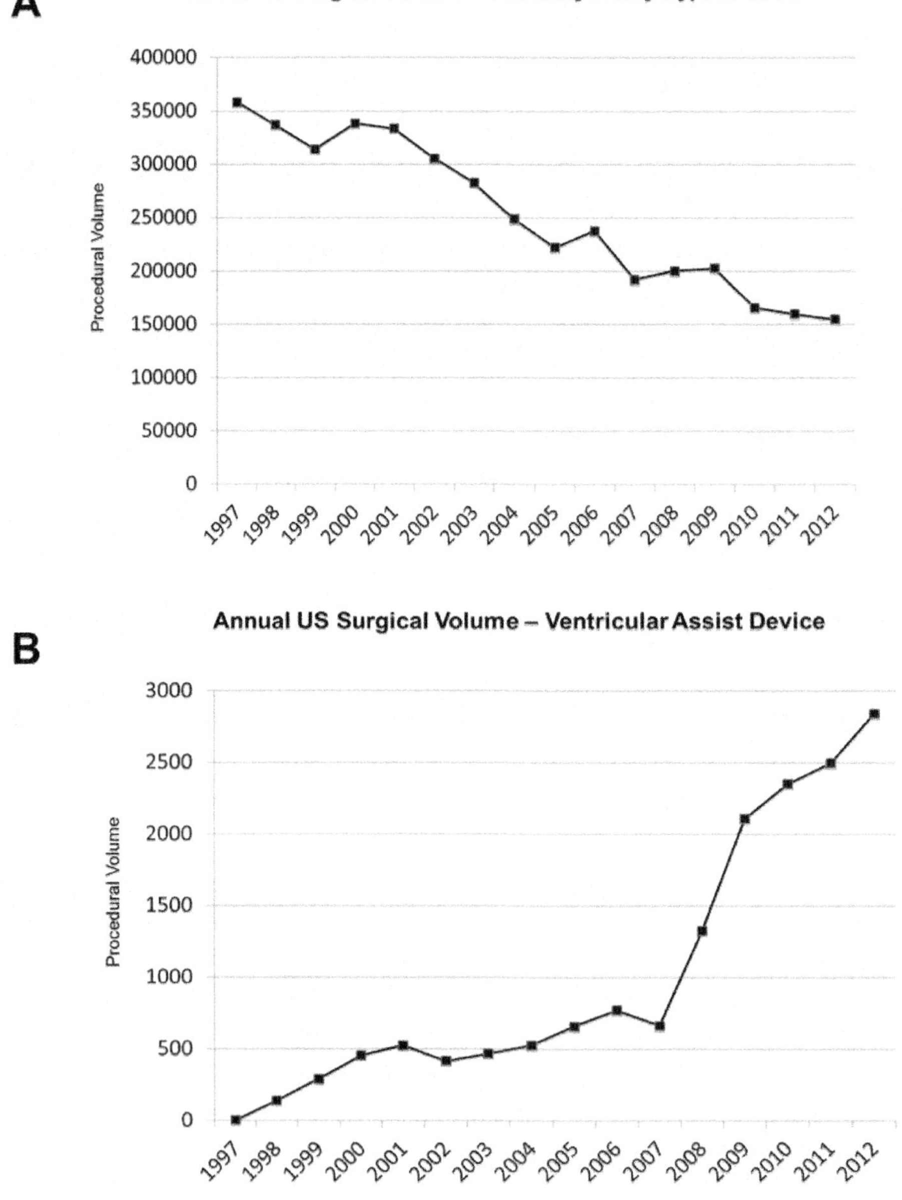

cardiac disease (Stehlik et al, 2012). Unfortunately, despite improvements in care and patient outcomes, restricted organ availability has always limited transplantation as a therapeutic option. While nearly 3,000 additional patients wait annually for a new heart in the US alone, the yearly wait list mortality still approaches 15%, and procedural volumes have remained largely stagnant for the past several decades (Colvin-Adams et al, 2013). Capitalizing on the imposing mismatch between organ supply and demand, mechanical circulatory support has since emerged as a palatable option for the advanced heart failure population (particularly those considered transplant-ineligible) and has led to influential and historic changes in cardiac surgical care.

The origins of MCS actually date back to the development of CPB. Seen as a potential option for cardiac support not only in the OR, but also in the ICU for patients with refractory shock, the National Institutes of Health established the Artificial Heart Program in 1964 and the clinical Ventricular Assist Device (VAD) program in the mid-1970s. VAD technology, like much of cardiac surgery, has seen substantial growth and monumental innovation. Little more than a decade after supplanting optimal medical therapy for patients with end-stage heart failure (Rose et al, 2001), remarkably a third-generation of durable left ventricular assist devices are now being implanted with increasing frequency worldwide. Figure 1B highlights the growth and exponentially increasing implantation rates of VADs in the US, while Figure 2 illustrates, in aggregate, the many historic developments that have influenced the epidemiology of cardiac surgical care.

NOVEL OPERATIONS, PATIENTS, AND PRIORITIES FOR CARDIAC CARE

Evolving Cardiac Surgeries

As previously alluded to, the increasing application of percutaneous techniques for obstructive coronary disease has resulted in declining rates of CABG. This epidemiologic finding has been demonstrated

Figure 2. Timeline of pivotal historic events central to the evolution of modern cardiac surgery

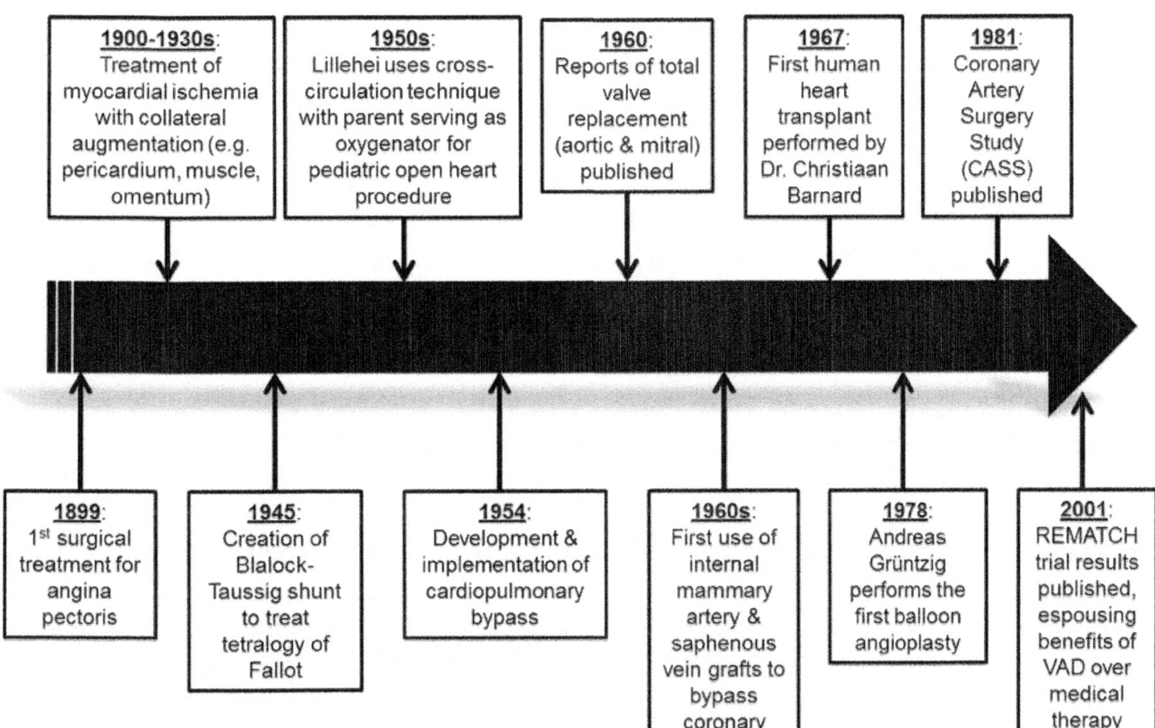

consistently across both North America and Europe (Head, Kieser, Flak, Huysmans, & Kappetein, 2013), and a recent review of US Department of Health and Human Services data supports the declining use of surgical coronary revascularization (Figure 1A). Looking at primary surgical procedures alone, CABG rates have remarkably decreased by more than fifty percent over the last decade and a half, dropping from over 350,000 cases per year in 1997 to just over 150,000 cases per year in 2012 (Agency for Healthcare Research and Quality, 2014).

At the same time, there has been a relatively slow, but consistent increase in cardiac valvular operations worldwide. Whether or not this trend will continue, given the rapid proliferation and implementation of transcatheter valve procedures, remains to be seen. Regardless, the development of these hybrid valve surgeries, along with an increasing interest in hybrid electrophysiologic and structural heart procedures – all using the combined expertise of cardiology subspecialists and cardiac surgeons – should greatly influence the future of the field (Gehi et al, 2013; Kirklin et al, 2014). Mechanical support for the failing heart, too, has already been mentioned as a rapid growth area for cardiac surgery. Reinforced by an expanding evidence-base highlighting significant morbidity, mortality, and quality-of-life benefits (Kirklin et al, 2014; Kirklin, Naftel, & Pagani, 2012; Grady et al, 2014), the use of these surgically implanted devices should continue to escalate and likewise motivate future surgical innovation.

Evolving Cardiac Patients

As the technologies and surgical techniques have evolved, so too have the patients who have benefited from these interventions. Across the board, there has been a steady increase in the average age of patients undergoing cardiac surgery (Agency for Healthcare Research and Quality, 2014). In Italy, for example, there has been a greater than 3-fold increase in the percentage of patients over the age of 80 years (Pierri, Capestro, Zingaro, & Torracca, 2010). Others have estimated that cardiovascular operative interventions performed on octo- and nano-generians may have increased by more than 24-fold over the past 2 decades (Friedrich et al, 2009). This parallels the well-documented current and predicted global escalation in our elderly census. In light of the ongoing increase in individual life expectancy, these surgical trends are likely to continue.

With older age comes a greater prevalence of medical comorbidities. Among these comorbid conditions include higher rates of hypertension, obesity, obstructive lung disease, and heart failure (Pierro et al, 2010). At the same time, patient frailty has also been increasingly acknowledged among cardiac surgical cohorts and has been shown to be a robust predictor of post-operative outcome (Afilalo et al, 2012). In aggregate, this evolving patient profile illustrates a group of individuals with cardiovascular disease who are at higher risk for complications than ever before.

The Importance of Cost

Increasingly, we also operate in an era that not only values patient outcomes, but also emphasizes the importance of care quality and fiscal responsibility. Not surprisingly, the cost of caring for cardiac surgical patients has escalated over time. While clearly influenced by a number of factors, hospital charges for CABG patients in our country, for instance, have increased by over 3-fold, rising from just over $48,000 in the late 1990s to over $150,000 per patient today (Agency for Healthcare Research and Quality, 2014). This increasing cost-of-care is not unique to the CABG population either, but rather has been described in association with numerous other cardiac operations. VAD care is another example of this. While demonstrable improvements in cost-effectiveness have been described, costs per quality adjusted life years after VAD implantation still remain unacceptably high (Rogers et al, 2012). A better and more thorough understanding of cost drivers, along with the simultaneous identification of potentially modifiable targets for cost improvement, should all be instrumental areas for future clinical investigation. Currently this evidence-base remains woefully incomplete.

EMERGING NEEDS IN THE POST-OPERATIVE CARDIOTHORACIC INTENSIVE CARE UNIT

The growing complexity of cardiac surgical care, along with an increasingly more challenging case-mix, has in turn led to an emerging set of unique needs for these patients. In particular, the need for more comprehensive postoperative intensive care appears paramount among these. In Canada, for example, the prevalence of ICU stays exceeding 72 hours after cardiac surgery has increased from 15.4% in 2001 to 21.1% in 2010 (Buth, Gainer, Legare, & Hirsch, 2014). Not only are patients requiring longer durations of ICU care, but also their care has become progressively more complicated. Among the reasons for this growing complexity include, but are not limited to: greater baseline operative risk, the emergence of novel technologies, the influence of non-cardiovascular organ dysfunction, and the growing armamentarium of supportive care therapies employed in the critical care environment. All of these, and others, have caused the cardiothoracic ICU to evolve from a place primarily focused on convalescent care, to a dynamic and sophisticated extension of the OR (Figure 3).

Figure 3. Balancing patient, operative, and resource changes has become pivotal for providing optimal post-operative cardiothoracic critical care. In addition, a focus on metrics such as patient outcome, cost-effectiveness, and quality must continue to be a part of evolving care delivery.

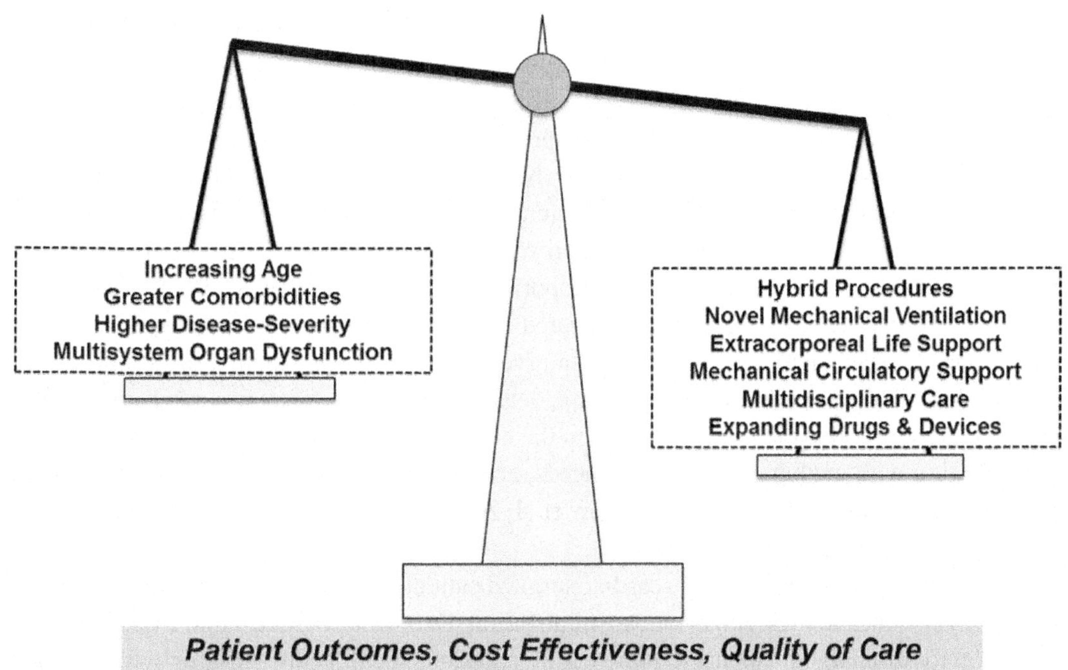

End-organ dysfunction, for instance, is an increasingly common finding among cardiac surgical cohorts managed in the ICU. Acute kidney injury has been reliably associated with greater risk for both post-operative morbidity and mortality (Mariscalco, Lorusso, Dominici, Renzulli, & Sala, 2011). An understanding of the etiologies for post-operative renal dysfunction, a careful appraisal of the available management options, and a comfort in the utility of renal replacement therapies is now vitally important for the care of the postoperative cardiac patient. Similarly, the employment of advanced mechanical ventilatory techniques, the measurement of invasive hemodynamics, and the effective utilization of an ever-expanding critical care pharmacopeia are also all key to the provision of timely and effective postoperative care in the contemporary era of cardiac surgery.

One particular area of increasing focus has been on the use of temporary mechanical circulatory support devices. Percutaneous LVADs, implantable paracorporeal devices, and even extra-corporeal membrane oxygenation (ECMO) now represent viable options within an ever-expanding cardiac critical care armamentarium for the emergent support of patients with refractory cardiogenic shock. Whether used as a bridge-to-recovery, bridge-to-decision, bridge-to-transplantation, or as a bridge to a more permanent device, rates of implantation have nonetheless been rising in historic fashion. A review of the Extracorporeal Life Support Organization (ELSO) registry (2014), as an example, demonstrates a steady increase over time in the placement of ECMO for circulatory collapse worldwide. Increasingly, these devices are also now being placed at the bedside, rather than in the OR. Management of MCS, therefore, creates a unique set of challenges for the cardiothoracic ICU team. Nurses, physicians, and other care providers must be well equipped to manage and trouble-shoot the equipment, and must be prepared to deal with the untoward sequelae of these devices including hemorrhage (Meyer et al, 2010), thrombosis (Starling et al, 2014), and hemolysis (J. Katz et al, 2015), to name a few. Specially trained perfusionists may also be required to assist in the bedside care of the MCS patient in the ICU.

The unique needs of postoperative cardiac care also bring to light many unanswered questions that require additional exploration. In particular, it appears increasingly imperative that we better define optimal staffing and structural needs for today's cardiothoracic ICU. From a staffing perspective, it remains unclear who should be primarily managing these critically ill individuals. Some have suggested that the operating cardiac surgeon, who intimately understands the pathology and the complexities of the recently completed surgery, may best manage these patients. Others instead advocate for management or co-management by critical care-trained specialists (i.e. intensivists) or even cardiac surgeons trained specifically in cardiovascular critical care (N. Katz, 2011). While no formal recommendations exist, the use of intensivist models of care are currently employed in the majority of other critical care environments, and have been associated with improved patient outcomes (Wilcox et al, 2013; Kogan et al, 2013). No matter the staffing method, it is important to understand that the goal of cardiothoracic critical care is to facilitate a rapid and uncomplicated recovery following cardiac surgery. This requires an anticipation of major challenges, proactive intervention, and the avoidance of complications and mistakes, all through the use of unique monitoring, detection, and early-response mechanisms. Those in the medical cardiac ICU have already recognized the challenges presented by an increasingly complex patient population with evolving critical care needs, and now support a tiered-system of ICU care led by uniquely trained cardiac intensivists (Morrow et al, 2012). Extension of this approach to the cardiothoracic ICU may very well follow.

The complexities and needs of today's cardiac surgical patients also don't end when they leave the ICU, and are not even isolated to their acute care hospitalization. Data would suggest that it has become much more common for discharged patients to now require additional health care services before returning to home. In the US, for example, home health referrals for individuals after cardiac surgery have increased from 26% to 33% over the last decade, and transfers to nursing homes or inpatient rehabilitation facilities have steadily risen from 11% to over 18% recently (Agency for Healthcare Research and Quality, 2014). This transition to home for an aging and increasingly frail population of surgical patients is a topic that warrants further attention. Its influence on quality of life, costs of care, and hospital recidivism all represent important focal points for future investigation.

CONCLUSION AND FUTURE DIRECTIONS

Compared with other surgical disciplines, the timeline of cardiac surgery has been a rather abbreviated one. Despite this brief history, however, the field has evolved considerably. Today's cardiac surgical patients are vastly different than ever before, and the operations themselves have changed dramatically over time. While coronary revascularization will always be a key component of contemporary cardiac surgical care, the more recent additions of hybrid cardiac procedures and an expanding armamentarium of novel MCS devices have each been increasingly instrumental in reshaping the field. In response to these epidemiologic changes, cardiac surgeons have been forced to rapidly expand their skill set, and likewise the postoperative ICUs have had to quickly adapt to a novel patient population with a burgeoning set of critical care needs (Figure 3).

It is also important to acknowledge that despite an escalating case-mix with increasing disease severity, cardiac surgical mortality has largely improved over time. While reasons for this are unclear, it is likely due at least in part to better operative techniques, the implementation of collaborative care models, more rigorous focus on patient outcomes and care quality, along with an expanding toolkit for treating postoperative critical illness. The chapters that follow will hope to shed additional light on the current and anticipated needs of the cardiac surgical patient, and will also help to identify future research priorities to support a slowly growing evidence-base.

REFERENCES

Afilalo, J., Mottillo, S., Eisenberg, M. J., Alexander, K. P., Noiseux, N., Perrault, L. P., & Bergman, H. et al. (2012). Addition of frailty and disability to cardiac surgery risk scores identifies elderly patients at high risk of mortality or major morbidity. *Circulation: Cardiovascular Quality and Outcomes*, *5*(2), 222–228. doi:10.1161/CIRCOUTCOMES.111.963157 PMID:22396586

Beck, C. S. (1935). The development of a new blood supply to the heart by operation. *Annals of Surgery*, *102*(5), 801–813. doi:10.1097/00000658-193511000-00001 PMID:17856670

Blalock, A., & Taussig, H. B. (1945). The surgical treatment of malformations of the heart in which there is pulmonary stenosis or pulmonary atresia. *Journal of the American Medical Association*, *128*(3), 189–202. doi:10.1001/jama.1945.02860200029009 PMID:6368878

Buth, K. J., Gainer, R. A., Legare, J. F., & Hirsch, G. M. (2014). The changing face of cardiac surgery: Practice patterns and outcomes 2001-2010. *The Canadian Journal of Cardiology*, *30*(2), 224–230. doi:10.1016/j.cjca.2013.10.020 PMID:24373760

Caine, N., Sharples, L. D., & Wallwork, J. (1999). Prospective study of health related quality of life before and after coronary artery bypass grafting: Outcomes at five years. *Heart (British Cardiac Society)*, *81*(4), 357–361. doi:10.1136/hrt.81.4.347 PMID:10092558

Colvin-Adams, M., Smith, J. M., Heubner, B. M., Skeans, M. A., Edwards, L. B., Waller, C., & Kasiske, B. L. et al. (2013). OPTN/SRTR 2011 Annual Data Report: Heart. *American Journal of Transplantation*, *13*(suppl 1), 119–148. doi:10.1111/ajt.12023 PMID:23237699

Detre, K., Murphy, M. L., & Hultgren, H. (1977). Effect of coronary bypass surgery on longevity in high and low risk patients. Report from the VA Cooperative Coronary Surgery Study. *Lancet*, *2*(8051), 1243–1245. doi:10.1016/S0140-6736(77)92659-9 PMID:73949

European Coronary Surgery Study Group. (1979). Coronary-artery bypass surgery in stable angina pectoris: Survival at two years. *Lancet*, *1*, 889–893. PMID:86665

Favaloro, R. G. (1969). Saphenous vein graft in the surgical treatment of coronary artery disease. Operative technique. *The Journal of Thoracic and Cardiovascular Surgery*, *58*, 178–185. PMID:5798222

Friedrich, I., Simm, A., Kötting, J., Thölen, F., Fischer, B., & Silber, R. E. (2009). Cardiac surgery in the elderly patient. *Deutsches Ärzteblatt International*, *106*, 416–422. PMID:19623310

Garrett, H. E., Dennies, E. W., & DeBakey, M. E. (1973). Aortocoronary bypass with saphenous vein graft. Seven-year follow-up. *Journal of the American Medical Association*, *223*(7), 792–794. doi:10.1001/jama.1973.03220070046012 PMID:4567689

Gasior, M., Zembala, M. O., Tajstra, M., Filipiak, K., Gierlotka, M., Hrapkowicz, T., & Zembala, M. et al. (2014). Hybrid revascularization for multivessel coronary artery disease. *Journal of the American College of Cardiology: Cardiovascular Interventions*, *7*, 1277–1283. PMID:25459040

Gehi, A. K., Mounsey, J. P., Pursell, I., Landers, M., Boyce, K., Chung, E. H., & Kiser, A. C. et al. (2013). Hybrid epicardial-endocardial ablation using a pericardioscopic technique for the treatment of atrial fibrillation. *Heart Rhythm*, *10*(1), 22–28. doi:10.1016/j.hrthm.2012.08.044 PMID:23064043

Gibbon, J. H. Jr. (1954). Application of a mechanical heart and lung apparatus to cardiac surgery. *Minnesota Medicine*, *37*, 171–180. PMID:13154149

Gibbons, R. J., Abrams, J., Chatterjee, K., Daley, J., Deedwania, P. C., Douglas, J. S., & Smith, S. C. Jr et al.. (2003). ACC/AHA 2002 guideline update for the management of patients with chronic stable angina – summary article: A report of the American College of Cardiology/American Heart Association Task Force on Practice Guidelines (Committee on the Management of Patients with Chronic Stable Angina). *Circulation*, *107*(1), 149–158. doi:10.1161/01.CIR.0000047041.66447.29 PMID:12515758

Grady, K. L., Naftel, D., Stevenson, L., Dew, M. A., Weidner, G., Pagani, F. D., & Young, J. et al. (2014). Overall quality of life improves to similar levels after mechanical circulatory support regardless of severity of heart failure before implantation. *The Journal of Heart and Lung Transplantation*, *33*(4), 412–421. doi:10.1016/j.healun.2013.10.017 PMID:24360203

Graham, M. M., Norris, C. M., Galbraith, P. D., Knudtson, M. L., & Ghali, W. A. (2006). Quality of life after coronary revascularization in the elderly. *European Heart Journal*, *27*(14), 1690–1698. doi:10.1093/eurheartj/ehl038 PMID:16717072

Gruntzig, A. (1978). Transluminal dilatation of coronary-artery stenosis. *Lancet*, *1*(8058), 263. doi:10.1016/S0140-6736(78)90500-7 PMID:74678

Harken, D. E. (1946). Foreign bodies in, and in relation to, thoracic blood vessels and heart, I: Techniques for approaching and removing foreign bodies from chambers of heart. *Surgery, Gynecology & Obstetrics*, *83*, 117–125. PMID:20988045

Harken, D. E., Black, H., Dickson, J. F. III, & Wilson, H. E. III. (1955). De-epicardialization: A simple, effective surgical treatment for angina pectoris. *Circulation*, *12*(6), 955–962. doi:10.1161/01.CIR.12.6.955 PMID:13270351

Head, S. J., Kieser, T. M., Falk, V., Huysmans, H. A., & Kappetein, A. P. (2013). Coronary artery bypass grafting: Part 1 – the evolution over the first 50 years. *European Heart Journal*, *34*(37), 2862–2872. doi:10.1093/eurheartj/eht330 PMID:24086085

Hlatky, M. A., Boothroyd, B. D., Bravata, D. M., Boersma, E., Booth, J., Brooks, M. M., & Pocock, S. J. et al. (2009). Coronary artery bypass surgery compared with percutaneous coronary interventions for multivessel disease: A collaborative analysis of individual patients data from ten randomised trials. *Lancet*, *373*(9670), 1190–1197. doi:10.1016/S0140-6736(09)60552-3 PMID:19303634

Katz, J. N., Jensen, B. C., Chang, P. P., Myers, S. L., Pagani, F. D., & Kirklin, J. K. (2015). A multicenter analysis of clinical hemolysis in patients supported with durable, long-term left ventricular assist device therapy. *The Journal of Heart and Lung Transplantation*, *34*(5), 701–709. doi:10.1016/j.healun.2014.10.002 PMID:25582036

Katz, N. M. (2011). The evolution of cardiothoracic critical care. *The Journal of Thoracic and Cardiovascular Surgery*, *141*(1), 3–6. doi:10.1016/j.jtcvs.2010.09.005 PMID:21168010

Key, J. A., Kergin, F. G., Martineau, Y., & Leckey, R. G. (1954). A method of supplementing the coronary circulation by a jejunal pedicle graft. *The Journal of Thoracic Surgery*, *28*, 320–330. PMID:13192879

Kirklin, J. K., Naftel, D. C., Pagani, F. D., Kormos, R. L., Stevenson, L., Miller, M., & Young, J. B. (2012). Long-term mechanical circulatory support (destination therapy): On track to compete with heart transplantation? *The Journal of Thoracic and Cardiovascular Surgery*, *144*(3), 584–603. doi:10.1016/j.jtcvs.2012.05.044 PMID:22795459

Kirklin, J. K., Naftel, D. C., Pagani, F. D., Kormos, R. L., Stevenson, L. W., Blume, E. D., & Young, J. B. et al. (2014). Sixth INTERMACS annual report: A 10,000-patient database. *The Journal of Heart and Lung Transplantation*, *33*(6), 555–564. doi:10.1016/j.healun.2014.04.010 PMID:24856259

Kogan, A., Preisman, S., Berkenstadt, H., Segal, E., Kassif, Y., Sternik, L., & Raanani, E. et al. (2013). Evaluation of the impact of a quality improvement program and intensivist-directed ICU team on mortality after cardiac surgery. *Journal of Cardiothoracic and Vascular Anesthesia*, *27*(6), 1194–1200. doi:10.1053/j.jvca.2013.02.028 PMID:24008163

Lillehei, C. W. (1955). Controlled cross circulation for direct-vision intracardiac surgery: Correction of ventricular septal defects, atrioventricularis cummuis, and tetralogy of Fallot. *Postgraduate Medical Journal*, *1*, 388–396.

Mariscalco, G., Lorusso, R., Dominici, C., Renzulli, A., & Sala, A. (2011). Acute kidney injury: A relevant complication after cardiac surgery. *The Annals of Thoracic Surgery*, *92*(4), 1539–1547. doi:10.1016/j.athoracsur.2011.04.123 PMID:21872837

Meyer, A. L., Malehsa, D., Bara, C., Budde, U., Slaughter, M. S., Haverich, A., & Streuber, M. (2010). Acquired von Willebrand syndrome in patients with an axial flow left ventricular assist device. *Circulation: Heart Failure*, *3*(6), 675–681. doi:10.1161/CIRCHEARTFAILURE.109.877597 PMID:20739614

Mohr, F. W., Morice, M. C., Kappetein, A. P., Feldman, T. E., Stahle, E., Colombo, A., & Serruys, P. W. et al. (2013). Coronary artery bypass graft surgery versus percutaneous coronary intervention in patients with three-vessel disease and left main coronary disease: 5-year follow-up of the randomised, clinical SYNTAX trial. *Lancet*, *381*(9867), 629–638. doi:10.1016/S0140-6736(13)60141-5 PMID:23439102

Moritz, A. R., Hudson, C. L., & Orgain, E. S. (1932). Augmentation of the extracardiac anastomoses of the coronary arteries through pericardial adhesions. *The Journal of Experimental Medicine*, *56*(6), 927–931. doi:10.1084/jem.56.6.927 PMID:19870113

Morrow, D. A., Fang, J. C., Fintel, D. J., Granger, C. B., Katz, J. N., Kushner, F. G., & Winkelman, C. et al. (2012). Evolution of critical care cardiology: Transformation of the cardiovascular intensive care unit and the emerging need for new medical staffing and training models. A scientific statement from the American Heart Association. *Circulation*, *126*(11), 1408–1428. doi:10.1161/CIR.0b013e31826890b0 PMID:22893607

National Heart, Lung, and Blood Institute Coronary Artery Surgery Study (CASS). (1981). A multi-center comparison of the effects of randomized medical and surgical treatment of mildly symptomatic patients with coronary artery disease, and a registry of consecutive patients undergoing coronary angiography. *Circulation*, *63*, I1-I81.

O'Shaughnessy, L. (1936). An experimental method of providing collateral circulation to the heart. *British Journal of Surgery*, *23*(91), 665–670. doi:10.1002/bjs.1800239122

Olearchyk, A.S., & Vasilii, I., & Kolesov. (1988). A pioneer of coronary revascularization by internal mammary-coronary artery grafting. *Journal of Cardiovascular and Thoracic Surgery*, *96*, 13–18. PMID:2898559

Pierri, M. D., Capestro, F., Zingaro, C., & Torracca, L. (2010). The changing face of cardiac surgery patients: An insight into a Mediterranean region. *European Journal of Cardio-Thoracic Surgery*, *38*(4), 407–413. doi:10.1016/j.ejcts.2010.02.040 PMID:20399675

Rogers, J. G., Bostic, R. R., Tong, K. B., Adamson, R., Russo, M., & Slaughter, M. S. (2012). Cost-effectiveness analysis of continuous-flow left ventricular assist devices as destination therapy. *Circulation: Heart Failure*, *5*(1), 10–16. doi:10.1161/CIRCHEARTFAILURE.111.962951 PMID:22052901

Rose, E. A., Gelijns, A. C., Moskowitz, A. J., Heitjan, D. F., Stevenson, L. W., Dembitsky, W., & Poirier, V. L. et al. (2001). Long-term use of a left ventricular assist device for end-stage heart failure. *The New England Journal of Medicine*, *345*, 1435–1443. PMID:11794191

Starling, R. C., Moazami, N., Silvestry, S. C., Ewald, G., Rogers, J. G., Milano, C. A., & Smedira, N. G. et al. (2014). Unexpected abrupt increase in left ventricular assist device thrombosis. *The New England Journal of Medicine*, *370*(1), 33–40. doi:10.1056/NEJMoa1313385 PMID:24283197

Stehlik, J., Edwards, L. B., Kucheryavaya, A. Y., Benden, C., Christie, J. D., Dipchand, A. I., & Hertz, M. I. et al. (2012). The Registry of the International Society for Heart and Lung Transplantation: 29th official adult heart transplant report – 2012. *The Journal of Heart and Lung Transplantation*, *31*(10), 1052–1064. doi:10.1016/j.healun.2012.08.002 PMID:22975095

Thorel, C. H. (1903). Pathologie der Kreislauforgane. *Ergebnisse der Allgemeinen Pathologie und Pathologischen Anatomie*, *9*, 559.

Weintraub, W. S., Grau-Sepulveda, M. V., Weiss, J. M., O'Brien, S. M., Peterson, E. D., Kolm, P., & Edwards, F. H. et al. (2012). Comparative effectiveness of revascularization strategies. *The New England Journal of Medicine*, *366*(16), 1467–1476. doi:10.1056/NEJMoa1110717 PMID:22452338

Wilcox, M. E., Chong, C. A., Niven, D. J., Rubenfeld, G. D., Rowan, K. M., Wunsch, H., & Fan, E. (2013). Do intensivist staffing patterns influence hospital mortality following ICU admission? A systematic review and meta-analyses. *Critical Care Medicine*, *421*(10), 2253–2274. doi:10.1097/CCM.0b013e318292313a PMID:23921275

ADDITIONAL READING

Aaronson, K. D., Slaughter, M. S., Miller, L. W., McGee, E. C., Cotts, W. G., Acker, M. A., & Boyce, S. W. et al. (2012). Use of an intrapericardial, continuous-flow, centrifugal pump in patients awaiting heart transplantation. *Circulation*, *25*(25), 3191–3200. doi:10.1161/CIRCULATIONAHA.111.058412 PMID:22619284

Alexander, J. H., Hafley, G., Harrington, R. A., Peterson, E. D., Ferguson, T. B. Jr, Lorenz, T. J., & Kouchoukos, N. T. et al.PREVENT IV Investigators. (2005). Efficacy and safety of edifoligide, an E2F transcription factor decoy, for prevention of vein graft failure following coronary artery bypass graft surgery: PREVENT IV: a randomized controlled trial. *Journal of the American Medical Association*, *294*(19), 2446–2454. doi:10.1001/jama.294.19.2446 PMID:16287955

Basra, S. S., Loyalka, P., & Kar, B. (2011). Current status of percutaneous ventricular assist devices for cardiogenic shock. *Current Opinion in Cardiology*, *26*(6), 548–554. doi:10.1097/HCO.0b013e32834b803c PMID:21926617

Cooley, D. A., & Frazier, O. H. (2010). The past 50 years of cardiovascular surgery. *Circulation*, *102*, IV-87–IV-93. PMID:11080137

Harken, D. E., Soroff, H. S., Taylor, W. J., Lefemine, A. A., Gupta, S. K., & Lunzer, S. (1960). Partial and complete prostheses in aortic insufficiency. *The Journal of Thoracic and Cardiovascular Surgery*, *40*, 744–762. PMID:13711583

Helman, D. N., & Rose, E. A. (2000). History of mechanical circulatory support. *Progress in Cardiovascular Diseases*, *43*(1), 1–4. doi:10.1053/pcad.2000.7194 PMID:10935552

Hickey, G. L., Grant, S. W., Murphy, G. J., Bhabra, M., Pagano, D., McAllister, K., & Bridgewater, B. et al. (2013). Dynamic trends in cardiac surgery: Why the logistic EuroSCORE is no longer suitable for contemporary cardiac surgery and implications for future risk models. *European Journal of Cardio-Thoracic Surgery*, *43*(6), 1146–1152. doi:10.1093/ejcts/ezs584 PMID:23152436

Katz, N. M. (2007). The emerging specialty of cardiothoracic surgical critical care: The leadership role of cardiothoracic surgeons on the multidisciplinary team. *The Journal of Thoracic and Cardiovascular Surgery*, *134*(5), 1109–1111. doi:10.1016/j.jtcvs.2007.07.032 PMID:17976436

Kumar, K., Zarychanski, R., Bell, D. D., Manji, R., Zivot, J., Menkis, A. H., & Arora, R. C. (2009). The impact of 24-hour in-house intensivists on a dedicated cardiac surgery intensive care unit. *The Annals of Thoracic Surgery*, *88*(4), 1153–1161. doi:10.1016/j.athoracsur.2009.04.070 PMID:19766800

Lee, D. H., Buth, K. J., Martin, B. J., Yip, A. M., & Hirsch, G. M. (2010). Frail patients are at increased risk for mortality and prolonged institutional care after cardiac surgery. *Circulation*, *121*(8), 973–978. doi:10.1161/CIRCULATIONAHA.108.841437 PMID:20159833

Miller, L. W., Pagani, F. D., Russell, S. D., John, R., Boyle, A. J., Aaronson, K. D., & Frazier, O. H. et al. (2007). Use of a continuous-flow device in patients awaiting a heart transplantation. *The New England Journal of Medicine*, *357*(9), 885–896. doi:10.1056/NEJMoa067758 PMID:17761592

Ngaage, D. L., Griffin, S., Guvendik, L., Cowen, M. E., & Cale, A. R. J. (2008). Changing operative characteristics of patients undergoing operations for coronary artery disease: Impact on early outcomes. *The Annals of Thoracic Surgery*, *86*(5), 1424–1430. doi:10.1016/j.athoracsur.2008.07.050 PMID:19049725

Rohde, S. L., Baker, R. A., Tully, P. J., Graham, S., Cullen, H., & Knight, J. L. (2010). Preoperative and intraoperative factors associated with long-term survival in octogenarian cardiac surgery patients. *The Annals of Thoracic Surgery*, *89*(1), 105–111. doi:10.1016/j.athoracsur.2009.10.006 PMID:20103215

Seco, M., & Edelman, B, J.J., Forrest, P., Ng, M., Wilson, M.K., Fraser, J., … Vallely, M.P. (. (2014). Geriatric cardiac surgery: Chronology vs. biology. *Heart Lung and Circulation*, *23*, 794–801. doi:10.1016/j.hlc.2014.04.008 PMID:24851829

Starr, A. (1960). Total mitral replacement: Fixation and thrombosis. *Surgical Forum*, *11*, 258–260.

Teuteberg, J. J., Stewart, G. C., Jessup, M., Kormos, R. L., Sun, B., Frazier, O. H., & Stevenson, L. W. et al. (2013). Implant strategies change over time and impact outcomes: Insights from the INTERMACS (Interagency Registry for Mechanically Assisted Circulatory Support). *Journal of the American College of Cardiology: Heart Failure*, *5*, 369–378. PMID:24621968

Tomey, M. I., Gidwani, U. K., & Sharma, S. K. (2013). Cardiac critical care after transcatheter aortic valve implantation. *Cardiology Clinics*, *31*(4), 607–618. doi:10.1016/j.ccl.2013.07.006 PMID:24188224 van Diepen, S., Granger, C. B., Jacka, M., Gilchrist, I. C., Morrow, D. A., & Katz, J. N. (2015). The unmet need for addressing cardiac issues in intensive care research. *Critical Care Medicine*, *43*(1), 128–134. doi:10.1097/CCM.0000000000000609 PMID:25243816

Velazquez, E. J., Lee, K. L., Deja, M. A., Jain, A., Sopko, G., Marchenko, A., & Rouleau, J. L. et al. (2011). Coronary-artery bypass surgery in patients with left ventricular dysfunction. *The New England Journal of Medicine*, *364*(17), 1607–1616. doi:10.1056/NEJMoa1100356 PMID:21463150

Wood, D. E. (2013). The future of cardiothoracic surgery: A view from North America. *European Journal of Cardio-Thoracic Surgery*, *43*(1), 241–243. doi:10.1093/ejcts/ezs423 PMID:23148076

Yusuf, S., Zucker, D., Peduzzi, P., Fisher, L. D., Takaro, T., & Kennedy, J. W. (1994, August). …Norris, R. Effect of coronary artery bypass graft surgery on survival: Overview of 10-year results from randomised trials by the Coronary Artery Bypass Graft Surgery Trialists Collaboration. *Lancet*, *344*(8922), 563–570. doi:10.1016/S0140-6736(94)91963-1 PMID:7914958

Chapter 2
Quality and Safety

Daniel Rubin
University of Chicago, USA

Avery Tung
University of Chicago, USA

ABSTRACT

Quality improvement is a goal of all institutions but effective quality improvement programs have been difficult to create and sustain. Cardiac surgery has long been a pioneer in the quality improvement process through protocolization, large database analysis, and evidence based research. This chapter will discuss the theoretical foundation for quality improvement in medicine, and address current quality improvement strategies in the cardiothoracic ICU including care bundles, large database review, and externally promulgated quality programs such as the Surgical Care Improvement Project (SCIP) or the Physician Quality Reporting Initiative (PQRS). Controversies from national quality improvement programs including SCIP, extended staffing, and the value of quality culture will be discussed.

INTRODUCTION

Cardiac surgery has been a high risk endeavor ever since its inception. Although John Gibbon is credited with developing the first artificial oxygenator, and his first procedure (an atrial-septal defect closure) was a success, the next 4 patients Dr. Gibbon operated on did not survive and Gibbon never again performed open heart surgery (Gott, 2005). Of the first 10 ventricular septal defects closed by the pioneering cardiac surgeon Walt Lillehei in 1954 only 6 survived (Moller, Shumway, & Gott, 2009). Although morbidity and mortality were significant when surgical techniques and post-operative care were still in their infancy, progressive refinement of surgical techniques, strategies for heart preservation, and advances in cardiopulmonary bypass and overall perioperative care have made cardiac surgery routine enough for overall coronary artery bypass graft (CABG) mortality to fall to 2% (Ferguson, 2012).

Physicians have taken advantage of these incremental improvements in cardiac surgery techniques by performing more difficult procedures on sicker patients. Combined coronary bypass and multiple valve procedures, mechanical assist device insertion, and minimally invasive cardiac surgery have dramatically increased both the complexity and risk of modern cardiac surgery. Patients undergoing these

DOI: 10.4018/978-1-4666-8603-8.ch002

procedures are routinely exposed to numerous therapeutic and diagnostic interventions that increase the risk of harm including central venous access, mechanical ventilation, and arterial pressure monitoring. Increasing numbers of consultants and medications also increase the complexity of care and raise the likelihood of adverse events.

That such complex care can be delivered so effectively is no accident. Cardiac surgery has a long history of focusing on quality improvement. In addition to frequent use of protocols and a limited set of procedures, cardiac surgeons have relied heavily on large clinical databases such as those created by the Society of Thoracic Surgeons (STS) and the New York State Department of Health to better understand risk factors and outcomes. The STS database in particular, to which 95% of cardiac surgeons send data, has been risk-adjusted for >20 years and has undergone multiple updates of the risk adjustment algorithm. Finally, government-sponsored initiatives such as the Surgical Care Improvement Program have led physicians to focus on quality and safety in care processes, including glycemic control, appropriate use of beta blockade and antibiotics, and best practices with respect to central line, and urinary catheter use. This chapter will discuss theoretical approaches to quality improvement, review current strategies for creating and maintaining quality and safety in the cardiac ICU, including safety culture, bundles, the influence of external quality programs, and large database analysis. Future strategies for maintaining and improving cardiac surgery quality will be discussed.

Theories of Quality

Organizations outside of medicine have developed two broad theoretical approaches to improving and maintaining quality performance. The first, a "one best way" approach, was first developed by the 20th century industrialist Frederick Taylor. In his 1911 book, The Principles of Scientific Management, Taylor argued that breaking a complex task into many smaller ones and then using comparative science to identify the "one best way" to perform each of them was the best route to optimal performance (Taylor, 1911). Among Taylor's examples were identifying the optimal weight for shoveling material by a worker (21 lbs), and using different sized shovels for different densities of material for optimal efficiency. Taylor believed that too much worker autonomy was bad for quality, and that emphasizing more managerial control was critical to improving quality. While "Taylorism" was controversial and led to strikes from skilled workers, Taylor was one of the first to focus on improving the system versus the individual workers.

The other approach was characterized by Dr. W. Edwards Deming, a physicist and statistician. Deming also emphasized system improvements, but unlike Taylor believed in worker input to quality improvement. As an example, Deming might seek a nurses understanding of how wrong medication errors occur in the ICU rather than just physician input. Such a "deep" understanding of workflow, Deming believed, was essential to optimizing complex systems. Among Deming's other recommendations were removing blame as a driver of quality and a culture that encourages the identification of errors and innovative solutions.

Today, organized medicine most commonly uses the Donabedian model, which incorporates elements from both Taylor and Deming. First described in 1966, the Donabedian model divides medical care into three distinct categories, structure, process and outcomes (Donabedian, 1966). These three categories are then used to identify areas to focus on for quality interventions and also to measure improvements in quality.

"Structure," describes the attributes of the settings in which care occurs. Examples of "attributes" that pertain to the cardiothoracic intensive care unit include the physical layout of the ICU, types of monitors, physician and nursing staffing models, and the presence of protocols. As an example of a structural issue, the location of patients at a significant distance from where care providers work may expose them to delayed diagnosis and therapeutic intervention. However, ensuring all patients on a service are in one unit may be difficult due to limited bed availability and nurse staffing ratios (Meyer & Massagli, 2001).

"Process," denotes actual task performance, and in medicine represents giving and receiving care, making the correct diagnosis, and instituting appropriate therapeutic interventions. Specific examples include removing central venous catheters when they are no longer needed and discontinuing antibiotics in a timely fashion.

"Outcomes," measure the effects of care on the health status of patients and populations. Because improved outcomes may not be directly related to the quality of care, outcomes can only be improved in the Donabedian model if they are directly tied to either a change in structure or process. One challenge with the Donabedian model is to accurately identify those structures and processes that can lead to improved outcomes. Improvements in outcomes can be especially difficult to measure due to variation in the severity of illness and the availability of risk adjusted models. Additionally, measuring outcomes data can be cumbersome and if the outcome that is to be measured is rare (ECMO cannula thrombosis) years may go by before meaningful data is collected.

CURRENT QUALITY IMPROVEMENT APPROACHES IN THE CARDIOTHORACIC ICU

The STS Database

One example of how cardiac surgery emphasizes safety is the development and ongoing maintenance of an extensive database of outcomes and risk factors for surgeons to benchmark themselves against. Originally developed in 1986 as a way to risk adjust for raw mortality statistics released by the Health Care Financing Administration(footnote), the Society for Thoracic Surgeons (STS) has since evolved into a national database of outcomes, patient characteristics and procedures that facilitate accurate prediction of operative mortality and morbidity. Known today as the STS National Adult Cardiac Surgery Database (STS NCD), this registry captures >95% of all cardiac surgical procedures performed in the United States, and serves as a model for the American College of Surgeons National Surgery Quality Improvement Program (NSQIP) or the National Anesthesia Clinical Outcomes Registry (NACOR). Centers participating in the STS national database submit risk factor and outcome data to the Database, which is maintained at the Duke Clinical Research institute. Data are then "harvested" quarterly from the Database, and risk adjusted performance is provided to each STS participant.(Figure 1) Reports contain individual, regional, and national outcome data, and range from 30-day mortality to re-intubation, renal failure, stroke, and other cardiac surgery complications. Comparisons to programs considered similar by case volume and procedure type are also provided.

The STS database is unusual in having extremely sophisticated risk adjustment. Models that adjust expected outcomes for patient comorbidities and perioperative variables are routinely updated for CABG and valve surgery, and combined CABG/valve surgery. Risk factors in the model include not only age and gender, but also comorbidities such as diabetes, renal failure and chronic lung disease, previous surgery, and surgical factors such as use of preoperative inotropes or an intra-aortic balloon pump. Access to the STS risk calculator for individual case outcome prediction is available on the internet, and allows providers and patients alike to estimate the risk for both mortality and outcomes such as renal failure, stroke, prolonged ventilation, and reoperation.

Partly due to their extensive experience and frequent updating of their risk model, the STS database has surprisingly good C statistics, ranging from 0.65 for reoperation to 0.8 for CABG mortality. Reports to providers include both odds ratios, risk adjusted rates, and observed/expected ratios for hospital and operative mortality. Because risk models may become outdated over time, calibration factors are provided to allow a provider to compare current to past performance. That calibration factors consistently demonstrate better risk adjusted outcomes over time suggests that cardiac surgical outcomes are improving over time.

The success of the STS NCD as a valid estimator of cardiac surgical outcomes suggests that outcome improvements may occur without nationally promulgated safety and quality programs. Although calibration factors consistently suggest better performance over time, considerable practice variability exists for even basic aspects of cardiac surgery such as the decision to transfuse (Snyder-Ramos et al., 2008), use pressors, (Butterworth, Legault, Royster, & Hammon, 1998), allow retrograde autologous priming (G. S. Murphy et al., 2006), or perform tracheostomy after failure to wean from mechanical ventilation (Hosseinian et al., 2014). Yet, most cardiac intensive care units have at least one formal protocol. In a 2011 Canadian survey of postoperative order sets, 84% of Canadian cardiac surgery ICUs had at least 1 formal protocol, with the most common care pathways being aspirin administration (91%), extubation (74%), analgesia (60%), or atrial fibrillation (57%) (Lamarche, Sirounis, & Arora, 2011). The survey noted that even though protocolization was frequent, their content varied significantly. Another older study found significant differences between two hospitals in the use of Lab tests, EKGs, and Chest X-Rays with no difference in length of stay or ICU mortality (Bell, Ostryzniuk, Verhoff, Spanier, & Roberts, 1998). Interestingly, the authors noted that the hospital with greater utilization of lab tests had higher costs and no better outcomes, suggesting that over-protocolization was possible. Taken together, these data suggest that many different routes to quality exist for cardiac surgery care, and that the content of any protocols may not be as important as other aspects of quality care such as a safety culture, adequate staffing, and strong communication.

Care Bundles

One strategy to maximize the impact of many small evidence based interventions targeting a common safety issue is to combine them into "bundles". This approach was initially developed by the Institute of healthcare improvement (IHI) to improve the reliability of evidence based process measures and improve patient outcomes. As defined by the IHI, a bundle is a small set of evidence based interventions for a defined patient segment/population and care setting resulting in better outcomes when implemented together. According to IHI guidelines, bundles should be limited to no more than three to five interventions to facilitate complete adoption, and each intervention should be independent so that omission of one does not affect the implementation of others. Even though each intervention is itself evidence based, the bundle strategy involves an "all or none" approach to ensure that all interventions are implemented (>95% compliance) (Nolan & Berwick, 2006). The "All or none," approach encourages system-wide changes to achieve all of the interventions and is a more sensitive measure for success.

One of the first formal bundles targeted the care of mechanically ventilated patients. Interventions chosen for this bundle included elevating the head of the bed to between 30-45 degrees, daily "sedation vacations," and assessment for readiness of extubation, prophylaxis against stress ulcers and deep venous thrombosis, and daily oral care with chlorhexidine (added in 2010). Some bundle elements were designed to allow regional/local variation in implementation such as choices for ulcer and DVT prophylaxis (Resar, 2012). As with many quality efforts in medicine, however, evidence supporting a link between process improvement and improved outcomes is difficult to interpret. Resar et al. performed the initial multi-institution study prospectively evaluating the effect of bundle implementation on VAP in 61 different hospitals (Resar et al., 2005). The intensive care units of the participating hospitals implemented/adopted the bundle according to their own methods but were encouraged to use multidisciplinary rounds, daily goals sheets and other non-specified faculty-recommended improvements. Only 35 ICU's (55%), including medical and surgical units, reported both compliance with the bundle and VAP rates but among full responders Resar found a strong negative correlation between VAP and bundle adherence. In the 21 units with $\geq$ 95% compliance, VAP rates decreased from 6.6 to 2.7 per 1000 ventilator days ($p < 0.001$ 59% reduction) with an average decrease of 44.5% for all units included in the analysis. .

More than a decade has passed since the development of the ventilator bundle and only one subsequent trial has evaluated both reported bundle adherence and the effectiveness of bundle implementation. Youngquist et al. described their experience in two ICU's which achieved full bundle adherence (>95% compliance with all four elements) after 6 months of adoption (Youngquist et al., 2007). Bundle implementation decreased VAP rates from 6.01/1000 mechanical ventilation (MV) days to 2.66/1000 MV days. Two other single institution studies did not measure bundle adherence but nonetheless found decreased VAP rates over a wide range of baseline incidences 8.2-3.3/1000 MV days in one study (Berriel-Cass, Adkins, Jones, & Fakih, 2006) and 13.3-8.3/1000 MV days in another (Unahalekhaka, Jamulitrat, Chongsuvivatwong, & Ovretveit, 2007). Current data suggest that outcomes may not improve if implementation is suboptimal. Pogorzelska et al. performed a survey of participating National Healthcare Safety Network (NHSN) hospitals adherence to the ventilator bundle and the reported VAP rates (Pogorzelska et al., 2011). Of the 250 hospitals that responded to the survey (415 ICU's) only 68% had a written policy regarding the bundle and only 66% of those ICU's actually monitored the implementation. Only 73 (39%) of ICUs responding to the survey reported full bundle adherence (>95% in all four elements) and only those ICUs reporting full adherence had lower VAP rates.

Another challenge with assessing the effectiveness of the VAP bundle is inconsistency in the definition of VAP. Skrupky et al. prospectively evaluated VAP rates using both administrative defined criteria (National Healthcare and Safety Network) and clinically oriented criteria (American College of Chest Physicians) (Skrupky, McConnell, Dallas, & Kollef, 2012). Over a 1 year period the incidence of VAP was 4% when ACCP criteria were used but only 0.6% with NHSN criteria. Even when only one diagnostic criteria is used at a single institution inter-observer variation can play a significant role in VAP rates due to the subjectivity of symptoms and frequency of nosocomial surveillance (Dodek, 2012). Furthermore, decreased VAP rates may not themselves translate into improvements in more tangible patient outcomes. Drakulovic et al. prospectively randomized 90 mechanically ventilated patients to the supine vs. the semi-recumbent position and found a large difference between clinically detected VAP rates (8% vs. 34%) (Drakulovic et al., 1999). However, outcomes such as length of ICU stay, duration of mechanical ventilation, or mortality did not differ.

Finally, care bundles must be continuously reevaluated in light of new evidence. As an example, stress ulcer prophylaxis for patients reduces GI bleeding, but also decreases the gastric pH, potentially leading to increased pneumonia risk due to bacterial colonization (Herzig et al., 2013). Other consensus guidelines for VAP prevention do not recommend routine stress ulcer prophylaxis in mechanically ventilated patients (Muscedere et al., 2008).

The ventilator bundle strategy is an example of a Taylor approach to care quality where the process of supportive care during mechanical ventilation is broken into its component parts, each part is optimized according to current evidence, and a protocol is created to reflect "best" practice. Although the effectiveness of the VAP bundle is unclear, many cardiothoracic ICUs use bundles similar to VAP for daily care protocols that do not require individualization such as glucose control, extubation, and antibiotic use.

CLABSI: A Bundle that Works!

An example of a care bundle that has clearly improved the quality of care in cardiothoracic ICU patients has been the effect of the central line insertion bundle on central line associated bloodstream infection (CLABSI) rates. Items in the CLABSI bundle relate to inserter hygiene (cap, gown, mask, hand hygiene, sterile gloves), patient hygiene (chlorhexidine scrub, full body drape), and organizational efforts (remove unneeded lines, avoid the femoral site).

Central lines are nearly ubiquitous in the cardiothoracic ICU and are routinely used for infusions of vasoactive medications, volume administration, and hemodynamic monitoring. The Centers for Disease Control estimates that in American ICUs central line use is as high as 15 million central venous catheter days per year. At an estimated CLABSI rate of 1 infection per 1000 catheter days, approximately 15,000 CLABSIs occur every year. Each CLABSI increases the length of stay by an estimated 19-22 days and costs by $34,508-56,167 (Dimick et al., 2001; Rello et al., 2000). The predicted mortality associated with CLABSI in intensive care units ranges from 0-35% depending on whether the study has controlled for the severity of the patients baseline critical illness (O'Grady et al., 2002).

The prevalence of CLABSI combined with the severity of associated cost, morbidity and mortality led in 2002 to the creation of multidisciplinary guidelines for insertion and management (O'Grady et al., 2002). The consensus statement consisted of five interventions, 1) improvement in educating and training health professionals involved with line insertion, 2) maximal sterile barrier precautions, 3) using 2% chlorhexidine for skin antisepsis, 4) avoiding routine replacement as a strategy to prevent infection, and 5) increased usage of antiseptic/antibiotic impregnated catheters. The effectiveness of these guidelines was first evaluated by Berenholtz et al. at Johns Hopkins who pursued a multi-pronged intervention in the surgical ICU (Berenholtz et al., 2004). The interventions included an education program to increase provider awareness about best practices, creation of a central line insertion cart to facilitate easier acquisition of materials, evaluating the clinical need for presence of central venous catheters daily on rounds, instituting a checklist performed during every insertion to ensure adherence to best practice guidelines and empowering nurses to halt the procedure if there is a violation of the guidelines. In Berenholz's study implementation of this intervention decreased CLABSI rates from 11.3/1,000 catheter days to 0/1,000 catheter days over a period of 4 years.

In a landmark follow-up study, Pronovost et al. examined the effect of this bundle on a large heterogeneous group of hospitals in Michigan (P. Pronovost et al., 2006). The five evidence based interventions in this study were 1) Hand washing prior to CVC placement 2) 2% Chlorhexadine solution for skin anti-sepsis 3) Full barrier precautions during insertion 4) Avoidance of the femoral site and a preference for subclavian insertion 5) Removal of unnecessary catheters as assessed daily on morning rounds in addition to a daily goals sheet to improve provider communication and a ventilator associated pneumonia bundle. A nurse observer was present during line insertion with a checklist to ensure compliance with all of the study interventions and empowered to stop insertion if any of these practices were violated. Significant emphasis was also placed upon improvements in the culture of the institution to improve staff education and promote safety by designating a team leader at each institution. Mean CLABSI rates decreased from 7.7/1000 catheter days prior to the intervention to 1.4/1000 catheter days by 16-18 months after study initiation.

Although impressive, this study suffered from lack of mechanistic clarity. Along with the bundle, an entire safety program was implemented contemporaneously, clouding the assessment of what intervention was most responsible for the benefit. In addition, no data on compliance with bundle interventions was available. Nevertheless, implementation of similar strategies has driven down the rate of CLABSI considerably, so much so that the United States Center for Disease Control's March 4, 2011 Morbidity and Mortality Weekly Report highlighted a dramatic drop in CLABSI over the 8 years following the Pronovost study ("Vital signs: central line-associated blood stream infections--United States, 2001, 2008, and 2009," 2011).

More recent data provide some clues regarding the relative importance of bundle elements for CLABSI prevention. In 1,071 ICUs participating in a CLABSI reduction program, Hsu et al. found that compliance with the chlorhexidine skin preparation, appropriate hand hygiene and full barrier precautions was highest (>90%), and that avoidance of the femoral insertion site (74%) and removing unnecessary lines/reviewing need (65%) were each independently associated with an increased risk of CLABSI (Hsu, Weeks, Yang, Sawyer, & Marsteller, 2014).

Another recent approach to reduction in CLABSI has been the development of simulation training for central venous catheter (CVC) insertion. CVC insertion is a technically complicated bedside procedure that has historically been taught at the bedside on actual patients. Simulation offers an opportunity to learn clinical skills and appropriate technique in a low stress environment before attempts on real patients. In early studies, simulation training improved resident comfort with CVC insertion and reduced arterial puncture and the number of needle passes, suggesting some benefit to learners (Barsuk, McGaghie, Cohen, O'Leary, & Wayne, 2009; Britt, Novosel, Britt & Sullivan 2009).

The effect of simulation on CLABSI reduction is unclear. Burden et al. studied the effect of a CVC simulation course on CLABSI rates after the CLABSI bundle described from Berenholz et al. had already been implemented (Burden et al., 2012). The intervention consisted of a didactic pre-course and four hour simulation session that included three hours of deliberate practice and completion of a simulated line insertion. Participants would complete the course when the supervising physician deemed them proficient. Although Burden et al. did find a decrease in CLABSI rates from 6.47 to 2.44/1000 catheter days ($P<0.05$) over a 4 year period, multiple other interventions were deployed during the study period which clouded the effectiveness of each individual intervention. Furthermore, the decrease in CLABSI rates did not match that seen in the Pronovost study. Simulation may offer additional benefits to the reduction in CLABSI in addition to decreases in mechanical complications but further research is needed to identify its impact in CLABSI reduction.

The experience with CLABSI reduction suggests that, regardless of mechanism, focusing on the technical process of line insertion and systematically optimizing each piece can pay major dividends. Whereas in the United States a CLABSI rate of 5 infections/1000 catheter days was once considered adequate performance, in 2014 CLABSI rates well under 1 are being routinely reported (Gozu, Clay, &

Younus, 2011; Lin et al., 2012; Ong et al., 2011). Such dramatic reductions in line infection may be partly responsible for the improvement in cardiac surgery outcomes reported by the STS database. Over the past decade identifying CLABSI as a preventable complication and using a systematic evidence-based approach has seen an impressive and sustained decrease in CLABSI rates.

Externally Promulgated Quality Programs (SCIP and PQRI)

An extension of the "care bundle" strategy for improving quality described above is to incentivize compliance with process measures on a nationwide scale. In the CTICU, the best examples of this approach are the national Surgical Care Improvement Program (SCIP) and Physician Quality Reporting Initiative (PQRI). Created in 2002 by the Center for Medicare & Medicaid Services (CMMS), the SCIP program was initially called the surgical infection project (SIP) and was targeted at appropriate perioperative antibiotic use. The SIP included 3 process measures: whether antibiotics had been given within 1 hour of incision, whether the appropriate antibiotic was chosen, and whether perioperative antibiotics had been discontinued within 24 hours of the end of surgery (Bratzler & Hunt, 2006).

A program to reduce surgical site infections would clearly have value to cardiac surgery. In such patients, surgical site infections result in sternal wound infections with considerable associated morbidity and mortality. Nationwide, the rate of superficial sternal wound infections, (skin, subcutaneous tissue and pectoralis fascia only), is 2-6%, and the rate of deep sternal wound infection is 0.25-4% depending on the type of cardiac surgery (Edwards, Engelman, Houck, Shahian, & Bridges, 2006). The associated mortality from superficial sternal wound infections is 5% and deep sternal wound infections is 8.1-48% (Kubota et al., 2013). The additional cost of a patient that develops a deep sternal wound infection has been estimated at $500,000, underscoring the impact of such a complication (Lee, Raman, & Song, 2010).

In early studies, SIP strategies have been somewhat effective at reducing surgical site infection rates. In a 2005 demonstration project involving over 50 participating hospitals significant improvements in adherence to the three SIP measures, were correlated with a 27% decrease in surgical site infections in patients undergoing coronary artery bypass or orthopedic surgery (Dellinger et al., 2005). Partly as a result of data such as these, 6 additional measures were added to the SIP program and the surgical care improvement project (SCIP) was born. Hospitals seeking greater Medicare reimbursement would be required to publically report their performance on these 9 measures. The SCIP program was initiated in July of 2006.

In the intervening 8 years since SCIP began, hospitals have markedly improved their performance in all SCIP measures. Performance in SCIP INF-1 (antibiotic administration < 1 hr), CARD-2 (perioperative beta blockade) and VTE-1 (prophylaxis ordered for DVT formation) are all >90% for most hospitals and other measures such as perioperative normothermia are not far behind.

In addition, however, accumulating evidence now suggests that the effect of improved SCIP performance is unclear. Current data suggest not only that performance on antibiotic measures do not correlate with outcome (Stulberg et al., 2010), but that performance on the DVT prophylaxis (Hawn et al., 2011), postoperative glucose (McDonnell, Alexanian, Junqueira, Cabral, & Lazar, 2013), and beta blockade measures (Bouri, Shun-Shin, Cole, Mayet, & Francis, 2014) did not correlate with their associated outcomes either. In some patients, harm may result, as noted by a recent vascular surgery report finding a 40% increase in surgical infection after implementation of SCIP measures (Dua et al., 2014).

Overall, widespread implementation of the SCIP program has not clearly led to improvement in cardiac surgery outcomes. As noted above, studies focusing on SCIP INF measures (excluding INF-4) have shown no consistent decrease in SSI's despite improved compliance (Hawn et al., 2013). Ingraham et al. only identified a small negative correlation between SSI and SCIP INF-2 (choice of antibiotic) when comparing all of the SCIP measures with outcomes (Ingraham et al., 2010).

Because performance on all SCIP measures have "topped out" at >90%, and perhaps because little data unequivocally link performance on process measures with improved outcomes, most SCIP measures will be retired in January 2015, along with process measures for pneumonia, heart failure, and heart attack. Instead, the focus of programs such as SCIP will be on outcomes, readmission rates, and measurable complications.

The only perioperative process measure that will remain is SCIP INF-4, which requires that all glucose measurements 18-24 hours after cardiac surgery be < 180 mg/dl. Unfortunately, the value of incrementally better performance on this measure is also uncertain. Studies evaluating the ability to achieve full compliance with the measure suggest an "unavoidable failure," rate between 6-10% despite the addition of intensive insulin protocols (M. A. Murphy et al., 2010; LaPar, Isbell, Kern, Ailawadi, & Kron 2014). Risk factors for SCIP failure include a pre-operative diagnosis of insulin requiring diabetes, high HbA1C levels and increased BMI (McDonnell et al., 2013). Nonetheless, patients who fail the measure have not had worse outcomes with respect to sternal wound infections, mortality or length of ICU stay (LaPar et al., 2014).

The other large, nationally promulgated quality programs focused on quality measures are the Physician Quality Reporting Initiative (PQRI) and the Medicare Value based purchasing initiative (VBP). Both programs incentivize physicians and hospitals to publically report their performance on pre-specified quality metrics to receive their full Medicare reimbursement. PQRS metrics exist for all specialties and in 2014 nineteen separate measures exist for cardiac surgery (Table 1). Most deal with process or outcome measures in either the pre or postoperative setting, and some are relevant to CTICU care. Among the PQRS measures relevant to postoperative ICU care are antibiotic discontinuation, prolonged mechanical ventilation, postoperative stroke, renal failure, and reoperation. For anesthesiologists, participation in the Anesthesia Quality Institute National Anesthesia Clinical Outcomes Registry allows reporting of several additional measures via the Qualified Clinical Data Registry pathway including central line complications and postoperative re-intubation.

Because PQRS metrics are continuously changing each year, definitive evidence of their benefit is lacking. But even if little direct benefit can be shown, a collateral benefit of PQRS reporting is to force physicians and hospitals to develop data gathering and analysis resources to feedback data to physicians.

CURRENT AND FUTURE QUALITY CONTROVERSIES

Staffing

Although a culture of safety is vital in delivering high quality Cardiac ICU care, an equally important aspect of ICU organization is appropriate levels of staffing.

No clear data identify the type or qualifications of attending staff that should deliver care in a cardiac surgery ICU. Early observational studies have argued that the presence of a board certified intensivist is associated with a decrease in length of stay and mortality (Pronovost et al., 1999). In that study, ICU staffing in Maryland hospitals was assessed using a questionnaire. The presence of daily ICU rounds by

Table 1. PQRS measures for cardiac surgery

PQRS Measure	
PQRS 20	Pre Op Antibiotic Timing
PQRS 21	Pre Op Antibiotic Selection
PQRS 43	CABG- IMA use
PQRS 44	CABG- Pre Op Beta Blocker
PQRS 45	Cardiac Surgery- Antibiotic Discontinued within 48 hr
PQRS 164	CABG- Prolonged Vent
PQRS 165	CABG- Deep Sternal Wound Infection
PQRS 166	CABG- Stroke
PQRS 167	CABG- Renal Failure
PQRS 168	CABG- Reoperation
PQRS 169	CABG- Antiplatelet medication prescribed at DC
PQRS 170	CABG- Beta blocker prescribed at DC
PQRS 171	CABG- Anti lipid prescribed at DC
STS 1	CABG- Prolonged postoperative length of stay
STS 2	CABG- Short postoperative length of stay
STS 3	CABG + Valve Surgery- Prolonged postoperative length of stay
STS 4	CABG + Valve Surgery- Short postoperative length of stay
STS 5	Isolated Valve Surgery- Prolonged postoperative length of stay
STS 6	Isolated Valve Surgery- Short postoperative length of stay

a board certified intensivist had a 3 fold reduction for in-hospital mortality in abdominal aortic surgery patients. The absence of daily rounds was associated with an increased risk of cardiac arrest, acute renal failure, septicemia, platelet transfusion, and re-intubation.

While several studies have found similar results to Pronovost, dissenting opinions exist (Park et al., 2014; Higgins et al., 2003). In a large prospective database of 123 ICUs, Levy et al. found no outcome benefit to management by critical care physicians, in fact observing that mortality rates were higher for patients cared for by intensivists (Levy et al., 2008). Another 2012 study comparing hospitalists and ICU management in a tertiary medical center found no difference in adjusted mortality or LOS between hospitalist and intensivist-led care teams (Wise et al., 2012). Another study of a transition between surgical and medical trained intensivists and cardiac surgeons found no difference in mortality or adherence to quality measures, but noted lower drug costs and a shorter LOS (Whitman et al., 2011).

Although the true value of dedicated attending ICU staff is incompletely understood, the presence of a dedicated intensivist is considered a quality metric for large health care purchasing consortiums such as the Leapfrog group. Since 2008, to achieve the highest safety rating hospitals must have an ICU physician present 8 hours a day, 7 days per week, exclusively provide ICU care, return >95% of pages within 5 minutes, and have a physician substitute able to respond to patients within 5 minutes in >95% of cases (Rockeymoore et al., 2003). The Leapfrog group estimates that this staffing model will improve mortality rates by 30-40% when compared to light intensity staffing. A significant deterrent to the adoption of this staffing model was the unknown cost associated with increased staffing.

If "high intensity" care is better than "low intensity" care, then an important recent controversy is whether even higher intensity care results in even better outcomes. One recent trend in critical care staffing is in house 24 hour intensivist coverage. Proponents of continuous in house intensivist coverage argue that faster evaluations of critically ill patients will lead to more rapid identification and treatment of acute life threatening complications, and more consistent medical decision making in the teaching environment. Detractors from 24-hr staffing cite increased cost and paucity of data to suggest actual improvement of outcomes. Currently, existing evidence has found mixed effects of 24 hour attending coverage on patient outcomes. In one 2008 study in a single academic center, 24-hr intensivist coverage improved adherence to process measures, decreased hospital length of stay, and increased staff and patient satisfaction (Gajic et al., 2008). Another multi-institutional study retrospectively reviewed 49 ICUs in 25 hospitals using the APACHE database that evaluated 24 hr in-house staffing on ICU mortality (Wallace, Angus, Barnato, Kramer, & Kahn, 2012). Staffing levels were obtained using a questionnaire sent to the APACHE clinical coordinators at the institution. In a mix of academic and non-academic ICUs covered by residents (N=25), nonintensivists (N=6) and nurse practitioners (N=1). Night time intensivist coverage improved mortality when compared to hospitals with low-intensity daytime coverage, but no effect on mortality was noted in hospitals that already had high intensity staffing during the day. Three recent retrospective studies examining the relationship between patterns of care and ICU mortality (Kerlin, Harhay, Kahn, & Halpern, 2014; Wilcox, Harrison, Short, Jonas, & Rowan 2014; van der Wilden et al., 2013) also found no effect of staffing patterns on mortality, although end of life care in ICU decedents may have been improved (Reineck, Wallace, Barnato, & Kahn, 2013).

Although the evidence is clear that a mortality effect of nighttime intensivist staffing is small if present, it remains unclear why additional nighttime staffing does not clearly improve mortality in ICU patients. Possibilities include inadequate supporting staff, inadequate attending notification (if the attending is not called about an event, it doesn't matter if he/she is in house) and safety concerns with active management of patients at night when nursing, pharmacy, and respiratory staff are at a low ebb. When the considerable cost of nighttime intensivist staffing and the adverse health effects of shift work on practitioners including depression, obesity (Di Lorenzo et al., 2003), cancer (Kubo et al., 2006), heart disease (Fujino et al., 2006), and divorce (White & Keith, 1990) then the incremental benefit of shift work becomes even more unclear.

Overall, it is clear that a well-functioning ICU needs not only a culture of safety but adequate nurse and physician staffing to optimize patient outcomes. While the literature is not consistent with respect to the subspecialty training of the ICU physician running the team, high intensity care is clearly better than low intensity care, a dedicated intensivist improves outcomes in most studies, and 24 hour in house attending coverage, while intuitively better, has failed to demonstrate benefit in current trials.

The Effects of Safety Culture

Culture is defined formally as a way of thinking, behaving, or working that exists in a place or organization (hospital) (Merriam Webster, 2014). A *safety* culture can be described as one that constantly thinks and works towards creating an environment that reduces/minimizes patient hazards and errors in patient care. Because many small organizations may coexist in a large hospital, many safety cultures may exist with differences in perspective. Operating room personnel, for example, may view care priorities such as checking lab values differently from CTICU staff.

In contrast to an approach where change is only instituted when an adverse event occurs, a safety culture constantly seeks out hazards that increase the risk of harm to patients and providers, and strives to eliminate those hazards. Primary components necessary to a safety culture include a robust reporting system for adverse events, near misses, or potential safety concerns, identifying unsafe practices, providing institutional leadership in safety initiatives, participating in continuing education, and encouraging teamwork (P. J. Pronovost et al., 2003).

Systematic approaches to create or enhance a safety culture have been proposed. The eight step Comprehensive Unit Safety Program (CUSP), proposed by Pronovost, begins by identifying the current presence or absence of safety culture elements via a survey and initiating a program of staff education on principles of safety culture (P. J. Pronovost et al., 2006). The next step involves identifying safety concerns identified by the staff, implementing a strategy for improvement and designing a method to measure the effectiveness of the intervention. Additionally, hospital executives must be meaningfully engaged in the effort. The final part of the project is to disseminate the results of the interventions using both quantifiable data and case reports to make the results more relatable and then to re-evaluate the safety culture to assess for change.(Table 2)

Evidence that improving safety culture leads to associated improvements in patient outcomes, however, is elusive. In one single institution ICU study, use of a nurse driven discharge summary focusing on medication reconciliation found that 94% of patients had at least one wrongly prescribed medication. At the end of the 24 week trial period, 10 orders per week were corrected by the survey and the approach was subsequently adopted throughout the institutions (P. Pronovost et al., 2003).

Huang et al. performed a comparative multi-center survey using the Safety Attitudes Questionnaire –ICU to evaluate the existing safety culture of 30 ICU's participating in the Project IMPACT Clinical database. Although the response rate was less than fifty percent, Huang found an odds ratio for mortality of 1.24 and a 15% increase in LOS for every 10% decrease in safety score (Huang et al., 2010). However this study only compared existing safety culture among different organizations and cannot say whether interventions to change safety culture would have benefit.

As with care bundles, 24-7 staffing and externally promulgated programs such as SCIP, it is unclear why the presence of a safety culture does not clearly result in improved outcomes. One possibility is that safety culture is difficult to measure, and that metrics such as "engaged hospital executives" fail to capture a true culture of quality and safety. Recent data does suggest some ways to more accurately

Table 2.

Step	Eight-Step CUSP
1	Evaluate current safety climate
2	Educate staff on the principles of safety
3	Identify areas of concern
4	Engage hospital executives for meaningful participation
5	Implement improvements projects
6	Record results (identify metrics)
7	Disseminate results/stories of improvement
8	Re-evaluate safety culture

(Pronovost, 2006)

measure hospital quality. In a 2013 review of the Medicare Inpatient file, Tsai examined predictors of readmission rates after CABG, AAA repair, Lobectomy, and Colectomy (Tsai, Joynt, Orav, Gawande, & Jha, 2013). Hospitals with lower readmission rates were more likely to be nonprofit & nonteaching, and did no better on surgical quality metrics, but lower mortality rates and higher volumes were both correlated with lower admission rates, suggesting a common factor for both observations. When a similar analysis was performed for nonsurgical patients, McCrum et al. found that hospitals that did better on 30-day mortality for heart failure, myocardial infarction, and pneumonia had lower medical, surgical, and overall mortality (McCrum, Joynt, Orav, Gawande, & Jha, 2013). Taken together, these data suggest that characteristics of hospitals with quality include higher volumes, lower admission rates, and better heart failure, myocardial infarction, and pneumonia care.

CONCLUSION

Cardiac surgery has a long history of employing quality improvement strategies to improve care. However, patients presenting for cardiac surgery continue to become sicker and surgeries continue to increase in complexity. Fortunately, caregivers have several well established tools to assist in optimizing care quality. Large databases with state of the art risk adjustment can be used to risk stratify patients and guide post-operative care. Nation-wide quality improvement metrics, such as SCIP and PQRS, incentivize physicians to develop data reporting abilities in their ICU and may help with feeding back performance improvements. Successes such as the CLABSI initiative demonstrate that meaningful improvement in quality is possible and sustainable. Finally, an increasing hospital and national quality push has increased awareness among all caregivers of the potential benefits of directly addressing care quality and boosted awareness of a safety culture. As Dr. Donabedian has observed, "Systems awareness and system design are important for health professionals, but are not enough. They are enabling mechanisms only. It is the ethical dimension of individuals that is essential to a system's success. Ultimately, the secret of quality is love. You have to love your patient, you have to love your profession, and you have to love your God. If you have love, you can then work backward to monitor and improve the system" (Best & Neuhauser, 2004).

REFERENCES

Barsuk, J. H., McGaghie, W. C., Cohen, E. R., O'Leary, K. J., & Wayne, D. B. (2009). Simulation-based mastery learning reduces complications during central venous catheter insertion in a medical intensive care unit. *Critical Care Medicine*, *37*(10), 2697–2701. doi:10.1097/CCM.0b013e3181a57bc1 PMID:19885989

Bell, D. D., Ostryzniuk, T., Verhoff, B., Spanier, A., & Roberts, D. E. (1998). Postoperative laboratory and imaging investigations in intensive care units following coronary artery bypass grafting: A comparison of two Canadian hospitals. *The Canadian Journal of Cardiology*, *14*(3), 379–384. PMID:9551032

Berenholtz, S. M., Pronovost, P. J., Lipsett, P. A., Hobson, D., Earsing, K., Farley, J. E., & Perl, T. M. et al. (2004). Eliminating catheter-related bloodstream infections in the intensive care unit. *Critical Care Medicine*, *32*(10), 2014–2020. doi:10.1097/01.CCM.0000142399.70913.2F PMID:15483409

Berriel-Cass, D., Adkins, F. W., Jones, P., & Fakih, M. G. (2006). Eliminating nosocomial infections at Ascension Health. *Joint Commission Journal on Quality and Patient Safety*, *32*(11), 612–620. PMID:17120920

Best, M., & Neuhauser, D. (2004). Avedis Donabedian: Father of quality assurance and poet. *Quality & Safety in Health Care*, *13*(6), 472–473. doi:10.1136/qshc.2004.012591 PMID:15576711

Bouri, S., Shun-Shin, M. J., Cole, G. D., Mayet, J., & Francis, D. P. (2014). Meta-analysis of secure randomised controlled trials of beta-blockade to prevent perioperative death in non-cardiac surgery. *Heart (British Cardiac Society)*, *100*(6), 456–464. doi:10.1136/heartjnl-2013-304262 PMID:23904357

Bratzler, D. W., & Hunt, D. R. (2006). The surgical infection prevention and surgical care improvement projects: National initiatives to improve outcomes for patients having surgery. *Clinical Infectious Diseases*, *43*(3), 322–330. doi:10.1086/505220 PMID:16804848

Britt, R. C., Novosel, T. J., Britt, L. D., & Sullivan, M. (2009). The impact of central line simulation before the ICU experience. *American Journal of Surgery*, *197*(4), 533–536. doi:10.1016/j.amjsurg.2008.11.016 PMID:19249739

Burden, A. R., Torjman, M. C., Dy, G. E., Jaffe, J. D., Littman, J. J., Nawar, F., & Reboli, A. C. et al. (2012). Prevention of central venous catheter-related bloodstream infections: Is it time to add simulation training to the prevention bundle? *Journal of Clinical Anesthesia*, *24*(7), 555–560. doi:10.1016/j.jclinane.2012.04.006 PMID:23101770

Butterworth, J. F. t., Legault, C., Royster, R. L., & Hammon, J. W. Jr. (1998). Factors that predict the use of positive inotropic drug support after cardiac valve surgery. *Anesthesia and Analgesia*, *86*(3), 461–467. PMID:9495394

Dellinger, E. P., Hausmann, S. M., Bratzler, D. W., Johnson, R. M., Daniel, D. M., Bunt, K. M., & Sugarman, J. R. et al. (2005). Hospitals collaborate to decrease surgical site infections. *American Journal of Surgery*, *190*(1), 9–15. doi:10.1016/j.amjsurg.2004.12.001 PMID:15972163

Di Lorenzo, L., De Pergola, G., Zocchetti, C., L'Abbate, N., Basso, A., Pannacciulli, N., & Soleo, L. et al. (2003). Effect of shift work on body mass index: Results of a study performed in 319 glucose-tolerant men working in a Southern Italian industry. *International Journal of Obesity and Related Metabolic Disorders*, *27*(11), 1353–1358. doi:10.1038/sj.ijo.0802419 PMID:14574346

Dimick, J. B., Pelz, R. K., Consunji, R., Swoboda, S. M., Hendrix, C. W., & Lipsett, P. A. (2001). Increased resource use associated with catheter-related bloodstream infection in the surgical intensive care unit. *Archives of Surgery*, *136*(2), 229–234. doi:10.1001/archsurg.136.2.229 PMID:11177147

Dodek, P. M. (2012). Ventilator-associated pneumonia--in the eyes of the beholder. *Critical Care Medicine*, *40*(1), 352–353. doi:10.1097/CCM.0b013e318232665b PMID:22179380

Donabedian, A. (1966). Evaluating the quality of medical care. *The Milbank Memorial Fund Quarterly*, *44*(3Suppl), 166–206. doi:10.2307/3348969 PMID:5338568

Drakulovic, M. B., Torres, A., Bauer, T. T., Nicolas, J. M., Nogue, S., & Ferrer, M. (1999). Supine body position as a risk factor for nosocomial pneumonia in mechanically ventilated patients: A randomised trial. *Lancet*, *354*(9193), 1851–1858. doi:10.1016/S0140-6736(98)12251-1 PMID:10584721

Dua, A., Desai, S. S., Seabrook, G. R., Brown, K. R., Lewis, B. D., Rossi, P. J., & Lee, C. J. et al. (2014). The effect of Surgical Care Improvement Project measures on national trends on surgical site infections in open vascular procedures. *Journal of Vascular Surgery*, *60*(6), 1635–1639. doi:10.1016/j.jvs.2014.08.072 PMID:25454105

Edwards, F. H., Engelman, R. M., Houck, P., Shahian, D. M., & Bridges, C. R. (2006). The Society of Thoracic Surgeons Practice Guideline Series: Antibiotic Prophylaxis in Cardiac Surgery, Part I: Duration. *The Annals of Thoracic Surgery*, *81*(1), 397–404. doi:10.1016/j.athoracsur.2005.06.034 PMID:16368422

Ferguson, T. B. Jr. (2012). Mortality in coronary artery bypass grafting: What's next? *Circulation*, *125*(20), 2409–2411. doi:10.1161/CIRCULATIONAHA.112.106856 PMID:22547672

Fujino, Y., Iso, H., Tamakoshi, A., Inaba, Y., Koizumi, A., Kubo, T., & Yoshimura, T. (2006). A prospective cohort study of shift work and risk of ischemic heart disease in Japanese male workers. *American Journal of Epidemiology*, *164*(2), 128–135. doi:10.1093/aje/kwj185 PMID:16707650

Gajic, O., Afessa, B., Hanson, A. C., Krpata, T., Yilmaz, M., Mohamed, S. F., & Wylam, M. E. et al. (2008). Effect of 24-hour mandatory versus on-demand critical care specialist presence on quality of care and family and provider satisfaction in the intensive care unit of a teaching hospital. *Critical Care Medicine*, *36*(1), 36–44. doi:10.1097/01.CCM.0000297887.84347.85 PMID:18007270

Gott, V. L. (2005). Lillehei, Lewis, and Wangensteen: The right mix for giant achievements in cardiac surgery. *The Annals of Thoracic Surgery*, *79*(6), S2210–S2213. doi:10.1016/j.athoracsur.2005.02.078 PMID:15919253

Gozu, A., Clay, C., & Younus, F. (2011). Hospital-wide reduction in central line-associated bloodstream infections: A tale of two small community hospitals. *Infection Control and Hospital Epidemiology*, *32*(6), 619–622. doi:10.1086/660098 PMID:21558777

Hawn, M. T., Richman, J. S., Vick, C. C., Deierhoi, R. J., Graham, L. A., Henderson, W. G., & Itani, K. M. (2013). Timing of surgical antibiotic prophylaxis and the risk of surgical site infection. *JAMA Surgery*, *148*(7), 649–657. doi:10.1001/jamasurg.2013.134 PMID:23552769

Hawn, M. T., Vick, C. C., Richman, J., Holman, W., Deierhoi, R. J., Graham, L. A., & Itani, K. M. et al. (2011). Surgical site infection prevention: Time to move beyond the surgical care improvement program. *Annals of Surgery*, *254*(3), 494–499, discussion 499–501. doi:10.1097/SLA.0b013e31822c6929 PMID:21817889

Herzig, S. J., Rothberg, M. B., Feinbloom, D. B., Howell, M. D., Ho, K. K., Ngo, L. H., & Marcantonio, E. R. (2013). Risk factors for nosocomial gastrointestinal bleeding and use of acid-suppressive medication in non-critically ill patients. *Journal of General Internal Medicine*, *28*(5), 683–690. doi:10.1007/s11606-012-2296-x PMID:23292499

Higgins, T. L., McGee, W. T., Steingrub, J. S., Rapoport, J., Lemeshow, S., & Teres, D. (2003). Early indicators of prolonged intensive care unit stay: Impact of illness severity, physician staffing, and pre-intensive care unit length of stay. *Critical Care Medicine*, *31*(1), 45–51. doi:10.1097/00003246-200301000-00007 PMID:12544992

Hosseinian, L., Chiang, Y., Itagaki, S., Polanco, A., Rhee, A., & Chikwe, J. (2014). Earlier versus later tracheostomy in patients with respiratory failure after cardiac surgery in the United States. *Journal of Cardiothoracic and Vascular Anesthesia*, *28*(3), 488–492. doi:10.1053/j.jvca.2013.07.023 PMID:24295717

Hsu, Y. J., Weeks, K., Yang, T., Sawyer, M. D., & Marsteller, J. A. (2014). Impact of self-reported guideline compliance: Bloodstream infection prevention in a national collaborative. *American Journal of Infection Control*, *42*(10Suppl), S191–S196. doi:10.1016/j.ajic.2014.05.010 PMID:25239709

Huang, D. T., Clermont, G., Kong, L., Weissfeld, L. A., Sexton, J. B., Rowan, K. M., & Angus, D. C. (2010). Intensive care unit safety culture and outcomes: A US multicenter study. *International Journal for Quality in Health Care*, *22*(3), 151–161. doi:10.1093/intqhc/mzq017 PMID:20382662

Ingraham, A. M., Cohen, M. E., Bilimoria, K. Y., Dimick, J. B., Richards, K. E., Raval, M. V., & Ko, C. Y. et al. (2010). Association of surgical care improvement project infection-related process measure compliance with risk-adjusted outcomes: Implications for quality measurement. *Journal of the American College of Surgeons*, *211*(6), 705–714. doi:10.1016/j.jamcollsurg.2010.09.006 PMID:21109157

Kerlin, M. P., Harhay, M. O., Kahn, J. M., & Halpern, S. D. (2014). Nighttime Intensivist Staffing, Mortality, and Limits on Life Support: A Retrospective Cohort Study. *Chest*. doi:10.1378/chest.14-0501 PMID:25321489

Kubo, T., Ozasa, K., Mikami, K., Wakai, K., Fujino, Y., Watanabe, Y., & Tamakoshi, A. et al. (2006). Prospective cohort study of the risk of prostate cancer among rotating-shift workers: Findings from the Japan collaborative cohort study. *American Journal of Epidemiology*, *164*(6), 549–555. doi:10.1093/aje/kwj232 PMID:16829554

Kubota, H., Miyata, H., Motomura, N., Ono, M., Takamoto, S., Harii, K., & Kyo, S. et al. (2013). Deep sternal wound infection after cardiac surgery. *Journal of Cardiothoracic Surgery*, *8*(1), 132. doi:10.1186/1749-8090-8-132 PMID:23688324

Lamarche, Y., Sirounis, D., & Arora, R. C. (2011). A survey of standardized management protocols after coronary artery bypass grafting surgery in Canadian intensive care units. *The Canadian Journal of Cardiology*, *27*(6), 705–710. doi:10.1016/j.cjca.2011.08.123 PMID:22019278

LaPar, D. J., Isbell, J. M., Kern, J. A., Ailawadi, G., & Kron, I. L. (2014). Surgical Care Improvement Project measure for postoperative glucose control should not be used as a measure of quality after cardiac surgery. *The Journal of Thoracic and Cardiovascular Surgery*, *147*(3), 1041–1048. doi:10.1016/j.jtcvs.2013.11.028 PMID:24418668

Lee, J. C., Raman, J., & Song, D. H. (2010). Primary sternal closure with titanium plate fixation: Plastic surgery effecting a paradigm shift. *Plastic and Reconstructive Surgery*, *125*(6), 1720–1724. doi:10.1097/PRS.0b013e3181d51292 PMID:20517097

Levy, M. M., Rapoport, J., Lemeshow, S., Chalfin, D. B., Phillips, G., & Danis, M. (2008). Association between critical care physician management and patient mortality in the intensive care unit. *Annals of Internal Medicine*, *148*(11), 801–809. doi:10.7326/0003-4819-148-11-200806030-00002 PMID:18519926

Lin, D. M., Weeks, K., Bauer, L., Combes, J. R., George, C. T., Goeschel, C. A., & Pham, J. C. et al. (2012). Eradicating central line-associated bloodstream infections statewide: The Hawaii experience. *American Journal of Medical Quality*, *27*(2), 124–129. doi:10.1177/1062860611414299 PMID:21918016

McCrum, M. L., Joynt, K. E., Orav, E. J., Gawande, A. A., & Jha, A. K. (2013). Mortality for publicly reported conditions and overall hospital mortality rates. *JAMA Internal Medicine*, *173*(14), 1351–1357. doi:10.1001/jamainternmed.2013.7049 PMID:23797306

McDonnell, M. E., Alexanian, S. M., Junqueira, A., Cabral, H., & Lazar, H. L. (2013). Relevance of the Surgical Care Improvement Project on glycemic control in patients undergoing cardiac surgery who receive continuous insulin infusions. *The Journal of Thoracic and Cardiovascular Surgery*, *145*(2), 590–594, discussion 595–597. doi:10.1016/j.jtcvs.2012.09.031 PMID:23062416

Meyer, G. S., & Massagli, M. P. (2001). The forgotten component of the quality triad: Can we still learn something from "structure"? *The Joint Commission Journal on Quality Improvement*, *27*(9), 484–493. PMID:11556257

Moller, J. H., Shumway, S. J., & Gott, V. L. (2009). The first open-heart repairs using extracorporeal circulation by cross-circulation: A 53-year follow-up. *The Annals of Thoracic Surgery*, *88*(3), 1044–1046. doi:10.1016/j.athoracsur.2009.05.077 PMID:19699962

Murphy, G. S., Szokol, J. W., Nitsun, M., Alspach, D. A., Avram, M. J., Vender, J. S., & Hoff, W. J. et al. (2006). Retrograde autologous priming of the cardiopulmonary bypass circuit: Safety and impact on postoperative outcomes. *Journal of Cardiothoracic and Vascular Anesthesia*, *20*(2), 156–161. doi:10.1053/j.jvca.2005.04.003 PMID:16616653

Murphy, M. A., Whitman, I., Campfield, A., Moxey, E., Haddad, M., & Whitman, G. (2010). Intense implementation of a strict insulin infusion protocol does not guarantee postoperative glycemic control. *Journal of the American College of Surgeons, 211*(4), 465-469. doi: 10.1016/j.jamcollsurg.2010.06.003

Muscedere, J., Dodek, P., Keenan, S., Fowler, R., Cook, D., & Heyland, D. (2008). Comprehensive evidence-based clinical practice guidelines for ventilator-associated pneumonia: Prevention. *Journal of Critical Care*, *23*(1), 126–137. doi:10.1016/j.jcrc.2007.11.014 PMID:18359430

Nolan, T., & Berwick, D. M. (2006). All-or-none measurement raises the bar on performance. *Journal of the American Medical Association*, *295*(10), 1168–1170. doi:10.1001/jama.295.10.1168 PMID:16522838

O'Grady, N. P., Alexander, M., Dellinger, E. P., Gerberding, J. L., Heard, S. O., Maki, D. G., & Weinstein, R. A. et al. (2002). Guidelines for the prevention of intravascular catheter-related infections. Centers for Disease Control and Prevention. *MMWR. Recommendations and Reports*, *51*(RR-10), 1–29. PMID:12233868

Ong, A., Dysert, K., Herbert, C., Laux, L., Granato, J., Crawford, J., & Cortes, V. et al. (2011). Trends in central line-associated bloodstream infections in a trauma-surgical intensive care unit. *Archives of Surgery*, *146*(3), 302–307. doi:10.1001/archsurg.2011.9 PMID:21422361

Park, C. M., Chun, H. K., Lee, D. S., Jeon, K., Suh, G. Y., & Jeong, J. C. (2014). Impact of a surgical intensivist on the clinical outcomes of patients admitted to a surgical intensive care unit. *Annals of Surgical Treatment and Research*, *86*(6), 319–324. doi:10.4174/astr.2014.86.6.319 PMID:24949324

Pogorzelska, M., Stone, P. W., Furuya, E. Y., Perencevich, E. N., Larson, E. L., Goldmann, D., & Dick, A. (2011). Impact of the ventilator bundle on ventilator-associated pneumonia in intensive care unit. *International Journal for Quality in Health Care*, *23*(5), 538–544. doi:10.1093/intqhc/mzr049 PMID:21821603

Pronovost, P., Needham, D., Berenholtz, S., Sinopoli, D., Chu, H., Cosgrove, S., & Goeschel, C. et al. (2006). An intervention to decrease catheter-related bloodstream infections in the ICU. *The New England Journal of Medicine*, *355*(26), 2725–2732. doi:10.1056/NEJMoa061115 PMID:17192537

Pronovost, P., Weast, B., Schwarz, M., Wyskiel, R. M., Prow, D., Milanovich, S. N., & Lipsett, P. et al. (2003). Medication reconciliation: A practical tool to reduce the risk of medication errors. *Journal of Critical Care*, *18*(4), 201–205. doi:10.1016/j.jcrc.2003.10.001 PMID:14691892

Pronovost, P. J., Jenckes, M. W., Dorman, T., Garrett, E., Breslow, M. J., Rosenfeld, B. A., & Bass, E. et al. (1999). Organizational characteristics of intensive care units related to outcomes of abdominal aortic surgery. *Journal of the American Medical Association*, *281*(14), 1310–1317. doi:10.1001/jama.281.14.1310 PMID:10208147

Pronovost, P. J., King, J., Holzmueller, C. G., Sawyer, M., Bivens, S., Michael, M., & Miller, M. et al. (2006). A web-based tool for the Comprehensive Unit-based Safety Program (CUSP). *Joint Commission Journal on Quality and Patient Safety*, *32*(3), 119–129. PMID:16617943

Pronovost, P. J., Weast, B., Holzmueller, C. G., Rosenstein, B. J., Kidwell, R. P., Haller, K. B., & Rubin, H. R. et al. (2003). Evaluation of the culture of safety: Survey of clinicians and managers in an academic medical center. *Quality & Safety in Health Care*, *12*(6), 405–410. doi:10.1136/qhc.12.6.405 PMID:14645754

Reineck, L. A., Wallace, D. J., Barnato, A. E., & Kahn, J. M. (2013). Nighttime intensivist staffing and the timing of death among ICU decedents: A retrospective cohort study. *Critical Care (London, England)*, *17*(5), R216. doi:10.1186/cc13033 PMID:24090194

Rello, J., Ochagavia, A., Sabanes, E., Roque, M., Mariscal, D., Reynaga, E., & Valles, J. (2000). Evaluation of outcome of intravenous catheter-related infections in critically ill patients. *American Journal of Respiratory and Critical Care Medicine*, *162*(3 Pt 1), 1027–1030. doi:10.1164/ajrccm.162.3.9911093 PMID:10988125

Resar, R., Pronovost, P., Haraden, C., Simmonds, T., Rainey, T., & Nolan, T. (2005). Using a bundle approach to improve ventilator care processes and reduce ventilator-associated pneumonia. *Joint Commission Journal on Quality and Patient Safety*, *31*(5), 243–248. PMID:15960014

Shahian, D. M., Edwards, F. H., Jacobs, J. P., Prager, R. L., Normand, S. L., Shewan, C. M., & Grover, F. L. et al. (2011). Public reporting of cardiac surgery performance: Part 2--implementation. *The Annals of Thoracic Surgery*, *92*(3Suppl), S12–S23. doi:10.1016/j.athoracsur.2011.06.101 PMID:21867788

Skrupky, L. P., McConnell, K., Dallas, J., & Kollef, M. H. (2012). A comparison of ventilator-associated pneumonia rates as identified according to the National Healthcare Safety Network and American College of Chest Physicians criteria. *Critical Care Medicine*, *40*(1), 281–284. doi:10.1097/CCM.0b013e31822d7913 PMID:21926609

Snyder-Ramos, S. A., Mohnle, P., Weng, Y. S., Bottiger, B. W., Kulier, A., Levin, J., & Mangano, D. T. (2008). The ongoing variability in blood transfusion practices in cardiac surgery. *Transfusion*, *48*(7), 1284–1299. doi:10.1111/j.1537-2995.2008.01666.x PMID:18422857

Stulberg, J. J., Delaney, C. P., Neuhauser, D. V., Aron, D. C., Fu, P., & Koroukian, S. M. (2010). Adherence to surgical care improvement project measures and the association with postoperative infections. *Journal of the American Medical Association*, *303*(24), 2479–2485. doi:10.1001/jama.2010.841 PMID:20571014

Tsai, T. C., Joynt, K. E., Orav, E. J., Gawande, A. A., & Jha, A. K. (2013). Variation in surgical-readmission rates and quality of hospital care. *The New England Journal of Medicine*, *369*(12), 1134–1142. doi:10.1056/NEJMsa1303118 PMID:24047062

Unahalekhaka, A., Jamulitrat, S., Chongsuvivatwong, V., & Ovretveit, J. (2007). Using a collaborative to reduce ventilator-associated pneumonia in Thailand. *Joint Commission Journal on Quality and Patient Safety*, *33*(7), 387–394. PMID:17711140

van der Wilden, G. M., Schmidt, U., Chang, Y., Bittner, E. A., Cobb, J. P., Velmahos, G. C., & King, D. R. et al. (2013). Implementation of 24/7 intensivist presence in the SICU: Effect on processes of care. *Journal of Trauma and Acute Care Surgery*, *74*(2), 563–567. doi:10.1097/TA.0b013e31827880a8 PMID:23354251

Vital signs: central line-associated blood stream infections--United States, 2001, 2008, and 2009. (2011). *MMWR Morbidity and Mortality Weekly Report, 60*(8), 243-248.

Wallace, D. J., Angus, D. C., Barnato, A. E., Kramer, A. A., & Kahn, J. M. (2012). Nighttime intensivist staffing and mortality among critically ill patients. *The New England Journal of Medicine*, *366*(22), 2093–2101. doi:10.1056/NEJMsa1201918 PMID:22612639

Whitman, G. J., Haddad, M., Hirose, H., Allen, J. G., Lusardi, M., & Murphy, M. A. (2011). Cardiothoracic surgeon management of postoperative cardiac critical care. *Archives of Surgery*, *146*(11), 1253–1260. doi:10.1001/archsurg.2011.298 PMID:22106316

Wilcox, M. E., Harrison, D. A., Short, A., Jonas, M., & Rowan, K. M. (2014). Comparing mortality among adult, general intensive care units in England with varying intensivist cover patterns: A retrospective cohort study. *Critical Care (London, England)*, *18*(4), 491. doi:10.1186/s13054-014-0491-3 PMID:25123141

Wise, K. R., Akopov, V. A., Williams, B. R. Jr, Ido, M. S., Leeper, K. V. Jr, & Dressler, D. D. (2012). Hospitalists and intensivists in the medical ICU: A prospective observational study comparing mortality and length of stay between two staffing models. *Journal of Hospital Medicine*, *7*(3), 183–189. doi:10.1002/jhm.972 PMID:22069304

Youngquist, P., Carroll, M., Farber, M., Macy, D., Madrid, P., Ronning, J., & Susag, A. (2007). Implementing a ventilator bundle in a community hospital. *Joint Commission Journal on Quality and Patient Safety*, *33*(4), 219–225. PMID:17441560

KEY TERMS AND DEFINITIONS

Avedis Donabedian M.D: An internal medicine physician known as, "the father of quality in healthcare," his systems based model divides healthcare into structure, process and outcomes to identify and measure quality improvement.

Outcome: In the Donabedian model measures the overall result of the care provided. Ideally outcomes are closely tied to any structural and process variables manipulated in the quality improvement process.

PQRS: Physician Quality Reporting System is a national quality improvement project using process and outcome measures.

Process: In the Donabedian model denotes application of health care practices to the patient. Examples are removal of central lines when they are no longer needed and appropriately prescribing anti-platelet medications in patients with coronary artery disease.

SCIP: The Surgical Care Improvement Project is a national quality improvement project designed to implement process measures to decrease surgical site infection, venous thromboembolism, cardiac and respiratory events.

Structure: In the Donabedian model describes the attributes of the setting in which patient care occurs. Examples are the location of the ICU, staffing models, and equipment used.

STS Database: Registry of outcomes from >95% of cardiac surgery procedures performed in the United States used for quality improvement in cardiac surgery and risk stratification.

W. Edwards Deming, Ph.D: Developed a theory of continuous quality improvement focusing on improvement in the system rather than the "worker," and the need for "profound knowledge" of system operations to impact quality.

Chapter 3
Education and Training

Jennifer Sandadi
Weill Cornell Medical College, USA

June M. Chan
Weill Cornell Medical College, USA

ABSTRACT

Education and training has been the cornerstone of medicine from the days of the Hippocratic oath. What began as an informal apprenticeship has become a standardized curriculum, with heavy influence from the education sciences, regulatory bodies and societal demands. As an area of rigorous study in its own right, physicians have a responsibility to understand education theory and their effective application in clinical practice in order to fulfill their professional obligations. This chapter will outline past and current education theory relevant to critical care practice; introduce ideas and suggestions to implement these theories, and present new and emerging paradigms that are set to change graduate medical education in the upcoming decades.

INTRODUCTION

"By my teaching, I will impart knowledge of this art to my own sons, and to my teacher's sons, and to disciples bound by an indenture and oath according to the medical laws..." – Hippocratic Oath

In the mid-1900s, a group of psychologists began to organize the educational process into a framework. Benjamin Bloom (1956) led the efforts by devising a classification for consecutive levels of comprehension and application. He based his taxonomy on three domains: Cognitive (knowledge), Psychomotor (skills) and Affective (attitudes). This system has been revised over the last fifty years to adapt with modernizing education theory (Anderson, Krathwohl, & Bloom, 2001). However, Bloom's core concepts remain clear - Educators should focus on three main objectives of the training process and their clinical application:

- **Knowledge:** What learned information is needed for success?
- **Skills:** What cognitive and psychomotor abilities are needed for success?
- **Attitude:** What defines professionalism in this field?

DOI: 10.4018/978-1-4666-8603-8.ch003

The word 'doctor' is derived from the Latin word '*docere*', first coined by Cicero meaning 'to teach' (I. Shapiro, 2001). A core responsibility of the physician is to foster the development of the next generation of doctors. Despite this time-honored obligation, formal instruction on education theory and its application in the real world is rarely encountered during post-graduate medical training (MacDougall & Drummond, 2005). A clear understanding of how we learn allows for more effective development of the knowledge, skills, values and behaviors essential to the practice of medicine. The goals of this chapter are threefold: to present an outline of past and current education theory relevant to critical care training, introduce ideas and suggestions to implement these theories into practice, and present new and emerging paradigms that are set to change graduate medical education in the upcoming decades.

KNOWLEDGE

"A genuine higher education for the professions will not be content with reflecting the professionally defined competencies, but will assert alternative modes of reasoning, action and reflection into the curriculum." – Ronald Barnett (1994)

Introduction

The body of modern medical knowledge is broad in scope and ever-changing. This ephemerality poses a particular challenge to educators, who must define what constitutes a suitable foundation for effective clinical practice, while maintaining the flexibility to integrate contemporary developments. The effective delivery of this knowledge requires a keen perception of the learner's needs, awareness of a range of learning styles, and the selection of the most appropriate teaching strategies. With the increasing emphasis on technology in clinical practice, teaching methods have similarly followed suit and are areas of ongoing development. This section aims to discuss the current issues in curriculum design, as well as how education theory may be applied in a practical intensive care-based setting.

Curriculum Design

Curriculum theory is an academic discipline in its own right (Anderson et al., 2001; Flinders & Thornton, 2004). While the definition of curriculum remains a subject of debate, there are four components that are common to most proposed definitions (J. Grant, Abdelrahmen, & Zachariah, 2013):

1. A syllabus defining the knowledge base,
2. A set of endpoints,
3. A process of teaching and learning,
4. The enactment of this knowledge in the real world.

As the blueprint for education within an institution, it is both a powerful manifesto yet fully dependent on its context – balancing the focus between content, process and outcomes, theory and implementation, teacher and student, individual and institution (see Figure 1).

Figure 1. Influences on curriculum design

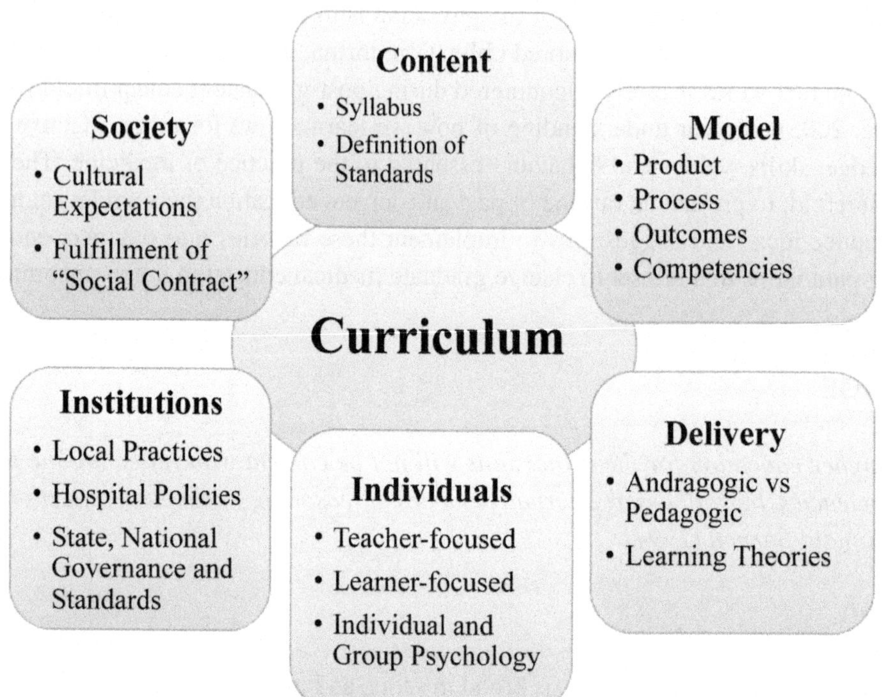

Tyler pioneered modern curriculum design in 1949 with a "product" model emphasizing structured outcomes and objectives as the basis for both learning and assessment (Tyler, 2013). The ability to form precise objectives and assess learners with efficiency and transparency made this model an attractive one to implement during the early introduction of standardized medical education in the early 1900s (Beck, 2004; I. Shapiro, 2001) and has subsequently influenced Western medical curriculum development for most of the twentieth century (Frank et al., 2010; MacDougall & Drummond, 2005). In the ensuring decades, this "product" model attracted criticism for being overly prescriptive and encouraging "learning by objective", to the detriment of other experiential learning (Kelly, 2009). Alternate models emerged alongside work on developmental psychology (as characterized by Piaget and Vygotsky) that were termed "process" based; that is, focusing on developing the cognitive mechanisms of attaining and applying knowledge to the clinical environment (Fish & Coles, 2005).

The erosion of heavily-structured objectives-based education, coupled with the cultural shift in the United States during the 1960s to 1980s, likely contributed to a notable decline in standardized test performance at the secondary and tertiary education level during that period (Carraccio, Wolfsthal, Englander, Ferentz, & Martin, 2002). This spurred a period of soul-searching amongst curriculum theorists, including notably Grant (1979), Harden (1999) and Spady (1994), who proposed the outcomes-based curriculum model and is the one upon which the current dominant standard for graduate medical education is based

Competence-based education arose during the 1970s, during a time where there was increasing demand for public accountability from the medical profession, and paralleled the formation of the Liaison Committee for Graduate Medical Education (later the Accreditation Council for Graduate Medical

Figure 2. Difference between Product, Process and Outcomes based models (with reference to work from (Kelly, 2009)

Note: Figure is made with reference to "The curriculum," (6 ed.), by A. V. Kelly, 2009, London: SAGE Publications.

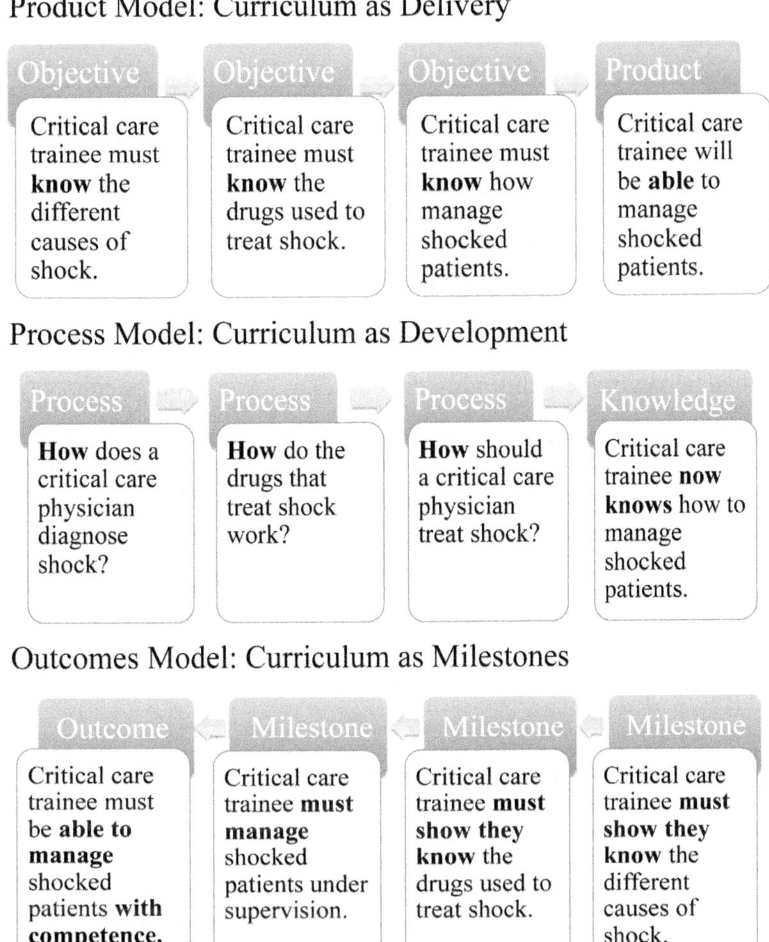

Education) (Carraccio et al., 2002). It was not until the 1990s, however, that this model saw formal adoption by international medical education bodies, first with the introduction of Tomorrow's Doctors by the General Medical Council (GMC) of the United Kingdom in 1993 (Iobst et al., 2010), (*Tomorrow's Doctors*, 1993). The new model was refocused on the learner's ability to demonstrate the appropriate application of knowledge in context, with emphasis on continuous formative assessment based on authentic representations of clinical work (Carraccio et al., 2002) (See Table 1).

Learning Theory and Its Influence on Curriculum Design

This evolution in curriculum theory has mirrored changes in learning models over the last century, reflecting the shifting socio-political landscape on which they are dependent. A selection of the predominant

Table 1. Structure-processed based versus Competency-based curriculum

Curriculum goals	Content	Outcomes
Curriculum driver	Teacher	Learner
Responsibility for content	Teacher	Learner and Teacher
Learning encounter	Knowledge acquisition	Knowledge application
Assessment	Single subjective	Multiple objective
Evaluation setting	Removed	Direct observation
Training period	Fixed time	Variable time

Note: Adapted from "Shifting paradigms: from Flexner to competencies," by C. Carraccio, S. D. Wolfsthal, R. Englander, K. Ferentz, C. Martin, 2002, Academic Medicine, 77(5), 361–367.

learning theories is presented in the table below (See Table 2). As the century progressed, the focus has shifted from individual behavioral conditioning encouraging lower order memory functions to socially based, integrative learning.

Many of these learning theories were developed with children as models and targets. In response, Knowles described several principles of adult learning in 1965, an approach termed "andragogy" (Knowles, Holton, & Swanson, 2011) ("adult-leading") as opposed to the prevailing pedagogic ("child-lead") approaches (See Table 3), and later described both as ends of a spectrum of teacher-learner directed learning (Merriam, Caffarella, & Baumgartner, 2007).

Table 2. Selected learning theories

Theory	Characteristic	Application
Behaviorism (1910s)	Knowledge is gained as a behavioral response to external stimuli.	• Rigorous, objective outcomes makes this suitable for psychomotor skills teaching • Positive / negative reinforcement by tutor can adversely impact learner
Cognitivism (1950s)	Knowledge is gained through understanding of mental processes	• Best for integrating knowledge with skills, values and attitudes • Understanding processes motivates adult learning • Social cognitivism allows sharing of mental models creating a coherent understanding of reality (e.g. in small group learning) • Focus on internal processing may de-emphasize the clinical environment in which the knowledge is based.
Constructivism (1970-80s)	Knowledge is gained by actively forming subjective representations of objective reality.	• Best for systems-based learning: integrating knowledge with skills, attitudes and clinical environment • Acknowledges individuality of learner and encourages self-directed learning • Social constructivism allows sharing of mental models allowing for different perspectives on applying this knowledge to the world (e.g. in problem-based learning) • Unsupportive educational environment can distort knowledge construction in the learner
Social Learning (1960s)	Knowledge is gained through interaction with role models and peers.	• Best for teaching attitudes and values • Collaborative learning provides multiple perspectives and improves socio-cultural competencies • Outcomes dependent on careful management of interpersonal dynamics

Note: Table data references "Human Learning," by J. E. Ormrod, 2002, Boston: Pearson and "Curriculum in Context," by J. Grant, M. Y. H. Abdelrahmen & A. Zachariah, 2013,

In K. Walsh (Ed.), Oxford Textbook of Medical Education (First edition), Oxford: Oxford University Press.

Table 3. Pedagogic vs. andragogic learning

Pedagogic Model		Andragogic Model	
Features	**Problems**	**Features**	**Problems**
• Needs Directing • One-way communication • Scheduled learning • Product driven	• Avoidance • Dependence on the educator for guidance • "Competitive" learning: focused on results, not the learning itself • Motivation	• Self-directing • Open communication • Continuous learning • Process driven	• Lack of structure • Missed content • Motivation

Note: Table data references: "A teaching model that promotes commitment, accountability, and responsibility." *by A. L. Beane, 1997, Educational Horizons, 76*(1), 45–52 *and "The Adult Learner," by M. S. Knowles, E. F. Holton, III & R. A. Swanson, 2011, Woburn:* Butterworth-Heinemann.

In the same way that a single descriptor cannot encompass the learning psychologies of all participants in a care team, adoption of a single education model will not meet the requirements of learners. By applying a variety of learning styles within a competency-based curriculum, educators allow for knowledge to be appropriately communicated, conceptualized and understood.

Education Theory and Its Practical Application in the Intensive Care Unit

There are a great number of suggested syllabuses for trainee education, some of which have been presented above. There is little guidance, however, on the practical application of the education sciences for teaching in ICU. In designing an education program for these trainees, it is important to integrate an understanding of the psychosocial influences that impact their ability to learn. While there are differences within each individual and institution, there are common experiences identifiable amongst residents in a modern ICU that can be summarized as (See Table 4):

1. Balancing Patient Care and Learning

Creating a culture of education within a busy, dynamic intensive care setting is challenging but is also rich in potential. It drives experiential learning through faculty leadership and diverse challenging clini-

Table 4. Barriers to learning in the Intensive Care Unit (Delva, Kirby, Schultz, & Godwin, 2004; Hoff, Pohl, & Bartfield, 2004; Nothnagle, Anandarajah, Goldman, & Reis, 2011)

Barrier to learning in the ICU	Proposed solutions
Balancing patient care with learning	• Creating a culture of education in the unit
Limited Access to learning	• E-learning resources • Self-directed learning • Establishing evidence-based protocols as guides to management
Satisfaction of achievement	• Encouraging trainee teaching and leadership

Note: Table data reference: "Assessing the relationship of learning approaches to workplace climate in clerkship and residency," by M. D. Delva, J. Kirby, K. Schultz, M. Godwin, 2004, Academic Medicine, 79(11), 1120–1126, "Creating a learning environment to produce competent residents: the roles of culture and context," by T. J. Hoff, H. Pohl, J. Bartfield, 2004, Academic Medicine, 79(6), 532–539, and "Struggling to Be Self-Directed: Residents - Paradoxical Beliefs About Learning.," by M. Nothnagle, G. Anandarajah, R. E. Goldman, and S. Reis, Academic Medicine, 86(12), 1539–1544.

Figure 3. Influences on the critical care trainee's participation in learning

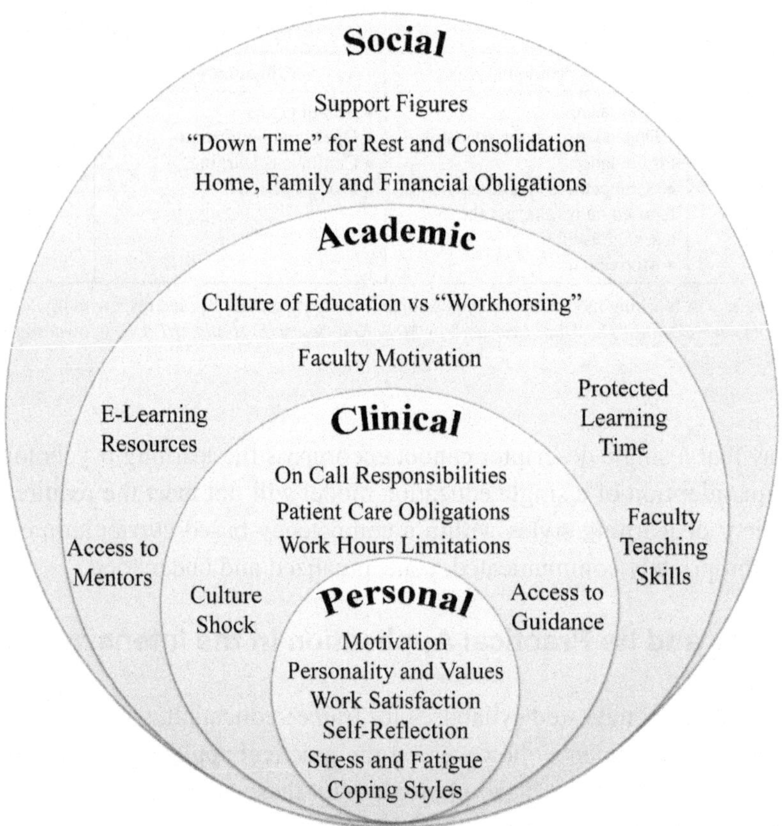

Box 1. Clinical vignette

The Challenges to Learning in an Intensive Care Unit
Dr. O is a third year critical care resident. She is particularly interested in learning the basic of bedside transthoracic echocardiography (TTE) and has made this one of her main learning goals for this rotation. She discussed his intentions with the critical care physician in charge of daily rounds, an expert in TTE within the faculty, who arranged to integrate it as a part of the daily physical exam that day as teaching. Shortly after rounds began, one of Dr. O's patients needed to be transported off-floor for an emergent radiological procedure. As the resident responsible for the patient, Dr. O accompanied and monitored the patient for the duration of their procedure. Due to its length, Dr. O misses most of the teaching rounds. According to the other members of the care team, it was a very informative session of hands-on TTE teaching. Dr. O returns to the critical care physician asking for another opportunity to review TTE. By then, the intensivist was attending to other tasks and was unable to oblige. "How about during tomorrow's rounds? It's my last day on service for a few weeks. We can go over TTE then." Dr. O is on call that night. She knows full well that as the only resident covering a busy unit overnight, she will be exhausted in the morning and probably in no shape to learn anything new. While technically she has the next day off as a part of work-hours regulations, this may be her only opportunity to learn from this particular intensivist and she is seriously considering breaking work-hours rules to attend.

cal situations (Teunissen et al., 2007), promotes team-based and shared learning (Stinson, Pearson, & Lucas, 2006) and provides a compass for self-directed and continuous learning for residents now and in their future career (Hoff et al., 2004).

The "routine" of a 24-hour intensive care work cycle provides a template for learning opportunities, which may be presented in multiple styles suitable for the individual strengths of participating faculty and trainees (see table 5).

The structure of current critical care teams is typically comprised of a small core group of clinicians, nurses, pharmacists and allied health practitioners. It follows that teaching in critical care also occurs most often in small groups. Small group learning principles are at the heart of most ICU-based education opportunities, and its core tenets of open communication, collaboration and group respect (Walton, 1997) have become a part of the broader culture of team-based medical practice. Faculty are leaders of the critical care team and often, by default, leaders in small group learning encounters. In order to be effective small group teachers, it is important to understand the principles governing small group learning. When applied correctly, it enhances team cohesion, facilitates free communication between faculty and resident, exposes team members to multiple perspectives and ideas, encourages residents to articulate and clarify their beliefs and ideas, and exercises the processes of integrating information and problem solving within a clinical care team (Edmunds & Brown, 2010; Steinert, 2004; Tiberius, 1999; Walton, 1997). Moreover, it allows the resident to monitor their own knowledge amongst their peers, promoting self-learning and independence. If improperly implemented, weaker group members may become isolated, and the group psychology may become dysfunctional, which may transfer into patient care (See Table 6).

Table 5. Daily teaching opportunities in the Intensive Care Unit

Routine	Example
Orientation	• Small Group: Learning the Equipment and Monitors, Didactics (Understanding Hemodynamics, Review of Evidence-based Protocols) • Scenario based training: Clinical vignettes • Simulation: Clinical vignettes, Application of unit protocols
Daily Rounds	• Small Group / Teams-based learning: Didactics (Clinical topics, operational and systems knowledge), Case-based discussion, Huddle coaching, Opportunistic learning / Rapid-fire teaching • Bedside teaching: Clinical examination, Point of Care Diagnostics • Role modeling: Communication, Collaboration, Leadership, Crisis Management, Resource Management
New Admissions	• Bedside teaching: Clinical Examination, Interpreting Monitors, Procedural Skills • Small Group: Case-based Discussion, Interpreting Hemodynamics • Role modeling: Communication, Collaboration, Leadership, Crisis Management, Resource Management
Protected teaching time	• Small Group: Didactics, Problem-based learning, Journal Club, Mortality & Morbidity, Quality Initiatives and Assurance, Game-based teaching: "Jeopardy", Competitive teams-led learning • Multidisciplinary team learning • Simulation • Self-directed learning
"Down time"	• Self-directed learning • E-learning • Reflection and Self-assessment • Rest and Consolidation

Table 6. Characteristics of small group learning

Positive characteristics	Negative characteristics
• Promotes teamwork and communication • Increased complexity and stimulation with group dynamics • Counteracts hierarchical culture outside of group learning • Knowledge is received and processed through multiple perspectives • Greater feedback opportunities	• Some participants may become overly dependent on their peers for problem solving • A broad spread of ability may lead to boredom for some, and others may feel out of their depth • Preparation burden for group leader • Time- and man-power intensive.

Note: Table data reference: "Small group methods in medical teaching," by H. Walton, 1997, Medical Education, 31(6), 459–464.

The key components to effective small group learning are interactivity, a collaborative group dynamic and structure (Walton, 1997). The group leader's role is central to maintaining these principles within their group. Whether it be lecture-based tutorials, role-play, bedside teaching or simulation-based teaching, the group leader should outline common goals and behavioral rules, recognize and respond to dysfunction in the group dynamic, and actively facilitate participation (Edmunds & Brown, 2010).

Tiberius (1990) described three broad sources of problems in small group learning, arising from dysfunctional structure, group interaction and motivation. Goals that are poorly delineated, irrelevant or communicated lead to inefficiency, apathy and poor preparation by the learners. Suggested strategies to manage problems in small group learning are detailed below (See Table 7).

2. Improving Access to Learning in the Critical Care Environment

Trainee participation in critical care learning may be limited physically by clinical distractions, on-call responsibilities and work-hours regulations. Stress and fatigue may also cognitively limit their ability to learn. "Culture shock" to the critical care environment and responsibilities may overwhelm the trainee's ability to cope with clinical demands, further compounding work-related stress. Solutions to this problem

Table 7. Common problems with small group learning

Problem	Example	Possible Solutions
Structure	Not getting through material	• Using goals as milestones • Set appropriate preparation material
	Not participating due to lack of background	• Send preparation materials ahead of time • Remind participants of the time and content of lesson
	Dissatisfaction with relevance	• Discuss group goals and tailor content to achieve these goals
Interaction	Domineering or disruptive group member	• Employ structured participation (go around the room) • Set ground rules • Privately address behavior
	Lack of participation	• Ensure group leader's authority is not overwhelming • Utilize techniques to enhance engagement (e.g. game-based teaching)
Motivation	Apathy	• Establish relevance of lesson • Reiterate educational impact of full participation • Utilize techniques to enhance engagement (e.g. game-based teaching)

Note: Table data reference: "Small Group Teaching," by R. G. Tiberius, 1999, London: Kogan Page Publishers.

are multifactorial and culture-dependent; below are examples of strategies that have been adapted from learning theory and modeled into principles emphasized by the ACGME ("ACGME Program Requirements for Graduate Medical Education in Anesthesiology Critical Care Medicine," 2013), and other graduate medical governance bodies (*The Trainee Doctor*, 2011).

I. Overcoming the Learning Curve

An important part of work-based learning is establishing a concrete place in the clinical environment for the learner (Teunissen et al., 2007). Orientation of junior trainees to the critical care environment should clearly delineate their dual roles: as clinicians with patient care responsibilities, and a specialist-in-training with expectations of meeting certain milestones and competencies. Orientation must therefore establish the physical space, the operational culture of the unit, and the cognitive and professional expectations of being a member of the critical care team. In doing so the trainee has a clear context in which to create education goals and to apply their newfound knowledge into practice (see Table 8).

II. Self-Directed Learning

Self-directed learning is a component of the ACGME Common Program Requirements (undefined author, 2013). While much is made of self-directed learning (SDL) in adult education theories, its practical application in graduate medical training continues to face several challenges. Nothnagle (Nothnagle et al., 2011) reports that even senior trainees often face difficulty with devising a structure and mustering the motivation to self-reflect, particularly in the face of stress and fatigue; there may also be a sense of guilt or inadequacy in seeking help for what they know conceptually but have little skill in. Residents appear to value guidance and direction from faculty to in order optimize self-directed learning rather than struggle alone.

The faculty's role in self-directed learning, therefore, is quite distinct from their role in small group learning. Whereas a group leader is a keeper and facilitator of knowledge, in self-directed learning the intensivist is a mentor, defined as one who enters a partnership with their mentee to help them achieve their personal and professional goals (Humphrey, 2010). The mentee remains the driver of self-directed learning and the mentor must take care to respect this role. Knowles (Knowles et al., 2011) described six assumptions about successful adult self-directed learning (See Table 9); using these assumptions as

Table 8. Domains of critical care orientation

Orientation Domain	Goal
Physical	• Establishes location of essential areas, equipment, personnel and sources of help
Cognitive	• Explicitly outline expected competencies at the end of training period • Formulate individualized learning goals to achieve these competencies • Reconcile informal "word-of-mouth" information with explicit curriculum • Review unit protocols and promote these as a guide for practice
Social	• Introduce team members • Outline aspects of unit culture important for practice • Provide positive role models, mentors and social support
Professional	• Provide avenues for resolving grievances and difficulties • Clearly establish clinical responsibilities • Outline assessment timelines

Table 9. Assumptions for successful adult learning

		Mentoring positives
Adults:	Are internally motivated	• Apply graded learning program • Avoid imposing own goals and agendas
	Apply their own life experiences to learning	• Facilitate self-reflection in processing learning modules • Establish rapport and communication with learner
	Are goal orientated	• Set clear curriculum • Facilitate formulation of clear learning goals
	Require relevance	• Provide meaning learning experiences • Case studies • Simulation
	Are practical	• Formulate difficult knowledge into a daily clinical context
	Like to be respected.	• Regard learner as colleague, not student • Encourage expression of opinion, ideas and feedback.

Note: Table data reference: "The Adult Learner," by M. S. Knowles, E. F. Holton, III & R. A. Swanson, 2011, Woburn: Butterworth-Heinemann.

a framework, practical assistance may be afforded by faculty to the mentee in setting their own learning milestones and reviewing their relevance, providing feedback through evaluation and self- and peer-reflection, and establishing protected time for progressively more independent, self-reflective learning.

III. E-Learning

The introduction of e-learning and education informatics has seen major developments in medical education since the 1990s, largely driven by the widening availability of computers and handheld devices, increasing multimedia capabilities and the growth of the internet (Choules, 2007; Liolios, 2008). Its popularity is due in part to its interactivity, entertainment value and easy access it allows to education resources outside the traditional clinical "classroom", especially at a time when access to both work hours and clinical experience is limited (Choules, 2007; Cook & McDonald, 2008; Ellaway & Masters, 2008). However, e-learning has also been notable for high initial cost of infrastructure, and limitations in hardware, implementation and usability (Childs, Blenkinsopp, Hall, & Walton, 2005; Cook, 2007) (See Table 10). It has also introduced learning problems that were not commonly seen with traditional teaching methods. An example of this is extraneous cognitive loading from poorly designed e-learning material, which can overwhelm the learner's information sensory and cognitive processing capacity, and lead to errors and inefficient learning (Young, van Merriënboer, Durning, & Cate, 2014).

E-learning is a powerful vehicle for an ever-expanding repertoire of teaching solutions; however, many of methods have yet to be validated with regard to their effectiveness (Cook, 2005). Broadly speaking, there are three main areas where e-learning is becoming heavily integrated with conventional techniques:

1. **Virtual Clinical Scenarios:** The rich palette of the Internet is ideally suited for building virtual clinical scenarios. A wide array of platforms exists, from complex software/hardware packages simulating entire virtual patient systems (Kononowicz & Hege, 2014; Seymour et al., 2002), simulated procedures (Ruiz, Mintzer, & Leipzig, 2006) to text-based, media-enhanced interactive case scenarios (Choules, 2007). Learning, knowledge retention and satisfaction are enhanced by engaging the trainee actively (Yoder & Hochevar, 2005) through interactivity, promoting an integration

Table 10. Characteristics of E-learning

Benefits	Disadvantages
• Accessible (site-independent, on-demand) • Flexible, Easily updated • Socially dynamic and Interactive • Standardizes course content • Allows for digital observation of learner online behavior • Allows for integration of outcomes assessment • Easy dissemination to larger audience without increasing time burden to teach	• Initial high cost • Hardware limitations, technology "creep" • Tech support • Chosen software platform may not work for everyone • Individual aversion to e-learning • Loss of team-building, emotional competence • Cognitive load

Note: Table data reference: "Web-based learning: pros, cons and controversies," by D. A. Cook, 2007, Clinical Medicine, 7(1), 37–42, "E-learning: is there anything special about the "E"?," by D. A. Cook and F. S. McDonald, 2008, Perspectives in Biology and Medicine, 51(1), 5–21, and "Introducing an online community into a clinical education setting: a pilot study of student and staff engagement and outcomes using blended learning," by K. Gray and J. Tobin, 2010, BMC Medical Education, 10(6).

of knowledge through problem solving and providing near-immediate feedback on performance. In the intensive care unit, where patients are often intolerant of minor physiological shifts, this is a potential solution to the ethical dilemmas of involving critical care patients in trainee education.

2. **Information and Media Sharing:** Blogs, wikis and podcasts ("Blog," n.d.; "Podcast," n.d.; "Wiki," n.d.) are online publications in common parlance today. The ability to widely and rapidly disseminate information makes e-learning an ideal platform for continuing medical education, online journal-club, and collaborative projects. It also allows for on-demand course materials, course evaluations and personal assessment. The responsiveness of internet-based platforms to the needs of end-users has lead to the development of new methods of information delivery, such as massive open online courses (MOOC), which combine content with access to expert opinion and interaction in a forum that can connect hundreds of thousand learners around world (Mehta, Hull, Young, & Stoller, 2013). Internet-based social media has unshackled peer interaction from the physical space and allowed spontaneous formation of interest groups spanning geographical boundaries, providing new social and experiential learning opportunities for the trainee (Grajales, Sheps, Ho, Novak-Lauscher, & Eysenbach, 2014).
3. **Milestones, Portfolios, and Credentialing:** Electronic credentialing is an evolving field in the era of competency based training with its emphasis on continuous assessment (Lipner, Hess, & Phillips, 2013). The ACGME has adopted a milestone system for assessing the trainee's path to competency ("The Anesthesiology Milestone Project," 2013); the use of the word "milestone" implying a clearly visible method of progressive formative evaluation. Online, real-time delivery of individualized assessment has allows for greater transparency and improved immediacy of results, thereby closing the loop of between educator feedback and change in trainee performance. The gathering of learning materials, assessment data and trainee-generated learning product in an education portfolio, and using this as a basis for teaching, is already well established as an effective form of competency-based and self-reflective learning (Buckley et al., 2009; Carraccio & Englander, 2004; Snadden & Thomas, 1998). The integration of e-learning technologies with individualized education portfolios improves engagement with learning and feedback mechanisms compared with traditional paper formats (Tochel et al., 2009). Building upon the electronic storage of competency milestones and the principles of life-long learning, Mehta (Mehta et al., 2013) described the concept of "digital badges", electronic credentials that document the competencies achieved by the trainee and follow them throughout their professional career as a form of electronic *curriculum vitae*.

Recent comparative work has shown at worst no inferiority of e-learning compared to traditional medical teaching (in terms of knowledge-based outcomes) for a broad range of critical care topics including difficult airway management (Bello et al., 2005), physiology (Dantas & Kemm, 2008), team skills (Cook, Dupras, Thompson, & Pankratz, 2005) and guidelines review (Cook et al., 2005), trainee reception of e-learning has been mixed to positive. Surveys conducted on the modern learner experience show that while they appreciate the attractiveness of interface and instant access to high-quality e-learning resources (Cochran, Edelman, Morris, & Saffle, 2008), personalized face-to-face teaching remains essential to their learning experience (Bell, Fonarow, Hays, & Mangione, 2000; Cook, 2007). This has given rise to the "blended" practice of using technology to introduce interactivity, interest and impact to a traditional small group model. This final trend highlights both the importance and limitations of e-learning within current education patterns, although as outlined above, new paradigms are emerging that may further enhance e-learning's role within a multimodal education program.

3. Residents and Fellows as Teachers

In the era of continuous competency assessments, residents and fellows are expected to constantly demonstrate their progressive transition to becoming a specialist physician. Teaching is a professional responsibility that is frequently delegated to trainees, starting from an early point in their career (Ruiz et al., 2006); in North America, residents and fellows are responsible for 20-70% of the clinical teaching received by medical students (Bensinger, Meah, & Smith, 2005). Resident and fellow teaching is an important consolidative activity in learning; it reinforces cognitive processes in accessing knowledge (Apter, Metzger, & Glassroth, 1988), enhances reflective learning (Busari, Scherpbier, Van Der Vleuten, & Essed, 2000), provides a sense of achievement and increases confidence (Busari et al., 2000; Morrison, Shapiro, & Harthill, 2005). It provides the trainee an opportunity for professional development and reproducing role model behavior (Busari & Scherpbier, 2004). Furthermore, faculty physicians are able to observe the processed end-result of their own teaching, thereby providing a mechanism of trainee assessment and feedback.

While trainees-as-teachers have arguably existed throughout the history of pedagogical medical education, it was not until the 1990s that explicit resident-as-teacher education curricula emerged in academic hospitals. It is now a component of specialist training in many teaching hospitals in the United States (Morrison et al., 2001), particularly within internal medicine and pediatric programs, and the rate of growth in the twenty years appears to be brisk (Bensinger et al., 2005). The rationale for developing a teaching skills course is three-fold: to empower the trainee-teacher, improve the quality and effectiveness of teaching, and to manage the internal conflict of their limitations as a trainee, their responsibilities as a clinician, and their emerging role as expert-in-training (Hill, Yu, Barrow, & Hattie, 2009). Integrating training in education principles early in residency is an investment in nurturing a cohort of specialist physician/teachers who can more effectively pass on their knowledge to the next generation.

Even in the absence of a formal education skills curriculum at their institution, intensivists can facilitate promoting trainees as teachers by recognizing the barriers to teaching in the critical care environment and overcoming them. Commonly reported problems include time management pressures, reluctance to mentor a student when their own need for supervision is unmet, and difficulties balancing critically-ill patient needs with teaching (Greenberg, Goldberg, & Jewett, 1984; Yedidia, Schwartz, Hirschkorn, & Lipkin, 1995).

Assessment of Knowledge

Assessment and feedback are the essential steps in adult reflective learning. Black and William (2004) describe two types of assessment events: formative and summative assessment (Black, Harrison, Lee, Marshall, & Wiliam, 2004). Formative assessment is a form of *a priori* feedback where a supervisor addresses specific areas of performance that could be improved. This information is then applied in the next educational encounter to further learning (Arends & Kilcher, 2010). By contrast, summative assessment is a post-priori review of performance and is commonly applied as an exit examination to confirm successful completion of learning objectives (see Table 11) (Wood, 2011).

Assessment of knowledge has traditionally been in the form of summative assessment (Cox, Irby, & Epstein, 2007). These were commonly in the form of written tests, the results of which were deemed accurate snapshots of a trainee's ability, and were collated into a final grade that summarized their performance against the curriculum expectation (Cox et al., 2007). While a clear role remains for summative assessment for the demonstration of competency in postgraduate medical training, the current trend now is to emphasize formative assessment as a tool for individualizing teaching (Rushton, 2005), which places responsibility on the assessors to create a test that not only encompasses content requisites but is valid in its representation of expected outcomes, relevant to the learner's understanding of the curriculum, and acceptable to all involved in the evaluation process (Van Der Vleuten, 1996). Formative assessment methods are known to increase trainee engagement with the assessment process and increases the reliability of results, and effectiveness of interventions based on these results (Schuwirth & Vleuten, 2011). However, the method and timing of assessment can also negatively impact learning by encourage last minute cramming, studying "to the test", and a superficial repetitious form of knowledge (Cox et al., 2007).

The over-reliance on written examination in modern medicine, particularly in the form of multiple-choice questions, is likely a vestige of the product-based approach to teaching, as well as its advantages in standardization, objectivity, time savings and cost. Careful design of the written test content can integrate clinical context, complex decision-making and subtle knowledge discrimination, albeit within an inflexible structure. Concerns over its absolute approach to right and wrong, and a tendency to rely on recall has lead to the development of alternate multiple choice answer formats that assess more subtle nuances in understanding and decision making (Bhakta, Tennant, Horton, Lawton, & Andrich, 2005; Charlin, Roy, Brailovsky, Goulet, & van der Vleuten, 2000).

Table 11. Differences between summative and formative assessment

	Summative Assessment	**Formative Assessment**
Timing	*Post-hoc*	*A priori*
Stakes	High	Low
Purpose	Summarizes achievements Sets standards	Monitors progress during training Provides feedback
Example	Specialist board examinations End of Year examination	In-training examination Weekly assignment

Note: Table data reference: "Assessment and Learning: differences and relationships between formative and summative assessment.," by W. Harlen and M. James, 1997, Assessment in Education: Principles, Policy & Practice, 4(3), 365–379

Traditional oral examinations remain a key barrier examination for specialist and sub-specialist medical bodies. In recent years, however, they have come under criticism for being unreliable, subjective and resource-intensive, and prone to racial, gender and language biases (Cox et al., 2007). However, it exercises several areas that are neglected in the written examination, including the integration of knowledge with professional and interpersonal competence, dynamic problem solving and defining the trainee's limits of knowledge (Memon, Joughin, & Memon, 2010). Moreover, Schuwirth argues that subjective data, such as concerning professionalism and non-technical preface, may be as useful as objective data in the assessment of medical trainees if the data is reliable and reproducible (Schuwirth & Van Der Vleuten, 2004). A structured approach has been advocated to improve test validity, reliability and minimize bias (Memon et al., 2010), the details of which are summarized in Table 12.

No one method of assessment can conclusively describe the trainee's knowledge, and one testing modality may be better suited to testing one domain of competency over another. The use of multiple methods of assessment spread out over multiple observations improves overall validity and reliability of results compared to single mode or encounter examinations (Norman, Van der Vleuten, & De Graaff, 1991; Van der Vleuten, Norman, & De Graaff, 1991). The ACGME describes nine features that improve the reliability, validity and applicability of post-graduate medical assessment programs (Swing, Clyman, Holmboe, & Williams, 2009):

1. Clear Purpose and Transparency
2. Blueprint
3. Milestones
4. Tools and Processes
5. Qualified Assessors
6. Assessor Training
7. Evaluation Committee
8. Leadership
9. Quality Improvement Process

By integrating greater range and flexibility in the design of assessment tools, more meaningful results can be obtained to feed back more effectively into the education plan of the trainee.

Table 12. Considerations for designing an improved oral examination

Quality End Points	Improvements
Validity	• Subject matter experts clearly establish what is being assessed. • Ensure assessment objectives are authentic and relevant to scope of practice.
Reliability	• Clearly determine and standardize a range of responses that encompasses what is being assessed. • Utilize formally trained examiners. • Review results using statistical methods to ensure reliability.
Fairness	• Utilize multiple examiners or observers to minimize judgment biases. • Examination items should be scrutinized by an appropriate group to minimize biases. • Variations in language and communication ability should be considered, but minimum acceptable standards for professional practice should be established.

Note: Adapted from "Oral assessment and postgraduate medical examinations: establishing conditions for validity, reliability and fairness" *by M. A. Memon, G. R. Joughin, M. Memon, 2010, Advances in Health Sciences Education, 15*(2), 277–289.

Giving Feedback

The process of feedback closes the educational loop by redirecting the results of assessment as new learning goals. Greater than merely an educational tool, effective feedback also enhances teacher-learner communication, indicates mutual respect, and promotes learner motivation (Ende, 1983). Conversely, poorly constructed feedback has little to no effect (or even a harmful effect) on the trainee's learning (Black & Wiliam, 1998).

Various models exist for giving feedback. Pendleton developed a set of "rules" (Pendleton, 1984) that didactically enforces reflection and balance in positive and negative feedback, as a counterweight to what was then a prevailing culture of what was perceived to be "destructive criticism" (Walsh, 2005). The increasing focus on learner-centered objective approaches to assessment lead to the development of alternative, more descriptive methods (See Table 13). In comparing the different models, it is evident that the key elements to effective feedback are very similar to the principles of adult learning (*see* Table 9): relevance, respect, collaboration and constructivism.

Knowledge: Summary Points

- Curriculum consists of the knowledge base, a set of end points, a method of teaching and learning, and the relationship of this knowledge with society and the world.
- Curriculum design has evolved over the last century from a content-based model to that which focuses on achieving competencies; that is, knowledge and skills applied in the clinical setting.
- Learning theory has progressively become more socially-based and learner focused, but the early models still have a role in the learning of specific areas of knowledge
- The critical care setting has many opportunities for education but also intrinsic barriers that can be overcome by promoting a culture of learning and education within the intensive care unit.

Table 13. Models for giving feedback

Pendleton's Rules (1984)	Agenda-Based Adaptation of descriptive feedback	Outcomes-Based Adaptation of Descriptive Feedback (SETGO method)
1. Establish learner's acceptance of feedback 2. Clarify and discuss material being assessed 3. Learner identifies strengths of performance 4. Observer identifies strengths of learner's performance 5. Learner identifies weaknesses in performance 6. Observer makes suggestions on improvements 7. Action plan for improvement is created based on discussion.	1. Identify learner's agenda 2. Discuss original desired outcomes 3. Encourage self-reflection and self assessment 4. Non-judgmental, balanced and supportive 360° feedback from all observers 5. Suggest alternative approaches to weaknesses 6. Rehearse suggestions through role play 7. Structure and summaries findings and lessons learned during assessment	1. Feedback with specific non-judgmental descriptors ("What I Saw") 2. Expand and facilitate discussion ("What Else did you see?") 3. Encourage reflection ("What do you Think?") 4. Clarify learning Goals before assessment 5. Offer suggestions of how to achieve these goals

Note: Adapted from "The Consultation," by D. Pendleton, 1984, Oxford: Oxford University Press, "The Calgary-Cambridge approach to communication skills teaching. 1. Agenda-led, outcome-based analysis of the consultation.," by J. D. Silverman, S. M. Kurtz, J. Draper 1996, Education for General Practice, (7), 288–299, and "The Calgary-Cambridge approach to communications skills teaching 2: The Set-Go method of descriptive feedback," by J. D. Silverman, J. Draper, S. M. Kurtz, 1997, Education for General Practice, (8), 16–23.

- The understanding of small-group learning principles and strategies is particularly relevant in critical care, which is formed in large part by small groups of trainees working and learning cooperatively.
- Trainee access to learning can be improved by promoting the use of E-learning and self-directed techniques, which are removed from the traditional clinical classroom but appears to be equally effective for learning.
- Promoting trainee as teachers is important for reflective learning, as well as the development of life-long teaching skills, which are invested into future specialist trainees.
- Assessment of trainees can be summative or formative. Both have different functions in the education curriculum. The current trend is towards continuous, formative assessment to feedback into learning.
- Effective feedback closes the education loop by redirecting assessment results into new learning goals, facilitates open communication and learner motivation.

SKILLS

"Knowing is not enough; we must apply. Willing is not enough; we must do." – Goethe

Introduction

The Association of American Medical Colleges defines a clinical skill as "any discrete and observable act within the overall process of patient care" ("Recommendations for Clinical Skills Curricula for Undergraduate Medical Education," 2005). Clinical skills relevant to intensive care can be broadly classified as technical skills and non-technical skills, with technical skills encompassing procedures and other complex motor tasks (See Table 14). The concept of non-technical skills is a relatively recent introduction in medicine but is well known in the aviation industry, where it is used to describe "cognitive, social and personal resource skills that complement technical skills, and contribute to safe and efficient task performance" (Flin, O'Connor, & Crichton, 2008). Effective skills acquisition and maintenance is an integral part of critical care medicine but adequate access to work-based experience is increasingly challenging and may no longer be relied upon as the only source for skills training (Kneebone et al., 2006). This section will examine the process models for procedural training, the developing field of non-technical skills training, skills supervision and assessment, and the role of simulation in skills acquisition.

Technical Skills

For decades the adage "See one, do one, teach one" comprised the informal curriculum for procedural skills training. This reflected the passive, behavioral models of learning that were dominant in the early to mid-20th century (See Table 15).

Common among these early models is the step-wise, passive exercise in skill progression, with reliance on repeated exposure in order to initially gain motor coordination, with awareness of clinical context appearing only after some familiarity has been achieved. The Dreyfus model gained traction in clinical education since its introduction through Benner's work in nursing training models in the 1980s

Table 14. Critical skills in Intensive Care

Technical Skills	Non-Technical Skills
Airway • Airway maneuvers • Airway devices • Intubation devices • Surgical airway **Breathing** • Oxygen delivery devices • Ventilator management • Bronchoscopy • Tube thoracostomy • Thoracocentesis **Circulation** • Arterial catheterization and care • Central venous catheterization and care • Pulmonary artery catheterization and care • Hemodynamic monitor interpretation • Cardioversion and defibrillation • Transvenous and transcutaneous pacing • Ventricular assist device management • Extracorporeal membrane oxygenation management • Pericardiocentesis **Point of care investigations** • Ultrasonography • Echocardiography	**Task Management** • Emergency planning and preparation • Prioritizing critically ill patients • Resource and bed flow management • Establishing evidence-based protocols, upholding standard of care, maintaining institutional guidelines **Team work** • Care coordination with critical care team and consulting medical and surgical services • Effective exchange of information • Leadership • Team player, team support **Situation Awareness** • Effectively gathering and monitoring of dynamic clinical data from multiple sources • Effective triaging of clinical data and its translation into action plans • Utilizing data to prepare for likely changes in patient or unit status **Decision making** • Efficiently identifying possible actions in response to an event • Efficient balancing of risks and benefits, and the selection of appropriate action • Monitoring and evaluating consequences of action **Documentation** • Daily patient record • Critical event record • Procedure records • Medical decision making documentation • Critical care time documentation • Billing compliance

Note: Adapted from "Guidelines for critical care medicine training and continuing medical education," by T. Dorman, P. B. Angood, D. C. Angus, T. P. Clemmer, N. H. Cohen, C. G. Durbin, Jr., 2004, Critical Care Medicine, 32(1), 263–272.

Table 15. Education models for Procedural Skills (Dave, 1970)

Dave (1970)	Simpson (1972)	Dreyfus (1986)
1. Imitation 2. Manipulation 3. Precision 4. Articulation 5. Naturalization	1. Perception / Awareness 2. Readiness 3. Guided response 4. Habitual mechanism 5. Complex response 6. Adaptation 7. Origination / Creation	1. Novice 2. Advanced beginner 3. Competent 4. Proficient 5. Expert

Note: Adapted from "Psychomotor levels," by D. H. Dave, 1970, In R. J. Armstrong (Ed.), Developing and writing educational objectives, Tucson: Educational Innovators Press, "The classification of educational objectives in the psychomotor domain.," by E. J. Simpson, 1972, Washington D. C.: Gryphon House, and "Mind over Machine: the power of human intuition and expertise in the age of the computer.," by H. L. Dreyfus and S. E. Dreyfus, 1986, Oxford: Basil Blackwell.

and introduces a cognitive element into the heretofore purely psychomotor concepts (Benner, 2004). It describes a linear progression from reflexive rule following, to contextual technical competence, through to the development of intuitive decision making while performing the task, implying the development of a deep, implicit knowledge coupled with the ability to dynamically analyze the task at hand. These traditional linear models of skills acquisition have come under some criticism for their overemphasis on psychomotor tasks (Kneebone, Nestel, Vincent, & Darzi, 2007) and lacking the accompanying social and cognitive elements that are essential to practice safety (Peña, 2010).

Modern curriculum design is now characterized by the delineation of clear objectives, a period of pre-clinical cognitive and psychomotor skills training, the introduction of these skills into the clinical arena, and the continuous involvement of subject matter experts (SMEs) to guide the teaching, evaluation and feedback process (Grantcharov & Reznick, 2008) (McLeod, Steinert, Trudel, & Gottesman, 2001) (See Table 16). In response to the move to competency-based education and increasing institutional and public demands for quality, safety and accountability, procedural skills education has rapidly evolved over the past two decades in complexity. Simulator and skills labs are now integral curricular components in procedure-critical specialties such as surgery (Reznick & MacRae, 2006), anesthesiology (Bould, Crabtree, & Naik, 2009) and intensive care (Barsuk, McGaghie, Cohen, O'Leary, & Wayne, 2009), and will be examined in detail later in this section.

Appropriate selection of curriculum and learning theory can be applied to compile a skills curriculum that responds to the needs of trainees within individual institutions and specialties. Evidence-based best practice, institutional protocols, local education resources, and the local needs of the group should guide skills training objectives (McGaghie, Issenberg, Petrusa, & Scalese, 2010). Procedural competency requires the mastery of skills in their clinical context; equal emphasis should be placed on both psychomotor skill and the related clinical contexts. A generic example of a skills curriculum is presented below, which is based on behavioral, cognitive and experiential learning models suited to the complexity of critical care setting (See Table 17).

Non-Technical Skills

The critical care setting is a high-acuity, rapidly changing environment that is unpredictable and marked by clinical uncertainty. Intensivists are expected to have the skills to manage patients and resources while maintaining a high standard of safety, quality and reliability. In his review, Reader (Reader, 2006) reported up to 50% of critical incidents in the ICU could be attributed to some form of non-technical skill deficit. In similar high-stakes industries such as the nuclear power and aviation industries, training in behavioral skills (termed "crew resource management") has been introduced to minimize errors and improve outcomes for the past four decades (Gordon, Darbyshire, & Baker, 2012; Toff, 2010). Medicine has had little formalized inclusion of non-technical skills training in clinical curriculum until the 1990s, when Gaba and colleagues introduced anesthesiology crisis resource management as a part of

Table 16. Three Phases of Clinical Skills Training

Pre-Training	Cognitive knowledge Psychomotor skills development Application of learning in skills lab/ simulator Direct observation and Expert Feedback
Clinical Exposure	Observation of procedure Direct observation Expert Feedback
Assessment and credentialing	

Table 17. Sample curriculum for central venous catheterization

Trainee will perform the insertion of internal jugular central venous catheters safely.		
Domain	**Competency**	**Learning goals**
Cognitive	Trainee should understand the anatomy, methods, indications, contraindications and complications of central venous catheterization.	• Anatomy and physiology • Ultrasound and radiologic anatomy • Differences between central vs. peripheral catheters • Infection control and sharps disposal • Complications of central line placement
Psychomotor	Trainee demonstrates technical ability in central venous catheterization.	• Introduction to central line kit • Sterile prep, gown, glove, hat and mask and drape • Seldinger technique • Ultrasound-needle skills • Guidewire management • Checking all lumens • Line fixation and dressings
Systems-level	Trainee demonstrates best practice in the care of central venous catheterization	• Preventing catheter-associated infection • Infection control and sharps disposal • Institutional protocols for central line placement

their simulation program (Gaba, Howard, Fish, Smith, & Sowb, 2001). Since then, formal non-technical skills development has expanded into the surgical, critical care, emergency medicine and obstetric environments (Baker, Gustafson, Beaubian, Salas, & Barach, 2005).

Part of the early difficulty in integrating non-technical skills training in a competency-based curriculum is due to the lack of objective assessment tools. Since then, several models have been described to allow for classification and evaluation. Flin and Glavin (1999) developed a taxonomy of non-technical skills from behavioral observations of anesthesiologists in the operating room environment (Patey, Flin, Fletcher, Maran, & Glavin, 2005), which has since been modified for surgeons (Crossley, Marriott, Purdie, & Beard, 2011). They proposed a framework of four broad categories and a behavioral rating scale allowing for evaluation of performance, which has been well validated in real-world usability trials (Fletcher et al., 2003). The main features are summarized in Table 18, and the full assessment tool can be accessed at http://www.abdn.ac.uk/iprc/ants/.

The other development that has allowed for the growth in non-technical skills training is the increasing accessibility and sophistication of simulators (Bradley, 2006; LeBlanc, 2012). Over the last two decades simulation-based education has become a complex area of study; while it cannot be reviewed in its entirety within this chapter, attention will be paid to its unique capabilities in medical education, strategies for the effective use of simulation in skills training, and outline its limitations.

Simulation and Skills Training

The concept of a "pre-trained novice" was made possible by the advent of medical simulators in the late 20th century (Van Sickle, Ritter, & Smith, 2006). Simulators can vary widely in design, complexity and cost, and include small bench top models (for practicing ultrasound-guided venous catheterization, for example), to virtual reality digital environments to a high-fidelity facsimile of a clinical environment (Palter & Grantcharov, 2010). Its introduction was largely driven by systems-level changes in health care, including work hours reform, the development of non-invasive critical care monitoring, changes

Table 18. Anesthesia Non-Technical Skills Assessment

Categories	Elements	Examples of Good and Bad Behavior
Task Management	• Planning and preparing • Prioritizing • Providing and maintaining standards • Identifying and utilizing resources	**Planning and Preparing:** *Good*: Communicates plan to team members *Bad*: Does not have emergency equipment
Team working	• Coordinating activities with team members • Exchanging information • Appropriately using authority and assertiveness • Supporting others	**Exchanging Information:** *Good:* Reports key events, confirms shared understanding *Bad*: Inadequate handover, does not include relevant people in communications
Situation Awareness	• Gathering information • Recognizing and understanding • Anticipating	**Anticipating:** *Good:* Takes action to avoid potential problems *Bad:* Does not consider potential problems, caught unaware
Decision making	• Identifying options • Balancing risks and selecting options • Re-evaluating	**Identifying options:** *Good:* Considers various options, asks for advice for difficult situations *Bad:* Jumps to one conclusion without considering alternatives

Note: Adapted from "Anaesthetists' non-technical skills," by R. Flin, R. Patey, R. Glavin, and N. Maran, 2010, British Journal of Anaesthesia, 105(1), 38–44.

in clinical practice leading to fewer procedures being performed, and an increasing cultural emphasis on patient safety (Kneebone et al., 2006; Palter & Grantcharov, 2010; Ziv, Wolpe, Small, & Glick, 2003). In bridging the gap between clinical exposure and the development of competency, simulation not only became a crucial teaching adjunct but a whole new teaching environment, where clinical scenarios could be controlled and repeated. It allowed for standardized assessment of trainees, and a closed loop feedback system where errors could be identified and corrected within the same teaching encounter (Kneebone et al., 2007). This is vitally useful in the critical care setting, where a small procedural error can cause devastating patient consequences.

Simulator encounters can be task-focused, or clinically-focused. Task trainers develop psychomotor procedural skills and equipment knowledge based on the principles of behavioral learning. By allowing for repetitive task processing, the initial steps on the learning curve can be taken in a safe, controlled environment, and problematic tasks may be repeated and analyzed to allow for focused attention (McGaghie, Issenberg, Petrusa, & Scalese, 2006). Rates of procedural skills acquisition correlate closely with experience in prior task training activities (Stefanidis et al., 2006) and this form of training is now a cornerstone of surgical procedural skills training (Sturm et al., 2008). Clinically-focused encounters are integrative exercises of non-technical skills and provide the context for procedural skills training. To facilitate the recreation of the various stimuli in clinical areas, these types of encounters often take place within high-fidelity simulated environments such as an operating theatre or trauma resuscitation area. This approach provides a social and cognitive framework for deeper understanding and integration of technical and non-technical skills. The immersive nature of clinically-focused simulation allows for risks and hazards to be introduced into training, allowing the trainee to incorporate familiar skills with clinical judgment and decision making (Gaba, 2004). Kneebone (2006) proposed an expansion of this model by combining a real human actor with a task simulator, further enhancing the clinical fidelity of the scenario by testing technical skills against stressors applied to trainee's professional and communication domains (Kneebone et al., 2006).

The task-focused encounter for technical skills should encourage the integration of the new task with the trainee's pre-existing knowledge. In these scenarios, the subject matter expert (SME) is a key learning resource for the trainee by providing the "gold standard" demonstration of the task and the cognitive processes behind it. While there is no one correct method of teaching, Miller's model of clinical competence (Miller, 1990) can be used as both a guide to teaching and assessment and has been used with success technical skills simulations (See Figure 4)

By contrast, the heavily social and experiential nature of non-technical skills training necessitates the establishment of clear learning outcomes prior to the creation of the simulation scenario itself (Salas, Wilson, Burke, & Priest, 2005). This maintains learning objectivity and minimizes distractions by the unfamiliar or lower-fidelity aspects of the simulator environment. Non-technical skills training typically requires multiple role players to generate the scenario; these may be trainees or standardized actors; regardless, all involved must be clear in their individual roles prior to the beginning of the lesson. The role of the SME is to evaluate and feedback rather than demonstrate, and guide the scenario from deviating too far from the learning objectives (Issenberg, 2006). Videography is becoming an essential tool for feedback in this setting, particularly as the repetition of complex social behaviors can be near-impossible even in a controlled simulator environment.

Figure 4. Miller's model of clinical competence
Note: Adapted from "The assessment of clinical skills/competence/performance," by G. E. Miller, 1990, Academic Medicine, 65(9), S63–67.

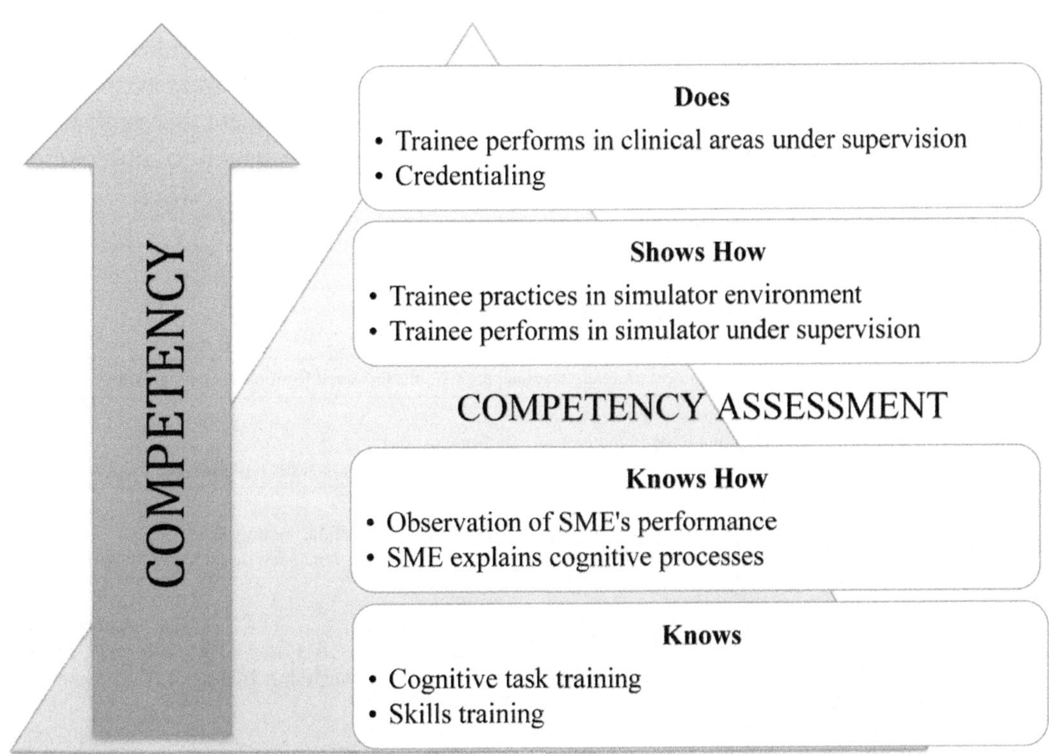

Despite the ubiquity of simulation in graduate medical education, there remain some limitations in its applicability and access. A review of simulation literature demonstrating the effectiveness and validity of simulation was limited by an over-representation of descriptive outcomes reporting, equivocal findings, varying methodologies and generally lacking in evidence base (Issenberg, McGaghie, Petrusa, Gordon, & Scalese, 2005; Sturm et al., 2008). Additional limitations of simulation training can be summarized in the table below (See Table 19). Despite the need for greater evidence of its efficacy and validity, simulation has intuitive benefits for skills training and patient safety, and deservedly takes on a core position in graduate medical training.

Supervision

The introduction of the procedure trainee into the critical care environment requires close supervision in order to optimize professional training and to safeguard patient safety (Kilminster, Cottrell, Grant, & Jolly, 2007) (Nasca, Day, & Amis, 2010). Supervision goes beyond merely observing the task and assuming legal responsibility; it encompasses the role of mentor, coach, observer and assessor (See Figure 5).

All procedures performed within the critical care environment by trainees are under the purview of the attending critical care physician, however it remains rare for ICUs to have 24/7 in-house attending physician supervision (Piquette, Fowler, & Slutsky, 2010). Farnan (2012) in his systematic review reported that enhanced attending supervision of trainees generally resulted in improved patient care and trainee education, particularly for invasive procedures and bedside patient assessment (Farnan et al., 2012), although there was no overall difference in patient mortality. The same group reported that the impact of increased attending night-time supervision was less conclusive and has been poorly studied (Farnan et al., 2012). More specific to the critical care environment, Piquette (2012) noted while that immediate, direct attending supervision improved medical trainee performance in critical care simulations compared to distant supervision by ICU fellows, it was at the expense of resident involvement in clinical tasks during real-world patient care (Piquette et al., 2010). Interestingly, these trainees did not show significant differences in unsupervised task independence on subsequent assessment. It implies the educational value of good supervision, perhaps allowing for a better quality of observational and cognitive learning.

Table 19. Limitations of simulator-based training

Transferability	• Simulation creating an "alternate reality" disconnected from professional practice
Resource burden	• High initial infrastructure cost • Ongoing costs of maintenance and support staff • Faculty development burden for SME* and supervisor skills training
Access	• Time-constraints on learner and SME • Physical separation from critical care unit is difficult during duty hours • Immersive learning may conflict with the attention demanded by critically ill patient care

* SME = Subject Matter Expert

Note: Table data references: "Features and uses of high-fidelity medical simulations that lead to effective learning: a BEME systematic review," *by S. B.* Issenberg, W. C. McGaghie, E. R. Petrusa, D. L. Gordon, and R. J. Scalese, 2005, *Medical Teacher, 27*(1), 10–28. "A systematic review of skills transfer after surgical simulation training," *by L. P. Sturm, J. A. Windsor, P. H. Cosman, P. Cregan, P. J. Hewett, G. J. Maddern, 2008, Annals of Surgery, 248*(2), 166–179.

Figure 5. Components of supervision

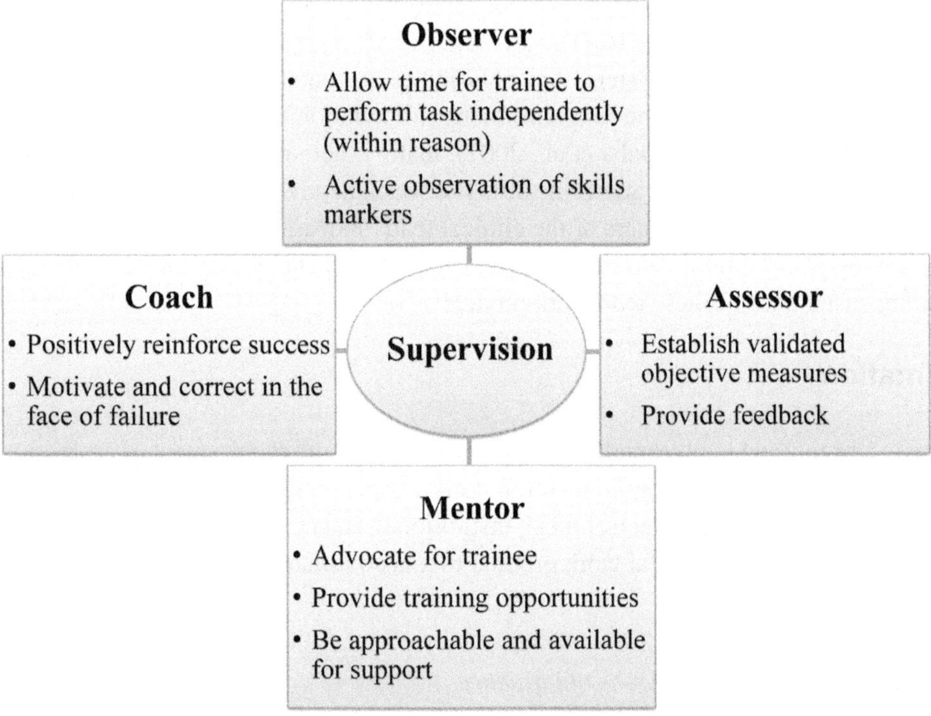

Skills Maintenance and Assessment

Tools that assist with maintenance and assessment of skills quality and standards include the use of clinical teamwork systems and checklists of competency objectives. The use of checklists in procedural skills training and evaluation is well-established, with several frameworks that are extensively studied and on the whole validated (McKinley et al., 2008). It clearly delineates the education and assessment goals, and forms a template for the "gold standard" of procedure thereby allowing standardization of performance and curriculum. Concerns have been raised over checklists leading to learning "by objective" and the knowledge deficits that can result from an overly-narrow design perspective (McKinley et al., 2008). Conversely, the use of well-designed checklists has the potential to expose the large "blind spot" in procedure skills training: task automation.

Behavioral learning models describe a degree of automation when a learner develops expertise with a procedure (H. L. Dreyfus & Dreyfus, 1986). The cognitive decisions that were explicitly made during the procedure are now disconnected from conscious awareness. Subsequently, this expert fails to pass on this sublimated information when teaching novices, leading to a knowledge gap that is perpetuated to another cohort of learners. Sullivan (M. E. Sullivan, Yates, Inaba, Lam, & Clark, 2014) describes the use of cognitive task analysis to capture the critical cognitive processes during procedural tasks as performed by experts. The rationale is that this implicit knowledge contributes significantly to what makes them an expert, and if it is explicitly documented (as a checklist, for example) it enables trainees access to expert knowledge and practice. Although cognitive task analysis is an emerging area of study in medicine, it has been well established and validated in military and there is evidence that this teaching model improves performance of novices (Clark & Estes, 1996). Its main limitation to generalized application is the time and resource burden to fully analyze and document the cognitive processes for a complex task (M. E. Sullivan et al., 2014).

The use of clinical teamwork systems has contributed to the successful exercise of non-technical skills in the clinical setting. Since the first introduction of aviation crew resource management training in anesthesia simulation in 1990 (Gaba et al., 2001), many other specialties have developed their own evidence-based teamwork systems (See Table 20). The social nature of this type of learning necessitates a collective "buy-in" from all members of the clinical team and significant investment in time and personnel. Leadership from administration and faculty can greatly influence the successful implementation and continuing sustenance of these teamwork models.

Documentation

Comprehensive, timely and legible medical documentation is a core requirement of professional medical practice and is a component of the communication skills competency as outlined by the ACGME. Medical documentation is the interface between clinical, institutional, financial, medico-legal and political forces in health care and is a visible clinical work product that is continuously under scrutiny (See Figure 6).

Figure 6. The medical document: Areas of influence

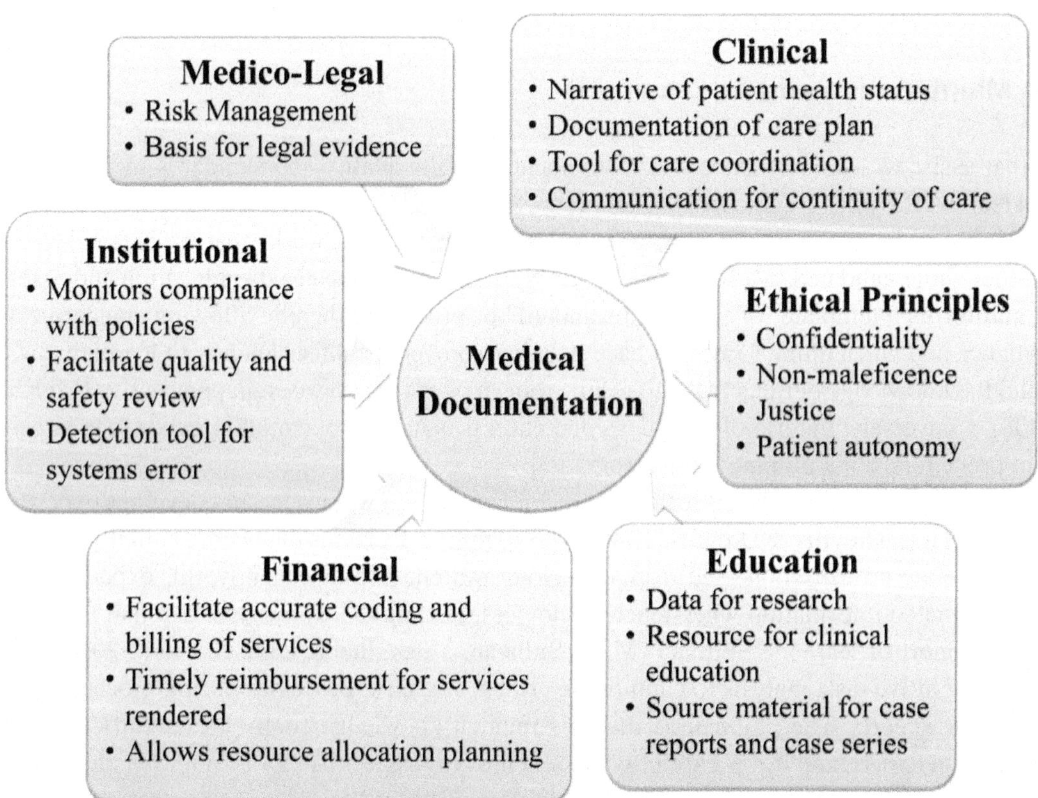

Table 20. Examples of health care teamwork systems

	Audience	Structure
Anesthesia Crisis Resource Management Program (1990) (Gaba et al., 2001)	• Anesthesiology • Operating room staff • Consulting physicians	• Based on commercial aviation critical incident training • Context-specific: teamwork during preset scenarios, focusing on ten core skills that can be applied in daily clinical practice and during crises • Evaluation through competencies via subjective and objective behavioral observations, and direct feedback • Three-day course with pre-reading material • Onsite training encompassing hands-on skills training, clinical event analysis, leadership and communication training, six hours of simulator scenario training with debriefing sessions. • Team-members rotate through different roles within scenarios, providing a 360° perspective on interpersonal operating room dynamics
MedTeams (1995) (Baker et al., 2005)	• Emergency Medicine • Emergency Nursing • Ancillary staff in the emergency department	• Proprietary teamwork system based on US Army helicopter pilot behavioral skills training • Context-specific: Teamwork during high-stakes uncertain situations where decisions are based on incomplete or conflicting data, focusing on five dimensions of effective teamwork based on needs-analysis data • Evaluation through objective behavioral checklists and rating scales and peer performance reviews • 14 hour classroom component with 6 month post-classroom clinical implementation phase • Classroom component encompasses behavioral training and feedback • Post-classroom phase provides regular mentoring, team-meetings, performance reviews and refresher courses.
Medical Team Management Program (2000) (Baker, Beaubien, Holtzman, Salas, & Barach, 2004)	• Physicians • Nurses • Laboratory technicians • Pharmacists • Ward clerks	• Based on US Air-Force fighter pilot crew resource management training • Generic context, applies to all inpatient and outpatient medical settings but designed for military medical settings • Instructors sourced from US military medical corps • Focuses on interdisciplinary team communication, command authority and local policy and regulations • Evaluation through knowledge testing, behavioral assessment and group feedback • Three-phase program of weeks-months duration - Phase 1: Internet-based pre-reading - Phase 2: Classroom group learning - Phase 3: Clinical practice and feedback, including a formal mechanism to reinforce training and assess progress.
Team Strategies and Tools to Enhance Performance and Patient Safety (2006) (Baker et al., 2005)	• Physicians • Nurses • Laboratory technicians • Pharmacists • Ward clerks	• Developed by the US Department of Defense and Agency for Healthcare Research and Quality • Generic context for all health care settings, inpatient and outpatient • Focuses on removing cultural barriers to teamwork between clinical care providers and creating a shared model for open information. • Provides framework for individually motivated sites to implement change • Evaluation through site-generated monitoring and feedback • Three-phase program lasting weeks-months - Phase 1: Assessment of organizational readiness, identifying leaders and barriers to implementation - Phase 2: Creation of location-specific action plans based on findings in phase 1, training of site-specific instructors to facilitate implementation. May encompass pre-training materials, simulation and group training as deemed most suitable for each institution - Phase 3: Sustaining skills learned through monitoring effectiveness and developing tools for continuing improvement

As a mode of communication between these different areas, the documentation of care should follow the same principles as verbal communication in the clinical setting: clear, accurate, concise and timely and context-appropriate. Despite its importance in health care, there is little to no guidance given to trainees in the essentials of medical documentation (Fakhry, 2000) (See Table 21). It is one of the earliest skills taught to medical students, often done so "on-the-job" by residents, which can propagate good as well as poor documentation practices. Furthermore, attending physicians "co-signing" a trainee note with only cursory review could lead to missed errors and the perpetuation of non-compliant practices. Critical care medicine poses even greater difficulties for medical documentation given the many changes in patient condition, the complexity of care and involvement of multiple consulting health care providers. These challenges make the case for the creation of explicit local guidelines for documentation, which should reflect local institutional and national regulatory requirements.

An additional layer of complexity is in considering the medical document as the basis for reimbursement. In the United States, third party insurers pay for services performed in the process of caring for the patient. The resultant diagnoses, procedures and services as documented in the medical record are coded into a numeric descriptor. Services, enumerated by the Current Procedural Terminology (CPT) system, are linked to the diagnosis justifying their treatment coded by the International Classification of Disease system (ICD, on version 10 as the time of writing) (Fakhry, 2000; M. J. Shapiro & Melendez, 2010). Financial charges are submitted based on these codes generated from the medical document. Due to its complexity and the sheer number of available codes describing individual specific services and diagnoses (the ICD-10-CM has over 150 000 codes) (Ramakrishnan, Hanauer, & Keller, 2010), billing and coding services have become a specialty field and rarely involves the physician except where accurate medical recordkeeping and CPT code selection is required. However, it is these physician responsibilities that are the most crucial in the reimbursement process. Inaccuracies in the medical record with subsequent errors in coding and billing of medical services not only results in loss of revenue but also constitutes fraud and abuse; this is clearly stated in federal legislation in reference to Medicare and other government funded health care programs (Fakhry, 2000).

The provision of critical care services has special considerations that intensivists, fellows and residents should be aware of as a part of their professional practice. While a comprehensive review is outside the scope of this chapter, the summary in Table 22 should provide some guidance for discussion and education.

Table 21. The essentials of medical documentation

- Legibility
- Identity of the provider, and the date of service
- Chief complaint
- Significant illnesses and medical conditions are indicated on the problem list
- Medication allergies are prominently noted in the medical record.
- Past medical history is easily identifiable.
- Appropriate notation concerning use of cigarettes, alcohol and recreational substances
- History and physical examination identifies appropriate subjective and objective information
- Laboratory studies
- Working diagnoses consistent with clinical findings
- Treatment plans consistent with diagnosis
- Encounter forms have a notation regarding follow-up care where indicated
- Length of visit, if counseling and care coordination is provided.
- Amendments, corrections and delayed entries should be clearly marked as such, with the original content maintained
- All orders must be signed, even telephone orders, otherwise on review it will be treated as if it was not performed

Note: Table data reference: "Guidelines for Medical Documentation," by the National Committee of Quality Assurance, 2006.

Table 22. Summary of CMS required documentation elements (Current as of April 2014)

Definitions of Critical Care Services (CPT 99291, 99292) • Critical illness = illness or injury acutely impairing one or more vital organ systems, such that there is a high probability of imminent or life-threatening deterioration • Critical care services = Physician's direct delivery of medical care for a critically injured patient, involving high complexity decision making to assess, manipulate and support vital organ system failure and/or to prevent further life threatening deterioration. • Failure to initiate these interventions on an urgent basis would likely result in sudden, clinically significant or life threatening deterioration in the patient's condition.
Requirements for documentation 1. Patient condition • Documentation of organ failure, or imminent risk of life-threatening deterioration • Relevant data supporting critically ill condition 2. Complexity of plan, e.g. • Ventilator management for acute respiratory failure • Dialysis for acute renal failure 3. Total time spent providing patient care • Total number of minutes where physician is immediately available to the patient, or Time in / Time out (minimum 30 minutes) • Exclude time for procedures billed separately 4. Activities involved • Review of tests and records • Discussion with care teams • Documentation • Patient care coordination • Exclude bundled critical care services: o Cardiac output and other physiological monitoring interpretation o Ventilator management o Gastric intubation o Chest X-ray interpretation o Blood gases interpretation, laboratory analysis of data stored in computers o Peripheral vascular access procedures o Temporary transcutaneous pacing • Be aware of procedures billed separately, e.g. o Cardiopulmonary resuscitation o Endotracheal intubation o Tracheostomy o Bronchoscopy o Arterial puncture and catheterization o Central venous catheterization o Intraosseous access o Tube thoracostomy o Temporary transvenous pacer o 12-Lead ECG interpretation o Elective electrical cardioversion • Be aware of situations requiring the use of modifiers, such as: o Resident involvement in procedures o Increased risk o Difficult procedure o Hemorrhage o Severe respiratory distress o Obesity 5. Details of discussion with health care proxy undertaken in order to facilitate patient care

Note: Table references: "Billing, coding, and documentation in the critical care environment.," by S. M. Fakhry, 2000, The Surgical Clinics of North America, 80(3), 1067–1083 and "Billing for Bedside Procedures.," by M. J. Shapiro and M. M. Melendez, 2010, In H. L. Frankel & B. P. deBoisblanc (Eds.), Bedside Procedures for the Intensivist. New York: Springer Science & Business.

Skills: Summary Points

- A clinical skill is any discrete, observable act within the process of patient care.
- Skills may be technical (focusing on psychomotor procedures) or non-technical (focusing on social cognitive tasks).
- Methods of learning procedural skills have moved away from repetitive motor training and now include explicit analysis of the cognitive processes involved with each step.
- The advent of simulation has allowed for the concept of the "pre-trained novice", with partial skills training prior to application in the clinical setting.
- Simulators may be task-focused for psychomotor skills training, or clinically-focused for the integration of technical skills into patient care and for non-technical skills training
- Supervision encompasses the role of mentor, coach, observer and assessor, and has value in education as a part of formative assessment.
- Implementation tools for technical and non-technical skills includes an array of checklists and clinical teamwork systems that have varying degrees of validation and reliability when used for assessment.
- Clinical Documentation is a vital skill that is rarely included in medical curricula; the specific complexities of critical care, coupled with its central role in health care should make this a point of educational focus.

ATTITUDES

"Personal and professional development is more than an isolated curriculum theme or strand, it is a way of approaching the entire course" – Jill Gordon

"...I know it when I see it..." – Justice Potter Stewart, Jacobellis v Ohio

Introduction

Professionalism is a core quality of a good physician and the basis of the social contract we hold with the community. In the past, it was seen as something that was observed and absorbed rather than explicitly taught, and nebulously defined within the same construct as ethics, morality and humanism (Cohen, 2007). Its formal introduction into the ACGME curriculum in 1999 and the subsequent movement towards a competency-based model of residency education has forced a more rigorous definition of professionalism to allow development of teaching strategies and assessment methods (Coulehan & Williams, 2000). Despite these efforts, there is still no agreed-upon definition of medical professionalism (see Table 23).

In broadly summarizing the sampling of definitions from an outcomes-based viewpoint, one can state that professionalism describes a set of desirable values and behaviors. These values and behaviors must meet the expectations of patients, fellow physicians, institutions and society of what is a "good" physician (S. R. Cruess & Cruess, 2012) (See Figure 7).

Faculty, charged with fulfilling this core curriculum component, must therefore develop strategies to assess the values and influence the behaviors of their residents and fellows. This is challenging on multiple levels. An individual's values are subjective, personal and influenced by their life experience.

Table 23. Definitions of professionalism

"Medical professionalism… is a set of observable behaviors [which are the] means to fulfill the profession's contract with society" *- J. J. Cohen (2007)*
"Professional competence is the habitual and judicious use of communication, knowledge, technical skills, clinical reasoning, emotions, values and reflection in daily practice for the benefit of the individual and the community being served" *– Epstein and Hundert (2002)*
"Medical professionalism is a belief system in which group members declare to each other, and the public, the shared competency standards and ethical values they promise to uphold in their work, and what the public and individual patients can and should expect from medical professionals" *– American Board of Medical Specialties* (Wynia, Papadakis, Sullivan, & Hafferty, 2014)
"Fellows must demonstrate a commitment to carrying out professional responsibilities and an adherence to ethical principles: Fellows must demonstrate competence in: • Compassion, integrity and respect for others • Responsiveness to patient needs • Respect for patient privacy and autonomy • Accountability to patients, society and the profession • Sensitivity and responsiveness to a diverse patient population, including diversity in gender, age, culture, race, religion, disabilities and sexual orientation; and, • Compliance with institutional departmental and program policies." *- ACGME (2014)*

Figure 7. Professional features of a "good" critical care physician

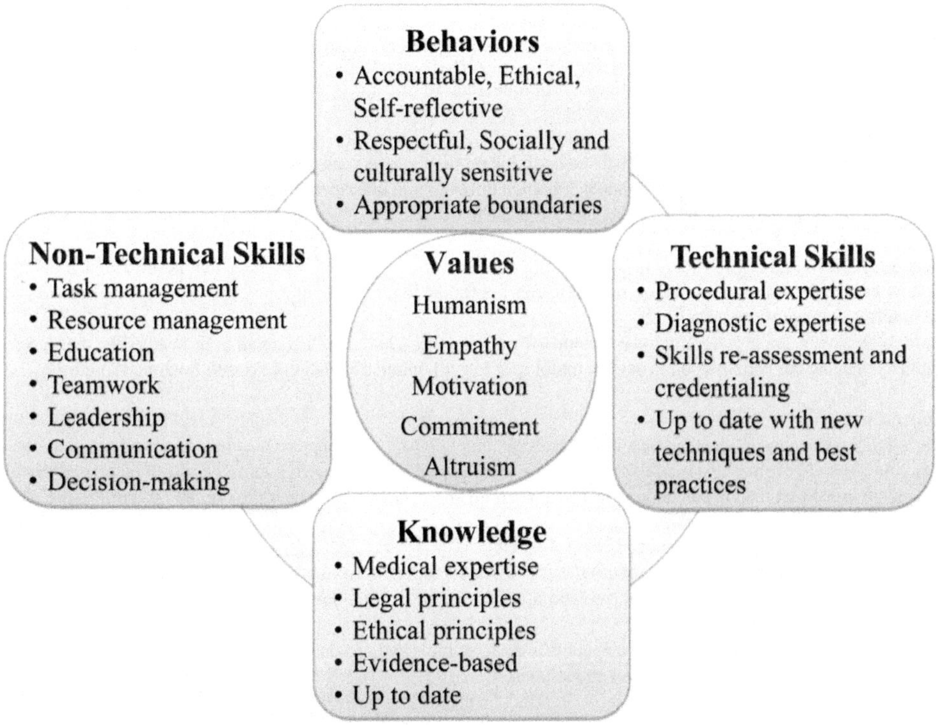

Behaviors
- Accountable, Ethical, Self-reflective
- Respectful, Socially and culturally sensitive
- Appropriate boundaries

Non-Technical Skills
- Task management
- Resource management
- Education
- Teamwork
- Leadership
- Communication
- Decision-making

Values

Humanism

Empathy

Motivation

Commitment

Altruism

Technical Skills
- Procedural expertise
- Diagnostic expertise
- Skills re-assessment and credentialing
- Up to date with new techniques and best practices

Knowledge
- Medical expertise
- Legal principles
- Ethical principles
- Evidence-based
- Up to date

Values are difficult to objectively measure and any attempts at directly commenting on an individual's values may be construed as confrontational and antagonistic. Values do, however, form a part of an individual's behavior, which may be observed and assessed by those around them.

The American Board of Medical Specialties (AMBS) takes the definition of professionalism one step further by describing it as a "belief system": that is, a motivational force subscribed to collectively by physicians to uphold the contract between their profession and society (Wynia et al., 2014). This relies on the uptake and propagation of shared beneficial values from one physician to another, further emphasizing the importance of the effective teaching and evaluation of trainee professionalism. When considered as a form of behavioral training, it becomes evident that teaching and evaluating professionalism is an expansion of the development of non-technical skills, discussed in the previous section. The primary difference, however, is that the teacher must recognize the insidious cultural factors pervasive in medical institutions that lead to unprofessional behavior, and what part they themselves play in this culture.

Box 2. Fictional case vignette

Professionalism
Dr. S is a critical care physician at an academic cancer center, responsible for patients who are often at the end stage of their disease. One such patient has been declining in the intensive care unit for several weeks despite aggressive therapy and is almost at the limits of care futility. He is incapacitated, has no advanced directive, and has a health care proxy (HCP) acting in his stead who wishes to continue aggressive treatment. The treating oncologist acknowledges there are some expensive salvage chemotherapy options that may extend life for several weeks. Dr. S, in her clinical assessment, feels that her patient would not survive the side effects and even with treatment is unlikely to survive beyond a few days at most. The patient's HCP is aggressively pushing for the chemotherapy to begin, but the patient's son feels he should have a dignified death and that this intensive level care is intrusive and dehumanizing. Dr. S has arranged a multidisciplinary meeting with the patient's HCP and his family to discuss the next steps in his care. Dr. C, the critical care fellow, has been invited to observe. **One Approach** Dr. C watches as Dr. S outlines the patient's clinical problems to his HCP and family. She, together with the oncologist, presents the treatment options, the pros and cons of each, and gives her opinion that despite any intervention the likelihood of imminent death is still high. The HCP interjects angrily, stating that it sounds like she is giving up on her loved one, and that she is the only one that seems to be advocating for his life. The patient's brother responds that being comatose and invasively monitored is not much of a life at all. Their interaction devolves into an antagonistic exchange, which Dr. S mediates by calling for quiet and to turn attention to her. Dr. S states that this level of exchange is not helpful to making decisions for her patient. She states that in the absence of any consensus from the HCP and family she will continue all current measures but thinks that any attempts at CPR or escalating pressors will be futile. She seeks the family's opinion of this plan. The HCP responds by saying she is not going to be the one to "pull the plug", and that "it's on all your heads if he dies". She walks out of the meeting angrily, leaving the patient's son to ask the oncologist to explain the treatment options to him one more time. **Alternate Approach** Dr. C watches as Dr. S introduces all the members of the meeting, and begins by inviting the patient's family to speak as she actively listened to their concerns. It becomes apparent that there was a lot of pre-existing simmering family conflict that has now come to the forefront. It is also revealed that the HCP is under considerable strain and is unwilling to bear the burden of "pulling the plug", but also does not want the patient to suffer needlessly. Dr. S reflects her observations to the group and invites the social worker and ethicist to offer their opinions. They outlined strategies to mitigate some the issues that are impacting patient care and offered to work with the family to resolve these. Dr. S, together with the oncologist, then outlined the patient's clinical status and reasonable management options, delivering this information in a way and context that his family can understand. The patient's HCP and family expressed increased understanding and satisfaction with the information presented. While they are not willing to make any concrete decisions about treatment, they agree together that a DNR is appropriate and that there should be specific limits on care escalation. They will work with social worker and ethicist to explore a possible consensus opinion about treatment withdrawal.

The Hidden Curriculum

The "hidden curriculum" refers to a socialization process during medical training, in which values are subliminally taught to trainees through the behavior of their peers and role models (S. W. Bloom, 1989; Hundert, Douglas-Steele, & Bickel, 1996; Mahood, 2011). This has most frequently been used to describe cultural factors within the hospital that ultimately lead to unprofessional and undesirable behavior through daily observations during training. While initially causing conflict with the idealism of early residency, these negative values are later subsumed into some trainee's own set of beliefs in a form of cultural acclimatization. Coulehan and Williams suggested that there are three behavioral responses to the conflict between idealist values and the hidden curriculum: abandoning the humanistic aspects of practice and becoming focused purely on technical skills and knowledge, distorting the negative culture into a framework that fits with the positive attributes that are explicitly taught, and overcoming the social indoctrination to successfully integrate the idealism into their professional practice (Coulehan & Williams, 2001). They contend that a majority of residents are in the second group, termed "non-reflective professionalism" (Coulehan & Williams, 2000). This is supported by work from Nagler, confirming that most residents can recite the desirable values and behaviors embodied in professionalism, but also have, at some point in their training, witnessed or engaged in unprofessional behavior themselves (Nagler et al., 2014). Hawryluck and Lingard have drawn similar conclusions in their reports of the hidden curriculum at work in the critical care setting, using direct observation and audio-capture to analyze team member interactions in the real world (Hawryluck, Espin, Garwood, Evans, & Lingard, 2002; Lingard et al., 2004). Sutcliffe posits that communication failures arising from these lapses into the hidden curriculum contributes to subsequent medical mishaps (Sutcliffe, Lewton, & Rosenthal, 2004).

Role Modeling

Role models, as described by Reed and Wright, are distinct from teachers (who impart knowledge and skills) or mentors (who work with mentees towards the successful achievement of their goals): they directly shape the values and behaviors of those around them through example and are therefore powerful teachers of professionalism (Reed & Wright, 2010; Reuler & Nardone, 1994).

Box 3. Fictional case vignette

The Hidden Curriculum
Dr. F is a fourth year critical care resident. He is caring for a patient who received a tricuspid and pulmonary valve replacement for infective endocarditis two days ago. The patient is extubated and is constantly complaining of pain despite the prescription of escalating doses of opioid analgesia.
Dr. F is approached by the nurse looking after the patient asking him to "please do something to shut that woman up – she's been driving me crazy with her whining". He reviews the analgesic dose history and notes that she has already received a large amount of opioid medications and asks his fellow for advice on how to treat her pain. The fellow replies "Oh, her? She's a druggie. You'll probably need a hammer to properly put her down. Just double the dose of whatever she's had and call for a pain consult – that way, she's their problem."
Dr. F orders the increased dose of pain medication, reviews her history on the electronic record and calls for a pain consultation. This was good advice – he *really* didn't want to deal that woman either.
The insidiousness of the hidden curriculum in hospital environments, particularly in stressful, high acuity areas, is such that no amount of explicit, formal teaching will alter its adverse influence unless these entrenched cultural practices are changed. Intensivists occupy a central role as the interface with all levels of the care team from student to allied health professionals to other specialty physicians, and are uniquely positioned to embody and propagate the best characteristics of their profession.

Broadly summarized, there are three stages to role modeling: self-reflection, social application and continuing development (S. R. Cruess & Cruess, 2012). Internal reflection requires self-awareness and honesty to allow a continuous cataloguing of one's own positive and negative beliefs and practices, and the discipline and willingness to improve upon them (Sambunjak, Straus, & Marusić, 2006) (See Table 24). Social application requires active translation those positive beliefs into behavior knowing others will observe them. Observers can implicitly or explicitly emulate, and can be encouraged to engage in their own self-reflection and develop their own skills in becoming good role models. Various authors have reported interactions between faculty and trainee that were consistently regarded as good role modeling were those that closely correlated with professionalism: respectful discourse with others, honest conduct, compassionate patient care, proficient clinical and communication skills, and genuine interest in their work and in their colleagues (Althouse, Stritter, & Steiner, 1999; Byszewski, Hendelman, McGuinty, & Moineau, 2012; Wright, 1996). Continuing development describes the propagation of good role modeling in one self through evaluation, and in others either informally through encouragement or formally through explicit teaching and faculty development.

Barriers to good role modeling include traits and behaviors such as impatience, disinterest, imposition of will and insensitivity. This is distinct from poor role models, who encourage unprofessional behavior in their observers through social conditioning. Lingard describes this in the perioperative context, where overt intimidation and frustration from senior team members had ripple effects through the other team members measured as observable negative behaviors (Lingard et al., 2004).

Strategies to promote good role models include self-reflection (see Table 25), formal professional development courses for faculty, fostering a cohesive faculty environment to facilitate peer role-modeling, acknowledgement of humanist behavior through honors and awards, and encouragement of their involvement in curriculum development. In creating more positive role models, a "critical mass" can be generated to overcome entrenched negative institutional practices.

Remediation

One of the greatest challenges in education is managing the struggling doctor. Academic departments devote significant amounts of time, effort and resources to a small group of trainees in difficulty (Hauer

Table 24. Influences on role modeling

	Positive role model	Negative role model
Personal factors	• Self-reflective but not self-centered • Altruistic • Applies humanist values • Personal stressors appropriately addressed and ameliorated	• Self-centered but unreflective • Humanist values does not translate into action • Unaddressed personal stressors, or inappropriate coping skills
Relational factors	• Open minded, considers others' point of view as equally valid • Congruent interests • Open communication • Respectful	• Closed minded, others' viewpoint invalid • Poorly matched personality • Communication gaps • Demeaning or abusive
Structural factors	• Continuity of interaction • Support and recognition from management • Makes time for interaction	• Lack of continuity • Minimal interaction • Unsupportive management • No time for interaction

Table 25. Strategies to improve role modeling

Encourage self-reflection • What makes a good role model? What makes a role model of mine a good one? • What aspects of my practice reflect these attributes of a good role model? • Which of my habits or behaviors are undesirable? o How can I change them, or avoid them in my daily practice? Self-awareness (not self-centeredness) with social interactions • Be conscious that you are always being observed. • Be aware of your own conduct, be it with patients, colleagues or junior staff. • Maintain clear communication with those around you, and be prepared to explain your actions.

et al., 2009). The rationale, first and foremost, is to preserving public safety; however, the subsequent objectives are less clear, depending on viewpoint, remediation may be seen as a threat of punishment, or as a higher level of assessment and feedback for trainee, the faculty and the teaching institution (Epstein & Hundert, 2002; Wu, Siewert, & Boiselle, 2010).

Poor performance is almost never attributable to merely one aspect of practice, but is a result of physical, psychological and socio-environmental factors that impair performance in the knowledge, skills and attitudes domains (See Figure 8). Some national governance bodies, including the General Medical Council (UK) together with the National Clinical Assessment Service (UK) have definitions of what constitutes a struggling trainee ("Managing Trainees in Difficulty," 2013), but few have clear guidelines for intervention and remediation.

Figure 8. Contributors to Poor Resident Performance

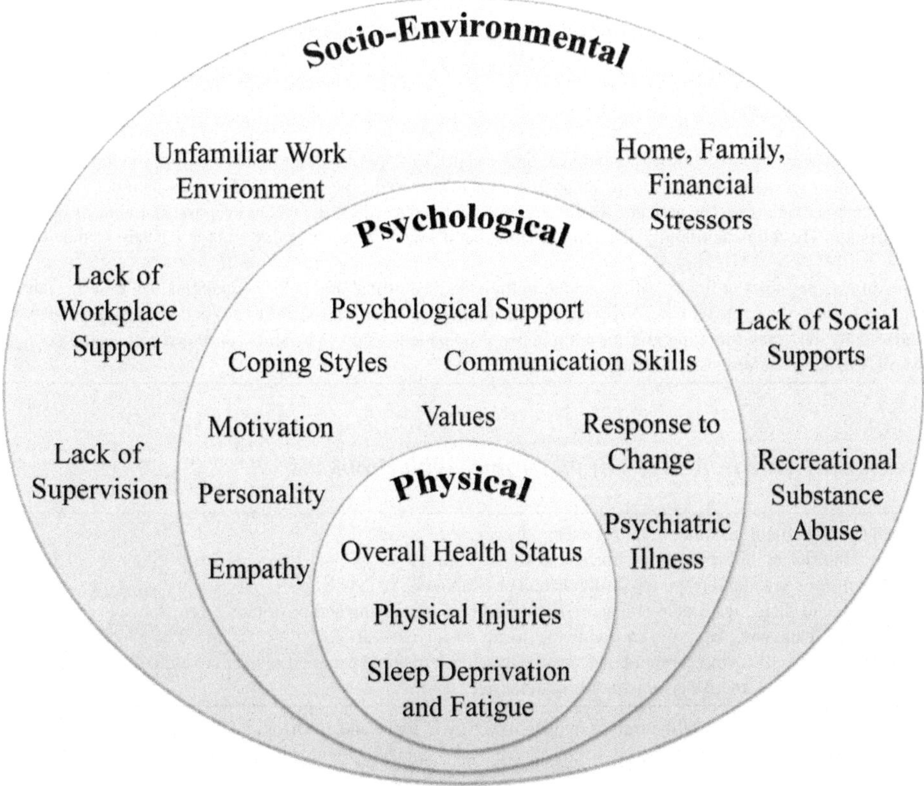

From the perspective of the ACGME curriculum, a struggling resident is deficient in one or more competencies. Internal medicine has produced the most research on identifying domains of resident difficulty using this definition. Dupras (2012) surveyed internal medicine program directors under the old ACGME curriculum and found up to 6.9% residents have demonstrated deficiencies (Dupras, Edson, Halvorsen, Hopkins, & McDonald, 2012). Perhaps unsurprisingly, the most reported problem area is in the patient care and medical knowledge domains, and over 76% of problem residents had deficiencies in more than one core competency. This finding was similar in surgical residency programs (Torbeck & Canal, 2009).

What are the markers for a resident in difficulty? Performance in in-training examinations and other scored knowledge exams could only prospectively identify less than 20% of problem residents. Identification of warning signs in residency application materials is unlikely (Dupras et al., 2012), although a negative or lukewarm dean's letter could have some correlation with future difficulties (Brenner, Mathai, Jain, & Mohl, 2010). Most problem trainees are identified through critical incidents direct observation and verbal reports from faculty and most trainees with problems typically become apparent early in training (Dupras et al., 2012; Yao & Wright, 2001). Paice (2004) describes generic attributes based on behavioral observation that can be displayed a trainee with problems (Paice & Orton, 2004) (See Table 26).

Box 4. Fictional case vignette

The Struggling Trainee
Dr. J is a PGY2 resident in her first critical care rotation. It is her third day in the ICU and she is on call. The ICU is very different to what she is used to. She is looking after fewer patients, but they all are so sick, have devices attached to them she's never seen before, and their condition is constantly changing. For much of the day she is trying to keep up and enact management plans from different consulting services. She has already had bad evaluations from her last two rotations saying that she wasn't keeping up with her work and was violating work hours. Her program director didn't offer much by way of concrete advice but did say that her work hours would be re-assessed next month to see if her organizational skills were still a problem. Nurses are constantly interrupting her work with other tasks and she just can't get anything finished before she has to do something else. By the time the other residents sign out to her, she feels completely overwhelmed. The fellow walks with her for patient rounds to summarize the management plans for the patients. She writes down her notes as best she can to keep track, and clear up as many of her questions up as possible. The fellow is friendly and approachable, but it's been such a long day and there is still so much work to do. After many hours of catching-up, she finally gets around to pulling the mediastinal drains for her patients. At least this part is easy – she's pulled lots of drains before. She starts with her VAD patient (the drain is an infection risk, after all) and frees up the maze of tubes on the chest. She wonders why the strange-looking inferior drain in her VAD patient seems to be stuck, and so she gives it a good strong pull. Shortly afterwards, the bedside alarms start sounding.

Table 26. Seven Early Warning Signs of the Trainee with Problems

1. "Disappearing act": Difficult to find or contact during the course of a work day
2. Low work rate: Inefficient, falls behind in clinical tasks
3. "Ward rage": Quick to anger and responds to slights real or imagined
4. Rigidity: Inflexible to changing clinical climate, difficulties in compromising and prioritizing, reluctance to ask for help
5. Bypass syndrome: Team members avoid involving the doctor during clinical care
6. Career problems: Difficulties with career choice, unable to achieve required examinations or credentials
7. Insight failure: Rejects constructive criticism, overly-defensive

Note: Table adapted from "Early signs of the trainee in difficulty.," by E. Paice and V. Orton, 2004, Hospital Medicine, 65(4), 238–240.

Approaches to remediation are necessarily personalized to the trainee and institutional-dependent in its enactment. Weinerth suggested a five-step model as a guide to goal-directed interventions that provides a simple, clear structure but overlooks several important processes in remediation (see table 27) (Zaas et al., 2013):

There are some limitations to Weinert's approach. The resident interview is not merely to communicate deficiencies and required improvements but the opportunity to establish the biopsychosocial influences on their difficulties and identifying the trainee's motivation to succeed. Furthermore, with objective assessments becoming the norm in medical education, preparation prior to the trainee interview is required not only to identify the deficiency and gather the evidence of underperformance, but also to establish the departmental resources available to assist the trainee with improvement. Just as a comprehensive medical history requires greater depth of approach than a physical review, the diagnosis of trainee problems and its successful remediation requires the full exercise of behavioral, cognitive and social approaches. An adaptation of Weinerth's model is suggested in Table 28.

Reported experience with remediation in post-graduate medicine is variable, largely due to broad spread of possible problem domains and the differences in remediation plans across different institutions. Dupras reported the most success in remediation for internal medicine trainees with deficiencies

Table 27. Weinerth's five-step policy for remediation

	Implementation
Identify deficiency	Relate to core competency, and specify observable behaviors that support this
Actions needed for improvement	Specify desired outcome and the measurable goals to achieve this, timeline for achievement
Determine criteria for success / failure	Identify modes assessment, time frame, and assessor.
Establish consequences of failure	Clearly outline all possible actions and outcomes with success, partial success and failure.
Proof of notification	Contract outlining remediation plan Resident signature, or witness, to document that the discussion took place

Note: Table adapted from "Constructive Corrective Action: Assessing and Developing Comprehensive Learning Plans for the Core Competencies.," by A. Zaas, K. Andolsek, J. L. Weinert, A. Nagler, R. Fortune, T. Tuck, and D. B. McNeil, 2013, Insight.

Box 5. Fictional case vignette

The Unprofessional Trainee

Dr. T is a critical care fellow who has been referred to you as a part of her remediation for unprofessional behavior. She has been at your ICU for three months, having transferred from an excellent residency program. She has an impressive bibliography and references in her CV, and the few times you have worked with her she has proven to have excellent clinical judgment and procedural skills.

She was recommended for remediation because of several complaints from nurses and patient family. These complaints document callous remarks about patients overheard by the nurse caring for the patient. Nurses also described a family meeting where a goals-of-care discussion was handled with insensitivity resulting in the family members walking out. This precipitated the intervention.

When questioned over the incident, Dr. T states that she feels she is an excellent doctor who always advocates for her patients. During this family meeting the health care proxy had unrealistic expectations of survival for their loved one. She said the family of this patient had to know he had no chance of surviving and that he was as good as dead. They would not agree to treatment withdrawal, a decision that was offensive to her: they were holding up an ICU bed that could go to someone who would benefit, instead of "this one who is unsalvageable".

Dr. T is offended that someone called her judgment into question and resents being in your office. She demands to know who it was that reported her so she could clear up the matter herself.

Table 28. Suggested model for remediation

Step	Implementation
Identify the problem	Identify the core competencies affected Detail the deficiencies Assess potential impact on trainee's development, on other co-trainees and faculty Misconduct: Need for involvement of legal or regulatory bodies
Gather evidence	Knowledge: Test scores Skills: Objective assessments, quality performance reviews Attitudes: Objective assessments, de-identified documented reports from team members
Establish baseline outcomes for success	Knowledge: Test scores, oral examination performance, competency milestones Skills: Supervised behavioral outcomes, competency milestones Attitudes: Observed behavioral outcomes, competency milestones
Identify resources available to assist with intervention	Knowledge: Tutors, Study program, Peer group study to assist with improving knowledge structures and cognitive processes Skills: Simulation, cognitive task analysis, coach/mentor, teamwork systems Attitudes: Simulation, non-technical skills training, psychologist, mentor/role model
Trainee interview	Establish non-threatening environment Outline problem to trainee Encourage trainee self-reflection for influencing factors Focused history on possible influences, if trainee not engaging Establish motivation for succeeding
Individualize remediation plan	Outline outcomes that need to be achieved Develop roadmap to these outcomes based on resident interview Outline assessments required, and their time frame Establish timeline for achievement of outcomes and review of progress Establish supervisors, mentors, assessors, and grievance officers involved in remediation.
Outline consequences of success / failure	Success: Mainstreaming with trainee group Partial success: Detail supervision requirements, outcomes and duration of probation Failure: Specify effect on duration of training, expulsion from program, trainee portfolio, references
Documentation	Document details of remediation plan and discussion Trainee does not have to agree with assessments, but must agree to participate in remediation Sign, date and file in trainee portfolio

Note: Table data references: "Constructive Corrective Action: Assessing and Developing Comprehensive Learning Plans for the Core Competencies.," by A. Zaas, K. Andolsek, J. L. Weinert, A. Nagler, R. Fortune, T. Tuck, and D. B. McNeil, 2013, Insight.

in the medical knowledge competency and the least with professionalism (Dupras et al., 2012), perhaps reflecting the more concrete interventions and outcomes achievable in the knowledge domain. These findings are consistent with the experience amongst surgical residents (Torbeck & Canal, 2009). More concerning is the lack of response to remediation in trainees who were deficient in professionalism, given that it was a relatively common cause of difficulty (Dupras et al., 2012).

The end point of remediation is binary: either the trainee returns to mainstream training, or they are dismissed from training. The stakes are high for individuals involved, and despite the efforts of academic faculty, not all trainees can be or are suitable for remediation. Conversely, a struggling trainee who has been appropriately mentored through remediation may prove to be successful when re-integrated into mainstream training, with the added experiential learning gained from remediation that could prove valuable to themselves and others in the future. As role models and gatekeepers to the profession, intensivists involved in the medical education have a responsibility to their profession to remain vigilant for those who are in difficulties, and make appropriate efforts to assist them to their fullest potential.

Attitudes: Summary Points

- Professionalism is a set of values, behaviors and social obligations that define good physicians.
- Values come from life experience and are difficult to objectively assess
- Values inform behaviors, which impact those around us. Behaviors can be observed and objectively assessed.
- Strong role models with humanist values can influence the values of others.
- Effective role modeling requires self-reflection and self-awareness with social interactions
- The Hidden Curriculum can negatively influence trainees, independent of what is taught about professionalism in the explicit curriculum.
- The trainee in difficulties often has multiple contributors to their struggles, and multiple competency areas are usually affected.
- There is little in interview materials that can predict a problem trainee.
- There are classic early warning signs that can help identify the problem trainee.
- Approaches to remediation should include objective evidence, multidisciplinary resources tailored to the problem domains, and a full diagnostic interview with the trainee.

REFERENCES

Accreditation Council for Graduate Medical Education. (2013). *Common Program Requirements*. Retrieved May 9, 2014 from https://www.acgme.org/acgmeweb/Portals/0/PFAssets/ProgramRequirements/CPRs2013.pdf

Accreditation Council for Graduate Medical Education. (2014). *Program Requirements for Graduate Medical Education in Anesthesiology Critical Care Medicine*. Retrieved May 9, 2014, from http://www.acgme.org/acgmeweb/Portals/0/PFAssets/ProgramRequirements/045_critical_care_anes_07012014_1-YR.pdf

Althouse, L. A., Stritter, F. T., & Steiner, B. D. (1999). Attitudes and Approaches of Influential Role Models in Clinical Education. *Advances in Health Sciences Education: Theory and Practice*, *4*(2), 111–122. doi:10.1023/A:1009768526142 PMID:12386424

Anderson, L. W., Krathwohl, D. R., & Bloom, B. S. (2001). *A taxonomy for learning, teaching, and assessing*. New York: Longman.

Apter, A., Metzger, R., & Glassroth, J. (1988). Residents' perceptions of their role as teachers. *Journal of Medical Education*, *63*(12), 900–905. PMID:3199418

Arends, D., & Kilcher, A. (2010). *Teaching for Student Learning*. New York: Routledge.

Baker, D., Gustafson, S., Beaubian, J., Salas, E., & Barach, P. (2005, July). Medical Teamwork and Patient Safety. *Agency for Health Care Research and Quality*. Rockville. Retrieved May 12, 2014, from http://www.ahrq.gov/research/findings/final-reports/medteam/index.html

Baker, D. P., Beaubien, M. J., Holtzman, A., Salas, E., & Barach, P. (2004). Medical team training: An initial assessment and future directions. Presented at the 19th annual meeting of the Society for Industrial and Organizational Psychology, Chicago.

Barnett, R. (1994). *The Limits of Competence*. Buckingham, UK: Open University Press.

Barsuk, J. H., McGaghie, W. C., Cohen, E. R., O'Leary, K. J., & Wayne, D. B. (2009). Simulation-based mastery learning reduces complications during central venous catheter insertion in a medical intensive care unit. *Critical Care Medicine*, *37*(10), 2697–2701. doi:10.1097/CCM.0b013e3181a57bc1 PMID:19885989

Beane, A. L. (1997). A teaching model that promotes commitment, accountability, and responsibility. *Educational Horizons*, *76*(1), 45–52.

Beck, A. H. (2004). The Flexner report and the standardization of American medical education. *Journal of the American Medical Association*, *291*(17), 2139–2140. doi:10.1001/jama.291.17.2139 PMID:15126445

Bell, D. S., Fonarow, G. C., Hays, R. D., & Mangione, C. M. (2000). Self-study from web-based and printed guideline materials. A randomized, controlled trial among resident physicians. *Annals of Internal Medicine*, *132*(12), 938–946. doi:10.7326/0003-4819-132-12-200006200-00003 PMID:10858176

Bello, G., Pennisi, M. A., Maviglia, R., Maggiore, S. M., Bocci, M. G., Montini, L., & Antonelli, M. (2005). Online vs live methods for teaching difficult airway management to anesthesiology residents. *Intensive Care Medicine*, *31*(4), 547–552. doi:10.1007/s00134-005-2561-0 PMID:15754200

Benner, P. (2004). Using the Dreyfus model of skill acquisition to describe and interpret skill acquisition and clinical judgment in nursing practice and education. *Bulletin of Science, Technology & Society*, *24*(3), 188–199. doi:10.1177/0270467604265061

Bensinger, L. D., Meah, Y. S., & Smith, L. G. (2005). Resident as teacher: The Mount Sinai experience and a review of the literature. *Mount Sinai Journal of Medicine: a Journal of Translational and Personalized Medicine*, *72*(5), 307–311. PMID:16184293

Bhakta, B., Tennant, A., Horton, M., Lawton, G., & Andrich, D. (2005). Using item response theory to explore the psychometric properties of extended matching questions examination in undergraduate medical education. *BMC Medical Education*, *5*(1), 9. doi:10.1186/1472-6920-5-9 PMID:15752421

Black, P., Harrison, C., Lee, C., Marshall, B., & Wiliam, D. (2004). Working Inside the Black Box: Assessment for Learning in the Classroom. *Phi Delta Kappan*, *86*(1), 8–21. doi:10.1177/003172170408600105

Black, P., & Wiliam, D. (1998). Assessment and Classroom Learning. *Assessment in Education: Principles, Policy & Practice*, *5*(1), 7–74. doi:10.1080/0969595980050102

Blog. (n.d.). Blog. *Merriam-Webster.com*. Retrieved May 11, 2014, from http://www.merriam-webster.com/dictionary/blog

Bloom, B. S., Engelhart, M. D., Furst, E. J., & Hill, W. H. (1956). *Taxonomy of educational objectives: Handbook I: Cognitive domain*. New York: David.

Bloom, S. W. (1989). The medical school as a social organization: The sources of resistance to change. *Medical Education, 23*(3), 228–241. doi:10.1111/j.1365-2923.1989.tb01538.x PMID:2725360

Bould, M. D., Crabtree, N. A., & Naik, V. N. (2009). Assessment of procedural skills in anaesthesia, *103*(4), 472–483. doi:10.1093/bja/aep241

Bradley, P. (2006). The history of simulation in medical education and possible future directions. *Medical Education, 40*(3), 254–262. doi:10.1111/j.1365-2929.2006.02394.x PMID:16483328

Brenner, A. M., Mathai, S., Jain, S., & Mohl, P. C. (2010). Can we predict "problem residents"? *Academic Medicine, 85*(7), 1147–1151. doi:10.1097/ACM.0b013e3181e1a85d PMID:20592510

Buckley, S. G., Coleman, J., Davison, I., Khan, K. S., Zamora, J., Malick, S., & Sayers, J. et al. (2009). The educational effects of portfolios on undergraduate student learning: A Best Evidence Medical Education (BEME) systematic review. BEME Guide No. 11. *Medical Teacher, 31*(4), 340–355. doi:10.1080/01421590902889897 PMID:19404891

Busari, J. O., & Scherpbier, A. J. (2004). Why residents should teach: A literature review. *Journal of Postgraduate Medicine, 50*(3), 205–210. PMID:15377808

Busari, J. O., Scherpbier, A. J. J. A., Van Der Vleuten, C. P. M., & Essed, G. E. (2000). Residents' perception of their role in teaching undergraduate students in the clinical setting. *Medical Teacher, 22*(4), 348–353. doi:10.1080/014215900409438

Byszewski, A., Hendelman, W., McGuinty, C., & Moineau, G. V. (2012). Wanted: Role models - medical students' perceptions of professionalism. *BMC Medical Education, 12*(1), 1–1. doi:10.1186/1472-6920-12-115 PMID:23153359

Carraccio, C., & Englander, R. (2004). Evaluating competence using a portfolio: A literature review and web-based application to the ACGME competencies. *Teaching and Learning in Medicine, 16*(4), 381–387. doi:10.1207/s15328015tlm1604_13 PMID:15582877

Carraccio, C., Wolfsthal, S. D., Englander, R., Ferentz, K., & Martin, C. (2002). Shifting paradigms: From Flexner to competencies. *Academic Medicine, 77*(5), 361–367. doi:10.1097/00001888-200205000-00003 PMID:12010689

Charlin, B., Roy, L., Brailovsky, C., Goulet, F., & van der Vleuten, C. (2000). The Script Concordance test: A tool to assess the reflective clinician. *Teaching and Learning in Medicine, 12*(4), 189–195. doi:10.1207/S15328015TLM1204_5 PMID:11273368

Childs, S., Blenkinsopp, E., Hall, A., & Walton, G. (2005). Effective e-learning for health professionals and students--barriers and their solutions. A systematic review of the literature--findings from the HeXL project. *Health Information and Libraries Journal, 22*(s2Suppl 2), 20–32. doi:10.1111/j.1470-3327.2005.00614.x PMID:16279973

Choules, A. P. (2007). The use of elearning in medical education: A review of the current situation. *Postgraduate Medical Journal, 83*(978), 212–216. doi:10.1136/pgmj.2006.054189 PMID:17403945

Clark, R. E., & Estes, F. (1996). Cognitive task analysis for training. *International Journal of Educational Research, 25*(5), 403–417. doi:10.1016/S0883-0355(97)81235-9

Cochran, A., Edelman, L. S., Morris, S. E., & Saffle, J. R. (2008). Learner satisfaction with Web-based learning as an adjunct to clinical experience in burn surgery. *Journal of Burn Care & Research; Official Publication of the American Burn Association, 29*(1), 222–226. doi:10.1097/BCR.0b013e31815ff2ac PMID:18182926

Cohen, J. J. (2007). Viewpoint: linking professionalism to humanism: what it means, why it matters. *Academic Medicine, 82*(11), 1029–1032. doi:10.1097/01.ACM.0000285307.17430.74 PMID:17971686

Cook, D. A. (2005). The Research We Still Are Not Doing: An Agenda for the Study of Computer-Based Learning. *Academic Medicine, 80*(6), 541–548. doi:10.1097/00001888-200506000-00005 PMID:15917356

Cook, D. A. (2007). Web-based learning: Pros, cons and controversies. *Clinical Medicine, 7*(1), 37–42. doi:10.7861/clinmedicine.7-1-37 PMID:17348573

Cook, D. A., Dupras, D. M., Thompson, W. G., & Pankratz, V. S. (2005). Web-based learning in residents' continuity clinics: A randomized, controlled trial. *Academic Medicine, 80*(1), 90–97. doi:10.1097/00001888-200501000-00022 PMID:15618102

Cook, D. A., & McDonald, F. S. (2008). E-learning: Is there anything special about the "E"? *Perspectives in Biology and Medicine, 51*(1), 5–21. doi:10.1353/pbm.2008.0007 PMID:18192762

Coulehan, J., & Williams, P. C. (2000). Professional Ethics and Social Activism. In D. Wear & J. Bickel (Eds.), *Educating For Professionalism: Creating A Culture Of Humanism In Medical Education*. Iowa City: University of Iowa Press.

Coulehan, J., & Williams, P. C. (2001). Vanquishing virtue: The impact of medical education. *Academic Medicine, 76*(6), 598–605. doi:10.1097/00001888-200106000-00008 PMID:11401802

Cox, M., Irby, D. M., & Epstein, R. M. (2007). Assessment in Medical Education. *The New England Journal of Medicine, 356*(4), 387–396. doi:10.1056/NEJMra054784 PMID:17251535

Crossley, J., Marriott, J., Purdie, H., & Beard, J. D. (2011). Prospective observational study to evaluate NOTSS (Non-Technical Skills for Surgeons) for assessing trainees' non-technical performance in the operating theatre. *British Journal of Surgery, 98*(7), 1010–1020. doi:10.1002/bjs.7478 PMID:21480195

Cruess, S. R., & Cruess, R. L. (2012). Teaching professionalism - Why, What and How. *Facts. Views & Vision in ObGyn, 4*(4), 259–265.

Dantas, A. M., & Kemm, R. E. (2008). A blended approach to active learning in a physiology laboratory-based subject facilitated by an e-learning component. *AJP: Advances in Physiology Education, 32*(1), 65–75. doi:10.1152/advan.00006.2007 PMID:18334571

Dave, D. H. (1970). Psychomotor levels. In R. J. Armstrong (Ed.), *Developing and writing educational objectives* (pp. 33–34). Tucson: Educational Innovators Press.

Delva, M. D., Kirby, J., Schultz, K., & Godwin, M. (2004). Assessing the relationship of learning approaches to workplace climate in clerkship and residency. *Academic Medicine, 79*(11), 1120–1126. doi:10.1097/00001888-200411000-00025 PMID:15504785

Dorman, T., Angood, P. B., Angus, D. C., Clemmer, T. P., Cohen, N. H., Durbin, C. G. Jr, & Napolitano, L. M. et al. (2004). Guidelines for critical care medicine training and continuing medical education. *Critical Care Medicine, 32*(1), 263–272. doi:10.1097/01.CCM.0000104916.33769.9A PMID:14707590

Dreyfus, H. L., & Dreyfus, S. E. (1986). *Mind over Machine: the power of human intuition and expertise in the age of the computer*. Oxford: Basil Blackwell.

Dupras, D. M., Edson, R. S., Halvorsen, A. J., Hopkins, R. H. Jr, & McDonald, F. S. (2012). "Problem residents": Prevalence, problems and remediation in the era of core competencies. *The American Journal of Medicine, 125*(4), 421–425. doi:10.1016/j.amjmed.2011.12.008 PMID:22444106

Edmunds, S., & Brown, G. (2010). Effective small group learning: AMEE Guide No. 48. *Medical Teacher, 32*(9), 715–726. doi:10.3109/0142159X.2010.505454 PMID:20795801

Ellaway, R., & Masters, K. (2008). AMEE Guide 32: e-Learning in medical education Part 1: Learning, teaching and assessment. *Medical Teacher, 30*(5), 455–473. doi:10.1080/01421590802108331 PMID:18576185

Ende, J. (1983). Feedback in clinical medical education. *Journal of the American Medical Association, 250*(6), 777–781. doi:10.1001/jama.1983.03340060055026 PMID:6876333

Epstein, R. M., & Hundert, E. M. (2002). Defining and assessing professional competence. *Journal of the American Medical Association, 287*(2), 226–235. doi:10.1001/jama.287.2.226 PMID:11779266

Fakhry, S. M. (2000). Billing, coding, and documentation in the critical care environment. *The Surgical Clinics of North America, 80*(3), 1067–1083. doi:10.1016/S0039-6109(05)70114-6 PMID:10897279

Farnan, J. M., Petty, L. A., Georgitis, E., Martin, S., Chiu, E., Prochaska, M., & Arora, V. M. (2012). A systematic review: The effect of clinical supervision on patient and residency education outcomes. *Academic Medicine: Journal of the Association of American Medical Colleges, 87*(4), 428–442. doi:10.1097/ACM.0b013e31824822cc PMID:22361801

Fish, D., & Coles, C. (2005). Clarifying curriculum aims: the practice of education, its nature and expertise. In *Medical Education: Developing A Curriculum For Practice*. Maidenhead: Open University Press.

Fletcher, G., Flin, R., McGeorge, P., Glavin, R., Maran, N., & Patey, R. (2003). Anaesthetists' Non-Technical Skills (ANTS): Evaluation of a behavioural marker system. *British Journal of Anaesthesia, 90*(5), 580–588. doi:10.1093/bja/aeg112 PMID:12697584

Flin, R., Patey, R., Glavin, R., & Maran, N. (2010). Anaesthetists' non-technical skills. *British Journal of Anaesthesia, 105*(1), 38–44. doi:10.1093/bja/aeq134 PMID:20522911

Flin, R. H., O'Connor, P., & Crichton, M. (2008). *Safety at the sharp end: a guide to non-technical skills*. Aldershot: Ashgate Publishing, Ltd.

Flinders, D. J., & Thornton, S. J. (2004). *The Curriculum Studies Reader*. Psychology Press.

Frank, J. R., Snell, L. S., Cate, O. T., Holmboe, E. S., Carraccio, C., Swing, S. R., & Harris, K. A. et al. (2010). Competency-based medical education: Theory to practice. *Medical Teacher*, *32*(8), 638–645. doi:10.3109/0142159X.2010.501190 PMID:20662574

Gaba, D. M. (2004). The future vision of simulation in health care. *Quality and Safety in Health Care*, *13*(suppl_1), i2–i10. doi:10.1136/qshc.2004.009878

Gaba, D. M., Howard, S. K., Fish, K. J., Smith, B. E., & Sowb, Y. A. (2001). Simulation-based training in anesthesia crisis resource management (ACRM): A decade of experience. *Simulation & Gaming*, *32*(2), 175–193. doi:10.1177/104687810103200206

Gordon, J. (2003). Fostering students' personal and professional development in medicine: A new framework for PPD. *Medical Education*, *37*(4), 341–349. doi:10.1046/j.1365-2923.2003.01470.x PMID:12654119

Gordon, M., Darbyshire, D., & Baker, P. (2012). Non-technical skills training to enhance patient safety: A systematic review. *Medical Education*, *46*(11), 1042–1054. doi:10.1111/j.1365-2923.2012.04343.x PMID:23078681

Grajales, F. J. III, Sheps, S., Ho, K., Novak-Lauscher, H., & Eysenbach, G. (2014). Social Media: A Review and Tutorial of Applications in Medicine and Health Care. *Journal of Medical Internet Research*, *16*(2), e13. doi:10.2196/jmir.2912 PMID:24518354

Grant, G. (1979). *On Competence*. San Francisco, USA: Jossey-Bass.

Grant, J., Abdelrahmen, M. Y. H., & Zachariah, A. (2013). Curriculum in Context. In K. Walsh (Ed.), *Oxford Textbook of Medical Education* (1st ed.). Oxford: Oxford University Press.

Grantcharov, T. P., & Reznick, R. K. (2008). Teaching procedural skills. *BMJ (Clinical Research Ed.)*, *336*(7653), 1129–1131. doi:10.1136/bmj.39517.686956.47 PMID:18483056

Gray, K., & Tobin, J. (2010). Introducing an online community into a clinical education setting: A pilot study of student and staff engagement and outcomes using blended learning. *BMC Medical Education*, *10*(6). doi:10.1186/1472-6920-10-6 PMID:20100354

Greenberg, L. W., Goldberg, R. M., & Jewett, L. S. (1984). Teaching in the clinical setting: Factors influencing residents' perceptions, confidence and behaviour. *Medical Education*, *18*(5), 360–365. doi:10.1111/j.1365-2923.1984.tb01283.x PMID:6472144

Harden, R. M., Crosby, J. R., & Davis, M. H. M. (1999). AMEE Guide No. 14: Outcome-based education: Part 5-From competency to meta-competency: a model for the specification of learning outcomes. *Medical Teacher*, *21*(6), 546–552. doi:10.1080/01421599978951 PMID:21281173

Harlen, W., & James, M. (1997). Assessment and Learning: Differences and relationships between formative and summative assessment. *Assessment in Education: Principles, Policy & Practice*, *4*(3), 365–379. doi:10.1080/0969594970040304

Hauer, K. E., Ciccone, A., Henzel, T. R., Katsufrakis, P., Miller, S. H., Norcross, W. A., & Irby, D. M. et al. (2009). Remediation of the deficiencies of physicians across the continuum from medical school to practice: A thematic review of the literature. *Academic Medicine: Journal of the Association of American Medical Colleges*, *84*(12), 1822–1832. doi:10.1097/ACM.0b013e3181bf3170 PMID:19940595

Hawryluck, L. A., Espin, S. L., Garwood, K. C., Evans, C. A., & Lingard, L. A. (2002). Pulling together and pushing apart: Tides of tension in the ICU team. *Academic Medicine*, *77*(10Suppl), S73–S76. doi:10.1097/00001888-200210001-00024 PMID:12377711

Hill, A. G., Yu, T.-C., Barrow, M., & Hattie, J. (2009). A systematic review of resident-as-teacher programmes. *Medical Education*, *43*(12), 1129–1140. doi:10.1111/j.1365-2923.2009.03523.x PMID:19930503

Hoff, T. J., Pohl, H., & Bartfield, J. (2004). Creating a learning environment to produce competent residents: The roles of culture and context. *Academic Medicine*, *79*(6), 532–539. doi:10.1097/00001888-200406000-00007 PMID:15165972

Humphrey, H. J. (2010). *Mentoring in Academic Medicine* (1st ed.). Philadelphia: American College of Physicians.

Hundert, E. M., Douglas-Steele, D., & Bickel, J. (1996). Context in medical education: The informal ethics curriculum. *Medical Education*, *30*(5), 353–364. doi:10.1111/j.1365-2923.1996.tb00847.x PMID:8949475

Iobst, W. F., Sherbino, J., Cate, O. T., Richardson, D. L., Dath, D., Swing, S. R., & Frank, J. R. et al. (2010). Competency-based medical education in postgraduate medical education. *Medical Teacher*, *32*(8), 651–656. doi:10.3109/0142159X.2010.500709 PMID:20662576

Issenberg, S. B. (2006). The scope of simulation-based healthcare education. *Simulation in Healthcare: the Journal of the Society for Simulation in Healthcare*, *1*(4), 203–208. doi:10.1097/01.SIH.0000246607.36504.5a PMID:19088590

Issenberg, S. B., McGaghie, W. C., Petrusa, E. R., Gordon, D. L., & Scalese, R. J. (2005). Features and uses of high-fidelity medical simulations that lead to effective learning: A BEME systematic review. *Medical Teacher*, *27*(1), 10–28. doi:10.1080/01421590500046924 PMID:16147767

Kelly, A. V. (2009). *The Curriculum* (6th ed.). London: SAGE Publications.

Kilminster, S., Cottrell, D., Grant, J., & Jolly, B. (2007). AMEE Guide No. 27: Effective educational and clinical supervision. *Medical Teacher*, *29*(1), 2–19. doi:10.1080/01421590701210907 PMID:17538823

Kneebone, R., Nestel, D., Wetzel, C., Black, S., Jacklin, R., Aggarwal, R., & Darzi, A. et al. (2006). The human face of simulation: Patient-focused simulation training. *Academic Medicine*, *81*(10), 919–924. doi:10.1097/01.ACM.0000238323.73623.c2 PMID:16985358

Kneebone, R. L., Nestel, D., Vincent, C., & Darzi, A. (2007). Complexity, risk and simulation in learning procedural skills. *Medical Education*, *41*(8), 808–814. doi:10.1111/j.1365-2923.2007.02799.x PMID:17661889

Knowles, M. S., Holton, E. F. III, & Swanson, R. A. (2011). *The Adult Learner* (7th ed.). Woburn: Butterworth-Heinemann.

Kononowicz, A. A., & Hege, I. (2014). Virtual patients as a practical realisation of the e-learning idea in medicine. In S. Soomro (Ed.), *E-learning Experiences and Future* (pp. 345–370). Intech; doi:10.5772/8803

LeBlanc, V. R. (2012). Review article: simulation in anesthesia: state of the science and looking forward. *Canadian Journal of Anesthesia/Journal Canadien D'anesthésie, 59*(2), 193–202. doi:10.1007/s12630-011-9638-8

Lingard, L., Espin, S., Whyte, S., Regehr, G., Baker, G. R., & Reznick, R. et al.. (2004). Communication failures in the operating room: An observational classification of recurrent types and effects. *Quality & Safety in Health Care, 13*(5), 330–334. doi:10.1136/qshc.2003.008425 PMID:15465935

Liolios, A. (2008). E-learning. In *Controversies in Intensive Care Medicine* (pp. 373–392). Berlin: Medizinisch Wissenschaftliche Verlagsgesellschaft.

Lipner, R. S., Hess, B. J., & Phillips, R. L. Jr. (2013). Specialty board certification in the United States: Issues and evidence. *The Journal of Continuing Education in the Health Professions, 33*(S1Suppl 1), S20–S35. doi:10.1002/chp.21203 PMID:24347150

MacDougall, J., & Drummond, M. J. (2005). The development of medical teachers: An enquiry into the learning histories of 10 experienced medical teachers. *Medical Education, 39*(12), 1213–1220. doi:10.1111/j.1365-2929.2005.02335.x PMID:16313580

Mahood, S. C. (2011). Medical education: Beware the hidden curriculum. *Canadian Family Physician Medecin de Famille Canadien, 57*(9), 983–985. PMID:21918135

Managing Trainees in Difficulty. (2013, October). Managing Trainees in Difficulty. *General Medical COuncil*. London. Retrieved May 12, 2014, from http://www.gmc-uk.org/Final_Appendix_5_Trainees_in_Difficulty.pdf_53816759.pdf

McGaghie, W. C., Issenberg, S. B., Petrusa, E. R., & Scalese, R. J. (2006). Effect of practice on standardised learning outcomes in simulation-based medical education. *Medical Education, 40*(8), 792–797. doi:10.1111/j.1365-2929.2006.02528.x PMID:16869926

McGaghie, W. C., Issenberg, S. B., Petrusa, E. R., & Scalese, R. J. (2010). A critical review of simulation-based medical education research: 2003-2009. *Medical Education, 44*(1), 50–63. doi:10.1111/j.1365-2923.2009.03547.x PMID:20078756

McKinley, R. K., Strand, J., Ward, L., Gray, T., Alun-Jones, T., & Miller, H. (2008). Checklists for assessment and certification of clinical procedural skills omit essential competencies: A systematic review. *Medical Education, 42*(4), 338–349. doi:10.1111/j.1365-2923.2007.02970.x PMID:18338987

McLeod, P. J., Steinert, Y., Trudel, J., & Gottesman, R. (2001). Seven principles for teaching procedural and technical skills. *Academic Medicine, 76*(10), 1080. doi:10.1097/00001888-200110000-00023 PMID:11597855

Mehta, N. B., Hull, A. L., Young, J. B., & Stoller, J. K. (2013). Just Imagine. *Academic Medicine, 88*(10), 1418–1423. doi:10.1097/ACM.0b013e3182a36a07 PMID:23969368

Memon, M. A., Joughin, G. R., & Memon, B. (2010). Oral assessment and postgraduate medical examinations: Establishing conditions for validity, reliability and fairness. *Advances in Health Sciences Education: Theory and Practice, 15*(2), 277–289. doi:10.1007/s10459-008-9111-9 PMID:18386152

Merriam, S. B., Caffarella, R. S., & Baumgartner, L. M. (2007). *Learning in Adulthood* (3rd ed.). San Francisco: Jossey-Bass.

Miller, G. E. (1990). The assessment of clinical skills/competence/performance. *Academic Medicine*, *65*(9), S63–S67. doi:10.1097/00001888-199009000-00045 PMID:2400509

Morrison, E. H., Friedland, J. A., Boker, J., Rucker, L., Hollingshead, J., & Murata, P. (2001). Residents-as-teachers training in US residency programs and offices of graduate medical education. *Academic Medicine: Journal of the Association of American Medical Colleges*, *76*(10Supplement), S1–S4. doi:10.1097/00001888-200110001-00002 PMID:11597856

Morrison, E. H., Shapiro, J. F., & Harthill, M. (2005). Resident doctors' understanding of their roles as clinical teachers. *Medical Education*, *39*(2), 137–144. doi:10.1111/j.1365-2929.2004.02063.x PMID:15679680

Nagler, A., Andolsek, K., Rudd, M., Sloane, R., Musick, D., & Basnight, L. (2014). The professionalism disconnect: Do entering residents identify yet participate in unprofessional behaviors? *BMC Medical Education*, *14*(1), 60. doi:10.1186/1472-6920-14-60 PMID:24674275

Nasca, T. J., Day, S. H., & Amis, E. S. Jr. (2010). The New Recommendations on Duty Hours from the ACGME Task Force. *The New England Journal of Medicine*, *363*(2), e3. doi:10.1056/NEJMsb1005800 PMID:20573917

National Committee of Quality Assurance. (2006). *Guidelines for Medical Documentation.* Retrieved May 2014, from http://www.ncqa.org/Portals/0/PolicyUpdates/Supplemental/Guidelines_Medical_Record_Review.pdf

Norman, G. R., Van der Vleuten, C. P., & De Graaff, E. (1991). Pitfalls in the pursuit of objectivity: Issues of validity, efficiency and acceptability. *Medical Education*, *25*(2), 119–126. doi:10.1111/j.1365-2923.1991.tb00037.x PMID:2023553

Nothnagle, M., Anandarajah, G., Goldman, R. E., & Reis, S. (2011). Struggling to Be Self-Directed: Residents - Paradoxical Beliefs About Learning. *Academic Medicine*, *86*(12), 1539–1544. doi:10.1097/ACM.0b013e3182359476 PMID:22030764

Ormrod, J. E. (2011). *Human Learning*. Boston: Pearson.

Paice, E., & Orton, V. (2004). Early signs of the trainee in difficulty. *Hospital Medicine (London, England)*, *65*(4), 238–240. doi:10.12968/hosp.2004.65.4.12739 PMID:15127680

Palter, V. N., & Grantcharov, T. P. (2010). Simulation in surgical education. *CMAJ: Canadian Medical Association Journal = Journal De l'Association Medicale Canadienne*, *182*(11), 1191–1196. doi:10.1503/cmaj.091743

Patey, R., Flin, R., Fletcher, G., Maran, N., & Glavin, R. (2005). Developing a Taxonomy of Anesthetists' Nontechnical Skills (ANTS). (K. Henricksen, J. B. Battles, & E. S. Marks, Eds.). Rockville: Advances in Patient Safety: From Research to Implementation (Volume 4: Programs, Tools, and Products).

Peña, A. (2010). The Dreyfus model of clinical problem-solving skills acquisition: A critical perspective. *Medical Education Online*, *15*(0). doi:10.3402/meo.v15i0.4846 PMID:20563279

Pendleton, D. (1984). *The Consultation*. Oxford: Oxford University Press.

Piquette, D., Fowler, R. A., & Slutsky, A. S. (2010). Impact of intensivist staffing on patient care and trainee education: A Canadian perspective. *American Journal of Respiratory and Critical Care Medicine*, *182*(4), 442–444. doi:10.1164/rccm.201006-0973ED PMID:20713639

Podcast. (n.d.). Podcast. *Merriam-Webster.com*. Retrieved May 11, 2014, from http://www.merriam-webster.com/dictionary/Podcast

Ramakrishnan, N., Hanauer, D., & Keller, B. (2010). Mining electronic health records. *Computer*, *43*(10), 77–81. doi:10.1109/MC.2010.292

Reader, T. (2006). Non-technical skills in the intensive care unit. *British Journal of Anaesthesia*, *96*(5), 551–559. doi:10.1093/bja/ael067 PMID:16567346

Recommendations for Clinical Skills Curricula for Undergraduate Medical Education. (2005, May 12). Recommendations for Clinical Skills Curricula for Undergraduate Medical Education. *Association of American Medical Colleges*. Retrieved May 12, 2014, from https://members.aamc.org/eweb/upload/Recommendations%20for%20Clinical%20Skills%20Curricula%202005.pdf

Reed, D. A., & Wright, S. M. (2010). Role Models in Medicine. In H. J. Humphrey (Ed.), *Mentoring in Academic Medicine*. Philadelphia: American College of Physicians.

Reuler, J. B., & Nardone, D. A. (1994). Role modeling in medical education. *The Western Journal of Medicine*, *160*(4), 335–337. PMID:8023482

Reznick, R. K., & MacRae, H. (2006). Teaching surgical skills--changes in the wind. *The New England Journal of Medicine*, *355*(25), 2664–2669. doi:10.1056/NEJMra054785 PMID:17182991

Ruiz, J. G., Mintzer, M. J., & Leipzig, R. M. (2006). The impact of E-learning in medical education. *Academic Medicine*, *81*(3), 207–212. doi:10.1097/00001888-200603000-00002 PMID:16501260

Rushton, A. (2005). Formative assessment: A key to deep learning? *Medical Teacher*, *27*(6), 509–513. doi:10.1080/01421590500129159 PMID:16199357

Salas, E., Wilson, K. A., Burke, C. S., & Priest, H. A. (2005). Using simulation-based training to improve patient safety: what does it take? *Joint Commission Journal on Quality and Patient Safety / Joint Commission Resources, 31*(7), 363–371.

Sambunjak, D., Straus, S. E., & Marusić, A. (2006). Mentoring in academic medicine: A systematic review. *Journal of the American Medical Association*, *296*(9), 1103–1115. doi:10.1001/jama.296.9.1103 PMID:16954490

Schuwirth, L. W. T., & Van Der Vleuten, C. P. M. (2004). Changing education, changing assessment, changing research? *Medical Education*, *38*(8), 805–812. doi:10.1111/j.1365-2929.2004.01851.x PMID:15271040

Schuwirth, L. W. T., & Vleuten, C. (2011). How to Design a Useful Test. In T. Swanwick (Ed.), *Understanding Medical Education* (p. 24). Oxford: Wiley-Blackwell.

Senge, P. M. (2010). *The Fifth Discipline: The Art and Practice of the Learning Organization* (2nd ed.). London: Random House.

Seymour, N. E., Gallagher, A. G., Roman, S. A., O'Brien, M. K., Bansal, V. K., Andersen, D. K., & Satava, R. M. (2002). Virtual reality training improves operating room performance: results of a randomized, double-blinded study. *Annals of Surgery, 236*(4), 458–63– discussion 463–4. doi:10.1097/01.SLA.0000028969.51489.B4

Shapiro, I. (2001). Doctor means teacher. *Academic Medicine, 76*(7), 711–711. doi:10.1097/00001888-200107000-00013 PMID:11448826

Shapiro, M. J., & Melendez, M. M. (2010). Billing for Bedside Procedures. In H. L. Frankel & B. P. deBoisblanc (Eds.), *Bedside Procedures for the Intensivist*. New York: Springer Science & Business. doi:10.1007/978-0-387-79830-1_17

Silverman, J. D., Draper, J., & Kurtz, S. M. (1997). The Calgary-Cambridge approach to communications skills teaching 2: The Set-Go method of descriptive feedback. *Education for General Practice*, (8), 16–23.

Silverman, J. D., Kurtz, S. M., & Draper, J. (1996). The Calgary-Cambridge approach to communication skills teaching. 1. Agenda-led, outcome-based analysis of the consultation. *Education for General Practice*, (7), 288–299.

Simpson, E. J. (1972). *The classification of educational objectives in the psychomotor domain*. Washington, D. C.: Gryphon House.

Snadden, D., & Thomas, M. (1998). The use of portfolio learning in medical education. *Medical Teacher, 20*(3), 192–199. doi:10.1080/01421599880904

Spady, W. G. (1994). *Outcome-based Education*. Arlington, USA: Amer Assn School Administrator.

Stefanidis, D., Korndorffer, J. R. Jr, Black, F. W., Dunne, J. B., Sierra, R., Touchard, C. L., & Scott, D. J. et al. (2006). Psychomotor testing predicts rate of skill acquisition for proficiency-based laparoscopic skills training. *Surgery, 140*(2), 252–262. doi:10.1016/j.surg.2006.04.002 PMID:16904977

Steinert, Y. (2004). Student perceptions of effective small group teaching. *Medical Education, 38*(3), 286–293. doi:10.1046/j.1365-2923.2004.01772.x PMID:14996338

Stinson, L., Pearson, D., & Lucas, B. (2006). Developing a learning culture: Twelve tips for individuals, teams and organizations. *Medical Teacher, 28*(4), 309–312. doi:10.1080/01421590600726433 PMID:16807167

Sturm, L. P., Windsor, J. A., Cosman, P. H., Cregan, P., Hewett, P. J., & Maddern, G. J. (2008). A systematic review of skills transfer after surgical simulation training. *Annals of Surgery, 248*(2), 166–179. doi:10.1097/SLA.0b013e318176bf24 PMID:18650625

Sullivan, M. E., Yates, K. A., Inaba, K., Lam, L., & Clark, R. E. (2014). The Use of Cognitive Task Analysis to Reveal the Instructional Limitations of Experts in the Teaching of Procedural Skills. *Academic Medicine, 89*(5), 811–816. doi:10.1097/ACM.0000000000000224 PMID:24667500

Sutcliffe, K. M., Lewton, E., & Rosenthal, M. M. (2004). Communication failures: An insidious contributor to medical mishaps. *Academic Medicine*, *79*(2), 186–194. doi:10.1097/00001888-200402000-00019 PMID:14744724

Swing, S. R. S., Clyman, S. G. S., Holmboe, E. S. E., & Williams, R. G. R. (2009). Advancing resident assessment in graduate medical education. *Journal of Graduate Medical Education*, *1*(2), 278–286. doi:10.4300/JGME-D-09-00010.1 PMID:21975993

Teunissen, P. W., Scheele, F., Scherpbier, A. J. J. A., van der Vleuten, C. P. M., Boor, K., van Luijk, S. J., & van Diemen-Steenvoorde, J. A. A. M. (2007). How residents learn: Qualitative evidence for the pivotal role of clinical activities. *Medical Education*, *41*(8), 763–770. doi:10.1111/j.1365-2923.2007.02778.x PMID:17661884

The Anesthesiology Milestone Project. (2013, December 13). The Anesthesiology Milestone Project. *Acgme*. Retrieved May 2014, from https://www.acgme.org/acgmeweb/Portals/0/PDFs/Milestones/AnesthesiologyMilestones.pdf

The Trainee Doctor. (2011). *The Trainee Doctor*. Manchester: General Medical Council.

Tiberius, R. G. (1999). *Small Group Teaching*. London: Kogan Page Publishers.

Tochel, C., Haig, A., Hesketh, A., Cadzow, A., Beggs, K., Colthart, I., & Peacock, H. (2009). The effectiveness of portfolios for post-graduate assessment and education: BEME Guide No 12. *Medical Teacher*, *31*(4), 299–318. doi:10.1080/01421590902883056 PMID:19404890

Toff, N. J. (2010). Human factors in anaesthesia: Lessons from aviation. *British Journal of Anaesthesia*, *105*(1), 21–25. doi:10.1093/bja/aeq127 PMID:20507856

Tomorrow's Doctors. (1993). *Tomorrow's Doctors*. London: General Medical Council.

Torbeck, L., & Canal, D. F. (2009). Remediation practices for surgery residents. *American Journal of Surgery*, *197*(3), 397–402. doi:10.1016/j.amjsurg.2008.10.008 PMID:19245922

Tyler, R. W. (2013). *Basic Principles of Curriculum and Instruction*. University of Chicago Press. doi:10.7208/chicago/9780226086644.001.0001

Van Der Vleuten, C. (1996). The assessment of professional competence: Developments, research and practical implications. *Advances in Health Sciences Education: Theory and Practice*, *1*(1), 41–67. doi:10.1007/BF00596229 PMID:24178994

Van der Vleuten, C. P., Norman, G. R., & De Graaff, E. (1991). Pitfalls in the pursuit of objectivity: Issues of reliability. *Medical Education*, *25*(2), 110–118. doi:10.1111/j.1365-2923.1991.tb00036.x PMID:2023552

Van Sickle, K. R., Ritter, E. M., & Smith, C. D. (2006). The pretrained novice: Using simulation-based training to improve learning in the operating room. *Surgical Innovation*, *13*(3), 198–204. doi:10.1177/1553350606293370 PMID:17056786

Walsh, K. (2005). The Rules. *BMJ: British Medical Journal*, *331*(7516), 574. doi:10.1136/bmj.331.7516.574

Walton, H. (1997). Small group methods in medical teaching. *Medical Education*, *31*(6), 459–464. doi:10.1046/j.1365-2923.1997.00703.x PMID:9463650

Wiki. (n.d.). Wiki. *Merriam-Webster.com*. Retrieved May 11, 2014, from http://www.merriam-webster.com/dictionary/wiki

Wood, D. F. (2011). Formative Assessment. In T. Swanwick (Ed.), *Understanding Medical Education* (pp. 259–270). Oxford: Wiley-Blackwell.

Wright, S. (1996). Examining what residents look for in their role models. *Academic Medicine*, *71*(3), 290–292. doi:10.1097/00001888-199603000-00024 PMID:8607931

Wu, J. S., Siewert, B., & Boiselle, P. M. (2010). Resident evaluation and remediation: A comprehensive approach. *Journal of Graduate Medical Education*, *2*(2), 242–245. doi:10.4300/JGME-D-10-00031.1 PMID:21975628

Wynia, M. K., Papadakis, M. A., Sullivan, W. M., & Hafferty, F. W. (2014). More Than a List of Values and Desired Behaviors. *Academic Medicine*, *89*(5), 712–714. doi:10.1097/ACM.0000000000000212 PMID:24667515

Yao, D. C., & Wright, S. M. (2001). The challenge of problem residents. *Journal of General Internal Medicine*, *16*(7), 486–492. doi:10.1046/j.1525-1497.2001.016007486.x PMID:11520388

Yedidia, M. J., Schwartz, M. D., Hirschkorn, C., & Lipkin, M. Jr. (1995). Learners as teachers. *Journal of General Internal Medicine*, *10*(11), 615–623. doi:10.1007/BF02602745 PMID:8583264

Yoder, J., & Hochevar, C. (2005). Encouraging Active Learning Can Improve Students' Performance on Examinations. *Teaching of Psychology*, *32*(2), 91–95. doi:10.1207/s15328023top3202_2

Young, J. Q., van Merriënboer, J., Durning, S., & Ten Cate, O. (2014). Cognitive Load Theory: Implications for medical education: AMEE Guide No. 86. *Medical Teacher*, *36*(5), 371–384. doi:10.3109/0142159X.2014.889290 PMID:24593808

Zaas, A., Andolsek, K., Weinerth, J. L., Nagler, A., Fortune, R., Tuck, T., & McNeil, D. B. (2013, October). Constructive Corrective Action: Assessing and Developing Comprehensive Learning Plans for the Core Competencies. *Insight*. Retrieved May 12, 2014, from http://www.im.org/Publications/Insight/Archives/2011/V9I2/Pages/corrective.aspx

Ziv, A., Wolpe, P. R., Small, S. D., & Glick, S. (2003). Simulation-based medical education: An ethical imperative. *Academic Medicine*, *78*(8), 783–788. doi:10.1097/00001888-200308000-00006 PMID:12915366

Chapter 4
Organization and Structure of the Cardiothoracic Intensive Care Unit

Michael H. Wall
University of Minnesota, USA

ABSTRACT

The purpose of this chapter is to emphasize and describe the team nature of critical care medicine in the Cardiothoracic Intensive Care Unit. The chapter will review the importance of various team members and discuss various staffing models (open vs closed, high intensity vs low intensity, etc.) on patient outcomes and cost. The chapter will also examine the roles of nurse practitioners and physician assistants (NP/PAs) in critical care, and will briefly review the growing role of the tele-ICU. Most studies support the concept that a multi-disciplinary ICU team, led by an intensivist, improves patient outcomes and decreases overall cost of care. The role of the tele-ICU and 24 hour in-house intensivist staffing in improving outcomes is controversial, and more research is needed in this area. Finally, a brief discussion of billing for critical care will be discussed.

INTRODUCTION

Modern critical care medicine is the ultimate team sport with all the members of the multidisciplinary critical care team contributing their expertise in the care of the critically ill patient. There is a large body of knowledge and evidence describing and supporting the team nature of critical care delivery.

The objective of this chapter is to review the organization and structure of the CT ICU team emphasizing the importance of the multidisciplinary nature of modern critical care delivery models, physician staffing models, the role of the tele-ICU, the growing field of critical care nurse practitioners and physician assistants (NP/PAs), and finally, will provide a brief overview of critical care billing practices.

DOI: 10.4018/978-1-4666-8603-8.ch004

HIGH-RELIABILITY ORGANIZATIONS (ICUs)

Because individual humans and teams can fail, the ideal ICU should be organized and structured in such a way to minimize failure and optimize patient care. Critical care is complex, dangerous, and time sensitive. Other industries such as coal mining, nuclear power, and commercial aviation are also complex, dangerous, and time sensitive, yet in these industries failure cannot be tolerated and the failure rate must be zero. How did these high risk high reliability organizations (HRO) accomplish this and how could this be applied to healthcare? Niedner et al (2013) in a fantastic review article describe how this could be done in a pediatric ICU. Several studies have shown that evidence based care is provided only about 50-60% of the time (McGlynn et al., 2003) and in 2000 the Institute of Medicine's (IOM) "To Err is Human" paper described the ICU (and the operating room) as an area most prone to errors and preventable harm (Kohn, Corrigan, & Donaldson, 2000). To put this in perspective, Larsen et al (2007) showed that in a 20-bed PICU it is estimated that there would be 1416 moderate and 44 serious adverse events per year! Clearly we have room to improve.

Reliability is expressed as the inverse of the failure rate. So if a process fails 1 in 10 times, the failure rate is 10% and the reliability level is 10^{-1}. 10^{-1} systems have very few processes, but rely on individual knowledge and individual work, and training and reminders (like signs in the locker and bathrooms). 10^{-2} systems are a bit better, such as using quality tools and evidence-based protocols (like central line insertion checklists). 10^{-3} systems begin to use even more standardized policies and procedures (Cady, 2008). [See Table 1] Of course the goal would be for all ICUs to perform at the level of six-sigma (3.4 errors in 1,000,000 opportunities), similar to the airline industry. How would we do it? Niedner et al

Table 1. Levels of Reliability

Level	Reliability	Success	Opportunities Per Failure	Real-World Example	Health Care Example
Chaotic	$<10^{-1}$	<90%	<10	Annual mortality if >90 years old	Achievement of best-practice processes in outpatient care
1	10^{-1}	90%	10	Mortality of climbing Mt. Everest	Achievement of best-practice processes in inpatient care
2	10^{-2}	99%	100	Mortality of Grand Prix racing	Deaths in risky surgery (American Society of Anesthesiologists grades 3-5)
3	10^{-3}	99.9%	1000	Helicopter crashes	Deaths in general surgery
4	10^{-4}	99.99%	10,000	Mortality of canoeing	Deaths in routine anesthesia
5	10^{-5}	99.999%	100,000	Chartered flight crashes	Deaths from blood transfusions
6	10^{-6}	99.9999%	1,000,000	Commercial airline crashes	—

Note. Levels of Reliability. Adapted from "The High-Reliability Pediatric Intensive Care Unit," by M.F. Niedner, S.E. Muething, and K.M. Sutcliffe, 2013, *Pediatric Clinics of North America, 60,* p. 564. Copyright 2013 by the Elsevier. Adapted with permission.

(2013) describe five processes that must all occur to transform an ICU (or anything in healthcare) to a HRO: 1) Preoccupation with failure, 2) Reluctance to simplify interpretations, 3) Sensitivity to operations, 4) Commitment to resilience, and 5) Flexible decision structures.

In HROs preoccupation with failure means that every small error and near-miss is evaluated and processes to improve are constantly being implemented and evaluated. Sensitivity to operations refers to ongoing attention and real-time data regarding front line operations, such as staffing, supervision, and support of a safety culture. Examples of reluctance to simplify include a culture where diversity in experience and opinion are actively encouraged and every near-miss is evaluated by a multidisciplinary team that is looking for system improvements to these problems. HROs rely on frontline workers' opinions and experience to improve process. Finally, a commitment to resilience means that errors and mistakes will happen, but because of the teamwork and safety culture that exist the team will anticipate failures, overcome them, and learn from them. All ICUs should be organized in such a way to embrace all of these principles of HROs and should all strive to become closer to a six-sigma organization every day (Niedner et al., 2013).

Teamwork and Team Service

The critical care team may consist of intensivists, fellows, residents, medical students, nurse practitioners, physician assistants, nurses, pharmacologists, nutritionists, physical therapists, medical assistants, housekeeping, and others. How does one get this team to work together? Manthous et al (2011) have written an outstanding review article on this topic focusing on four factors that have been shown to impact non-medical team performance that I will briefly review: 1) Leadership style, 2) Psychological safety, 3) Transactional memory, and 4) Mutual accountability. It is interesting how many of these factors are also crucial to making an ICU a six-sigma HRO! Leadership is important for all intensivists, not just medical directors and service chiefs. There are many different leadership styles, but a common model divides into autocratic or transactional and democratic or transformational. It is likely that the situation will determine which style works best. For example, in a rapidly deteriorating patient the autocratic style is probably best. But to develop a HRO where the safety culture is paramount using a democratic or transformational style where the leader seeks out and encourages all members of the team to participate in decision making as needed. Psychological safety is essential in HROs because it allows all members of the team to present different views and question decisions without worrying about being embarrassed in public or fearing retribution. Unfortunately, many physicians exclusively use an autocratic leadership style, which is not effective in enhancing psychological safety. Something as minor as asking each team member to comment on their thoughts for each patient on rounds before the final daily plan is made is one easy way to improve psychological safety. Transactive Memory is a concept that states that the more teams work together and share knowledge and experiences, the better they will function and trust each other as a team. Simulation exercises may be one way to improve transactive memory. Hunziker et al (2009) showed an improvement in CPR performance in teams that had trained together vs teams that had not. Finally, mutual accountability refers to the willingness to accept responsibility for one's actions, and also holding others on the team accountable (Hunziker et al., 2009). A study of top performing academic medical centers found that accountability was key in their success (Keroack et al., 2007). How can these important concepts be implemented in our ICUs? I agree with Manthous et al (2011) who recommended that we should include formal education about teams and leadership for our fellows and residents (and medical students). We should encourage team building exercises along with didactics. They also recommend that formal studies be done to evaluate teamwork and leadership in the performance and outcomes of critical care teams.

TEAM MEMBERS

There are many members of the team. In this section I will review some aspects of the roles and importance of many members of the team.

Nurse Practitioners and Physician Assistants

Due to the shortage of intensivists and resident work hour restrictions the roles of NP/PAs in the ICU have been expanding. Costa et al (2009) in retrospective cohort database from 2009-2010 and an ICU survey found that 72% of the ICUs reported NP/PAs participating in care of ICU patients. Previous surveys have shown that 24% of PAs and 68% of NPs reported working in ICUs. Costa et al (2014) showed that in 29 mixed medical-surgical ICUs in 22 hospitals where NP/PAs worked in the ICU, the Acute Physiology Scores were lower (42.4 vs 46.7, $p<0.001$), and the rate of mechanical ventilation was lower (38.8 vs 44.2, $p<0.001$) when compared to ICUs without NP/PAs. There was no difference in unadjusted and adjusted mortality [adjusted relative risk: 1.10 (95% CI: 0.92-1.31)] which was consistent in all subgroups. This is consistent with other single center studies that showed no difference in outcomes (Costa, Wallace, Barnato, & Kahn, 2014). There are some studies that have shown some improvements in specific outcomes—cost, compliance with bundles, et cetera (Moote, Krsek, Kleinpell, & Todd, 2011). Studies have shown that compliance with evidence based bundles, guidelines, and improved nursing communication (and teamwork) may be responsible for these improvements (Gracias et al., 2008). Several studies have evaluated the role of NP/PAs in trauma ICUs (Collins et al., 2014). These studies have shown that trauma ICU services where NP/PAs were involved had reduced LOS, reduced direct patient costs, improved documentation, and no changes in other quality metrics (D. S. Morris et al., 2012). Collins et al (2014) evaluated the impact of acute care NPs (ACNPs) on a trauma ICU step down service. They found that the addition of ACNPs decreased the hospital LOS from 7.2 to 6.8 days. In addition, there was a $9,000 per patient savings or a $27.8 million dollar per year reduction of charges. Further, a survey showed that 100% of intensivists and staff nurses felt the addition of ACNPs was beneficial and improved flow and communication. Although large multi-center studies are lacking, it appears that the addition of experienced NP/PAs to an ICU service has a very positive effect on morale, communication, and is cost effective. Gershengorn has also written a recent extensive review on this topic (Gershengorn, Johnson, & Factor, 2012).

Critical Care Nursing

Kelly et al (2014) recently showed that ICU nursing staffing, work environment, education, and experience is associated with mortality. Many previous studies on this topic have been inconclusive and have had other methodological problems, which limits conclusions. Kelly et al (2014) evaluated 55,155 older patients being mechanically ventilated that were admitted to 303 hospitals in 4 states (CA, FL, NJ, PA). They then used logistic regression for the effect of ICU nursing variables on 30d mortality after adjusting for patient, hospital, and physician. They found that after adjustment, nursing education with a BS and a better working nurse environment were associated with a decrease in 30d mortality [odds ratios and 95% confidence intervals 0.98 (0.97-0.99), 0.89 (0.81-0.89) respectively]. This translates into ICUs with a better environment had an 11% lower odds ratio for 30d mortality. Further, they found that each 10% increase in the percent of nurses with a BS is associated with a 2% decrease in the odds of 30d mortality. Staffing levels and nurse experience were not associated with mortality. The authors conclude that improving the ICU work environment and hiring more BS trained ICU nurses may improve outcomes. Again, the "work environment" is essential to transition the ICU into a HRO.

Another important part of becoming a HRO is for all leaders to understand what the front line workers actually do. Douglas et al (2013) have reported a detailed evaluation of the unique work nurses perform in the ICU. They performed a total of 147 hours of direct real-time observation in 4 different ICUs at one rural tertiary care community hospital. This study showed that 75% of ICU nurses' time was spent on patient care activities, about 50% of this time was spent on direct patient care (including documentation), 20% on care coordination, 28% on non-patient care, and 2% on indirect patient care. It was also observed that on average nurses performed about 129 activities per hour, averaging a switch between tasks every 29 seconds (Douglas et al., 2013)! What is also surprising is that only 3% of the ICU RNs' time was spent in conversation with ICU doctors and only 2% of their time was spent on bedside rounds with the ICU team. It is no surprise that poor communication with the ICU team is a common problem in many ICUs. I think this type of data is important to know prior to (and after) making changes to the ICU RN workload such as implementation of an electronic health record or new bundles such as oral care, pressure ulcer prevention, et cetera.

Pharmacologists

Preslaski et al (2013) have written an excellent review of the role of the pharmacist as a member of the multidisciplinary ICU team. In my opinion they are an absolutely indispensable part of the team! In 2000 the Society of Critical Care Medicine and American College of Clinical Pharmacy published a position paper describing fundamental, desirable, and optimal activities (Rudis & Brandl, 2000). Fundamental services are those that must be provided to all patients. Desirable activities add things needed for the care of the ICU patient and optimal activities are those needed to optimize outcomes (and required to for the ICU to become an HRO). Unfortunately, two surveys published in 2006, 2007, and 2011 have all showed that fundamental services are being provided <70% of the time, and desirable and optimal services are being provided <1 time per week. This is unfortunate because Bond et al (2007) studied almost 3 million patients across 888 hospitals and showed that hospital mortality decreased as pharmacy staffing improved and pharmacists performed fundamental or desirable services. It is interesting to ponder the effect on mortality if optimal services were provided daily to all patients in every ICU!

The Infectious Diseases Society of America and the Society for Healthcare Epidemiology of America clearly state that pharmacists should be involved in the multidisciplinary antibiotic teams, based on numerous studies showing improved outcomes with pharmacy involvement. For example, pharmacist involvement has decreased length of stay and mortality when they are involved with restricted antibiotic administration, surgical prophylaxis, vancomycin, aminoglycoside dosing, community acquired infections, nosocomial infections, and in sepsis (Preslaski et al., 2013).

Clinical pharmacists have made similar improvements in the management of anticoagulation in the ICU. Again numerous studies have shown that time to achieve target aPTT is shorter, length of stay, mortality, transfusion, number of supratherapeutic INRs and re-admission rates are lower when clinical pharmacists and nursing are independently directing anticoagulation using predefined clinical protocols and pathways (Preslaski et al., 2013).

Similarly studies have shown that pharmacist driven sedation and analgesic protocols have shortened duration of mechanical ventilation, ICU, and hospital LOS. In addition, use of these protocols has increased the time patients were at the goal level of sedation while decreasing drug costs (Preslaski et al., 2013).

Draper et al (2008) showed that more non-compliant AHA-ACLS interventions took place when a pharmacist was not a member of the code team (59.3% vs 31.9% p=0.03). Most of the errors were due to medication errors.

Finally, there is no question that clinical pharmacists decrease the number of adverse drug events (ADEs). Leape et al (1999) reported that the addition of a pharmacist to the ICU team was associated with a decrease of order writing ADE (10.4 vs 3.5 per 1000 patient days, p<0.001) and preventable ADEs (33 vs 11.6 per 1000 patient days, p<0.001). Other studies have shown that increasing pharmacy staffing from one to five pharmacists per 100 beds reduced ADEs by 48%, and were associated with reduced mortality (Bond & Raehl, 2007).

It is obvious to me that clinical pharmacists improve safety and quality and outcomes in ICU patients. Involvement of ICU clinical pharmacists providing fundamental, desirable and optimal services 7 days a week is an absolutely essential part of the multidisciplinary ICU team for the ICU to become a HRO.

Physical Therapy

Over the last several years there has been growing evidence that supports using less sedation and more physical activity (commonly referred to as "early mobilization") in all ICU patients. Implementation of early mobilization in the ICU requires the expertise of physical (and occupational) therapists, and in the best ICUs they have been added to the multidisciplinary ICU team. Pawlik and Kress (2013) have written an outstanding review on this topic that I will briefly summarize. Several papers have been published describing early mobilization teams that are needed to provide this service. The composition of the teams vary, but to ambulate a patient who is intubated, mechanically ventilated, connected to one or more infusion/nutrition pumps, et cetera takes more than one person! Teams have included: ICU nurses, respiratory therapists, occupational therapists, nursing/rehabilitation assistants, and of course physical therapists. Schweickert et al (2009) in a relatively early study of early mobilization showed that in mechanically ventilated patients who were mobilized early (1.5 days after intubation) vs mobilized late (7.4 days) had improved functional outcomes and increased ventilator free days even though 95% of patients in both groups received mobilization. Morris et al (2008) also showed that early mobilization decreased ICU and hospital LOS. Morris also showed that the cost of the additional members of the mobilization team was about $250,000, but the costs of the intervention group were $500,000 less than the control group. Thus, similar to clinical pharmacist support it appears that the addition of additional members to the ICU team with specialty expertise will improve outcomes—and when looking at the total cost of care for the entre hospitalization may actually save money, even though the individual "siloed" budget for physical therapy (or pharmacy) actually gets worse. Pawlick and Kress (2013) review numerous other studies of early mobilization (and early mobilization teams) that have also shown improvements in ICU team work, culture, multidisciplinary collaboration, and adherence to guidelines such as sedation interruptions. It is interesting to note that similar findings are seen with the addition of clinical pharmacists, and all of these help to improve the "culture" of the ICU, again which is necessary for ICUs to become HROs. Pawklik and Kress (2013) also discuss what is needed to prepare physical therapists to work in the ICU. Studies have shown that physical therapists with >7 years of experience are better suited to work with complex patients in the ICU, but as of 2013 the American Board of Physical Therapy specialties does not offer board certification in acute or critical care physical therapy. Although some hospitals have described competencies for critical care physical therapists, there are no formal training programs, residencies, or fellowships available to train physical therapists with an interest in this growing and important field.

Finally, there is a growing body of evidence that as long as 5 years after recovering from ARDs patients have decreased functional activity, quality of life, and some adverse physiological outcomes, and it is unclear what effect early mobilization and longer term physical therapy after hospital discharge will have on these outcomes. It is known that outpatient rehab programs improve functional capacity and decrease re-admissions after admission for COPD, and improve mortality and quality of life in patients with coronary artery disease and congestive heart failure. It is possible that similar programs following ICU admission may have similar outcomes and more research does need to be done in this area.

Palliative Care

Providing palliative care is a core competency of intensivists. However, extremely complex patients or those not responding to treatment may benefit from a palliative care specialist. Numerous mostly single center studies have shown that early use palliative care services, triggered by ICU specific criterion have increased palliative care involvement, improved patient family and intensivist satisfaction and decreased costs. Nelson et al (2013) recently published a review article describing the selection, implementation and use of screening criterion for palliative care consultation.

Most criterion used triggers focused on family request for consultation, communication problems with the patient or family, and those patients with a high risk of ICU or hospital mortality. Nelson et al (2013) recommend that because each ICU is different, screening criterion should be selected by stakeholders in each ICU and a standard process for implementation of the screening tool, and the impact of the tool should be followed (Nelson et al., 2013). O'Mahony et al (2010) published a study comparing the integration of a palliative care nurse within the ICU team on rounds and with a standardized sign-out to an ICU without such a service. Patients who were in the integrated palliative care model had a formal palliative care consultation happen sooner (2.8 vs 15.5 days, p-0.018), had fewer tests done, and received higher doses of pain medication. They also had more formalized advanced directives and had life prolonging treatments stopped earlier. Most importantly, the addition of the palliative care nurse to the team seemed to improve the multidisciplinary culture of the team and seemed to provide improved communication to the patients.

In summary, similar to clinical pharmacists and physical therapists, the addition of palliative care specialists to the ICU team seems to improve team work, culture, and patient outcomes.

ICU PHYSICIAN STAFFING MODELS

There are literally dozens of articles that have been written on this topic. Garland et al (2013) has written a recent review that summarizes this complex area. In the following sections, I will highlight recent studies that have examined high vs low intensity staffing, 24-hour in-house coverage, staffing ratios and briefly touch on telemedicine.

Closed vs Open ICUs

Closed ICUs are those in which an intensivist is the primary physician directing the care of the patient in the ICU. This model is commonly used in Medical ICUs at academic medical centers in the US and Europe. Open ICUs are those in which multiple specialists care for the patient with or without involvement of an intensivist. Semi-open or semi-closed models also exist where patients are "co-managed" by an intensivist and another physician. This model is quite common in surgical ICUs in academic medical centers in the US and is the model most commonly used in academic cardiothoracic surgical ICUs in the US.

Because the definition of open vs closed does not adequately describe the care model, several studies have compared "high intensity" ICUs where care is transferred to an intensivist or there is mandatory intensivist consultation vs "low intensity" where there is no intensivist involvement. Young et al (2000) and Pronovost et al (2002) both published systematic reviews that concluded high intensity intensivist led care decreased ICU and hospital mortality when compared to low intensity ICUs. However, Levy et al (2008) published a study of 101,000 patients in 123 ICUs using the SCCM's Project Impact data that have showed adjusted hospital mortality was higher in high intensity ICUs (odds ratio 1.42, $p<0.001$). Rubenfeld and Angus (2008) in an editorial entitled "Are Intensivists Safe?" examined the differences between these three systematic reviews. It is interesting that the North American and European guidelines both recommend a high intensity model, ideally with 24-hour in-hospital intensivists (De Lange, Van Aken, & Burchardi, 2002).

Because of these conflicting findings and guideline recommendations, Wilcox et al (2013) performed a systematic review and meta-analyses on fifty-two studies that examined intensivists staffing (high vs low intensity) and ICU or hospital mortality. All 52 trials were observational and involved trials from 13 countries and a variety of ICUs (MICU, PICU, SICU, mixed) from mostly academic medical centers. This study showed that high intensity staffing was associated with decreased ICU and hospital mortality and length of stay. The study also showed that within a high intensity model, 24-hour in-house intensivists did not reduce ICU or hospital mortality. Further this benefit was most beneficial in surgical (risk ratio 0.84; 95% CI 0.44-1.6) and combined medical surgical ICUs (risk ratio 0.76; 95% CI 0.66 – 0.83) vs medical ICUs (risk ration 1.1; 95% CI 0.83-1.5). Furthermore, hospital mortality varied by decade with pooled risk ratios 1980 – 89 (risk ratio 0.74), 1990 – 1999 (risk ratio 0.96), 2000-2009 (risk ratio 0.7) and 2010 – 2012 (risk ratio 1.2).

In an excellent editorial, Capanni et al (2013), pointed out the strengths and weakness of this article. Specifically they suggest that the reason there was no difference seen with 24-hour in-house coverage in high intensity units could be because 49 of the 52 studies were done in academic health centers and there were residents, fellows, and NP/PAs already in the ICU at night. This is an important observation since there is a shortage of intensivists and night work contributes to intensivist burn out.

24-Hour In-House Intensivists

This topic is also controversial because it is recommended by numerous subspecialty societies based on limited observational data, even though the most recent meta-analysis by Wilcox et al (2013) does not support it, and because of the shortage of intensivists, it is almost impossible (and expensive) to provide. Five recent additional studies deserve to be discussed. Gajic et al (2008) showed that the addition of 24-

hour in-house intensivists in a high intensity medical ICU (that already had ICUs in-house at night) did not decrease ICU (10.2% vs 10.4% p=0.83) or hospital (17% vs 19% p=0.33) mortality OR/ICU LOS. It also did not improve family satisfaction. It did however increase intensivist burnout.

Garland et al (2012) used an alternating cross-over design in two closed high intensity ICUs (one academic ICU with house staff in house and one community ICU without house staff). Again, there was no improvement in outcomes or family satisfaction, but there were negative effects related to burn out.

Wallace et al (2012) evaluated 49 ICUs that were participating in the APACHE database project. They found that the addition of a nighttime intensivist improves outcomes in low intensity ICUs (odds ratio 0.62, p=0.04) but not in high intensity ICUs (odds ratio 1.08, p=0.78) consistent with Wilcox et al (2013). Kerlin et al (2013) recently reported the first truly randomized prospective trial of 24-hour in-house intensivist coverage in a closed, high intensity MICU at an academic medical center. Intensivists randomly covered seven blocks of nights vs control when they were available by phone. 1,598 patients were studied. The presence of 24-hour in-house intensivists did not decrease ICU LOS (rate ratio 0.98, 95% CI 0.88 – 1.09; P=0.72) or ICU mortality (relative risk 1.07; 95% CI 0.50 – 1.28). It is important to emphasize that this took place in a well-run closed high intensity ICU with residents and fellows in-house at night.

Finally, Kumar et al (2014) evaluated the effect of adding 24-hour in-house intensivist coverage to a high intensity cardiothoracic surgical ICU in patients admitted for more than 48 hours. A previous study by this same group showed that addition of 24-hour coverage reduced blood use, duration of mechanical ventilation and hospital LOS, but did not decrease OR mortality. This study showed similar findings. There was no difference in ICU or 30-day mortality or ICU LOS. Hospital LOS was shorter (12.3 vs 11.0; p<0.01). The 24-hour group also had less transfusions (80.8% vs 65.7%; p<0.001), less sepsis (4.7% vs 0.7%, p<0.01), and less renal failure (22.55 vs 12.5%; p<0.01).

Based on the above studies it is clear that 24-hour coverage does improve many secondary outcomes, but it does not appear to improve mortality. However, most of these studies were under powered to show a mortality benefit, did not look at the effects of 30 day (or longer) mortality or morbidity, and were done in high intensity ICUs. More studies will need to be done to prove 24-hour coverage improves mortality in high intensity models.

Intensivist/Patient Ratios

Ward et al (2013) recently published a statement from the Society of Critical Care Medicine task force on ICU staffing. The task force conducted a review of published literature, held an expert roundtable conference, and an iterative consensus process of the effect of staffing rations (in closed high intensity ICUs) on outcomes. They concluded that the following seven principles should be used when determining an institution's staffing levels: 1) Proper staffing impacts patient care; 2) Large caseloads prolong rounds, limiting time for other work; 3) Staffing decisions need to factor "surge" capacity; 4) Staffing should be routinely reassessed; 5) High staff turnover may be an indicator of excess workload; 6) Other staffing models could be used to decrease the workload of intensivists; 7) In closed academic medical ICUs physician patient staffing levels greater than 1:14 negatively impact education, staff well-being and patient care. This paper also provides a staffing tool that can be used to estimate intensivist staffing needs.

Somewhat related to physician:patient staffing rations is the question of how many intensivists are needed to form a well-functioning ICU group. Reed et al (2014) reported the effects of the number of intensivist FTEs and National Surgical Quality Improvement Program (NSQIP) quality measures. The number of supervised intensivists varied from 8 to 2 over the study period. There was a significant decline in FTEs in 2010. Before 2010 there were an average of 6.6 ± 0.55 vs post decline there was an average of 4.0 ± 1.0 (p=0.0027). Post decline the ICU was often covered by non-intensivists. The period post-decline was associated with an increased risk of mechanical ventilation for > 48 hours (odds ratio 0.94 vs 1.87; p=0.0086) and venous thromboembolism (odds ratio 0.84 vs 1.43; p=0.027). There was no difference in mortality. The quality indicators returned to baseline after full staffing with intensivists was re-established. The authors opine that having an adequate number of intensivists is needed to assure policies, procedures, and protocols are followed. Adherence to these policies improves things that occur outside the walls of the ICU, like venous thromboembolism. They further comment (and I agree) that there must be strong institutional commitment to a fully staffed (surgical in this case) ICU service.

Hand-offs

Due to resident work hour restrictions and some units having 24-hour intensivist models, multiple hand-offs happen every day in all ICUs. There is a large number of studies that have shown associations between hand-offs and medical errors. However, there is another point of view that a "fresh set of eyes" will discover an error (or make a new diagnosis) that was missed. Amaral et al (2014) evaluated the effect of hand-offs by nighttime cross-coverage fellows in an academic mixed medical surgical high intensity closed ICU. In an evaluation of 689 ICU patients admitted for >48 hours they noticed that hand-offs/cross-coverage decreased ICU mortality (odds ratio 0.77; 95% CI 0.60-0.99; p=0.04). Fellows also increased nighttime decision making, transfusions, and pain medicine administration. The authors suggest that a "second look" by fellows may mitigate cognitive errors and actually improve patient safety. In an accompanying editorial, Halpern (2014) comments that although the post-test probability that cross-coverage truly saves lives is quite low—it is certainly possible that "new providers with fresh perspectives in the care of complex patients could yield benefits." Definitely more research on various staffing models and hand-offs need to be done.

Tele-ICU

Another method of providing intensivist coverage is tele-ICU, where a remote ICU team usually consisting of an intensivist, ICU nurses, and some also include software that analyzes data and can act as an early warning system. Hundreds of hospitals in the US have implemented these expensive systems in spite of conflicting evidence supporting their use. Young et al (2011) recently reported a systematic review and meta-analysis on the patient outcomes of telemedicine. They evaluated 13 studies from 35 ICUs. All of the studies were observational and all used before vs after design. The studies included 41,774 patients. Tele-ICU was associated with a decrease in ICU mortality (odds ratio 0.88; 98% CI 0.66-0.77; p=0.02), but not hospital mortality (odds ratio 0.82; 95% CI 0.65-1.03; P=0.08). Tele-ICU was also associated with a decrease in ICU LOS but not hospital LOS. The authors comment that there was huge variation in how tele-ICU was defined, the hospitals it was used in (academic vs community), and the type and staffing model (open vs closed, high vs low intensity) of the ICU it was used in. Based on this study the authors were not able to provide recommendations for which hospitals, ICUSs, or patients are likely to benefit the most from this technology.

Yager et al (2012) evaluated the impact and feasibility of tele-ICU communication in the pediatric ICU. In this study the intensivist was on call from home and was available for telecommunication. 56 episodes of communication were evaluated. Telecommunication allowed visual patient assessment, communication with the patient's family, and communication with the entire ICU team, which could not have happened over the telephone alone. Importantly, medical management was changed 32% of the time. The authors commented that tele-communication is feasible, improves team communication, and at least in this study led to changes in management.

Finally Kruklitis et al (2014) have written an excellent review article on the clinical and financial implications for implementation a tele-ICU program. They conclude that the vast majority of research on tele-ICU has shown improvements in mortality, LOS, and cost. In addition, they point out that tele-ICU improves compliance with evidence-based bundles and protocols which are also likely to improve outcome. The authors also perform a very thorough evaluation of the financial impacts of such a system. They conclude that even though installation and yearly operations costs are enormous ($7,000,000 initially and $3,000,000 per year at University of Massachusetts Medical Center) the cost savings to the hospital and payors was $25,000,000 and $13,000,000 per year respectively. This is clearly enough money to pay for the initial capital expense and ongoing operating costs.

BILLING

For an exhaustive review of critical care billing I refer readers to the excellent SCCM monograph edited by Sample and (*Coding and Billing for Critical Care, A Practice Tool*). I will briefly review adult critical care billing in this section. There are two adult critical care codes 99291—for 30-74 minutes, and 99252—for each additional 30 minutes before 74 minutes. 99291 can be used once per day by a group or individual physician for the total time, even if it is not continuous. 99252 is used for time greater than 74 minutes per day. Medicare regulations are clear: providers are not required to be present at the bedside to bill for critical care services. Providers may bill for time spent reviewing patient data, case planning with consultants, writing notes, and discussing patient issues with family members. Providers may bill for their services when they are "immediately available" and in the same unit or floor as the patient. CMS defines critical care as the "direct delivery by physician(s) of medical care for a critically ill or injured patient." This generally must include all three of the collowing criterion: 1) Impairment of one or more organ systems with a high probability of imminent or life-threatening deterioration; 2) Complex decision making to treat or prevent single or multiple organ system failure; 3) Time as described above.

If the initial visit is less than 30 minutes, or the patient is not critically ill then the following evaluation and management codes (E/M) should be used:

99221/level 1 initial hospital care 30 minutes face time
99222/level 2 initial hospital care 50 minutes face time
99223/level 3 initial hospital care 70 minutes face time

There are strict criterion that must be followed to qualify and use these billing codes. See page 73 (*Coding and Billing for Critical Care, A Practice Tool*).

For follow up visits of patients who do not meet critical care codes subsequent hospital visit E/M codes should be used:

99231/level 1 subsequent hospital visit 15 minutes face time
99232/level 2 subsequent hospital visit 25 minutes face time
99233/level 3 subsequent hospital visit 35 minutes face time

Additional codes can be used for placement of arterial, central, and PICC lines and for a variety of procedures such as intubation, bronchoscopy, thoracentesis, etc. The reader is referred to *Coding and Billing for Critical Care* for a complete discussion.

FUTURE RESEARCH DIRECTIONS

As I have pointed out in each section much more research needs to be done in all areas in this chapter. Specifically, I think more research needs to be done on how to change the culture of ICUs to become more like HROs. Research needs to be done in how best to train leadership skills during residency and fellowship training.

Much more needs to be done on the longer term outcomes of early mobilization and mobility teams looking at functional outcomes and who benefits the most. Ideally, large studies on the role of 24-hour intensivist models adequately powered to evaluate mortality and costs should be done along with similar studies performed with tele-ICU in both low and high intensity staffing models.

CONCLUSION

Our goal should be to make the ICUs into HROs. To do this, we are going to have to learn and apply leadership and team work skills to build a safety culture that must be present in HROs. I think all ICUs should be staffed in the high intensity staffing model during the daytime. I am not sure that 24 hour staffing is needed in academic medical centers that are staffed 24/7 by fellows, residents, and NP/PAs. The care team model works and has many benefits and I believe NP/PAs should be involved in all ICUs. Further, we should have clinical pharmacologists, physical therapists, and palliative care specialists on all of our ICU teams and these services should be provided 7 days a week. If we do all this we can improve short and long term outcomes for our patients.

REFERENCES

Bond, C. A., & Raehl, C. L. (2007). Clinical pharmacy services, pharmacy staffing, and hospital mortality rates. *Pharmacotherapy*, *27*(4), 481–493. doi:10.1592/phco.27.4.481 PMID:17381374

Cady, R. F. (2008). "Becoming a high reliability organization-operational advice for hospital leaders" report. *JONA'S Healthcare Law, Ethics and Regulation*, *10*, 33. doi:10.1097/01.NHL.0000300780.65358.e0 PMID:18525400

Capanni, F., & Checkley, W. (2013). Differences in hospital mortality by ICU staffing models: You cannot always get what you want, but sometimes you get what you need. *Critical Care Medicine*, *41*(10), 2433–2434. doi:10.1097/CCM.0b013e31829cb0aa PMID:24060770

Collins, N., Miller, R., Kapu, A., Martin, R., Morton, M., Forrester, M., & Wilkinson, L. et al. (2014). Outcomes of adding acute care nurse practitioners to a Level I trauma service with the goal of decreased length of stay and improved physician and nursing satisfaction. *J Trauma Acute Care Surg*, *76*(2), 353–357. doi:10.1097/TA.0000000000000097 PMID:24398767

Costa, D. K., Wallace, D. J., Barnato, A. E., & Kahn, J. M. (2014). Nurse practitioner/physician assistant staffing and critical care mortality. *Chest*, *146*(6), 1566–1573. doi:10.1378/chest.14-0566 PMID:25167081

De Lange, S., Van Aken, H., & Burchardi, H. (2002). European Society of Intensive Care Medicine statement: Intensive care medicine in Europe--structure, organisation and training guidelines of the Multidisciplinary Joint Committee of Intensive Care Medicine (MJCICM) of the European Union of Medical Specialists (UEMS). *Intensive Care Medicine*, *28*(11), 1505–1511. doi:10.1007/s00134-002-1504-2 PMID:12583367

Douglas, S., Cartmill, R., Brown, R., Hoonakker, P., Slagle, J., Schultz Van Roy, K., & Carayon, P. et al. (2013). The work of adult and pediatric intensive care unit nurses. *Nursing Research*, *62*(1), 50–58. doi:10.1097/NNR.0b013e318270714b PMID:23222843

Draper, H. M., & Eppert, J. A. (2008). Association of pharmacist presence on compliance with advanced cardiac life support guidelines during in-hospital cardiac arrest. *The Annals of Pharmacotherapy*, *42*(4), 469–474. doi:10.1345/aph.1K475 PMID:18349308

Gajic, O., Afessa, B., Hanson, A. C., Krpata, T., Yilmaz, M., Mohamed, S. F., & Wylam, M. E. et al. (2008). Effect of 24-hour mandatory versus on-demand critical care specialist presence on quality of care and family and provider satisfaction in the intensive care unit of a teaching hospital. *Critical Care Medicine*, *36*(1), 36–44. doi:10.1097/01.CCM.0000297887.84347.85 PMID:18007270

Garland, A., & Gershengorn, H. B. (2013). Staffing in ICUs: Physicians and alternative staffing models. *Chest*, *143*(1), 214–221. doi:10.1378/chest.12-1531 PMID:23276844

Garland, A., Roberts, D., & Graff, L. (2012). Twenty-four-hour intensivist presence: A pilot study of effects on intensive care unit patients, families, doctors, and nurses. *American Journal of Respiratory and Critical Care Medicine*, *185*(7), 738–743. doi:10.1164/rccm.201109-1734OC PMID:22246176

Gershengorn, H. B., Johnson, M. P., & Factor, P. (2012). The use of nonphysician providers in adult intensive care units. *American Journal of Respiratory and Critical Care Medicine*, *185*(6), 600–605. doi:10.1164/rccm.201107-1261CP PMID:22135345

Gracias, V. H., Sicoutris, C. P., Stawicki, S. P., Meredith, D. M., Horan, A. D., Gupta, R., & Schwab, C. W. et al. (2008). Critical care nurse practitioners improve compliance with clinical practice guidelines in "semiclosed" surgical intensive care unit. *Journal of Nursing Care Quality*, *23*(4), 338–344. doi:10.1097/01.NCQ.0000323286.56397.8c PMID:18521045

Halpern, S. D. (2014). Cross-coverage in the intensive care unit: More than meets the "i"? *American Journal of Respiratory and Critical Care Medicine*, *189*(11), 1297–1298. doi:10.1164/rccm.201405-0801ED PMID:24881934

Hunziker, S., Tschan, F., Semmer, N. K., Zobrist, R., Spychiger, M., Breuer, M., & Marsch, S. C. et al. (2009). Hands-on time during cardiopulmonary resuscitation is affected by the process of teambuilding: A prospective randomised simulator-based trial. *BMC Emergency Medicine*, *9*(1), 3. doi:10.1186/1471-227X-9-3 PMID:19216796

Kajdacsy-Balla Amaral, A. C., Barros, B. S., Barros, C. C., Innes, C., Pinto, R., & Rubenfeld, G. D. (2014). Nighttime cross-coverage is associated with decreased intensive care unit mortality. A single-center study. *American Journal of Respiratory and Critical Care Medicine*, *189*(11), 1395–1401. doi:10.1164/rccm.201312-2181OC PMID:24779652

Kelly, D. M., Kutney-Lee, A., McHugh, M. D., Sloane, D. M., & Aiken, L. H. (2014). Impact of critical care nursing on 30-day mortality of mechanically ventilated older adults. *Critical Care Medicine*, *42*(5), 1089–1095. doi:10.1097/CCM.0000000000000127 PMID:24368346

Kerlin, M. P., Small, D. S., Cooney, E., Fuchs, B. D., Bellini, L. M., Mikkelsen, M. E., & Halpern, S. D. et al. (2013). A randomized trial of nighttime physician staffing in an intensive care unit. *The New England Journal of Medicine*, *368*(23), 2201–2209. doi:10.1056/NEJMoa1302854 PMID:23688301

Keroack, M. A., Youngberg, B. J., Cerese, J. L., Krsek, C., Prellwitz, L. W., & Trevelyan, E. W. (2007). Organizational factors associated with high performance in quality and safety in academic medical centers. *Academic Medicine*, *82*(12), 1178–1186. doi:10.1097/ACM.0b013e318159e1ff PMID:18046123

Kohn, L. T., Corrigan, J. M., & Donaldson, M. S. (2000). *To err is human: building a safer health system* (p. 287). Washington, D.C.: National Academy Press.

Kruklitis, R. J., Tracy, J. A., & McCambridge, M. M. (2014). Clinical and financial considerations for implementing an ICU telemedicine program. *Chest*, *145*(6), 1392–1396. doi:10.1378/chest.13-0868 PMID:24889437

Kumar, K., Singal, R., Manji, R. A., Zarychanski, R., Bell, D. D., Freed, D. H., & Arora, R. C. (2014). The benefits of 24/7 in-house intensivist coverage for prolonged-stay cardiac surgery patients. *The Journal of Thoracic and Cardiovascular Surgery*, *148*(1), 290–297.e296. doi:10.1016/j.jtcvs.2014.02.074 PMID:24703332

Larsen, G. Y., Donaldson, A. E., Parker, H. B., & Grant, M. J. (2007). Preventable harm occurring to critically ill children. *Pediatric Critical Care Medicine*, *8*(4), 331–336. doi:10.1097/01.PCC.0000263042.73539.99 PMID:17417126

Leape, L. L., Cullen, D. J., Clapp, M. D., Burdick, E., Demonaco, H. J., Erickson, J. I., & Bates, D. W. (1999). Pharmacist participation on physician rounds and adverse drug events in the intensive care unit. *Journal of the American Medical Association*, *282*(3), 267–270. doi:10.1001/jama.282.3.267 PMID:10422996

Levy, M. M., Rapoport, J., Lemeshow, S., Chalfin, D. B., Phillips, G., & Danis, M. (2008). Association between critical care physician management and patient mortality in the intensive care unit. *Annals of Internal Medicine*, *148*(11), 801–809. doi:10.7326/0003-4819-148-11-200806030-00002 PMID:18519926

Manthous, C. A., & Hollingshead, A. B. (2011). Team science and critical care. *American Journal of Respiratory and Critical Care Medicine*, *184*(1), 17–25. doi:10.1164/rccm.201101-0185CI PMID:21471081

McGlynn, E. A., Asch, S. M., Adams, J., Keesey, J., Hicks, J., DeCristofaro, A., & Kerr, E. A. (2003). The quality of health care delivered to adults in the United States. *The New England Journal of Medicine*, *348*(26), 2635–2645. doi:10.1056/NEJMsa022615 PMID:12826639

Moote, M., Krsek, C., Kleinpell, R., & Todd, B. (2011). Physician assistant and nurse practitioner utilization in academic medical centers. *American Journal of Medical Quality*, *26*(6), 452–460. doi:10.1177/1062860611402984 PMID:21555487

Morris, D. S., Reilly, P., Rohrbach, J., Telford, G., Kim, P., & Sims, C. A. (2012). The influence of unit-based nurse practitioners on hospital outcomes and readmission rates for patients with trauma. *J Trauma Acute Care Surg*, *73*(2), 474–478. doi:10.1097/TA.0b013e31825882bb PMID:22846959

Morris, P. E., Goad, A., Thompson, C., Taylor, K., Harry, B., Passmore, L., & Haponik, E. et al. (2008). Early intensive care unit mobility therapy in the treatment of acute respiratory failure. *Critical Care Medicine*, *36*(8), 2238–2243. doi:10.1097/CCM.0b013e318180b90e PMID:18596631

Nelson, J. E., Curtis, J. R., Mulkerin, C., Campbell, M., Lustbader, D. R., Mosenthal, A. C., & Weissman, D. E. et al. (2013). Choosing and using screening criteria for palliative care consultation in the ICU: A report from the Improving Palliative Care in the ICU (IPAL-ICU) Advisory Board. *Critical Care Medicine*, *41*(10), 2318–2327. doi:10.1097/CCM.0b013e31828cf12c PMID:23939349

Niedner, M. F., Muething, S. E., & Sutcliffe, K. M. (2013). The high-reliability pediatric intensive care unit. *Pediatric Clinics of North America*, *60*(3), 563–580. doi:10.1016/j.pcl.2013.02.005 PMID:23639655

O'Mahony, S., McHenry, J., Blank, A. E., Snow, D., Eti Karakas, S., Santoro, G., & Kvetan, V. et al. (2010). Preliminary report of the integration of a palliative care team into an intensive care unit. *Palliative Medicine*, *24*(2), 154–165. doi:10.1177/0269216309346540 PMID:19825893

Pawlik, A. J., & Kress, J. P. (2013). Issues affecting the delivery of physical therapy services for individuals with critical illness. *Physical Therapy*, *93*(2), 256–265. doi:10.2522/ptj.20110445 PMID:23162041

Preslaski, C. R., Lat, I., MacLaren, R., & Poston, J. (2013). Pharmacist contributions as members of the multidisciplinary ICU team. *Chest*, *144*(5), 1687–1695. doi:10.1378/chest.12-1615 PMID:24189862

Pronovost, P. J., Angus, D. C., Dorman, T., Robinson, K. A., Dremsizov, T. T., & Young, T. L. (2002). Physician staffing patterns and clinical outcomes in critically ill patients: A systematic review. *Journal of the American Medical Association*, *288*(17), 2151–2162. doi:10.1001/jama.288.17.2151 PMID:12413375

Reed, C. R., Fogel, S. L., Collier, B. R., Bradburn, E. H., Baker, C. C., & Hamill, M. E. (2014). Higher surgical critical care staffing levels are associated with improved National Surgical Quality Improvement Program quality measures. *J Trauma Acute Care Surg, 77*(1), 83-88; discussion 88. doi: 10.1097/TA.0000000000000279

Rubenfeld, G. D., & Angus, D. C. (2008). Are intensivists safe? *Annals of Internal Medicine*, *148*(11), 877–879. doi:10.7326/0003-4819-148-11-200806030-00010 PMID:18519933

Rudis, M. I., & Brandl, K. M. (2000). Position paper on critical care pharmacy services. Society of Critical Care Medicine and American College of Clinical Pharmacy Task Force on Critical Care Pharmacy Services. *Critical Care Medicine*, *28*(11), 3746–3750. doi:10.1097/00003246-200011000-00037 PMID:11098984

Schweickert, W. D., Pohlman, M. C., Pohlman, A. S., Nigos, C., Pawlik, A. J., Esbrook, C. L., & Kress, J. P. et al. (2009). Early physical and occupational therapy in mechanically ventilated, critically ill patients: A randomised controlled trial. *Lancet*, *373*(9678), 1874–1882. doi:10.1016/S0140-6736(09)60658-9 PMID:19446324

Wallace, D. J., Angus, D. C., Barnato, A. E., Kramer, A. A., & Kahn, J. M. (2012). Nighttime intensivist staffing and mortality among critically ill patients. *The New England Journal of Medicine*, *366*(22), 2093–2101. doi:10.1056/NEJMsa1201918 PMID:22612639

Ward, N. S., Afessa, B., Kleinpell, R., Tisherman, S., Ries, M., Howell, M., & Kahn, J. et al. (2013). Intensivist/patient ratios in closed ICUs: A statement from the Society of Critical Care Medicine Taskforce on ICU Staffing. *Critical Care Medicine*, *41*(2), 638–645. doi:10.1097/CCM.0b013e3182741478 PMID:23263586

Wilcox, M. E., Chong, C. A., Niven, D. J., Rubenfeld, G. D., Rowan, K. M., Wunsch, H., & Fan, E. (2013). Do intensivist staffing patterns influence hospital mortality following ICU admission? A systematic review and meta-analyses. *Critical Care Medicine*, *41*(10), 2253–2274. doi:10.1097/CCM.0b013e318292313a PMID:23921275

Yager, P. H., Cummings, B. M., Whalen, M. J., & Noviski, N. (2012). Nighttime telecommunication between remote staff intensivists and bedside personnel in a pediatric intensive care unit: A retrospective study. *Critical Care Medicine*, *40*(9), 2700–2703. doi:10.1097/CCM.0b013e3182591dab PMID:22732287

Young, L. B., Chan, P. S., Lu, X., Nallamothu, B. K., Sasson, C., & Cram, P. M. (2011). Impact of telemedicine intensive care unit coverage on patient outcomes: A systematic review and meta-analysis. *Archives of Internal Medicine*, *171*(6), 498–506. doi:10.1001/archinternmed.2011.61 PMID:21444842

Young, M. P., & Birkmeyer, J. D. (2000). Potential reduction in mortality rates using an intensivist model to manage intensive care units. *Effective Clinical Practice*, *3*, 284–289. PMID:11151525

ADDITIONAL READING

Afessa, B. (2010). Tele-intensive care unit: The horse out of the barn. *Critical Care Medicine*, *38*(1), 292–293. doi:10.1097/CCM.0b013e3181b9d4dc PMID:20023465

American Medical Association. (2012). *Current Procedural Terminology: CPT 2013*. Chicago, IL: American Medical Association.

American Medical Association. (2012). *ICD-9 CM: 2013 Code Book for Physicians*. Chicago, IL: American Medical Association.

American Society of Health-System Pharmacists. (2010). ASHP statement on the pharmacist's role in antimicrobial stewardship and infection prevention and control. *American Journal of Health-System Pharmacy*, *67*(7), 575–577. doi:10.2146/sp100001 PMID:20237387

Angus, D. C., Shorr, A. F., White, A., Dremsizov, T. T., Schmitz, R. J., Kelley, M. A., & Critical Care, S. et al. (2006). Critical care delivery in the United States: Distribution of services and compliance with Leapfrog recommendations. *Critical Care Medicine*, *34*(4), 1016–1024. doi:10.1097/01.CCM.0000206105.05626.15 PMID:16505703

Bray, K., Wren, I., Baldwin, A., St Ledger, U., Gibson, V., Goodman, S., & Walsh, D. (2010). Standards for nurse staffing in critical care units determined by: The British Association of Critical Care Nurses, The Critical Care Networks National Nurse Leads, Royal College of Nursing Critical Care and In-flight Forum. *Nursing in Critical Care*, *15*(3), 109–111. doi:10.1111/j.1478-5153.2010.00392.x PMID:20500648

Centers for Medicare and Medicaid Services. 1997 Documentation Guidelines for Evaluation and Management Services. Retrieved December 26, 2014, from http://www.cms.gov/outreach-and-education/medicare-learning-network-mln/mlnedwebguide/downloads/97docguidelines.pdf

Centers for Medicare and Medicaid Services. Critical Care Visits and Neonatal Intensive Care (Codes 99291 – 99292). Retrieved December 26, 2014, from http://www.cms.gov/Regulations-and-Guidance/Guidance/Transmittals/downloads/r1548cp.pdf

Centers for Medicare and Medicaid Services. Medicare Claims Processing Manual [IOM 100-04]. Retrieved December 26, 2014, from http://www.cms.gov/regulationsandguidance/guidance/manuals/internet-only-manuals-ioms-items/cms018912.html

Centers for Medicare and Medicaid Services. Medicare Enrollment Application--Physicians and Non-Physician Practitioners [Form CMS 855i]. Retrieved December 26, 2014, from http://www.cms.gov/Medicare/CMS-Forms/CMS-Forms/downloads/cms855i.pdf

Gawande, A. (2007). The checklist: If something so simple can transform intensive care, what else can it do? *New Yorker (New York, N.Y.)*, 86–101. PMID:18084821

Gawande, A. (2010). *The Checklist Manifesto: How to Get Things Right*. New York, NY: Penguin.

Gosselink, R., Bott, J., Johnson, M., Dean, E., Nava, S., Norrenberg, M., & Vincent, J. L. et al. (2008). Physiotherapy for adult patients with critical illness: Recommendations of the European Respiratory Society and European Society of Intensive Care Medicine Task Force on Physiotherapy for Critically Ill Patients. *Intensive Care Medicine*, *34*(7), 1188–1199. doi:10.1007/s00134-008-1026-7 PMID:18283429

Harris, K. (2006). Critical Care Competency Program Development and Implementation. *Acute Care Perspectives*, *15*, 16–19.

Haupt, M. T., Bekes, C. E., Brilli, R. J., Carl, L. C., Gray, A. W., Jastremski, M. S., & Md, M. H. et al. (2003). Guidelines on critical care services and personnel: Recommendations based on a system of categorization of three levels of care. *Critical Care Medicine*, *31*(11), 2677–2683. doi:10.1097/01.CCM.0000094227.89800.93 PMID:14605541

Institute for Healthcare Improvement. (2011). *Improvement Leader's Guide to Sustainability and Spread*. Cambridge, MA.

Institute for Healthcare Improvement. (2011). How-to Guide: Sustainability and Spread. Cambridge, MA.

Institute of Medicine (IOM). (2001). *Crossing the Quality Chasm: A New Health System for the 21st Century*. Washington, D.C. Institute of Medicine (IOM). (2010). The future of nursing: the Institute of Medicine (IOM) issues report. The future of nursing: leading change, advancing health. *The Prairie Rose*, *79*(4), 6.

Kleinpell, R. M. (2014). ICU workforce: Revisiting nurse staffing. *Critical Care Medicine*, *42*(5), 1291–1292. doi:10.1097/CCM.0000000000000202 PMID:24736341

Kleinpell, R. M., Ely, E. W., & Grabenkort, R. (2008). Nurse practitioners and physician assistants in the intensive care unit: An evidence-based review. *Critical Care Medicine*, *36*(10), 2888–2897. doi:10.1097/CCM.0b013e318186ba8c PMID:18766097

Landrigan, C. P., Rothschild, J. M., Cronin, J. W., Kaushal, R., Burdick, E., Katz, J. T., & Czeisler, C. A. et al. (2004). Effect of reducing interns' work hours on serious medical errors in intensive care units. *The New England Journal of Medicine*, *351*(18), 1838–1848. doi:10.1056/NEJMoa041406 PMID:15509817

Lanken, P. N., Terry, P. B., Delisser, H. M., Fahy, B. F., Hansen-Flaschen, J., Heffner, J. E., & Yankaskas, J. R. et al. (2008). An official American Thoracic Society clinical policy statement: Palliative care for patients with respiratory diseases and critical illnesses. *American Journal of Respiratory and Critical Care Medicine*, *177*(8), 912–927. doi:10.1164/rccm.200605-587ST PMID:18390964

Nolan, T., Resar, R., Haraden, C., & Griffin, F. (2004). Improving the Reliatbility of Health Care. *IHI Innovation Series White Paper*.

Pastores, S. M., O'Connor, M. F., Kleinpell, R. M., Napolitano, L., Ward, N., Bailey, H., & Coopersmith, C. M. et al. (2011). The Accreditation Council for Graduate Medical Education resident duty hour new standards: History, changes, and impact on staffing of intensive care units. *Critical Care Medicine*, *39*(11), 2540–2549. doi:10.1097/CCM.0b013e318225776f PMID:21705890

Patterson, K., Grenny, J., McMillan, R., & Switzler, A. (2002). *Crucial Conversations: Tools for Talking when Stakes are High*. New York, NY: Mc-Graw-Hill.

Pronovost, P., Needham, D., Berenholtz, S., Sinopoli, D., Chu, H., Cosgrove, S., & Goeschel, C. et al. (2006). An intervention to decrease catheter-related bloodstream infections in the ICU. *The New England Journal of Medicine*, *355*(26), 2725–2732. doi:10.1056/NEJMoa061115 PMID:17192537

Rhodes, A., Moreno, R. P., Azoulay, E., Capuzzo, M., Chiche, J. D., Eddleston, J., & Valentin, A. et al. (2012). Prospectively defined indicators to improve the safety and quality of care for critically ill patients: A report from the Task Force on Safety and Quality of the European Society of Intensive Care Medicine (ESICM). *Intensive Care Medicine*, *38*(4), 598–605. doi:10.1007/s00134-011-2462-3 PMID:22278594

Selecky, P. A., Eliasson, C. A., Hall, R. I., Schneider, R. F., Varkey, B., & McCaffree, D. R. (2005). Palliative and end-of-life care for patients with cardiopulmonary diseases: American College of Chest Physicians position statement. *Chest*, *128*(5), 3599–3610. doi:10.1378/chest.128.5.3599 PMID:16304319

Siegal, E. M., Dressler, D. D., Dichter, J. R., Gorman, M. J., & Lipsett, P. A. (2012). Training a hospitalist workforce to address the intensivist shortage in American hospitals: A position paper from the Society of Hospital Medicine and the Society of Critical Care Medicine. *Critical Care Medicine*, *40*(6), 1952–1956. doi:10.1097/CCM.0b013e318258eef7 PMID:22610197

Sutcliffe, K. M. (2011). High reliability organizations (HROs). *Best Practice & Research. Clinical Anaesthesiology*, *25*(2), 133–144. doi:10.1016/j.bpa.2011.03.001 PMID:21550539

The American Association of Critical-Care Nurses. (2005). AACN Standards for Establishing and Sustaining Healthy Work Environments: A Journey to Excellence. *American Journal of Critical Care*, *14*(3), 187–197. PMID:15840893

The Leapfrog Group. ICU Physician Staffing. Retrieved October 19, 2014, from http://www.leapfroggroup.org/media/file/Leapfrog-ICU_Physician_Staffing_Fact_Sheet.pdf

Truog, R. D., Campbell, M. L., Curtis, J. R., Haas, C. E., Luce, J. M., Rubenfeld, G. D., & Kaufman, D. C. et al. (2008). Recommendations for end-of-life care in the intensive care unit: A consensus statement by the American College [corrected] of Critical Care Medicine. *Critical Care Medicine*, *36*(3), 953–963. doi:10.1097/CCM.0B013E3181659096 PMID:18431285

Valentin, A., & Ferdinande, P. (2011). Recommendations on basic requirements for intensive care units: Structural and organizational aspects. *Intensive Care Medicine*, *37*(10), 1575–1587. doi:10.1007/s00134-011-2300-7 PMID:21918847

KEY TERMS AND DEFINITIONS

Closed ICU: ICUs where care is transferred to a specialist, usually but not always an intensivist.

Critical Care Team: This consists of all members of the team which can include: intensivists, medical students, residents, fellows, NP/PAs, nurses, clinical pharmacologists, physical therapists, social workers, unit assistants, housekeepers, respiratory therapists, palliative care specialists.

High Intensity Staffing Model: An ICU that has all care provided by an intensivist or mandatory consultation by an intensivist.

High-Reliability Organization (HRO): High risk and high reliability organizations that are committed to a zero failure rate.

Low Intensity Staffing Model: An ICU where intensivists are only used if specifically consulted.

Open ICU: ICUs where care is provided by many consultants and generalists. Intensivists may or may not be involved in care.

Team Science: The study of successful teams and leadership strategy that could be applied to critical care teams.

Tele-ICU: A staffing model when a team (usually an intensivist and ICU RN) monitors patients usually from a remote location. These teams usually have no direct patient contact, and often are supported by software that analyzes data and provides an "early warning" system.

Chapter 5
Palliative Care

May Hua
Columbia University, USA

ABSTRACT

Palliative care is a specialty of medicine that focuses on improving quality of life for patients with serious illness and their families. As the limitations of intensive care and the long-term sequelae of critical illness continue to be delimited, the role of palliative care for patients that are unable to achieve their original goals of care, as well as for survivors of critical illness, is changing and expanding. The purpose of this chapter is to introduce readers to the specialty of palliative care and its potential benefits for critically ill patients, and to present some of the issues related to the delivery of palliative care in surgical units.

INTRODUCTION

When patients are admitted to the intensive care unit (ICU), the goal of care is most often to rescue and to cure. While this is achievable for the majority of patients, 9% of patients die during their hospitalization (Lilly, 2011). For these patients, the goals of care need to be transitioned, an undertaking that requires the patient, family and all participating members of the care team to agree to these changes. Because of this, the provision of end-of-life care in the ICU is often inadequate, with multiple barriers arising from the patient and family, clinicians and institutional factors (Nelson, 2006b). While patients that die in the ICU have obvious palliative care needs, there is increasing evidence delineating the long-term outcomes of critical illness, with survivors of critical illness being at risk for increased morbidity and mortality and debilitating symptomatology (Herridge; Hofhuis, 2008; Pandharipande, 2013; Wunsch, 2014; Wunsch, 2010). As it becomes clearer that both ICU patients and survivors of critical illness are at risk of having significant symptoms and poor outcomes, it becomes increasingly pressing to determine how to provide the requisite care to meet these needs.

The use of palliative care is one approach that is being advocated to address these concerns. This chapter reviews what palliative care is, evidence for the benefit of palliative care in the ICU setting, models for delivering palliative care in the ICU, barriers to implementing palliative care, particular challenges related to the setting of surgical critical care and discusses future directions for improving the delivery of palliative care and end-of-life care to the surgical patient.

DOI: 10.4018/978-1-4666-8603-8.ch005

I. WHAT IS PALLIATIVE CARE?

Traditionally, the goal of medicine has been to cure disease. Hospice and palliative medicine differ in that the goal is to improve quality of life. Palliative care is defined by the World Health Organization as "an approach that improves the quality of life of patients and their families facing the problems associated with life-threatening illness, through the prevention and relief of suffering by means of early identification and impeccable assessment and treatment of pain and other problems, physical, psychosocial and spiritual." As a specialty, palliative care arose out of the hospice movement. Hospice is a model of care for patients with limited life expectancy that focuses on palliation and symptom management, and often requires patients to forego curative therapies. Hospice is most often provided in a patient's home, but can also be provided in hospice inpatient facilities. Unlike hospice, palliative care is appropriate for patients with serious illness at any time in the course of their disease, does not require patients to give up curative treatments, and can be provided in conjunction with other aggressive therapies.

Because the goal of palliative care is to improve quality of life and relieve suffering and stress associated with having a serious illness, the delivery of palliative care may involve many different domains that are utilized based on an individual's specific needs. The use of palliative care addresses various needs for critically ill patients and their families including: 1) symptom management (e.g. pain, nausea, fatigue, thirst, depression, anxiety, existential distress), 2) conflict resolution (conflict between family members, or between the family and the medical team), 3) spiritual support, and 4) complex decision-making regarding goals of care. In the ICU, the role of palliative care has traditionally been as a part of delivering end-of-life care for patients who die in the ICU. However, there is an expanding role for palliative care in the management of patients who may survive their illness but are at risk for having significant symptomatology, such as patients with chronic critical illness.

A. Models for Delivering Palliative Care in the ICU

The two models of delivering palliative care in the ICU are the integrative and consultative models. With the integrative approach, principles of palliative care are woven into routine care, and palliative care is delivered by the primary team, whereas with the consultative approach, palliative care is provided by a specialized palliative care consultation team. These models can co-exist, and reflect the distinction between generalist and specialist palliative care (Quill, 2013). Generalist palliative care is delivered by primary providers, and includes basic pain and symptom management, as well as basic discussions regarding prognosis and goals of care. Specialized palliative care may be required for refractory pain and symptom management, conflict resolution and complex decision-making (Quill, 2013). Each model has its benefits and drawbacks, and which model is optimal likely depends on the characteristics of an individual ICU. Benefits of the integrative model are that there does not need to be additional staffing in order to deliver palliative care, there is less fragmentation of care, and it may decrease conflict associated with having another consulting team. With the consultative model, there is less variability in clinicians' education and their palliative care skill set, and in situations of conflict resolution, the introduction of an impartial party may be helpful. There is a greater body of evidence demonstrating the benefits of specialized palliative care, as a systematic review of communication interventions showed that a consultative approach had better outcomes than an integrative approach (Scheunemann, 2011). However, there is an existing workforce shortage of palliative care physicians (Lupu, 2010), and estimates of the need for palliative care consultation likely outstrips what the current palliative care workforce can provide (Hua, 2014). Consequently, a sustainable model of palliative care delivery in ICUs is likely to be one that is mixed, combining both approaches.

II. EVIDENCE FOR PALLIATIVE CARE IN THE ICU

A. Palliative Care Needs in Critically Ill Patients

In the U.S., admission to an ICU is associated with high in-hospital mortality (Lilly, 2011), and it is estimated that approximately 14% of ICU patients meet screening criteria for palliative care consultation (Hua, 2014). In addition to the large volume of patients with end-of-life care needs, ICU patients may have a substantial symptom burden. Of chronic critically ill patients who were able to report symptoms, 90% endorsed having significant symptoms with uncontrolled pain, psychological distress and dyspnea being most prominent (Nelson, 2004). Cancer patients in the ICU experienced moderate to severe pain, discomfort and anxiety (Delgado-Guay, 2009; Nelson, 2001), and quality of life for patients who die in the ICU is poorer than for those who die at home (Wright, 2010).

Although death frequently occurs during or after an ICU stay, there is also evidence that an ICU admission is a marker of poor long-term prognosis. Survivors of critical illness, particularly those who received mechanical ventilation, have increased 3-year mortality, the bulk of which is concentrated in the first 6 months after hospital discharge (Wunsch, 2010). ICU survivors have also been shown to have significant symptomatology with long-term functional disability, sleep disorders, post-traumatic stress disorder, increased risk of developing a psychological diagnosis and decreased health-related quality of life (Davydow, 2008; Herridge, 2003; Herridge; Hofhuis, 2008; Lee, 2009; Wunsch, 2014). Together, this constellation of symptoms is beginning to carry the label of a post-intensive care syndrome (Harvey, 2012; Mehlhorn, 2014). Furthermore, patients with chronic critical illness who survived to hospital discharge are also known to have a high burden of palliative care needs, with approximately 90% of patients having at least one need (Baldwin, 2013).

Surgical ICU patients, are often perceived to be healthier and to have improved outcomes in comparison to non-surgical ICU patients; of surgical ICU patients, cardiac surgical patients also have lower mortality, with estimates of short-term mortality ranging between 3-4% (Mosenthal, 2012; Nashef, 2012; Shahian, 2012). However, the palliative care needs of patients with surgical critical illness may not differ greatly from their non-surgical counterparts. Mortality remains high for patients with longer ICU stays (Laupland, 2006; Lipsett, 2000), and surgical patients represent a significant portion of the chronic critically ill, a population well-known to be at high-risk for poor outcomes. In a study of the chronic critically ill, 25% of patients transferred to long-term acute care hospitals were surgical, with cardiac surgery patients representing over half of these patients (Kahn, 2013). Furthermore, a study estimating the need for palliative care consultation did not find a significant difference in the percentage of patients meeting screening criteria for palliative care consultation in surgical units in comparison to medical units, but did find that patients in surgical units were significantly less likely to have limitations on treatment placed (Hua, 2014). Thus, the surgical critically ill population may be at higher risk for having unmet palliative care needs.

B. Benefits of Palliative Care in the ICU

The importance of palliative care in the ICU setting has been accepted and supported by multiple societies, including the American College of Critical Care Medicine and the American Thoracic Society (Lanken, 2008; Truog, 2008). The integration of specialized palliative care in the ICU has been associated with increased rates of formalized advanced directives, increased use of hospice and decreased use of non-beneficial life-sustaining therapies (O'Mahony, 2010). Furthermore, palliative care may also improve costs and resource use. The use of palliative care has been associated with decreased direct costs at the end of life in a generalized hospital setting (Morrison, 2011; Morrison, 2008; Penrod, 2010), and both proactive palliative care consultation and ethics consultations in selected ICU patients were associated with decreased hospital length of stay and decreased use of non-beneficial life-sustaining therapies, without an increase in mortality (Campbell, 2003; Schneiderman, 2003). These outcomes are noteworthy, as non-aggressive care and a family/patient-centered approach to dying are associated with a better quality of death and improved family satisfaction with end-of-life decision making (Gries, 2008; Mularski, 2005). Adequate end-of-life care is highly desired by patients and their families, who may prefer to avoid aggressive and burdensome care in the setting of a poor prognosis (Fried, 2002; Nelson, 2010).

III. BARRIERS TO DELIVERY OF PALLIATIVE CARE

Despite the benefits of palliative care, there are multiple barriers stemming from the culture of the ICU, patients, families, clinicians and institutional factors that ultimately result in the under-utilization of palliative care (Nelson, 2006b).

A. Culture of the ICU

The ICU is the most technologically advanced practice setting in the hospital, where routine care involves the use of machines and medications to monitor and replace organ function for the heart, the lungs, and the kidneys in order to keep patients alive. When a patient is admitted to the ICU, all the stakeholders involved, including the patient, family members and clinicians, often start with the goal of staving off death and "rescuing" the patient. Because of this focus, expectations and hopes are high, and this can lead to a sense of failure, particularly for clinicians, when patients are unable to be "saved" (Nelson, 2006a). When these goals cannot be met, it must first be recognized and accepted by clinicians and families before the goals of care can be changed to providing high-quality end-of-life care. The need for this transition often delays the onset of high-quality end-of-life and palliative care.

B. Patient and Family Members

In a survey of ICU directors, barriers stemming from the patient and family members were rated as the largest barriers to the provision of adequate end-of-life care in the ICU (Nelson, 2006b). These included unrealistic expectations about the patient's prognosis or the effectiveness of therapies, the inability of patients to participate in treatment discussions, a lack of advanced directives and disagreements within families about goals of care (Aslakson, 2012; Nelson, 2006b). Some of the dissonance between families' and clinicians' perceptions may come from a distrust of clinicians' abilities to accurately prognosticate, and family members relying on their own knowledge of a patient to form their own prognosis (Boyd, 2010; Zier, 2012).

C. Clinician and Institutional Factors

Clinicians and institutional factors also present barriers to the delivery of end-of-life and palliative care. In this domain, the most significant barriers reported were that clinicians may not have adequate skills in communication regarding end-of-life care or in techniques for withdrawing or withholding life-sustaining treatment, that there are competing demands for clinicians' time, and that communication with families and other involved clinicians about appropriate goals of care can be deficient (Aslakson, 2012; Friedenberg, 2012; Nelson, 2006b). Barriers that arise from institutional factors include the lack of a palliative care service or palliative care consultants, inadequate support services for family and the lack of a continuity of care due to changes in clinician staffing (Nelson, 2006b).

Many barriers to the adequate delivery of end-of-life care and palliative care have been elicited, but overall, those related to the patient and family (lack of patient involvement in end-of-life care decisions, a lack of advanced directives and unrealistic expectations) have been consistently rated as major barriers, whereas clinician and institutional factors were not reported to be as significant (Friedenberg, 2012; Nelson, 2006b). However, the generalizability of barriers to end-of-life and palliative care may be questionable, as perceived barriers have been shown to differ by level of training, discipline and institution (Friedenberg, 2012). This suggests that to some degree, models and interventions to improve the delivery of palliative care and end-of-life care in the ICU may need to be tailored to specific institutions.

IV. ISSUES SPECIFIC TO CARDIOTHORACIC CRITICAL CARE

A. Surgical Critical Illness

Surgical critical illness differs from non-surgical critical illness in several ways that may impact efforts to initiate end-of-life care or palliative care. First, surgeons are less likely to operate on patients with a do-not-resuscitate order and advanced directives, which may make surgical patients less likely to have them (Bradley, 2010b). Second, unlike many non-surgical patients who are admitted to the ICU for worsening of a chronic condition, surgical patients are often healthier with an acute illness that requires emergent surgery (e.g. trauma), or are undergoing a procedure that is meant to be curative (e.g. aortic valve replacement), or are receiving therapy that is intended to cure their chronic illness (e.g. heart transplantation). Most often, patients, families and surgeons start with a goal of "beating a disease" and this leads to high hopes for recovery (Mosenthal, 2012). This may be particularly pronounced in situations where patients and families have approached surgeons specifically with the intention of "fixing" the problem, and have not yet begun to entertain the possibility that this goal may not be achievable. Consequently, it may be harder to come to terms with a failure of therapy and there needs to be time for all parties to adjust to the idea that the initial goals may not be met.

B. The Surgical Contract

Surgeons are often perceived as an impediment to the initiation of palliative care and end-of-life care for critically ill patients (Schwarze, 2010). This is explained in part by the complexity of the relationship between the surgeon and a patient, which begins pre-operatively, prior to the onset of any acute critical illness. The idea of a surgical contract, or surgical "buy-in" refers to a process where surgeons, often informally, negotiate a commitment to postoperative care prior to undergoing high-risk surgical procedures (Schwarze, 2010). Surgeons make a commitment to patient when they decide to operate, and they expect a similar commitment from the patient to undergo the post-operative care that they believe is necessary for recovery. As a consequence, surgeons may then feel betrayed or disappointed when approached by families with request to withdraw life-sustaining treatment at a time that they may feel is premature, and they may be unwilling to agree to the withdrawal and may negotiate with families and other caregivers about continuing to pursue aggressive care (Schwarze, 2010). Surgeons also often feel a sense of personal responsibility for adverse postoperative outcomes, and have described feelings of guilt with poor outcomes that may be accentuated when that outcome was unexpected, or when the outcome may involve a surgical error (Schwarze, 2010; Schwarze, 2012). This is compounded by the fact that surgeons are taught to view death as a "failure" (Mosenthal, 2006). While these pre-operative discussions seem to document the risks inherent in the procedure and the potential need for intensive care, the possibility of requiring prolonged life-sustaining treatment is not often discussed, and patients' preferences regarding these treatments are not elicited (Pecanac, 2014). Awareness of the intricacies of this relationship and its existence as a backdrop for post-operative decision-making is crucial for intensivists as they negotiate goals of care between surgeons, patients and families.

C. Lack of Formal Education in Palliative Care for Surgeons

Until recently, education in palliative care was not emphasized as a part of surgical training. This is problematic, as surgeons are unlikely to involve palliative care for symptom management and unfamiliarity with palliative care services has been associated with decreased referral rates to palliative care (Snow, 2009; Tilden, 2009). 84% of surgical residents surveyed did not report receiving any training in palliative care during residency, and informal training in palliative care was also infrequent, where only 50% of surgical residents reported discussing death and dying with a surgical attending (Brasel, 2004; Galante, 2005). Furthermore, surgical residents lacked skills in basic symptom management, as less than half of a group surveyed were proficient in the treatment of cancer-related pain, and competency did not improve as these residents progressed through their training (Brasel, 2004). These deficiencies may correlate to patient outcomes, as a lack of education in end-of-life care has been shown to be associated with decreased willingness to place limitations on care (Forte, 2012). Also, in a study of palliative care in the ICU, nurse ratings' of the quality of death were lowest for patients cared for by surgical intensivists, and patients cared for by surgical intensivists were significantly less likely to have indicators of palliative care documented in their medical charts (Kross, 2014). As surgeons may be unaware of what palliative care is and its benefits, it is not surprising that surgeons may be more likely to only involve palliative care at the end-of-life (Tilden, 2009).

D. Conflict between Surgeons and ICU Clinicians

With surgical patients, there is always another highly-invested clinician involved whose relationship with the patient exists prior to the onset of critical illness, and this creates an extra layer of potential conflict that surrounds decision-making. Surgeons are perceived by ICU clinicians as an impediment to end-of-life and palliative care (Schwarze, 2010), and surgeons perceive conflict frequently with ICU clinicians, with approximately 40% of surveyed surgeons reporting that they experienced conflict with intensivists or nurses during the care of one of their patients (Paul Olson, 2013). Much of this conflict may revolve around prognostication, which is often at the center of discussion regarding appropriate goals of care. In a cross-sectional survey, the majority of surgeons were satisfied with their own communication regarding prognosis to patients and families, but less than a quarter of ICU physicians and less than 5% of ICU nurses reported being satisfied with the surgeon's communication of prognosis (Aslakson, 2010). Furthermore, ICU physicians reported having fewer opportunities to communicate with surgeons regarding their concerns about prognosis, and did not report feeling that their comments were valued (Aslakson, 2010). This additional layer of conflict complicates the process of addressing goals of care, and consequently, may hinder the initiation of palliative care and end-of-life care.

E. Staffing Model

Many surgical patients are cared for in open units, with surgeons retaining primary responsibility for the patient's care. Organizational aspects of this particular staffing model present unique challenges to decision-making and palliative care. First, it may be ambiguous which clinician, the surgeon or the intensivist, is responsible for leading discussions regarding goals of care and for coordinating care. Also, the presence of the surgical team in the ICU may vary throughout the day, leading to fragmentation of communication and the overall care plan (Mosenthal, 2012). Lastly, with regards to quality improvement, it may be more difficult to effect cultural changes or implement interventions to improve palliative care and end-of-life care in open units in comparison to closed units (Mosenthal, 2006).

F. Mechanical Circulatory Support Devices

Although the ICU has always represented a forefront of medicine where technology is employed to provide life support and prolong life, the advent of mechanical circulatory support devices (MCSD) such as the ventricular assist device (VAD) and extracorporeal membrane oxygenation (ECMO) adds a new layer of complexity to the provision of palliative care and end-of-life care in a cardiothoracic ICU. These patients are at increased risk for having palliative care needs, and being considered as a candidate for a VAD or having had a cardiac arrest have been suggested as triggers for palliative care consultation (Norton, 2007; Weissman, 2011). Patients requiring mechanical circulatory support are at high risk of mortality, may suffer devastating complications (e.g. stroke, limb ischemia, life-threatening bleeding), and often require complex decision-making regarding goals of care. As an example, consider a patient who receives a VAD as a bridge-to-transplant and then suffers a large stroke that precludes transplantation. While the initial goal of VAD therapy was to support the patient until transplantation, this goal is no longer applicable, and new goals of care need to be defined. In the case of ECMO, goals of care also may rapidly change, particularly if the patient's condition has not improved and continuing care becomes futile. The role of palliative care consultations for ECMO patients has yet to be well-defined (Abrams, 2014), but may be particularly helpful in situations with high prognostic uncertainty and medical complexity (Doorenbos, 2013).

The use of MCSD also may complicate withdrawal of life-sustaining therapy at the end of life. Families may have difficulty with the concept of discontinuing device support, and clinicians may also be reluctant due to ethical and legal concerns (Swetz, 2011). There are also technical issues with discontinuing MCSD, requiring staff to be familiar with each specific device and the proper method of discontinuing support to avoid causing the device to alarm, which may cause distress to families. Consequently, having a protocol in place for device withdrawal has been advocated (Brush, 2010; MacIver, 2005).

V. METHODS TO IMPROVE DELIVERY OF PALLIATIVE CARE IN THE CARDIOTHORACIC ICU

General recommendations for developing and integrating palliative care in a surgical ICU setting have been proposed with three steps outlined: 1) form an interdisciplinary workgroup of key stakeholders to lead the effort to implement palliative care, 2) choose a model for implementing palliative care and 3) implement screening triggers for palliative care consultation (Mosenthal, 2012). To start, the workgroup should be comprised of representatives from the leadership of all involved parties, including intensivists, surgeons, cardiologists, critical care nurses, palliative care specialists, and if possible, hospital leadership. For the second step, the needs and resources for palliative care that are particular to the institution should be assessed to determine how much each model (consultative, integrative, or mixed) should be employed. For the integrative model, one particular approach has been described where a palliative care intervention is implemented for all patients, irrespective of prognosis (Table 1) (Mosenthal, 2006). This has the advantage of not being concerned with prognostication, which is problematic for clinicians and may be difficult for families to accept (Meadow, 2011; Zier, 2012).

In order to facilitate use of the consultative model, choosing appropriate screening triggers for palliative care consultation is recommended. It is estimated that approximately 14% of all ICU patients meet published triggers for palliative care consultation (Hua, 2014). However, whether or not this strategy is feasible in the setting of a cardiothoracic ICU is not known. Triggers have been developed specifically for use in a surgical ICU setting, but when implemented, they failed to increase the number of palliative care consultations (Bradley, 2010a). This may have been secondary to the triggers occurring infrequently or surgeons being unwilling to involve palliative care consultants. Triggers may be more useful in a cardiothoracic ICU if they target specific populations, (e.g. transplant patients, VAD patients, ECMO patients), or if referral is mandated upon meeting a trigger (Mosenthal, 2012).

Changing culture is also a vital component of improving the delivery of palliative care in a cardiothoracic ICU. Surgeons and intensivists may require education about the role of palliative care to understand that palliative care can be provided in conjunction with aggressive therapies. In particular for surgeons, this may be necessary to alleviate fears that palliative care is simply "death care," or that they will lose control of decision-making regarding goals of care. However, for this type of change to occur, the provision of high-quality palliative care must be viewed as being equally important to "rescuing" patients and emphasized as an important goal by the leadership of all key stakeholders.

Table 1. Checklist of a palliative care intervention in a surgical/trauma intensive care unit(Mosenthal, 2006)*

Intervention	Goal
1. Bereavement and psychosocial support for patients and families within 24 hours of admission to the surgical ICU	To establish a supportive relationship with families early on, which can aid future discussions and decision-making if needed
2. Interdisciplinary palliative care assessment within 24 hours of admission - Assessment of pain and symptoms - Assessment of psychosocial, spiritual and bereavement needs of family - Identify surrogate decision maker - Solicit and clarify advanced directives - Assessment of likely outcome and prognosis (discharge from ICU, discharge from hospital) from the current illness with regards to mortality and quality of life	Focus on symptom management and relief, identify conflicts related to goals of care early
3. Family meeting with physician and nurse within 72 hours of admission to the surgical ICU	To communicate information to families regarding outcomes, address goals of care and model shared decision-making
4. Comprehensive palliative care plan by 72 hours	To document a palliative care plan for all patients who remain in the ICU for ≥ 3 days, including pain and symptom management, goals of care, family support and ongoing communication, irrespective of prognosis To institute limitations in care if appropriate
5. Implementation of Palliative Care Standing Order Set for patients who are identified as imminently dying	To facilitate a standardized delivery of palliative care measures for dying patients
6. Integration of palliative care performance into morbidity and mortality conferences and peer review	To raise awareness of the importance of high-quality palliative care by making the quality of palliative care delivery and the quality of death a formal part of quality improvement

*Adapted from Mosenthal and Murphy.

VI. FUTURE DIRECTIONS

Research in several particular domains is crucial to improving palliative care and end-of-life care for critically ill surgical patients. Different models of delivering palliative care and methods for successful implementation in a cardiothoracic ICU setting require further study, as few successful models have been reported. Approaches that account for the differences in trajectories of illness for cardiac surgical patients, organizational differences in the ICU and the reality of the surgical contract need to be developed and examined to determine their efficacy. Another area that merits investigation is how to improve education in generalist palliative care for both surgeons and intensivists. As consultants are unlikely to be able to fully meet the palliative care needs of cardiothoracic ICU patients, enhancing the palliative care skill set of "front-line" clinicians will not only improve palliative care for patients, but increase the involvement of specialist palliative care when appropriate. Also, there is a need to standardize the manner in which the quality and effectiveness of palliative care in ICUs is measured. If palliative care in the ICU is to be improved, outcomes and measurements that can reliably differentiate high-quality from low-quality palliative care need to be developed and employed consistently. Lastly, given the increasing use of MCSD, this group of patients at high-risk of having palliative care needs will continue to pose a challenge for ICU clinicians. Identifying the palliative care needs of this particular patient population is a necessary first step towards understanding how these needs may be met.

VII. CONCLUSION

Palliative care in the ICU is appropriate for patients with significant symptomatology, psychological or spiritual distress or conflict regarding goals of care. Adequate delivery of palliative care for all patients is likely to involve a combination of basic palliative care that is delivered by ICU clinicians, and specialized palliative care that is delivered by palliative care consultants. In cardiothoracic surgical units, particular challenges exist to the delivery of palliative care that relate to the surgical ethos of rescuing the patient, the involvement of another clinician that is deeply invested in the patient's outcome and the perceptions of cardiac surgical patients as being relatively healthy and more robust by both families and clinicians. In particular, the population of patients requiring mechanical circulatory support represents a group of patients that are potentially high-risk for having palliative care needs. Efforts to improve palliative care delivery to cardiac surgical critically ill patients should focus on the continuing education of surgeons and intensivists as to what palliative care is and its potential benefits, determining which model of palliative care delivery is most appropriate for cardiac surgical patients, and studying the implementation of these models, and defining the role of palliative care for particular high-risk populations.

REFERENCES

Abrams, D. C., Prager, K., Blinderman, C. D., Burkart, K. M., & Brodie, D. (2014). Ethical dilemmas encountered with the use of extracorporeal membrane oxygenation in adults. *Chest*, *145*(4), 876–882. doi:10.1378/chest.13-1138 PMID:24687709

Aslakson, R. A., Wyskiel, R., Shaeffer, D., Zyra, M., Ahuja, N., Nelson, J. E., & Pronovost, P. J. (2010). Surgical intensive care unit clinician estimates of the adequacy of communication regarding patient prognosis. *Critical Care (London, England)*, *14*(6), R218. doi:10.1186/cc9346 PMID:21114837

Aslakson, R. A., Wyskiel, R., Thornton, I., Copley, C., Shaffer, D., Zyra, M., & Pronovost, P. J. et al. (2012). Nurse-perceived barriers to effective communication regarding prognosis and optimal end-of-life care for surgical ICU patients: A qualitative exploration. *Journal of Palliative Medicine*, *15*(8), 910–915. doi:10.1089/jpm.2011.0481 PMID:22676315

Baldwin, M. R., Wunsch, H., Reyfman, P. A., Narain, W. R., Blinderman, C. D., Schluger, N. W., & Bach, P. (2013). *High Burden of Palliative Needs among Older ICU Survivors Transferred to Post-Acute Care Facilities: A Single Center Study*. Ann Am Thorac Soc. doi:10.1513/AnnalsATS.201303-039OC

Boyd, E. A., Lo, B., Evans, L. R., Malvar, G., Apatira, L., Luce, J. M., & White, D. B. (2010). "It's not just what the doctor tells me:" factors that influence surrogate decision-makers' perceptions of prognosis. *Critical Care Medicine*, *38*(5), 1270–1275. doi:10.1097/CCM.0b013e3181d8a217 PMID:20228686

Bradley, C., Weaver, J., & Brasel, K. (2010a). Addressing access to palliative care services in the surgical intensive care unit. *Surgery*, *147*(6), 871–877. doi:10.1016/j.surg.2009.11.005 PMID:20097397

Bradley, C. T., Brasel, K. J., & Schwarze, M. L. (2010b). Physician attitudes regarding advance directives for high-risk surgical patients: A qualitative analysis. *Surgery*, *148*(2), 209–216. doi:10.1016/j.surg.2010.05.020 PMID:20580048

Brasel, K. J., & Weissman, D. E. (2004). Palliative care education for surgeons. *Journal of the American College of Surgeons*, *199*(3), 495–499. doi:10.1016/j.jamcollsurg.2004.06.004 PMID:15325621

Brush, S., Budge, D., Alharethi, R., McCormick, A. J., MacPherson, J. E., Reid, B. B., & Kfoury, A. G. et al. (2010). End-of-life decision making and implementation in recipients of a destination left ventricular assist device. *The Journal of Heart and Lung Transplantation*, *29*(12), 1337–1341. doi:10.1016/j.healun.2010.07.001 PMID:20817564

Campbell, M. L., & Guzman, J. A. (2003). Impact of a proactive approach to improve end-of-life care in a medical ICU. *Chest*, *123*(1), 266–271. doi:10.1378/chest.123.1.266 PMID:12527629

Davydow, D. S., Gifford, J. M., Desai, S. V., Needham, D. M., & Bienvenu, O. J. (2008). Posttraumatic stress disorder in general intensive care unit survivors: A systematic review. *General Hospital Psychiatry*, *30*(5), 421–434. doi:10.1016/j.genhosppsych.2008.05.006 PMID:18774425

Delgado-Guay, M. O., Parsons, H. A., Li, Z., Palmer, L. J., & Bruera, E. (2009). Symptom distress, interventions, and outcomes of intensive care unit cancer patients referred to a palliative care consult team. *Cancer*, *115*(2), 437–445. doi:10.1002/cncr.24017 PMID:19107768

Doorenbos, A. Z., Starks, H., Bourget, E., McMullan, D. M., Lewis-Newby, M., Rue, T. C., & Wilfond, B. S. et al. (2013). Examining palliative care team involvement in automatic consultations for children on extracorporeal life support in the pediatric intensive care unit. *Journal of Palliative Medicine*, *16*(5), 492–495. doi:10.1089/jpm.2012.0536 PMID:23540309

Forte, D. N., Vincent, J. L., Velasco, I. T., & Park, M. (2012). Association between education in EOL care and variability in EOL practice: A survey of ICU physicians. *Intensive Care Medicine*, *38*(3), 404–412. doi:10.1007/s00134-011-2400-4 PMID:22222566

Fried, T. R., Bradley, E. H., Towle, V. R., & Allore, H. (2002). Understanding the treatment preferences of seriously ill patients. *The New England Journal of Medicine*, *346*(14), 1061–1066. doi:10.1056/NEJMsa012528 PMID:11932474

Friedenberg, A. S., Levy, M. M., Ross, S., & Evans, L. E. (2012). Barriers to end-of-life care in the intensive care unit: Perceptions vary by level of training, discipline, and institution. *Journal of Palliative Medicine*, *15*(4), 404–411. doi:10.1089/jpm.2011.0261 PMID:22468773

Galante, J. M., Bowles, T. L., Khatri, V. P., Schneider, P. D., Goodnight, J. E. Jr, & Bold, R. J. (2005). Experience and attitudes of surgeons toward palliation in cancer. *Archives of Surgery*, *140*(9), 873–878, discussion 878–880. doi:10.1001/archsurg.140.9.873 PMID:16172296

Gries, C. J., Curtis, J. R., Wall, R. J., & Engelberg, R. A. (2008). Family member satisfaction with end-of-life decision making in the ICU. *Chest, 133*(3), 704-712. doi: chest.07-1773 [pii] 10.1378/chest.07-1773

Harvey, M. A. (2012). The truth about consequences--post-intensive care syndrome in intensive care unit survivors and their families. *Critical Care Medicine*, *40*(8), 2506–2507. doi:10.1097/CCM.0b013e318258e943 PMID:22809925

Herridge, M. S., Cheung, A. M., Tansey, C. M., Matte-Martyn, A., Diaz-Granados, N., Al-Saidi, F., & Slutsky, A. S. et al. (2003). One-year outcomes in survivors of the acute respiratory distress syndrome. *The New England Journal of Medicine*, *348*(8), 683–693. doi:10.1056/NEJMoa022450 PMID:12594312

Herridge, M. S., Tansey, C. M., Matte, A., Tomlinson, G., Diaz-Granados, N., Cooper, A., & Cheung, A. M. et al. (2011, April 07). Cheung, A. M. Functional disability 5 years after acute respiratory distress syndrome. *The New England Journal of Medicine*, *364*(14), 1293–1304. doi:10.1056/NEJMoa1011802 PMID:21470008

Hofhuis, J. G., Spronk, P. E., van Stel, H. F., Schrijvers, G. J., Rommes, J. H., & Bakker, J. (2008). The impact of critical illness on perceived health-related quality of life during ICU treatment, hospital stay, and after hospital discharge: A long-term follow-up study. *Chest*, *133*(2), 377–385. doi:10.1378/chest.07-1217 PMID:17925419

Hua, M. S., Li, G., Blinderman, C. D., & Wunsch, H. (2014). Estimates of the Need for Palliative Care Consultation across United States Intensive Care Units Using a Trigger-based Model. *American Journal of Respiratory and Critical Care Medicine*, *189*(4), 428–436. doi:10.1164/rccm.201307-1229OC PMID:24261961

Kahn, J. M., Werner, R. M., David, G., Ten Have, T. R., Benson, N. M., & Asch, D. A. (2013). Effectiveness of long-term acute care hospitalization in elderly patients with chronic critical illness. *Medical Care*, *51*(1), 4–10. doi:10.1097/MLR.0b013e31826528a7 PMID:22874500

Kross, E. K., Engelberg, R. A., Downey, L., Cuschieri, J., Hallman, M. R., Longstreth, W. T. Jr, & Curtis, J. R. et al. (2014). Differences in end-of-life care in the ICU across patients cared for by medicine, surgery, neurology, and neurosurgery physicians. *Chest*, *145*(2), 313–321. doi:10.1378/chest.13-1351 PMID:24114410

Lanken, P. N., Terry, P. B., Delisser, H. M., Fahy, B. F., Hansen-Flaschen, J., & Heffner, J. E. et al. Force, A. T. S. E.-o.-L. C. T. (2008). An official American Thoracic Society clinical policy statement: Palliative care for patients with respiratory diseases and critical illnesses. *American Journal of Respiratory and Critical Care Medicine*, *177*(8), 912–927. doi:10.1164/rccm.200605-587ST PMID:18390964

Laupland, K. B., Kirkpatrick, A. W., Kortbeek, J. B., & Zuege, D. J. (2006). Long-term mortality outcome associated with prolonged admission to the ICU. *Chest*, *129*(4), 954–959. doi:10.1378/chest.129.4.954 PMID:16608944

Lee, C. M., Herridge, M. S., Gabor, J. Y., Tansey, C. M., Matte, A., & Hanly, P. J. (2009). Chronic sleep disorders in survivors of the acute respiratory distress syndrome. *Intensive Care Medicine*, *35*(2), 314–320. doi:10.1007/s00134-008-1277-3 PMID:18802684

Lilly, C. M., Zuckerman, I. H., Badawi, O., & Riker, R. R. (2011). Benchmark data from more than 240,000 adults that reflect the current practice of critical care in the United States. *Chest*, *140*(5), 1232–1242. doi:10.1378/chest.11-0718 PMID:21868469

Lipsett, P. A., Swoboda, S. M., Dickerson, J., Ylitalo, M., Gordon, T., Breslow, M., & Rosenfeld, B. et al. (2000). Survival and functional outcome after prolonged intensive care unit stay. *Annals of Surgery*, *231*(2), 262–268. doi:10.1097/00000658-200002000-00016 PMID:10674619

Lupu, D. (2010). Estimate of current hospice and palliative medicine physician workforce shortage. *Journal of Pain and Symptom Management*, *40*(6), 899–911. doi:10.1016/j.jpainsymman.2010.07.004 PMID:21145468

MacIver, J., & Ross, H. J. (2005). Withdrawal of ventricular assist device support. *Journal of Palliative Care*, *21*(3), 151–156. PMID:16334969

Meadow, W., Pohlman, A., Frain, L., Ren, Y., Kress, J. P., Teuteberg, W., & Hall, J. (2011). Power and limitations of daily prognostications of death in the medical intensive care unit. *Critical Care Medicine*, *39*(3), 474–479. doi:10.1097/CCM.0b013e318205df9b PMID:21150582

Mehlhorn, J., Freytag, A., Schmidt, K., Brunkhorst, F. M., Graf, J., Troitzsch, U., & Gensichen, J. et al. (2014). Rehabilitation Interventions for Postintensive Care Syndrome: A Systematic Review. *Critical Care Medicine*, *42*(5), 1263–1271. doi:10.1097/CCM.0000000000000148 PMID:24413580

Morrison, R. S., Dietrich, J., Ladwig, S., Quill, T., Sacco, J., Tangeman, J., & Meier, D. E. (2011). Palliative care consultation teams cut hospital costs for Medicaid beneficiaries. *Health Affairs*, *30*(3), 454–463. doi:10.1377/hlthaff.2010.0929 PMID:21383364

Morrison, R. S., Penrod, J. D., Cassel, J. B., Caust-Ellenbogen, M., Litke, A., & Spragens, L. et al.. (2008). Cost savings associated with US hospital palliative care consultation programs. *Archives of Internal Medicine*, *168*(16), 1783–1790. doi:10.1001/archinte.168.16.1783 PMID:18779466

Mosenthal, A. C., & Murphy, P. A. (2006). Interdisciplinary model for palliative care in the trauma and surgical intensive care unit: Robert Wood Johnson Foundation Demonstration Project for Improving Palliative Care in the Intensive Care Unit. *Critical Care Medicine*, *34*(11Suppl), S399–S403. doi:10.1097/01.CCM.0000237044.79166.E1 PMID:17057605

Mosenthal, A. C., Weissman, D. E., Curtis, J. R., Hays, R. M., Lustbader, D. R., Mulkerin, C., & Nelson, J. E. et al. (2012). Integrating palliative care in the surgical and trauma intensive care unit: A report from the Improving Palliative Care in the Intensive Care Unit (IPAL-ICU) Project Advisory Board and the Center to Advance Palliative Care. *Critical Care Medicine*, *40*(4), 1199–1206. doi:10.1097/CCM.0b013e31823bc8e7 PMID:22080644

Mularski, R. A., Heine, C. E., Osborne, M. L., Ganzini, L., & Curtis, J. R. (2005). Quality of dying in the ICU: Ratings by family members. *Chest*, *128*(1), 280–287. doi:10.1378/chest.128.1.280 PMID:16002947

Nashef, S. A., Roques, F., Sharples, L. D., Nilsson, J., Smith, C., Goldstone, A. R., & Lockowandt, U. (2012). EuroSCORE II. *European Journal of Cardio-Thoracic Surgery, 41*(4), 734-744; discussion 744-735. doi: 10.1093/ejcts/ezs043

Nelson, J. E. (2006a). Identifying and overcoming the barriers to high-quality palliative care in the intensive care unit. *Critical Care Medicine*, *34*(11Suppl), S324–S331. doi:10.1097/01.CCM.0000237249.39179.B1 PMID:17057594

Nelson, J. E., Angus, D. C., Weissfeld, L. A., Puntillo, K. A., Danis, M., & Deal, D. et al. Critical Care Peer Workgroup of the Promoting Excellence in End-of-Life Care, P. (2006b). End-of-life care for the critically ill: A national intensive care unit survey. *Critical Care Medicine*, *34*(10), 2547–2553. doi:10.1097/01.CCM.0000239233.63425.1D PMID:16932230

Nelson, J. E., Meier, D. E., Litke, A., Natale, D. A., Siegel, R. E., & Morrison, R. S. (2004). The symptom burden of chronic critical illness. *Crit Care Med, 32*(7), 1527-1534. doi: 00003246-200407000-00010 [pii]

Nelson, J. E., Meier, D. E., Oei, E. J., Nierman, D. M., Senzel, R. S., Manfredi, P. L., & Morrison, R. S. et al. (2001). Self-reported symptom experience of critically ill cancer patients receiving intensive care. *Critical Care Medicine, 29*(2), 277–282. doi:10.1097/00003246-200102000-00010 PMID:11246306

Nelson, J. E., Puntillo, K. A., Pronovost, P. J., Walker, A. S., McAdam, J. L., Ilaoa, D., & Penrod, J. (2010). In their own words: Patients and families define high-quality palliative care in the intensive care unit. *Critical Care Medicine, 38*(3), 808–818. doi:10.1097/CCM.0b013e3181c5887c PMID:20198726

Norton, S. A., Hogan, L. A., Holloway, R. G., Temkin-Greener, H., Buckley, M. J., & Quill, T. E. (2007). Proactive palliative care in the medical intensive care unit: Effects on length of stay for selected high-risk patients. *Critical Care Medicine, 35*(6), 1530–1535. doi:10.1097/01.CCM.0000266533.06543.0C PMID:17452930

O'Mahony, S., McHenry, J., Blank, A. E., Snow, D., Eti Karakas, S., Santoro, G., & Kvetan, V. et al. (2010). Preliminary report of the integration of a palliative care team into an intensive care unit. *Palliative Medicine, 24*(2), 154–165. doi:10.1177/0269216309346540 PMID:19825893

Pandharipande, P. P., Girard, T. D., Jackson, J. C., Morandi, A., Thompson, J. L., Pun, B. T., & Ely, E. W. et al. (2013). Long-term cognitive impairment after critical illness. *The New England Journal of Medicine, 369*(14), 1306–1316. doi:10.1056/NEJMoa1301372 PMID:24088092

Paul Olson, T. J., Brasel, K. J., Redmann, A. J., Alexander, G. C., & Schwarze, M. L. (2013). Surgeon-reported conflict with intensivists about postoperative goals of care. *JAMA Surgery, 148*(1), 29–35. doi:10.1001/jamasurgery.2013.403 PMID:23324837

Pecanac, K. E., Kehler, J. M., Brasel, K. J., Cooper, Z., Steffens, N. M., McKneally, M. F., & Schwarze, M. L. (2014). It's big surgery: Preoperative expressions of risk, responsibility, and commitment to treatment after high-risk operations. *Annals of Surgery, 259*(3), 458–463. doi:10.1097/SLA.0000000000000314 PMID:24253139

Penrod, J. D., Deb, P., Dellenbaugh, C., Burgess, J. F. Jr, Zhu, C. W., Christiansen, C. L., & Morrison, R. S. et al. (2010). Hospital-based palliative care consultation: Effects on hospital cost. *Journal of Palliative Medicine, 13*(8), 973–979. doi:10.1089/jpm.2010.0038 PMID:20642361

Quill, T. E., & Abernethy, A. P. (2013). Generalist plus Specialist Palliative Care - Creating a More Sustainable Model. *The New England Journal of Medicine, 368*(13), 1173–1175. doi:10.1056/NEJMp1215620 PMID:23465068

Scheunemann, L. P., McDevitt, M., Carson, S. S., & Hanson, L. C. (2011). Randomized, controlled trials of interventions to improve communication in intensive care: A systematic review. *Chest, 139*(3), 543–554. doi:10.1378/chest.10-0595 PMID:21106660

Schneiderman, L. J., Gilmer, T., Teetzel, H. D., Dugan, D. O., Blustein, J., Cranford, R., & Young, E. W. et al. (2003). Effect of ethics consultations on nonbeneficial life-sustaining treatments in the intensive care setting: A randomized controlled trial. *Journal of the American Medical Association*, *290*(9), 1166–1172. doi:10.1001/jama.290.9.1166 PMID:12952998

Schwarze, M. L., Bradley, C. T., & Brasel, K. J. (2010). Surgical "buy-in": The contractual relationship between surgeons and patients that influences decisions regarding life-supporting therapy. *Critical Care Medicine*, *38*(3), 843–848. doi:10.1097/CCM.0b013e3181cc466b PMID:20048678

Schwarze, M. L., Redmann, A. J., Brasel, K. J., & Alexander, G. C. (2012). The role of surgeon error in withdrawal of postoperative life support. *Annals of Surgery*, *256*(1), 10–15. doi:10.1097/SLA.0b013e3182580de5 PMID:22584696

Shahian, D. M., O'Brien, S. M., Sheng, S., Grover, F. L., Mayer, J. E., Jacobs, J. P., & Edwards, F. H. et al. (2012). Predictors of long-term survival after coronary artery bypass grafting surgery: Results from the Society of Thoracic Surgeons Adult Cardiac Surgery Database (the ASCERT study). *Circulation*, *125*(12), 1491–1500. doi:10.1161/CIRCULATIONAHA.111.066902 PMID:22361330

Snow, C. E., Varela, B. R., Pardi, D. A., Adelman, R. D., Said, S., & Reid, M. C. (2009). Identifying factors affecting utilization of an inpatient palliative care service: A physician survey. *Journal of Palliative Medicine*, *12*(3), 231–237. doi:10.1089/jpm.2008.0235 PMID:19254200

Swetz, K. M., Ottenberg, A. L., Freeman, M. R., & Mueller, P. S. (2011). Palliative care and end-of-life issues in patients treated with left ventricular assist devices as destination therapy. *Current Heart Failure Reports*, *8*(3), 212–218. doi:10.1007/s11897-011-0060-x PMID:21538039

Tilden, L. B., Williams, B. R., Tucker, R. O., MacLennan, P. A., & Ritchie, C. S. (2009). Surgeons' attitudes and practices in the utilization of palliative and supportive care services for patients with a sudden advanced illness. *Journal of Palliative Medicine*, *12*(11), 1037–1042. doi:10.1089/jpm.2009.0120 PMID:19663713

Truog, R. D., Campbell, M. L., Curtis, J. R., Haas, C. E., Luce, J. M., Rubenfeld, G. D., & Kaufman, D. C. et al. (2008). Recommendations for end-of-life care in the intensive care unit: A consensus statement by the American College [corrected] of Critical Care Medicine. *Critical Care Medicine*, *36*(3), 953–963. doi:10.1097/CCM.0B013E3181659096 PMID:18431285

Weissman, D. E., & Meier, D. E. (2011). Identifying patients in need of a palliative care assessment in the hospital setting: A consensus report from the Center to Advance Palliative Care. *Journal of Palliative Medicine*, *14*(1), 17–23. doi:10.1089/jpm.2010.0347 PMID:21133809

Wright, A. A., Keating, N. L., Balboni, T. A., Matulonis, U. A., Block, S. D., & Prigerson, H. G. (2010). Place of death: Correlations with quality of life of patients with cancer and predictors of bereaved caregivers' mental health. *Journal of Clinical Oncology*, *28*(29), 4457–4464. doi:10.1200/JCO.2009.26.3863 PMID:20837950

Wunsch, H., Christiansen, C. F., Johansen, M. B., Olsen, M., Ali, N., Angus, D. C., & Sorensen, H. T. (2014). Psychiatric diagnoses and psychoactive medication use among nonsurgical critically ill patients receiving mechanical ventilation. *Journal of the American Medical Association*, *311*(11), 1133–1142. doi:10.1001/jama.2014.2137 PMID:24643603

Wunsch, H., Guerra, C., Barnato, A. E., Angus, D. C., Li, G., & Linde-Zwirble, W. T. (2010). Three-year outcomes for Medicare beneficiaries who survive intensive care. *Journal of the American Medical Association*, *303*(9), 849–856. doi:10.1001/jama.2010.216 PMID:20197531

Zier, L. S., Sottile, P. D., Hong, S. Y., Weissfield, L. A., & White, D. B. (2012). Surrogate decision makers' interpretation of prognostic information: A mixed-methods study. *Annals of Internal Medicine*, *156*(5), 360–366. doi:10.7326/0003-4819-156-5-201203060-00008 PMID:22393131

ADDITIONAL READING

Aslakson, R., Cheng, J., Vollenweider, D., Galusca, D., Smith, T. J., & Pronovost, P. J. (2014). Evidence-based palliative care in the intensive care unit: A systematic review of interventions. *Journal of Palliative Medicine*, *17*(2), 219–235. doi:10.1089/jpm.2013.0409 PMID:24517300

Baggs, J. G., Norton, S. A., Schmitt, M. H., Dombeck, M. T., Sellers, C. R., & Quinn, J. R. (2007). Intensive care unit cultures and end-of-life decision making. *Journal of Critical Care*, *22*(2), 159–168. doi:10.1016/j.jcrc.2006.09.008 PMID:17548028

Bradley, C. T., & Brasel, K. J. (2009). Developing guidelines that identify patients who would benefit from palliative care services in the surgical intensive care unit. *Critical Care Medicine*, *37*(3), 946–950. doi:10.1097/CCM.0b013e3181968f68 PMID:19237901

Campbell, M. L., & Guzman, J. A. (2003). Impact of a proactive approach to improve end-of-life care in a medical ICU. *Chest*, *123*(1), 266–271. doi:10.1378/chest.123.1.266 PMID:12527629

Campbell, M. L., & Guzman, J. A. (2004). A proactive approach to improve end-of-life care in a medical intensive care unit for patients with terminal dementia. *Critical Care Medicine*, *32*(9), 1839–1843. doi:10.1097/01.CCM.0000138560.56577.88 PMID:15343010

Carlet, J., Thijs, L. G., Antonelli, M., Cassell, J., Cox, P., Hill, N., & Thompson, B. T. et al. (2004). Challenges in end-of-life care in the ICU. Statement of the 5th International Consensus Conference in Critical Care: Brussels, Belgium, April 2003. *Intensive Care Medicine*, *30*(5), 770–784. doi:10.1007/s00134-004-2241-5 PMID:15098087

Curtis, J. R., Engelberg, R. A., Wenrich, M. D., Shannon, S. E., Treece, P. D., & Rubenfeld, G. D. (2005). Missed opportunities during family conferences about end-of-life care in the intensive care unit. *American Journal of Respiratory and Critical Care Medicine*, *171*(8), 844–849. doi:10.1164/rccm.200409-1267OC PMID:15640361

Curtis, J. R., Nielsen, E. L., Treece, P. D., Downey, L., Dotolo, D., Shannon, S. E., & Engelberg, R. A. et al. (2011). Effect of a quality-improvement intervention on end-of-life care in the intensive care unit: A randomized trial. *American Journal of Respiratory and Critical Care Medicine, 183*(3), 348–355. doi:10.1164/rccm.201006-1004OC PMID:20833820

DeCato, T. W., Engelberg, R. A., Downey, L., Nielsen, E. L., Treece, P. D., Back, A. L., & Curtis, J. R. et al. (2013). Hospital variation and temporal trends in palliative and end-of-life care in the ICU. *Critical Care Medicine, 41*(6), 1405–1411. doi:10.1097/CCM.0b013e318287f289 PMID:23518869

Goldsmith, B., Dietrich, J., Du, Q., & Morrison, R. S. (2008). Variability in access to hospital palliative care in the United States. *Journal of Palliative Medicine, 11*(8), 1094–1102. doi:10.1089/jpm.2008.0053 PMID:18831653

Hartog, C. S., Peschel, I., Schwarzkopf, D., Curtis, J. R., Westermann, I., Kabisch, B., & Reinhart, K. et al. (2014). Are written advance directives helpful to guide end-of-life therapy in the intensive care unit? A retrospective matched-cohort study. *Journal of Critical Care, 29*(1), 128–133. doi:10.1016/j.jcrc.2013.08.024 PMID:24331948

Heyland, D. K., Dodek, P., Rocker, G., Groll, D., Gafni, A., Pichora, D., . . . Canadian Researchers End-of-Life, N. (2006). What matters most in end-of-life care: perceptions of seriously ill patients and their family members. *CMAJ: Canadian Medical Association Journal, 174*(5), 627-633. doi: 10.1503/cmaj.050626

Johnson, S. K., Bautista, C. A., Hong, S. Y., Weissfeld, L., & White, D. B. (2011). An empirical study of surrogates' preferred level of control over value-laden life support decisions in intensive care units. *American Journal of Respiratory and Critical Care Medicine, 183*(7), 915–921. doi:10.1164/rccm.201008-1214OC PMID:21037019

Kapo, J., & Siegel, M. D. (2013). Penguins and palliative care: Facilitating cultural change in the ICU. *Critical Care Medicine, 41*(10), 2443–2444. doi:10.1097/CCM.0b013e31829136f3 PMID:24060776

Khandelwal, N., & Curtis, J. R. (2014). Clinical and economic implications of timing of limitations in life support. *Critical Care Medicine, 42*(2), 455–456. doi:10.1097/CCM.0b013e3182a522de PMID:24434447

Lau, B. D., Aslakson, R. A., Wilson, R. F., Fawole, O. A., Apostol, C. C., Martinez, K. A., & Dy, S. E. et al. (2014). Methods for improving the quality of palliative care delivery: A systematic review. *The American Journal of Hospice & Palliative Care, 31*(2), 202–210. doi:10.1177/1049909113482039 PMID:23532404

Lautrette, A., Darmon, M., Megarbane, B., Joly, L. M., Chevret, S., Adrie, C., & Azoulay, E. et al. (2007). A communication strategy and brochure for relatives of patients dying in the ICU. *The New England Journal of Medicine, 356*(5), 469–478. doi:10.1056/NEJMoa063446 PMID:17267907

Lee Char, S. J., Evans, L. R., Malvar, G. L., & White, D. B. (2010). A randomized trial of two methods to disclose prognosis to surrogate decision makers in intensive care units. *American Journal of Respiratory and Critical Care Medicine, 182*(7), 905–909. doi:10.1164/rccm.201002-0262OC PMID:20538959

Meissner, A., Genga, K. R., Studart, F. S., Settmacher, U., Hofmann, G., Reinhart, K., & Sakr, Y. (2010). Epidemiology of and factors associated with end-of-life decisions in a surgical intensive care unit. *Critical Care Medicine, 38*(4), 1060–1068. doi:10.1097/CCM.0b013e3181cd1110 PMID:20068464

Mularski, R. A., Heine, C. E., Osborne, M. L., Ganzini, L., & Curtis, J. R. (2005). Quality of dying in the ICU: Ratings by family members. *Chest, 128*(1), 280–287. doi:10.1378/chest.128.1.280 PMID:16002947

Nelson, J. E., Bassett, R., Boss, R. D., Brasel, K. J., Campbell, M. L., Cortez, T. B., & Weissman, D. E. et al. (2010). Models for structuring a clinical initiative to enhance palliative care in the intensive care unit: A report from the IPAL-ICU Project (Improving Palliative Care in the ICU). *Critical Care Medicine, 38*(9), 1765–1772. doi:10.1097/CCM.0b013e3181e8ad23 PMID:20562699

Nelson, J. E., Cox, C. E., Hope, A. A., & Carson, S. S. (2010). Chronic critical illness. *American Journal of Respiratory and Critical Care Medicine, 182*(4), 446–454. doi:10.1164/rccm.201002-0210CI PMID:20448093

Nelson, J. E., Curtis, J. R., Mulkerin, C., Campbell, M., Lustbader, D. R., Mosenthal, A. C., & Weissman, D. E. et al.Improving Palliative Care in the. (2013). Choosing and Using Screening Criteria for Palliative Care Consultation in the ICU: A Report From the Improving Palliative Care in the ICU (IPAL-ICU) Advisory Board*. *Critical Care Medicine, 41*(10), 2318–2327. doi:10.1097/CCM.0b013e31828cf12c PMID:23939349

Norton, S. A., Hogan, L. A., Holloway, R. G., Temkin-Greener, H., Buckley, M. J., & Quill, T. E. (2007). Proactive palliative care in the medical intensive care unit: Effects on length of stay for selected high-risk patients. *Critical Care Medicine, 35*(6), 1530–1535. doi:10.1097/01.CCM.0000266533.06543.0C PMID:17452930

Penrod, J. D., Pronovost, P. J., Livote, E. E., Puntillo, K. A., Walker, A. S., Wallenstein, S., & Nelson, J. E. et al. (2012). Meeting standards of high-quality intensive care unit palliative care: Clinical performance and predictors. *Critical Care Medicine, 40*(4), 1105–1112. doi:10.1097/CCM.0b013e3182374a50 PMID:22202706

Puntillo, K., Nelson, J. E., Weissman, D., Curtis, R., Weiss, S., Frontera, J., & Campbell, M. et al. (2014). Palliative care in the ICU: Relief of pain, dyspnea, and thirst--a report from the IPAL-ICU Advisory Board. *Intensive Care Medicine, 40*(2), 235–248. doi:10.1007/s00134-013-3153-z PMID:24275901

The SUPPORT Principal Investigators. (1995). A controlled trial to improve care for seriously ill hospitalized patients. The study to understand prognoses and preferences for outcomes and risks of treatments (SUPPORT). *JAMA, 274*(20), 1591-1598.

Zalenski, R., Courage, C., Edelen, A., Waselewsky, D., Krayem, H., Latozas, J., & Kaufman, D. (2014). *Evaluation of screening criteria for palliative care consultation in the MICU: a multihospital analysis.* BMJ Support Palliat Care; doi:10.1136/bmjspcare-2013-000570

KEY TERMS AND DEFINITIONS

Consultative Model: A model of delivering palliative care using the services of a palliative care consultation service.

End-of-Life Care: Care, including pain and symptom management and family support, that is provided to patients at the end of their life, often when death is imminent.

Generalist Palliative Care: Basic palliative care, including pain and symptom management, prognosis and discussions regarding goals of care, that is to be performed by primary providers.

Integrative Model: A model of delivering palliative by incorporating principles of palliative care into routine ICU care.

Mixed Model: A model of delivering palliative care that combines the integrative and consultative models.

Palliative Care: A discipline of medicine that focuses on improving quality of life through the management of symptoms including pain, nausea, anxiety, psychological and spiritual distress for patients with serious illness.

Specialized Palliative Care: Advanced palliative care, including complex and refractory pain and symptom management, conflict resolution and complex decision-making that is performed by palliative care consultants.

Surgical Buy-In: A contract, often informally made, between a surgeon and a patient whereby both parties commit to undergo a surgical procedure and its attendant postoperative course.

Surgical Critical Illness: A trajectory of critical illness more commonly seen with surgical patients, where previously healthy patients suddenly become acutely and critically ill.

Triggers for Palliative Care Consultation: Screening criteria used to identify patients at high-risk of having palliative care needs for referral for palliative care consultation.

Chapter 6
Ethics

Natalia S. Ivascu
Weill Cornell Medical College, USA

Sheida Tabaie
Weill Cornell Medical College, USA

Ellen C. Meltzer
Weill Cornell Medical College, USA

ABSTRACT

In all areas of medicine physicians are confronted with a myriad ethical problems. It is important that intensivists are well versed on ethical issues that commonly arise in the critical care setting. This chapter will serve to provide a review of common topics, including informed consent, decision-making capacity, and surrogate decision-making. It will also highlight special circumstances related to cardiac surgical critical care, including ethical concerns associated with emerging technologies in cardiac care.

INTRODUCTION

Patients undergoing surgery and those that are critically ill are vulnerable and require special consideration. This chapter will provide a brief overview of ethical principles and discuss common ethical issues that arise during the care of cardiac surgical patients. It concludes by exploring contemporary and emerging ethical problems associated with technological advances in life sustaining therapies.

BACKGROUND

Basic Principles of Medical Ethics

Several decades ago, Beauchamp and Childress described a framework to address ethical issues that arise in medical care (Beauchamp, 1979). It consists of four central principles: beneficence, non-maleficence, autonomy and justice. While there are limitations to relying solely on these four principles to address the range of issues encountered in the care of the critically ill, they do provide a foundation for contemporary medical ethics.

DOI: 10.4018/978-1-4666-8603-8.ch006

Beneficence

Beneficence is the desire to act in the best interest of the patient. The core of medical practice is the desire to heal or, at the least, to ease the suffering of a patient. Physicians should consider whether treatments and procedures truly offer the potential for benefit, and counter this against any potential for burden. The modern practice of medicine can make this calculation more complex.

Non-Maleficence

The well-known primary principle of the ethical practice of medicine is the admonition by Hippoctrates "primum non nocere" – "first do no harm." This principle can be especially important when considering highly invasive surgery, such as cardiac surgery. Again, the potential burdens and benefits of the intervention should be fully explored to ensure a reasonable balance,

Autonomy

The principle of autonomy is the right of an individual to govern decisions made about his or her own body. Autonomy is the fundamental groundwork for the informed consent process.

Justice

The principle of justice refers to fairness in the distribution of healthcare resources, as well as respect for the governing laws. Justice is usually invoked when discussing access to treatments that are limited by availability or cost.

Informed Consent

Obtaining consent for a surgery or invasive procedure is frequently focused on the signing of a consent form. However, the informed consent process is far more complex. The written documentation of permission is the result of a frank and open conversation between practioner and patient. The groundwork to the modern standard of informed consent was laid a century ago. The landmark case, Schloendorf vs. The Society of the New York Hospital, is often cited as the turning point in the doctor patient relationship. The patient, Ms. Schloendorf, presented for an examination under anesthesia to investigate a fibroid uterus. The court transcripts note her explicit refusal of surgery before she was placed under anesthesia (Chevernak, 2014). After she was unconscious, the surgeon performed an examination, and upon diagnosing a tumor, proceeded to perform a hysterectomy. The patient sued, and Judge Benjamin Cardozo found in favor of the defendant and stated in his opinion that "*...every human being of adult years and sound mind has a right to determine what shall be done with his body; and a surgeon who performs an operation without his patient's consent commits an assault, for which he is liable in damage, except in cases of emergency, where the patient is unconscious and where it is necessary to operate before consent can be obtained*" (Chevernak, 2014). In the (then) largely paternalistic medical environment, this was a dramatic shift. In addition to elevating the requirements for permission to perform invasive procedures, it marked a move toward honoring patients' autonomy. Many decades after the Schloendorf case, the informed consent standards were again legally challenged by cases in which patients suffered complications that had not been disclosed prior to surgery. Up until this point, the accepted practice was the "professional practice standard," which is what an appropriately experienced physician in the community would tell the patient about the condition, the therapeutic options available, and the generalized risks and benefits of each therapy. The last vestiges of paternalism were cast off with the rejection of the professional practice standard. What emerged was a new requirement to reveal to patients all risks and complications, even those with little probability of occurring.

The modern standard for informed consent includes three key elements: The patient should 1) be given adequate information regarding the nature and purpose of proposed treatments (risks, benefits, and alternatives), 2) be free from coercion, and 3) have medical decision-making capacity.

Decision Making Capacity

The terms "competence" and "capacity" are frequently interchanged; however, in the strictest sense, they are not equivalent. Competence refers to a legal determination of one's ability to enjoy the rights and responsibilities of adulthood. An individual over the age of 18 that is deemed incompetent must fall under the guardianship of another adult and cannot make decisions for himself be it financial, legal, or medical. Capacity more appropriately describes the ability of a person to make a medical decision for himself.

A major distinction separating capacity from competence is that capacity is a temporally and situationally specific designation. The question of capacity encompasses one particular decision at one particular time. The temporal aspect is easiest to understand. Many things may occur in the care of a patient that impairs their decision-making capacity, such as sedation or anesthesia. Certainly a healthy patient arriving from home to the operating room is likely to retain their decision making capacity; however, while under anesthesia the patient is no longer able to make decisions. Other factors affecting capacity may come into play in the intensive care unit, including critical illness, delirium, hypoxemia, metabolic derangement, etc.

There are four main elements of capacity: 1) ability to <u>communicate</u> a choice, 2) ability to <u>understand</u> the relevant information, 3) <u>appreciation</u> of the nature of the condition, and the risk and benefits of proposed treatment, 4) ability to <u>rationally</u> manipulate the given information (Applebaum, 2007). Communication does not have to be done verbally. Every effort should be made to attempt to communicate effectively with intubated or tracheotomized patients. Writing, letter boards, and lip-reading with specialized lip-reading interpreters have been utilized in these circumstances (Meltzer, 2012). The ability to understand information is often equated with cognitive function, but one should exercise great caution with this interpretation. Approximately one-third of learning disabled patients and almost 50% of Alzheimer's patients retain the capacity to make medical decisions (Sessums, 2011). The mini-mental status exam has a poor correlation with capacity determination, except on the extremes of the scored scaling system (Sessums, 2011). When patients come to a decision that differs from medical recommendation, it is critical to elicit the reason behind the patient's decision. In doing so, incorrect perceptions of risks/benefits or side effects can be dispelled. Most importantly, if a patient can rationally explain how he has come to a decision then it must be honored, even if it conflicts with medical advice. When a patient fails to meet these four elements of capacity, an alternative decision maker must be sought.

Surrogate Decision Makers

In the event that a patient loses capacity, the best alternative is an advanced directive outlining what the patient would want in this event. When that is not available, it is beneficial if the patient has previously completed a health care proxy (HCP) form appointing a health care agent (HCA) to speak on his behalf. The requirements for a health care agent or health care power-of-attorney vary from state to state. A HCA has the legal authority to make medical decisions for an incapacitated patient. Ideally, the HCA should be familiar with the patient's values and expressed wishes regarding specific health decisions. When a specific preference is not known, the HCA is asked to use substituted judgment to say what he believes the patient would decide in the given situation. If this, too, is unknown, then the HCA is expected to make a decision that is in the best interest of the patient.

Often, critically ill patients facing life-determining decisions have not completed a HCP designating a HCA. In this event, a surrogate decision maker must be identified. The legal standing for surrogates varies between states. The most recent compilation of state-by-state criteria is in table 1. However, changes have occurred since 2009, such as the Family Health Care Decisions Act that was passed in New York in 2010. This act newly empowered surrogate decision makers to direct the withdrawal or withholding of life-sustaining treatment. In addition, same sex domestic partners were elevated in rank order of priority to be on par with opposite sex spouses (Swidler, 2010).

Witholding and Withdrawing Life Sustaining Therapies

Most deaths in the ICU occur after a decision to withhold or withdraw life-supporting therapies. Withholding life-sustaining therapy refers to situations in which a medical intervention is *not* performed even though death is likely to follow, such as CPR, intubation, or dialysis. Withdrawing life-sustaining therapy refers to *stopping* currently provided care. The decision to limit or remove life-sustaining therapy is generally made when the patient has a minimal chance of recovery or the burden of treatment outweighs the

Table 1. Spectrum of ethical care at the end of life

	Withhold LST	Withdraw LST	Palliative Sedation	Physician Aid in Dying	Euthanasia
Cause of death	Underlying disease	Underlying disease	Underlying disease[a]	Intervention prescribed by physician and used by patient	Intervention used by physician
Intent/goal of intervention	Avoid burdensome intervention	Remove burdensome intervention	Relieve symptoms	Termination fo patient's life	Termination of patient's life
Legal?	Yes[b]	Yes[b]	Yes	Limited by jurisdiction[c]	No
Abrbreviation: LST, life-sustaining treatment.					
[a] Note "double effect."					
[b] Several states limit the power of surrogate decision makers regarding LSTs					
[c] Legal only in states of Oregon, Washington, Montana, and Vermont in the United States					

Table taken from Swetz KM, Mansel JK. Ethical Issues and Palliative Care in the Cardiovascular Intensive Care Unit. *Cardiol Clin* 2013; 31: 657-668.

potential benefits. It is important to recognize that withholding and withdrawal are morally equivalent actions, and that withdrawal of life-sustaining therapy is not assisted suicide or euthanasia. This is because there is no intention to end life by removing or limiting a technology; rather, the goal is to allow the underlying disease process and the dying process to progress naturally. Without the intent to harm, there is no criminal act. Table 1 outlines the spectrum of ethical care at the end of life (Swetz, 2013).

One example, in the cardiac population, is end-of-life decision-making with cardiac pacemakers and automatic internal debrillators (AICDs). A patient or his surrogate has the authority to request deactivation/ discontinuation of cardiac pacemakers and AICDs if continuation of these devices serves to prolong the dying process and/or is no longer consistent with the patient's goals of care (Kramer, 2012). Regardless of the duration or dependency on the device, these devices may legally and ethically be discontinued if this is consistent with the goal of care (Pellegrino, 2005). For many physicians, concerns about futility, often leads to consideration of withholding or withdrawing life-sustaining therapy.

Futility and Futility Disputes

Futility is an amorphous concept fraught with controversy in the public arena. Experts have defined medical futility combining both a quantitative and qualitative approach, as "the unacceptable likelihood of achieving an effect that the patient has the capacity to appreciate as a benefit" (Schneiderman, 2011). Edmund Pellegrino's analysis of withdrawal of life-sustaining therapy incorporates these two components. The quantitative aspect of futility, which lies within the domain of the physician, addresses the effectiveness of the therapy. The qualitative aspect of futility, which lies within the domain of the patient, addresses the subjective benefit of such therapy (Lampert, 2010). Thus, medical futility cannot be decided without the input of both the patient and the physician. Take the example of patient X, a 76-year-old male with non-ischemic cardiomyopathy secondary to chemotherapy for a primary hematologic cancer. He is admitted to the cardiothoracic ICU in decompensated heart failure refractory to medical management. Patient X has failed multiple lines of chemotherapy, but his disease has progressed slowly. Per his oncologist, he could possibly live a year or longer. A left ventricular assist device (LVAD) is offered as a bridge to destination, given that he is not a candidate for heart transplant secondary to his cancer. Patient X refuses. Although a LVAD would provide Patient X with more time, he offers a capacitated refusal, relaying that he finds the burden of living with the LVAD to be overwhelming and disproportionate to the potential benefits. Thus, qualitative futility has been established because, despite the LVAD being a potentially effective therapy, the patient does not feel it provides sufficient benefit.

In this example, withholding life-sustaining therapy as per Patient X's wishes may, or may not, seem ethically ambiguous to you, however it is important to recognize that your colleagues may not always feel comfortable with withholding (or withdrawal) of life-sustaining therapy. In a study from Germany, Jox and colleagues investigated the attitudes of clinicians regarding the definition of futility, communication surrounding futility, and the continuation of life-sustaining therapy despite recognition of futility. The reasons for continuing futile life-sustaining therapy were largely emotional, stemming from clinicians' feelings of guilt, grief, fear of legal consequences, and concerns about the family's reaction (Jox, 2012). It is important to be sensitive to those around you and to support colleagues, in addition to patients and families, when facing difficult decisions.

Situations may arise in which surrogates for critically ill or dying patients wish to continue providing life-sustaining therapies and invasive interventions, even though they offer the patient no benefit and may have prospect for harm. Conflict, often termed a futility dispute, may develop between the clinical team and the surrogate regarding the plan of care. These situations are complicated and can be frustrating for all involved. We suggest trying to anticipate in advance the prospect for a futility dispute to develop so that steps, such as providing frequent clinical updates and ensuring the surrogate is receiving consistent messages about the patient's poor prognosis, can be taken to mitigate the conflict. When conflict does develop, the following might serve to be helpful.

First, ensure that all members of the clinical team, including consultants, are in agreement about the patient's prognosis and what the options are for care. Inconsistent messages can provide a surrogate with false hope and also generate mistrust of the clinical team. Next, ensure that the surrogate has an accurate understanding of the patient's clinical situation. Then, rather than offer discrete options for care, such as "do everything", "do nothing", or "perform CPR" or "issue a do not resuscitate (DNR) order", engage the surrogate in a broader discussion about goals of care. It can be helpful to elicit whether the patient ever expressed any preferences about their medical care or what they might want, given the current clinical situation. Helping to frame this as a discussion of what *the patient* would want can help to alleviate the surrogate of the burden of medical decision-making. Finally, once the surrogate has articulated a goal of care, i.e. a goal of comfort or a goal to reduce suffering, then craft a plan in conjunction with the surrogate that will serve to achieve this goal. For example, if the goal is to provide comfort, then explain that medications will be provided for palliation and that CPR would be inconsistent with this objective. Depending on your institution, medical ethics, palliative care, and/or pastoral care may be consulted to assist you with this process.

Specific Religious Issues Regarding Withdrawl of Life-Sustaining Therapy

It is often difficult to initiate a discussion of goals of care and end-of-life care with a patient or surrogate. Some understanding of the patient's religious background can aid in providing a framework for this discussion. It is important to note, however, that while a patient may identify himself as a member of a particular religious community, he may not ascribe to all beliefs set forth by that religion. As such, one should proceed cautiously and without presumption when addressing withdrawal of life-sustaining therapies. Below is a brief comment regarding the viewpoints of several, major religions to familiarize the reader. This is meant only as a brief introduction for the critical care practitioner, and not as a comprehensive religious review. It is advised that all patients and surrogates are asked whether they follow a particular religious tradition and whether a member of their own clergy or hospital pastoral care might be a source of support. In addition, local ethics consultation service may also provide assistance.

Christian: Catholic/Orthodox Christian

The Catholic and Orthodox Christian perspectives begin with the principle that the intentional, direct, or voluntary killing of another human being is always wrong. To that end, removing life-sustaining therapies with the intension of ending life is also impermissible and morally equivalent to euthanasia or suicide. However, removing such treatments in the event that they are futile, or that the burden of treatment outweighs the potential benefit, is ethically permissible as a resignation of an inevitable death. One careful distinction in these faiths is that the burden of life is not the same thing as the burden of treatment. As such, if a particular treatment is painful and shows little potential benefit, a Catholic or Orthodox Christian can in good conscience forgo that care. However, the intolerability of a difficult or limited life is not justification to terminate life-sustaining measures (Donovan, 1997).

Christian: Evangelical Protestant

There are many other denominations within the Christian faith and this description may not be all encompassing. In general, Evangelical Protestants accept that death is an inevitable end to a human's existence on Earth. They generally hold that all medical options should be exhausted in the defense of life. Once the medical personnel believe that battle has been lost, however, the faith would not object to allowing death to occur. They accept withdrawal of treatment to sustain life with the intention to allow death to occur. It is important for treating clinicians to keep in mind the strongly held belief that judgment in the eyes of God will come with their death. Family members may be conflicted about resigning to death if they fear that forgiveness and peace with God has not yet been obtained (Ankeny, 2005).

Orthodox Jewish

Orthodox Judaism views life as precious and sacred to the end. The defense of life is intended to trump any other mandate. Jewish law, or "Halacha", implores physicians to do anything possible to save a patient, no matter how briefly the patient may survive. Food, fluids, and oxygen may never be withheld even if artificial means are necessary. When death approaches and is clearly inevitable, the person is considered to be "a Goses". A "Goses" is a person actively in the process of dying whose soul has not yet departed. Any action to hasten the death of a Gosses is akin to murder, however palliation and provisions for comfort while dying are allowed, even if they accelerate the process. For example, administration of pain medication is permissible even if respirations are depressed, as long as the intention is only to palliate and not to hasten death (Brenner, 2002; Baeke, 2005; Steinberg, 2003).

Islam

Muslims derive their moral directives from four sources in order of importance: the Koran, the Sunnah, the consensus of the learned, and wisdom. Life is seen as a gift from God, and the central Islamic prophet has been quoted as saying, "seek treatment, for every illness God created a treatment." As such, if there is any hope for recovery, discontinuation of treatment is not permissible. Islamic law forbids any form of euthanasia. A strict interpretation of the law would not allow for withdrawal of life-support, owing to the impossibility of knowing with certainty the outcome of treatment. A modern interpretation does advocate for avoiding prolongation of suffering when there is no hope of survival. However, withholding food and hydration is permitted as this is seen as distinct from the removal of artificial life support (Alsolamy, 2014).

Hindu

There is no central authority or text to dictate the beliefs of the Hindu faith. Traditionally, Hinduism identifies suicide as morally intolerable. Yet modern Hindu practice is generally supportive of stopping life-support in futile situations. There may be a wide variety of views in common practice.

Buddhist

Although suicide and murder are prohibited in Buddhist traditions, ending one's life to help others is a practice ascribed to even Buddha himself. As believers in reincarnation, the impact of death is received differently than that in other faiths. Of primary importance is to die in a calm, conscious state, as this is thought to provide for the most favorable rebirth. There is no clear consensus on Buddhist approach to ending life-support, but in general they do not advocate for the prolonging of life or the hastening of death (Chaicharoen, 1998). A unique feature of Buddhism is the belief that the mind is not the same as the brain. Thus, while the heart remains beating, Buddhists may not easily accept brain death as the death of the person. Buddhists would generally accept palliative care, but with the aim of preserving consciousness while making the patient comfortable (Chan, 2012).

FUTURE RESEARCH DIRECTIONS

Emerging Technologies

Advances in mechanical circulatory support (MCS) and increasing use of extracorporeal life support (ECSL) and left ventricular assist devices (LVAD) have given rise new arenas for ethical debate. While these therapies do have the potential to save the lives of patients who otherwise would certainly die from cardiac failure, they are invasive and burdensome and require careful consideration, if not before initiation of therapy, then certainly after the patient is stabilized (Meltzer, 2014).

Emergency ECLS

Failed cardiopulmonary resuscitation (CPR) has generally been synonymous with certain death. Many cardiac surgery centers, however, now have the capability to rapidly place a patient with cardiac failure on ECLS and maintain oxygenation and perfusion in spite of a failing heart. Despite being a highly invasive procedure, in these circumstances ECLS is often initiated without explicit informed consent by invoking the emergency presumption (i.e. the presumption that a patient would want to receive potentially life saving therapies unless he or his surrogate specifically noted otherwise).. The urgency, which is the very essence of an emergency intervention, prohibits a long and detailed conversation with the patient's surrogate and family. The intention of emergency ECLS is to provide a "bridge to decision." Maintenance on ECLS can prevent secondary organ failure while allowing time to assess neurologic recovery. ECLS may even allow for an opportunity for the patient to regain capacity to make decisions for themselves regarding advanced therapies, such as long-term assist devices or heart transplantation. Advance directives rarely, if ever, address such a specific situation and generally offer little guidance in the emergency setting (Shah, 2014).

Termination of LVAD Support

In spite of technologic advances, heart failure is a progressive and terminal condition. ECLS has been very successful at improving both quality and duration of life in this setting. However, there may come a time at which the patient no longer wishes to continue LVAD support. Depending on the patient's underlying function, termination of LVAD support has a variable outcome, ranging from sudden death to pulmonary congestion with gradual deterioration. The decision to stop a LVAD should be made in concert with a palliative care plan to ensure the comfort and dignity of the patient. The LVAD is a supportive therapy, not a replacement therapy. As such, it is ethically permissible to withdraw such support when the patient or, if necessary, the patient's proxy determines that ongoing treatment would be futile. As with any withdrawal of life-sustaining therapy, local institutional guidelines should be consulted prior to discontinuation.

CONCLUSION

Ethical issues commonly arise in the intensive care unit, particularly concerning including informed consent, decision-making capacity, and surrogate decision-making. Cardiac surgery patients may be incapacitated and unable to make decisions for themselves. They may be ill for prolonged periods of time and questions regarding withholding and withdrawal of life-sustaining therapy may arise. Understanding the legal as well as ethical responsibilities regarding decision-making for this vulnerable population is a cornerstone of critical care. Ethics consultation may serve to assist you in clarifying goals of care and mediating futility disputes.

REFERENCES

Alsolamy, S. (2014). Islamic views on artificial nutrition and hydration in terminally ill patients. *Bioethics*, *28*(2), 96–99. doi:10.1111/j.1467-8519.2012.01996.x PMID:22845721

Ankeny, R. A., Clifford, R., Jordens, C. F. C., Kerridge, I. H., & Benson, R. (2005). Religious perspectives on withdrawal of treatment from patients with multiple organ failure. *The Medical Journal of Australia*, *183*, 616–621. PMID:16336148

Applebaum, P. S. (2007). Assessment of Patients' Competence to Consent to Treatment. *The New England Journal of Medicine*, *357*(18), 1834–1840. doi:10.1056/NEJMcp074045 PMID:17978292

Baeke, G., Wils, J. P., & Broeckaert, B. (2005). 'There is a time to be born and a time to die' (Ecclesiastes 3:2a): Jewish perspectives on euthanasia. *Journal of Religion and Health*, *50*(4), 778–795. doi:10.1007/s10943-011-9465-9 PMID:21253848

Beachamp, T. L., & Childress, J. F. (1979). *Principles of Biomedical Ethics*. New York, NY: Oxford University Press, Incorporated.

Brenner, D. S. (2002). *Embracing life & facing death: a Jewish guide to palliative care*. New York, NY: CLAL.

Chaicharoen, P., & Ratanakul, P. (1998). Letting-Go or Killing: Thai Buddhist Perspectives on Euthanasia. *Journal of Asian and International Bioethics*, *8*, 37–40.

Chan, R. W., & Hegney, D. (2012). Buddhism and medical futility. *Bioethical Inquiry*, *9*(4), 433–438. doi:10.1007/s11673-012-9392-9 PMID:23188402

Chevernak, J., McCullough, L. B., & Chevernak, F. A. (2014). Surgery Without Consent or Miscommunication? A New Look at a Landmark Legal Case. *American Journal of Obstetrics and Gynecology*, *212*(5), 586–590. doi:10.1016/j.ajog.2014.06.062 PMID:24995772

Donovan, G. K. (1997). Decisions at the end of life: Catholic tradition. *Christ.*, *3*(3), 188–203. doi:10.1093/cb/3.3.188 PMID:11655313

Jox, R. J., Schaider, A., Marckmann, G., & Borasio, G. D. (2012). Medical futility at the end of life: The perspectives of intensive care and palliative care clinicians. *Journal of Medical Ethics*, *38*(9), 540–545. doi:10.1136/medethics-2011-100479 PMID:22562948

Kramer, D. B., Mitchell, S. L., & Brock, D. W. (2012). Deactivation of Pacemakers and Implantable Cardioverter-Defibrillators. *Progress in Cardiovascular Diseases*, *55*(3), 290–299. doi:10.1016/j.pcad.2012.09.003 PMID:23217433

Lampert, R., Hayes, D. L., Annas, G. J., Farley, M. A., Goldstein, N. E., Hamilton, R. M., & Zellner, R. et al. (2010). HRS Expert Consensus Statement on the Management of Cardiovascular Implantable Electronic Devices (CIEDs) in patients nearing end of life or requesting withdrawal of therapy. *Heart Rhythm*, *7*(7), 1008–1026. doi:10.1016/j.hrthm.2010.04.033 PMID:20471915

Meltzer, E. C., Gallagher, J. J., Suppes, A., & Fins, J. J. (2012). Lip-reading and the ventilated patient. *Critical Care Medicine*, *40*(5), 1529–1531. doi:10.1097/CCM.0b013e318241e56c PMID:22430239

Meltzer, E. C., Ivascu, N. S., Acres, C. A., Stark, M., Kirkpatrick, J. N., Paul, S., & Fins, J. J. et al. (2014). Extracorporeal membrane oxygenation in adults: A grief review and ethical prconsiderations for non-specialist health providers and hospitalists. *Journal of Hospital Medicine*, *9*(12), 808–813. doi:10.1002/jhm.2262 PMID:25332093

Pellegrino, E. D. (2005). Futility in medical decisions: The word and the concept. *HEC Forum*, *17*(4), 308–318. doi:10.1007/s10730-005-5156-9 PMID:16637443

Schneiderman, L. J. (2011). Defining medical futility and improving medical care. *Journal of Bioethical Inquiry*, *8*(2), 123–131. doi:10.1007/s11673-011-9293-3 PMID:21765643

Sessums, L. L., Zembruzuska, H., & Jackson, J. L. (2011). Does this patient have decision-making capacity? *Journal of the American Medical Association*, *306*(4), 420–427. doi:10.1001/jama.2011.1023 PMID:21791691

Shah, K. B., Levenson, J. L., & Mehra, M. R. (2014). Emergent use of mechanical circulatory support devices: Ethical dilemmas. *Current Opinion in Cardiology*, *29*(3), 281–284. doi:10.1097/HCO.0000000000000058 PMID:24686401

Steinberg, A. (2003). *Encyclopedia of Jewish medical ethics: a compilation of Jewish medical law on all topics of medical interest*. Jerusalem, New York: Feldheim Publishers.

Swetz, K. M., & Mansel, J. K. (2013). Ethical Issues and Palliative Care in the Cardiovascular Intensive Care Unit. *Cardiology Clinics*, *31*(4), 657–668. doi:10.1016/j.ccl.2013.07.013 PMID:24188227

Swidler, R. N. (2010). The Family Health Care Decisions Act: A Summary of Key Provisions. *Health Law Journal*, *15*(1), 32–35.

KEY TERMS AND DEFINITIONS

Autonomy: The right of persons to make decisions about their fate.

Beneficence: The desire to act in the patient's best interest.

Health Care Agent: A person legal appointed by a patient to make medical decisions should the patient lose capacity.

Heath Care Proxy: A form that an patient completes to legally empowers another individual, ie the health care agent, to make medical decisions should the patient lose capacity.

Justice: The principle of fairness in distribution of resources.

Non-Maleficence: The desire to avoid harm.

Surrogate: A person selected to serve as a decision maker for an incapacitated patient when a health care agent has not been previously appointed. The surrogate is determined by proximity as next-of-kin.

Withdrawal of Life-Sustaining Therapy: The removal of medications or machines, without which a patient is not expected to survive.

Withholding Life-Sustaining Therapy: The decision not to provide a medical therapy, without which the patient is not expected to survive.

Section 2

Preoperative Assessment and Optimization

Chapter 7
Acute Coronary Syndrome

Brandon W. Calenda
Icahn School of Medicine at Mount Sinai, USA

Umesh K. Gidwani
Icahn School of Medicine at Mount Sinai, USA

ABSTRACT

Acute coronary syndrome (ACS) is a common and sometimes lethal event, usually precipitated by sudden rupture and thrombosis of an atherosclerotic plaque. Patients presenting with ACS can be rapidly risk stratified based on signs, symptoms, electrocardiogram, and biomarkers. There is a new generation of potent and reliable antiplatelet drugs, which in concert with anticoagulation and rapid revascularization, can preserve myocardium and save lives. When choosing how to revascularize, hemodynamically stable patients with diabetes mellitus and complex coronary disease benefit more from coronary artery bypass grafting rather than percutaneous coronary intervention. Despite optimal treatment, ACS can result in deadly complications such as cardiogenic shock. Supportive care is paramount, but despite its widespread use, the utility of intraaortic balloon counterpulsation is uncertain. In the future, advanced coronary imaging may enhance preventative care, novel molecular targets will help expand treatment options, and cell-based regenerative therapies may aid myocardial recovery after acute coronary syndrome.

INTRODUCTION

This chapter aims to provide the reader with an in-depth, evidence-based understanding of the principles behind the current understanding and management of acute coronary syndrome. The mechanisms of plaque rupture and thrombosis are explored in some depth, as these are key to understanding principles of pharmacologic therapy. A discussion on risk stratification follows, as does the basis for choosing between treatment modalities. The most important decision is whether to pursue a conservative or early-invasive treatment strategy, and this directly follows from individualized risk stratification. An evidence-based review of pharmacologic agents follows, with a focus on several of the newer antiplatelet agents, which are beginning to replace clopidogrel as mainstays of therapy. This is followed by a discussion of revascularization strategies and the factors which would make a patient a better candidate for coronary artery bypass grafting (CABG) versus percutaneous coronary intervention (PCI). Post-ACS care is es-

DOI: 10.4018/978-1-4666-8603-8.ch007

sential, as there are a number of potentially lethal complications which can be anticipated and managed to varying degrees. Finally, the discussion looks to the horizon of acute coronary syndrome care and potential future therapies.

Chapter Objectives

By the end of the chapter, the reader will be able to:

- Understand basic mechanisms of ACS at the molecular and cellular level
- Risk stratify patients with ACS and use this assessment to appropriately tailor therapy
- Understand the mechanisms and clinical evidence underlying the use of current antiplatelet, anticoagulant, and adjunctive medications in treatment of ACS
- Individualize the optimal choice and timing of coronary revascularization
- Anticipate and treat complications of acute coronary syndrome
- Appreciate the frontiers and limitations of advanced coronary imaging, new therapeutic targets, and regenerative myocardial stem cell treatments

BACKGROUND

Epidemiology

Despite recent advances in prevention and therapy, acute coronary syndrome (ACS) – a broad term which includes unstable angina (UA), non-ST segment elevation myocardial infarction (NSTEMI), ST segment elevation myocardial infarction (STEMI) and sudden cardiac death due to myocardial infarction - remains a tremendous source of morbidity and mortality. Current estimates suggest that there will be 515,000 new acute myocardial infarctions (AMI) and 205,000 recurrent AMIs in 2014 in the United States, with significant associated mortality (American Heart Association, 2014). Coronary disease accounted for roughly 15% of all deaths in the United States in 2010, a third of which were caused by acute MI. This equates to one death every 83 seconds due to acute MI (Alexander, et al., 2011)

Overall death rates due to coronary disease declined 59% in the period from 1950 to 1999. This decline in mortality correlated with modest improvements in modifiable risk factors as well as advances in medical therapy. Development and use of evidence-based medical therapies such as aspirin, novel anti-platelet agents, beta blockers, and revascularization have helped decrease in-hospital mortality from AMI (McGovern, et al., 2001). Despite this progress, acute coronary syndrome represents a common and dangerous phenomenon, requiring rapid diagnosis and treatment.

Pathogenesis

With a few notable exceptions (see Table 3), acute coronary syndromes develop in the setting of existing atherosclerotic plaques which are typically not flow-limiting prior to rupture. In contrast to larger, more fibrotic and occlusive lesions, which tend to cause stable angina, these "softer," non-occlusive plaques are more prone to sudden rupture and resultant thrombosis, leading to ACS (Libby, 2013).

"The Vulnerable Plaque"

Because such plaques are not flow limiting, they tend to be angiographically mild, with a mean stenosis of about 50%. The search for characteristics and behavior of "the vulnerable plaque" – i.e., one prone to rupture and cause large infarctions – has yielded several insights. High-risk plaques tend to be high in lipid content and covered by a thin fibrous cap. They have a high-burden of inflammation, macrophage infiltration, and neovascularization with vaso vasorum. Finally, they tend to display "positive remodeling," in which plaque grows outwards through the external elastic membrane, rather than inwards, resulting in a large plaque with only mild angiographic stenosis (Moreno, 2010). Table 1 contrasts characteristics of a high-risk, vulnerable plaque to those lesions which are lower-risk for rupture.

Acute coronary syndrome occurs when disruption of such a plaque leads to acute thrombosis. Plaque disruption results most commonly from plaque rupture (the most common mechanism), plaque erosion, or calcified nodule (rare) (Jia, et al., 2013). Typical precipitants for plaque disruption include mechanical stress from tachycardia and hypertension as well as inflammatory stress leading to breakdown of the fibrous cap. Exposure of tissue factor within the plaque to the bloodstream activates the clotting cascade, and exposure of sub-endothelial collagen recruits platelets and initiates their activation and aggregation. The result is a platelet-thrombin clot. These pathways of coagulation, platelet activation and aggregation represent the principal targets for ACS treatment. Occasionally, ACS may be caused by non-atherothrombotic events (see Table 2), requiring an individualized approach.

The significance of this intra-coronary thrombosis depends upon the balance between platelet and endothelial-derived vasodilators (nitric oxide, prostacyclin) and vasoconstrictors (thromboxane, serotonin, thrombin). In innocuous cases, the inflammatory and thrombotic cascade will attenuate, the vessel will dilate, coronary blood flow will continue, the thrombus will eventually degrade or be incorporated into the plaque, and the event may not manifest clinically.

Conversely, unchecked platelet aggregation and impaired vasodilation may result in significant ischemia. In most cases, the extent of ischemia is what distinguishes unstable angina, NSTEMI, and STEMI. Unstable angina and NSTEMI typically result from partially occlusive thrombosis and transient ischemia, with the latter resulting in cardiac myocyte necrosis. STEMI, on the other hand, is usually caused by a 100% occlusive thrombus, resulting in prolonged ischemia and transmural infarction.

Table 1. Contrasting attributes of high and low-risk plaques

	High-risk plaque	Low-risk plaque
Fibrous cap	Thin	Thick
Remodeling	"Positive" – growth away from lumen	"Negative/constrictive" – growth into lumen
Lipid core	Large, necrotic	Less necrosis
Inflammation	High	Low
Location	Proximal coronary arteries, near branch points	Variable
Neovascularization	Prominent	Minimal
Angiography	Non-obstructive	Obstructive (>50%)
Risk of rupture	High	Low
Clinical correlate	Possible ACS	Stable angina Superficial erosions

Table 2. Non-atherothrombotic causes of acute coronary syndromes

Causes of ACS not due to atherothrombosis
Coronary vasospasm, especially with cocaine use
Spontaneous coronary dissection
Atrial or ventricular thromboembolism to coronaries
Coronary thrombus in situ due to hypercoagulable stable
Vasculitis
Myocardial bridging

Table 3. The Killip classification

Killip Class	Key Findings
I	No signs of heart failure
II	Rales < 1/3 up posterior lung fields SBP > 90 mmHg
III	Rales > 1/3 up posterior lung fields SBP > 90 mmHg
IV	Cardiogenic shock SBP < 90 mmHg

History and Clinical Presentation

The initial patient evaluation should be focused on estimating the likelihood that the patient's symptoms are coronary in origin and excluding alternate diagnoses. ACS is most often heralded by the development of new or progressive chest discomfort. When an individual experiences predictable, exertional chest discomfort which abates with rest or nitroglycerin, this is referred to as stable angina, and is not considered a form of ACS. Conversely, chest pain of increasing frequency, duration, severity, or occurring at rest is characteristic of unstable angina or acute myocardial infarction.

It is important to note that many individuals may have ACS without experiencing significant chest discomfort. Certain populations, particularly the elderly, females, and diabetics often experience atypical symptoms such as dyspnea, nausea, vomiting, presyncope, or generalized fatigue or malaise. Inferior wall, "diaphragmatic" infarcts may also present with symptoms which may appear to be gastrointestinal in nature. In an at-risk patient, such symptoms should be considered possible "anginal equivalents," requiring the same evaluation as more traditional chest pain.

RISK STRATIFICATION

Once ACS is suspected, the physician must estimate likelihood of adverse outcomes, as this will dictate further management. High-risk patients are more likely to benefit from more aggressive pharmacotherapy and an early-invasive strategy. Patients can be rapidly risk stratified using a combination of physical exam, electrocardiography, serum biomarkers, and integrated risk calculators.

Physical Exam

Signs and symptoms of acute heart failure indicate high risk for complications. Symptoms of orthopnea and dyspnea are often historical clues to acute heart failure. Physical exam should carefully evaluate for signs such as elevated jugular venous pressure, tachycardia, the presence of an S3, rales, pleural effusions, cool extremities and lower extremity edema. The Killip score is an easy-to-use method of classifying patients with ACS based entirely on physical exam findings of heart failure and systolic blood pressure (SBP) (see Table 3). It has been shown to be predictive of both short and long-term mortality in STEMI and NSTEMI. In fact, a Killip score of III/IV has been shown to be the most powerful predictor of mortality in a large study of patients presenting with NSTEMI (Khot, et al., 2003). In an age of ever-advancing technology, the bedside exam remains essential in the evaluation and triage of patients with acute coronary syndrome.

Electrocardiography and Biomarkers

In patients with suspected ACS, an electrocardiogram (ECG) should be performed immediately. The ECG is most valuable for its ability to immediately distinguish between ST elevation MI (STEMI) and non-ST elevation MI (NSTEMI) or unstable angina. In the absence of absolute contraindications, patients with STEMI should proceed to emergent revascularization, while those with NSTEMI/UA generally do not. Detailed treatment strategies follow later in this chapter.

The ECG provides prognostic information beyond ST elevations. The presence of ST depressions and the quantitative depth of depressions have been established as markers of elevated risk in ACS compared with those without ST changes. In the PARAGON study, for example, those with ST depressions > 2 mm were 5.7 times more likely to die within one year compared with those without ST depressions (Kaul, et al., 2003). Another prospective trial identified the presence of ST segment depressions greater than 1mm as an independent predictor of both in-hospital and five-year mortality in ACS, regardless of treatment strategy (Mueller, Neumann, Perach, Perruchoud, & Buettner, 2004)

Serum markers of cardiac necrosis are also useful both for establishing the diagnosis of acute myocardial infarction and identifying higher-risk patients. Using current assays, troponin levels typically become detectable approximately six hours after the onset of myocyte necrosis. New, "high-sensitivity" troponin assays (not currently approved in the United States) promise to offer more rapid detection and superior negative predictive value. In the future, patients may be effectively "ruled out" for myocardial infarction with two negative high-sensitivity troponins drawn just two hours apart.

Prospective trials have demonstrated a clear correlation between quantitative troponin levels and short-term risk. When the clinical presentation is consistent with ACS, even low-level elevations (above 0.1 ng/mL) should be considered a marker of elevated risk and predictive of benefit from an early-invasive approach (Morrow, et al., 2001). Furthermore, the combination of both elevated troponin and ST depressions identifies a particularly high-risk group in the setting of UA/NSTEMI (Kaul, et al., 2003).

Predictive Models for Risk Stratification

Several prognostic scoring systems are available which integrate history, physical exam, ECG, and biomarkers to estimate the patient's risk of serious complications due to ACS. The goal is to identify those who are considered high-risk and therefore most likely to benefit from aggressive therapy and an early invasive approach. Risk stratification should not be considered a static, one-time event on admission, but rather as a dynamic process requiring continuous reassessment.

The two most widely-accepted and well-validated prognostic scoring systems are the TIMI risk score and the GRACE score. The TIMI risk score was developed from TIMI (Thrombolysis In Myocardial Infarction, the academic research organization) clinical trial data and has been prospectively validated. It is easily calculated at the bedside using seven variables and can predict risk of death, MI, or need for urgent revascularization at 14 days (see Table 4, and Figure 1). It is also useful in identifying those who will benefit most from an early invasive treatment strategy, the use of GP IIb/IIIa inhibitors, and the preferential use of enoxaparin over unfractionated heparin (Antman, et al., 2000).

Table 4. The TIMI Risk Score

Age ≥ 65 yr
Three or more CAD risk factors
Known CAD (> 50% stenosis)
ST segment deviation
Two or more anginal events in previous 24 hours
Use of aspirin in last 7 days
Elevated serum biomarkers

Figure 1. TIMI Risk Score and 14-day risk of death, MI, need for urgent revascularization

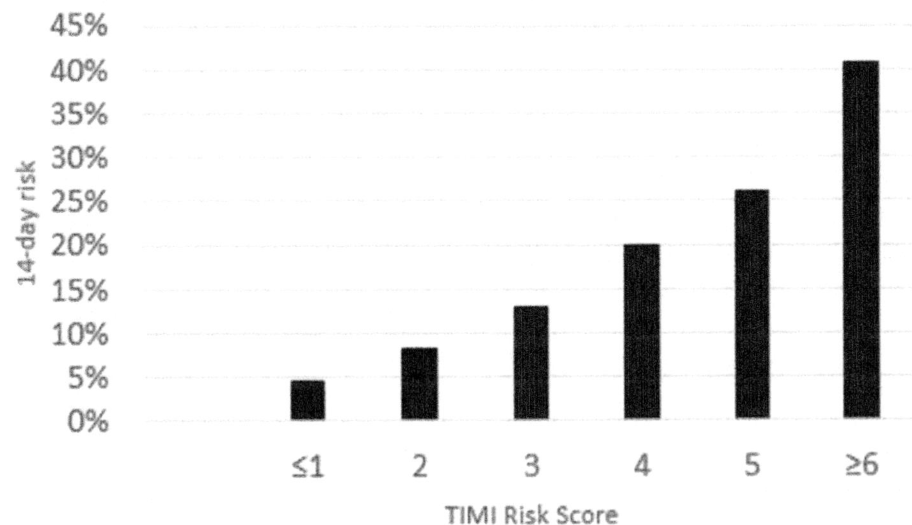

A new, "Dynamic TIMI score" can also be used to synthesize the TIMI risk score on admission with clinical variables based on the patient's hospital course. Incorporating the development of in-hospital MI, arrhythmia, major bleed, stroke, congestive heart failure, recurrent ischemia and renal failure, this score has been prospectively validated and shown to predict one-year mortality. A higher Dynamic TIMI risk score, calculated after admission or at discharge, helps identify higher-risk people who may require closer monitoring or additional interventions (Amin, et al., 2013).

Another well-validated clinical risk assessment is the Global Registry of Acute Cardiac Events (GRACE) model. In contrast with the TIMI score, GRACE is used to estimate all-cause mortality at six months post-discharge, and was derived from an international registry, rather than clinical trial data.

Proponents argue that this enhances its real-world applicability (Eagle, et al., 2004). It uses a combination of medical history, findings at initial presentation, and in-hospital treatment to create a score. Via a nomogram, this score translates into predicted six-month mortality.

Ultimately, the goal of risk stratification is to identify patients at high risk of complications, who are typically the most likely to benefit from aggressive medical therapy and early invasive treatment. One must remember that the above risk calculators are derived from population data. It is imperative for the physician to use these calculators only as tools to assist in the unique risk assessment of each individual patient.

TREATMENT OVERVIEW

Optimal treatment depends upon risk stratification. Those with STEMI are at highest risk and require emergent angiography and revascularization with concurrent dual antiplatelet therapy and parenteral anticoagulation. Those with UA/NSTEMI who are hemodynamically or electrically unstable should also proceed to urgent angiography. Relatively stable patients with UA/NSTEMI who are high-risk based on TIMI or GRACE scores will benefit from an "early invasive" strategy of angiography and revascularization, simultaneous with dual antiplatelet therapy and anticoagulation. Lower-risk UA/NSTEMI patients can be observed with dual antiplatelet therapy alone, pending further risk stratification. In the absence of contraindications, optimal dual antiplatelet therapy consists of aspirin and newer agents such as ticagrelor or prasugrel, rather than clopidogrel.

PHARMACOTHERAPY: ANTIPLATELET AGENTS

Overview

Antiplatelet therapy has evolved dramatically in the last several years. While aspirin remains a mainstay, clopidogrel has demonstrated significant shortcomings as a result of marked inter-patient variability. Clopidogrel is gradually being replaced in the guidelines as a first-line agent by a new generation of more potent and reliable P2Y-12 inhibitors such as ticagrelor and prasugrel. A new, fast-acting, intravenous P2Y-12 inhibitor, cangrelor, has also joined the arsenal, though it currently lacks a clear niche. Table 5 summarizes the attributes of commonly-used antiplatelet agents. Below is a review of pharmacology, indications, and evidence for the most common drugs used in the treatment of ACS. The abundance of new, powerful agents has brought with it unanswered questions regarding their safety. Special attention is paid here to the perioperative uses of antiplatelet medications in the setting of possible coronary artery bypass graft (CABG) surgery. Figure 2 provides an overview of therapeutic targets of antiplatelet drugs.

Aspirin

Aspirin irreversibly inhibits the enzyme cyclooxygenase 1 (COX-1), blocking thromboxane A2 (TXA2) synthesis in platelets. TXA2 is integral to platelet activation and aggregation, and is also a local vasoconstrictor. For years, aspirin has been the mainstay of treatment for acute coronary syndromes. In 1990, the RISC study was published, in which aspirin 75 mg daily was administered to patients with UA/

Table 5. Characteristics of common antiplatelet agents

	Aspirin	Clopidogrel	Prasugrel	Ticagrelor	Cangrelor	Eptifibatide
Route	Oral	Oral	Oral	Oral	IV	IV
Loading dose	325 mg	600 mg	60 mg	180 mg	30 μg/kg	180 mcg/kg
Daily dose	81 mg	75 mg	10 mg	90 mg BID	4 μg/kg/min	2 mcg/kg/min
Prodrug?	No	Yes	Yes	No	No	No
Metabolism	GI esterases	Hepatic CYP2C19	GI esterases	Hepatic	Plasma	Renal excretion
Time to peak effect	1-2 hours	2-4 hours	30 min	1.5 hours	30 min	15 min
Duration of effect	7-10 days	3-10 days	5-10 days	3-4 days	1 hour	4-6 hours
Unique Concerns	n/a	Variable efficacy	Major bleeding	Dyspnea, Bleeding	n/a	Bleeding, Thrombocytopenia
Timing pre-CABG	Continue	Surgeon-Dependent	Hold at least 7 days prior	Hold at least 5 days prior	Hold at least 1 hour prior	Hold at least 4 to 6 hours prior
Approved for Clinicalal Use in USA	Yes	Yes	Yes	Yes	No	Yes

NSTEMI. The results were astounding: compared with placebo, the relative risk of death/MI was 0.43, 0.31, and 0.36 at 5 days, 1 month, and 3 months, respectively (RISC Group, 1990). It has continued to demonstrate efficacy in both acute treatment and secondary prevention. Current recommendations are for a loading dose of 162-325 mg (in the rapidly absorbable form) in the setting of suspected ACS, and a daily dose of 81 mg (preferably enteric coated) thereafter for secondary prevention. Higher maintenance doses have shown a higher risk of bleeding with diminishing benefit (Berger, et al., 2012).

Well-controlled trials are lacking to determine the safety and efficacy of aspirin prior to CABG surgery, particularly in the setting of ACS. The best available data seems to suggest that perioperative aspirin use may decrease in-hospital post-operative mortality without an attendant increase in significant bleeding (Bybee, et al., 2005). The risk of bleeding can be further minimized by maintaining the daily dose of aspirin less than 325 mg (Sun, et al., 2008). Thus it is generally recommended to continue aspirin perioperatively, particularly in the setting of ACS.

Clopidogrel

Clopidogrel is a thienopyridine and an irreversible inhibitor of the adenosine diphosphate (ADP) P2Y-12 receptor blocker. Its efficacy was first demonstrated in the CURE trial, which randomized patients with ACS to aspirin vs. aspirin and clopidogrel. The dual anti-platelet therapy showed 20% relative risk reduction in composite outcomes at one year compared to aspirin alone (The Clopidogrel in Unstable Angina to Prevent Recurrent Events Trial Investigators, 2001). Those who underwent percutaneous coronary intervention (PCI) showed additional benefit from the addition of clopidogrel. Dual anti-platelet therapy is now a cornerstone of ACS treatment.

The major shortcoming of clopidogrel is its wide inter-patient variability. Clopidogrel is a prodrug which requires two-step hepatic conversion (primarily via cytochrome-P (CYP) enzymes) to generate the active metabolite. Individual, genetic variations in hepatic prodrug metabolism leads to marked vari-

Figure 2. Targets of Antiplatelet Therapy. Adapted from Storey, RF: New P2Y12 Inhibitors. Heart 2011. Used with permission from BMJ Publishing Group Ltd.

Platelet activation and site of action of various antiplatelet agents

Upon exposure of injured endothelium, platelets bind to von Willebrand factor (vWF) and exposed collagen via glycoprotein (GP) VI and GP IB alpha, leading to platelet activation. This causes a conformational change in the platelet shape and degranulation of dense and alpha granules, leading to release of adenosine disphosphate (ADP), thromboxane A2 (TxA2), and various proinflammatory mediators.

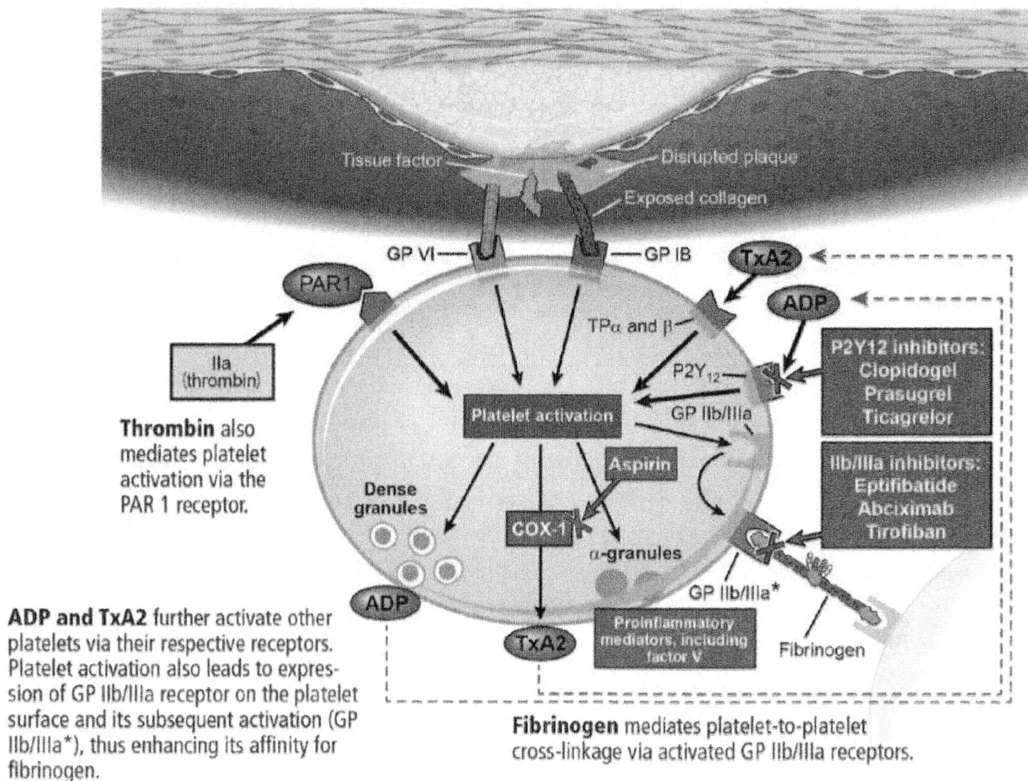

ability in pharmacokinetics and bioavailability of the active metabolite. A substantial subset of patients do not manifest appropriate platelet inhibition after dosing and are deemed clopidogrel "non-responders" (also erroneously referred to as "resistant"). Despite this variability, the current guidelines do not support genetic testing, and only tepidly acknowledge that platelet reactivity testing "may be considered" in the appropriate clinical scenario, such as recurrent events while on clopidogrel (Wright, et al., 2011). It remains to be seen exactly how platelet reactivity testing will fit into future management of ACS.

Optimal dosing of clopidogrel in ACS necessitates a minimum "loading dose" of 300 mg. Yet up to 30% of individuals may not manifest appropriate platelet inhibition in response to this dose. Larger loading doses have been shown to markedly improve platelet inhibition and outcomes (Gurbel, et al., 2005). The large CURRENT-OASIS 7 trial demonstrated modest additive reduction in adverse cardiovascular outcomes with a loading dose of 600 mg at the cost of a marginal increase of major bleeding (Mehta, et al., 2010). The optimal loading dose of clopidogrel remains somewhat controversial, but a minimum of 300 mg is standard of care, and 600 mg seems to offer additional protection against recurrent ischemia.

There is heterogeneous evidence surrounding perioperative use of clopidogrel. The majority of studies have been retrospective and confounded by the inclusion of both elective CABG and urgent CABG in the setting of ACS. Existing AHA/ACCF guidelines suggest stopping clopidogrel at least five days prior to CABG based on an observed increase in mortality and reoperation in those continuing clopidogrel perioperatively. At the same time, there is clear data that continuation of clopidogrel is associated with reduction in perioperative MI, and a large number of urgent CABG surgeries are performed on clopidogrel safely (Nijjer, Watson, Athanasiou, & Malik, 2011). Given the limitations of the data, surgeons should individualize perioperative use of clopidogrel based upon urgency of revascularization, risk of recurrent MI, and their own experience and comfort level with surgery in the setting of dual antiplatelet therapy.

Prasugrel

Prasugrel is a newer thienepyridine and an irreversible inhibitor of the ADP P2Y-12 receptor. While chemically similar to clopidogrel, it requires only a single-step conversion to its active metabolite, primarily via intestinal esterases rather than CYP enzymes. As a result, it has substantially less inter-patient variability than clopidogrel. Developed to be a more potent and predictable platelet inhibitor than clopidogrel, its efficacy was demonstrated in the TRITON-TIMI 38 study, which randomized patients with ACS undergoing PCI to prasugrel vs. clopidogrel. The prasugrel group showed marked reduction in the composite endpoint of cardiovascular death, MI or ischemic stroke, but with a concomitant increased risk of major bleeding. The bleeding risk was particularly high in those greater than 75 years old, females, those with low BMI, history of stroke/TIA (Wiviott, et al., 2007). This led to an FDA "black box warning" delineating the above risks and contraindications to prasugrel's use. There was no difference in overall mortality.

In addition to serious concerns regarding bleeding, some question prasugrel's efficacy. Unlike aspirin and ticagrelor, prasugrel did not impact overall mortality. Furthermore, the comparison group in TRITON-TIMI 38 was given a loading dose of only 300 mg clopidogrel, which is generally inferior to a loading dose of 600 mg with respect to ischemic outcomes (see above). Unfortunately, such a trial is unlikely to be repeated with a higher dose of clopidogrel.

The role of prasugrel in CABG was examined in a follow-up of the TRITON-TIMI 38 cohort. Among those who underwent subsequent CABG, those treated with prasugrel showed significantly better survival compared to those with clopidogrel (Smith, et al., 2012). Interestingly, this was despite significantly greater bleeding in the prasugrel group. It should be noted that these were largely elective CABG (85%), most of them were performed more than 90 days after the index ACS diagnosis, and the drug was consistently stopped one to seven days prior to surgery. Of course, one cannot extrapolate this data to urgent CABG after acute MI. Surgeons should anticipate significantly greater bleeding if the patient has been taking prasugrel, and factor this into the risk/benefit assessment when choosing optimal timing for post-ACS bypass grafting.

Ticagrelor

Ticagrelor is a novel oral inhibitor of the ADP P2Y12 receptor. It is molecularly distinct from prasugrel and clopidogrel and is itself an active drug, rather than a prodrug. As such, it displays more rapid onset of action, has a shorter half-life, demonstrates reversible platelet inhibition, and is not dependent upon the variable metabolism of hepatic CYP enzymes. It also has a unique, secondary effect of blocking local serotonin reuptake, which may lead to pleiotropic effects beyond simple platelet inhibition.

Ticagrelor was compared head-to-head with clopidogrel in ACS in the PLATO trial. This was a very large, randomized trial in which patients with STEMI and UA/NSTEMI were randomized to either aspirin and clopidogrel or aspirin and ticagrelor. In addition to decreasing all-cause mortality by 24%, those treated with ticagrelor had a 16% relative risk reduction in the composite endpoint of cardiovascular death, MI or stroke. There was no difference in overall bleeding outcomes, but ticagrelor had significantly higher rates of non-CABG related major bleeding (Wallentin, et al., 2009). Interestingly, ticagrelor was also associated with dyspnea (more than 10% of patients). The mechanism of this has yet to be fully elucidated, though it may be related to its effect on adenosine reuptake.

The PLATO trial has attracted much scrutiny as a result of geographically heterogeneous outcomes: those in North America overall experienced harms from ticagrelor, in contrast with those worldwide. Further statistical analysis has postulated that this may have been from chance alone, as the North American group represented less than 10% of the overall study population. A second explanation is that those in North America were more likely to receive a daily dose of aspirin 325 mg (rather than 81 mg) while receiving ticagrelor. This seems to markedly increase risk of bleeding and may account for the regional variation (Mahaffey, et al., 2011). It has been proposed that high-dose aspirin may attenuate some pleiotropic, cardioprotective effects of ticagrelor. As a result, it is strongly recommended that those receiving ticagrelor take no more than 81 mg of aspirin daily.

Those who underwent CABG during the PLATO study period showed decreased mortality and a non-significant trend towards decreased CABG-related bleeding with ticagrelor compared to clopidogrel (Varenhorst, et al., 2012). The trend towards decreased bleeding seems consistent among follow-up studies. One comparison of clopidogrel versus ticagrelor pre-CABG (in setting of ACS) showed no differences in bleeding if the study drug was held at least 2 days prior to surgery. However, if either drug was held only 0 to 1 days before surgery, there was a strong trend towards increased bleeding in the ticagrelor patients (Hansson, Rexius, Dellborg, Albertsson, & Jeppsson, 2014). With its shorter half-life and reversible platelet inhibition, ticagrelor seems to be at least equivalent to clopidogrel with respect to surgical bleeding outcomes, provided that the drug is held at least 2 days prior to CABG. However, current ACC/AHA guidelines recommend holding ticagrelor for a minimum of 5 days prior to CABG (Hillis, et al., 2011).

Cangrelor

Like ticagrelor, cangrelor is a directly-acting, reversible inhibitor of the P2Y12 receptor. It differs from ticagrelor, and indeed all of the above agents, in one significant respect: it is administered intravenously and rapidly achieves therapeutic levels. The evidence supporting cangrelor in acute coronary syndromes is rather modest, but its rapid onset and IV administration may offer the drug a niche in the treatment of ACS.

Two major trials have demonstrated that cangrelor was neither superior to a loading dose of clopidogrel 600 mg nor to placebo in the setting of high-risk ACS proceeding to PCI (Harrington, et al., 2009); (Bhatt, et al., 2009). A subsequent third trial examined cangrelor versus clopidogrel loading prior to PCI (either in ACS or elective PCI) and showed no difference in mortality. There was a reduction in peri-procedural ischemic events with no significant differences in bleeding (Bhatt, et al., 2013).

Cangrelor appears to be a relatively safe and effective antiplatelet agent, but not more so than clopidogrel. Its role in the future treatment for ACS remains to be elucidated. It is currently approved and in use in Europe, but has not been approved for use in the United States. Cangrelor may find a niche in temporary situations where longer-acting P2Y12 inhibitors are unacceptable. In fact, cangrelor has been demonstrated to be a safe and effective "bridge" to CABG in patients hospitalized after ACS and previously treated with coronary stents and an oral P2Y12 inhibitor (Angiolillo, et al., 2012).

GP IIb/IIIa Inhibitors: Eptifibatide and Abciximab

Eptifibatide is a reversible inhibitor of platelet glycoprotein IIb/IIIa (GP IIb/IIIa). It remains popular, though use has declined markedly in recent years. Abciximab is a monoclonal antibody to GPIIb/IIIa. This receptor is responsible for the aggregation of activated platelets. Like cangrelor, eptifibatide and abciximab are administered intravenously and have a rather short duration of action. GP IIb/IIIa inhibitors were more widely used in ACS prior to the development of current dual antiplatelet therapy with P2Y12 inhibitors and prior to the development of bivalirudin. More recently, evidence and guidelines support their only in those high-risk patients who undergo primary PCI for ACS, and even then, their use is ideally restricted to use in the catheterization lab as needed, rather than early and "upstream" (Giugliano, et al., 2009). Risks such as bleeding and profound thrombocytopenia tend to outweigh anti-ischemic effects in patients treated non-invasively.

A small number of case reports support the idea that eptifibatide may potentially be used safely as a "bridge" in situations where longer-acting, oral antiplatelet therapy must be temporarily discontinued (Ben Morrison, Horst, Brown, Bell, & Daniels, 2012). However, this has not been rigorously studied, and should be interpreted with caution.

PHARMACOTHERAPY: ANTICOAGULANTS

Blockade at various steps of the clotting cascade has long been an integral part of the treatment of acute coronary syndrome. While parenteral anticoagulation has been overshadowed in recent years by antiplatelet therapy, it retains an important role in attenuating acute thrombosis. Bivalirudin, an intravenous direct thrombin inhibitor, continues to grow in popularity. The novel oral anticoagulants, whose use is rapidly expanding for stroke prophylaxis in atrial fibrillation, have an unclear role in the treatment of ACS.

Unfractionated and Low Molecular Weight Heparin

Unfractionated heparin (UFH) has been a mainstay of treatment in ACS for years. It induces a conformational change in anti-thrombin III, leading to rapid inactivation of thrombin and factors IXa and Xa. Large trials in the 1990's demonstrated heterogeneous results, with an unclear effect on mortality. However, studies do consistently show that UFH reduces reinfarction, and typically only causes minor bleeding (Magee, Campbell, Moher, & Rowe, 2008). UFH is looked upon favorably by many clinicians due to its long history of safe use, short half-life, and easy reversibility with protamine sulfate. Thrombocytopenia associated with its use is the biggest concern. It is widely used during PCI, where it can be closely titrated to goal activated clotting time (ACT), a rapid point-of-care test. However, UFH's efficacy and role have been not rigorously tested since the advent of dual anti-platelet therapy.

Multiple studies have demonstrated the superiority of low-molecular weight heparin (LMWH) over UFH in ACS. LMWH outperforms UFH in terms of ischemic outcomes, but at the cost of greater bleeding (Singh, Gupta, & Vacek, 2014) and lower risk of thrombocytopenia. Its relative lack of reversibility and longer half-life make it potentially higher-risk than UFH in those with higher bleeding risks or an imminent procedure. It also frequently requires dose adjustment or outright avoidance in advanced renal dysfunction.

Fondaparinux

Fondaparinux indirectly inhibits factor Xa by means of antithrombin. It is administered subcutaneously and reaches peak effect within two hours. Fondaparinux has been shown to slightly outperform both UFH and LMWH in ACS. A very important caveat, however, is that in both studies, those undergoing PCI had more thrombotic complications with fondaparinux (Singh, Gupta, & Vacek, 2014). Therefore, fondaparinux should be reserved for those ACS patients who are being treated non-invasively.

Bivalirudin

Bivalirudin is an intravenous, direct thrombin inhibitor. Despite tremendous cost, its popularity has grown as it continues to outperform other anticoagulants in a majority of clinical trials. Direct comparisons between bivalirudin and UFH have been difficult to interpret due to variable use of GP IIb/IIIa inhibitors, but seem to favor bivalirudin in those undergoing early invasive treatment (Singh, Gupta, & Vacek, 2014). However, more recent head-to-head data have clouded the picture and indicate that heparin may in fact be superior (Shahzad & Stables, 2014). In practice, bivalirudin is often administered in the catheterization lab periprocedurally. However, indications may be expanding. Recent evidence suggests there may be substantial benefit to bivalirudin started prior to arrival at the hospital for STEMI and PCI, as compared to standard care (Steg, et al., 2013). While cost remains an obstacle, we foresee that bivalirudin will continue to be a popular agent in the short to intermediate term. Based on the continued uncertainty regarding efficacy compared to heparin, further studies may be conducted comparing these agents; however, any definitive results will not be at hand for several years (Schulz, et al., 2013).

Novel Oral Anticoagulants

In recent years, several non-vitamin K antagonist oral anticoagulants have come to market, primarily for stroke prophylaxis in atrial fibrillation or treatment of acute venous thromboembolism. In an attempt to broaden indications, all three agents have been tested against placebo in acute coronary syndromes. Thus far, results have been discouraging. However, they may find a future role in the treatment of patients with atrial fibrillation and acute coronary syndrome.

Standard treatment plus rivaroxaban, a direct factor Xa inhibitor, reduced serious cardiovascular outcomes but increased major bleeding, including intracranial hemorrhage (Mega, et al., 2012). When apixaban, another direct factor Xa inhibitor, was added to standard therapy in ACS, there was no difference in ischemic events or death, but there was a significant increase in bleeding, including fatal and intracranial bleeding (Alexander, et al., 2011). Similarly, the addition of dabigatran, a direct thrombin inhibitor, to dual antiplatelet therapy after ACS resulted in higher incidence of major bleeding. The study was not designed to detect clinical ischemic endpoints (Oldgren, et al., 2011).

In short, none of the novel oral anticoagulants can currently be recommended for the treatment of acute coronary syndrome. The observed increased bleeding from these drugs, in the setting of biochemical irreversibility, gives them a very unfavorable safety profile. Multiple new studies are underway to help determine their role in treatment of ACS. If effective reversal agents are developed and further trials demonstrate improvement in outcomes, they may yet find a treatment niche, particularly in those requiring chronic anticoagulation in addition to anti-platelet therapy.

PHARMACOTHERAPY: ADJUNCT AGENTS

Beta-Blockers

It has long been held that early administration of beta-blockers, in the absence of contraindications such as shock or pulmonary edema, is beneficial in the setting of acute coronary syndrome. The traditionally proposed mechanism is a decrease in heart rate and blood pressure, leading to reduced cardiac oxygen demand, thereby optimizing oxygen balance and potentially reducing infarct size. More recent imaging studies suggest beta-blockers may also help attenuate the local inflammatory response in acute MI. While overall evidence for beta blockers has been mixed, one large meta-analysis of early IV beta-blockade in ACS found a significant decrease in in-hospital mortality, re-infarction, and ventricular arrhythmias (Chatterjee, et al., 2013). Early (within six hours) IV metoprolol in the setting of STEMI has been shown to decrease infarct size as well as a composite endpoint of death, shock, and arrhythmia (Ibanez, et al., 2013). Thus, in patients with acute coronary syndrome and no signs of acute heart failure, early beta-blockers are likely beneficial, and should preferentially be administered intravenously.

Renin-Angiotensin Blockers

The importance of the renin-angiotensin system (RAAS) in the peri-MI period is well-established. Numerous clinical trials have demonstrated mortality benefit with the use of angiotensin converting enzyme (ACE) inhibitors as well as angiotensin receptor blockers (ARBs). Initiation of an ACE inhibitor or ARB post-MI carries a class I indication for both STEMI and NSTEMI, regardless of ejection fraction (Wright, et al., 2011). More downstream RAAS inhibition may be considered in select patients. The use of eplerونone, an aldosterone inhibitor, has been shown to reduce mortality and secondary outcomes in those with reduced ejection fraction after MI (Pitt, et al., 2003). This is rarely administered in the acute setting.

Statins

Statins, particularly in high doses, appear to be beneficial in the setting of acute coronary syndrome. Patients seem to derive benefit whether the statin is started as a new medication or continued prior statin therapy. Conversely, abrupt cessation of statin therapy in the setting of ACS is associated with higher mortality (Fonarow, et al., 2005). Furthermore, intensive statin therapy has been shown to be superior to moderate therapy in preventing recurrent events (Cannon, et al., 2004). Statins are well-known to have pleiotropic effect besides lipid lowering, and they are thought to help stabilize “vulnerable” plaques by decreasing macrophage infiltration and thickening the fibrous cap by increasing smooth muscle and collagen deposition. Despite potential for side-effects such as myositis or elevated transaminases, statins are recommended early and at high doses for patients experiencing an acute coronary syndrome.

REVASCULARIZATION

STEMI

The decision of whom and when to revascularize are based upon the previously discussed risk stratification. Those presenting with STEMI are considered to be at highest risk. They have complete occlusion and require emergent revascularization, usually via percutaneous coronary intervention (PCI), and preferably within 90 minutes or less from time of first presentation ("door to balloon time"). If, due to facility or transportation limitations, PCI cannot be performed within 90 minutes, thrombolysis should be performed, particularly if symptoms have been present for less than 12 hours. Patients should subsequently be transferred to a PCI-capable facility post-thrombolysis. Regardless of whether PCI or thrombolysis is chosen, treatment should also consist of dual antiplatelet therapy and anticoagulation with either unfractionated heparin or bivalirudin (O'Gara, et al., 2013).

STEMI and Cardiogenic Shock

Cardiogenic shock post-STEMI is a unique situation. Though benefits of revascularization in this setting extend for up to 54 hours post-MI, emergent revascularization seems to offer the best outcomes. In the SHOCK trial, patients with STEMI and cardiogenic shock who underwent emergent revascularization had improved six-month survival over those with delayed revascularization (Hochman, et al., 1999). Current guidelines for STEMI and cardiogenic shock now emphasize angiography immediately after initial resuscitation (O'Gara, et al., 2013). The ultimate choice between PCI and CABG depends largely on complexity of coronary anatomy, as discussed below. Intraaortic balloon counterpulsation (IABP) is discussed in more depth below, but it is worth noting that its use has been downgraded to a class II indication in recent guidelines (O'Gara, et al., 2013).

STEMI and CABG

Though PCI can typically be performed much more rapidly than CABG, there are limited circumstances in which CABG may be optimal treatment for STEMI. Patients with STEMI should be considered for urgent CABG if they experience failure of PCI, have known complex coronary anatomy unsuitable for PCI, or need urgent surgical repair of a mechanical complication, such as papillary muscle rupture. In the SHOCK trial, survival was similar between those with cardiogenic shock who underwent emergent PCI and emergent CABG, even though median time to intervention was three times higher for CABG (0.9 versus 2.7 hours) (White, et al., 2005). Appropriate antiplatelet therapy should not be withheld for impending CABG, though timing of surgery and the surgeon's comfort level should guide selection and timing of antiplatelet agents. In clinical practice, the vast majority of patients with STEMI have their "culprit lesion" rapidly revascularized with PCI before being evaluated for CABG.

UA/NSTEMI

The decision of when to proceed to angiography with intent to revascularize in the setting of UA/NSTEMI is dependent upon risk-stratification. In general, high-risk patients benefit from an early-invasive strategy. One can be considered high-risk based on signs of hemodynamic or electrical instability, refractory symptoms, high TIMI risk score, or high GRACE score. Those who are hemodynamically or electrically unstable or those with severe, refractory angina are considered at very high risk and should proceed to angiography as soon as possible (Anderson, et al., 2007).

For stable but high-risk patients, multiple randomized trials have demonstrated a benefit to the early invasive approach. Those with higher TIMI ($\geq$3) and GRACE (>140) scores seem to derive the most benefit. These patients do not derive additional benefit from immediate angiography, though angiography and revascularization within 24 hours appears to be superior to a delay of 36 hours or more (Wright, et al., 2011). Between presentation and intervention, patients should be treated with appropriate dual antiplatelet therapy as well as parenteral anticoagulation.

CABG vs. PCI

When angiography in the setting of UA/NSTEMI reveals complex coronary disease, ideally, a multidisciplinary 'heart team' should confer to determine the optimal modality for revascularization. Clinical features such as diabetes mellitus, complex multi-vessel coronary disease, left main coronary artery disease and possibly left ventricular dysfunction favor CABG over PCI. See figure 3, and Tables 6 and 7 for a summary of recommendations.

The angiographic complexity of coronary disease can be quantified and used to guide decision making via the SYNTAX score, a powerful tool which identifies those with coronary anatomy which would make PCI unfavorable (Serruys, et al., 2009). The risk of cardiac surgery can be estimated with

Figure 3. Appropriateness criteria for CABG or PCI in those requiring revascularization. A: appropriate, U: uncertain, I:inappropriate. From Smith, 2009: Journal of Thoracic and Cardiovascular Surgery. Used with permission from Elsevier.

	CABG			PCI		
	No diabetes and normal LVEF	Diabetes	Depressed LVEF	No diabetes and normal LVEF	Diabetes	Depressed LVEF
Two vessel coronary artery disease with proximal LAD stenosis	A	A	A	A	A	A
Three vessel coronary artery disease	A	A	A	U	U	U
Isolated left main stenosis	A	A	A	I	I	I
Left main stenosis and additional coronary artery disease	A	A	A	I	I	I

Table 6. Treatment recommendations based on SYNTAX score without left main disease

Anatomy	SYNTAX Score	Recommendation
3VCAD	>22	CABG
3VCAD	<22	CABG or PCI
2VCAD w/ proximal LAD	<22	CABG or PCI

Table 7. Treatment recommendations based on SYNTAX score with left main disease

Anatomy	SYNTAX score	Recommendation
Any Left Main (LM)	>33	CABG
Any LM	<33	CABG or PCI

clinical risk predictors such as the Society for Thoracic Surgery (STS) score or EuroSCORE (Nilsson, Algotsson, Hoglund, Luhrs, & Brandt, 2004). Together, the team can integrate SYNTAX score, global surgical risk, comorbidities, and patient preference to arrive at an optimal means for revascularization.

Ultimately, the optimal revascularization technique for multi-vessel CAD depends more upon the complexity of disease than the number of stenosis. Three-vessel coronary artery disease (3VCAD) may be amenable to PCI if the overall anatomy is not markedly complex (SYNTAX score 0-22). However, those who underwent PCI with intermediate (22-32) or high (≥33) SYNTAX score have consistently shown worse outcomes (Mohr, et al., 2013). See Table 6 for a summary of recommendations in complex coronary disease, excluding left main disease.

The presence of unprotected left main coronary artery disease (ULMD) is defined as significant luminal stenosis without patent bypass grafts to its downstream branches. It is associated with high-mortality rates (up to 50% at 3 years) if not revascularized (Deb, et al., 2013). The decision of how best to revascularize ULMD is often not straightforward, but again depends on the overall complexity of coronary disease (See Table 7). Here the SYNTAX score threshold for obligatory CABG appears to be slightly higher than that seen in multi-vessel CAD: those with SYNTAX scores > 33 had worse outcomes with PCI (Mohr, et al., 2013).

In addition to left main disease and complex multi-vessel coronary disease, diabetes mellitus (DM) is a powerful factor in determining optimal revascularization technique. Those with diabetes and multivessel coronary disease have repeatedly shown better outcomes with CABG than with PCI, most recently in the FREEDOM study. All-cause mortality and composite cardiovascular outcomes were significantly lower in those who underwent CABG compared to PCI, though the PCI group did experience a lower risk of stroke (Farkouh, et al., 2011). Thus, in the absence of contraindications, current evidence favors CABG over PCI in stable patients with diabetes mellitus and multi-vessel CAD.

The presence of left ventricular dysfunction does not dramatically favor either CABG or PCI, as those with significant heart failure are often underrepresented in major revascularization trials. In the STITCH trial, patients with heart failure and CAD were randomized to either medical therapy or CABG. There was no difference in 5-year all-cause mortality, though those receiving CABG did have reduced incidence of cardiovascular-related death and hospitalization. Those with three-vessel CAD and LM or proximal LAD stenosis tended to do better with CABG (Velazquez, et al., 2011). While supporting a role for CABG in ischemic heart failure, the STITCH trial did not compare CABG and PCI. There is prospective registry data that seems to favor CABG over PCI in CAD and heart failure, but randomized trials are lacking (Nagendran, et al., 2013). However, one can reasonably conclude that greater complexity of coronary disease may favor CABG in patients with left ventricular dysfunction, as it does in the larger population.

In summary, the decision of whether to revascularize via PCI or CABG is often not straightforward. In such situations, the importance of a detailed discussion between patients and the heart team cannot be overemphasized. When angiography for UA/NSTEMI reveals multi-vessel disease, there is an obligation to pause and have a detailed discussion of risks and benefits of each proposed course of action. The presence of diabetes mellitus, complex multi-vessel coronary disease, and/or left main coronary artery disease should prompt serious consideration of CABG over PCI.

POST-MI CARE

Timely revascularization and appropriate medical therapy help minimize ischemia and prevent complications. The short-term sequelae of acute coronary syndrome are dependent upon the extent of myocardial necrosis and can often be anticipated in advance. Key diagnostic and management points are discussed here.

Ventricular Arrhythmias and Sudden Cardiac Death

Acute Management

Ischemic and/or scarred myocardium presents an excellent electrical substrate for life-threatening ventricular arrhythmias. Ventricular fibrillation (VF) and polymorphic ventricular tachycardia (VT) are commonly seen in the early post-MI period. Acutely, in addition to guideline-based antiarrhythmic treatment (including beta-blockers, if not contraindicated), or ACLS (as needed), it is essential to assess for recurrent ischemia, to correct any electrolyte abnormalities or metabolic acidosis, to remove non-essential arrhythmogenic agents such inotropes or vasopressors, and to reduce autonomic tone with pain control and sedation as necessary.

ICDs and Prevention of Sudden Cardiac Death

In the weeks and months following an acute MI, those with left ventricular dysfunction remain at particularly high risk for sustained VT, VF, and sudden cardiac death (SCD). Current guidelines give a class I indication to placement of an implantable cardioverter-defibrillator (ICD) in the post-MI period given the following conditions:

- Primary prevention of sudden cardiac death post-MI in patients with an ejection fraction less than 35% and New York Heart Association (NYHA) Class II-III functional status
- Primary prevention of sudden cardiac death post-MI in patients with an ejection fraction less than 30%, with NYHA Class I functional status.
- Secondary prevention of VT/VF post-MI with ejection fraction less than 40%

These recommendations are contingent upon a reasonable life expectancy (usually more than one year) and persistent left ventricular dysfunction despite optimal medical therapy for at least 40 days post-MI (Epstein, et al., 2013b).

Early ICD placement (i.e. less than 40 days post-MI) has not been demonstrated to be superior to standard medical therapy (Hohnloser, et al., 2004). In fact, despite a reduction in arrhythmic death, those with early ICD placement consistently experience an increase in non-arrhythmic cardiac death which negates the benefits of the ICD (Steinbeck, et al., 2009). Yet these patients remain at high risk for SCD, especially in the first month. It is often difficult to risk-stratify for SCD in the early post-MI period, and it is particularly difficult to predict who will not recover LV function and become ICD-eligible. Optimal management of patients in this 40-day window period remains controversial.

In addition to maximizing beta-blockade, a wearable cardioverter-defibrillator (WCD) may represent a safe, non-invasive means of protecting this population from SCD. While randomized trials are still needed, two retrospective trials suggest that WCDs can effectively treat ventricular arrhythmias in the early post-MI patient. In one large registry, the majority of shocks occurred within the first 30 days post-MI, 1.6% of all patients received appropriate shocks, and 1.1% received an inappropriate shock (Epstein, et al., 2013a). In another retrospective study of patients acutely revascularized post-MI, 1.3% of patients were appropriately shocked, and the use of a WCD was associated with reduced mortality compared to a matched registry (Zishiri, et al., 2013). A large prospective trial is currently underway, and cost-effectiveness studies are needed, but the current data suggests that there is a small but substantial subset (approximately 1-2%) of patients who receive life-saving therapy from WCDs.

Cardiogenic Shock and Intra-Aortic Balloon Counterpulsation

Acute infarction of a large amount of myocardium can lead to rapid decrease in cardiac output, tissue hypoperfusion, and end-organ damage. The presence of cardiogenic shock can worsen cardiac ischemia, leading to a deadly positive feedback loop. In addition to revascularization and inotropes, patients are often temporized with placement of an intra-aortic balloon pump (IABP). Rapidly implantable in the catheterization lab or even at the bedside, the IABP inflates in the descending aorta during diastole and deflates during systole to augment coronary perfusion pressure and decrease left ventricular afterload, respectively.

Registry data and older clinical trials suggest the IABP is both safe and effective, particularly post-PCI (Ohman, et al., 1994). However, recent clinical trials have cast doubt on its efficacy. The IABP SHOCK-II trial demonstrated no benefit in 30-day mortality between those receiving IABP versus standard therapy in cardiogenic shock post-MI (Thiele, et al., Intraaortic Balloon Support for Myocardial Infarction with Cardiogenic Shock, 2012). This was confirmed at 6 and 12 month follow-up (Thiele, et al., 2013). This trial generally included patients undergoing PCI with subsequent IABP placement, and had a very small number of surgical patients enrolled. Results may not be generalizable to those undergoing surgical revascularization or those with IABP for other indications such as ventricular arrhythmia or acute mitral valve dysfunction. Furthermore, many patients enrolled were concurrently receiving intravenous catecholamine support. This may have obscured the potential benefit of using IABPs as an alternative to catecholamines in the setting of cardiogenic shock post-MI. IABPs should be used with discretion and, like vasopressors and inotropes, with the understanding that they may not improve mortality. Cases of refractory cardiogenic shock may necessitate placement of temporary or durable ventricular assist devices, or in some cases, extracorporeal membrane oxygenation. These interventions are discussed in more depth elsewhere.

Conduction Blocks

Acute ischemia of the conduction system can lead to a variety of conduction blocks. The most dangerous are high-grade atrioventricular blocks resulting from infarction of His-Purkinje system tissue. Infarcts arising from the right coronary system are particularly high-risk for bradyarrhythmias. Presence of complete heart block, Mobitz II second degree heart block, or symptomatic bradycardia necessitate trans-venous pacemaker insertion.

Recurrent Ischemia

While improvements in medical therapy and revascularization techniques have decreased the incidence of reinfarction, any signs of recurrent angina after revascularization should prompt an expedient evaluation for signs of recurrent ischemia. Stent thrombosis can be a devastating early complication that must be recognized and treated emergently.

Mechanical Complications

Large areas of infarcted myocardium can result in loss of mechanical strength and structural breakdown of the heart. Ventricular septal rupture and papillary muscle rupture are surgical emergencies which can result in rapidly progressive congestive heart failure. Ventricular pseudoaneurysm or free wall rupture can result in cardiac tamponade and are immediately life-threatening. More chronically, ventricular aneurysms can result in ventricular thrombus and/or persistent ST-segment elevation on electrocardiogram.

Pericarditis

Post-MI pericarditis can be acute or chronic. Acute pericarditis is an extension of inflammation from the infarcted myocardium into the pericardium. The presence of a friction rub may help distinguish this pain from recurrent angina. In the weeks post-MI, an immune-related inflammatory response can also cause pericarditis (Dressler's syndrome). Both forms of pericarditis can be treated with colchicine or high-dose aspirin, in the absence of contraindications.

FUTURE RESEARCH DIRECTIONS

Advanced Imaging and Prevention

Intracoronary imaging is developing rapidly in hopes of improving upon the crude, stenosis-based risk stratification of angiographic lesions. Defining the composition of plaques, rather than just their shape, could lead to identification of high-risk or "vulnerable" plaques before they rupture, potentially preventing a large number of acute myocardial infarctions. At present, intravascular ultrasound (IVUS) and optical coherence tomography (OCT) are some of the leading invasive technologies able to define plaque composition. IVUS is particularly effective at determining plaque components and morphology, where OCT is able to very accurately measure the thickness of the fibrous cap (Moreno, 2010). Together with the rapidly expanding computer tomography angiography (CTA) of the coronaries, in the future it may be possible to fully define morphology and content of coronary plaques. Whether this will translate to actual prevention of coronary events remains to be seen. There is no convincing evidence to suggest that prophylactic stenting of vulnerable lesions will improve outcomes. The factors which lead to acute plaque rupture and thrombosis tend to be complex and systemic, and defy our simplistic notions of localized lesions. Accordingly, attention to risk factors and aggressive optimal medical therapy are the current therapy of choice for vulnerable lesions.

Ultimately, high-risk plaque features may best serve as warning signs and motivation to maximize medical therapy, rather than indication for prophylactic invasive treatment. In fact, a renewed emphasis on preventative care is growing in cardiology, and various forms of advanced imaging have been proposed as means of detecting high-risk coronary disease before it becomes an acute coronary syndrome. Non-invasive plaque detection, for example, of the coronaries, carotids, and superficial femoral artery (SFA) was recently shown to be a better predictor of coronary events than the Framingham Score (Fuster, 2013). Detection of global, systemic atherosclerotic disease may ultimately help detect high-risk individuals and serve as motivation to intensify lifestyle and medical therapy. This is emblematic of a gradual shift away from the search for a focal, "vulnerable plaque," to the more holistic identification of "the vulnerable patient."

Anti-Inflammatory Therapy

Increasing recognition of the centrality of inflammation in acute coronary syndrome has led to a renewed interest in the role of anti-inflammatory therapy in ACS. While glucocorticoids and non-steroidal anti-inflammatory drugs (NSAIDs) increase adverse outcomes, there are newly appreciated molecular targets which may represent targets of future therapy. Multi-protein complexes known as "inflammasomes" activate numerous pro-inflammatory pathways and appear to partially mediate ischemia and reperfusion injury in acute myocardial infarction. Efforts are underway to further elucidate the mechanisms and to examine whether targeted anti-inflammatory agents may improve outcomes in acute coronary syndromes (Takahashi, 2014). The new focus on inflammation is evident in the fact that colchicine, a drug in use for at least 2000 years, is now being re-examined as a potential adjunctive treatment for acute myocardial infarction.

Cell-Based Regenerative therapy ("Stem Cell Therapy")

In recent years, an increased understanding of stem and progenitor cell biology has led to hopes that intracoronary or intramyocardially administered cell therapy could lead to generation of viable cardiomyocytes. Potential regeneration of myocardium, rather than scar formation and myocardial fibrosis, would be a groundbreaking paradigm shift. However, multiple clinical trials in humans of intracoronary injection of autologous bone marrow mononuclear cells have shown only modest (5% or less) effects on left ventricular ejection fraction (LVEF), with minimal appreciable clinical benefit (de Jong, Houtgraff, Samiei, Boersma, & Duckers, 2014). Whether the cardiac environment post-MI is able to support differentiation to viable myocytes remains an open question. Advances in stem cell technology should allow for incremental improvements, but this is unlikely to become an effective treatment modality in the near future.

CONCLUSION

Acute coronary syndromes remain a tremendous source of morbidity and mortality. Early risk stratification is essential to individualizing medications and revascularization strategies in order to optimize outcomes. An ever-expanding arsenal of antiplatelet and antithrombotic drugs is at our disposal, in addition to progressively advanced techniques in revascularization. Along with novel therapeutic targets and agents, greater emphasis on prevention of acute coronary syndrome will likely be the focus of the future.

REFERENCES

Alexander, J., Lopes, R., James, S., Kilaru, R., He, Y., Mohan, P., & Atar, D. et al. (2011). Apixaban with Antiplatelet Therapy after Acute Coronary Syndrome. *The New England Journal of Medicine*, *365*(8), 699–708. doi:10.1056/NEJMoa1105819 PMID:21780946

American Heart Association. (2014). AHA Statistical Update: Heart Disease and Stroke Statistics - 2014 Update. *Circulation*, *129*, e28–e292. doi:10.1161/01.cir.0000441139.02102.80 PMID:24352519

Amin, S., Morrow, D., Braunwald, E., Sloan, S., Contant, C., Murphy, S., & Antman, E. (2013). Dynamic TIMI risk score for STEMI. *Journal of the American Heart Association*, *2*(1), e003269. doi:10.1161/JAHA.112.003269 PMID:23525425

Anderson, J., Adams, C., Antman, E., Bridges, C., Califf, R., Casey, D. E., & Wright, R. S. et al. (2007). ACC/AHA 2007 guidelines for the Management of Patients With Unstable Angina/Non-ST-Elevation Myocardial Infarction. *Circulation*, *116*(7), e148–e304. doi:10.1161/CIRCULATIONAHA.107.181940 PMID:17679616

Angiolillo, D., Firstenberg, M., Price, M., Tummala, P., Hutyra, M., Welsby, I., & Topol, E. et al. (2012). Bridging Antiplatelet Therapy With Cangrelor in Patients Undergoing Cardiac Surgery. *Journal of the American Medical Association*, *307*(3), 265–274. doi:10.1001/jama.2011.2002 PMID:22253393

Antman, E. M., Cohen, M., Bernink, P., McCabe, C. H., Horacek, T., Papuchis, G., & Braunwald, E. et al. (2000). The TIMI Risk Score for Unstable Angina / Non-ST Elevation MI. *Journal of the American Medical Association*, *284*(7), 835–842. doi:10.1001/jama.284.7.835 PMID:10938172

Ben Morrison, T., Horst, B., Brown, M., Bell, M., & Daniels, P. (2012). Bridging with glycoprotein IIb/IIIa inhibitors for periprocedural management of antiplatelet therapy in patients with drug eluting stents. *Catheterization and Cardiovascular Interventions*, *79*(4), 575–582. doi:10.1002/ccd.23172 PMID:22448399

Berger, J., Sallum, R., Katona, B., Maya, J., Ranganathan, G., Xu, Y., & Mwamburi, M. (2012). Is there an association between aspirin dosing and cardiac and bleeding events after treatment of acute coronary syndrome? A systematic review of the literature. *American Heart Journal*, *164*(2), 153–162. doi:10.1016/j.ahj.2012.04.001 PMID:22877800

Bhatt, D. L., Lincoff, A. M., Gibson, C. M., Stone, G. W., McNulty, S., Montalescot, G., & Mahaffey, K. W. et al. (2009). Intravenous platelet blockade with cangrelor during PCI. *The New England Journal of Medicine*, *361*(24), 2330–2341. doi:10.1056/NEJMoa0908629 PMID:19915222

Bhatt, D. L., Stone, G. W., Mahaffey, K. W., Gibson, C. M., Steg, P. G., Hamm, C. W., & Radke, P. W. et al. (2013). Effect of Platelet Inhibition with Cangrelor during PCI on Ischemic Events. *The New England Journal of Medicine*, *368*(14), 1303–1313. PMID:23473369

Boersma, E., Pieper, K. S., Steyerberg, E. W., Wilcox, R. G., Chang, W.-C., Lee, K. L., & Simoons, M. L. et al. (2000). Predictors of Outcome in Patients With Acute Coronary Syndromes Without Persistent ST-Segment Elevation. *Circulation*, *101*(22), 2557–2567. doi:10.1161/01.CIR.101.22.2557 PMID:10840005

Bybee, K. A., Powell, B. D., Valeti, U., Rosales, A. G., Kopecky, S. L., Mullany, C., & Wright, R. S. (2005). Preoperative Aspirin Therapy Is Associated With Improved Postoperative Outcomes in Patients Undergoing Coronary Artery Bypass Grafting. *Circulation*, *112*(9suppl), I-286–I292. PMID:16159833

Cannon, C. P., Braunwald, E., McCabe, C. H., Rader, D. J., Rouleau, J. L., Belder, R., & Skene, A. M. et al. (2004). Intensive versus Moderate Lipid Lowering with Statins after Acute Coronary Syndromes. *The New England Journal of Medicine*, *350*(15), 1495–1504. doi:10.1056/NEJMoa040583 PMID:15007110

Chatterjee, S., Chaudhuri, D., Vedanthan, R., Fuster, V., Ibanez, B., & Sripal Bangalore, D. M. (2013). Early intravenous beta-blockers in patients with acute coronary syndrome - A meta-analysis of randomized trials. *International Journal of Cardiology*, *168*(2), 915–921. doi:10.1016/j.ijcard.2012.10.050 PMID:23168009

Cuisset, T., Frere, C., Quilici, J., Morange, P.-E., Nait-Saidi, L., Carvajal, J., & Aless, M.-C. et al. (2006). Benefit of a 600-mg Loading Dose of Clopidogrel on Platelet Reactivity and Clinical Outcomes in Patients With Non–ST-Segment Elevation Acute Coronary Syndrome Undergoing Coronary Stenting. *Journal of the American College of Cardiology*, *48*(7), 1339–1345. doi:10.1016/j.jacc.2006.06.049 PMID:17010792

Cullen, L., Mueller, C., Parsonage, W., Wildi, K., Greenslade, J., Twerenbold, R., & Mosimann, T. et al. (2013). Validation of high-sensitivity troponin I in a 2-hour diagnostic strategy to assess 30-day outcomes in emergency department patients with possible acute coronary syndrome. *Journal of the American College of Cardiology*, *62*(14), 1242–1249. doi:10.1016/j.jacc.2013.02.078 PMID:23583250

de Jong, R., Houtgraff, J., Samiei, S., Boersma, E., & Duckers, H. (2014). Intracoronary stem cell infusion after acute myocardial infarction: A meta-analysis and update on clinical trials. *Circulation: Cardiovascular Interventions*, *7*(2), 156–167. doi:10.1161/CIRCINTERVENTIONS.113.001009 PMID:24668227

Deb, S., Wijeysunera, H. C., Ko, D. T., Tsubota, H., Hill, S., & Fremes, S. E. (2013). Coronary Artery Bypass Graft Surgery vs. Percutaneous Interventions in Coronary Revascularization: A Systematic Review. *Journal of the American Medical Association*, *310*(19), 2086–2095. doi:10.1001/jama.2013.281718 PMID:24240936

Dismore, J., & Dib, N. (2010). Stem Cell Therapy for the Treatment of Acute Myocardial Infarction. *Cardiology Clinics*, *28*(1), 127–138. doi:10.1016/j.ccl.2009.09.004 PMID:19962054

Eagle, K., Lim, M., Dabbous, O., Pieper, K., Goldberg, R., VandeWerf, F., & Fox, K. et al.for the GRACE Investigators. (2004). A Validated Prediction Model for All Forms of Acute Coronary Syndrome. *Journal of the American Medical Association*, *291*(22), 2727–2733. doi:10.1001/jama.291.22.2727 PMID:15187054

Epstein, A., Abraham, W., Bianco, N., Kern, K., Mirro, M., Rao, S., & Szymkiewicz, S. et al. (2013). Wearable Cardioverter-Defibrillator Use in Patients Perceived to Be at High Risk Early Post-Myocardial Infarction. *Journal of the American College of Cardiology*, *62*(21), 2000–2007. doi:10.1016/j.jacc.2013.05.086 PMID:23916930

Epstein, A., DiMarco, J., Ellenbogen, K., Estes, N., Freedman, R., Gettes, L., & Sweeney, M. et al. (2013). 2012 ACCF/AHA/HRS Focused Update Incorporated Into the ACCF/AHA/HRS 2008 Guidelines for Device-Based Therapy of Cardiac Rhythm Abnormalities. *Journal of the American College of Cardiology*, 6–e75. PMID:23265327

Farkouh, M., Domanski, M., Sleeper, L., Siami, F., Dangas, G., Mack, M., & Fuster, V. et al. (2011). Strategies for multivessel revascularization in patients with diabetes. *The New England Journal of Medicine*, *367*(25), 2375–2384. doi:10.1056/NEJMoa1211585 PMID:23121323

Fonarow, G. C., Wright, R. S., Spencer, F. A., Fredrick, P. D., Dong, W., Every, N., & French, W. J. (2005). Effect of statin use within the first 24 hours of admission for acute myocardial infarction on early morbidity and mortality. *The American Journal of Cardiology*, *96*(5), 611–616. doi:10.1016/j.amjcard.2005.04.029 PMID:16125480

Fuster, V. (2013). *Subclinical Athersclerotic Burden: High-Risk Population.* American College of Cardiology Scientific Sessions.

Giugliano, R., White, J., Bode, C., Armstrong, P., Montalescot, G., Lewis, B., & Newby, L. et al. (2009). Early versus Delayed, Provisional Eptifibatide in Acute Coronary Syndromes. *The New England Journal of Medicine*, *360*(21), 2176–2190. doi:10.1056/NEJMoa0901316 PMID:19332455

Gurbel, P. A., Bliden, K. P., Hayes, K. M., Yoho, J. A., Herzog, W. R., & Tantry, U. S. (2005). The Relation of Dosing to Clopidogrel Responsiveness and the Incidence of High Post-Treatment Platelet Aggregation in Patients Undergoing Coronary Stenting. *Journal of the American College of Cardiology*, *45*(9), 1392–1396. doi:10.1016/j.jacc.2005.01.030 PMID:15862408

Hansson, E. C., Rexius, H., Dellborg, M., Albertsson, P., & Jeppsson, A. (2014). Coronary artery bypass grafting-related bleeding complications in real-life acute coronary syndrome patients treated with clopidogrel or ticagrelor. *European Journal of Cardio-Thoracic Surgery*, *46*(4), 699–705. doi:10.1093/ejcts/ezt662 PMID:24482383

Harrington, R. A., Mc, G. W., Nulty, S., White, H. D., Lincoff, A. M., Gibson, C. M., & Kleiman, N. S. et al. (2009). Platelet inhibition with cangrelor in patients undergoing PCI. *The New England Journal of Medicine*, *361*(24), 2318–2329. doi:10.1056/NEJMoa0908628 PMID:19915221

Hillis, L., Smith, P., Anderson, J., Bittl, J., Bridges, C., Byrne, J., & Puskas, J. et al. (2011). 2011 ACCF/AHA guideline for Coronary Artery Bypass Graft Surgery. *Circulation*, *124*(23), e652–e735. doi:10.1161/CIR.0b013e31823c074e PMID:22064599

Hochman, J., Sleeper, L., Webb, J., Sanborn, T., White, H., Talley, J., & LeJemtel, T. et al. (1999). Early Revascularization in Acute Myocardial Infarction Complicated by Cardiogenic Shock. *The New England Journal of Medicine*, *341*(9), 625–634. doi:10.1056/NEJM199908263410901 PMID:10460813

Hohnloser, S., Kuck, K., Dorian, P., Roberts, R., Hampton, J., Hatala, R., & Connoly, S. et al. (2004). Prophylactic use of an implantable cardioverter-defibrillator after acute myocardial infarction. *The New England Journal of Medicine*, *351*(24), 2481–2488. doi:10.1056/NEJMoa041489 PMID:15590950

Ibanez, B., Macaya, C., Sánchez-Brunete, V., Pizarro, G., Fernández-Friera, L., Mateos, A., & Fuster, V. et al. (2013). Effect of Early Metoprolol on Infarct Size in ST-Segment-Elevation Myocardial Infarction Patients Undergoing Primary Percutaneous Coronary Intervention. *Circulation*, *128*(14), 1495–1503. doi:10.1161/CIRCULATIONAHA.113.003653 PMID:24002794

Jia, H., Abtahian, F., Aguirre, A., Lee, S., Chia, S., Lowe, H., & Jang, I. et al. (2013). In Vivo Diagnosis of Plaque Erosion and Calcified Nodule in Patients With Acute Coronary Syndrome by Intravascular Optical Coherence Tomography. *Journal of the American College of Cardiology*, *62*(19), 1748–1758. doi:10.1016/j.jacc.2013.05.071 PMID:23810884

Kaul, P., Newby, L. K., Fu, Y., Hasselblad, V., Mahaffey, K., Christenson, R., & Armstrong, P. et al. (2003). Troponin T and Quantitative ST-Segment Depression Offer Complementary Prognostic Information in the Risk Stratification of Acute Coronary Syndrome Patients. *Journal of the American College of Cardiology*, *41*(3), 371–380. doi:10.1016/S0735-1097(02)02824-3 PMID:12575962

Khot, U., Jia, G., Moliterno, D., Lincoff, A., Khot, M., Harrington, R., & Topol, E. (2003). Prognostic Importance of Physical Examination for Heart Failure in Non–ST-Elevation Acute Coronary Syndromes. *Journal of the American Medical Association*, *290*(16), 2174–2181. doi:10.1001/jama.290.16.2174 PMID:14570953

Libby, P. (2013). Mechanisms of Acute Coronary Syndromes and Their Implications for Therapy. *The New England Journal of Medicine*, *368*(21), 2004–2013. doi:10.1056/NEJMra1216063 PMID:23697515

Magee, K., Campbell, S. G., Moher, D., & Rowe, B. H. (2008). Heparin versus placebo for acute coronary syndromes. *Cochrane Database of Systematic Reviews*, CD003462. PMID:18425889

Mahaffey, K. W., Wojdyla, D. M., Carroll, K., Becker, R. C., Storey, R. F., Angiolillo, D. J., & Wallentin, L. et al. (2011). Ticagrelor Compared With Clopidogrel by Geographic Region in the Platelet Inhibition and Patient Outcomes (PLATO) Trial. *Circulation*, *124*(5), 544–554. doi:10.1161/CIRCULATIONAHA.111.047498 PMID:21709065

McGovern, P. G., Jacobs, D. R. Jr, Shahar, E., Arnett, D. K., Folsom, A. R., Blackburn, H., & Luepker, R. (2001). Trends in Acute Coronary Heart Disease Mortality, Morbidity, and Medical Care From 1985 Through 1997. *Circulation*, *104*(1), 19–24. doi:10.1161/01.CIR.104.1.19 PMID:11435332

Mega, J. L., Braunwald, E., Wiviott, S. D., Bassand, J.-P., Bhatt, D. L., Bode, C., & Sun, X. et al. (2012). Rivaroxaban in Patients with a Recent Acute Coronary Syndrome. *The New England Journal of Medicine*, *366*(1), 9–19. doi:10.1056/NEJMoa1112277 PMID:22077192

Mehta, S., Tanguay, J.-F., Eikelboom, J. W., Jolly, S. S., Joyner, C. D., Granger, C. B., & Yusuf, S. et al. (2010). Double-dose versus standard-dose clopidogrel and high-dose versus low-dose aspirin in individuals undergoing percutaneous coronary intervention for acute coronary syndromes (CURRENT-OASIS 7): A randomised factorial trial. *Lancet*, *376*(9748), 1233–1243. doi:10.1016/S0140-6736(10)61088-4 PMID:20817281

Mohr, F. W., Morice, M.-C., Keppetein, A. P., Feldman, T. E., Stahle, E., Colombo, A., & Serruys, P. W. et al. (2013). Coronary artery bypass graft surgery versus percutaneous coronary intevention in patients with three-vessel disease and lef tmain cornoary disease: 5 -year follow-up of the randomised, clinical SYNTAX trial. *Lancet*, *381*(9748), 629–638. PMID:23439102

Moreno, P. R. (2010). Vulnerable Plaque: Definition, Diagnosis, and Treatment. *Cardiology Clinics*, *28*(1), 1–30. doi:10.1016/j.ccl.2009.09.008 PMID:19962047

Morrow, D., Cannon, C., Rifai, N., Frey, M., Vicari, N., Lakkis, N., & Braunwald, E. et al. (2001). Ability of minor elevations of troponins I and T to predict benefit from an early invasive strategy in patients with unstable angina and non-ST elevation myocardial infarction: Results from a randomized trial. *Journal of the American Medical Association*, *286*(19), 2405–2412. doi:10.1001/jama.286.19.2405 PMID:11712935

Mueller, C., Neumann, F.-J., Perach, W., Perruchoud, A., & Buettner, H. (2004). Prognostic value of the admission electrocardiogram in patients with unstable angina/non–ST-segment elevation myocardial infarction treated with very early revascularization. *The American Journal of Medicine*, *117*(3), 145–150. doi:10.1016/j.amjmed.2004.02.034 PMID:15276591

Nagendran, J., Norris, C. M., Graham, M. M., Ross, D. B., MacArthur, R. G., Kieser, T. M., & Meyer, S. R. et al. (2013). Coronary Revascularization for Patients With Severe Left Ventricular Dysfunction. *The Annals of Thoracic Surgery*, *96*(6), 2038–2044. doi:10.1016/j.athoracsur.2013.06.052 PMID:23968761

Nijjer, S., Watson, G., Athanasiou, T., & Malik, I. (2011). Safety of clopidogrel being continued until the time of coronary artery bypass grafting in patients with acute coronary sundrome: A meta-analysis of 34 studies. *European Heart Journal*, *32*(23), 2970–2988. doi:10.1093/eurheartj/ehr151 PMID:21609973

Nilsson, J., Algotsson, L., Hoglund, P., Luhrs, C., & Brandt, J. (2004). Early mortality in coronary bypass surgery: The EuroSCORE versus The Society of Thoracic Surgeons risk algorithm. *The Annals of Thoracic Surgery*, *77*(4), 1235–1239. doi:10.1016/j.athoracsur.2003.08.034 PMID:15063242

O'Gara, P., Kushner, F. G., Ascheim, D. D., Casey, D. E., Chung, M. K., Lemos, J. A., & Zhao, D. et al. (2013). 2013 ACCF/AHA Guideline for the Management of ST-Elevation Myocardial Infarction. *Journal of the American College of Cardiology*, *61*(4), e78–e140. doi:10.1016/j.jacc.2012.11.019 PMID:23256914

Ohman, E. M., George, B. S., White, C. J., Kern, M. J., Gurbel, P. A., Freedman, R. J., & Frey, M. J. et al.The Randomized IABP Study Group. (1994). Use of Aortic Counterpulsation to Improve Sustained Coronary Artery Patency During Acute Myocardial Infarction. *Circulation*, *90*(2), 792–799. doi:10.1161/01.CIR.90.2.792 PMID:8044950

Oldgren, J., Budaj, A., Granger, C. B., Khder, Y., Roberts, J., Siegbahn, A., & Frans Van de Werf, L. W. et al. (2011). Dabigatran vs. placebo in patietns with acute coronary syndromes on dual antiplatelet therapy: A randomized, double-blind, phase II trial. *European Heart Journal*, *32*(22), 2781–2789. doi:10.1093/eurheartj/ehr113 PMID:21551462

Pitt, B., Remme, W., Zannad, F., Neaton, J., Martinez, F., Roniker, B., & Gatlin, M. et al. (2003). Eplerenone, a Selective Aldosterone Blocker, in Patients with Left Ventricle Dysfunction after Myocardial Infarction. *The New England Journal of Medicine*, *348*(14), 1309–1321. doi:10.1056/NEJMoa030207 PMID:12668699

RISC Group. (1990). Risk of myocardial infarction and death during treatment with low dose aspirin and intravenous heparin in men with unstable coronary artery disease. *Lancet*, *336*(8719), 827–830. doi:10.1016/0140-6736(90)92336-G PMID:1976875

Schulz, S., Kastrati, A., Ferenc, M., Massberg, S., Birkmeier, K., Laugwitz, K., & Neumann, F. et al. (2013). One-year outcomes with abciximab and unfractionated heparin versus bivalirudin during percutaneous coronary interventions in patients with non-ST-segment elevation myocardial infarction: Updated results from the ISAR-REACT 4 trial. *EuroIntervention*, *9*(4), 430–436. doi:10.4244/EIJV9I4A71 PMID:23455033

Serruys, P. W., Morice, M.-C., Keppetein, A. P., Colombo, A., Holmes, D. R., Mack, M. J., & Mohr, F. et al. (2009). Percutaneous Coronary Intervention versus Coronary-Artery Bypass Grafting for Severe Coronary Artery Disease. *The New England Journal of Medicine*, *360*(10), 961–972. doi:10.1056/NEJMoa0804626 PMID:19228612

Shahzad, A., & Stables, R. (2014). *HEAT PPCI: How Effective are Antithrombotic Therapies in PPCI.* American College of Cardiology Scientific Sessions.

Singh, D., Gupta, K., & Vacek, J. L. (2014). Anticoagulation and antiplatelet therapy in acute coronary syndromes. *Cleveland Clinic Journal of Medicine*, *81*(2), 103–114. doi:10.3949/ccjm.81a.13016 PMID:24493493

Smith, P. K., Goodnough, L. T., Levy, J. H., Poston, R. S., Short, M. A., Weerakkody, G. J., & LeNarz, L. A. (2012). Mortality Benefit With Prasugrel in the TRITON-TIMI 38 Coronary Artery Bypass Grafting Cohort: Risk-Adjusted Retrospective Data Analysis. *Journal of the American College of Cardiology*, *60*(5), 388–396. doi:10.1016/j.jacc.2012.03.030 PMID:22633653

Steg, P., van'tHof, A., Hamm, C., Clemmensen, P., Lapostelle, F., Coste, P., & Goldstein, P. et al. (2013). Bivalirudin Started during Emergency Transport for Primary PCI. *The New England Journal of Medicine*, *369*(23), 2207–2217. doi:10.1056/NEJMoa1311096 PMID:24171490

Steinbeck, G., Andrensen, D., Seidl, K., Brachmann, J., Hoffman, E., Wojciechowski, D., & Senges, J. et al. (2009). Defibrillator Implantation Early after Myocardial Infarction. *The New England Journal of Medicine*, *361*(15), 1427–1436. doi:10.1056/NEJMoa0901889 PMID:19812399

Sun, J., Whitlock, R., Cheng, J., Eikelboom, J., Thabane, L., Crowther, M., & Teoh, K. (2008). The effect of pre-operative aspirin on bleeding, transfusion, myocardial infarction, and mortality in coronary artery bypass surgery: A systematic review of randomized and observational studies. *European Heart Journal*, *29*(8), 1057–1071. doi:10.1093/eurheartj/ehn104 PMID:18346962

Takahashi, M. (2014). NLRP3 Inflammasome as a Novel Player in Myocardial Infarction. *International Heart Journal*, *55*(2), 101–105. doi:10.1536/ihj.13-388 PMID:24632952

The Clopidogrel in Unstable Angina to Prevent Recurrent Events Trial Investigators. (2001). Effects of Clopidogrel in Addition to Aspirin in Patients with Acute Coronary Syndromes without ST-Segment Elevation. *The New England Journal of Medicine*, *345*(7), 494–502. doi:10.1056/NEJMoa010746 PMID:11519503

Thiele, H., Zeymer, U., Neumann, F.-J., Ferenc, M., Olbrich, H.-G., Hausleiter, J., & Schuler, G. et al. (2013). Intra-aortic balloon counterpulsation in acute myocardial infarction complicated by cardiogenic shock (IABP-SHOCK II): Final 12 month results of a randomised, open-label trial. *Lancet*, *382*(9905), 1638–1645. doi:10.1016/S0140-6736(13)61783-3 PMID:24011548

Thiele, H., Zeymer, U., Neumann, F.-J., Ferenc, M., Olbrich, H.-G., Hausleiter, J., & Werdan, K. et al. (2012). Intraaortic Balloon Support for Myocardial Infarction with Cardiogenic Shock. *The New England Journal of Medicine*, *367*(14), 1287–1296. doi:10.1056/NEJMoa1208410 PMID:22920912

Varenhorst, C., Alstrom, U., Scirica, B., Hogue, C., Asenblad, N., Storey, R., & Held, C. et al. (2012). Factors Contributing to the Lower Mortality With Ticagrelor Compared with Clopidogrel in Patients Undergoing Coronary Artery Bypass Surgery. *Journal of the American College of Cardiology*, *60*(17), 1623–20. PMID:23021325

Velazquez, E. J., Lee, K. L., Deja, M. A., Jain, A., Sopko, G., Marchenko, A., & Rouleau, J. et al. (2011). Coronary-Artery Bypass Surgery in Patients with Left Ventricular Dysfunction. *The New England Journal of Medicine*, *364*(17), 1607–1616. doi:10.1056/NEJMoa1100356 PMID:21463150

Wallentin, L., Becker, R. C., Budaj, A., Cannon, C. P., Emanuelsson, H., Held, C., & Harrington, R. A. et al. (2009). Ticagrelor versus Clopidogrel in Patients with Acute Coronary Syndromes. *The New England Journal of Medicine*, *361*(11), 1045–1057. doi:10.1056/NEJMoa0904327 PMID:19717846

White, H., Assmann, S. F., Sanborn, T. A., Jacobs, A. K., Webb, J. G., Sleeper, L. A., & Hochman, J. S. et al. (2005). Comparison of Percutaneous Coronary Intervention and Coronary Artery Bypass Graft After Acute Myocardial Infarction Complicated by Cardiogenic Shock. *Circulation*, *112*(13), 1992–2001. doi:10.1161/CIRCULATIONAHA.105.540948 PMID:16186436

Wiviott, S., Braunwald, E., McCabe, C., Montalescot, G., Ruzyllo, W., Gottlieb, S., & Antman, E. et al. (2007). Prasugrel versus clopidogrel in patients with acute coronary syndromes. *The New England Journal of Medicine*, *357*(20), 2001–2015. doi:10.1056/NEJMoa0706482 PMID:17982182

Wright, R. S., Anderson, J. L., Adams, C. D., Bridges, C. R., Casey, D. E. Jr, Ettinger, S. M., & Zidar, J. P. et al. (2011). ACCF/AHA Focused Update of the Guidelines for the Management of Patients With Unstable Angina/Non–ST-Elevation Myocardial Infarction (Updating the 2007 Guideline). *Journal of the American College of Cardiology*, *57*(19), 1920–1959. doi:10.1016/j.jacc.2011.02.009 PMID:21450428

Zishiri, E., William, S., Cronin, E., Blackstone, E., Ellis, S., Roselli, E., & Chung, M. et al. (2013). Early Risk of Mortaliy After Coronary Artery Revascularization in Patients with Left Ventricular Dysfunction and Potential Role of the Wearable Cardioverter Defibrillator. *Circulation: Arrhythmia and Electrophysiology*, *6*(1), 117–128. doi:10.1161/CIRCEP.112.973552 PMID:23275233

ADDITIONAL READING

Ahrens, I., Bode, C., & Zirlik, A. (2014). Anticoagulation during and after acute coronary syndrome. *Hamostaseologie*, *34*(1), 72–77. doi:10.5482/HAMO-13-09-0048 PMID:24337310

Alexopoulos, G., Galati, A., Xanthopoulou, I., Mavronasiou, E., Kassimis, G., Theodoropoulos, K. C., & Davlouros, P. et al. (2012). Ticagrelor versus prasugrel in acute coronary syndrome patients with high on-clopidogrel platelet reactivity following percutaneous coronary intervention: A pharmacodynamics study. *Journal of the American College of Cardiology*, *60*(3), 193–199. doi:10.1016/j.jacc.2012.03.050 PMID:22789884

Bandstein, N., Ljung, R., Johansson, M., Holzmann, M.J. (2014). Undetectable High Sensitivity Cardiac Troponin T Level in the Emergency Department and Risk of Myocardial Infarction. *Journal of the American College of Cardiology, doi: . Journal of the American College of Cardiology.2014.03.017*10.1016/j

Berger, J. S. (2013). Aspirin, clopidogrel, and ticagrelor in acute coronary syndromes. *The American Journal of Cardiology*, *112*(5), 737–745. doi:10.1016/j.amjcard.2013.04.055 PMID:23751937

Birnbaum, Y., Wilson, J. M., Fiol, M., de Luna, A. B., Eskola, M., & Nikus, K. (2014). ECG Diagnosis and Classification of Acute Coronary Syndrome. *Annals of Non-Invasive Electrocardiography*, *19*(1), 4–14. doi:10.1111/anec.12130 PMID:24382164

Boersma, E., Pieper, K. S., Steyerberg, E. W., Wilcox, R. G., Chang, W.-C., Lee, K. L., & Simoons, M. L. et al. (2000). Predictors of Outcome in Patients With Acute Coronary Syndromes Without Persistent ST-Segment Elevation. *Circulation*, *101*(22), 2557–2567. doi:10.1161/01.CIR.101.22.2557 PMID:10840005

Bonello, L., Laine, M., Kipson, N., Mancini, J., Helal, O., Fromonot, J., & Guieu, R. et al. (2014). Ticagrelor increases adenosine plasma concentration in patients with an acute coronary syndrome. *Journal of the American College of Cardiology*, *63*(9), 872–877. doi:10.1016/j.jacc.2013.09.067 PMID:24291273

Christiansen, S., & Autschbach, R. (2010). Results and treatment strategy for patients undergoing emergent coronary artery bypass grafting. *Annals of Thoracic and Cardiovascular Surgery*, *16*(3), 168–173. PMID:20930677

Chung, M. K. (2014). The Role of the Wearable Cardioverter-Defibrillator in Clinical Practice. *Cardiology Clinics*, *32*(2), 253–270. doi:10.1016/j.ccl.2013.11.002 PMID:24793801

Cuisset, T., Frere, C., Quilici, J., Morange, P.-E., Nait-Saidi, L., Carvajal, J., & Aless, M.-C. et al. (2006). Benefit of a 600-mg Loading Dose of Clopidogrel on Platelet Reactivity and Clinical Outcomes in Patients With Non–ST-Segment Elevation Acute Coronary Syndrome Undergoing Coronary Stenting. *Journal of the American College of Cardiology*, *48*(7), 1339–1345. doi:10.1016/j.jacc.2006.06.049 PMID:17010792

Dominguez-Rodriguez, A., Abreu-Gonzalez, P., & Reiter, R. J. (2014). Cardioprotection and pharmacological therapies in acute myocardial infarction: Challenges in the current era. *World Journal of Cardiology*, *6*(3), 100–106. doi:10.4330/wjc.v6.i3.100 PMID:24669291

Everett, B., Pradhan, A. D., Solomon, D. H., Paynter, N., MacFadyen, J., Zaharris, E., & Ridker, P. M. et al. (2013). Rationale and design of the Cardiovascular Inflammation Reduction Trial: A test of the inflammatory hypothesis of atherothrombosis. *American Heart Journal*, *2*(166), 199–207.e15. doi:10.1016/j.ahj.2013.03.018 PMID:23895801

Feldman, T. (2009). The SYNTAX Score in Practice: An Aid for Patient Selection for Complex PCI. *Catheterization and Cardiovascular Interventions*, *73*(5), 618–619. doi:10.1002/ccd.22043 PMID:19309708

Firstenburg, M., Dyke, C. M., Angiolillo, A., Ramaiahm, C., Price, M., Brtko, M., & Topol, E. J. et al. (2013). Safety and efficacy of cangrelor, an intravenous, short-acting platelet inhibitor in patients requiring coronary artery bypass surgery. *The Heart Surgery Forum*, *16*(2), E60–E69. doi:10.1532/HSF98.20121103 PMID:23625478

Fujii, K., Hao, H., Ohyanagi, M., & Masuyama, T. (2013). Intracoronary Imaging for Detecting Vulnerable Plaque. *Circulation Journal*, *77*(3), 588–595. doi:10.1253/circj.CJ-12-1599 PMID:23370454

Kolte, D., Khera, S., Aronow, W. S., Mujib, M., Palaniswamy, C., Sule, S., & Fonarow, G. C. et al. (2014). Trends in incidence, management, and outcomes of cardiogenic shock complicating ST-elevation myocardial infarction in the United States. *Journal of the American Heart Association*, *3*(1), e000590. doi:10.1161/JAHA.113.000590 PMID:24419737

Mylotte, D., Morice, M. C., Eltchaninoff, H., Garot, L., Louvard, Y., Lefevre, T., & Garot, P. (2013). Primary percutaneous coronary intervention in patients with acute myocardial infarction, resuscitated cardiac arrest, and cardiogenic shock: The role of primary multivessel revascularization. *Journal of the American College of Cardiology: Cardiovascular Interventions*, *2*(6), 115–125. PMID:23352816

Oldgren, J., Wallentin, L., Alexander, J. H., James, S., Jonelid, B., Steg, G., & Sundstrom, J. (2013). New oral anticoagulations in addition to single or dual antiplatelet therapy after an acute coronary syndrome: A systematic review and meta-analysis. *European Heart Journal*, *34*(22), 1670–1680. doi:10.1093/eurheartj/eht049 PMID:23470494

Patel, M. R., Dehmer, G. J., Hirshfeld, J. W., Smith, P. K., & Spertus, J. A. (2012). 2012 Appropriate Use Criteria for Coronary Revascularization Focused Update. *Journal of the American College of Cardiology*, *59*(9), 857–881. doi:10.1016/j.jacc.2011.12.001 PMID:22296741

Perrier, S., Kindo, M., Gerelli, S., & Mazzucotelli, J. (2013). Coronary artery bypass grafting or percutaneous revascularization in acute myocardial infarction? *Interactive Cardiovascular and Thoracic Surgery*, *17*(6), 1015–1019. doi:10.1093/icvts/ivt381 PMID:23962854

Pickett, A. M., Taylor, D. A., & Ackman, M. L. (2010). Prolonged infusion of eptifibatide as bridge therapy between bare-metal stent insertion and cardiovascular surgery: Case report and review of the literature. *Pharmacotherapy*, *30*(4), 127e–133e. doi:10.1592/phco.30.4.420 PMID:20334463

Ridker, P. M., Thuren, T., Zalewski, A., & Libby, P. (2011). Interleukin-1β inhibition and the prevention of recurrent cardiovascular events: Rationale and Design of the Canakinumab Anti-inflammatory Thrombosis Outcomes Study (CANTOS). *American Heart Journal*, *4*(162), 597–605. doi:10.1016/j.ahj.2011.06.012 PMID:21982649

Sanidas, E., & Dangas, G. (2013). Evolution of intravascular assessment of coronary anatomy and physiology: From ultrasound imaging to optical and flow assessment. *European Journal of Clinical Investigation*, *43*(9), 996–1008. doi:10.1111/eci.12119 PMID:23827051

Serebruany, V. L., Sibbing, D., & DiNicolantonio, J. J. (2014). Dyspnea and reversibility of antiplatelet agents: Ticagrelor, elinogrel, cangrelor, and beyond. *Cardiology*, *127*(1), 20–24. doi:10.1159/000354876 PMID:24192670

Shahzad, A., Cooper, R. M., & Stables, R. H. (2013). Antithrombotic therapy in PCI: Why not heparin? *EuroIntervention*, *9*(4), 423–426. doi:10.4244/EIJV9I4A69 PMID:23965346

Smith, P. K. (2009). Treatment Selection for coronary artery disease: The collision of a belief system with evidence. *The Journal of Thoracic and Cardiovascular Surgery*, *137*(5), 1050–1053. doi:10.1016/j.jtcvs.2009.03.043 PMID:19379965

Stone, G. W., Witzenbichler, B., Guagliumi, G., Peruga, J. Z., Brodie, B. R., Dudek, D., & Mehran, R. et al. (2008). Bivalirudin during primary PCI in acute myocardial infarction. *The New England Journal of Medicine*, *358*(21), 2218–2230. doi:10.1056/NEJMoa0708191 PMID:18499566

Storey, RF. (2009). Pharmacology and clinical trials of reversibly-binding P2Y12 inhibitors. *Thrombosis and Haemostasis*, *105*(Suppl 1), S75-S81.

Tamis-Holland, J. E., & O'Gara, P. (2014). Highlights From the 2013 ACCF/AHA Guidelines for the Management of ST-Elevation Myocardial Infarction and Beyond. *Clinical Cardiology*, *4*(37), 252–259. doi:10.1002/clc.22258 PMID:24523153

Thompson, P. L., Nidorf, S. M., & Eikelboom, J. (2013). Targeting the Unstable Plaque in Acute Coronary Syndromes. *Clinical Therapeutics*, *8*(35), 1099–1107. doi:10.1016/j.clinthera.2013.07.332 PMID:23973042

Trenk, D., Stone, G. W., Gawaz, M., Kastrati, A., Angiolillo, D. J., Muller, U., & Neumann, F. J. et al. (2012). A randomized trial of prasugrel versus clopidogrel in patients with high platelet reactivity on clopidogrel after elective percutaneous coronary intervention with implantation of drug-eluting stents: Results of the TRIGGER-PCI (Testing Platelet Reactiivity In Patients Undergoing Elective Stent Placement on Clopoidogrel to Guide Alternative Therapy With Prasugrel) study. *Journal of the American College of Cardiology*, *59*(24), 2159–2164. doi:10.1016/j.jacc.2012.02.026 PMID:22520250

Zei, P. C. (2013). Is the Wearable Cardioverter-Defibrillator the Answer for Early Post-Myocardial Infarction Patients at Risk for Sudden Death? Mind the Gap. *Journal of the American College of Cardiology*, *62*(21), 2008–2009. doi:10.1016/j.jacc.2013.07.022 PMID:23916931

KEY TERMS AND DEFINITIONS

Early Invasive Strategy: An approach to treatment of acute coronary syndrome which favors early angiography and revascularization; tends to be most appropriate in higher-risk patients.

Killip Score: A prognostic score for acute coronary syndrome based on signs and symptoms of acute heart failure.

NSTEMI: Non-ST elevation myocardial infarction, resulting from subtotal coronary occlusion and ischemia.

Stem Cells: pluripotent cells which can be delivered to the coronaries in hopes that they will differentiate into cardiomyocytes, facilitating myocardial regeneration.

STEMI: ST elevation myocardial infarction, resulting from sudden, complete coronary occlusion, and corresponding to transmural infarction.

SYNTAX Score: A way to quantitate complexity of coronary anatomy which has been shown to predict sub-optimal outcomes in PCI; can help guide decision between CABG and PCI.

TIMI Score: A prognostic score for acute coronary syndrome based on historical points, ECG, and biomarkers.

Vulnerable Plaque: An atherosclerotic plaque which is prone to rupture, characterized by high lipid burden, a thin fibrous cap, and significant inflammatory burden.

Chapter 8
Valvular Heart Disease

Christine M. Lennon
Weill Cornell Medical Center, USA

Alexander C. P. Fort
Weill Cornell Medical Center, USA

Shawn Hansberry
Weill Cornell Medical Center, USA

ABSTRACT

Valvular heart disease is a common cardiovascular disorder, with an estimated prevalence of 2.5% in the United States. The disease is particularly burdensome in adults over 75 years of age, with 13.3% having moderate to severe disease of the aortic or mitral valve. As populations grow older, diagnostic capabilities improve, and health care becomes more accessible, the number of patients with valvular heart disease undergoing both cardiac and non-cardiac surgery will continue to grow. The preoperative assessment and optimization of these patients is a complex task involving multiple specialists, including internists, cardiologists, intensivists, cardiothoracic surgeons, and anesthesiologists. As newer therapeutic options are offered to patients with numerous comorbidities, the preoperative management of these patients will require a sophisticated multimodal approach. The purpose of this chapter is to summarize the preoperative assessment and optimization of patients with valvular heart disease undergoing cardiac and non-cardiac surgery.

INTRODUCTION

The modern cardiothoracic intensive care unit is a dynamic place. As the scope of cardiothoracic surgery has expanded over the last century, specialists with a specific understanding of complex cardiac anatomy, physiology, and cardiovascular imaging have been needed to manage these patients perioperatively. With the arrival of endovascular approaches to the treatment of major vascular and cardiac pathology, the patient populations served in these intensive care units have changed dramatically. These technological advances have allowed higher-risk and elderly patients to undergo procedures they otherwise would not be candidates for via traditional open approaches.

DOI: 10.4018/978-1-4666-8603-8.ch008

Over the last decade, the population characteristics of cardiothoracic patients and the landscape of cardiac procedures have changed. For example, a Canadian study by Buth et al. reviewed all adult patients undergoing cardiac surgery at a single cardiothoracic surgical center between 2001 and 2010. Over the study period, annual case volume decreased by 13%, with a drop in isolated CABG rates, an increase in isolated valve procedures, and an increase in other cardiac procedures including combined valvular and non-CABG procedures, open aortic surgery, and ventricular assist device insertion (Buth, Gainer, Legare, & Hirsch, 2014). Valvular surgery is a growing field, and a thorough understanding of structural anatomy, hemodynamic perturbations, and co-morbidities must be understood to manage these complex patients.

BACKGROUND

The preoperative assessment of patients with valvular heart disease is vital to anesthetic and surgical planning. General principles include a thorough evaluation of the severity of valvular disease, the degree of impaired myocardial function, and associated comorbidities. The preoperative assessment should start with a thorough history and physical. The history should focus on functional capacity, cardiac reserve, symptoms of congestive heart failure, and symptoms of coronary ischemia. On physical exam, congestive heart failure is evidenced by jugular venous distension, peripheral edema, third and fourth heart sounds, crackles, and rales. Every patient should receive an electrocardiogram (EKG) and chest radiograph (CXR) as part of the preoperative workup. A complete transthoracic echocardiogram (TTE) is indicated in all patients with suspected valvular disease, and periodic repeat studies are indicated at intervals dependent on the type and severity of valvular disease. Based on findings in the aforementioned tests, advanced testing can be performed, which may include transesophageal echocardiography (TEE), three dimensional echocardiography, cardiac catherization, stress testing, cardiac magnetic resonance imaging (CMR), and computed tomography (CT).

In 2014 the ACC/AHA published a new classification system for valvular heart disease (VHD). This new system is similar to the staging system for heart failure that was published by the AHA/ACC in 2013, and is based upon four stages of disease progression. Table 1 describes these four stages (Nishimura et al., 2014).

Table 1. Stages of Progression of VHD

Stage	Definition	Description
A	At risk	Patients with risk factors for development of VHD
B	Progressive	Patients with progressive VHD (mild-to-moderate severity and asymptomatic
C	Asymptomatic severe	Asymptomatic patients who have the criteria for severe VHD: C1: Asymptomatic patients with severe VHD in whom the left or right ventricle remains compensated C2: Asymptomatic patients with severe VHD, with decompensation of the left or right ventricle
D	Symptomatic severe	Patients who have developed symptoms as a result of VHD

Table taken from 2014 ACC/AHA Valvular Heart Disease Guidelines (Nishimura et al., 2014).
VHD indicates valvular heart disease.

Optimization of patients with valvular heart disease continues to be a controversial topic. There still exists conflicting evidence regarding the use of medical management in valvular heart disease, especially related to beta-blockers and statins. Optimization is highly dependent on the type of valvular lesion, the planned surgery, and any comorbidities. A prospective single-center study of 3826 patients undergoing cardiac surgery showed that frailty was a risk factor for postoperative complications and an independent predictor of in-hospital mortality, institutional discharge, and reduced midterm survival (Lee, Buth, Martin, Yip, & Hirsch, 2010). Recent literature also suggests that this elderly population might be more prone to the psychological stresses of cardiac surgery. A prospective multicenter cohort study by Williams et al. examined preoperative anxiety and depression in 148 patients over 70 years of age undergoing major cardiac surgery. Although only 7% patients reported high levels of anxiety, the study found that anxiety remained an independent predictor of postoperative mortality or major morbidity (Williams et al., 2013).

The 2014 AHA/ACC guidelines present a novel approach to assessment and therapeutic planning for patients with valvular heart disease with their recommendations for a "Heart Valve Team" and "Heart Valve Centers of Excellence." This team, comprised of a cardiologist and surgeon as well as an interventionalist, anesthesiologist, and imaging specialist for complex cases, would serve to provide thorough planning for the most severe cases of VHD. Part of the reason for the development of such a comprehensive team of specialists is the emergence of less invasive surgical techniques such as the transcatheter aortic valve replacement (TAVR), a procedure currently indicated in patients with the highest surgical risk, and one which requires a multidisciplinary approach to perioperative planning. The preoperative assessment of surgical or interventional risk in all patients with VHD is based on a new scoring system presented in Table 2 that includes the Society of Thoracic Surgeons (STS) predicted risk of mortality (PROM) calculator, an assessment of frailty, major organ system compromise, and procedure-specific impediments (Nishimura et al., 2014). This assessment, along with a full risk and benefit discussion, should be shared with potential surgical or interventional candidates.

AORTIC STENOSIS

Background

Although traditionally aortic stenosis (AS) was considered the most common valvular disease in the United States and Europe, recent epidemiologic studies show that it may be the second most common after mitral regurgitation (MR). Estimated prevalence of AS in patients over 75 years of age is 2.8% (Nkomo et al., 2006). A thorough pre-operative workup should be performed when evaluating an AS patient for surgery, as the burden of disease in these patients can be severe. Unlike other valvular lesions, rates of sudden cardiac death are high in patients with severe AS, with a reported incidence of 1% per year (Pellikka et al., 2005).

Diagnosis

Initial evaluation includes a history and physical examination, EKG, CXR, and TTE. While classic teaching describes a triad of symptomology that includes syncope, angina, and dyspnea in patients with severe disease, patients with mild to moderate AS generally have minimal symptoms due to LV com-

Table 2. Risk Assessment Combining STS Risk Estimate, Frailty, Major Organ System Dysfunction, and Procedure-Specific Impediments

	Low Risk (Must Meet ALL Criteria in This Column)	Intermediate Risk (Any 1 Criterion in This Column)	High Risk (Any 1 Criterion in This Column)	Prohibitive Risk (Any 1 Criterion in This Column)
STS PROM *	<4% AND	4% to 8% OR	>8% OR	Predicted risk with surgery of death or major morbidity (all-cause) >50% at 1 y OR
Frailty **	None AND	1 Index (mild) OR	≥2 Indices (moderate to severe) OR	
Major organ system compromise not to be improved postoperatively ***	None AND	1 Organ system OR	No more than 2 organ systems OR	≥3 Organ systems OR
Procedure-specific impediment ****	None	Possible procedure-specific impediment	Possible procedure-specific impediment	Severe procedure-specific impediment

Table taken from 2014 ACC/AHA Valvular Heart Disease Guidelines (Nishimura et al., 2014).

*Use of the STS PROM to predict risk in a given institution with reasonable reliability is appropriate only if institutional outcomes are within 1 standard deviation of STS average observed/expected ratio for the procedure in question.

**Seven frailty indices: Katz Activities of Daily Living (independence in feeding, bathing, dressing, transferring, toileting, and urinary incontinence) and independence in ambulation (no walking aid or assist required or 5-meter walk in <6 s). Other scoring systems can be applied to calculate no, mild-, or moderate-to-severe frailty.

***Examples of major organ system compromise: Cardiac- severe LV systolic or diastolic dysfunction or RV dysfunction, fixed pulmonary hypertension; CKD stage 3 or worse; pulmonary dysfunction with FEV1<50% or $DLCO_2$<50% of predicted; CNS dysfunction (dementia, Alzheimer's disease, Parkinson's disease, CVA with persistent physical limitation); GI dysfunction- Crohn's disease, ulcerative colitis, nutritional impairment, or serum albumin <3.0; cancer- active malignancy; and liver- any history of cirrhosis, variceal bleeding, or elevated INR in the absence of VKA therapy.

****Examples: tracheostomy present, heavily calcified ascending aorta, chest malformation, arterial coronary graft adherent to posterior chest wall, or radiation damage.

CKD indicates chronic kidney disease; CNS, central nervous system; CVA, stroke; $DLCO_2$, diffusion capacity for carbon dioxide; FEV1, forced expiratory volume in 1 s; GI, gastrointestinal; INR, international normalized ratio; LV, left ventricular; PROM, predicted risk of mortality; RV, right ventricular; STS, Society of Thoracic Surgeons; and VKA, vitamin K antagonist.

pensation. On physical examination, findings may include a crescendo-decrescendo systolic murmur that radiates to the base of the neck, an S4 gallop if sinus rhythm is maintained, and pulsus parvus et tardus (a slow-to-rise and delayed carotid pulse). EKG may show signs of left ventricular hypertrophy, left atrial enlargement, left bundle branch block, and non-specific ST and T waves changes. CXR is generally non-specific and may show a boot-shaped heart due to concentric left ventricular hypertrophy, calcification of the aortic valve (typically found in the lateral view), and post-stenotic aortic root dilation.

The staging of AS is an important aspect of therapeutic planning and requires evaluating the severity of disease via TTE. Table 3 describes the new staging system for AS as described in the 2014 ACC/AHA Valvular Heart Disease Guidelines, and is based on valve anatomy, valve hemodynamics, hemodynamic consequences, and symptoms. As in all valvular lesions, the new guidelines consist of four stages (A-D) that are based on valve anatomy, valve hemodynamics, hemodynamic consequences, and patient symptoms. The new staging system for AS replaces the former, which staged AS as mild, moderate, or severe. Of note is the definition of severe stenosis, which correlates with a peak aortic valve velocity of > 4.0 m/s or a mean aortic valve gradient > 40 mm Hg in patients with normal forward flow and an aortic valve area < 1.0 cm^2 in patients with low forward flow. The new guidelines have also broken down severe symptomatic AS into subgroups to take into account low-flow/low-gradient lesions. Class I evidence as to the timing of surgical intervention recommends valve replacement in patients with

Table 3. Stages of AS

Stage	Definition	Valve Anatomy	Valve hemodynamics	Hemodynamic Consequences	Symptoms
A	At risk of AS	-Bicuspid AV (or other congenital anomaly) -AV sclerosis	-Aortic V_{max} <2 m/s	-None	-None
B	Progressive AS	-Mild-to-moderate leaflet calcification of a bicuspid or trileaflet valve with some reduction in systolic motion or -Rheumatic valve changes with commissural fusion	-**Mild AS**: aortic valve V_{max} 2.0-2.9 m/s or mean ΔP <20 mm Hg -**Moderate AS**: Aortic V_{max} 3.0-3.9 m/s or mean ΔP 20-39 mm Hg	-Early LV diastolic dysfunction may be present -Normal LVEF	-None
C: Asymptomatic severe AS					
C1	Asymptomatic severe AS	-Severe leaflet calcification or congenital stenosis with severely reduced leaflet opening	-Aortic V_{max} ≥ 4m/s or mean ΔP ≥ 40 mm Hg -AVA typically is ≤ 1.0 cm^2 (or AVAi ≤ 0.6 cm^2/m^2) -Very severe AS is an aortic V_{max} ≥ 5 m/s or mean ΔP ≥ 60 mm Hg	-LV diastolic dysfunction -Mild LV hypertrophy -Normal LVEF	-None: Exercise testing is reasonable to confirm symptom status
C2	Asymptomatic severe AS with LV dysfunction	-Severe leaflet calcification or congenital stenosis with severely reduced leaflet opening	-Aortic V_{max} ≥ 4m/s or mean ΔP ≥ 40 mm Hg -AVA typically is ≤ 1.0 cm^2 (or AVAi ≤ 0.6 cm^2/m^2)	-LVEF <50%	-None
D: Symptomatic severe AS					
D1	Symptomatic severe high-gradient AS	-Severe leaflet calcification or congenital stenosis with severely reduced leaflet opening	-Aortic V_{max} ≥ 4m/s or mean ΔP ≥ 40 mm Hg -AVA typically ≤ 1.0 cm^2 (or AVAi ≤ 0.6 cm^2/m^2) but may be larger with mixed AS/AR	-LV diastolic dysfunction -LV hypertrophy -Pulmonary hypertension may be present	-Exertional dyspnea or decreased exercise tolerance -Exertional angina -Exertional syncope or presyncope
D2	Symptomatic severe low-flow/low-gradient AS with reduced LVEF	-Severe trileaflet calcification with severely reduced leaflet motion	-AVA ≤ 1.0 cm^2 with resting aortic V_{max} < 4 m/s or mean ΔP < 40 mm Hg -Dobutamine stress echocardiography shows AVA ≤ 1.0 cm^2 with V_{max} ≥ 4 m/s at any flow rate	-LV diastolic dysfunction -LV hypertrophy -LVEF < 50%	-HF -Angina -Syncope or presyncope

continued on following page

Table 3. Continued

Stage	Definition	Valve Anatomy	Valve hemodynamics	Hemodynamic Consequences	Symptoms
D3	Symptomatic severe low-gradient AS with normal LVEF or paradoxical low-flow severe AS	-Severe trileaflet calcification with severely reduced leaflet motion	-AVA $\leq$ 1.0 cm^2 with aortic V_{max} < 4 m/s or mean ΔP < 40 mm Hg -Indexed AVA $\leq$ 0.6 cm^2/m^2 and -Stroke volume index <35 mL/m^2 -Measured when patient is normotensive (systolic BP < 140 mm Hg)	-Increased LV relative wall thickness -Small LV chamber with low stroke volume -Restrictive diastolic filling -LVEF $\geq$ 50%	-Angina -Syncope or presyncope

Table taken from 2014 ACC/AHA Valvular Heart Disease Guidelines (Nishimura et al., 2014).

AR indicates aortic regurgitation; AS, aortic stenosis; AVA, aortic valve area; AVAi, aortic valve area indexed to body surface area; BP, blood pressure; HF, heart failure; LV, left ventricular; LVEF, left ventricular ejection fraction; ΔP, pressure gradient; V_{max}, maximum aortic velocity.

symptomatic severe high-gradient AS, asymptomatic severe AS with a LVEF <50%, and severe AS if undergoing another cardiac surgical procedure. Figure 1 shows all indications for AVR regardless of level of evidence in patients with AS (Nishimura et al., 2014).

Arrows show the decision pathways that result in a recommendation for AVR. Periodic monitoring is indicated for all patients in whom AVR is not yet indicated, including those with asymptomatic AS (stage D or C) and those with low-gradient AS (stage D2 or D3) who do not meet the criteria for intervention.

*AVR should be considered with stage D3 AS only if valve obstruction is the most likely cause of symptoms, stroke volume index is <35 mL/m^2, indexed AVA is $\leq$ 0.6 cm^2/m^2, and data are recorded when the patient is normotensive (SBP < 140 mm Hg).

AS indicates aortic stenosis; AVA, aortic valve area; AVR, aortic valve replacement by either surgical or transcatheter approach; BP, blood pressure; DSE, dobutamine stress echocardiography; ETT, exercise treadmill test; LVEF, left ventricular ejection fraction; ΔP_{mean}, mean pressure gradient; and V_{max}, maximum velocity.

Preoperative stress testing in patients with AS is important given the high incidence of ischemic heart disease in this patient population (Exadactylos, Sugrue, & Oakley, 1984). The type of stress testing varies with the severity of disease. As a general rule, exercise stress testing should never be performed in patients with symptomatic severe AS, given the high likelihood of ischemic disease and the risk of cardiovascular collapse with exertion (Nishimura et al., 2014). Invasive cardiovascular testing via catheterization is frequently performed in patients with severe AS undergoing high risk surgery and in patients with AS undergoing cardiac surgery, regardless of their AS stage.

Optimization

Medical optimization in patients with AS is focused on blood pressure control, treatment of heart failure symptoms, and statin therapy. Hypertension adds to the total left ventricular afterload. Antihypertensive options include beta-blockers, ACE inhibitors, and diuretics. Beta-blockers have the added benefit of slowing the heart rate to maximize flow across the stenotic valve, but also may negatively affect inotropy.

Figure 1. Indications for AVR in patients with AS
Figure taken from 2014 ACC/AHA Valvular Heart Disease Guidelines (Nishimura et al., 2014).

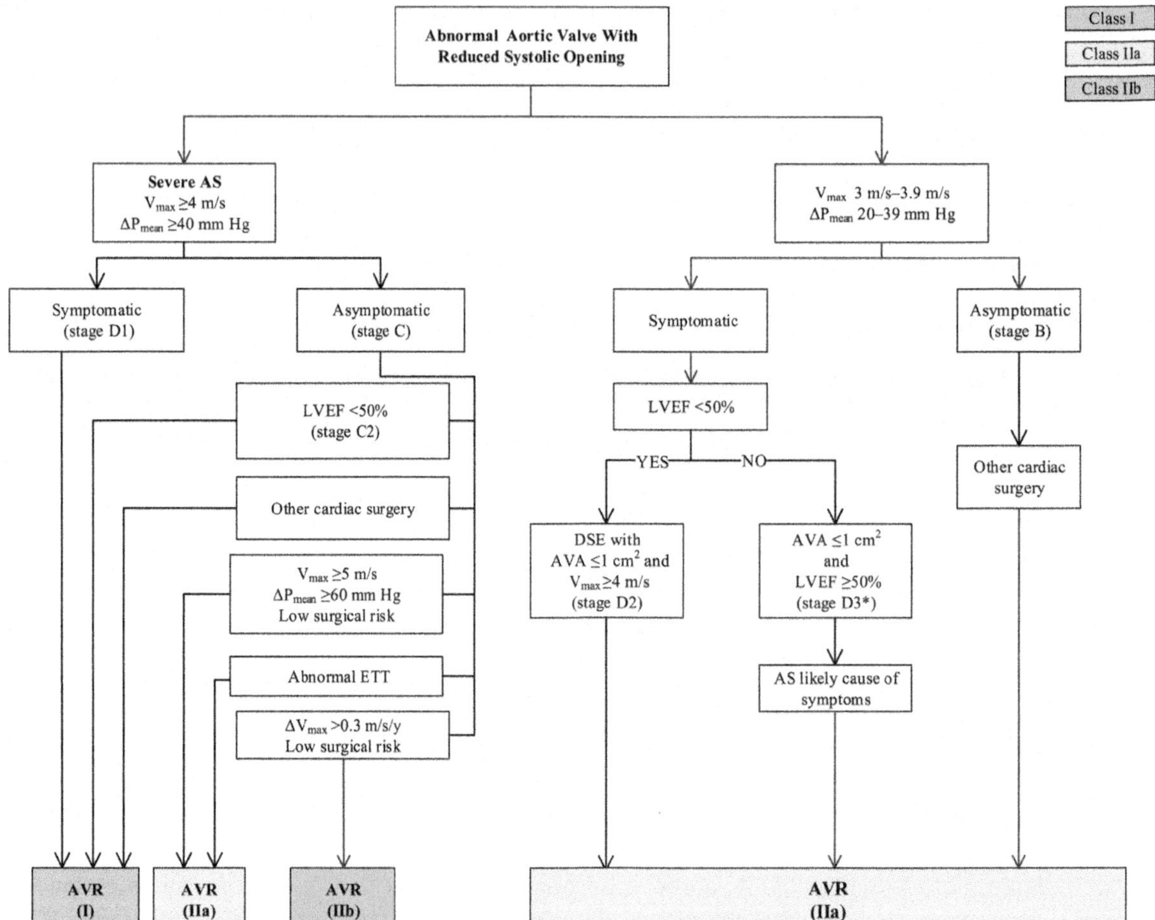

Given the dependence of preload on cardiac output in AS, diuretics should be used with caution in patients with small LV volumes noted on echocardiography. Regardless of pharmacologic choice, careful titration of antihypertensives is required so as to avoid hypotension, which can result in syncope and coronary ischemia. Decompensated heart failure in patients with AS is one of the few instances when short acting, potent vasodilators such as sodium nitroprusside may be indicated in order to diminish LV filling pressures and thereby augment LV function and cardiac output (Carabello & Paulus, 2009; Khot et al., 2003).

Statins (HMG-CoA reductase inhibitors) have been well studied in the management of AS. Histological studies have consistently shown that degenerative aortic valves share common features with atherosclerosis such as inflammation, atherogenic lipid deposition, extracellular matrix remodeling, calcification, and bone tissue. A recent review article that studied the current literature on statins found that the majority of retrospective studies supported the use of statins in slowing disease progression, whereas the majority of prospective studies did not share this finding (Parolari et al., 2009). A recent large randomized double-blind placebo-controlled clinical trial showed that in 269 patients with mild to moderate AS, rosuvastatin 40mg daily did not reduce the progression of AS, a finding that was later corroborated via a large randomized controlled trial (Chan, Teo, Dumesnil, Ni, & Tam, 2010; Rossebø et al., 2008). The ACC/AHA suggest that statin therapy is class III (no benefit) and level of evidence A in the prevention of AS progression for patients with mild to moderate disease (stage B to D) (Nishimura et al., 2014). Although data suggests that statins do not affect disease progression, given the high incidence of comorbidities in this patient population such as hypercholesterolemia and ischemic heart disease along with evidence that lowering cholesterol may decrease ischemic events in patients with AS, a broad clinical picture should be considered when deciding whether to initiate statin therapy (Rossebø et al., 2008).

AORTIC REGURGITATION

Background

Aortic regurgitation (AR) is a common disease in the United States, with an estimated prevalence of roughly 13% in men and 8.5% in women (Singh et al., 1999). AR can be divided into acute and chronic subgroups. As with all valvular lesions, preoperative evaluation should include a thorough history and physical, EKG, CXR, and TTE, as well as possible TEE, cardiac catherization, stress testing, and CMR.

Diagnosis

Chronic AR is most commonly initially identified by clinical examination. Generally, mild and moderate AR are relatively asymptomatic stages. Symptoms of AR typically commence once the degree of regurgitation becomes severe. Common patient complaints predominately relate to symptoms of congestive heart failure, and include exertional dyspnea, paroxysmal nocturnal dyspnea, orthopnea, and generalized fatigue. On physical exam, common findings include a blowing decrescendo diastolic murmur traditionally noted at the right sternal border, an S3 gallop, a displaced point of maximal impulse (PMI), and a "water-hammer' or "Corrigan's pulse," which is a rapidly increasing and collapsing pulse noted peripherally or in the carotid artery respectively. Classically an Austin Flint murmur (a mid-diastolic or presystolic rumble with multiple proposed etiologies) is noted with severe AR (Landzberg et al., 1992). Blood pressure measurements may show widened pulse pressure or decreased diastolic blood pressure.

Although TTE is the cornerstone of pre-operative diagnostic testing, an evaluation using multiple modalities may be employed. EKG may show evidence of LV enlargement, supraventricular arrhythmias, or ventricular arrhythmias. CXR classically shows an enlarged cardiac silhouette. Stress testing, cardiac MRI, and left heart catherization may be indicated in the workup of AR when symptoms and TTE findings do not correlate (Nishimura et al., 2014). Coronary artery disease is less common in AR than it is in AS, with one study showing an incidence of 14% in a cohort of patients with isolated severe AR (Timmermans, Willems, Piessens, & De Geest, 1988). Stress testing or coronary angiography should be considered in confirming the lack of symptoms in patients with AR and in those patients with symptoms of or known risk factors for myocardial ischemia (Nishimura et al., 2014; Timmermans et al., 1988).

The staging of chronic AR based on the 2014 AHA/ACC guidelines is presented in table 4. Class I evidence regarding indications for surgical intervention for AR includes symptomatic severe AR regardless of LV function, asymptomatic chronic severe AR with LVEF <50%, and severe AR if undergoing another cardiac surgery. Figure 2 shows all indications for surgical intervention regardless of level of evidence (Nishimura et al. 2014).

Table 4. Stages of Chronic AR

Stage	Definition	Valve Anatomy	Valve Hemodynamics	Hemodynamic Consequences	Symptoms
A	At risk	-Bicuspid AV (or other congenital valve anomaly) -AV sclerosis -Disease of aortic sinuses or ascending aorta -History of rheumatic fever or known rheumatic heart disease -IE	-AR severity: none or trace	-None	-None
B	Progressive	-Mild-to-moderate calcification of a trileaflet valve, bicuspid AV (or other congenital anomaly) -Dilated aortic sinuses -Rheumatic valve changes -Previous IE	**-Mild AR:** -Jet width < 25% of LOVT -Vena contracta < 0.3 cm -RVol < 30 mL/beat -RF < 30% -ERO < 0.10 cm^2 -Angiography grade 1+ **-Moderate AR:** -Jet width 25%-64% of LVOT -Vena contracta 0.3-0.6 cm RVol 30-59 mL/beat -RF 30%-49% -ERO 0.10-0.29 cm^2 -Angiography grade 2+	-Normal LV systolic function -Normal LV volume or mild LV dilation	-None
C	Asymptomatic severe	-Calcific aortic valve disease -Bicuspid valve (or other congenital abnormality) -Dilated aortic sinuses or ascending aorta -Rheumatic valve changes -IE with abnormal leaflet closure or perforation	**-Severe AR:** -Jet width ≥ 65% of LVOT -Vena contracta > 0.6 cm -Holodiastolic flow reversal in the proximal abdominal aorta -RVol ≥ 60 mL/beat -RF ≥ 50% -ERO ≥ 0.3 cm^2 -Angiography grade 3+ to 4+ -In addition, diagnosis of chronic severe AT requires evidence of LV dilation	-C1: Normal LVEF (≥ 50%) and mild-to-moderate LV dilation (LVESD ≤ 50mm) -C2: Abnormal LV systolic function with depressed LVEF (< 50%) or severe LV dilatation (LVESD > 50mm or indexed LVESD > 25 mm/m^2)	-None; exercise testing is reasonable to confirm symptom status

continued on following page

Table 4. Continued

Stage	Definition	Valve Anatomy	Valve Hemodynamics	Hemodynamic Consequences	Symptoms
D	Symptomatic severe	-Calcific valve disease -Bicuspid valve (or other congenital abnormality) -Dilated aortic sinuses or ascending aorta -Rheumatic valve changes -Previous IE with abnormal leaflet closure or perforation	**-Severe AR:** -Doppler jet width ≥ 65% of LVOT -Vena contracta > 0.6 cm -Holodiastolic flow reversal in the proximal abdominal aorta -RVol ≥ 60 mL/beat -RF ≥ 50% -ERO ≥ 0.3 cm^2 -Angiography grade 3+ to 4+ -In addition, diagnosis of chronic severe AR requires evidence of LV dilation	-Symptomatic severe AR may occur with normal systolic function (LVEF ≥ 50%), mild-to-moderate LV dysfunction (LVEF 40% to 50%), or severe LV dysfunction (LVEF < 40%) -Moderate-to-severe LV dilation is present	-Exertional dyspnea or angina or more severe HF symptoms

Table taken from 2014 ACC/AHA Valvular Heart Disease Guidelines (Nishimura et al., 2014).

AR indicates aortic regurgitation; ERO, effective regurgitant orifice; HF, heart failure; IE, infective endocarditis; LV, left ventricular; LVEF, left ventricular ejection fraction; LVESD, left ventricular end-systolic dimension; LVOT, left ventricular outflow tract; RF, regurgitant fraction; RVol, regurgitant volume.

Optimization

Pre-operative optimization of chronic AR has traditionally focused on afterload reduction, preload reduction, and ensuring adequate contractility, with the ultimate goal of symptom improvement and preservation of left ventricular function. When deciding upon medical therapy for patients with AR, treatment should to be tailored to the determinants of the regurgitant volume. The two major determinants that can be treated medically are the duration of diastole and the transvalvular diastolic pressure gradient, while a third determinant, the regurgitant orifice area, is fixed and can only be treated surgically (Levine & Gaasch, 1996). Indirectly, the treatment of these determinants will protect against myocardial ischemia and LV failure. Increased LV mass due to volume overload, decreased diastolic aortic pressures, and decreased diastolic filling times due to prolonged systolic ejection all promote myocardial ischemia. Despite the clear pathophysiologic link between AR and coronary artery disease, a retrospective study of 198 patients with severe AR found that roughly 14% had coronary artery stenosis greater than 50% via angiography, which is substantially less than that found in other valvular lesions such as AS (Timmermans et al., 1988).

Afterload and preload reduction through vasodilator therapy is indicated in patients with symptomatic severe AR, LV dysfunction, or significant LV dilatation (Glower, 2003; Evangelista, Tornos, Sambola, Permanyer-Miralda, & Soler-Soler, 2005). Both venodilators and arterial dilators can accomplish these therapeutic goals. The benefits of arterial vasodilators and venodilators are distinct; arterial vasodilators augment forward flow by reducing regurgitant volume, while venodilators work predominately on preload reduction with resultant decreases in end diastolic volumes and pressures (Boon & Bloomfield, 2002). Pharmacologic treatment options to achieve these goals include calcium channel blockers, alpha

Figure 2. Indications for AVR in chronic AR
Figure taken from 2014 ACC/AHA Valvular Heart Disease Guidelines (Nishimura et al., 2014).
AR indicates aortic regurgitation; AVR, aortic valve replacement (valve repair may be appropriate in selected patients); ERO, effective regurgitant orifice; LV, left ventricular; LVEDD, left ventricular end-diastolic dimension; LVEF, left ventricular ejection fraction; LVESD, left ventricular end-systolic dimension; RF, regurgitant fraction; and RVol, regurgitant volume.

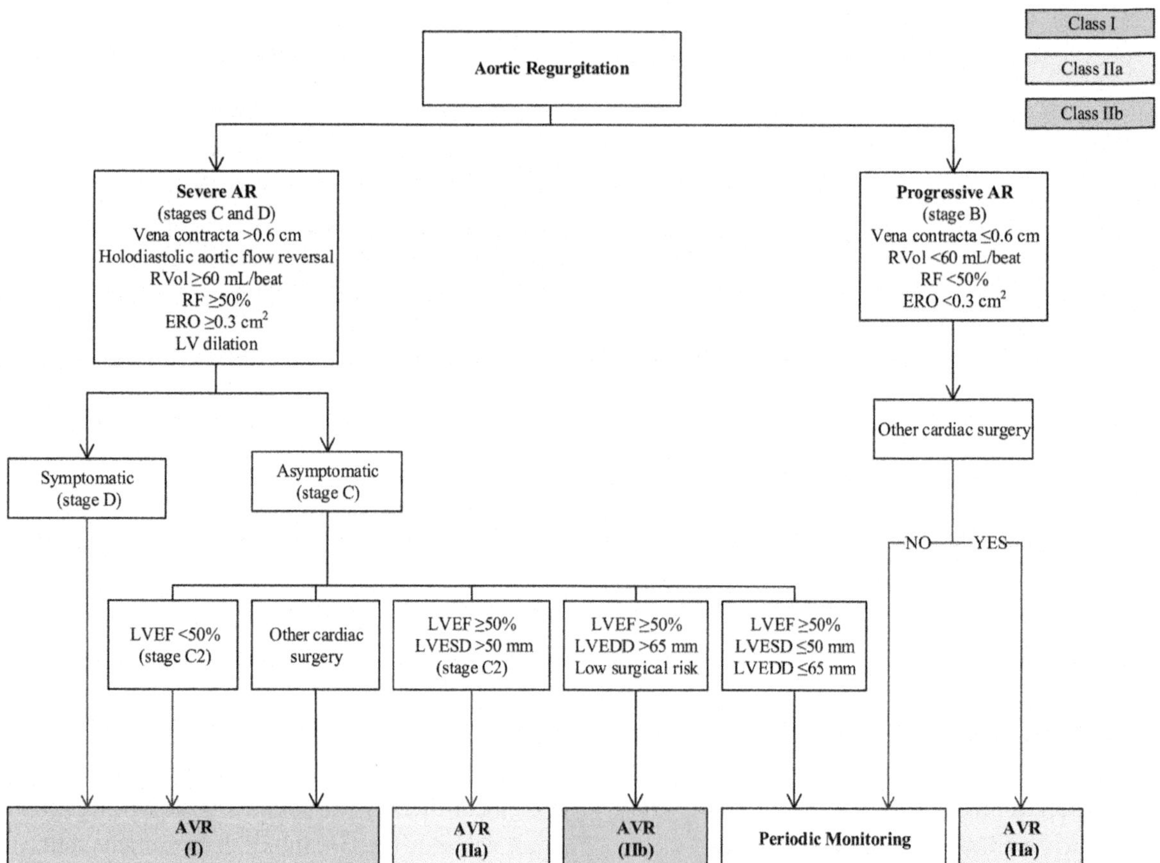

blockers, and angiotensin-converting enzyme inhibitors (ACEI's). The calcium channel blocker nifedipine has been extensively studied in the treatment of AR. A prospective randomized trial showed that nifedipine treatment in asymptomatic patients with chronic severe AR and normal LV function either reduced or delayed the need for aortic valve replacement (Scognamiglio, Rahimtoola, Fasoli, Nistri, & Volta, 1994). Despite the historic use of these medications in the management of AR, recent studies have shown confounding results related to the effectiveness of afterload reduction. A recent prospective randomized controlled trial showed that in patients with asymptomatic severe AR and normal LV function, long-term pharmacotherapy with either enalapril or nifedipine did not result in improvement in either the time to aortic valve replacement of the percentage of patients who needed an aortic valve replacement (Evangelista et al., 2005). The controversy regarding vasodilators was further demonstrated by a systematic review that showed inconsistent results among 8 studies comparing vasodilators to placebo or no therapy, and a more recent meta-analysis which did show positive effect on LV remodeling after assessing 7 studies (Mahajerin, Gurm, Tsai, Chan, & Nallamothu, 2007; Shah et al., 2012.) Despite these mixed findings, the 2014 AHA/ACC guidelines recommend treatment of afterload in patients with chronic AR to a goal systolic blood pressure less than 140 mm Hg with dihidropyridine calcium channel blockers, ACEI's, or angiotensin-receptor blockers (ARB's). This recommendation was labeled class I (treatment should be administered) and level of evidence B (Nishimura et al., 2014).

In general, excessive beta blockade should be avoided in patients with significant AR, especially when the onset is acute. Decreased heart rate and increased diastolic filling time prolongs the time for regurgitant flow. However, in that chronic AR produces a sympathetically driven heart failure state, beta blockers could theoretically minimize LV remodeling and myocardial dysfunction. This hypothesis was tested in an observational study of 756 patients with severe AR, with the results showing a statistically significant survival benefit at 1 and 5 years in those patients taking beta blockers (Sampat et al., 2009). The 2014 AHA/ACC guidelines recommend beta blockers in patients with symptomatic severe AR and/or LV dysfunction, with a treatment effect listed as class IIa (reasonable to administer treatment) and level B evidence (Nishimura et al., 2014). Importantly, whether or not vasodilator therapy or beta-blockade is employed, chronic vasodilator therapy should be continued during the preoperative period to prevent rebound hypertension unless otherwise contraindicated.

Acute AR is generally a surgical emergency resulting from trauma, endocarditis, aortic dissection, or iatrogenic injury from percutaneous interventions (Nishimura et al., 2014; Glower, 2003). Symptoms of AR can develop in a matter of hours to days, and predominately consist of dyspnea due to acute pulmonary edema from LV overload and chest pain from coronary ischemia due to the high workload on the LV coupled with the decreased coronary perfusion pressure from a diminished diastolic blood pressure. In cases of suspected acute AR, a TTE is vital in determining management.

Optimization of acute AR consists of afterload reduction with a short acting vasodilator, such as sodium nitroprusside, and inotropic support with an agent such as dobutamine to assist the decompensated left ventricle. As opposed to chronic AR, beta blockade is relatively contraindicated in these patients, as cardiac output and minimization of regurgitant flow is highly dependent on a relatively higher heart rate and shorter diastolic filling time. In cases of acute AR due to aortic dissection, a risk-benefit analysis should be conducted by the treating clinician as to whether beta-blockers should be employed pharmacologically.

MITRAL STENOSIS

Background

Mitral stenosis (MS) affects 0.1% of Americans, and the historic majority has been attributed to rheumatic fever caused by the group A hemolytic streptococcus, *S. pyogenes* (Vuyisile, Gardin, Skelton, Gottdiener, & Enriquez-Sarano, 2006). Up to 40% of individuals diagnosed with rheumatic heart disease develop isolated mitral stenosis. Despite an equal infection rate between men and women, women tend to have a higher rate of stenosis, with male:female ratio estimated to be 1:2 (Bonow et al. 2006). The connection between the systemic streptococcal bacterial infection and the targeted tissue injury of rheumatic heart disease is believed to occur via the M protein antigen. The M protein, which is a component of the bacterial cell wall, is highly antigenic and stimulates a robust inflammatory reaction (Stollerman, 2001). Because the M protein naturally exists on cardiac fibers as well, the heart valve is a target of antibody-mediated antigenic cross-reactivity. It is this inflammatory reaction that is believed to be the cause of rheumatic valvular disease; however, the reason why the mitral valve is particularly vulnerable to this reaction compared to other valves is not well understood.

In rheumatic heart disease, the mitral valve leaflets begin to fuse over time as a result of chronic inflammation of the endocardium. As the disease progresses, commissural fusion advances and the valve aperture narrows, causing free flow from the left atrium into the left ventricle to be impeded during diastole. This increased pressure gradient leads to decreased left ventricular end-diastolic volume (LVEDV) and left ventricular end-diastolic pressure (LVEDP), resulting in decreased stroke volume (Carabello, 2005). The result is an increased pressure gradient across the valve, leading to elevated left atrial pressures and ultimately, with severely advanced disease, pulmonary congestion and hypertension. In late stages, left heart failure may lead to right heart failure if left untreated.

As medicine has advanced, the incidence of MS has decreased in the developed world. Theories have attributed this decline to the increasing use of antibiotics; however, it has been shown that the decline began nearly two decades prior the widespread use of penicillin (Massel, Chute, Walker, & Kurkland, 1988). Other less common, non-rheumatologic etiologies of MS are senile mitral annular calcification (MAC) and congenital stenosis. As one ages, annular and leaflet calcifications accumulate and disrupt diastolic blood flow. In addition, decreases in both annular relaxation and leaflet mobility further contribute to stenosis. One study found the occurrence of MAC in patients diagnosed with MS was as high as 18.5% (Akram, Chan, McAuliffe, & Chenzbraun, 2009). It was found that the degree of stenosis and symptoms at the time of diagnosis were less severe when compared to rheumatic MS, but there was a higher observed degree of left ventricular hypertrophy (LVH) in MAC.

The natural history of the disease and its physiologic implications are important to understand, as they dictate the timing of intervention. After the initial inflammatory insult, it can take decades until a patient starts to become symptomatic (Horstkotte, Niehues, & Strauer, 1991). Some have estimated a rate of narrowing of 0.09 cm^2 each year after infection (Sagie et al., 1996). When the cross-sectional area is reduced from a normal mitral valve area (MVA) of 4-5 cm^2 to around 2.5 cm^2, symptoms may begin to appear on exertion or during other periods of hemodynamic stress such as pregnancy. Symptoms at rest typically are seen when the MVA is less than 1.5 cm^2 (Kaplan, 2008). The 2014 AHA/ACC staging system for MS is summarized in Table 5. Based on these parameters, recommendations for surgeons and interventionists have been created, with varying degrees of evidence, regarding when, and in whom, repair or replacement of the mitral valve would be appropriate. These recommendations are summarized in Figure 3.

Diagnosis

As in other valvular disease, the diagnosis starts with eliciting a thorough history and physical exam. MS symptoms mimic those of left ventricular failure; initial symptoms are typically dyspnea on exertion, worsening exercise tolerance and orthopnea. Palpitations may be a symptom of atrial fibrillation, which can occur in up to 39% of individuals with MS (Wood, 1954). Cardiac auscultation can reveal a loud first heart sound (S1) during systole (mitral valve closure) followed by an opening snap (mitral valve opening) and mid-diastolic rumbling murmur. Lung auscultation may reveal rales from pulmonary vascular congestion. Other findings in severe disease may be signs of right heart failure such as jugular venous distention and ascites.

Table 5. Stages of MS

Stage	Definition	Valve Anatomy	Valve Hemodynamics	Hemodynamic consequences	Symptoms
A	At risk of MS	Mild valve doming during diastole	Normal transmitral flow velocity	None	None
B	Progressive	-Rheumatic valve changes with commissural fusion and diastolic doming of the mitral valve leaflets -Planimetered MVA > 1.5 cm^2	-Increased transmitral flow velocities -MVA > 1.5 cm^2 -Diastolic pressure half-time < 150 ms	-Mild-moderate LA enlargement -Normal pulmonary pressure at rest	None
C	Severe (asymptomatic)	-Rheumatic valve changes with commissural fusion and diastolic doming of the mitral valve leaflets -Planimetered MVA ≤ 1.5 cm^2 (MVA ≤ 1.0 cm^2 with very severe MS)	-MVA ≤ 1.5 cm^2 (MVA ≤ 1.0 cm^2 with very severe MS) -Diastolic pressure half-time ≥ 150 ms (Diastolic pressure half-time ≥ 220 ms with very severe MS)	-Severe LA enlargement -Elevated PASP > 30 mm Hg	None
D	Severe (symptomatic)	Rheumatic valve changes with commissural fusion and diastolic doming of the mitral valve leaflets Planimetered MVA ≤ 1.5 cm^2	-MVA ≤ 1.5 cm^2 (MVA ≤ 1.0 cm^2 with very severe MS) -Diastolic pressure half-time ≥ 150 ms (Diastolic pressure half-time ≥ 220 ms with very severe MS)	-Severe LA enlargement -Elevated PASP > 30 mm Hg	-Decreased exercise tolerance -Exertional dyspnea

Table taken from 2014 ACC/AHA Valvular Heart Disease Guidelines (Nishimura et al, 2014).
LA indicates left atrial; LV, left ventricular; MS, mitral stenosis; MVA, mitral valve area; and PASP, pulmonary artery systolic pressure.

Initial testing typically includes an EKG, CXR and TTE. EKG may reveal left ventricular hypertrophy, atrial fibrillation, and/or the appearance of a broad, bi-lobed P wave (*p mitrale*), which is a marker of left atrial dilation. CXR is useful to detect pulmonary vascular congestion or more subtle left atrial dilation. Various studies have examined the utility of using inflammatory markers such as C-reactive protein in the diagnostic process, but their utility has yet to be fully understood (Ucer et al., 2008).

TTE enables the physician to non-invasively evaluate valvular appearance and pressure gradients throughout the heart with the assistance of doppler hemodynamic measurements. The 2014 AHA/ACC staging guidelines are based on various echocardiographic measurements, including estimations of the valve area based on planimetry and diastolic pressure half-time, examination of left atrial enlargement, and pulmonary artery systolic pressures (PASP), as well as patient symptoms. Because the diastolic pressure half-time can vary depending on changes in the CO and HR, planimetry is generally regarded as a more accurate means of measuring valve area (Carabello, 2005). Because TTE has a low sensitivity for identifying a LA thrombus, prior to any intervention, a TTE is recommended to better visualize the LA

Figure 3. Indications for intervention in rheumatic MS
Figure taken from 2014 ACC/AHA Valvular Heart Disease Guidelines (Nishimura et al., 2014).
AF indicates atrial fibrillation; LA, left atrial; MR, mitral regurgitation; MS, mitral stenosis; MVA, mitral valve area; MVR, mitral valve surgery (repair or replacement); NYHA, New York Heart Association; PCWP, pulmonary capillary wedge pressure; PMBC, percutaneous mitral balloon commissurotomy; and T ½, pressure half-time.

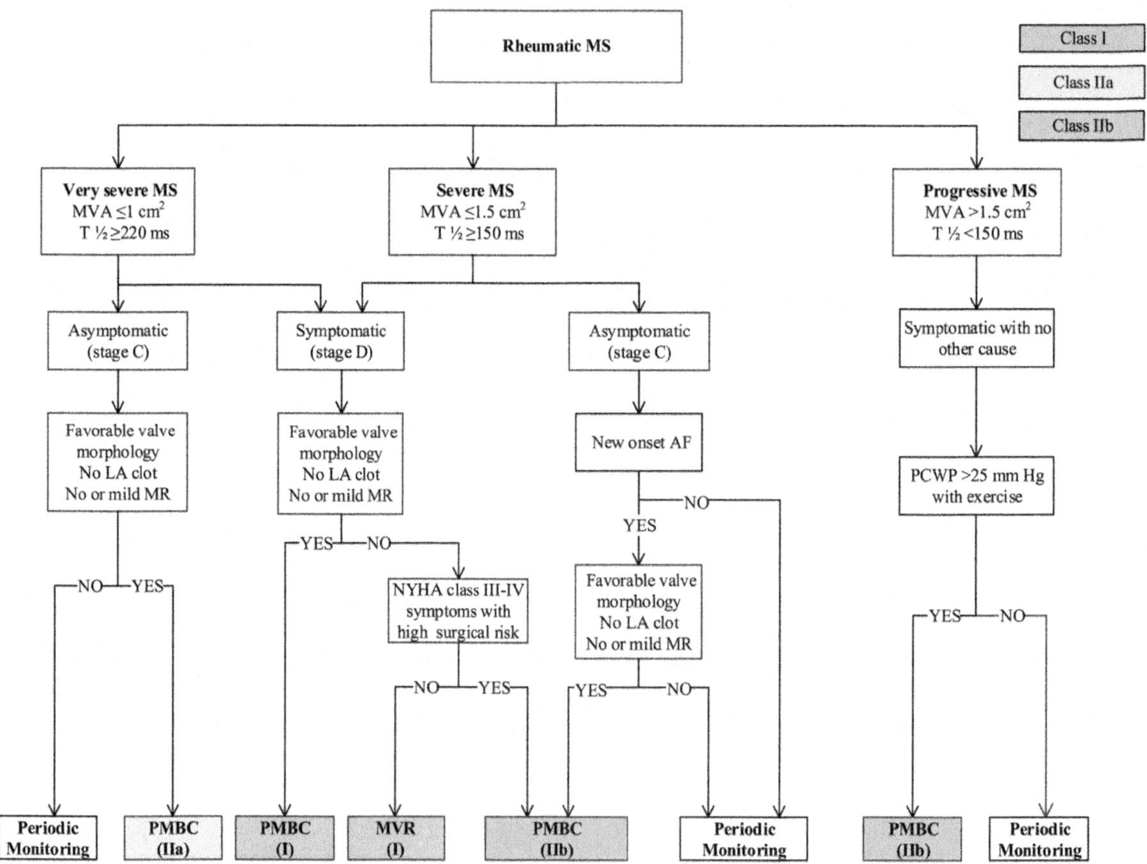

in order to identify thrombi and reduce the risk of embolization. This recommendation holds true even in the presence of long-term anticoagulation because of a 10% risk of thrombus presence (Manning, Reis, & Douglas, 1992). If the echocardiography data is discordant with patient symptoms (i.e. unimpressive resting TTE but complaints of reduced exercise tolerance), stress testing with echocardiography or invasive catheterization is the next logical step. During exercise, the increase in trans-mitral gradient causes greater LA pressures and subsequent pulmonary hypertension, resulting in symptomatic exacerbation.

Optimization

Medical therapy for mitral stenosis generally revolves around rate control and anticoagulation for those not in sinus rhythm. If atrial fibrillation has a resultant rapid ventricular response, a diminished diastolic time leads to a decrease in LVEDV and cardiac output. For this reason, significant hemodynamic changes during rapid atrial fibrillation in patients with MS can be a critical clinical issue (Kaplan 2008). There is a subset of data that suggests using AV nodal blocking agents (beta or calcium channel blockers) can benefit these patients (Wood, 1954). Since the side effects of these drugs are typically minimal, initiation of blockade is encouraged if no major contraindications exist. In patients with mitral stenosis who are acutely hemodynamically unstable and unable to be medically managed, standard ACLS algorithms should be followed and cardioversion may be needed. There is weak evidence for the use of beta blockers in those who have severe MS with symptomatic exertion, given that the only randomized controlled trial disproves any performance benefit (Stoll et al., 1995). However, the AHA/ACC guidelines point to case studies possibly showing some benefit, thus giving beta-blockers for exertional symptomatic improvement a class IIb recommendation.

Rheumatic mitral valve disease has a higher incidence of embolic events than any other acquired valve abnormality because of relative left atrial stasis. Early studies found that the incidence of embolic events ranges from 9-27% (Wood, 1956; Ellis & Harken, 1961), while others observed a lower rate ranging between 1.5-4.7% per year (Deverall, Olley, Smith, Watson, & Whitaker, 1968). Regardless, patients with mitral stenosis are considered "high risk" compared to those without valvular disease. Patients with coexisting left atrial thrombosis, long-standing atrial fibrillation, paroxysmal atrial fibrillation, or prior embolic events have an even greater embolization risk. The 2014 AHA/ACC guidelines suggest that these latter high-risk patients benefit from treatment with vitamin K antagonists, such as warfarin (level of evidence B) (Nishimura et al., 2014). The National Study for Prevention of Embolism in Atrial Fibrillation (NASPEAF) trial found that a dual-therapy regimen using the antiplatelet drug triflusal (600mg/day) and moderate-intensity anticoagulation with warfarin (target 2.2; range 1.9-2.5) versus monotherapy anticoagulation (INR 2.0-3.0) conferred a risk reduction of embolic events (systemic embolism, vascular death, stroke) in MS patients with and without a history of embolic events by 69% and 48%, respectively.

MITRAL REGURGITATION

Background

Mitral regurgitation is believed to be the most common form of valvular heart disease in the United States, with a prevalence of 1.7% (Vuyisile, 2006). Like mitral stenosis, rheumatic heart disease can also lead to mitral regurgitation (MR). MR has a variety of causes that can be divided into primary (organic) and secondary (functional). Primary causes of MR are those that result from dysfunction of the leaflets or subvalvular structures (the chordae) leading to insufficiency. Mitral valve degeneration is the most common primary chronic cause of MR, and is due to myxomatous degeneration of the leaflets leading to mitral valve prolapse (De Bonis, Maisano, La Canna, & Alfieri, 2012). Mitral valve degeneration can be an isolated disease, in that degeneration only happens at the level of the mitral valve, or it can be part of a systemic connective tissue disorder such as Ehlers-Danlos or Marfan's syndrome. Other examples of primary disease are congenital, papillary muscle rupture, trauma or infectious endocarditis (typically from *S. aureus* endocarditis). Secondary MR is due to remodeling of the left ventricle secondary to idiopathic or ischemic causes. The LV remodeling displaces the papillary muscles apically and posteriorly, causing traction on the chordae and disrupting the coaptation of the mitral valve leaflets, which ultimately leads to regurgitant flow (Yiu, Enriquez-Sarano, Tribouilloy, & Tajik, 2000). It has been found that moderate and severe primary MR have yearly mortality rates of 3% and 6% respectively (Enriquez-Sarano, Akins, & Vahanian, 2009).

Chronic causes of MR lead to left ventricular and atrial remodeling (dilation and eccentric hypertrophy), with the atrium acting as a systolic "pop-off" for the increasing end-diastolic volume of the left ventricle. Initially the LV may have a higher calculated ejection fraction (EF) because the higher ventricular preload increases the ventricular contractility in a manner described by the Frank-Starling curve (Kaplan, 2008). At first, these physiologic changes are met with adaptation, but as the disease progresses and chamber pressures begin to elevate, the LV compensation ceases and symptoms begin to appear. This is why some have determined an EF of 60% to be the tipping point for severe disease despite a seemingly "normal" EF (Vahanian et al., 2012). Acute causes of MR (e.g. papillary muscle rupture) are often met with symptoms in the acute phase because the heart does not have time to adapt. The low "afterload" of the left atrium causes retrograde flow from the left ventricle and elevation of atrial, pulmonary, and in severe cases, right heart pressures.

Diagnosis

As in mitral stenosis, MR can progress to severe disease before symptoms start to develop. In the case of chronic MR, patients may unknowingly reduce their activity level to compensate for the symptomatic progression. The symptoms of MS and MR are alike in that they occur secondary to elevations in left heart pressures, ultimately causing pulmonary hypertension and right heart failure. Initial symptoms include exertional dyspnea, orthopnea, and paroxysmal nocturnal dyspnea due to elevated pulmonary pressures and reduced systemic cardiac output. Acute MR, often seen in the setting of myocardial infarction, is not tolerated well and typically necessitates intervention because of patient decompensation.

Diagnosis starts by obtaining a detailed history and physical exam. Important historical details may underline the possibility of mitral regurgitation such as timeline of symptoms, personal or family history of mitral valve prolapse or connective tissue disorders, rheumatic fever, recurrent or current infection, coronary risk factors, and exercise tolerance. Stress should be placed on the time course of the development of symptoms, because the etiology and treatment of acute and chronic MR are quite different. For example, a patient who has been admitted for an acute MI who develops sudden hypoxemia with signs of pulmonary edema may have decompensated left heart failure secondary to acute MR from papillary rupture. The physical exam may be notable for a holosystolic murmur best heard at the apex radiating to the axilla, with or without a preceding mid-systolic click signaling the presence of MVP. In severe, acute decompensated cases, the left ventricular and atrial pressures approach equalization, resulting in a minimal holosystolic murmur (or none at all). The same reasoning illustrates why doppler flow evaluation of severe MR may underestimate the lesion severity because of chamber pressure equilibration (Vahanian et al., 2012). Diagnostic testing should include EKG and CXR, which can show similar findings to those in MS. On the EKG, one may identify *p mitrale*, atrial fibrillation or left ventricular hypertrophy. On CXR, there may also be signs of left atrial and left ventricular enlargement (the latter of which is not typically a finding in MS, given that the LV is usually normal in structure and function). While these findings are typical for chronic causes of MR due to eccentric cardiac dilation and remodeling, acute causes may not share these findings. In instances of acute ischemia, there may be ST elevations on EKG. Depending on the severity of decreased forward cardiac output, the patient may present with hypotension or shock.

As in other valvular diseases, TTE is the cornerstone of diagnostic evaluation of patients with suspected MR. Echocardiographic observations were integrated into 2014 AHA/ACC guidelines, which stratify disease progression of both primary and secondary MR. In primary MR, the utilized criteria include anatomy and behavior of the chordae and leaflets, valve hemodynamics (mitral valve regurgitant characteristics, regurgitant volume and fraction, effective regurgitant orifice area), and hemodynamic consequences (LA enlargement, pulmonary pressure elevation and LV ejection fraction) (Table 6). There has been a focus on replacing estimations of the severity of the regurgitant jet by planimetry with the *vena contracta*, which is the narrow part of the jet and a more accurate method of measurement (Vahanian et al., 2012). Secondary MR grading (Table 7) focuses on signs of ischemia or infarction such as regional wall motion abnormalities and mitral annular dilation, because the chordae and leaflets are often normal in these cases. Most important in grading are signs of decompensated LV function (reduced EF, dilated left atrium with atrial fibrillation, pulmonary hypertension, etc.) and the presence of symptoms, as they are generally indicators of poor prognosis.

Despite TTE being a useful tool for diagnosis and surgical planning, some patients may have TTE findings discordant with their symptoms. These individuals may benefit from stress echocardiography or catheterization, where real-time elevations of ventricular, atrial, and pulmonary pressures can be measured. There stands a chance that these exertional symptoms may be pulmonary in origin and not a result of the valvular disease. Given its higher sensitivity with identifying perivalvular lesions, TEE, while more invasive, may be warranted if the suspected etiology is IE.

Optimization

The medical management for MR depends on the etiology of dysfunction and the time course of disease. In chronic primary MR, the goal should be to optimize "forward" cardiac output by reducing afterload through the use of vasodilators. This recommendation is only made in individuals with symptomatic disease or initial signs of heart failure (e.g. EF<60%) and who are not going to be operated on (Nishimura et al., 2014). Essentially, standard heart failure therapies should not be withheld (i.e. beta blockers, ACE inhibitors, diuretics, etc.) if the gold standard (repair or replacement) will not be immediate (level of evidence B). While acutely managing patients with MR in the intensive care unit, fast acting and easily titratable intravenous drugs such as calcium channel blockers (nicardipine) or nitroprusside can accomplish this in order to bridge to surgery if indicated (Nishimura at al., 2014). If the patient is increasingly decompensating, an intra-aortic balloon pump can be used to reduce LV afterload and promote forward flow.

It is crucial to understand the timing of intervention necessary to optimize the prognosis of patients with MR. In symptomatic patients or those with degenerative severe MR with early signs of failure (e.g. EF<60%), surgical intervention should be pursued, as it can restore a patient's normal life expectancy back to baseline (De Bonis et al., 2012). Regarding secondary MR, guidelines on intervention are less clear and are still under investigation. The presence of irreversible cardiac damage and tissue remodeling may cause the operative morbidity and mortality to outweigh the survival benefit. Treating clinicians must take into consideration patient comorbidities and the predictive probability of an adequate repair in order to avoid repair failure and increased morbidity and mortality associated with re-operation. Indications for surgical correction of MR are summarized in Figure 4.

Table 6. Stages of Primary MR

Grade	Definition	Valve Anatomy	Valve Hemodynamics	Hemodynamic Consequences	Symptoms
A	At risk of MR	-Mild mitral valve prolapse with normal coaptation -Mild valve thickening and leaflet restriction	-No MR jet or small central jet area < 20% LA on Doppler -Small vena contracta < 0.3 cm	None	None
B	Progressive MR	-Severe mitral valve prolapse with normal coaptation -Rheumatic valve changes with leaflet restriction and loss of central coaptation -Prior IE	-Central jet MR 20-40% LA or late systolic eccentric jet MR -Vena contracta < 0.7 cm -Regurgitant volume < 60 mL -Regurgitant fraction < 50% -ERO < 0.40 cm^2 -Angiographic grade 1-2+	-Mild LA enlargement -No LV enlargement -Normal pulmonary pressure	None
C	Severe MR (asymptomatic)	-Severe mitral valve prolapse with loss of coaptation or flail leaflet -Rheumatic valve changes with leaflet restriction and loss of central coaptation -Prior IE -Thickening of leaflets with radiation heart disease	-Central jet MR > 40% LA or holosystolic eccentric jet MR -Vena contracta ≥ 0.7 cm -Regurgitant volume ≥ 60 mL -Regurgitant fraction ≥ 50% -ERO ≥ 0.40 cm^2 -Angiographic grade 3-4+	-Moderate or severe LA enlargement -LV enlargement -Pulmonary HTN may be present at rest or with exercise -**C1**: LVEF >-60% and LVESD < 40 mm -**C2**: LVEF ≤ 60% and LVESD ≥ 40 mm	None
D	Severe MR (symptomatic)	-Severe mitral valve prolapse with loss of coaptation or flail leaflet -Rheumatic valve changes with leaflet restriction and loss of central coaptation -Prior IE -Thickening of leaflets with radiation heart disease	-Central jet MR > 40% -LA or holosystolic eccentric jet MR -Vena contracta ≥ 0.7 cm -Regurgitant volume ≥ 60mL -Regurgitant fraction ≥ 50% -ERO ≥ 0.40 cm^2 -Angiographic grade 3-4+	-Moderate or severe LA enlargement -LV enlargement -Pulmonary HTN	-Decreased exercise tolerance -Exertional dyspnea

Table taken from 2014 ACC/AHA Valvular Heart Disease Guidelines (Nishimura et al., 2014).

ERO indicated effective regurgitant orifice; IE, infective endocarditis; LA, left atrium/atrial; LV, left ventricular; LVEF, left ventricular ejection fraction; LVESD; left ventricular end-systolic dimension; and MR, mitral regurgitation.

Table 7. Stages of Secondary MR

Grade	Definition	Valve Anatomy	Valve Hemodynamics	Associated Cardiac Findings	Symptoms
A	At risk for MR	Normal valve leaflets, chords, annulus in a patient with coronary disease or cardiomyopathy	-No MR jet or small central jet area <20% LA on Doppler -Small vena contracta < 0.30 cm	-Normal or mildly dilated LV size with fixed (infarction) or inducible (ischemia) regional wall abnormalities -Primary myocardial disease with LV dilation and systolic dysfunction	Symptoms due to coronary ischemia or HR may be present that respond to revascularization and appropriate medical therapy
B	Progressive MR	-Regional wall motion abnormalities with mild tethering of mitral leaflet -Annular dilation with mild loss of central coaptation of the mitral leaflets	-ERO < 0.20 cm^2 -Regurgitant volume < 30 mL -Regurgitant fraction < 50%	-Regional wall motion abnormalities with reduced LV systolic function -LV dilation and systolic dysfunction due to primary myocardial disease	Symptoms due to coronary ischemia or HR may be present that respond to revascularization and appropriate medical therapy
C	Severe MR (asymptomatic)	-Regional wall motion abnormalities and/or LV dilation with severe tethering of mitral leaflet -Annular dilation with severe loss of central coaptation of the mitral leaflets	-ERO ≥ 0.20 cm^2 -Regurgitant volume ≥ 30 mL -Regurgitant fraction ≥ 50%	-Regional wall motion abnormalities with reduced LV systolic function -LV dilation and systolic dysfunction due to primary myocardial disease	Symptoms due to coronary ischemia or HR may be present that respond to revascularization and appropriate medical therapy
D	Severe MR (symptomatic)	-Regional wall motion abnormalities and/or LV dilation with severe tethering of mitral leaflet -Annular dilation with severe loss of central coaptation of the mitral leaflets	-ERO ≥ 0.20 cm^2 -Regurgitant volume ≥ 30 mL -Regurgitant fraction ≥ 50%	-Regional wall motion abnormalities with reduced LV systolic function -LV dilation and systolic dysfunction due to primary myocardial disease	-HF symptoms due to MR persist even after revascularization and optimization of medical therapy -Decreased exercise tolerance -Exertional dyspnea

Table taken from 2014 ACC/AHA Valvular Heart Disease Guidelines (Nishimura et al., 2014).

2D indicates 2-dimensional; ERO, effective regurgitant orifice; HF, heart failure; LA, left atrium; LV, left ventricular; MR, mitral regurgitation; and TTE, transthoracic echocardiogram.

Figure 4. Indications for surgery for MR

Figure taken from 2014 ACC/AHA Valvular Heart Disease Guidelines (Nishimura et al., 2014). AF indicates atrial fibrillation; CAD, coronary artery disease; CRT, cardiac resynchronization therapy; ERO, effective regurgitant orifice; HF, heart failure; LV, left ventricular; LVEF, left ventricular ejection fraction; LVESD, left ventricular end-systolic dimension; MR, mitral regurgitation; MV, mitral valve; MVR, mitral valve replacement; NYHA, New York Heart Association; PASP, pulmonary artery systolic pressure; RF, regurgitant fraction; RVol, regurgitant volume; and Rx, therapy.

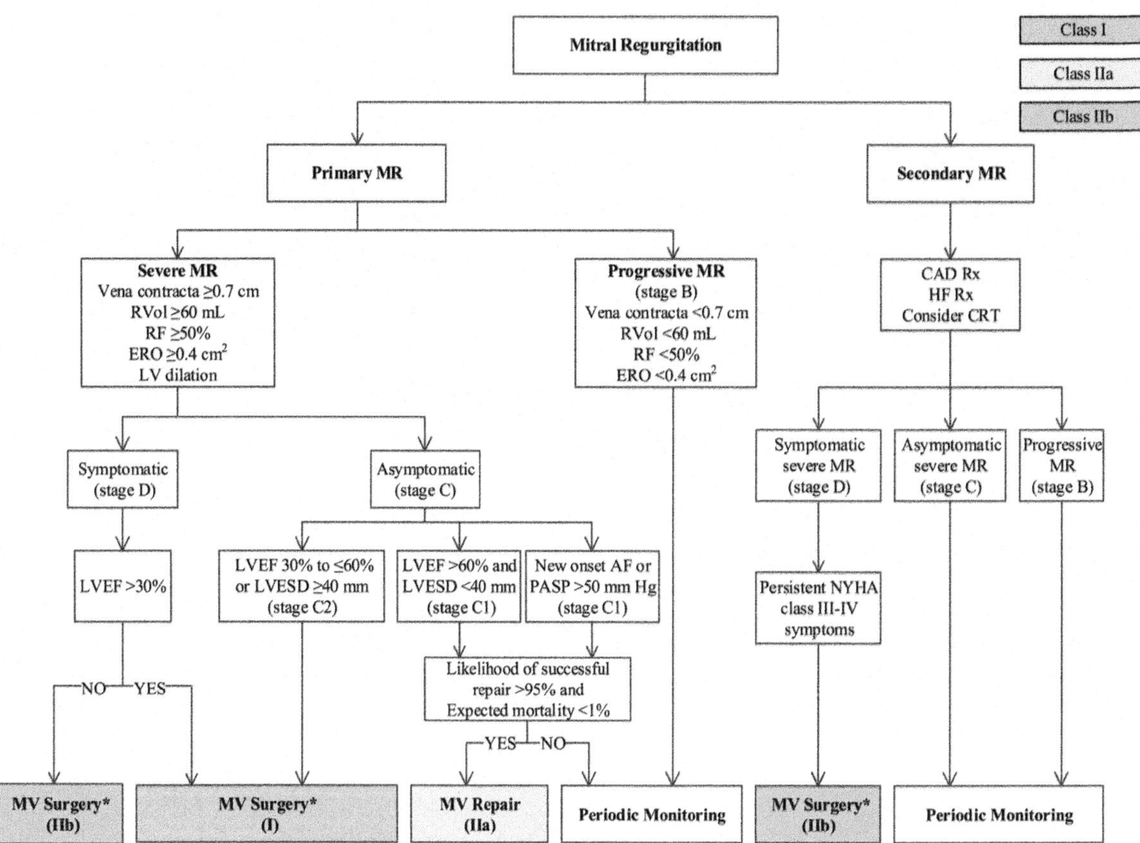

PULMONIC STENOSIS

Background

Pulmonic valve disease comprises a small proportion of valvular heart disease. While similar in structure to the aortic valve, the pulmonic valve is thinner because its environment is a lower pressure system (Lancellotti et al., 2013). Pulmonic stenosis is present in 10% of patients diagnosed with congenital heart disease (Snellen et al., 1968). Patients are typically diagnosed in childhood. The level of the stenotic lesion can be described as a valvular, supravalvular or subvalvular location. At the level of the valve, there are three described main subtypes. The first subtype is characterized by dome-shaped, fibrosed, mobile leaflets causing a narrowed central aperture. The second subcategory is less common and features a dysplastic, thickened, poorly mobile valve with no commissural fusion; this is often seen in Noonan's syndrome. Lastly, 20% of PS cases involve a bicuspid valve (Keith, Rowe, & Vlad, 1978) and in some instances, a unicuspid valve (Warnes et al., 2008). Unlike other valvular diseases, calcific disease is quite rare. Subvalvular stenosis can be seen in tetralogy of Fallot where the right ventricular outflow tract is hypertrophied, termed primary infundibular pulmonic stenosis (IPS). While primary IPS is generally considered rare (in those with TOF or not), secondary formation of IPS from the increased pressure in the right ventricle from pulmonic valve stenosis is relatively common (Snellen et al., 1968). Supravalvular causes of stenosis such as pulmonary artery stenosis can be found postoperatively in those patients who have had native valve repairs or stenosis of prosthetic valves. Early studies have shown that progression of mild to moderate disease is relatively uncommon, and surgical treatment is often reserved only for progression. After surgical treatment of the severely stenotic valve, it has been observed that IPS slowly regresses to baseline over the course of months to years (Snellen et al, 1968).

Diagnosis

Patients often present at a young age with an asymptomatic murmur, given the congenital predominance of pulmonary stenosis. With the coexistence of a right to left shunt, exertional dyspnea or cyanosis can be observed. With right ventricular hypertension, the increased atrial pressure may perpetuate the existence of a patent foramen ovale or atrial septal defect (Snellen et al, 2008). The most important initial tool is cardiac auscultation, which can reveal splitting of the second heart sound, an early (mild-moderate stenosis) or holosystolic (moderate to severe stenosis) right sided heart murmur, or an S4 heart sound signifying atrial contraction against a firm and hypertrophied right ventricle. There may be a prominent "A" jugular venous wave with severe disease; otherwise, there are rarely signs of right ventricular failure unless severe disease is present. EKG can show right atrial dilation or right ventricular hypertrophy when there is a high peak gradient (> 60 mm Hg) (Warnes et al., 2008). The RVH on EKG can be seen to improve after surgical treatment as the RVOT thickening regresses back to baseline over the course of months to years (Snellen et al., 1968). CXR may show a dilated RA, PA dilation or "Chen's sign," which is left lung base vascular fullness because of preferential blood flow to the left PA with PS (Warnes et al., 2008).

As in other cardiac diseases, echocardiography with Doppler studies is needed to characterize the lesion and grade the disease in order to determine the next steps in management. The AHA/ACC guidelines outline how to identify severe pulmonary stenosis and its staging criteria (Table 7). During these studies, atrial septal defects may also be identified, which can be repaired if surgery is indicated. Cardiac catheterization, while not necessary for diagnosis, can be an important tool for more accurately diagnosing the right-sided pressure gradients and dictating exactly when surgery should be carried out (Warnes et al., 2008). As in other valvular diseases, exercise tests are indicated if the objective measurements do not correlate with patient symptoms.

Optimization

When disease is mild (peak instantaneous valvular gradient < 30 mm Hg), progression of the disease is rare, and the only management necessary is serial TTE exams every 5 years if patients remain asymptomatic. For gradients > 30 mm Hg in an asymptomatic individual, TTE should be repeated every 2-5 years (Warnes et al, 2008).

While surgical intervention is covered by the 2008 AHA/ACC guidelines, Class I indications recommend balloon valvotomy in the symptomatic individual with domed morphology with peak Doppler gradients > 50 mm Hg or 30 mm Hg with mild pulmonic regurgitation. Asymptomatic individuals may also meet operative criteria when peak pressures > 60 mm Hg or 40 mm Hg with regurgitant disease. Surgical valvotomy is indicated for patients with supravalvular and subvalvular stenosis (Bouzaz, Kilner, & Gatzoulis, 2005). Medical management is generally supportive for the side effects of the disease. Anecdotally, some have shown that exertional dyspnea in patients with certain subvalvular obstructions may benefit from increased diastolic filling time with the use of beta-blockers, but the data is limited to case reports (Arai et al., 2001). Right-sided heart failure generally requires surgical intervention, but medical management with diuretics can be used as a temporizing measure.

PULMONIC REGURGITATION

Background

Mild pulmonic regurgitation (PR) is not uncommon in asymptomatic individuals with normal pulmonic valves, and is reported to be as high as 78% (Bouzaz et al., 2005). Moderate PR can be seen in individuals with pulmonary hypertension. However, severe PR is always pathologic. Commonly, PR can occur postoperatively in patients who have had valvotomy for PS or tetralogy of Fallot repair. Patients who have had trans-annular repair for TOF experience a particularly high incidence of postoperative PR, so much so that the use of this surgical approach has been declining. As medicine continues to advance, more individuals will live to adulthood and may suffer from such post-operative issues. If untreated, significant PR can lead to right heart failure and significant morbidity and mortality. It has been reported that 32% of adults who have had TOF repair have tricuspid regurgitation from either PR or tricuspid annulus disease (Bouzaz et al., 2005); as TR progresses in these individuals, it can contribute to postoperative ventricular tachycardia and increase the risk of sudden cardiac death. Other causes of PR include rheumatic heart disease, carcinoid syndrome, congenital absence of the pulmonary valve and infective endocarditis.

Diagnosis

Most individuals with mild to moderate PR live an uneventful life without any sequelae, as this can be a normal finding on echocardiography. With isolated significant PR, individuals can often live until their third decade without significant symptoms. As the right ventricle becomes hypertrophic and dilated, symptoms of right heart failure begin to emerge and irreversible myocardial damage may develop. Because right heart failure predisposes individuals to arrhythmias (i.e. ventricular tachycardia), presentation can be sudden cardiac death. On physical exam, a decrescendo diastolic murmur may be heard over the left lower sternal border. QRS prolongation on EKG can suggest right ventricular enlargement, which has been shown to correlate with worsening hypertrophy and is a risk factor for sudden cardiac death (Gatzoulis et al., 2000). CXR can show RA enlargement, and possibly dilation of the pulmonary artery (Beatriz et al., 2005).

The 2014 AHA/ACC guidelines outline the role of echocardiography and symptomatic progression in the diagnosis of severe PR (Table 8). Volume overload can be observed by the RVOT being filled by the regurgitant color jet. The regurgitant jet differs from normal individuals in that is occurs throughout diastole, not just a brief portion, and the color jet is much wider. However, if the lesion is severe enough, as in mitral regurgitation, there can be a quick equalization of pressure on both sides of the

Table 8. Stages of Severe Pulmonic Stenosis

Stage	Definition	Valve Anatomy	Valve Hemodynamics	Hemodynamic Consequences	Symptoms
C, D	Severe PS	-Thickened, distorted, possibly calcified leaflets with systolic doming and/or reduced excursion -Other anatomic abnormalities may be present, such as narrowed RVOT	Vmax > 4 m/s; peak instantaneous gradient > 64 mm Hg	-RVH -Possible RV, RA enlargement -Post-stenotic enlargement of main PA	None or variable and dependent on severity of obstruction

Table taken from 2014 AHA/ACC Valvular Heart Disease Guidelines (Nishimura et al., 2014).

PA indicates pulmonary artery; PS, pulmonic stenosis; RA, right atrium; RV, right ventricle; RVH, right ventricular hypertrophy; RVOT, right ventricular outflow tract; and Vmax, maximal pulmonic valve jet velocity.

pulmonic valve and the regurgitant jet may be quite brief (Lancellotti et al., 2013). While visualization of the pulmonic valve leaflets may be limited using both TTE and TEE, paradoxical ventricular septal motion can be seen and is a sign of RV overload (Bouzaz et al., 2005). Stress testing also has value in the individual with discordant symptoms and TTE findings. Once a patient has a diagnosis of severe PR, the only therapy available is replacement of the valve.

Optimization

Much like other regurgitant valvular diseases, medical therapy is typically a temporizing management technique. Diuretics can be used to alleviate symptoms of heart failure; however, the goal in treating severe PR is to replace the pulmonary valve before irreversible heart disease and failure occur. Elective repair should be encouraged as long as echocardiography supports the diagnosis in order to improve prognosis.

TRICUSPID STENOSIS

Background

Tricuspid valve disease is a common disorder that is usually clinically silent unless severe disease is present. Tricuspid disease can be divided into stenotic and regurgitant lesions; however, it is not uncommon to have elements of both. In general, regurgitant lesions are much more common than stenotic lesions. A review of 363 patients undergoing tricuspid valve replacement at a single center showed that 74% of lesions were purely regurgitant, 23% were mixed, and 2% were purely stenotic (Hauck, Freeman, Ackermann, Danielson, & Edwards, 1988). Isolated tricuspid stenosis is a rare phenomenon, as the vast majority TS cases also exhibit some degree of TR.

The etiology of tricuspid stenosis (TS) includes rheumatic disease, congenital stenosis or atresia, carcinoid syndrome, bacterial endocarditis, pacemaker and AICD lead scarring, and both primary and metastatic tumors (Nishimura et al., 2014; Taira et al., 2006). Historically, the most common cause of TS has been post-inflammatory changes due to rheumatic heart disease (Hauck et al., 1988). Importantly, tricuspid stenosis rarely exists without other valvular lesions, especially mitral and aortic valve disease (Roguin, Rinkevich, Milo, Markiewicz, & Reisner, 1998). As such, the signs and symptoms of TS may be overshadowed by those of left-sided heart lesions.

Diagnosis

As with all valvular lesions, the workup should include a history and physical, EKG, CXR, TTE, and possibly a TEE or right heart catheterization. Symptoms, which usually occur with severe disease, include generalized fatigue, abdominal bloating, and palpitations if arrhythmias are present. Physical exam findings may include jugular venous distention, peripheral edema, hepatosplenomegaly with right upper quadrant tenderness, ascites, and anasarca. Chest auscultation may reveal an opening snap followed by a high-pitched diastolic rumble heard best at the left sternal border. As mitral valve disease may also present concomitantly, the opening snap of TS may be overshadowed by or indistinguishable from the opening snap of MS. The murmur of TS typically becomes more pronounced with maneuvers that increase venous return such as inspiration and leg raise, while becoming more blunted with maneuvers that decrease venous return such as valsalva. A prominent *a* wave may be noted on examination of jugular venous pulsations in patients who remain in normal sinus rhythm. EKG findings include evidence of right atrial enlargement and supraventricular arrhythmias, most commonly atrial fibrillation. CXR may show evidence of right atrial or superior vena cava enlargement and pleural effusions if left sided valvular disease coexists. Given the risk of hepatic dysfunction, laboratory evaluation of synthetic liver function should be performed in patients with advanced disease.

The stages of TS in Table 9 are in accordance with the 2014 AHA/ACC Valvular Heart Disease guidelines. A mean pressure gradient > 5 mm Hg is commonly found in cases of severe TS; however, this has not been included in the formal staging due to effects of heart rate, cardiac output, and respirophasic variations on the calculated gradient. Surgical management is generally indicated for symptomatic isolated severe lesions or if a severe lesion is present at the time of correction of a left-sided valvular disorder (Nishimura et al., 2014).

Optimization

Very little evidence-based research exists relating to the medical optimization of TS. Management is focused mainly on relieving symptoms of volume overload, optimizing associated left sided heart disease,

Table 9. Stages of Severe PR

Stage	Definition	Valve Anatomy	Valve Hemodynamics	Hemodynamic Consequences	Symptoms
C, D	Severe PR	Distorted or absent leaflets, annular dilation	-Color jet fills RVOT -CW jet density and contour; dense laminar flow with steep deceleration slope; may terminate abruptly	-Paradoxical septal motion (volume overload pattern) -RV enlargement	None or variable and dependent on cause of PR and RV function

Table taken from 2014 AHA/ACC Valvular Heart Disease Guidelines (Nishimura et al., 2014).

CW indicates continuous wave; PR, pulmonic regurgitation; RV, right ventricular; and RVOT, right ventricular outflow tract.

and maintaining normal sinus rhythm. The goals of therapy can be achieved by the use of diuretics, cardiac glycosides, beta blockers and anti-arrhythmics. Maintenance of sinus rhythm is important to maximize ventricular filling through the stenotic lesion. The 2014 AHA/ACC guidelines suggest loop diuretics as useful agents in the treatment of right sided heart failure symptoms due to severe TS (Nishimura et al., 2014). Regardless of the choice of diuretic, therapy should be closely monitored, as stenotic lesions promote low-output states that can be further exacerbated by intravascular volume depletion.

TRICUSPID REGURGITATION

Background

The etiology of tricuspid regurgitation (TR) is much broader than TS, and can be divided into lesions that are primary (anatomically abnormal valve) or functional (anatomically normal valve). Etiologies of an anatomically abnormal valve causing TR include rheumatic heart disease, myxomatous degeneration, floppy valves, congenital abnormalities (most commonly Ebstein's anomaly, ASD, or VSD), carcinoid syndrome, prolapse from papillary muscle dysfunction, radiation, biopsy-related trauma, chest wall trauma, pacemaker or AICD leads, and infective endocarditis. TR with an anatomically normal valve results from right ventricular pressure or volume overload due to various causes including primary RV dysfunction, primary pulmonary hypertension, chronic obstructive pulmonary disease, pulmonary thomboemboli, and left-sided heart disease (Nishimura et al., 2014; Waller, 1987; Rogers & Bolling, 2009). Similarly to TS, the most common etiology of TR has been post-inflammatory changes associated with rheumatic heart disease (Hauck et al., 1988).

Diagnosis

As in TS, the workup of TR should include a history and physical, EKG, CXR and TTE. The most recent guidelines from the AHA/ACC also recommend considering a TEE, CMR, 3-D echocardiography, or right heart catheterization, especially when suspicion of RV dysfunction is present, as these patients are prone to disease progression (Nishimura et al., 2014; Nath, Forster, & Heidenreich, 2004). Stress testing may be indicated in the asymptomatic patient in whom suspicion of severe disease is high and early recognition of severe disease would lead to surgical correction (Nishimura et al., 2014). Symptoms of TR may include generalized fatigue, decreased exercise tolerance, abdominal bloating, anorexia, and palpitations. Physical examination findings consist of jugular venous distention with a prominent regurgitant *j* wave, a high-pitched pansystolic murmur noted at the left sternal border that increases with inspiration, an S3 sound that increases with inspiration, an increased P2 sound if pulmonary hypertension is present, hepatosplenomegaly with systolic pulsatility noted at the liver edge, and peripheral edema. As disease progression occurs, patients may appear cachectic with evidence of jaundice. EKG findings include evidence of right atrial enlargement and atrial fibrillation. CXR findings may include evidence of right ventricular or atrial enlargement, pleural effusions if left sided valvular disease is present, azygous vein dilatation, and upward displacement of the diaphragm due to abdominal ascites. Laboratory evaluation of liver function should be performed in patients with advanced disease. Invasive testing via right heart catheterization should be considered when more accurate estimates of pulmonary artery systolic pressure or pulmonary vascular resistance are necessary for therapeutic planning (Nishimura et al., 2014).

The stages of TR in Table 10 are in accordance with the 2014 AHA/ACC guidelines. Current class I guidelines recommend surgical correction of severe symptomatic or asymptomatic TR regardless of etiology if left-sided valvular surgery is performed (Nishimura et al., 2014).

Optimization

The preoperative optimization of patients with TR involves the treatment of the underlying cause of right ventricular failure, and as such, usually involves concomitant evaluation and treatment of left-sided heart disease. There is limited evidence-based research regarding specific medical therapies for the treatment of TR. Current guidelines from the AHA/ACC recommend diuretics in the treatment of severe TR with evidence of heart failure (Nishimura et al., 2014). If ventricular function is poor, medications tailored to the preservation of function, such as beta blockers, ACEI's, and ARB's should be considered. Cardiac revascularization for RV ischemia or LV ischemia causing ventricular dysfunction should be considered. Management of systemic hypertension should be employed in cases of functional TR so as to limit the effects of increased left-sided pressures on the degree of regurgitation. Other therapies to treat underlying causes of functional TR, such as COPD, primary pulmonary hypertension, pulmonary hypertension secondary to obstructive sleep apnea, and pulmonary thromboemboli, can be employed as well.

INFECTIVE ENDOCARDITIS

Background

Infective endocarditis (IE) is a serious disease that carries a high risk of mortality and complications. It is characterized by the development of a vegetative lesion caused by a microbial infection on the endocardial surface of the heart. This lesion is composed of a collection of platelets, fibrin, microorganisms, and inflammatory cells. The mechanism of pathogenesis is most often a combination of endothelial valvular damage coupled with introduction of microbes into the bloodstream, resulting in a localized vegetation on the valvular endothelium, which is normally resistant to colonization by bacteria. IE has historically been classified as "acute" or "subacute-chronic" on the basis of the timing of the development of symptoms and the rapidity of disease progression, with most cases in the modern era presenting as acute disease (Mylonakis & Calderwood, 2001; Hoen & Duval, 2013). In the modern era, it is now

Table 10. Stages of Severe TS

Stage	Definition	Valve Anatomy	Valve Hemodynamics	Hemodynamic Consequences	Symptoms
C, D	Severe TS	Thickened, distorted, calcified leaflets	-$T_{1/2} \geq 190$ ms -Valve area ≤ 1.0 cm^2	-RA/IVC enlargement	-None or variable and dependent on severity of associated valve disease and degree of obstruction

Table taken from 2014 ACC/AHA Valvular Heart Disease Guidelines (Nishimura et al., 2014).
IVC indicates inferior vena cava; RA, right atrium; $T^{1/2}$; pressure half-time; and TS, tricuspid stenosis.

classified according to underlying cardiac comorbidities, location of the lesion, presence of intracardiac devices or prosthetic valves, or the mode of acquisition, with some overlap of these classifications (Hoen & Duval, 2013). Since Sir William Osler first analyzed a series of cases of infective endocarditis in 1885 (Osler, 1885), the incidence of the disease has not changed significantly. However, epidemiological patterns have changed over time, and mortality has decreased along with therapeutic advances in the areas of antibiotic therapy, microbiologic diagnosis, imaging modalities and surgical treatment. Despite these advances, mortality today remains high, with in-hospital mortality around 20% (Murdoch et al., 2009) and 5-year mortality rate around 40% (Bannay et al., 2011). There has been some recent evidence to suggest that mortality may be significantly lowered by treating patients with a management-based team approach at a specialized heart valve centers, and these results need to be borne out in future studies (Botelho-Nevers et al., 2009; Tattevin, Donal, & Revest, 2010).

Epidemiology/Risk Factors

The incidence of infective endocarditis is difficult to define precisely, as classifications are variable, and the incidence of predisposing variables such as rheumatic heart disease and IV drug use differs over time and between regions. Generally, incidence varies from 3-10 episodes/100,000 person-years depending on geographic location. In the United States, there are approximately 10,000-15,000 new cases of IE per year. This incidence has not changed significantly over recent decades, despite advances in health care. However, the epidemiological pattern of IE in developing countries has changed over time as a result of increasing life expectancy, changing risk factors, and an increase in nosocomial cases (Tleyjeh et al., 2007; Thuny, Grisoli, Collart, Habib, & Raoult, 2012).

Independent non-cardiac risk factors that may predispose to the development of IE include male sex, advanced age, history of intravenous drug use, poor dentition or oral infection, chronic hemodialysis, the presence of an indwelling intravascular device, and diabetes mellitus. Approximately three-fourths of patients who develop IE have some preexisting structural cardiac abnormality. Cardiac comorbid conditions that are considered risk factors include valvular heart disease (including rheumatic heart disease, mitral valve prolapse/mitral regurgitation, aortic valve disease, and other valvular abnormalities), unrepaired congenital heart disease (ventricular septal defect, patent ductus arteriosus, coarctation of the aorta, and tetralogy of Fallot), the presence of prosthetic heart valves, the presence of intracardiac devices, and a prior history of infective endocarditis.

Microbiology

A variety of microorganisms may cause infective endocarditis, with staphylococcus and streptococcus species accounting for 80% of cases. Staphylococcus and streptococcus account for equal proportions of cases of community-acquired IE, whereas staphylococcus accounts for most cases of healthcare-associated IE. Other less common causative organisms include enterococci, fungi, bacteria in the HACEK group (haemophilus species, *Aggregatibacter* (formerly *Actinobacillus*) *actinomycetemcomitans, Cardiobacterium hominis, Eikenella corrodens*, and *Kingella kingae*), and non-HACEK gram-negative bacteria. In cases of IE with negative blood cultures (10% of cases), causative organisms are likely to be fastidious microorganisms such as bartonella species, brucella species, Coxiella burnetti (the agent that causes Q fever) and HACEK organisms (Murdoch et al., 2009).

Table 11. Stages of TR

Stage	Definition	Valve Anatomy	Valve Hemodynamics*	Hemodynamic Consequences	Symptoms
A	At risk of TR	**Primary** -Mild rheumatic change -Mild prolapse -Other (e.g., IE with vegetation, early carcinoid deposition, radiation) -Intra-annular RV pacemaker or ICD lead -Postcardiac transplant (biopsy related) **Functional** -Normal -Early annular dilation	-No or trace TR	-None	-None or in relation to other left heart or pulmonary/ pulmonary vascular disease
B	Progressive TR	**Primary** -Progressive leaflet deterioration/destruction -Moderate-to-severe prolapse, limited chordal rupture **Functional** -Early annular dilation -Moderate leaflet tethering	**Mild TR** -Central jet area < 5.0 cm^2 -Vena contracta width no defined -CW jet density and contour: soft and parabolic -Hepatic vein flow: systolic dominance **Moderate TR** -Central jet area 5-10 cm^2 -Vena contracta width not defined but < 0.70 cm -CW jet density and contour: dense, variable contour -Hepatic vein flow: systolic blunting	**Mild TR** -RV/RA/IVC size normal **Moderate TR** -No RV enlargement -No or mild RA enlargement -No or mild IVC enlargement with normal respirophasic variation -Normal RA pressure	-None or in relation to other left heart or pulmonary/ pulmonary vascular disease
C	Asymptomatic, severe TR	**Primary** -Flail or grossly distorted leaflets **Functional** -Severe annular dilation (> 40 mm or > 21 mm/m^2) -Marked leaflet tethering	-Central jet area >10 cm^2 Vena contracta width > 0.7 cm -CW jet density and contour: dense, triangular with early peak -Hepatic vein flow: systolic reversal	-RV/RA/IVC dilated with decreased IVC respirophasic variation -Elevated RA pressure with "c-V" waves -Diastolic interventricular septal flattening may be present	-None or in relation to other left heart or pulmonary/ pulmonary vascular disease
D	Symptomatic, Severe TR	**Primary** -Flail or grossly distorted leaflets **Functional** -Severe annular dilation (> 40 mm or > 21 mm/m^2) -Marked leaflet tethering	-Central jet area > 10 cm^2 Vena contracta width > 0.7 cm -CW jet density and contour: dense, triangular with early peak -Hepatic vein flow: systolic reversal	-RV/RA/IVC dilated with decreased IVC respirophasic variation -Elevated RA pressure with "c-V" waves -Diastolic interventricular septal flattening -Reduced RV systolic function in late phase	-Fatigue, palpitations, dyspnea, abdominal bloating, anorexia, edema

Table taken from 2014 ACC/AHA Valvular Heart Disease Guidelines (Nishimura et al., 2014).

*Several valve hemodynamic criteria are provided for assessment of severity of TR, but not all criteria for each category will necessarily be present in every patient. Categorization of severity of TR as mild, moderate, or severe also depends on image quality and integration of these parameters with clinical findings. CW indicated continuous waves; ICD, implantable cardioverter-defibrillator; IE, infective endocarditis; IVC, inferior vena cava; RA, right atrium; RV, right ventricle; and TR, tricuspid regurgitation.

Prosthetic valve endocarditis (PVE) differs from native valve endocarditis in its presentation and microbiologic features. PVE may present early after valve replacement (within 2 months) or late after surgery (after 2 months). Microorganisms associated with early infection may be introduced directly by contamination during surgery, or indirectly via hematogenous spread after surgery. The microorganisms most commonly associated with early PVE are hospital-acquired organisms; these include *Staphylococcus aureus*, coagulase-negative staphylococci, gram-negative bacilli, and fungi. Microorganisms most commonly associated with late PVE, especially cases presenting more than 12 months after surgery, are usually caused by the same organisms that cause native valve endocarditis. Coxiella burnetii has a unique predisposition to cause PVE, although it is a relatively rare cause of native valve endocarditis (Wang et al., 2007).

Clinical Manifestations/Diagnosis

The diagnosis of infective endocarditis is generally based upon a combination of factors, including history and physical examination, blood cultures and other laboratory studies, echocardiography, EKG, and CXR. Infective endocarditis in the modern age usually presents acutely rather than chronically. Fever is a common presenting symptom, occurring in more than 80% of cases. Onset of a new heart murmur is a presenting sign in about 50% of cases, and worsening of an existing heart murmur occurs in about 20% of cases. Less frequent signs include hematuria, splenomegaly, splinter hemorrhages, Janeway's lesions, Roth's spots, and conjunctival hemorrhage. Patients may also prevent with signs of advanced disease including sepsis, meningitis, heart failure, septic pulmonary emboli, stroke, acute peripheral arterial occlusion, and renal failure. Elevated inflammatory markers (erythrocyte sedimentation rate, C-reactive protein) may be seen in about two-thirds of cases. Leukocytosis and anemia may be seen in about half of all presenting cases (Murdoch et al., 2009).

Establishing the diagnosis of infective endocarditis is relatively straightforward in the setting of positive blood cultures and evidence of endocardial involvement, but in the case of negative blood cultures and/or lack of obvious cardiac pathology, the diagnosis is more difficult to make and may be delayed. In 1994, the Duke criteria were proposed as a standardized algorithm to diagnose endocarditis based upon microbiological data and echocardiographic imaging (Durack, Lukes, & Bright, 1994). These criteria were validated in several independent series. In 2000 the criteria were refined to more accurately detect endocarditis in the setting of negative blood cultures and Staphylococcus aureus bacteremia (Li et al., 2000). Diagnosis is made based on the fulfillment of set numbers of major and minor clinical criteria (see Table 12 and Table 13). The Duke criteria have sensitivity and specificity greater than 80%, but they should not be used as a replacement for clinical judgment.

Identification of the causative organism is crucial in establishing the diagnosis of endocarditis and guiding antimicrobial therapy. In patients with underlying risk factors and unexplained fever for more than 48 hours, or in patients with newly-diagnosed left-sided valve regurgitation, at least 2-3 sets of blood cultures should be obtained from separate peripheral sites (ideally not from an indwelling vascular catheter) before starting antibiotic therapy (Nishimura et al., 2014). Identification of the causative pathogen is successful in about 90% of cases when 3 blood cultures are obtained. Culture-negative endocarditis should be considered in any patient with persistent fever and one or more findings consistent with endocarditis. Culture-negative endocarditis usually occurs when blood cultures have been drawn

Table 12. Modified Duke criteria for diagnosis of infective endocarditis

Definite IE
• Pathologic criteria
• Microorganism: demonstrated by culture or histology in a vegetation, or in a vegetation that has embolized, or in an intracardiac abscess **OR**
• Pathologic lesions: vegetation or intracardiac abscess, confirmed by histology showing active endocarditis
• Clinical criteria (using definitions listed in part B)
• 2 major criteria **OR**
• 1 major and 3 minor criteria **OR**
• 5 minor criteria
Possible IE
• 1 major criterion and 1 minor criterion **OR**
• 3 minor criteria
Rejected IE
• Firm alternate diagnosis for manifestations of endocarditis **OR**
• Resolution of manifestations of endocarditis, with antibiotic therapy for four days or less **OR**
• No pathologic evidence of infective endocarditis at surgery or autopsy after antibiotic therapy for four days or less
• Does not meet criteria for possible infective endocarditis, as above

Table taken from Li et al., 2000.
IE: infective endocarditis.

after the initiation of antibiotics, or in the case of endocarditis caused by obligate intracellular bacteria, fungi, or fastidious organisms. Isolation of these organisms requires culture on specialized media, and growth may be slow, so microbiologic diagnosis is often delayed. To address these issues, some institutions have implemented protocols to standardize the timing and type of laboratory tests that are sent for any patient with suspected endocarditis, which include multiple sets of aerobic and anaerobic blood cultures, as well as a serum sample for detection of rheumatoid factor and estimation of specific antibodies for *Coxiella burnetti, Bartonella* spp, *Brucella* spp, *Chlamydia* spp, *Mycoplasma pneumonia, Legionella pneumophilia*, and *Aspergillus* spp. However, the benefit of immediate serological detection should be considered, especially in low-prevalence areas. Causative organisms may also be identified by examination of tissue obtained during surgical valve excision, either by tissue culture or with the use of histochemical stains or immunohistochemical analysis (Thuny et al., 2012). Finally, PCR (polymerase chain reaction) has been validated as a modality for detection of pathogens in explanted valve tissue, and it shows promise for detection of pathogens obtained from blood. Broad-range PCR techniques may be used to identify bacterial or fungal pathogens from blood, but they are susceptible to contamination and false-positive results. Recently, the sequencing of complete genome sequences for specific pathogens and the development of real-time PCR assays has led to improvements in speed and accuracy of pathogen determination, and it has been proposed that pathogen identification via PCR be included as one of the Duke criteria. However, it must be recognized that PCR may produce a false-positive result by amplification of non-viable microorganisms after a clinical cure has been achieved, and so the amplified DNA results must be correlated with the clinical picture (Fenollar & Raoult, 2007).

Table 13. Major and minor criteria for the diagnosis of infective endocarditis

Major criteria
• Positive blood cultures for IE
o Typical microorganism for infective endocarditis from two separate blood cultures
▪ Viridans streptococci
▪ *Streptococcus gallolyticus* (formerly *S. bovis*), including nutritional variant strains (*Granulicatella* spp and *Abiotrophia defectiva*)
▪ HACEK group: *Haemophilus* spp, *Aggregatibacter* (formerly *Actinobacillus actinomycete comitants*), *Cardiobacterium hominis*, *Eikenella* spp, and *Kingella kingae*
▪ *Staphylococcus aureus*
▪ Community-acquired enterococci, in the absence of a primary focus; **OR**
o Persistently positive blood culture, defined as recovery of a microorganism consistent with IE from:
▪ Blood cultures drawn more than 12 hours apart **OR**
▪ All of three or a majority of four or more separate blood cultures, with first and last drawn at least one hour apart
o Single positive blood culture for Coxiella burnetii or antiphase I IgG antibody titer > 1:800
• Evidence of endocardial involvement
o Positive echocardiogram for IE
▪ TEE recommended in patients with prosthetic valves, rated at least "possible IE" by clinical criteria, or complicated IE (paravalvular abscess); TTE as first test in other patients
▪ Definition of positive echocardiogram
• Oscillating intracardiac mass, on valve or supporting structures, or in the path of regurgitant jets, or on implanted material, in the absence of an alternative anatomic explanation **OR**
• Abscess **OR**
• New partial dehiscence of prosthetic valve
o New valvular regurgitation
▪ Increase or change in preexisting murmur not sufficient
Minor criteria
• Predisposition: predisposing heart condition or intravenous drug use
• Fever: 38.0°C (100°F)
• Vascular phenomena: major arterial emboli, septic pulmonary infarcts, mycotic aneurysm, intracranial hemorrhage, conjunctival hemorrhages, Janeway lesions
• Immunologic phenomena: glomerulonephritis, Osler's nodes, Roth spots, rheumatoid factor
• Microbiologic evidence: positive blood culture but not meeting major criterion as noted previously (excluding single positive cultures for coagulase-negative staphylococci and organisms that do not cause endocarditis) **OR** serologic evidence of active infection with organism consistent with IE
• Echocardiographic minor criteria eliminated

Table taken from Li et al., 2000.
IE: infective endocarditis, TEE: transesophageal echocardiography, TTE: transthoracic echocardiography

Transthoracic echocardiography is generally recommended as the initial imaging study in all patients with suspected endocarditis to identify vegetations, characterize the hemodynamic severity of valvular lesions, assess ventricular function and pulmonary pressures, and detect complications (Nishimura et al., 2014). In low-risk patients, a normal TTE is a fast, non-invasive way of confirming that endocarditis is unlikely. Furthermore, TTE is better than transesophageal echocardiography for detection of anterior cardiac abscesses and for assessment of hemodynamic consequences of valve dysfunction (Thuny et al., 2012). Transesophageal echocardiography has higher sensitivity and specificity than TTE, and thus should be performed in cases of nondiagnostic TTE, the presence of intracardiac leads or devices, the development or suspicion of complications such as significant regurgitation or perivalvular abscess, or negative TTE associated with high clinical suspicion (e.g. bacteremia due to an organism known to be a common cause of IE, or persistent fever without bacteremia or a new murmur in patients with prosthetic valves) (Nishimura et al., 2014).

In patients with small or absent vegetations or with challenging anatomy, neither TTE nor TEE may be sufficient to make a definitive diagnosis, and the use of new and innovative imaging modalities may be helpful. 3-D echocardiography has preliminarily been shown to be slightly more effective than 2-D echocardiography in identifying vegetations and complications such as abscesses, perforations, and ruptured chordae (Hansalia et al., 2009). Cardiac CT scan has also been shown to be useful in providing information about valvular abscesses and pseudoaneurysms, and it is recommended in the setting of suspected paravalvular infections when the anatomy cannot be clearly demonstrated by echocardiography (Feuchtner et al., 2009; Nishimura et al., 2014). Although PET-CT scans are not usually as accurate in identifying vegetations as echocardiography, some studies have reported that this modality may be useful in detecting aortic root infections and pacing system infections in the setting of negative or equivocal echocardiography. PET-CT can also be extremely useful in the detection of silent peripheral embolic events and infectious metastases, early detection of which has been shown to confer a therapeutic effect in about a quarter of cases of infective endocarditis (Thuny et al., 2012; Van Reit et al., 2010). Finally, performing systematic cerebral MRI in patients with suspected endocarditis may be of value in detecting subclinical cerebrovascular complications, and has been shown to result in modification diagnostic classification as well as therapeutic and surgical plans (Duval et al., 2010). Further study needs to be undertaken in order to clarify the best practices regarding the use of these various imaging modalities.

Repeat imaging (TTE and/or TEE) should be performed in cases with initially negative findings if infective endocarditis continues to be suspected (Hoen & Duval, 2013). Repeat imaging is also indicated for reevaluation of patients with endocarditis who have had a change in clinical signs or symptoms (e.g. a new murmur, embolism, abscess, heart failure, atrioventricular heart block, or persistent fever) and in patients at high risk of complications (e.g. extensive infected tissue or large vegetation seen on initial echocardiogram or staphylococcal, enterococcal or fungal infections) (Nishimura et al., 2014). Figure 5 summarizes all recommendations for imaging studies in native and prosthetic valve endocarditis according to the 2014 AHA/ACC guidelines.

Because of the complex nature of establishing the diagnosis of IE in some patients as well as the high morbidity and mortality associated with the disease, these patients should evaluated in a systematic way using a management-based approach. It has been demonstrated that patients with suspected IE who were treated with a standardized diagnostic and therapeutic protocol experience significantly lower mortality, better compliance with antimicrobial therapy, and lower incidence of complications such as renal failure than patients who were treated without a standardized protocol (Botelho-Nevers et al., 2009). Thus, current AHA/ACC guidelines recommend that patients with suspected IE be evaluated and managed with consultation of a multispecialty Heart Valve team including an infectious disease specialist, cardiologist, and cardiac surgeon. In surgically managed patients, this team should also include a cardiac anesthesiologist (Nishimura et al., 2014).

Figure 5. Recommendations for imaging studies in NVE and PVE
*Figure taken from 2014 ACC/AHA Valvular Heart Disease Guidelines (Nishimura et al., 2014). *Repeat TEE and/or TTE recommended for reevaluation of patients with IE and a change in clinical signs or symptoms and in patients at high risk of complications. CT indicates computed tomography; IE, infective endocarditis; NVE, native valve endocarditis; PVE, prosthetic valve endocarditis; S. aureus, Staphylococcus aureus ; TEE, transesophageal echocardiography; and TTE, transthoracic echocardiography.*

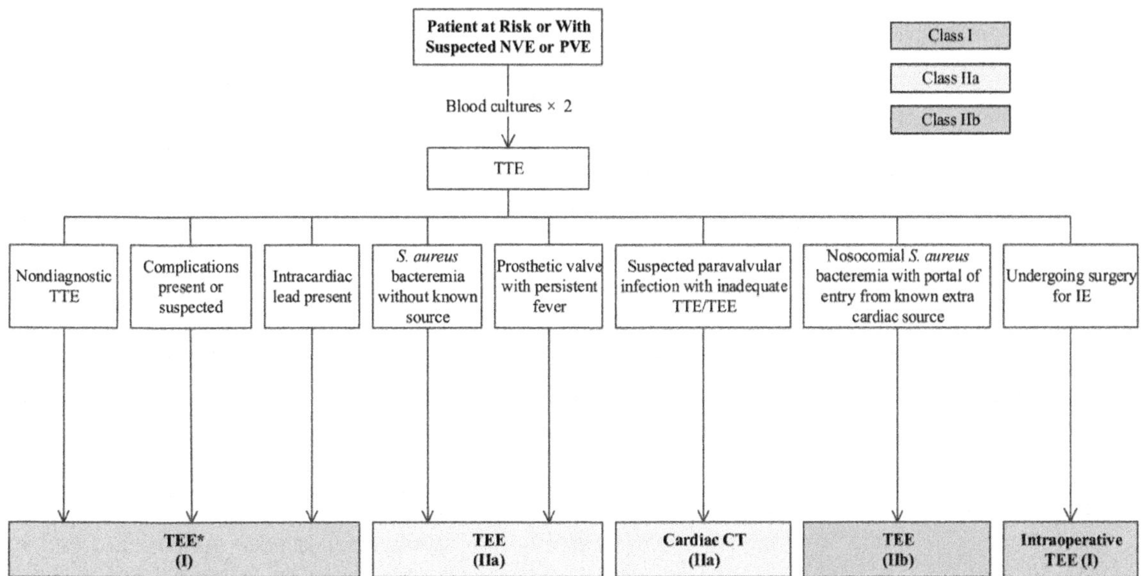

Treatment

Because delayed or inappropriate antibiotic therapy can result in increased morbidity and mortality, antibiotics should be initiated promptly after microbiological sampling in patients with suspected or confirmed endocarditis. Antibiotic regimens must be designed to provide bactericidal concentrations of drug throughout the course of treatment based on in vitro determination of the minimum inhibitory concentration, as bacteriostatic agents are ineffective in endocarditis. Prolonged parenteral administration of a single agent or combination of agents is recommended. The duration of treatment must be long enough to allow for the eradication of all microorganisms concentrated within the valvular vegetation. Antibiotic therapy is often initiated on an empiric basis and then modified as culture and sensitivity results become available. Empiric antibiotic therapy should provide coverage for the most likely causative organisms, including staphylococcus (methicillin-sensitive and resistant), streptococcus, and enterococcus. In general, many experts recommend using a combination of agents that are active against the cell wall (β-lactams or glycopeptides) with or without an aminoglycoside (gentamycin) for most cases of infectious endocarditis (Thuny et al., 2012). For native-valve endocarditis due to common microorganisms, recommended treatment duration ranges from 2 to 6 weeks, depending on the pathogen and the site of valvular infection. For prosthetic valve endocarditis, duration of treatment is usually 6 weeks. Guidelines for appropriate antibiotic regimens are published and updated regularly by professional societies, and much in terms of specific antibiotic regimens is outside of the scope of this chapter due to the constantly changing nature of pathogens and resistance (Hoen & Duval, 2013).

Because morbidity and mortality in endocarditis have remained high despite the availability of new and potent antibiotics, much effort has been made in recent years to identify synergistic combinations of antibiotics that may result in increased efficacy and decreased toxicity. However, few synergistic combinations of antibiotics have been globally validated in in vitro models, experimental IE models, and human clinical trials. The addition of aminoglycosides to an antibiotic with activity against gram-positive bacteria often results in synergistic interaction in vitro, and it is the combination most commonly recommended. However, in the few randomized trials that have evaluated this, the addition of an aminoglycoside to a β-lactam was shown to result in synergy clinically only in the case of enterococcal infective endocarditis (Le & Bayer, 2003). Although traditional guidelines for enterococcal endocarditis have recommended combination treatment with a cell wall-active antibiotic agent plus an aminoglycoside, a prospective single-center cohort study noted favorable outcomes in patients treated with a shorter course of aminoglycoside plus a longer/traditional course of a cell wall-active agent. Thus, reducing the aminoglycoside component to approximately 2 weeks may maintain clinical efficacy while reducing potential toxicity such as kidney injury in this population (Olaison & Schadewitz, 2002). It has also been demonstrated in two multicenter prospective cohort studies that patients with enterococcal endocarditis may be effectively treated with double β-lactam therapy (ampicillin plus a third-generation cephalosporin), which may reduce nephrotoxic complications associated with aminoglycosides (Gavaldà et al., 2007; Fernández-Hidalgo et al., 2013). Combination therapy for carefully selected cases of streptococcus viridans endocarditis with a cell wall-active agent plus an aminoglycoside has been shown to be effective, and allows the duration of therapy to be reduced to only two weeks, making outpatient treatment feasible (Wilson et al., 1981; Francioli, Ruch, & Stamboulian, 1995; Sexton et al., 1998). Finally, combination therapy for cases of right-sided endocarditis from Staphylococcus aureus with nafcillin and an aminoglycoside has been demonstrated to be effective (Chambers, Miller, & Newman, 1988). Despite widespread use, there exists very little evidence from human trials that synergistic combination therapy for the treatment of left-sided *Staphylococcus aureus* endocarditis is clinically beneficial. Additionally, no randomized trials have demonstrated clinical benefit of combination therapy with vancomycin plus an aminoglycoside (Le & Bayer, 2003).

Patients who develop endocarditis and have been taking oral anticoagulant therapy for prosthetic valves or for other reasons are at increased risk for intracerebral hemorrhage due to bleeding from emboli, and the risk of embolism is not decreased with anticoagulation (Mylonakis & Calderwood, 2001). As such, anticoagulant therapy with vitamin K antagonists should be temporarily discontinued in patients with endocarditis who develop central nervous system symptoms compatible with embolism or stroke, regardless of the other indications for anticoagulation. Temporary discontinuation of anticoagulation may also be considered in any patient receiving vitamin K antagonists at the time of diagnosis of endocarditis, at the discretion of the treating physician (Nishimura et al., 2014). Generally, patients who are on anticoagulation for a prosthetic valve and develop endocarditis are cautiously continued on anticoagulant therapy during treatment unless CNS complications develop. However, indirect evidence from uncontrolled studies suggests that patients with prosthetic valve endocarditis caused by Staph. aureus may be at higher risk of CNS hemorrhage, and cessation of anticoagulant therapy should especially be considered in these patients. If surgical intervention is planned in any patient, oral anticoagulation may be discontinued and bridged with heparin to allow for rapid reversal at the time of surgery (Mylonakis & Calderwood, 2001).

The rate of early valve replacement or repair (during initial hospitalization and before completion of a full therapeutic course of antibiotics) has increased over the past several decades to approximately

50%. There has been general consensus that indications for early surgery for native valves include heart failure, uncontrolled infection, and prevention of embolic events. The trend towards reduced mortality and complications with early surgery has been suggested in many observational and retrospective studies, but results have been inconsistent, likely due to bias inherent in these observational series. For example, selection bias may occur, where treatment groups differ in baseline characteristics or clinical features of disease based on investigators assigning treatment groups without randomization. This selection bias may be reduced using propensity score analysis, where the conditional probability of valve surgery given the observed confounders is matched on or adjusted for. Additionally, survivor treatment bias may be present, where patients who live longer are more likely to undergo surgery because they have more time to be selected for surgery than those who die earlier. Survivor bias may be reduced by consideration of surgery as a time-dependent covariate, or by a match on the follow-up time between surgically treated and non-surgically treated patients. Finally, hidden bias, or unaccounted-for patient characteristics that may affect both the decision to treat and the outcome, can play a role in skewing the results of observational studies (Hoen & Duval, 2013). Some investigators have attempted to control for these biases in meta-analyses by standardizing methods and introducing controls for the most important sources of bias. The trend towards decreased long-term mortality in patients with left-sided infective endocarditis has been confirmed in these studies (Bannay et al., 2011; Lalani et al., 2010). One randomized prospective trial of adults with left-sided native valve endocarditis and a large vegetation demonstrated decreased rates of systemic embolization in the group randomized to early surgery (within 48 hours of randomization) compared to the group assigned to conventional treatment, but no differences were observed in in-hospital mortality or 6-month mortality. However, the patients included in this study were comparatively young with a low incidence of comorbidities and low mortality, so it is unclear whether these results may be extrapolated to the general population (Kang et al., 2012). There is a dearth of randomized trials investigating the role of surgical management, and so present practice guidelines are based largely on the results of observational/retrospective series and expert opinion (Thuny et al., 2012).

The most recent recommendations from the 2014 AHA/ACC guidelines emphasize the importance of the involvement of a multispecialty Heart Valve Team when making decisions about the timing of surgical intervention. Specifically, early surgery for endocarditis is recommended in patients who present with valvular dysfunction resulting in symptoms of heart failure. Early surgery is also indicated in cases of uncontrolled infection, including endocarditis caused by difficult-to-treat pathogens (*Staphylococcus aureus*, fungus, or other highly resistant organisms), annular or aortic abscess, destructive penetrating lesions, heart block, or persistent bacteremia or fevers lasting longer than 5 to 7 days after the initiation of appropriate antibiotics. Early surgery is recommended in patients who present with recurrent emboli and persistent vegetations despite appropriate antibiotic therapy, as well as in patients with native valve endocarditis who exhibit mobile vegetations greater than 10 mm in length, with or without clinical evidence of embolic phenomena. Surgery is indicated for patients with prosthetic valve endocarditis and relapsing infection (defined as recurrence of bacteremia after a complete course of appropriate antibiotics and subsequently negative blood cultures) without other identifiable source for portal of infection. Finally, complete removal of pacemaker or defibrillator systems, including all leads and the generator, is recommended as part of the early management plan in patients with endocarditis with documented infection of the device or leads, in patients with endocarditis caused by Staphylococcus aureus or fungi even without evidence of device or lead infection, and in patients undergoing valve surgery for endocarditis (Nishimura et al., 2014). Figure 6 summarizes all recommendations for diagnosis and treatment of infective endocarditis according to the 2014 AHA/ACC guidelines.

Figure 6. Diagnosis and treatment of IE

Figure taken from 2014 ACC/AHA Valvular Heart Disease Guidelines (Nishimura et al., 2014). HF indicates heart failure; ICD, implantable cardioverter-defibrillator; IE, infective endocarditis; NVE, native valve endocarditis; PVE, prosthetic valve endocarditis; Rx, therapy; S. aureus, Staphylococcus aureus; TEE, transesophageal echocardiography; TTE, transthoracic echocardiography; and VKA, vitamin K antagonist.

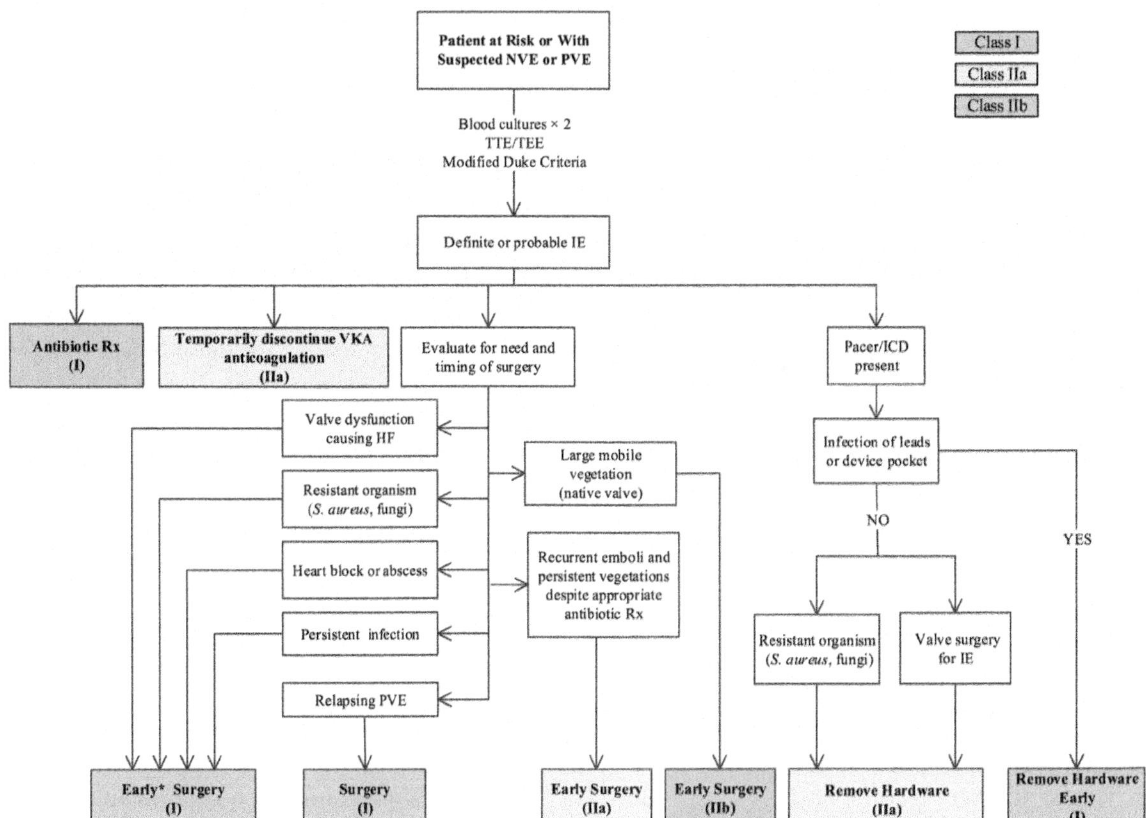

Complications

Cardiac complications and neurologic complications are the most common causes of major morbidity and mortality in infective endocarditis. Congestive heart failure occurs in approximately 50% of cases, and is the leading cause of mortality from endocarditis. CHF may result from infection-induced valvular or prosthesis damage, or much less commonly, from embolism of fragments of vegetations causing myocardial infarction. CHF is more frequently associated with aortic valve infection than with mitral valve infection, and it is observed more frequently in cases where the infection extends beyond the valve annulus (Mylonakis & Calderwood, 2001). Hemodynamic failure may also be caused by the development of septic shock, which is most likely to occur during the acute phase of *Staphylococcus aureus* bacteremia (Mourvillier et al., 2004). Neurologic complications are the most serious extracardiac complications of endocarditis, occurring at a rate of 15 to 40% in various case series, and may be the initial presenting symptom of endocarditis in some patients. Neurologic complications include ischemic and hemorrhagic stroke, transient ischemic attack, silent cerebral embolism, mycotic aneurysm, brain abscess, and meningitis. Cerebral embolism is more likely to occur when vegetations are large, mobile, and located on the mitral valve, or when *Staphylococcus aureus* is the causative agent (Mylonakis & Calderwood, 2001, Hoen & Duval, 2013). The rate of cerebral embolic events decreases rapidly once antimicrobial therapy has been started; analysis from a large multicenter cohort study found that the crude incidence of stroke in patients receiving appropriate antimicrobial therapy was 4.82/1000 patient days in the first week of therapy, fell to 1.71 patient days in the second week, and continued to decline further throughout the course of therapy (Dickerman et al., 2007). Acute renal failure may result from cardiogenic or septic shock leading to acute tubular necrosis or from the administration of nephrotoxic drugs or contrast agents. Septic embolism may involve the spleen, kidney, liver, and iliac or mesenteric arteries. Splenic abscess may result from direct seeding of the spleen or bacteremic seeding of a previously infarcted area, and may be a cause of prolonged fever (Mylonakis & Calderwood, 2001).

CONCLUSION

The preoperative assessment and optimization of patients with valvular heart disease is a complex task. As newer therapeutic options are offered to patients with numerous comorbidities, specialized "Heart Valve Teams" and "Heart Valve Centers of Excellence" have come into the forefront in an attempt to standardize medical optimization and therapeutic approaches according to evidence-based medicine. Multiple specialists, including internists, cardiologists, intensivists, cardiothoracic surgeons, and anesthesiologists will be integral in the assessment and optimization of these patients.

REFERENCES

Akram, M. R., Chan, T., McAuliffe, S., & Chenzbraun, A. (2008). Non-rheumatic annular mitral stenosis: Prevalence and characteristics. *European Journal of Echocardiography*, *10*(1), 103–105. doi:10.1093/ejechocard/jen179 PMID:18579487

Arai, N., Matsumoto, A., Nishikawa, N., Yonekura, K., Eto, Y., Kuwada, Y., & Aoyahi, T. et al. (2001). Beta-blocker therapy improved symptoms and exercise capacity in a patient with dynamic intra-right ventricular obstruction an atypical form of double-chambered right ventricle. *Journal of the American Society of Echocardiography*, *14*(6), 650–653. doi:10.1067/mje.2001.110782 PMID:11391298

Bannay, A., Hoen, B., Duval, X., Obadia, J., Selton-Suty, C., Le Moing, V., & Alla, F. et al.AEPEI Study Group. (2011). The impact of valve surgery on short- and long-term mortality in left-sided infective endocarditis: Do differences in methodological approaches explain previous conflicting results? *European Heart Journal*, *32*(16), 2003–2015. doi:10.1093/eurheartj/ehp008 PMID:19208650

Boon, N. A., & Bloomfield, P. (2002). The medical management of valvar heart disease. *Heart (British Cardiac Society)*, *87*(4), 395–400. doi:10.1136/heart.87.4.395 PMID:11907022

Botelho-Nevers, E., Thuny, F., Casalta, J. P., Richet, H., Gouriet, F., Collart, F., & Raoult, D. et al. (2009). Dramatic reduction in infective endocarditis-related mortality with a management-based approach. *Archives of Internal Medicine*, *169*(14), 1290–1298. doi:10.1001/archinternmed.2009.192 PMID:19636030

Bouzas, B., Kilner, P. J., & Gatzoulis, M. A. (2005). Pulmonary regurgitation: Not a benign lesion. *European Heart Journal*, *26*(5), 433–439. doi:10.1093/eurheartj/ehi091 PMID:15640261

Buth, K. J., Gainer, R. A., Legare, J. F., & Hirsch, G. M. (2014). The changing face of cardiac surgery: Practice patterns and outcomes 2001-2010. *The Canadian Journal of Cardiology*, *30*(2), 224–230. doi:10.1016/j.cjca.2013.10.020 PMID:24373760

Cabell, C. H., Jollis, J. G., Peterson, G. E., Corey, G. R., Anderson, D. J., Sexton, D. J., & Fowler, V. G. et al. (2002). Changing patient characteristics and the effect on mortality in endocarditis. *Archives of Internal Medicine*, *162*(1), 90–94. doi:10.1001/archinte.162.1.90 PMID:11784225

Carabello, B. A. (2005). Modern management of mitral stenosis. *Circulation*, *112*(3), 432–437. doi:10.1161/CIRCULATIONAHA.104.532498 PMID:16027271

Carabello, B. A., & Paulus, W. J. (2009). Aortic stenosis. *Lancet*, *373*(9667), 956–966. doi:10.1016/S0140-6736(09)60211-7 PMID:19232707

Chambers, H. F., Miller, R. T., & Newman, M. D. (1988). Right-sided Staphylococcus aureus endocarditis in intravenous drug abusers: Two-week combination therapy. *Annals of Internal Medicine*, *109*(8), 619–624. doi:10.7326/0003-4819-109-8-619 PMID:3421575

Chan, K. L., Teo, K., Dumesnil, J. G., Ni, A., & Tam, J. (2010). Effect of lipid lowering with rosuvastatin on progression of aortic stenosis. *Circulation*, *121*(2), 306–314. doi:10.1161/CIRCULATIONAHA.109.900027 PMID:20048204

Crawford, M. H., Souchek, J., Oprian, C. A., Miller, D. C., Rahimtoola, S., Giacomini, J. C., & Hammermeister, K. E. et al.Department of Veterans Affairs Cooperative Study on Valvular Heart Disease. (1990). Determinants of survival and left ventricular performance after mitral surgery. *Circulation*, *81*(4), 1173–1181. doi:10.1161/01.CIR.81.4.1173 PMID:2317900

De Bonis, M., Maisano, F., La Canna, G., & Alfieri, O. (2012). Treatment and management of mitral regurgitation. *Nature Reviews. Cardiology*, *9*(3), 133–144. doi:10.1038/nrcardio.2011.169 PMID:22105677

Deverall, P. B., Olley, P. M., Smith, D. R., Watson, D. A., & Whitaker, W. (1968). Incidence of systemic embolism before and after mitral valvotomy. *Thorax*, *23*(5), 530–536. doi:10.1136/thx.23.5.530 PMID:5680237

Dickerman, S. A., Abrutyn, E., Barsic, B., Bouza, E., Cecchi, E., Moreno, A., & Cabell, C. H. et al. (2007). The relationship between the initiation of antimicrobial therapy and the incidence of stroke in infective endocarditis: An analysis from the ICE Prospective Cohort Study (ICE-PCS). *American Heart Journal*, *154*(6), 1086–1094. doi:10.1016/j.ahj.2007.07.023 PMID:18035080

Durack, D. T., Lukes, A. S., & Bright, D. K.Duke Endocarditis Service. (1994). New criteria for diagnosis of infective endocarditis: Utilization of specific echocardiographic findings. *The American Journal of Medicine*, *96*(3), 200–209. doi:10.1016/0002-9343(94)90143-0 PMID:8154507

Duval, X., Iung, B., Klein, I., Brochet, E., Thabut, G., Arnoult, F., & Leport, C. et al. (2010). Effect of early cerebral magnetic resonance imaging on clinical decisions in infective endocarditis: A prospective study. *Annals of Internal Medicine*, *152*(8), 497–504. doi:10.7326/0003-4819-152-8-201004200-00006 PMID:20404380

Ellis, L. B., & Harken, D. E. (1961). Arterial embolization in relation to mitral valvuloplasty. *American Heart Journal*, *62*(5), 611–620. doi:10.1016/0002-8703(61)90369-6 PMID:13889996

Erniquez-Sarano, M., Akins, C. W., & Vahanian, A. (2009). Mitral regurgitation. *Lancet*, *373*(9672), 1382–1394. doi:10.1016/S0140-6736(09)60692-9 PMID:19356795

Evangelista, A., Tornos, P., Sambola, A., Permanyer-Miralda, G., & Soler-Soler, J. (2005). Long-term vasodilator therapy in patients with severe aortic regurgitation. *The New England Journal of Medicine*, *353*(13), 1342–1349. doi:10.1056/NEJMoa050666 PMID:16192479

Exadactylos, N., Sugrue, D. D., & Oakley, C. M. (1984). Prevalence of coronary artery disease in patients with isolated aortic stenosis. *British Heart Journal*, *51*(2), 121–124. doi:10.1136/hrt.51.2.121 PMID:6691863

Fenollar, F., & Raoult, D. (2007). Molecular diagnosis of bloodstream infections caused by non cultivable bacteria. *International Journal of Antimicrobial Agents*, *30*(suppl 1), S7–S15. doi:10.1016/j.ijantimicag.2007.06.024 PMID:17707613

Fernández-Hidalgo, N., Almirante, B., Gavaldà, J., Gurgui, M., Peña, C., de Alarcón, A., & Pahissa, A. et al. (2013). Ampicillin plus ceftriaxone is as effective as ampicillin plus gentamycin for treating Enterococcus faecalis infective endocarditis. *Clinical Infectious Diseases*, *56*(9), 1261–1268. doi:10.1093/cid/cit052 PMID:23392394

Feuchtner, G. M., Stolzmann, P., Dichtl, W., Schertler, T., Bonatti, J., Scheffel, H., & Alkadhi, H. et al. (2009). Multislice computed tomography in infective endocarditis: Comparison with transesophageal echocardiography and intraoperative findings. *Journal of the American College of Cardiology*, *53*(5), 436–444. doi:10.1016/j.jacc.2008.01.077 PMID:19179202

Francioli, P., Ruch, W., & Stamboulian, D. (1995). Treatment of streptococcal endocarditis with a single daily dose of ceftriaxone and netilmicin for 14 days: A prospective multicenter study. *Clinical Infectious Diseases*, *21*(6), 1406–1410. doi:10.1093/clinids/21.6.1406 PMID:8749624

Gatzoulis, M. A., Balaji, S., Webber, S. A., Siu, S. C., Hokanson, J. S., Poile, C., & Redington, A. N. et al. (2000). Risk factors for arrhythmia and sudden cardiac death late after repair of tetralogy of Fallot: A multicentre study. *Lancet*, *356*(9254), 975–981. doi:10.1016/S0140-6736(00)02714-8 PMID:11041398

Gavaldà, J., Len, O., Miró, J. M., Muñoz, P., Montejo, M., Alarcón, A., & Pahissa, A. et al. (2007). Brief communication: Treatment of Enterococcus faecalis endocarditis with ampicillin plus ceftriaxone. *Annals of Internal Medicine*, *146*(8), 574–579. doi:10.7326/0003-4819-146-8-200704170-00008 PMID:17438316

Glower, D. D. (2003). Management of chronic aortic regurgitation. *Current Treatment Options in Cardiovascular Medicine*, *5*(6), 511–520. doi:10.1007/s11936-003-0040-x PMID:14575628

Hansalia, S., Biswas, M., Dutta, R., Hage, F. G., Hsiung, M. C., Nanda, N. C., & Yin, W. et al. (2009). The value of live/real time three-dimensional transesophageal echocardiography in the assessment of valvular vegetations. *Echocardiography (Mount Kisco, N.Y.), 26*(10), 1264–1273. doi:10.1111/j.1540-8175.2009.01042.x PMID:19929872

Hauck, A. J., Freeman, D. P., Ackermann, D. M., Danielson, G. K., & Edwards, W. D. (1988). Surgical pathology of the tricuspid valve: A study of 363 cases spanning 25 years. *Mayo Clinic Proceedings, 63*(9), 851–863. doi:10.1016/S0025-6196(12)62687-1 PMID:3045434

Hoen, B., & Duval, X. (2013). Infective endocarditis. *The New England Journal of Medicine, 368*(15), 1425–1433. doi:10.1056/NEJMcp1206782 PMID:23574121

Horstkotte, D., Niehues, R., & Strauer, E. (1991). Pathomorphological aspects, aetiology and natural history of acquired mitral valve stenosis. *European Heart Journal, 12*(suppl B), 55–60. doi:10.1093/eurheartj/12.suppl_B.55 PMID:1936027

Kang, D., Kim, Y., Kim, S., Sun, B. J., Kim, D., Yun, S., & Sohn, D. et al. (2012). Early surgery versus conventional treatment for infective endocarditis. *The New England Journal of Medicine, 366*(26), 2466–2473. doi:10.1056/NEJMoa1112843 PMID:22738096

Kaplan, J. A. (2008). *Essentials of Cardiac Anesthesia*. Philadelphia, PA: Saunders.

Keith, J. D., Rowe, R. D., & Vlad, P. (1978). *Heart Disease in Infancy and Childhood* (3rd ed.). New York, NY: MacMillan.

Khot, U. N., Novaro, G. M., Popović, Z. B., Mills, R. M., Thomas, J. D., Tuzcu, E. M., & Francis, G. S. et al. (2003). Nitroprusside in critically ill patients with left ventricular dysfunction and aortic stenosis. *The New England Journal of Medicine, 348*(18), 1756–1763. doi:10.1056/NEJMoa022021 PMID:12724481

Lalani, T., Cabell, C. H., Benjamin, D. K., Lasca, O., Naber, C., Fowler, V. G. Jr, & Wang, A. et al. (2010). Analysis of the impact of early surgery on in-hospital mortality of native valve endocarditis: Use of propensity score and instrumental variable methods to adjust for treatment-selection bias. *Circulation, 121*(8), 1005–1013. doi:10.1161/CIRCULATIONAHA.109.864488 PMID:20159831

Lancellotti, P., Tribouilloy, C., Hagendorff, A., Popescu, B. A., Edvardsen, T., Pierard, L. A., Badano, L., & Zamorano, J. L. (2013). Recommendations for the echocardiographic assessment of native valvular regurgitation: An executive summary from the European Association of Cardiovascular Imaging. *European Heart Journal – Cardiovascular Imaging, 14*(7), 611-644.

Landzberg, J. S., Pflugfelder, P. W., Cassidy, M. M., Schiller, N. S., Higgins, C. B., & Cheitlin, M. D. (1992). Etiology of the Austin Flint murmur. *Journal of the American College of Cardiology, 20*(2), 408–413. doi:10.1016/0735-1097(92)90110-9 PMID:1634679

Le, T., & Bayer, A. S. (2003). Combination antibiotic therapy for infective endocarditis. *Clinical Infectious Diseases, 36*(5), 615–621. doi:10.1086/367661 PMID:12594643

Lee, D. H., Buth, K. J., Martin, B. J., Yip, A. M., & Hirsch, G. M. (2010). Frail patients are at increased risk for mortality and prolonged institutional care after cardiac surgery. *Circulation, 121*(8), 973–978. doi:10.1161/CIRCULATIONAHA.108.841437 PMID:20159833

Levine, H. J., & Gaasch, W. H. (1996). Vasoactive drugs in chronic regurgitant lesions of the mitral and aortic valves. *Journal of the American College of Cardiology*, *28*(5), 1083–1091. doi:10.1016/S0735-1097(96)00288-4 PMID:8890799

Li, J. S., Sexton, D. J., Mick, N., Nettles, R., Fowler, V. G., Ryan, T., & Corey, G. R. et al. (2000). Proposed modifications to the Duke criteria for the diagnosis of infective endocarditis. *Clinical Infectious Diseases*, *30*(4), 633–638. doi:10.1086/313753 PMID:10770721

Mahajerin, A., Gurm, H. S., Tsai, T. T., Chan, P. S., & Nallamothu, B. K. (2007). Vasodilator therapy in patients with aortic insufficiency: A systematic review. *American Heart Journal*, *153*(4), 454–461. doi:10.1016/j.ahj.2007.01.006 PMID:17383279

Manning, W. J., Reis, G. J., & Douglas, P. S. (1992). Use of transoesophageal echocardiography to detect left atrial thrombi before percutaneous balloon dilation of the mitral valve: A prospective study. *British Heart Journal*, *67*(2), 170–173. doi:10.1136/hrt.67.2.170 PMID:1540437

Massell, B. F., Chute, C. G., Walker, A. M., & Kurland, G. S. (1988). Penicillin and the marked decrease in morbidity and mortality from rheumatic fever in the United States. *The New England Journal of Medicine*, *318*(5), 280–286. doi:10.1056/NEJM198802043180504 PMID:3336421

Mittnacht, A., Fanshawe, M., & Konstadt, S. (2008). Anesthetic considerations in the patient with valvular heart disease undergoing noncardiac surgery. *Seminars in Cardiothoracic and Vascular Anesthesia*, *12*(1), 33–59. doi:10.1177/1089253208316442 PMID:18397904

Moreillon, P., & Que, Y. (2004). Infective endocarditis. *Lancet*, *363*(9403), 139–149. doi:10.1016/S0140-6736(03)15266-X PMID:14726169

Mourvillier, B., Trouillet, J. L., Timsit, J. F., Baudot, J., Chastre, J., Régnier, B., & Wolff, M. et al. (2004). Infective endocarditis in the intensive care unit: Clinical spectrum and prognostic factors in 228 consecutive patients. *Intensive Care Medicine*, *30*(11), 2046–2052. doi:10.1007/s00134-004-2436-9 PMID:15372147

Murdoch, D. R., Corey, G. R., Hoen, B., Miró, J. M., Fowler, V. G., Bayer, A. S., & Cabell, C. H. et al. (2009). Clinical presentation, etiology, and outcome of infective endocarditis in the 21st century: The international collaboration on endocarditis-prospective cohort study. *Archives of Internal Medicine*, *169*(5), 463–473. doi:10.1001/archinternmed.2008.603 PMID:19273776

Mylonakis, E., & Calderwood, S. B. (2001). Infective Endocarditis in Adults. *The New England Journal of Medicine*, *345*(18), 1318–1330. doi:10.1056/NEJMra010082 PMID:11794152

Nath, J., Forster, E., & Heidenreich, P. A. (2004). Impact of tricuspid regurgitation on long-term survival. *Journal of the American College of Cardiology*, *43*(3), 405–409. doi:10.1016/j.jacc.2003.09.036 PMID:15013122

Nishimura, R. A., Otto, C. M., Bonow, R. O., Carabello, B. A., Erwin, J. P. III, Guyton, R. A., & Thomas, J. D. et al. (2014). 2014 AHA/ACC guideline for the management of patients with valvular heart disease: Executive summary: A report of the American College of Cardiology/American Heart Association task force on practice guidelines. *Journal of the American College of Cardiology*, *63*(22), 2438–2488. doi:10.1016/j.jacc.2014.02.537 PMID:24603192

Nkomo, V. T., Gardin, J. M., Skelton, T. N., Gottdiener, J. S., Scott, C. G., & Enriques-Sarano, M. (2006). Burden of valvular heart disease: A population-based study. *Lancet*, *368*(9540), 1005–1011. doi:10.1016/S0140-6736(06)69208-8 PMID:16980116

Olaison, L., & Schadewitz, K. (2002). Enterococcal endocarditis in Sweden, 1995-1999: Can shorter therapy with aminoglycosides be used? *Clinical Infectious Diseases*, *34*(2), 159–166. doi:10.1086/338233 PMID:11740702

Osler, W. (1885). The Gulstonian lectures, on malignant endocarditis. *British Medical Journal*, *1*(1263), 522–526. doi:10.1136/bmj.1.1263.522 PMID:20751196

Parolari, A., Loardi, C., Mussoni, L., Cavallotti, L., Camera, M., Biglioli, P., & Alamanni, F. et al. (2009). Nonrheumatic calcific aortic stenosis: An overview from basic science to pharmacological prevention. *European Journal of Cardio-Thoracic Surgery*, *35*(3), 493–504. doi:10.1016/j.ejcts.2008.11.033 PMID:19162497

Pellikka, P. A., Sarano, M. E., Nishimura, R. A., Malouf, J. F., Bailey, K. R., Scott, C. G., & Tajik, A. J. et al. (2005). Outcome of 622 adults with asymptomatic, hemodynamically significant aortic stenosis during prolonged follow-up. *Circulation*, *111*(24), 3290–3295. doi:10.1161/CIRCULATIONAHA.104.495903 PMID:15956131

Perez-Gomez, F., Salvador, A., Zumalde, J., Iriarte, J. A., Berjon, J., Alegria, E., & Fernandez, C. et al. (2006). Effect of antithrombotic therapy in patients with mitral stenosis and atrial fibrillation: A sub-analysis of NASPEAF randomized trial. *European Heart Journal*, *27*(8), 960–967. doi:10.1093/eurheartj/ehi667 PMID:16330464

Rogers, J. H., & Bolling, S. F. (2009). The tricuspid valve: Current perspective and evolving management of tricuspid regurgitation. *Circulation*, *119*(20), 2718–2725. doi:10.1161/CIRCULATIONAHA.108.842773 PMID:19470900

Roguin, A., Rinkevich, D., Milo, S., Markiewicz, W., & Reisner, S. A. (1998). Long-term follow-up of patients with severe rheumatic tricuspid stenosis. *American Heart Journal*, *136*(1), 103–108. doi:10.1016/S0002-8703(98)70189-9 PMID:9665226

Rossebø, A. B., Pedersen, T. R., Boman, K., Brudi, P., Chambers, J. B., Egstrup, K., & Willenheimer, R. et al. (2008). Intensive lipid lowering with simvastatin and ezetimibe in aortic stenosis. *The New England Journal of Medicine*, *359*(13), 1343–1356. doi:10.1056/NEJMoa0804602 PMID:18765433

Sagie, A., Freitas, N., Padial, L. R., Leavitt, M., Weyman, A. E., & Levine, R. A. (1996). Doppler echocardiographic assessment of long-term progression of mitral stenosis in 103 patients: Valve area and right heart disease. *Journal of the American College of Cardiology*, *28*(2), 472–479. doi:10.1016/0735-1097(96)00153-2 PMID:8800128

Sampat, U., Varadarajan, P., Turk, R., Kamath, A., Khandhar, S., & Pai, R. G. (2009). Effect of beta-blocker therapy on survival in patients with severe aortic regurgitation. *Journal of the American College of Cardiology*, *54*(5), 452–457. doi:10.1016/j.jacc.2009.02.077 PMID:19628121

Scognamiglio, R., Rahimtoola, S. H., Fasoli, G., Nistri, S., & Volta, S. D. (1994). Nifedipine in asymptomatic patients with severe aortic regurgitation and normal left ventricular function. *The New England Journal of Medicine*, *331*(1), 689–694. doi:10.1056/NEJM199409153311101 PMID:8058074

Sedgwick, J. F., & Burstow, D. J. (2012). Update on echocardiography in the management of infective endocarditis. *Current Infectious Disease Reports*, *14*(2), 373–380. doi:10.1007/s11908-012-0262-8 PMID:22544484

Sexton, D. J., Tenenbaum, M. J., Wilson, W. R., Steckelberg, J. M., Tice, A. D., Gilbert, D., & Durack, D. T. et al.Endocarditis Treatment Consortium Group. (1998). Ceftriaxone once daily for four weeks compared with ceftriaxone plus gentamycin once daily for two weeks for treatment of endocarditis due to penicillin-susceptible streptococci. *Clinical Infectious Diseases*, *27*(6), 1470–1474. doi:10.1086/515038 PMID:9868662

Shah, R. M., Singh, M., Bhuriya, R., Molnar, J., Arora, R. R., & Khosla, S. (2012). Favorable effects of vasodilators on left ventricular remodeling in asymptomatic patients with chronic moderate-severe aortic regurgitation and normal ejection fraction: A meta-analysis of clinical trials. *Clinical Cardiology*, *35*(10), 619–625. doi:10.1002/clc.22019 PMID:22707241

Singh, J. P., Evans, J. C., Levy, D., Larson, M. G., Freed, L. A., Fuller, D. L., & Benjamin, E. J. et al. (1999). Prevalence and clinical determinants of mitral, tricuspid, and aortic regurgitation (the Framingham Heart Study). *The American Journal of Cardiology*, *83*(6), 897–902. doi:10.1016/S0002-9149(98)01064-9 PMID:10190406

Snellen, H. A., Hartman, H., Buis-Liem, T. N., Kole, E. H., & Rohmer, J. (1968). Pulmonic Stenosis. *Circulation*, *38*(1S5suppl V), V93–V101. doi:10.1161/01.CIR.38.1S5.V-93 PMID:4889601

Stollerman, G. H. (2001). Rheumatic fever in the 21st century. *Clinical Infectious Diseases*, *33*(6), 806–814. doi:10.1086/322665 PMID:11512086

Taira, K., Suzuki, A., Fujino, A., Watanabe, T., Ogyu, A., & Ashikawa, K. (2006). Tricuspid valve stenosis related to subvalvular adhesion of pacemaker lead: A case report. *Journal of Cardiology*, *47*(6), 301–306. PMID:16800373

Tattevin, P., Donal, E., & Revest, M. (2010). Can we really achieve a 1-year mortality rate lower than 10% in patients with infective endocarditis? *Archives of Internal Medicine*, *170*(2), 211–212. PMID:20101020

Thuny, F., Grisoli, D., Collart, F., Habib, G., & Raoult, D. (2012). Management of infective endocarditis: Challenges and perspectives. *Lancet*, *379*(9819), 965–975. doi:10.1016/S0140-6736(11)60755-1 PMID:22317840

Timmermans, P., Willems, J. L., Piessens, J., & De Geest, H. (1988). Angina pectoris and coronary artery disease in severe aortic regurgitation. *The American Journal of Cardiology*, *61*(10), 826–829. doi:10.1016/0002-9149(88)91074-0 PMID:3354447

Tleyjeh, I. M., Abdel-Latif, A., Rahbi, H., Scott, C. G., Bailey, K. R., Steckelbert, J. M., & Baddour, L. M. et al. (2007). A systematic review of population-based studies of infective endocarditis. *Chest*, *132*(3), 1025–1035. doi:10.1378/chest.06-2048 PMID:17873196

Ucer, E., Gungor, B., Erdinler, I. C., Akyol, A., Alper, A. T., Eksik, A., & Ulufer, T. et al. (2008). High sensitivity CRP levels predict atrial tachyarrhythmias in rheumatic mitral stenosis. *Annals of Noninvasive Electrocardiology*, *13*(1), 31–38. doi:10.1111/j.1542-474X.2007.00198.x PMID:18234004

Vahanian, A., Alfieri, O., Andreotti, F., Antunes, M. J., Barón-Esquivias, G., Baumgartner, H., & Zembala, M. et al. (2012). Guidelines on the management of valvular heart disease (version 2012): The Joint Task Force on the Management of Valvular Heart Disease of the European Society of Cardiology (ESC) and the European Association for Cardio-Thoracic Surgery (EACTS). *European Journal of Cardio-Thoracic Surgery*, *42*(4), S1–S44. doi:10.1093/ejcts/ezs455 PMID:22922698

Van Reit, J., Hill, E. E., Gheysens, O., Dymarkowski, S., Herregods, M., Herijgers, P., & Mortelmans, L. et al. (2010). ^{18}F-FDG PET/CT for early detection of embolism and metastatic infection in patients with infective endocarditis. *European Journal of Nuclear Medicine and Molecular Imaging*, *37*(6), 1189–1197. doi:10.1007/s00259-010-1380-x PMID:20204357

Vuyisile, N. T., & Gardin, J. M. (2006). Burden of valvular heart diseases: A population-based study. *Lancet*, *368*(9540), 1005–1011. doi:10.1016/S0140-6736(06)69208-8 PMID:16980116

Waller, B. F. (1987). Etiology of pure tricuspid regurgitation. *Cardiovascular Clinics*, *17*(2), 53–95. PMID:3536106

Wang, A., Athan, E., Pappas, P. A., Fowler, V. G., Olaison, L., Paré, C., & Cabell, C. H. et al. (2007). Contemporary clinical profile and outcome of prosthetic valve endocarditis. *Journal of the American Medical Association*, *297*(12), 1354–1361. doi:10.1001/jama.297.12.1354 PMID:17392239

Warnes, C. A., Williams, R. G., Bashore, T. M., Child, J. S., Connolly, H. M., Dearani, J. A., & Webb, G. D. et al. (2008). ACC/AHA 2008 guidelines for the management of adults with congenital heart disease: Executive summary. *Journal of the American College of Cardiology*, *52*(23), e143–e263. doi:10.1016/j.jacc.2008.10.001 PMID:19038677

Williams, J. B., Alexander, K. P., Morin, J. F., Langlois, Y., Noiseux, N., Perrault, L. P., & Afilalo, J. et al. (2013). Preoperative anxiety as a predictor of mortality and major morbidity in patients aged > 70 years undergoing cardiac surgery. *The American Journal of Cardiology*, *111*(1), 137–142. doi:10.1016/j.amjcard.2012.08.060 PMID:23245838

Wilson, W. R., Thompson, R. L., Wilkowske, C. J., Washington, J. A. II, Giuliani, E. R., & Geraci, J. E. (1981). Short-term therapy for streptococcal infective endocarditis: Combined intramuscular administration of penicillin and streptomycin. *Clinical Infectious Diseases*, *245*(4), 360–363. PMID:7452862

Wood, P. (1954). An appreciation of mitral stenosis. *British Medical Journal*, *1*(4879), 1051–1063. doi:10.1136/bmj.1.4870.1051 PMID:13149899

Wood, P. (1956). *Disease of the heart and circulation*. Philadelphia, PA: Lippincott.

Yiu, S., Enriquez-Sarano, M., Tribouilloy, C., & Tajik, A. J. (2000). Determinants of the degree of functional mitral regurgitation in patients with systolic left ventricular dysfunction: A quantitative clinical study. *Circulation*, *102*(12), 1400–1406. doi:10.1161/01.CIR.102.12.1400 PMID:10993859

ADDITIONAL READING

Akram, M. R., Chan, T., McAuliffe, S., & Chenzbraun, A. (2008). Non-rheumatic annular mitral stenosis: Prevalence and characteristics. *European Journal of Echocardiography*, *10*(1), 103–105. doi:10.1093/ejechocard/jen179 PMID:18579487

Arai, N., Matsumoto, A., Nishikawa, N., Yonekura, K., Eto, Y., Kuwada, Y., & Aoyahi, T. et al. (2001). Beta-blocker therapy improved symptoms and exercise capacity in a patient with dynamic intra-right ventricular obstruction an atypical form of double-chambered right ventricle. *Journal of the American Society of Echocardiography*, *14*(6), 650–653. doi:10.1067/mje.2001.110782 PMID:11391298

Boon, N. A., & Bloomfield, P. (2002). The medical management of valvar heart disease. *Heart (British Cardiac Society)*, *87*(4), 395–400. doi:10.1136/heart.87.4.395 PMID:11907022

Botelho-Nevers, E., Thuny, F., Casalta, J. P., Richet, H., Gouriet, F., Collart, F., & Raoult, D. et al. (2009). Dramatic reduction in infective endocarditis-related mortality with a management-based approach. *Archives of Internal Medicine*, *169*(14), 1290–1298. doi:10.1001/archinternmed.2009.192 PMID:19636030

Bouzas, B., Kilner, P. J., & Gatzoulis, M. A. (2005). Pulmonary regurgitation: Not a benign lesion. *European Heart Journal*, *26*(5), 433–439. doi:10.1093/eurheartj/ehi091 PMID:15640261

Carabello, B. A. (2005). Modern management of mitral stenosis. *Circulation*, *112*(3), 432–437. doi:10.1161/CIRCULATIONAHA.104.532498 PMID:16027271

Carabello, B. A., & Paulus, W. J. (2009). Aortic stenosis. *Lancet*, *373*(9667), 956–966. doi:10.1016/S0140-6736(09)60211-7 PMID:19232707

De Bonis, M., Maisano, F., La Canna, G., & Alfieri, O. (2012). Treatment and management of mitral regurgitation. *Nature Reviews. Cardiology*, *9*(3), 133–144. doi:10.1038/nrcardio.2011.169 PMID:22105677

Durack, D. T., Lukes, A. S., & Bright, D. K.Duke Endocarditis Service. (1994). New criteria for diagnosis of infective endocarditis: Utilization of specific echocardiographic findings. *The American Journal of Medicine*, *96*(3), 200–209. doi:10.1016/0002-9343(94)90143-0 PMID:8154507

Erniquez-Sarano, M., Akins, C. W., & Vahanian, A. (2009). Mitral regurgitation. *Lancet*, *373*(9672), 1382–1394. doi:10.1016/S0140-6736(09)60692-9 PMID:19356795

Evangelista, A., Tornos, P., Sambola, A., Permanyer-Miralda, G., & Soler-Soler, J. (2005). Long-term vasodilator therapy in patients with severe aortic regurgitation. *The New England Journal of Medicine*, *353*(13), 1342–1349. doi:10.1056/NEJMoa050666 PMID:16192479

Hoen, B., & Duval, X. (2013). Infective endocarditis. *The New England Journal of Medicine*, *368*(15), 1425–1433. doi:10.1056/NEJMcp1206782 PMID:23574121

Kang, D., Kim, Y., Kim, S., Sun, B. J., Kim, D., Yun, S., & Sohn, D. et al. (2012). Early surgery versus conventional treatment for infective endocarditis. *The New England Journal of Medicine*, *366*(26), 2466–2473. doi:10.1056/NEJMoa1112843 PMID:22738096

Khot, U. N., Novaro, G. M., Popović, Z. B., Mills, R. M., Thomas, J. D., Tuzcu, E. M., & Francis, G. S. et al. (2003). Nitroprusside in critically ill patients with left ventricular dysfunction and aortic stenosis. *The New England Journal of Medicine*, *348*(18), 1756–1763. doi:10.1056/NEJMoa022021 PMID:12724481

Li, J. S., Sexton, D. J., Mick, N., Nettles, R., Fowler, V. G., Ryan, T., & Corey, G. R. et al. (2000). Proposed modifications to the Duke criteria for the diagnosis of infective endocarditis. *Clinical Infectious Diseases*, *30*(4), 633–638. doi:10.1086/313753 PMID:10770721

Mittnacht, A., Fanshawe, M., & Konstadt, S. (2008). Anesthetic considerations in the patient with valvular heart disease undergoing noncardiac surgery. *Seminars in Cardiothoracic and Vascular Anesthesia*, *12*(1), 33–59. doi:10.1177/1089253208316442 PMID:18397904

Moreillon, P., & Que, Y. (2004). Infective endocarditis. *Lancet*, *363*(9403), 139–149. doi:10.1016/S0140-6736(03)15266-X PMID:14726169

Murdoch, D. R., Corey, G. R., Hoen, B., Miró, J. M., Fowler, V. G., Bayer, A. S., & Cabell, C. H. et al. (2009). Clinical presentation, etiology, and outcome of infective endocarditis in the 21st century: The international collaboration on endocarditis-prospective cohort study. *Archives of Internal Medicine*, *169*(5), 463–473. doi:10.1001/archinternmed.2008.603 PMID:19273776

Mylonakis, E., & Calderwood, S. B. (2001). Infective Endocarditis in Adults. *The New England Journal of Medicine*, *345*(18), 1318–1330. doi:10.1056/NEJMra010082 PMID:11794152

Nishimura, R. A., Otto, C. M., Bonow, R. O., Carabello, B. A., Erwin, J. P. III, Guyton, R. A., & Thomas, J. D. et al. (2014). 2014 AHA/ACC guideline for the management of patients with valvular heart disease: Executive summary: A report of the American College of Cardiology/American Heart Association task force on practice guidelines. *Journal of the American College of Cardiology*, *63*(22), 2438–2488. doi:10.1016/j.jacc.2014.02.537 PMID:24603192

Perez-Gomez, F., Salvador, A., Zumalde, J., Iriarte, J. A., Berjon, J., Alegria, E., & Fernandez, C. et al. (2006). Effect of antithrombotic therapy in patients with mitral stenosis and atrial fibrillation: A sub-analysis of NASPEAF randomized trial. *European Heart Journal*, *27*(8), 960–967. doi:10.1093/eurheartj/ehi667 PMID:16330464

Rogers, J. H., & Bolling, S. F. (2009). The tricuspid valve: Current perspective and evolving management of tricuspid regurgitation. *Circulation*, *119*(20), 2718–2725. doi:10.1161/CIRCULATIONAHA.108.842773 PMID:19470900

Rossebø, A. B., Pedersen, T. R., Boman, K., Brudi, P., Chambers, J. B., Egstrup, K., & Willenheimer, R. et al. (2008). Intensive lipid lowering with simvastatin and ezetimibe in aortic stenosis. *The New England Journal of Medicine*, *359*(13), 1343–1356. doi:10.1056/NEJMoa0804602 PMID:18765433

Sampat, U., Varadarajan, P., Turk, R., Kamath, A., Khandhar, S., & Pai, R. G. (2009). Effect of beta-blocker therapy on survival in patients with severe aortic regurgitation. *Journal of the American College of Cardiology*, *54*(5), 452–457. doi:10.1016/j.jacc.2009.02.077 PMID:19628121

Shah, R. M., Singh, M., Bhuriya, R., Molnar, J., Arora, R. R., & Khosla, S. (2012). Favorable effects of vasodilators on left ventricular remodeling in asymptomatic patients with chronic moderate-severe aortic regurgitation and normal ejection fraction: A meta-analysis of clinical trials. *Clinical Cardiology*, *35*(10), 619–625. doi:10.1002/clc.22019 PMID:22707241

Snellen, H. A., Hartman, H., Buis-Liem, T. N., Kole, E. H., & Rohmer, J. (1968). Pulmonic Stenosis. *Circulation*, *38*(1S5suppl V), V93–V101. doi:10.1161/01.CIR.38.1S5.V-93 PMID:4889601

Thuny, F., Grisoli, D., Collart, F., Habib, G., & Raoult, D. (2012). Management of infective endocarditis: Challenges and perspectives. *Lancet*, *379*(9819), 965–975. doi:10.1016/S0140-6736(11)60755-1 PMID:22317840

Vuyisile, N. T., & Gardin, J. M. (2006). Burden of valvular heart diseases: A population-based study. *Lancet*, *368*(9540), 1005–1011. doi:10.1016/S0140-6736(06)69208-8 PMID:16980116

Wang, A., Athan, E., Pappas, P. A., Fowler, V. G., Olaison, L., Paré, C., & Cabell, C. H. et al. (2007). Contemporary clinical profile and outcome of prosthetic valve endocarditis. *Journal of the American Medical Association*, *297*(12), 1354–1361. doi:10.1001/jama.297.12.1354 PMID:17392239

Warnes, C. A., Williams, R. G., Bashore, T. M., Child, J. S., Connolly, H. M., Dearani, J. A., & Webb, G. D. et al. (2008). ACC/AHA 2008 guidelines for the management of adults with congenital heart disease: Executive summary. *Journal of the American College of Cardiology*, *52*(23), e143–e263. doi:10.1016/j.jacc.2008.10.001 PMID:19038677

Chapter 9
Advanced Heart Failure Management and Selection for Advanced Therapies

Alexander Papolos
Icahn School of Medicine at Mount Sinai, USA

Elrond Teo
Emory University Hospital, USA

Nishant A. Gandhi
Icahn School of Medicine at Mount Sinai, USA

Raymond Bietry
Icahn School of Medicine at Mount Sinai, USA

ABSTRACT

Advancements in the field of heart failure have significantly improved both mortality and the quality of life of millions. However, heart failure generally remains a chronic disease with an insidious progression to organ failure despite optimal medical treatment. Early consideration of advanced therapies such as mechanical circulatory support and cardiac transplantation in advanced heart failure is essential. The purpose of this chapter is to assist the reader in the identification of patients with advanced heart failure that have not yet developed irreversible end-organ dysfunction, as interventions in this narrow therapeutic window results in improved post-surgical outcomes.

INTRODUCTION

Heart failure is a multifaceted clinical syndrome of impaired cardiac function in which the heart fails to meet the metabolic demands of the body. Today an estimated 5 million Americans are living with heart failure, and current projections estimate this will increase 25% by 2030 (Go et al., 2013). In 2011, heart failure was the second most common reason for hospitalization among Americans aged 65-85 (Pfuntner, Wier, & Stockes, 2013). Not only is heart failure a menace to public health, but in 2013 the economic burden associated with its treatment was approximated to be $32 billion (Go et al., 2013).

Large randomized controlled trials have provided a robust armament of pharmacological and electrophysiological therapies to improve both mortality and quality of life. Unfortunately, events such as life threatening arrhythmias, clinical decompensation, and progressive end-organ damage remain common

DOI: 10.4018/978-1-4666-8603-8.ch009

among patients with heart failure. Thus, early consideration of mechanical circulatory support and cardiac transplant must be made in patients at increased risk of morbidity and mortality despite adequate medical therapy.

Objectives

1. Understand guideline directed therapy for heart failure.
2. Identify the patient refractory to medical therapy.
3. Understand the role of pre-surgical optimization prior to surgery for advanced therapies.

Heart Failure Pathogenesis

Heart failure is a progressive disease of deteriorating cardiac function. The inciting event that initiates progressive decline may be acute, such as with myocardial infarction, or insidious in nature as seen in structural, hypertensive, metabolic, infectious, genetic, toxic, and tachyarrhythmic induced cardiomyopathies. Regardless of etiology, suboptimal pump function stimulates compensatory homeostatic neurohormonal mechanisms that lead to myocardial damage, fibrosis, and negative remodeling that further beget disease progression.

Thus, when patients are found to have undifferentiated cardiomyopathy, it is paramount to determine the underlying etiology. There are a myriad of diseases associated with the development of cardiomyopathy as outlined in Table 1 (Table of common cardiomyopathies by etiology.), however specific attention should be made to those that are potentially reversible. The first step in delineating an etiology begins with obtaining a comprehensive history. Ischemic cardiomyopathy should be strongly considered in all patients, particularly those with risk factors or known coronary artery disease. History of cancer should prompt suspicion for infiltrative disease as seen with amyloidosis in multiple myeloma, as well as the effects of treatment with cardiotoxic therapies such as anthracyclines or chest radiation. Elements

Table 1. Etiologies of cardiomyopathy

Category	Example
Ischemic	Coronary artery disease, coronary embolus, coronary dissection
Infectious	HIV, Lyme, Coxsackie, Chagas, rheumatic
Hereditary	Arrhythmogenic right ventricle, ventricular non-compaction, hypertrophic, mitochondrial disorders, glycogen storage disorders, muscular dystrophy
Valvular	Mitral regurgitation, aortic regurgitation, aortic stenosis
Congenital	Ventricular septal defect, tetralogy of fallot, transposition
Autoimmune	Systemic lupus erythematosus, giant cell myocarditis, scleroderma, rheumatoid arthritis, hypersensitivity myocarditis, endocardial fibroelastosis
Toxin	Alcohol, cocaine, anthracyclines, amphetamines, antiretrovirals
Arrhythmias	Tachycardia induced
Infiltrative	Amyloidosis, hemochromatosis, sarcoidosis
Nurtritional	Thiamine deficiency
Misc	Takotsubo, peripartum, radiation, thyrotoxicosis, sleep apnea

of the review of systems, social, and or family history may suggest infectious, toxic-metabolic, and or autoimmune etiologies that must be considered (HIV, Lyme, Chagas, alcohol, cocaine, thyrotoxicosis, tachycardic, systemic lupus erythematosus, giant cell myocarditis, sarcoidosis, hemochromatosis, thiamine deficiency etc.).

Cardiac ischemia is by far the most common etiology, and responsible for approximately 70% of advanced cardiomyopathies (Bortman, Sellanes, Odell, Ring, & Olivari, 1994). The diagnosis of ischemic cardiomyopathy generally requires coronary evaluation by cardiac catheterization, and can potentially be improved by revascularization. In terms of non-invasive imaging; echocardiography can help establish the severity of the disease as well as providing insight in the etiology. Cardiac MRI can help elucidate many conditions that must be entertained when presented with an undifferentiated cardiomyopathy; ischemic, hypertrophic, myocarditis, arrhythmogenic right ventricle, sarcoidosis, amyloidosis, hemochromatosis, chagas, and non-compaction (Francois, Schiebler, & Reeder, 2010). Treatment of any reversible cause is an important consideration in all cases, and should be done in conjunction with initiation of medical therapies.

Medical management of chronic systolic heart failure

The best-described neurohormonal mechanisms implicated in heart failure are the sympathetic nervous system and renin-angiotensin system (RAS). Together, these physiologic feedback loops work in concert to maintain tissue perfusion by potentiating inotropy, chronotropy, fluid retention, and vascular tone. While necessary to maintain the metabolic demands of the body during acute cardiovascular decompensation, unabated activation of these mechanisms invariably leads to progressive cardiac dysfunction, and as such are the primary targets of standard pharmacotherapy. The cumulative effect of these therapies has significantly improved the overall prognosis in heart failure.

Angiotensin Converting Enzyme Inhibitors (ACEI) block the RAS by inhibiting renin-mediated conversion of angiotensin-I to angiotensin-II, which acts as a potent vasoconstrictor and promotes sodium retention (directly and by stimulating aldosterone secretion). ACEIs have been shown to reverse negative remodeling, improve heart failure symptoms, prevent hospitalizations, and reduce mortality in patients with heart failure with reduced ejection fraction (HFrEF) (Sayer & Bhat, 2014). Pooled data of placebo controlled trials using ACEIs in patients with New York Heart Association (NYHA) class I-IV symptoms have shown that they incur a 23% relative risk reduction (RRR) in all cause mortality (Garg & Yusuf, 1995). Multiple studies have proven the efficacy of ACEIs, leading to the ACC/AHA recommendation that all patients with HFrEF receive ACEI therapy (Yancy et al., 2013).

ACEIs should be started at low doses and slowly titrated as blood pressure, renal function, and serum potassium permit. An increase in creatinine of up to 30% is expected and is typically transient in nature. Cardiovascular efficacy has been shown to be dose related, and thus moderate-high dose regimens are optimal (Packer et al., 1999). There is no data to support the use of one particular ACEI over another. Adverse effects of ACEI include hypotension, hyperkalemia, and renal insufficiency due to reduced transglomerular pressure (secondary to decreased efferent glomerular arterial vascular tone). A significant number of patients will develop dry cough, and those hypersensitive to increased levels of bradykinin may develop angioedema.

Angiotensin Receptor Blockers (ARB) are an alternative type of RAS antagonist generally used in patients with HFrEF that can't tolerate an ACEI. ARBs inhibit angiotensin-II from activating angiotensin type-I receptors, which is the predominate receptor subtype associated with cardiovascular dysfunction in

Figure 1. Effect of guideline directed therapy on 5-year survival in a theoretical 65 year old man with NYHA/AHA III-B ischemic cardiomyopathy and ejection fraction of 30% as per the Seattle Heart Failure Model. ACEI: Angiotensin Converting Enzyme Inhibitors; BB: Beta blockers, AA: Aldosterone antagonists, ICD: Implantable Cardioverter-Defibrillator

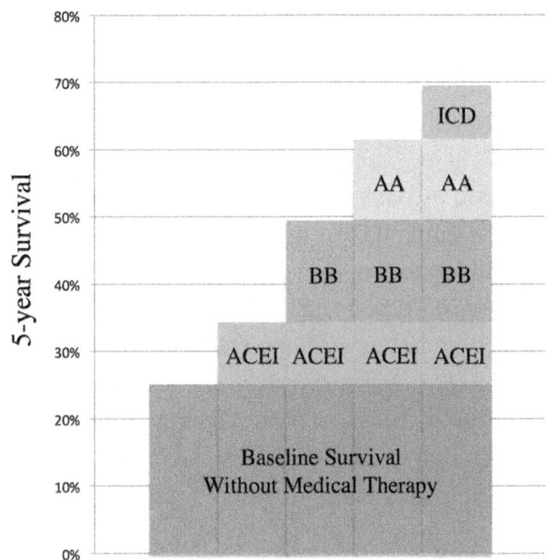

Effect of guideline directed therapy on 5-year survival in a theoretical 65 year old man with NYHA/AHA class III-B ischemic cardiomyopathy and ejection fraction of 30% as per the Seattle Heart Failure Model.
ACEI: Angiotensin Converting Enzyme Inhibitors; BB: Beta blockers, AA: Aldosterone antagonists, ICD: Implantable Cardioverter-Defibrillator

heart failure (Sayer & Bhat, 2014). Many studies have demonstrated that ARBs have comparable effects as ACEIs in reversing cardiac remodeling, improving heart failure symptoms, preventing hospitalizations, and reducing all-cause mortality (Maggioni et al., 2002).

ARBs should be started at low doses and slowly uptitrated. Similar to ACEIs; renal function, blood pressure, and potassium levels should be monitored regularly during initiation and dosage adjustment. Dual-RAS inhibition through the use of ARBs in combination with ACEIs has been shown to reduce mortality; however, the combination of ACEI with aldosterone antagonists is preferred due to superior outcomes (McMurray et al., 2003).

Beta blockers (BB) inhibit the sympathetic nervous systems deleterious effects on myocardial function and cardiac remodeling. Myocardial beta-1 adrenergic receptor activation triggers the protein kinase-A signaling cascade, ultimately improving myocardial calcium handling and increases inotropy, chronotropy, and lusitropy. In heart failure, the myocardium is subjected to persistent adrenergic tone that results in negative feedback mechanisms that uncouple the beta-1 adrenergic response, which clinically manifests as decompensated heart failure, cardiac remodeling, arrhythmogensis, and apoptosis. BBs work to inhibit the cardiotoxic effects of prolonged adrenergic stimulation.

Unlike the numerous ACEIs and ARBs that exhibit a class effect and are considered interchangeable, clinical trials have demonstrated that the efficacy of BBs in heart failure are drug specific. The three BBs shown to decrease mortality in NYHA class II-IV HFrEF are metoprolol succincate, bisoprolol (both competitive antagonists of the beta-1 adrenergic receptor), and carvedilol (a competitive antagonist of alpha-1, beta-1, and beta-2 adrenergic receptors). Most striking of these trials was the U.S. Carvedilol trial in which NYHA class II-III patients with HFrEF on diuretics, digitalis, and ACEIs were randomized to receive carvedilol vs. placebo. The trial was terminated early due to superiority, at which point the carvedilol arm demonstrated a RRR in mortality of 65% (Packer et al., 1996). Furthermore, the MOCHA study demonstrated that carvedilol produces dose-related improvements in LV function, mortality, and rate of hospitalization, providing evidence supporting the use of high-dose regiments (Bristow et al., 1996).

In heart failure, titration of BBs should be done slowly, at intervals of no less than 2-weeks as sudden adrenergic inhibition can lead to worsening fluid retention, reduced inotropy, and clinical decompensation. Typical adverse effects of BBs are orthostatic hypotension, bradycardia, varying degrees of heart block, and use is not recommended in asthmatics with active bronchospasm.

Aldosterone antagonists are the third class of neurohormonal antagonists used in the management of heart failure. Aldosterone is a mineralocorticoid produced and released by the adrenal cortex upon stimulation by the RAS (via angiotensin type-I receptor stimulation), and to a lesser degree by hyperkalemia, ACTH, and the sympathetic nervous system. The effect of aldosterone is to increase sodium and water reabsorption in exchange for potassium within the kidney. Aldosterone antagonists such as spironolactone and epleranone are classified as potassium sparing diuretics. However, the beneficial effects of these medications are not limited to their effects on sodium and water handling, as aldosterone induces the expression of several genes implicated in vascular and myocardial extracellular remodeling (Sayer & Bhat, 2014).

The RALES trial demonstrated that the use of spironolactone in addition to standard therapy with ACEIs and diuretics in patients with NYHA class III-IV HFrEF led to a 30% RRR in all-cause mortality (Pitt et al., 1999). Slightly more impressive was the EMPHASIS-HF trial in which NYHA class II patients with HFrEF on diuretics, BBs, ACEIs, and or ARBs were randomized to epleranone vs. placebo. The results of which found that epleranone incurred a 24% RRR in mortality, and 42% RRR in heart failure hospitalization (Zannad et al., 2011).

Aldosterone antagonists should not be used in patients with GFR < 30mL/min or serum potassium > 5.5 mmol/L, and titration of the medications should be performed with close observation of renal function and serum potassium in all patients. Painful gynecomastia has been reported in up to 10% of patients with spironolactone, an adverse effect that is not observed with epleranone.

Hydralazine and isosorbide dinitrate has been shown to have additional benefits in certain populations. Early hemodynamic studies using the combination of the arterialdilator hydralaize (H) and venodilator isosorbide dinitrite (ISDN) in patients with NYHA class II-IV HFrEF described significant increases in cardiac output, and reduction in both ventricular filling pressures and systemic vascular resistance (SVR) (Pierpont et al., 1978). Subsequent trials comparing ACEIs and H-ISDN showed that ACEIs were more efficacious in terms of mortality among caucasians, while no difference was observed in African Americans (Carson, Ziesche, Johnson, & Cohn, 1999). Racial discordance in medical efficacy fueled the A-HeFT trial, in which self-identified African Americans with NYHA class III-IV HFrEF on optimal medical therapy were randomized to receive H-ISDN vs placebo. Addition of H-ISDN resulted in a 43% RRR in mortality, suggesting that self-identified race is likely a crude phenotypic marker of patients who may respond favorably to vasodilator therapy (Taylor et al., 2004). This has led to the current ACCF/AHA guideline that all African American patients with heart failure on optimal medical therapy (including BB, ACEI or ARB) or patients of any race who cannot tolerate ACE or ARBs be treated with H-ISDN (Yancy et al., 2013).

Digitalis is a cardiac glycoside that impairs myocardial sodium potassium-ATPase activity to increase the intracellular calcium concentration. Thereby, the drug improves inotropy and potentiates vagal tone. Digitalis has been shown to reduce rates of hospitalization and alleviate symptoms of heart failure; however, it has not been shown to improve mortality (Rekha, Gorlin, Smith, & Yusuf, 1997). Common adverse reactions are arrhythmias such as heart block, as well as neurologic and gastrointestinal complaints.

Diuretics are a common component of most heart failure regimens, and function to counter excessive and symptomatic sodium and fluid retention. There are many subclasses of diuretic, however in the treatment of heart failure the two most commonly uses are loop and thiazide diuretics.

Loop diuretics (Furosemide, Bumetanide, Torsmide, and Ethacrynic acid) block the sodium-potassium-chloride transporter of renaltubular epithelial cells in the thick ascending limb of the loop of Henle. The diuretic response to loop diuretics is concentration dependent. A minimal renaltubular luminal concentration of loop must be met, following which a dose-dependant diuresis will occur.

Thiazide diuretics (chlorothiazide, hydrochlorothiazide, chlorthalidone, indapamide, and metolazone) block the sodium-chloride transporter of the distal convoluted tubule. Thiazides are not as potent as loop diuretics; however, the two classes can be used in conjunction when diuresis is refractory to a loop alone, a strategy called sequential nephron blockade.

Patients on diuretics must be monitored for electrolyte abnormalities and renal insufficiency. Loop diuretics are associated with ototoxicity in a dose-dependant manner, which may manifest as tinnitus and varying degrees of hearing impairment. These adverse effects are typically reversible and more common with intravenous administration.

Neprilysin-inhibitors are a promising new category of therapy for heart failure. Neprilysin is an endogenous endopeptidase that degrades several vasoactive proteins, such as bradykinin, adrenomedullin, and natriuretic peptides. In the PARADIGM-HF trial of patients with NYHA class II-IV HFrEF, inhibition of neprilysin in combination with the ARB Valsartan resulted in a 20% risk reduction is cardiovascular death (NNT=32) when compared to optimal medical therapy (McMurray et al., 2014).

Neprilysin inhibition is currently under investigation by the Food and Drug Administration for clinical use, but shows great promise as a new therapy.

Initiation and titration of the medications described above is the cornerstone of medical therapy for patients with HFrEF. Whenever possible, drugs known to have adverse effects should be avoided and or discontinued. The 2013 ACCF/AHA heart failure guidelines recognize most antiarrhythmics, calcium channel blockers (other than amlodipine), nonsteroidal anti-inflammatories, and thiazolidinediones as potentially harmful medications (Yancy et al., 2013).

Implantable Cardioverter-Defibrillator (ICD) and Cardiac Resynchronization Therapy (CRT)

Sudden cardiac death (SCD) due to malignant arrhythmias is a common cause of mortality in patients with heart failure. The role of primary prevention of SCD with ICD therapy in patients with ischemic and non-ischemic HFrEF was accessed in the SCD-HeFT trial, the results of which found that ICD placement led to a 23% RRR in all cause mortality (Bardy et al., 2005). Accordingly, current guidelines support the use of ICDs in patients with HFrEF with an LVEF $\leq$35% in symptomatic patients or an LVEF $\leq$30% in asymptomatic ischemic cardiomyopathy who are at least 40 days post-MI, while on chronic optimal medical therapy, if the patient's life expectancy is greater than one year (Yancy et al., 2013).

Conduction abnormalities that disrupt the natural propagation of electrical signals involved in myocardial contraction and relaxation are common in heart failure and place the heart at a mechanical disadvantage. Cardiac resynchronization therapy via biventricular pacing has been shown to decrease mortality, reduce hospitalization rates, improve functional status, and reverse cardiac remodeling (Sutton et al., 2006). In one of the largest CRT trials, patients with NYHA class II-III HFrEF on optimal medical therapy with QRS complex duration >120ms were randomized to CRT with ICD vs ICD alone. The RRR of all-cause mortality in the CRT-ICD group was 25%. Of note, subgroup analysis revealed that patients with QRS duration >150ms benefited most (Tang et al., 2010). Currently the strongest indication for CRT is among NYHA class II-IV HFrEF with left bundle branch block and QRS complex duration >150msec. However, CRT may be useful in patients with HFrEF that lack left bundle morphology and have QRS duration >120msec, albeit at a lower level of evidence and with less benefit (Yancy et al., 2013). Furthermore, the BLOCK-HF trial supports the use of biventricular pacing in patients with mild-moderate HFrEF and concomitant high-degree atrio-ventricular block necessitating pacemaker implantation (Curtis et al., 2013).

Non-Pharmacologic Therapy of Chronic Heart Failure

Central and obstructive sleep apnea are common comorbidities observed in up to half of all patients with HFrEF (Krawczyk, et al., 2013). Sleep apnea should be suspected in patients that are obese, snore, have witnessed apneic episodes, complain of daytime somnolence, or have large neck diameter. Such patients should be referred for polysomnography, as recurrent episodes of apnea result in tissue hypoxia and surges of sympathetic output associated with hypertension, tachycardia, and negative cardiac remodeling. The use of nocturnal continue positive airway pressure respiration (CPAP) in patients with HFrEF is associated with improved cardiac function, decreased sympathetic activity, and improved quality of life among patients with obstructive sleep apnea (Mansfield, Gollogly, Kaye, Richardson, Bergin, & Naughton, 2004). Similarly, CPAP for the treatment of central sleep apnea has been shown to improve both cardiac function and cardiac transplant-free survival (Arzt et al., 2007).

Obesity is associated with a multitude of negative cardiovascular effects, including a known association with the development of heart failure. This risk was quantified in a reanalysis of the Framingham Heart Study that showed that every body-mass index (BMI) unit above normal increased the odds of developing heart failure by 5-7% (Kenchaiah, 2002). The role of bariatric surgery in these patients remain unclear, as patients with heart failure are at a much higher risk of surgical complications (Benotti et al., 2014).

In regard to lifestyle education that can be provided to patients, current recommendations advocate that physical activity is a safe and effective modality to improve NYHA functional class in patients with heart failure (Yancy et al., 2013). A meta-analysis of randomized control trials found that exercise reduced heart failure-related hospitalization and improved quality of life (Davies, et al., 2010). In terms of diet, common practice and current guidelines recommend 2g salt and 1.5-2L fluid restrictions as a reasonable nonpharmological therapy to reduce symptoms of congestion. However, while this strategy conceptually makes sense, current evidence is conflicting to support this recommendation.

Medical Management of Acute Decompensated Heart Failure

The aim of therapy in patients with acute decompensated heart failure is to optimize the volume status, improve cardiac output, and manage any reversible etiology that may have precipitated the clinical picture. Patients should initially be assessed by their hemodynamic profile, using clinical and ancillary information to determine both their volume and perfusion status.

Evaluation of the volume status defines the patient as either "wet" or "dry". Volume overloaded patients will provide a history of weight gain, lower extremity edema, chest congestion, dyspnea, orthopnea, paroxysmal nocturnal dyspnea, and decreased exercise tolerance. On examination, these patients may exhibit elevated jugular venous pressure, hepato-jugular reflex, pulmonary rales, regurgitant murmurs, an S3 gallop, ascites, a palpable and or pulsatile liver, and lower extremity edema. Ancillary testing such as cephalized congestion on chest X-ray, elevated serum brain naturetic peptide, or IVC dilation on echocardiogram further support volume overload physiology. The absence of these features is consistent with a "dry" or euvolemic profile.

Evaluation of tissue perfusion determines if the patient is classified as either "warm" or "cold". A patient is said to be "cold" if there is evidence of end organ dysfunction secondary to poor tissue perfusion. The first clinical signs of hypoperfusion are reflexive tachycardia if the patient is chronotropicaly competent, and narrowing of the pulse pressure, which signifying elevated systemic vascular resistance (SVR). In low flow states the cardiovascular system will preferentially perfuse the "vital organs", and cardiac output (CO) will be shunted away from the renal and integumentary systems, resulting in oliguria,

Figure 2. Hemodynamic profiles in acute decompensated heart failure by perfusion and volume status with corresponding treatment options. PCWP: pulmonary capillary wedge pressure

	Warm	Cold
Dry	Normal Cardiac Output Normal Systemic Vascular Resistance Normal PCWP Rx: Titration of Guideline Directed Therapy	Low Cardiac Output High Systemic Vascular Resistance Normal PCWP Rx: Inotropes
Wet	Normal Cardiac Output Normal Systemic Vascular Resistance High PCWP Rx: Diuresis +/- Vasodilators	Low Cardiac Output High Systemic Vascular Resistance High PCWP Rx: Inotropic Support and Diuresis

PCWP: pulmonary capillary wedge pressure

and cool clammy skin. Further hypoperfusion is poorly tolerated, and patients will become fatigued and lethargic. In addition to these clinical findings, pertinent labs such as serum lactate, mixed venous oxygen saturation, and glomerular filtration may reflect if the metabolic demand of the body are not being met.

In volume-overloaded patients, the goal is to reduce cardiac filling pressures while maintaining tissue perfusion. This is generally done with the use of diuretics. However, if there is an inadequate response, mechanical removal with ultrafiltration or hemodialysis may be considered. In patients without hypotension, classified as "warm and wet", vasodilators such as intravenous nitroglycerin, nitroprusside, or nesiritide can further improve symptoms and facilitate diuresis. Vasodilators reduce cardiac filling pressures and SVR, which effectively improves CO and reduces myocardial oxygen demand (MOD). Nitroglycerin is a rapidly acting and potent vasodilator, that at low infusion rates functions largely as a venodilator, lowering ventricular filling pressures, alleviating congestion, and reduce both MOD and mean arterial pressure (MAP). At high infusion rates, nitroglycerin will also cause arterial dilatation, reducing SVR to improve CO while reducing MOD at the cost of further reduction in MAP. Nitroprusside is a balanced veno-arterialdilator with rapid onset of action; its use is temporally limited to 24-48hrs secondary to the production of the toxic metabolites cyanide and thiocyanate. Nesiritide is a recombinant human B-type natriuretic peptide that acts as a balanced veno-arterialdilator with natriuretic properties. The overall effect is increased CO and reduction in both MAP and MOD, much like nitroprusside.

Overloaded patients with evidence of hypoperfusion usually will not benefit from optimization of volume status alone. These "cold and wet" patients generally require hemodynamic support. The choice of agent is not universally agreed upon, however an understanding of the pharmacologic effects of each agent can assist in choosing an initial agent (Table 2, Hemodynamic effect and dosing of common inotropic and vasoactive medications used in heart failure. B: beta-adrenergic agonist; α: alpha-adrenergic agonist, BNP: B-type natriuretic peptide, CO: cardiac output, SVR: systemic vascular resistance, PVR: pulmonary vascular resistance, MAP: mean arterial pressure, MOD: myocardial oxygen demand.).

"Cold and wet" patients without hypotension can be managed with either a vasodilator as noted above, or in cases where CO is suspected to be severely reduced, through the use of a vasodilator with inotropic properties such as milrinone. This "ino-dilator" is a phosphodiesterase-3 inhibitor that blocks

Table 2. Inotropic and vasoactive infusions

Agent	Dose	Mechanism	Inotropy	CO	SVR	PVR	MAO	MOD
Milrinone	0.375-0.75 mcg/Kg/min	PDE-3 Inhibitor	↑	↑↑	↓↓	↓↓	↓	↑
Dobutamine	1-10 mcg/Kg/min	B-1, B-2, α-1	↑↑	↑↑	↓	≈	≈	↑↑
Dopamine	1-3 mcg/Kg/min	Dopamine-1	≈	≈	↓	≈	↓	≈
	3-10 mcg/Kg/min	B-1>α-1	↑	↑	↑	≈	↑	↑
	10-20 mcg/Kg/min	B-1<α-1	↑	↑	↑↑	≈	↑↑	↑↑
Epinephrine	2-10 mcg/Kg/min	B-1, B-2, α-1	↑↑	↑↑	↑↑	≈	↑↑	↑↑
Norepinephrine	2-10 mcg/Kg/min	B-1, α-1	↑↑	↑↑	↑↑	≈	↑↑	↑↑
Nitroprusside	0.5-5 mcg/Kg/min	Nitric Oxide	≈	↑	↓↓	≈	↓	↓
Nitroglycerin	10-200 mcg/Kg/min	Nitric Oxide	≈	↑	↓↓	≈	↓	↓
Nesiritide	0.015-0.03 mcg/Kg/min	BNP	≈	↑	↓↓	≈	↓	↓

B: beta-adrenergic agonist; α: alpha-adrenergic agonist; BNP: B-type natriuretic peptide.

intracellular degradation of cAMP. This results in increased myocardial inotropy and lusitropy, whereas in the vasculature this produces relaxation of smooth muscle and thus decreased systemic and pulmonary vascular resistance (PVR). The use of a pulmonary artery catheter can further support the use of a vasodilator with the demonstration of elevated SVR.

Patients with borderline blood pressure may benefit more from an inotrope without significant vasodilatory effects. Dobutamine is a sympathomimetic amine that predominantly stimulates beta-1 adrenergic receptors (ARs) with mild beta-2 and alpha-1 activity. The net effect of which is increased inotropy, chronotropy, and minimal peripheral vasodilatation. As opposed to milrinone, the predominant effect of dobutamine is that of an inotrope with weak vasodilatory properties.

Patients with significant hypotension will require inotropic support in conjunction with peripheral vasoconstriction. Dopamine is catecholamine that's cardiovascular effect varies greatly in a dose-dependant manor. At low doses (1-3 mcg/Kg/min) it will primarily stimulate dopamine-1 receptors in the renal and splanchnic arteries, resulting in increased renal perfusion. Moderate doses (3-10 mcg/Kg/min) will begin to partially stimulate myocardial beta-1 ARs and activate the sympathetic nervous system causing release of norepinephrine, a net effect of increased inotropy, chronotropy, and SVR, leading to increased MAP and MOD. At high doses (10-20 mcg/Kg/min) the predominant effect is on vascular alpha-1 ARs, increasing SVR, MAP, and MOD to a greater degree. Epinephrine has potent beta-1 activity with moderate beta-2 and alpha-1 effects. At low to medium infusion rates epinephrine is relatively SVR neutral, increasing CO through both inotropic and chronotropic potentiation. At higher concentrations vasoconstrictive alpha-1 activity outweighs the vasodilator effects of beta-2 stimulation, greatly elevating SVR, MAP, and MOD. Norepinephrine preferentially stimulates beta-1 and alpha-1 ARs to increase inotropy, chronotropy, and SVR, which is why it is a commonly used agent in septic shock. Use of inotropes and vasoconstrictors that directly stimulate the myocardium may be limited by tachyarrhythmias and or myocardial ischemia, and as such should be used at the lowest possible dose for the shortest duration of time clinically feasible.

Beyond inotropic support, patients may require additional mechanical support either while awaiting myocardial recovery or as a bridge to more durable support with heart transplantation or a ventricular assist device. There are multiple forms of mechanical support with variable features; temporary or durable support, extracorporeal or intracorporeal circulation, partial or full hemodynamic support, and surgical or percutaneous placement. An intraaortic balloon pump (IABP) is a temporary form of percutaneous support that augments coronary perfusion and reduces afterload with balloon counterpulsation. It is readily available and can even be placed at the bedside, but overall it provides a minimal degree of cardiac support (0.5-1L/min) and was not shown to have a mortality benefit in a recent trial (Sayer, Baker, Parks, 2012, & Prondzinsky et al., 2012). There are other forms of percutaneous devices such as Impella (Abiomed, Danvers, MA) and TandemHeart (CardiacAssist, Inc., Pittsburgh, PA) that can be placed in the cardiac catheterization lab and provide greater degrees of support, however, these have not demonstrated benefits in overall survival (Westaby, Anastasiadis, & Wieselthaler, 2012).

Extracorporeal membrane oxygenation (ECMO) can emergently provide rapid and complete respiratory and cardiovascular support. It involves surgically placed peripheral catheters, typically in the femoral artery and vein, which then creates an extracorporal circuit of blood flow with an external oxygenator (Smedira et, al., 2001). ECMO provides salvage therapy and hemodynamic stabilization, but may increase left ventricle afterload and impair myocardial recovery.

Surgical implantation of ventricular assist devices offer the benefit of direct cannulation, unloading of the affected ventricle, and complete hemodynamic support. Temporary devices such as the CentriMag (Thoratec, Pleasanton, CA) can be used for weeks, allowing time for assessment of myocardial recovery or the need to upgrade to more durable support or cardiac transplantation.

Features and Characteristics of the Advanced Heart Failure Patient

The patients with acute decompensated heart failure who do not stabilize and remain tenuous on inotropes or temporary mechanical support are readily identified as having advanced heart failure and may benefit from durable mechanical support or transplantation. A greater challenge is to identify the ambulatory heart failure patient who is at a high risk to progress with refractory symptoms and an increased risk of mortality. Traditionally, patients are classified by New York Heart Association (NYHA) Functional class as a means to classify the severity of symptoms (The Criteria Committee of the New York Heart Association, 1994). The NYHA class designates a patient based on their stated functional capacity and places the patient in a category from I-IV. This classification scheme has been shown to correlate with increased mortality, but has many limitations in clinical practice (Madsen, Hansen, Stokholm, Brons, Husum, & Mortensen, 1994). The typical chronic heart failure patient will often have periods of clinical improvement between exacerbations. Thus, although a patient may clinically improve by NYHA class for a period of time, there is often an overall clinical deterioration that can be under-recognized.

Another useful classification scheme is the ACC/AHA staging of heart failure that reflects the progressive nature of heart failure. The stages from A-D reflect the natural course of the disease from patients at risk of developing heart failure to the refractory patient requiring advanced intervention.

There is no standard criteria to identify the ACC/AHA stage D heart failure patient, but there are multiple signs that suggest a patient has refractory symptoms with increased mortality and may benefit from advanced therapies.

Evidence to identify the advanced (ACC-AHA stage D) heart failure patient can be seen in a variety of clinical markers. Recurrent hospitalizations are a strong and consistent marker of increased mortality. In one study, patients have a median survival of 2.4 years after their first hospitalization for heart failure (Setoguchi, Stevenson, & Schneeweiss, 2007). Mortality furthers increases after each subsequent hospitalization, with a median survival of only 0.6 years after a fourth hospitalization.

Functional limitations can be objectively measured, and offer additional prognostic information. Severe impairment can be identified by history or in the clinic with the use of a six minute walk test. The use of cardiopulmonary exercise testing to measure peak oxygen uptake (VO2) provides objective and reproducible information that can predict increased mortality and define the severity of heart failure. A peak oxygen consumption of $\leq$ 10 mL/kg/min is associated with a 65% 1 year survival, compared to an 87% 1 year survival with a VO2 > 14 (Lang, Piergiuseppe, & Mancini, 2007). Peak oxygen consumption is a continuous variable that is affected by age, medications, and gender and should be interpreted in the context of a particular patient; however guidelines generally define a peak VO2 < 12 to 14 mL/kg/min as suggestive of advanced heart failure warranting consideration of advanced therapies (Yancy et al., 2013).

Requirements and intolerance of medical therapy are also important markers of mortality in advanced heart failure. Increasing diuretic doses are seen in late stages of heart failure and are associated with increased mortality (Eshaghian, Horwich, & Fonarow, 2006). Similarly, intolerance of neurohormonal blockade is predictive of increased mortality. Intolerance of angiotensin-converting enzyme inhibitors was associated with a 57% risk of mortality over a median 8.5 month follow-up compared to a 22%

mortality in patients on therapy (Kittleson, et al., 2003). Further, when patients are chronically dependent on inotropes, their survival is extremely poor with 50% mortality at 6 months (Stevenson, 2003).

Risk of mortality is also seen in progressive end organ function. The development of progressive renal dysfunction is a strong predictor of increased mortality. The ADHERE registry found an associated increased in-hospital mortality in patients with a BUN >43, a systolic blood pressure of < 115 mmHg, and a serum creatinine of > 2.75. The presence of all three markers at admission is associated with a 21.94% risk of in-hospital mortality, compared to a risk of only 2.14% in the lowest risk cohort.

Ultimately these are a few important, but not comprehensive, examples of ominous markers of increased mortality in heart failure. Over 100 individual factors have been identified, but no single factor is sufficient to fully predict the patient's prognosis. This has led to the development of several predictive models that combine individual signs into a comprehensive score to assist in risk stratification. The Heart Failure Survival Score is a predictive model that uses 7 clinical characteristics to stratify patients into low, medium and high risk categories (Aaronson, Schwartz, Chen, Wong, Goin, & Mancini, 1997). It incorporates the following variables:

- Ischemic etiology of cardiomyopathy
- Resting heart rate
- Left ventricular ejection fraction
- Mean blood pressure
- Intraventricular conduction delay
- Peak oxygen consumption (VO2)
- Serum sodium

Unfortunately as is the limitation of most models, the HFSS may not be applicable to current patients since it was derived prior to the broad use of current therapies including beta-blockers and biventricular pacemakers.

The Seattle Heart Failure Model is another validated risk predictor that was initially derived from the PRAISE cohort, but has been validated in multiple other cohorts, and recently updated in 2013 (Levy et al., 2006). It is a multivariate risk model that uses multiple clinical features including demographics, etiology, laboratory findings, and medication use to predict survival.

Patients with heart failure under consideration for advanced therapies should also be considered by their INTERMACS profile. The Interagency Registry for mechanically Assisted Circulatory Support (INTERMACS) has developed a profile with 7 classifications within the NYHA class III-IV or ACC/AHA stage D patient. Most patients referred for mechanical support are INTERMACS 1-4. In 2012, 16.6% of patients who underwent MCS were INTERMACS 1, which are patients in critical cardiogenic shock with estimated hours of survival without intervention (Kirklin et al., 2013). Predictably, these patients have a poor survival and longer hospitalization when compared to patients with a higher INTERMACS profile (Boyle et al., 2011). This supports the need for early identification of the at risk patient with an overall increased mortality, before the progression of disease leads to increased peri-operative mortality.

Evaluation and Optimization Prior to Surgery for Advanced Therapies

Beyond identification of patients who will benefit from advanced therapies, clinicians are challenged to identify the narrow therapeutic window that avoids patients who are too sick to benefit. Chronic heart failure can lead to multi-organ dysfunction, and it is often difficult to determine which comorbidities will reverse with treatment of heart failure. A multidisciplinary approach to assess end-organ function, nutrition, social support, and psychological well-being is necessary to identify and optimize patients prior to surgery.

Heart failure can affect every organ, however renal dysfunction is a common and crucial comorbidity in patients with advanced heart failure. Patients with known pre-operative renal dysfunction have poorer post-surgical survival after implantation for mechanical circulatory support (Sandner et al., 2009). The pre-operative challenge is to differentiate the patients with reversible renal dysfunction due to advanced heart failure and renal dysfunction that is independent of the heart condition.

There is a complex interaction between the pathophysiology of heart failure and renal dysfunction described as cardiorenal syndrome. Renal injury is thought to be induced by a variety of factors including poor forward flow from a reduced cardiac output, renal congestion from elevated venous pressure, adverse neurohormonal signaling, and exacerbated by medications including diuretics and ACE inhibitors (Ronco, Haapio, House, Anavekar, & Bellomo, 2008).

The pre-operative management of renal dysfunction in heart failure primarily involves hemodynamic optimization and evaluation to exclude intrinsic renal disease. Demonstration of improvement in renal function with increased forward flow and optimization of right atrial pressures to avoid venous congestion as well as excluding intrinsic renal disease are typically performed, although evidence is lacking to support that these interventions change outcomes. Advanced and irreversible renal insufficiency is a relative contraindication to advanced therapies, particularly in patients who are not candidates for cardiac transplantation.

Right heart catheterization is routinely performed on all patients undergoing consideration for advanced therapies. The goal of the procedure is to provide a hemodynamic assessment to demonstrate the severity of the cardiac disease as well as provide information on right ventricular function and severity of pulmonary hypertension. The presence of pulmonary hypertension is common in potential heart transplant patients and can predispose patients to early post-operative right heart failure. Markers of increased risk of RV failure include pulmonary artery systolic pressures of > 50 mmHg, and elevated transpulmonary gradient of > 15 mmHg, or an elevated pulmonary vascular resistance of > 3 woods units. These findings all demonstrate an abnormal pulmonary vasculature response to chronically elevated pulmonary venous hypertension due to heart failure (Guazzi & Borlaug, 2012). It is important to differentiate if this elevated pressure is reversible or fixed. Reversible hypertension is likely due to endothelial dysfunction and can be demonstrated with a reduction in the PVR and TPG with a vasodilator challenge. Fixed pulmonary hypertension is suggestive of pulmonary arteriolar remodeling and is considered a relative contraindication for cardiac transplant when the PVR is > 5 woods units or the TPG is > 16-20 mmHg (Mehra, Jessup, Gronda, & Costanzo, 2006). Continued ventricular unloading with inotropic or mechanical support can occasionally demonstrate reversibility despite a lack of response with acute therapy, so continued support and re-measurement of hemodynamics should be considered in non-responders.

Frailty is another important factor to evaluate prior to surgery. Patients being considered for advanced therapies are often of advanced age with comorbid disease. In the setting of their cardiac disease they are often home bound, relatively immobile, cachectic with muscle wasting, and with global neurologic impairments due to poor cardiac output. This cumulative process is defined as frailty, and is readily identified by most clinicians despite the lack of a widely accepted definition. The presence of frailty has consistently been shown to predict adverse outcomes (Flint, Matlock, Lindenfeld, & Allen, 2012). Measurements such a grip strength and gait speed are useful objectives measurements for a clinical feature that is typically assessed by clinical gestalt. Ongoing research is still needed to help determine which patients with a frail phenotype will reverse with improvement in cardiac function with advanced therapies.

Other comorbidities that reduce the likelihood of overall survival need to be considered prior to consideration for advanced therapies. Advanced age, obesity, recent history of malignancy with risk of recurrence, diabetes with end-organ damage, recent tobacco use, and peripheral vascular disease all impact survival (Mehra, et al., 2006). Although many of these patients may not be eligible for cardiac transplantation listing, consideration for mechanical support as destination therapy should still be considered.

The candidacy of a patient for advanced therapies rests upon the recognition of advanced heart failure and consideration of their comorbid conditions. The first decision to be made is if the patient is appropriate for cardiac transplantation. If the patient can be listed for cardiac transplantation, bridging strategies including inotropic use and mechanical support can then be considered based on the expected wait time to transplantation. Given the national rise in wait times, there has been a growing role of mechanical circulatory support in patients listed for heart transplantation (Schulze, Kitada, Clerkin, Jin, & Mancini, 2014). If a patient is not a candidate for cardiac transplantation, mechanical support can still be considered as destination therapy (Rose et al., 2001). Although there has been growing enthusiasm and utility of destination therapy Left ventricular assist devices (LVAD), The center for Medicare and Medicaid Services (CMS) has provided strict conditions that patients must meet to be meet to be eligible for LVAD as destination therapy. All patients with advanced left ventricular failure must not be a candidate for cardiac transplantation, have an left ventricular ejection fraction of < 25%, have class IV heart failure symptoms despite optimal medical therapy for 60 of the last 90 days, and have a peak oxygen consumption of < 12 ml/kg/min or be dependent on inotropic therapy (Phurrough, Farrell, Ulrich, & Long, 2003).

CONCLUSION

There has been remarkable progress in the medical management of heart failure. Prompt and comprehensive medical therapies have greatly improved the outlook of this chronic and progressive disease. For many patients who have progressed beyond the point of pharmacologic treatment, mechanical support devices and cardiac transplantation can prolong survival in the appropriate patient population. Early identification and referral of the patient who has progressed to end-stage disease is necessary to prevent the development of irreversible end-organ dysfunction and increased mortality.

REFERENCES

Aaronson, K., Schwartz, J., Chen, T., Wong, K., Goin, J., & Mancini, D. (1997). Development and prospective validation of a clinical index to predict survival in ambulatory patients referred for cardiac transplant evaluation. *Circulation*, *95*(12), 2660–2667. doi:10.1161/01.CIR.95.12.2660 PMID:9193435

Arzt, M., Floras, J., Logan, A., Kimoff, J., Series, F., Morrison, D., & Bradley, D. et al. (2007). Suppression of central sleep apnea by continuous positive airway pressure and transplant-free survival in heart failure: A post hoc analysis of the Canadian Continuous Positive Airway Pressure for Patients with Central Sleep Apnea and Heart Failure Trial (CANPAP). *Circulation*, *115*(25), 3173–3180. doi:10.1161/CIRCULATIONAHA.106.683482 PMID:17562959

Bardy, G., Lee, K., Mark, D., Poole, J., Packer, D., Boineau, R., & Ip, J. et al. (2005). Amiodarone or an Implantable Cardioverter–Defibrillator for Congestive Heart Failure. *The New England Journal of Medicine*, *352*(3), 225–237. doi:10.1056/NEJMoa043399 PMID:15659722

Benotti, P., Wood, G., Winegar, D., Petrick, A., Still, C., Argyropoulos, G., & Gerhard, G. (2014). Risk Factors Associated With Mortality After Roux-en-Y Gastric Bypass Surgery. *Annals of Surgery*, *259*(1), 123–130. doi:10.1097/SLA.0b013e31828a0ee4 PMID:23470583

Bortman, G., Sellanes, M., Odell, D., Ring, W., & Olivari, M. (1994). Discrepancy between pre- and post-transplant diagnosis of end-stage dilated cardiomyopathy. *The American Journal of Cardiology*, *74*(9), 921–924. doi:10.1016/0002-9149(94)90587-8 PMID:7977122

Boyle, A., Ascheim, D., Russo, M., Kormos, R., John, R., Naka, Y., & Teuteberg, J. et al. (2011). Clinical outcomes for continuous-flow left ventricular assist device patients stratified by pre-operative INTERMACS classification. *The Journal of Heart and Lung Transplantation*, *30*(4), 402–407. doi:10.1016/j.healun.2010.10.016 PMID:21168346

Bristow, M., Gilbert, E., Abraham, W., Fowler, M., Hershberger, R., Kubo, S., & Shusterman, N. et al. (1996). Carvedilol produces dose-related improvements in left ventricular function and survival in subjects with chronic heart failure. MOCHA Investigators. *Circulation*, *94*(11), 2807–2816. doi:10.1161/01.CIR.94.11.2807 PMID:8941106

Carson, P., Ziesche, S., Johnson, G., & Cohn, J. (1999). Racial differences in response to therapy for heart failure: analysis of the vasodilator-heart failure trials: Vasodilator-Heart Failure Trial Study Group. *Journal of Cardiac Failure*, *5*(3), 178–187. doi:10.1016/S1071-9164(99)90001-5 PMID:10496190

Curtis, A., Worley, S., Adamson, P., Chung, E., Niazi, I., Sherfesee, L., & Sutton, M. et al. (2013). Biventricular pacing for atrioventricular block and systolic dysfunction. *The New England Journal of Medicine*, *368*(17), 1585–1593. doi:10.1056/NEJMoa1210356 PMID:23614585

Davies, E., Moxham, T., Rees, K., Singh, S., Coats, A., Ebrahim, S., & Taylor, S. et al. (2010). Exercise training for systolic heart failure: Cochrane systematic review and meta-analysis. *European Journal of Heart Failure*, *12*(7), 706–715. doi:10.1093/eurjhf/hfq056 PMID:20494922

Eshaghian, S., Horwich, T., & Fonarow, G. (2006). Relation of Loop Diuretic Dose to Mortality in Advanced Heart Failure. *The American Journal of Cardiology*, *97*(12), 1759–1764. doi:10.1016/j.amjcard.2005.12.072 PMID:16765130

Flint, K., Matlock, D., Lindenfeld, J., & Allen, L. (2012). Frailty and the Selection of Patients for Destination Therapy Left Ventricular Assist Device. *Circulation: Heart Failure*, *5*(2), 286–293. doi:10.1161/CIRCHEARTFAILURE.111.963215 PMID:22438521

Francois, C., Schiebler, M., & Reeder, S. (2010). Cardiac MRI evaluation of nonischemic cardiomyopathies. *Journal of Magnetic Resonance Imaging*, *31*(3), 518–530. doi:10.1002/jmri.22030 PMID:20187194

Garg, R., & Yusuf, S. (1995). Overview of randomized trials of angiotensin-converting enzyme inhibitors on mortality and morbidity in patients with heart failure. Collaborative Group on ACE Inhibitor Trials. *Journal of the American Medical Association*, *273*(18), 1450–1456. doi:10.1001/jama.1995.03520420066040 PMID:7654275

Go, A., Mozaffarian, D., Roger, V., Benjamin, E., Berry, J., Borden, W., & Turner, M. et al. (2013). Heart Disease and Stroke Statistics-2013 Update: A report from the American Heart Association. *Circulation*, *127*(1), e6–e245. PMID:23239837

Guazzi, M., & Borlaug, B. (2012). Pulmonary Hypertension Due to Left Heart Disease. *Circulation*, *126*(8), 975–990. doi:10.1161/CIRCULATIONAHA.111.085761 PMID:22908015

Kenchaiah, S., Evans, J., Levy, D., Wilson, P., Benjamin, E., Larson, M., & Vasan, R. et al. (2002). Obesity and the risk of heart failure. *The New England Journal of Medicine*, *347*(5), 305–313. doi:10.1056/NEJMoa020245 PMID:12151467

Kirklin, J., Naftel, D., Kormos, R., Stevenson, L., Pagani, F., Ph, D., & Young, J. et al. (2013). Fifth INTERMACS annual report: Risk factor analysis from more than 6,000 mechanical circulatory support patients. *The Journal of Heart and Lung Transplantation*, *32*(2), 141–156. doi:10.1016/j.healun.2012.12.004 PMID:23352390

Kittleson, M., Hurwitz, S., Shah, M., Nohria, A., Lewis, E., Givertz, M., & Stevenson, L. et al. (2003). Development of circulatory-renal limitations to angiotensin-converting enzyme inhibitors identifies patients with severe heart failure and early mortality. *Journal of the American College of Cardiology*, *41*(11), 2029–2035. doi:10.1016/S0735-1097(03)00417-0 PMID:12798577

Krawczyk, M., Flinta, I., Garncarek, M., Jankowska, E., Banasiak, W., Germany, R., & Ponikowski, P. et al. (2013). Sleep disordered breathing in patients with heart failure. *Cardiology Journal*, *20*(4), 345–355. doi:10.5603/CJ.2013.0092 PMID:23913452

Lang, C., Piergiuseppe, A., & Mancini, D. (2007). Prognostic Significance and Measurement of Exercise-Derived Hemodynamic Variables in Patients With Heart Failure. *Journal of Cardiac Failure*, *13*(8), 672–697. doi:10.1016/j.cardfail.2007.05.004 PMID:17923361

Levy, W., Mozaffarian, D., Linker, D., Sutradhar, S., Anker, S., Cropp, A., & Packer, M. et al. (2006). The Seattle Heart Failure Model. Prediction of Survival in Heart Failure. *Heart Failure*, *133*(11), 1424–1433. PMID:16534009

Madsen, B., Hansen, J., Stokholm, K., Brons, J., Husum, D., & Mortensen, L. (1994). Chronic congestive heart failure. Description and survival of 190 consecutive patients with a diagnosis of chronic congestive heart failure based on clinical signs and symptoms. *European Heart Journal*, *15*(3), 303–310. PMID:8013501

Maggioni, A., Anand, I., Gottlieb, S., Latini, R., Tognoni, G., & Cohn, J. (2002). Effects of valsartan on morbidity and mortality in patients with heart failure not receiving angiotensin-converting enzyme inhibitors. *Journal of the American College of Cardiology*, *40*(8), 1414–1421. doi:10.1016/S0735-1097(02)02304-5 PMID:12392830

Mansfield, D., Gollogly, C., Kaye, D., Richardson, M., Bergin, P., & Naughton, M. (2004). Controlled Trial of Continuous Positive Airway Pressure in Obstructive Sleep Apnea and Heart Failure. *American Journal of Respiratory and Critical Care Medicine*, *169*(3), 361–366. doi:10.1164/rccm.200306-752OC PMID:14597482

McMurray, J., Ostergren, J., Swedberg, K., Granger, C., Held, P., Michelson, E., & Pfeffer, M. et al. (2003). Effects of candesartan in patients with chronic heart failure and reduced left-ventricular systolic function taking angiotensin-converting-enzyme inhibitors: The CHARM-Added trial. *Lancet*, *362*(9386), 767–771. doi:10.1016/S0140-6736(03)14283-3 PMID:13678869

McMurray, J., Packer, M., Desai, A., Gong, J., Lefkowitz, M., Rizkala, A., & Zile, M. et al. (2014). Angiotensin-neprilysin inhibition versus enalapril in heart failure. *The New England Journal of Medicine*, *371*(11), 993–1004. doi:10.1056/NEJMoa1409077 PMID:25176015

Mehra, M., Jessup, M., Gronda, E., & Costanzo, M. (2006). Rationale and Process: International Society for Heart and Lung Transplantation Guidelines for the Care of Cardiac Transplant Candidates—2006. *The Journal of Heart and Lung Transplantation*, *25*(9), 1001–1002. doi:10.1016/j.healun.2006.06.006 PMID:16962462

Packer, M., Bristow, M., Cohn, J., Colucci, W., Fowler, M., Gilbert, E., & Shusterman, N. (1996). The effect of carvedilol on morbidity and mortality in patients with chronic heart failure. US carvedilol heart failure study group. *The New England Journal of Medicine*, *334*(21), 1349–1355. doi:10.1056/NEJM199605233342101 PMID:8614419

Packer, M., Poole-Wilson, P., Armstrong, P., Cleland, J., Horowitz, J., Massie, B., & Uretsky, B. et al. (1999). Comparative effects of low and high doses of the angiotensin-converting enzyme inhibitor, lisinopril, on morbidity and mortality in chronic heart failure. ATLAS Study Group. *Circulation*, *100*(23), 2312–2318. doi:10.1161/01.CIR.100.23.2312 PMID:10587334

Pfuntner, A., Wier, L. M., & Stocks, C. (2013). Most Frequent Conditions in U.S. Hospitals, 2011. *HCUP Statistical Brief #162. Agency for Healthcare Research and Quality*, Retrieved May 25, 2015, from http://www.hcup-us.ahrq.gov/reports/statbriefs/sb162.pdf

Phurrough, S., Farrell, J., Ulrich, M., & Long, K. (2003). *Decision Memo for Ventricular Assist Devices as Destination Therapy (CAG-00119N).* Retrieved May 25, 2015, from http://www.cms.gov/medicare-coverage-database/details/nca-decision-memo.aspx?ncaid=79&ncaname=ventricular+assist+devices+as+destination+therapy&ncdid=246&ispopup=y&bc=aaaaaaaaeaaa&

Pierpont, L., Cohn, J., & Franciosa, J. (1978). Combined oral hydralazine-nitrate therapy in left ventricular failure: Hemodynamic equivalency to sodium nitroprusside. *American College of Chest Physicians*, *73*(1), 8–13. PMID:620563

Pitt, B., Zannad, F., Remme, W., Cody, R., Castaigne, A., Perez, A., & Wittes, J. et al. (1999). The effect of spironolactone on morbidity and mortality in patients with severe heart failure. *The New England Journal of Medicine*, *341*(10), 709–717. doi:10.1056/NEJM199909023411001 PMID:10471456

Prondzinsky, R., Lemm, H., Swyter, M., Wegener, N., Unverzagt, S., Carter, J., & Buerke, M. et al. (2010). Intra-aortic balloon counterpulsation in patients with acute myocardial infarction complicated by cardiogenic shock: The prospective, randomized IABP SHOCK Trial for attenuation of multiorgan dysfunction syndrome. *Critical Care Medicine*, *38*(1), 152–160. doi:10.1097/CCM.0b013e3181b78671 PMID:19770739

Rathore, S., Wang, Y., & Krumholz, M. (2002). Sex-based differences in the effect of digoxin for the treatment of heart failure. *The New England Journal of Medicine*, *347*(18), 1403–1411. doi:10.1056/NEJMoa021266 PMID:12409542

Rekha, G., Gorlin, R., Smith, T., & Yusuf, S. (1997). The effect of digoxin on mortality and morbidity in patients with heart failure. *The New England Journal of Medicine*, *336*(8), 525–533. doi:10.1056/NEJM199702203360801 PMID:9036306

Ronco, C., Haapio, M., House, A., Anavekar, N., & Bellomo, R. (2008). Cardiorenal Syndrome. *Journal of the American College of Cardiology*, *52*(19), 1527–1539. doi:10.1016/j.jacc.2008.07.051 PMID:19007588

Rose, E., Gelijns, A., Moskowitz, A., Heitjan, D., Stevenson, L., Dembitsky, W., & Meier, P. et al. (2001). Long-Term Use of a Left Ventricular Assist Device for End-Stage Heart Failure. *The New England Journal of Medicine*, *345*(20), 1435–1443. doi:10.1056/NEJMoa012175 PMID:11794191

Sandner, S. E., Zimpfer, D., Zrunek, P., Rajek, A., Schima, H., Dunkler, D., & Wieselthaler, G. M. et al. (2009). Renal function and outcome after continuous flow left ventricular assist device implantation. *The Annals of Thoracic Surgery*, *87*(4), 1072–1078. doi:10.1016/j.athoracsur.2009.01.022 PMID:19324130

Sayer, G., Baker, J., & Parks, K. (2012). Heart rescue: The role of mechanical circulatory support in the management of severe refractory cardiogenic shock. *Current Opinion in Critical Care*, *18*(5), 409–416. doi:10.1097/MCC.0b013e328357f1e6 PMID:22895213

Sayer, G., & Bhat, G. (2014). The renin-angiotensin-aldosterone system and heart failure. *Cardiology Clinics*, *32*(1), 21–32. doi:10.1016/j.ccl.2013.09.002 PMID:24286576

Schulze, C., Kitada, S., Clerkin, K., Jin, Z., & Mancini, D. (2014). Regional Differences in Recipient Waitlist Time and Pre- and Post-Transplant Mortality After the 2006 United Network for Organ Sharing Policy Changes in the Donor Heart Allocation Algorithm. *Journal of the American College of Cardiology: Heart Failure*, *2*(2), 166–177. PMID:24720925

Setoguchi, S., Stevenson, L., & Schneeweiss, S. (2007). Repeated hospitalizations predict mortality in the community population with heart failure. *American Heart Journal*, *154*(2), 260–266. doi:10.1016/j.ahj.2007.01.041 PMID:17643574

Smedira, N., Moazami, N., Golding, C., McCarthy, P., Apperson-Hansen, C., Blackstone, E., & Cosgrove, D. (2001). Clinical experience with 202 adults receiving extracorporeal membrane oxygenation for cardiac failure: Survival at five years. *The Journal of Thoracic and Cardiovascular Surgery*, *122*(1), 92–102. doi:10.1067/mtc.2001.114351 PMID:11436041

Stevenson, L. (2003). Clinical use of inotropic therapy for heart failure: looking backward or forward? Part II: chronic inotropic therapy. *Circulation*, *108*(4), 492–497. doi:10.1161/01.CIR.0000078349.43742.8A PMID:12885733

Sutton, M., Plappert, T., Hilpisch, K., Abraham, W., Hayes, D., & Chinchoy, E. (2006). Sustained reverse left ventricular structural remodeling with cardiac resynchronization at one year is a function of etiology: Quantitative Doppler echocardiographic evidence from the Multicenter InSync Randomized Clinical Evaluation (MIRACLE). *Circulation*, *113*(2), 266–272. doi:10.1161/CIRCULATIONAHA.104.520817 PMID:16401777

Tang, A., Wells, G., Taljic, M., Arnold, M., Sheldon, R., Connolly, S., & Rouleau, J. et al. (2010). Cardiac resynchronization therapy for mild-to-moderate heart failure. *The New England Journal of Medicine*, *363*(25), 2385–2395. doi:10.1056/NEJMoa1009540 PMID:21073365

Taylor, A., Ziesche, S., Yancy, C., Carson, P., D'Agostino, R. Jr, Ferdinand, K., & Cohn, J. et al. (2004). Combination of isosorbide dinitrate and hydralazine in blacks with heart failure. *The New England Journal of Medicine*, *351*(20), 2049–2057. doi:10.1056/NEJMoa042934 PMID:15533851

The Criteria Committee of the New York Heart Association. (1994). *Nomenclature and criteria for diagnosis of diseases of the heart and great vessels* (9th ed.). Boston, MA.

Westaby, S., Anastasiadis, K., & Wieselthaler, G. (2012). Cardiogenic shock in ACS. Part 2: Role of mechanical circulatory support. *Nature Reviews. Cardiology*, *9*(4), 195–208. doi:10.1038/nrcardio.2011.205 PMID:22231716

Yancy, C., Jessup, M., Bozkurt, B., Butler, J., Casey, D., Drazner, M. H., & Wilkoff, B. L. et al. (2013). ACCF/AHA Guideline for the Management of Heart Failure: Executive Summary: A Report of the American College of Cardiology Foundation/American Heart Association Task Force on Practice Guidelines. *Circulation*, *128*(16), 1810–1852. doi:10.1161/CIR.0b013e31829e8807 PMID:23741057

Zannad, F., McMurray, J., Krum, H., Van Veldhuisen, D., Sweedberg, K., Shi, H., & Pitt, B. et al. (2011). Eplerenone in patients with systolic heart failure and mild symptoms. *The New England Journal of Medicine*, *364*(1), 11–21. doi:10.1056/NEJMoa1009492 PMID:21073363

ADDITIONAL READING

Baran, D., & Jaiswal, A. (2014). Management of the ACC/AHA Stage D patient: Mechanical circulatory support. *Cardiology Clinics*, *32*(1), 113–124. doi:10.1016/j.ccl.2013.09.013 PMID:24286582

Birks, E. J. (2011). A Changing Trend Toward Destination Therapy. *Texas Heart Institute Journal*, *38*(5), 552–554. PMID:22163133

Flint, K. M., Matlock, D. D., Lindenfeld, J., & Allen, L. (2012). Frailty and the selection of patients for destination therapy left ventricular assist device. *Circulation: Heart Failure*, *5*(2), 286–293. doi:10.1161/CIRCHEARTFAILURE.111.963215 PMID:22438521

Mehra, M., Jessup, M., Gronda, E., & Costanzo, M. (2006). Rationale and Process: International Society for Heart and Lung Transplantation Guidelines for the Care of Cardiac Transplant Candidates—2006. *The Journal of Heart and Lung Transplantation*, *25*(9), 1001–1002. doi:10.1016/j.healun.2006.06.006 PMID:16962462

Nohria, A., Lewis, E., & Stevenson, L. W. (2002). Medical management of advanced heart failure. *Journal of the American Medical Association*, *287*(5), 628–640. doi:10.1001/jama.287.5.628 PMID:11829703

Reynolds, H. R., & Hochman, J. S. (2008). Cardiogenic shock: Current concepts and improving outcomes. *Circulation*, *117*(5), 686–697. doi:10.1161/CIRCULATIONAHA.106.613596 PMID:18250279

Ronco, C., Haapio, M., House, A., Anavekar, N., & Bellomo, R. (2008). Cardiorenal Syndrome. *Journal of the American College of Cardiology*, *52*(19), 1527–1539. doi:10.1016/j.jacc.2008.07.051 PMID:19007588

Westaby, S., Anastasiadis, K., & Wieselthaler, G. (2012). Cardiogenic shock in ACS. Part 2: Role of mechanical circulatory support. *Nature Reviews. Cardiology*, *9*(10), 195–208. doi:10.1038/nrcardio.2011.205 PMID:22231716

Yancy, C., Jessup, M., Bozkurt, B., Butler, J., Casey, D., Drazner, M., & Wilkoff, B. et al. (2013). 2013 ACCF/AHA Guideline for the Management of Heart Failure: Executive Summary: A Report of the American College of Cardiology Foundation/American Heart Association Task Force on Practice Guidelines. *Circulation*, *128*(16), 1810–1852. doi:10.1161/CIR.0b013e31829e8807 PMID:23741057

KEY TERMS AND DEFINITIONS

Cardiac Index: The cardiac output indexed to body surface area (L/min/m^2).

Cardiac Output: The volume of blood ejected by the heart per minute (L/min).

Guideline Directed Therapy: The comprehensive and evidenced based use of pharmacologic, behavioral, and device therapies as recommended by consensus guidelines.

Inotropes: Medications that increase cardiac output with direct effect on myocardial function.

Neurohormonal Blockade: Medications that target the mechanisms of disease progression in heart failure. The most common targets include the sympathetic nervous system and the renin-angiotensin system.

Pulmonary Vascular Resistance: The resistance to blood flow by the pulmonary circulation. Can be calculated as PVR= (Mean pulmonary arterial pressure- Pulmonary Capillary Wedge pressure)/ Cardiac output. Typically expressed in Woods Units.

Systemic Vascular Resistance: The resistance to blood flow by the peripheral circulation. Can be calculated by 80 x (Mean arterial pressure-Mean right atrial pressure) / Cardiac output. Typically expressed as dyn·s/cm5.

Transpulmonary Gradient: The difference between the mean pulmonary arterial pressure and the pulmonary capillary wedge pressure.

Vasodilators: Medications that dilate blood vessels and reduce vascular resistance.

Section 3

Pharmacology in the Cardiothoracic ICU

Chapter 10
Antiarrhythmics, Inotropes, and Vasopressors

Bethany R. Tellor
Barnes-Jewish Hospital, USA

Keki R. Balsara
Washington University School of Medicine, USA

ABSTRACT

Arrhythmias, low cardiac output syndromes, and low blood pressure are commonly faced complications in the cardiothoracic surgery patient. In order to provide appropriate clinical management, one must identify underlying etiologies while recognizing and understanding available treatment options. The objective of this chapter is to review common agents utilized to manage arrhythmias and maintain hemodynamic stability following cardiac surgery. Mechanisms of action, key clinical pearls and relevant literature pertaining to each agent will be discussed.

BACKGROUND

One of the most common complications following cardiac or thoracic surgery includes cardiac arrhythmias. Postoperative atrial fibrillation has been associated with significant morbidity and mortality as well as increased cost and hospital length of stay. Nearly 30% of patients undergoing any form of chest surgery develop postoperative arrhythmias. Atrial fibrillation is the most common with ventricular ectopy being less common. Cardiac dysrhythmias can broadly be categorized into two categories – chronic and acute. Chronic arrhythmias have multiple treatment options including pharmacological therapy, internal defibrillators and surgery. Acute arrhythmias are more commonly managed medically.

Low cardiac output syndrome occurring during or post cardiopulmonary bypass (CPB) is also common and may be a result of reperfusion injury, inflammatory and coagulation cascade activation, or direct ischemic insult. Additionally, many patients have underlying cardiac dysfunction or heart failure, contributing to low output states after surgery. As with any critically ill patient, shock states may also develop in the postoperative period due to hypovolemia, cardiogenic or obstructive causes, distributive causes such as sepsis, or an overlapping variety of each.

DOI: 10.4018/978-1-4666-8603-8.ch010

These complications require most patients to be supported in the short-term with some form of antiarrythmic, inotrope and/or vasopressor. While many older generation antiarrhythmic agents are available, postoperative arrhythmias are often managed with amiodarone, lidocaine, β –blockers, calcium channel blockers, or a combination of these therapies. In order to augment cardiac output (CO) or vascular tone in shock states, inotropic and vasopressor agents are administered. In this chapter, differences in mechanism of action, adrenergic receptor selectivity, adverse effects, and clinical features that influence the selection of an agent will be discussed. There is a high degree of variability in the use of specific therapy that will be discussed; the choice is often driven by clinical context, expert opinion, and clinician preference.

ANTIARRHYTHMIC AGENTS

Antiarrhythmic drugs exert their action by blocking sodium, potassium or calcium. They are classified as either Class IA (prolong action potential), IB (shorten action potential), IC (slow conduction), II (block beta adrenergic receptors), III (prolong repolarization), and IV (blocker calcium channels) (Table 1.) While a number of medications exist in each category, most intensive care units use a handful of medications with which they have familiarity. Guidelines related to the pharmacological management of perioperative atrial fibrillation for cardiothoracic surgery patients highlight the use of β –blockers and amiodarone (Martinez, 2005a; Martinez 2005b; Frendl, 2014).

β-Blockers

Class II agents largely include all β -blockers. While a number are commercially available, the most commonly utilized include metoprolol, carvedilol, atenolol and esmolol. These agents can be utilized in

Table 1. Vaughn-Williams Classification of Antiarrhythmic Agents

Classification	Agents	Primary Ion Blockade/Effect
1a	**Disopyramide** **Quinidine** **Procainamide**	Na^+ Increased refractory period
1b	**Lidocaine** **Mexiletine**	Na^+ Decreased refractory period
1c	**Flecainide** **Propafenone**	Na^+ No effect on refractory period
II	**Metoprolol** **Atenolol** **Esmolol**	Ca^{2+} (through β-receptor blockade) Increased refractory period Decreased atrioventricular conduction
III	**Amiodarone** **Dronedarone** **Sotalol** **Dofetilide**	K^+ Increased refractory period
IV	**Verapamil** **Diltiazem**	Ca^{2+} Increased refractory period Decreased atrioventricular conduction

the acute treatment of arrhythmias, or can be used for long-term prevention. Due to their mechanism of action and their effects on both β -1 and β -2 receptors, they can treat a spectrum of problems including rhythms, blood pressure and other disorders. Arrhythmias due to adrenergic stimulation respond very well to β -blocker therapy and they are considered first line therapy for rate control after cardiac surgery (Martinez, 2005a). Conversely, while good for rate control, β -blockers are not first line therapy for conversion of atrial fibrillation/flutter to normal sinus rhythm. There is no evidence to support the use of β-blockers aside from sotalol as primary prevention for atrial fibrillation. There is some evidence as supported by a meta analysis of seven randomized trials that beta blockers might have some benefit in dysrhythmia prevention in chronic heart failure patients.

Amiodarone

Amiodarone is a class III agent that is increasingly being utilized for a wide variety of arrhythmias. It is important to note that it is common for atrial fibrillation to persist or recur during the loading phase of therapy due to the delay in onset. Amiodarone may interfere with the hepatic metabolism of other medications such as digoxin or warfarin and has been associated with numerous adverse effects. Clinically important noncardiovascular toxicities include thyroid (3-20%), pulmonary (< 3%), hepatic (15%), dermatologic (25-75%), and neurologic (3-30%) abnormalities (Zimetbaum, 2007).

Amiodarone has demonstrated efficacy in atrial fibrillation/flutter, re-entrant tachyarrhythmias, ventricular fibrillation and ventricular tachycardia (Mitchell, 2005a). In general, amiodarone's efficacy equals or exceeds that of all other antiarrhythmic agents and is in the range of 60-80% for most supraventricular tachyarrhythmias and 40-60% for ventricular tachyarrythmias. Moreover, a meta-analysis looking at more than 6500 patients treated with amiodarone following acute MI or chronic heart failure demonstrated improved survival. This was true for patients with hypertrophic cardiomyopathy, nonischemic dilated cardiomyopathy, ventricular arrhythmias following MI and ventricular arrhythmias following resuscitation after cardiac arrest (Amiodarone Trials Meta-Analysis Investigators, 1997; Bardy, 2005; Bokhari, 2004). As demonstrated in the Canadian trial of atrial fibrillation, the AFFIRM trial and the SAFE-T trial, nearly two-thirds of patients treated with amiodarone achieved and maintained sinus rhythm long-term (Roy, 2000; Wyse, 2002; Singh, 2005). Amiodarone is perhaps the best studied and most effective drug for the prevention of atrial fibrillation. Prophylactic amiodarone following heart surgery has been shown to decrease the incidence of post-operative atrial fibrillation and has proven to be more effective than class I antiarrythmics and sotalol in maintaining sinus rhythm in patients with recurrent atrial fibrillation (Mitchell, 2005b).

Lidocaine

Lidocaine is a class IB agent. It acts on sodium channels and has a rapid onset and offset. It is typically used in the treatment of ventricular arrhythmias. It is administered as an IV infusion and has demonstrated efficacy in improved survival in patients resuscitated following VF arrest. More recent studies have demonstrated that it is less effective than other medications, most notably amiodarone, in the treatment of ventricular dysrhythmia following surgery or cardiac arrest (Dorian, 2002). Lidocaine is typically used as short-term therapy, however it is important to note adverse effects. Serious effects such as seizures, psychosis, and respiratory arrest may be seen with larger doses and supratherapeutic drug concentrations. Drowsiness, disorientation, and agitation are described to a lesser degree (Harrison, 1974).

While long-term survival with either rate or rhythm control is similar, controversy regarding which strategy is best still remains. Many attempt to re-establish sinus rhythm to improve symptoms and reduce the need for anticoagulation. The safety and efficacy of a number of antiarrhythmics was examined in a 2012 meta-analysis which looked at 56 trials (n=20,771) in which an antiarrhythmic drug used to treat atrial fibrillation was compared against placebo, untreated controls or another antiarrhythmic (Lafuente-Lafuente, 2012). Compared to placebo, class IA, IC, II, and III lowered the rate of atrial fibrillation. Of note, it did appear that there was a higher incidence of mortality with class IA drugs and a proarrhythmic effect with all drugs except amiodarone.

VASOACTIVE AGENTS

Inotropes

Inotropic agents are used to improve myocardial contractility in patients presenting with low CO in order to maintain systemic perfusion and preserve end-organ function. Inotropes may be initiated in patients with heart failure with reduced ejection fraction, (Yancy, 2013; McMurray, 2012), patients with septic shock and myocardial dysfunction (Dellinger, 2013), and in patients with low cardiac output syndromes occurring during or post cardiopulmonary bypass (CPB) (St Andre, 2005). Inotropes are often used until the acute precipitating event has resolved or until definitive therapy is established (e.g., mechanical circulatory support, heart transplantation, coronary revascularization, palliative therapy). Therapy is guided by achievement of hemodynamic parameters such as cardiac index or central or mixed venous oxygenation saturation and by clinical signs of perfusion.

Vasoactive agents with inotropic properties include dobutamine, milrinone, dopamine, epinephrine, levosimendan, and isoproterenol (Table 2). Through different mechanisms of action, all agents influence calcium sensitivity or release in order to improve the contractile force of the myocardium and increase CO. Dobutamine, dopamine, epinephrine, and isoproterenol directly stimulate β_1-adrenergic receptors expressed on cardiac myocytes. Stimulation of these receptors activates adenylate cyclase, leading to increased intracellular cyclic adenosine monophosphate (cAMP) production, calcium channel activation, and facilitation of the actin-myosin-troponin system. Without directly stimulating adrenergic receptors, milrinone increases myocardial contractility by preventing intracellular enzymatic degradation of cAMP through inhibition of phosphodiesterase, while levosimendan binds to cardiac troponin C to increase cardiac myocyte calcium responsiveness. Additionally, both agents decrease afterload through direct vasodilatory properties; milrinone displays cAMP-mediated vasodilation in vascular smooth muscle cells while levosimendan opens ATP-dependent potassium channels (Overgaard, 2008; Hollenberg, 2011).

Dobutamine

Dobutamine increases CO and decreases left ventricular filling pressure and left ventricular end-diastolic volume, allowing for more efficient ventricular function (Sonnenblick, 1979). It is a potent inotrope binding to β_1 receptors predominately and to a lesser degree, β_2 and α_1. The α_1 – mediated vasoconstriction is likely offset by a decrease in peripheral vascular resistance (PVR) occurring through direct β_2 receptor stimulation, explaining why significant changes in blood pressure are uncommon (Ruffolo, 1987). Tolerance may develop after a few days (Unverferth, 1980) while tachyarrythmias and worsened

Table 2. Vasopressor and Inotrope Agents: Receptor Activity and Standard Dose Range

Drug	Receptor Activity					Continuous Infusion Dose Range
	α_1	β_1	β_2	DA	V_1, V_2	
Dobutamine	+	+++++	+++	-	-	2 - 20 mcg/kg/min
Milrinone	-	-	-	-	-	0.375 - 0.75 mcg/kg/min
Dopamine	+++	++++	++	+++++	-	1 - 20 mcg/kg/min
Epinephrine	+++++	++++	+++	-	-	0.02 - 0.2 mcg/kg/min
Levosimendan	-	-	-	-	-	0.05 - 0.2 mcg/kg/min
Isoproterenol	-	+++++	+++++	-	-	0.02 - 0.1 mcg/kg/min
Norepinephrine	+++++	+++	++	-	-	0.02 - 3 mcg/kg/min
Vasopressin	-	-	-	-	+++	0.02 - 0.04 units/min
Phenylephrine	+++++	-	-	-	-	0.5 - 10 mcg/kg/min
DA = Dopamine, V_1, V_2 = vasopressin, + through +++++ = minimal to maximal relative receptor affinity, - = no significant receptor affinity						

myocardial ischemia may result from increases in heart rate (HR) and myocardial oxygen consumption. Dobutamine has shown to produce a proportional increase in coronary blood flow, which may negate potential coronary constrictive effects seen in the setting of increased myocardial oxygen consumption (Fowler, 1984).

The use of dobutamine in cardiac surgery has been associated with increased morbidity and mortality (Fellahi, 2008; Nielsen, 2014). Perioperative dobutamine administration, based on physician judgment and preference, was associated with increased ventricular arrhythmias, use of an intraaortic ballon pump, and myocardial infarction (MI) after propensity score stratification in a small cohort study of 657 cardiac surgery patients (Fellahi, 2008). Furthermore, a recent nonrandomized observational study including a propensity-matched cohort of over 6,000 patients, demonstrated perioperative inotropes (mainly dobutamine and milrinone) to be associated with higher one year mortality (11%) compared to no inotropic therapy (4.2%). Inotropes were also independently associated with postoperative MI, stroke, and renal replacement therapy (Neilsen, 2014). Similarly, mortality rates of 14% and 12% have been noted in patients with decompensated heart failure receiving dobutamine or milrinone (Abraham, 2005). No randomized trials have been powered to show dobutamine increases morbidity and mortality in cardiac surgery patients, however the risk of harmful long-term effects should not be overlooked

Milrinone

Milrinone increases HR, stroke volume (SV), and CO while decreasing systemic vascular resistance and left ventricular filling pressures (Colucci, 1986). It has potent pulmonary vasodilator effects and is often preferred in patients with right heart failure. This agent may be useful in the setting of down regulated adrenergic receptors seen in patients with chronic heart failure or in patients recently treated with long term β-blockers (Bristow, 2001). Unlike dobutamine, limited data suggests that milrinone retains hemodynamic effects in the setting of β-blockade and advantages of continued β-blocker use with milrinone have been postulated (Jennings, 2009). It is important to consider a patient's renal function when using milrinone as the half-life of approximately 2.5 hours in normal renal function is significantly prolonged.

The accumulation of milrinone in this setting can lead to profound hypotension. Like dobutamine, the risk of arrhythmias is of concern while myocardial oxygen consumption may be lower (Baim, 1989). In the OPTIME-CHF trial (Cuffe, 2002), 4.6% of patients with acute decompensated heart failure who received milrinone for 48 hours experienced new atrial arrhythmias compared to with 1.5% of patients who received placebo ($p = 0.004$). Sustained hypotension was also more frequent in patients receiving milrinone [10.7% vs. 3.2% ($p < 0.001$)].

In cardiac surgery, milrinone has been identified as an independent predictor of postoperative atrial fibrillation (Fleming, 2008). A recent meta-analysis found no difference in mortality between cardiac surgery patients who received milrinone and patients who received other agents. A sensitivity analysis of included trials with low risk of bias actually noted a trend towards increased mortality (Majure, 2013). Furthermore, milrinone has not shown to reduce length of hospital stay or mortality in heart failure patients when added to standard care (Cuffe, 2002; Majure 2013). Like dobutamine, there is evidence to suggest that although milrinone improves hemodynamics in the short-term, the use of this agent must be weighed with the potential risk of harmful long-term outcomes.

Dopamine

Dopamine displays dose-dependent pharmacological effects. It acts on dopaminergic receptors, leading to vasodilation in renal and mesenteric beds at lower doses (< 3 mcg/kg/min) (Hoogenberg, 1998). Increased contractility and HR occur via β_1 receptor activation at intermediate doses (3-10 mcg/kg/min), while α_1 mediated vasoconstriction occurs at higher doses (10-20 mcg/kg/min) (Overguard, 2008). The direct natriuretic effects seen through its action on renal tubules providing "renal protection" is controversial as this has not shown to protect patients from renal dysfunction or increase glomerular filtration rate (Bellomo, 2000). In the ROSE HF trial (Chen, 2013), 360 hospitalized patients with acute heart failure and renal dysfunction were randomized to receive low-dose dopamine, nesiritide or placebo. Neither dopamine nor nesiritide improved renal function when added to diuretic therapy.

A large randomized trial in patients with shock compared dopamine to norepinephrine and found no difference in mortality. Of note, more arrhythmic events occurred in patients receiving dopamine and a subgroup analysis showed that dopamine was associated with an increased rate of death at 28 days among patients with cardiogenic shock (De Baker, 2010). Dopamine may also be associated with increased rates of death in patients with septic shock (De Backer, 2012). Due to these findings, the Surviving Sepsis Guidelines do not recommend use of this agent as first line therapy in septic shock or for renal protection (Dellinger, 2013). There is limited data discussing the use of this agent in cardiac surgery.

Epinephrine

Epinephrine increases mean arterial pressure by increasing both CO and PVR (Hollenberg, 2011). It has potent α_1, β_1, and β_2 activity. Like dopamine, a dose dependent receptor activity response occurs; higher doses will provide more α activity while lower doses provide more β activity. It also causes pulmonary vasoconstriction and increased right ventricular afterload (Aviado, 1957). When compared to norepinephrine and doubtamine, epinephrine infusion has been associated with an increase in lactate levels and decreased splanchnic flow (Levy, 1997; Annane, 2007). It may also cause hyperglycemia.

A randomized trial comparing epinephrine to the combination of dobutamine and norepinephrine in 330 patients with septic shock, found no difference in mortality at 28 days (Annane, 2007). However, this study did not meet their expected sample size. It has been considered a second-line agent in patients with septic shock failing to respond to other therapies (Dellinger, 2013). Epinephrine is commonly used after cardiac surgery with CPB to overcome myocardial stunning although limited data support the use. In patients receiving epinephrine or dobutamine after coronary artery bypass surgery, dobutamine increased HR to a great degree but both drugs were shown to have similar effects on mean arterial pressure, central venous pressure, pulmonary artery occlusion pressure, systemic vascular resistance, pulmonary vascular resistance, and left-ventricular stroke (Butterworth, 1992). Long-term data assessing morbidity and mortality with this agent are lacking.

Levosimenden

Levosimenden increases HR, SV and CO while decreasing pulmonary capillary wedge pressure, mean pulmonary artery pressures, and PVR (Nieminen, 2000). In comparison to dobutamine, improvement in cardiac index and PCWP in heart failure patients were more profound with levosidmenden after 48 hours of therapy, although hypotension was more frequent (Bergh, 2010). The elimination half-life of levosimendan is approximately 1 hour whereas that of its metabolite, OR-1896, is 70 to 80 hours (Kivikko, 2002). The vasodilatory properties and lasting hemodynamic effects are thought to be mediated by OR-1896 which is slowly eliminated over two weeks (Kivikko, 2002; Erdei, 2006). The long-term effects of the metabolite should be considered, especially in patients with shock.

Reductions in morality have been suggested in select cardiac surgery patients receiving levosimendan (Maharaj, 2011; Harrison, 2013), but have not been shown in patients with acute decompensated heart failure (Mebazaa, 2007; Packer, 2013). A recent meta- analysis investigating the effects of levosimendan in 1,155 cardiac surgery patients from 14 randomized controlled trials showed a reduction in mortality in patients with an ejection fraction of <40%. Reductions in the need for dialysis, myocardial injury, and postoperative atrial fibrillation were also seen (Harrison, 2013). Interest in the use of this agent in cardiac surgery patients, particularly those with a reduced ejection fraction, is growing. Levosimenden is currently not approved in the United States.

Isoproterenol

Isoproterenol has a very low affinity for α receptors and potent affinity for β_1, and β_2. It reduces pulmonary arterial pressures (Aviado, 1957) and produces comparable increases in CO as dobutamine with greater positive chronotropic effects (Sonnenblick, 1979). A greater reflex in increased HR may be seen, secondary to greater decreases in PVR (Ruffolo, 1987). It has historically been used as the mainstay of therapy for chronotropy post heart transplantation (Stinson, 1975) and is often utilized for bradycardia and transient complete heart block following cardiac surgery. The role of this agent in cardiogenic shock is less recognized.

Although there are several inotropic agents available, definitive evidence guiding therapy is sparse. There is considerable inter-hospital variability in the use of inotropic agents in heart failure and cardiac surgery patients (Allen, 2014; Williams, 2011). Available evidence highlights the uncertainties pertaining to utilization and duration of these agents and the need for new therapies. Although novel inotropic agents with new mechanism of action are currently in clinical development (Francis, 2014), methods used to evaluate their safety and efficacy will likely be challenging. Inotropes can increase myocardial oxygen consumption, induce atrial or ventricular arrhythmias, lead to infarct expansion, and cause hypotension. It is prudent to consider patient specific factors such as renal function, the need for afterload reduction, and concomitant medications when deciding inotrope use and duration.

VASOPRESSORS

Vasopressor agents are used when hypotension persists despite adequate fluid resuscitation in patients with circulatory shock. Vasopressors are most commonly used in vasodilatory shock but may also be needed in other forms of shock to maintain perfusion. Therapy is guided by effectiveness in achieving blood pressure restoration, typically a mean arterial pressure (MAP) of $\geq$ 60 or 65 mmgHg. Vasoactive agents with vasoconstriction properties include norepinephrine, vasopressin, epinephrine, dopamine, and phenylephrine (Table 2). Agents that stimulate α-1 receptors, lead to activation of a regulatory G protein that acts through a series of intracellular steps to ultimately increase the release of calcium from the sarcoplasmic reticulum (SR), leading to vascular smooth muscle constriction (Overguard, 2008). Adrenergic agents are typically chosen first line due to their rapid onset of action and short half-life, allowing for easy titration. Vasopressin acts through vasopressin receptors to produce its effects.

Norepinephrine

Norepinephrine increases blood pressure without significantly impacting CO and SV as it is a potent α_1-adrenergic receptor agonist with minimal β activity (Hollenberg, 2011). It may decrease renal, splanchnic, or peripheral blood flow in the setting of low flow states (Woolsey, 2005). Catecholamine agents with α- properties like norepinephrine may result in increased pulmonary pressures, increasing the workload of the right side of the heart. This is important to consider in patients with pulmonary hypertension or RV failure. Norepinephrine is recommended as the first line vasopressor according to the Surviving Sepsis Guidelines as data has suggested it may be a safer agent when compared to dopamine for septic shock (Dellinger, 2013; De Baker, 2010; De Baker, 2012).

Vasopressin

Vasopressin binds to vasopressin receptors in vascular smooth muscle, the pituitary gland, and renal collecting duct. Stimulation of V_{1a} mediates constriction of vascular smooth muscle. Like norepinephrine, there is evidence to suggest that vasopressin has adverse effects on splanchnic perfusion and metabolism (Woolsey, 2005). Vasopressin is thought to cause less direct coronary and cerebral vasoconstriction than catecholamines, and is often utilized to augment the effects of norepinephrine (Holmes, 2001). Adding low dose vasopressin to norepinephrine may be associated with survival benefit in patients with lower norepinephrine requirements (Russell, 2008). At this time, vasopressin is recommended to be added to norepinephrine to decrease norepinephrine dosage or increase MAP in patients with septic shock (Dellinger, 2013). Vasopressin may be a particularly attractive agent in cardiac surgery patients presenting with pulmonary hypertension or RV failure (Tayama, 2007; Vida, 2005). Furthermore, postcardiotomy vasopressin deficiency has been described (Morales, 2000; Argenziano, 1997), suggesting that certain cardiac surgery patients may benefit from use of this agent.

Phenylephrine

Phenylephrine displays potent selective α_1 -adrenergic activity. Its rapid onset of action, short duration, and primary vascular effects make it an ideal agent to use as a rapid bolus for correction of sudden hypotension. It may have a place in patients with obstructive hypertrophic cardiomyopathy to decrease the outflow tract gradient or in patients with severe arrhythmias. A significant reflex bradycardia may be seen secondary to absent effects on HR so it should not be used in patients with cardiogenic shock. In septic shock, phenylephrine is only recommended in certain circumstances (e.g. serious arrhythmias associated with norepinephrine, high CO with persistently low blood pressure, salvage therapy) (Dellinger, 2013).

The choice of a vasopressor agent will likely be driven by the clinical situation, including patient specific factors. Underlying conditions occurring in critically ill patients like hypoxia or acidosis may disrupt adrenergic receptor binding of vasoactive agents (Modest, 1995; Li, 1995). Norepinephrine, vasopressin, dopamine, and epinephrine may decreases splanchnic flow (Woolsey, 2005), agents with β activity may provoke or contribute to arrhythmias, while the risk of bradycardia may discourage the use of phenylephrine. Overall, there is a lack of randomized trials adequately powered to show long term morbidity and mortality outcomes of one agent versus another.

CONCLUSION

Complications related to cardiac rhythms and hemodynamic instability are commonly seen when providing care to cardiothoracic surgery patients. Although treatment of the underlying cause is most important, pharmacological therapy may be utilized in the short-term to maintain hemodynamic stability and prevent further complications. In the acute postoperative setting, a combined comprehensive approach including rate and rhythm control may be worthwhile in most patients. Overall, there is paucity of data regarding the ideal vasoactive agent and the effects of such therapy on long-term outcomes. Pharmacologic management should be aimed at short-term hemodynamic stabilization and based on the clinical context of the patient.

REFERENCES

Abraham, W. T., Adams, K. F., Fonarow, G. C., Costanzo, M. R., Berkowitz, R. L., LeJemtel, T. H., & Wynne, J. et al. (2005). In-hospital mortality in patients with acute decompensated heart failure requiring intravenous vasoactive medications: An Analysis from the Acute Decompensated Heart Failure National Registry (ADHERE). *Journal of the American College of Cardiology*, *46*(1), 57–64. doi:10.1016/j.jacc.2005.03.051 PMID:15992636

Allen, L. A., Fonarow, G. C., Grau-Sepulveda, M. V., Hernandez, A. F., Peterson, P. N., Partovian, C., & Krumholz, H. M. et al. (2014). Hospital variation in intravenous inotrope use for patients hospitalized with heart failure: Insights from Get With The Guidelines. *Circulation: Heart Failure*, *7*(2), 251–260. doi:10.1161/CIRCHEARTFAILURE.113.000761 PMID:24488983

Amiodarone Trials Meta-Analysis Investigators. (1997). Effect of prophylactic amiodarone on mortality after acute myocardial infaction and in congestive heart failure: Meta-analysis of individual data from 6500 patients in randomized trials. *Lancet*, *350*(9089), 1417–1424. doi:10.1016/S0140-6736(97)05281-1 PMID:9371164

Annane, D., Vignon, P., Renault, A., Bollaert, P., Charpentier, C., Martin, C., & Bellissant, E. et al. (2007). Norepinephrine plus dobutamine versus epinephrine alone for management of septic shock: A randomised trial. *Lancet*, *370*(9588), 676–684. doi:10.1016/S0140-6736(07)61344-0 PMID:17720019

Argenziano, M., Choudhri, A. F., Oz, M. C., Rose, E. A., Smith, C. R., & Landry, D. W. (1997). A prospective randomized trial of arginine vasopressin in the treatment of vasodilatory shock after left ventricular assist device placement. *Circulation*, *96*(9suppl), II-286–II-290. PMID:9386112

Aviado, D. M. Jr, & Schmidt, C. F. (1957). Effects of sympathomimetic drugs on pulmonary circulation: With special reference to a new pulmonary vasodilator. *The Journal of Pharmacology and Experimental Therapeutics*, *120*(4), 512–527. PMID:13476376

Baim, D. S. (1989). Effect of phosphodiesterase inhibition on myocardial oxygen consumption and coronary blood flow. *The American Journal of Cardiology*, *63*(2), 23A–26A. doi:10.1016/0002-9149(89)90388-3 PMID:2521267

Bardy, G. H., Lee, K. L., Mark, D. B., Poole, J. E., Packer, D. L., Boineau, R., & Ip, J. H. et al. (2005). Amiodarone or an implantable cardioverter-defibrillator for congestive heart failure. *The New England Journal of Medicine*, *352*(3), 225–237. doi:10.1056/NEJMoa043399 PMID:15659722

Bellomo, R., Chapman, M., Finfer, S., Hickling, K., & Myburgh, J. (2000). Low-dose dopamine in patients with early renal dysfunction: A placebo-controlled randomised trial. Australian and New Zealand Intensive Care Society (ANZICS) Clinical Trials Group. *Lancet*, *356*(9248), 2139–2143. doi:10.1016/S0140-6736(00)03495-4 PMID:11191541

Bergh, C. H., Andersson, B., Dahlström, U., Forfang, K., Kivikko, M., Sarapohja, T., & Wikström, G. et al. (2010). Intravenous levosimendan vs. dobutamine in acute decompensated heart failure patients on beta-blockers. *European Journal of Heart Failure*, *12*(4), 404–410. doi:10.1093/eurjhf/hfq032 PMID:20335355

Bokhari, F., Newman, D., Greene, M., Korley, V., Mangat, I., & Dorian, P. (2004). Long-term comparison of the implantable cardioverter defibrillator versus amiodarone: Eleven year follow-up of a subset of patients in the Canadian Implantable Defibrillator Study (CIDS). *Circulation*, *110*(2), 112–116. doi:10.1161/01.CIR.0000134957.51747.6E PMID:15238454

Bristow, M. R., Shakar, S. F., Linseman, J. V., & Lowes, B. D. (2001). Inotropes and β-blockers: Is there a need for new guidelines? *Journal of Cardiac Failure*, *7*(2Suppl 1), 8–12. doi:10.1054/jcaf.2001.26655 PMID:11605160

Butterworth, J. F. IV, Prielipp, R. C., Royster, R. L., Spray, B. J., Kon, N. D., Wallenhaupt, S. L., & Zaloga, G. P. (1992). Dobutamine increases heart rate more than epinephrine in patients recovering from aortocoronary bypass surgery. *Journal of Cardiothoracic and Vascular Anesthesia*, *6*(5), 535–541. doi:10.1016/1053-0770(92)90095-O PMID:1421064

Chen, H. H., Anstrom, K. J., Givertz, M. M., Stevenson, L. W., Semigran, M. J., Goldsmith, S. R., & Redfield, M. M. et al. (2013). Low-dose dopamine or low-dose nesiritide in acute heart failure with renal dysfunction: The ROSE acute heart failure randomized trial. *Journal of the American Medical Association*, *310*(23), 2533–2543. doi:10.1001/jama.2013.282190 PMID:24247300

Colucci, W. S., Wright, R. F., Jaski, B. E., Fifer, M. A., & Braunwald, E. (1986). Milrinone and dobutamine in severe heart failure: Differing hemodynamic effects and individual patient responsiveness. *Circulation*, *73*(3 Pt 2), III175–III183. PMID:3510774

Cuffe, M.S., Califf, R.M., Adams, K.F. Jr, Benza, R., Bourge, R., & Colucci, W.S., … Outcomes of a Prospective Trial of Intravenous Milrinone for Exacerbations of Chronic Heart Failure (OPTIME-CHF) Investigators. (2002). Outcomes of a Prospective Trial of Intravenous Milrinone for Exacerbations of Chronic Heart Failure I. Short-term intravenous milrinone for acute exacerbation of chronic heart failure: A randomized controlled trial. *Journal of the American Medical Association*, *287*(12), 1541–1547. doi:10.1001/jama.287.12.1541 PMID:11911756

Day, N. P., Phu, N. H., Bethell, D. P., Mai, N. T., Chau, T. T., Hien, T. T., & White, N. J. (1996). The effects of dopamine and adrenaline infusions on acid-base balance and systemic haemodynamics in severe infection. *Lancet*, *348*(9022), 219–223. doi:10.1016/S0140-6736(96)09096-4 PMID:8684198

De Backer, D., Aldecoa, C., Njimi, H., & Vincent, J. L. (2012). Dopamine versus norepinephrine in the treatment of septic shock: A meta-analysis*. *Critical Care Medicine*, *40*(3), 725–730. doi:10.1097/CCM.0b013e31823778ee PMID:22036860

De Backer, D., Biston, P., Devriendt, J., Madl, C., Chochrad, D., Aldecoa, C., & Vincent, J.-L. et al. (2010). Comparison of dopamine and norepinephrine in the treatment of shock. *The New England Journal of Medicine*, *362*(9), 779–789. doi:10.1056/NEJMoa0907118 PMID:20200382

Dellinger, R. P., Levy, M. M., Rhodes, A., Annane, D., Gerlach, H., Opal, S. M., & Moreno, R. et al. (2013). Surviving sepsis campaign: international guidelines for management of severe sepsis and septic shock: 2012. *Critical Care Medicine*, *41*(2), 580–637. doi:10.1097/CCM.0b013e31827e83af PMID:23353941

Dorian, P., Cass, D., Schwartz, B., Cooper, R., Gelaznikas, R., & Barr, A. (2002). Amiodarone as compared with lidocaine for shock-resistant ventricular fibrillation. *The New England Journal of Medicine*, *346*(12), 884–890. doi:10.1056/NEJMoa013029 PMID:11907287

Erdei, N., Papp, Z., Pollesello, P., Edes, I., & Bagi, Z. (2006). The levosimendan metabolite OR-1896 elicits vasodilation by activating the K(ATP) and BK(Ca) channels in rat isolated arterioles. *British Journal of Pharmacology*, *148*(5), 696–702. doi:10.1038/sj.bjp.0706781 PMID:16715115

Fellahi, J. L., Parienti, J. J., Hanouz, J. L., Plaud, B., Riou, B., & Ouattara, A. (2008). Perioperative use of dobutamine in cardiac surgery and adverse cardiac outcome: Propensity-adjusted analyses. *Anesthesiology*, *108*(6), 979–987. doi:10.1097/ALN.0b013e318173026f PMID:18497597

Fleming, G. A., Murray, K. T., Yu, C., Byrne, J. G., Greelish, J. P., Petracek, M. R., & Pretorius, M. et al. (2008). Milrinone use is associated with postoperative atrial fibrillation after cardiac surgery. *Circulation*, *118*(16), 1619–1625. doi:10.1161/CIRCULATIONAHA.108.790162 PMID:18824641

Fowler, M. B., Alderman, E. L., Oesterle, S. N., Derby, G., Daughters, G. T., Stinson, E. B., & Miller, D. C. et al. (1984). Dobutamine and dopamine after cardiac surgery: Greater augmentation of myocardial blood flow with dobutamine. *Circulation*, *70*(3 Pt 2), I103–I111. PMID:6744557

Francis, G. S., Bartos, J. A., & Adatya, S. (2014). Inotropes. *Journal of the American College of Cardiology*, *63*(20), 2069–2078. doi:10.1016/j.jacc.2014.01.016 PMID:24530672

Frendl, G., Sodickson, A.C., Chung, M.K., Waldo, A.L., Gersh, B.J., & Tisdale, J.E., …American Association for Thoracic Surgery. (2014). (2014). AATS guidelines for the prevention and management of perioperative atrial fibrillation and flutter for thoracic surgical procedures. *The Journal of Thoracic and Cardiovascular Surgery*, *148*(3), e153–e193.

Harrison, D. C., & Collinsworth, K. A. (1974). Antiarrhythmic actions of lidocaine. *Annual Review of Medicine*, *25*(1), 143–148. doi:10.1146/annurev.me.25.020174.001043 PMID:4596228

Harrison, R. W., Hasselblad, V., Mehta, R. H., Levin, R., Harrington, R. A., & Alexander, J. H. (2013). Effect of levosimendan on survival and adverse events after cardiac surgery: A meta-analysis. *Journal of Cardiovascular and Vascular Anesthesia*, *27*(6), 1224–1232. doi:10.1053/j.jvca.2013.03.027 PMID:24050857

Hollenberg, S. M. (2011). Vasoactive Drugs in Circulatory Shock. *American Journal of Respiratory and Critical Care Medicine*, *183*(7), 847–855. doi:10.1164/rccm.201006-0972CI PMID:21097695

Holmes, C. L., Patel, B. M., Russell, J. A., & Walley, K. R. (2001). Physiology of vasopressin relevant to management of septic shock. *Chest*, *120*(3), 989–1002. doi:10.1378/chest.120.3.989 PMID:11555538

Hoogenberg, K., Smit, A. J., & Girbes, A. R. (1998). Effects of low-dose dopamine on renal and systemic hemodynamics during incremental norepinephrine infusion in healthy volunteers. *Critical Care Medicine*, *26*(2), 260–265. doi:10.1097/00003246-199802000-00022 PMID:9468162

Jennings, D. L., & Thompson, M. L. (2009). Use of combination therapy with a beta-blocker and milrinone in patients with advanced heart failure. *The Annals of Pharmacotherapy*, *43*(11), 1872–1876. doi:10.1345/aph.1M357 PMID:19789358

Kivikko, M., Antila, S., Eha, J., Lehtonen, L., & Pentikäinen, P. J. (2002). Pharmacodynamics and safety of a new calcium sensitizer, levosimendan, and its metabolites during an extended infusion in patients with severe heart failure. *Journal of Clinical Pharmacology*, *42*(1), 43–51. doi:10.1177/0091270002042001005 PMID:11808823

Lafuente-Lafuente, C., Longas-Tejero, M. A., Bergman, J. F., & Belmin, J. (2012). Antiarrhythmics for maintaining sinus rhythm after cardioversion of atrial fibrillation. *Cochrane Database of Systematic Reviews*, *5*, CD005049. PMID:22592700

Levy, B., Bollaert, P. E., Charpentier, C., Nace, L., Audibert, G., Bauer, P., & Larcan, A. et al. (1997). Comparison of norepinephrine and dobutamine to epinephrine for hemodynamics, lactate metabolism, and gastric tonometric variables in septic shock: A prospective, randomized study. *Intensive Care Medicine*, *23*(3), 282–287. doi:10.1007/s001340050329 PMID:9083230

Li, H. T., Long, C. S., Rokosh, D. G., Honbo, N. Y., & Karliner, J. S. (1995). Chronic hypoxia differentially regulates alpha 1-adrenergic receptor subtype mRNAs and inhibits alpha 1-adrenergic receptor-stimulated cardiac hypertrophy and signaling. *Circulation*, *92*(4), 918–925. doi:10.1161/01.CIR.92.4.918 PMID:7641375

Maharaj, R., & Metaxa, V. (2011). Levosimendan and mortality after coronary revascularisation: A meta-analysis of randomised controlled trials. *Critical Care (London, England)*, *15*(3), R140. doi:10.1186/cc10263 PMID:21651806

Majure, D. T., Greco, T., Greco, M., Ponschab, M., Biondi-Zoccai, G., Zangrillo, A., & Landoni, G. (2013). Meta-analysis of randomized trials of effect of milrinone on mortality in cardiac surgery: An update. *Journal of Cardiothoracic and Vascular Anesthesia*, *27*(2), 220–229. doi:10.1053/j.jvca.2012.08.005 PMID:23063100

Martinez, E.A., Bass, E.B., & Zimetbaum, P., & American College of Chest Physicians. (2005b). Pharmacologic control of rhythm: American College of Chest Physicians guidelines for the prevention and management of postoperative atrial fibrillation after cardiac surgery. *Chest*, *128*(2Suppl), 48S–55S.

Martinez, E. A., Epstein, A. E., & Bass, E. B. (2005a). Pharmacologic control of ventricular rate: American College of Chest Physicians guidelines for the prevention and management of postoperative atrial fibrillation after cardiac surgery. *Chest*, *128*(2Suppl), 56S–60S. doi:10.1378/chest.128.2_suppl.56S PMID:16167666

McMurray, J. J., Adamopoulos, S., Anker, S. D., Auricchio, A., Böhm, M., Dickstein, K., & Ponikowski, P. et al. (2012). ESC guidelines for the diagnosis and treatment of acute and chronic heart failure 2012: The Task Force for the Diagnosis and Treatment of Acute and Chronic Heart Failure 2012 of the European Society of Cardiology. Developed in collaboration with the Heart Failure Association (HFA) of the ESC. *European Heart Journal*, *33*(14), 1787–1847. doi:10.1093/eurheartj/ehs104 PMID:22611136

Mebazaa, A., Nieminen, M. S., Packer, M., Cohen-Solal, A., Kleber, F. X., Pocock, S. J., & SURVIVE Investigators, et al.. (2007). Levosimendan vs dobutamine for patients with acute decompensated heart failure: The SURVIVE randomized trial. *Journal of the American Medical Association*, *297*(17), 1883–1891. doi:10.1001/jama.297.17.1883 PMID:17473298

Mitchell, L. B., Exner, D. V., Wyse, D. G., Connolly, C. J., Prystai, G. D., Bayes, A. J., & Maitland, A. et al. (2005). Prophylactic oral amiodarone for the prevention of arrhythmias that begin early after revascularization, valve replacement or repair: PAPABEAR: a randomized controlled trial. *Journal of the American Medical Association*, *294*(24), 3093–3100. doi:10.1001/jama.294.24.3093 PMID:16380589

Mitchell, L. B., Exner, D. V., Wyse, D. G., Connolly, C. J., Prystai, G. D., Bayes, A. J., & Maitland, A. et al. (2005). Prophylactic oral amiodarone for the prevention of arrhythmias that begin early after revascularization, valve replacement or repair: PAPABEAR: a randomized controlled trial. *Journal of the American Medical Association*, *294*(24), 3093–3100. doi:10.1001/jama.294.24.3093 PMID:16380589

Modest, V. E., & Butterworth, J. F. IV. (1995). Effect of pH and lidocaine on beta adrenergic receptor binding: Interaction during resuscitation? *Chest*, *108*(5), 1373–1379. doi:10.1378/chest.108.5.1373 PMID:7587445

Morales, D. L., Gregg, D., Helman, D. N., Williams, M. R., Naka, Y., Landry, D. W., & Oz, M. C. (2000). Arginine vasopressin in the treatment of 50 patients with postcardiotomy vasodilatory shock. *The Annals of Thoracic Surgery*, *69*(1), 102–106. doi:10.1016/S0003-4975(99)01197-2 PMID:10654495

Nielsen, D. V., Hansen, M. K., Johnsen, S. P., Hansen, M., Hindsholm, K., & Jakobsen, C. J. (2014). Health outcomes with and without use of inotropic therapy in cardiac surgery: Results of a propensity score-matched analysis. *Anesthesiology*, *120*(5), 1098–1108. doi:10.1097/ALN.0000000000000224 PMID:24614322

Nieminen, M. S., Akkila, J., Hasenfuss, G., Kleber, F. X., Lehtonen, L. A., Mitrovic, V., & Remme, W. J. et al. (2000). Hemodynamic and neurohumoral effects of continuous infusion of levosimendan in patients with congestive heart failure. *Journal of the American College of Cardiology*, *36*(6), 1903–1912. doi:10.1016/S0735-1097(00)00961-X PMID:11092663

Overgaard, C. B., & Dzavik, V. (2008). Inotropes and Vasopressors. *Circulation*, *118*(10), 1047–1056. doi:10.1161/CIRCULATIONAHA.107.728840 PMID:18765387

Packer, M., Colucci, W., Fisher, L., Massie, B. M., Teerlink, J. R., Young, J., & Sarapohja, T. et al. (2013). Effect of levosimendan on the short-term clinical course of patients with acutel decompensated heart failure. *Journal of American College Cardiology Heart Failure*, *1*(2), 103–111. doi:10.1016/j.jchf.2012.12.004 PMID:24621834

Roy, D., Talajic, M., Dorian, P., Connolly, S., Eisenberg, M. J., Green, M., & Thibault, B. et al. (2000). Amiodarone to prevent recurrence of atrial fibrillation. Canadian Trial of Atrial Fibrillation Investigators. *The New England Journal of Medicine*, *342*(13), 913–920. doi:10.1056/NEJM200003303421302 PMID:10738049

Ruffolo, R. R. Jr. (1987). The pharmacology of dobutamine. *The American Journal of the Medical Sciences*, *294*(4), 244–248. doi:10.1097/00000441-198710000-00005 PMID:3310640

Russell, J. A., Walley, K. R., Singer, J., Gordon, A. C., Hébert, P. C., Cooper, D. J., & Ayers, D. et al. (2008). Vasopressin versus norepinephrine infusion in patients with septic shock. *The New England Journal of Medicine*, *358*(9), 877–887. doi:10.1056/NEJMoa067373 PMID:18305265

Singh, B. N., Singh, S. N., Reda, D. J., Tang, X. C., Lopez, B., Harris, C. L., & Ezekowitz, M. D. et al. (2005). Amiodarone versus sotalol for atrial fibrillation. *The New England Journal of Medicine*, *352*(18), 1861–1872. doi:10.1056/NEJMoa041705 PMID:15872201

Sonnenblick, E. H., Frishman, W. H., & LeJemtel, T. H. (1979). Dobutamine: A new synthetic cardioactive sympathetic amine. *The New England Journal of Medicine*, *300*(1), 17–22. doi:10.1056/NEJM197901043000105 PMID:362214

St André, A. C., & DelRossi, A. (2005). Hemodynamic management of patients in the first 24 hours after cardiac surgery. *Critical Care Medicine*, *33*(9), 2082–2093. doi:10.1097/01.CCM.0000178355.96817.81 PMID:16148484

Stinson, E. B., Caves, P. K., Griepp, R. B., Oyer, P. E., Rider, A. K., & Shumway, N. E. (1975). Hemodynamic observations in the early period after human heart transplantation. *The Journal of Thoracic and Cardiovascular Surgery*, *69*(2), 264–270. PMID:1089847

Tayama, E., Ueda, T., Shojima, T., Akasu, K., Oda, T., Fukunaga, S., & Aoyagi, S. et al. (2007). Arginine vasopressin is an ideal drug after cardiac surgery for the management of low systemic vascular resistant hypotension concomitant with pulmonary hypertension. *Interactive Cardiovascular and Thoracic Surgery*, *6*(6), 715–719. doi:10.1510/icvts.2007.159624 PMID:17704123

Unverferth, D. A., Blanford, M., Kates, R. E., & Leier, C. V. (1980). Tolerance to dobutamine after a 72 hour continuous infusion. *The American Journal of Medicine*, *69*(2), 262–266. doi:10.1016/0002-9343(80)90387-3 PMID:7405947

Vida, V. L., Mack, R., & Castaneda, A. R. (2005). The role of vasopressin in treating systemic inflammatory syndrome complicated by right ventricular failure. *Cardiology in the Young*, *15*(1), 88–90. doi:10.1017/S1047951105000193 PMID:15831170

Williams, J. B., Hernandez, A. F., Li, S., Dokholyan, R. S., O'Brien, S. M., Smith, P. K., & Peterson, E. D. et al. (2011). Postoperative inotrope and vasopressor use following CABG: Outcome data from the CAPS-care study. *Journal of Cardiac Surgery*, *26*(6), 572–578. doi:10.1111/j.1540-8191.2011.01301.x PMID:21951076

Woolsey, C. A., & Coopersmith, C. M. (2006). Vasoactive drugs and the gut: Is there anything new*? Current Opinion in Critical Care*, *12*(2), 155–159. doi:10.1097/01.ccx.0000216584.72427.e4 PMID:16543793

Wyse, D. G., Waldo, A. L., DiMarco, J. P., Domanski, M. J., Rosenberg, Y., & Schron, E. B. (2002). A Comparison of Rate Control and Rhythm Control in Patients with Atrial Fibrillation. *The New England Journal of Medicine*, *347*(23), 1825–1833. doi:10.1056/NEJMoa021328 PMID:12466506

Yancy, C.W., Jessup, M., Bozkurt, B., Butler, J., Casey, D.E. Jr, & Drazner, M.H., … American College of Cardiology Foundation; American Heart Association Task Force on Practice Guidelines. (2013). ACCF/AHA guideline for the management of heart failure: A report of the American College of Cardiology Foundation/American Heart Association Task Force on Practice Guidelines. *Journal of the American College of Cardiology*, *62*(16), e147–e239. doi:10.1016/j.jacc.2013.05.019 PMID:23747642

Zimetbaum, P. (2007). Amiodarone for atrial fibrillation. *The New England Journal of Medicine*, *356*(9), 935–941. doi:10.1056/NEJMct065916 PMID:17329700

ADDITIONAL READING

Annane, D., Vignon, P., Renault, A., Bollaert, P., Charpentier, C., Martin, C., & Bellissant, E. et al. (2007). Norepinephrine plus dobutamine versus epinephrine alone for management of septic shock: A randomised trial. *Lancet*, *370*(9588), 676–684. doi:10.1016/S0140-6736(07)61344-0 PMID:17720019

Francis, G. S., Bartos, J. A., & Adatya, S. (2014). Inotropes. *Journal of the American College of Cardiology*, *63*(20), 2069–2078. doi:10.1016/j.jacc.2014.01.016 PMID:24530672

Harrison, R. W., Hasselblad, V., Mehta, R. H., Levin, R., Harrington, R. A., & Alexander, J. H. (2013). Effect of levosimendan on survival and adverse events after cardiac surgery: A meta-analysis. *J Cardiovascular and Vascular Anesthesia*, *27*(6), 1224–1232. doi:10.1053/j.jvca.2013.03.027 PMID:24050857

Hollenberg, S. M. (2011). Vasoactive Drugs in Circulatory Shock. *American Journal of Respiratory and Critical Care Medicine*, *183*(7), 847–855. doi:10.1164/rccm.201006-0972CI PMID:21097695

Martinez, E. A., Epstein, A. E., & Bass, E. B. (2005a). Pharmacologic control of ventricular rate: American College of Chest Physicians guidelines for the prevention and management of postoperative atrial fibrillation after cardiac surgery. *Chest*, *128*(2Suppl), 56S–60S. doi:10.1378/chest.128.2_suppl.56S PMID:16167666

Nielsen, D. V., Hansen, M. K., Johnsen, S. P., Hansen, M., Hindsholm, K., & Jakobsen, C. J. (2014). Health outcomes with and without use of inotropic therapy in cardiac surgery: Results of a propensity score-matched analysis. *Anesthesiology*, *120*(5), 1098–1108. doi:10.1097/ALN.0000000000000224 PMID:24614322

Russell, J. A., Walley, K. R., Singer, J., Gordon, A. C., Hébert, P. C., Cooper, D. J., & Ayers, D. et al. (2008). Vasopressin versus norepinephrine infusion in patients with septic shock. *The New England Journal of Medicine*, *358*(9), 877–887. doi:10.1056/NEJMoa067373 PMID:18305265

Wyse, D. G., Waldo, A. L., DiMarco, J. P., Domanski, M. J., Rosenberg, Y., & Schron, E. B. (2002). A Comparison of Rate Control and Rhythm Control in Patients with Atrial Fibrillation. *The New England Journal of Medicine*, *347*(23), 1825–1833. doi:10.1056/NEJMoa021328 PMID:12466506

Chapter 11
Anticoagulation Options

Michael Mazzeffi
University of Maryland, USA

Ashleigh Lowery
University of Maryland, USA

ABSTRACT

There are multiple indications for anticoagulation in the cardiac surgery intensive care unit including cardiac valve replacement, mechanical circulatory pumps (ECMO and ventricular assist devices), deep vein thrombosis prophylaxis, treatment of heparin-induced thrombocytopenia, and treatment of other thrombotic conditions including pulmonary embolism. Anticoagulant medications broadly fall into two categories: antiplatelet drugs and inhibitors of protein clotting factors. In this chapter we will review anticoagulant medications, therapeutic drug monitoring, common indications for anticoagulation, and the risks associated with anticoagulation after cardiac surgery.

INTRODUCTION

Human blood has the remarkable ability to transform from its normal fluid state to a semi-solid state known as clot. Over thousands of years, evolution selected for this highly specialized mechanism, which limits blood loss during injury and leads to wound healing. In a simplified paradigm coagulation can be thought of as primary and secondary. Primary coagulation occurs when a platelet plug adheres to a site of endothelial injury and secondary coagulation occurs when blood proteins solidify the plug creating a clot.

Although coagulation is a highly adaptive mechanism, it can also be pathologic. For example clots in coronary arteries, pulmonary arteries, or cerebral arteries can lead to permanent organ injury or death. Virchow described the classic triad for clot formation as: endothelial injury, changes in blood flow (stasis), and hypercoagulability. Because cardiac surgery often requires implantation of artificial surfaces (cardiac valves, graft material etc.) patients are at risk for pathologic clotting. Cardiac surgery also leads to disruption of the normal endothelium, stasis (due to immobility), and altered levels of common coagulant and anticoagulant factors.

DOI: 10.4018/978-1-4666-8603-8.ch011

This chapter will review anticoagulant drugs that are commonly used in the cardiac surgery intensive care unit, therapeutic monitoring for these drugs, indications for anticoagulation, and the risks associated with anticoagulation after cardiac surgery.

Background

Anticoagulation management is a frequent issue in cardiac surgery critical care. There are a bevy of drugs available to today's intensive care unit (ICU) practitioner allowing for maximal benefit and minimal risk when an anticoagulant is properly selected, dosed, and monitored. Available drugs work through different pathways, have different pharmacokinetic profiles, and have different routes of administration making them best suited for particular clinical scenarios. They also carry different levels of risk depending on a patient's hepatic and renal function. For these reasons, ICU practitioners must be facile in managing the various anticoagulant medications that are available.

Anti-platelet drugs are used frequently in the cardiac surgery ICU, particularly in patients who have had coronary artery bypass graft (CABG) surgery, aortic replacement surgery, or bioprosthetic cardiac valve replacement. Almost all of these patients require aspirin and select patients receive dual anti-platelet therapy, typically with a thienopyridine drug.

Drugs that inhibit protein coagulation factors are also used in the cardiac surgery ICU for mechanical valve replacement, mechanical circulatory support devices or ECMO, prolonged atrial fibrillation in high-risk patients, heparin induced thrombocytopenia (HIT), pulmonary embolism, and certain bioprosthetic valves. Recently novel oral anticoagulant drugs have become available which will likely change future anticoagulation practices (eg: apixiban, dabigatran, and rivaroxaban).

STATE OF THE ART APPROACHES

Anti-Platelet Drugs

Aspirin

Acetylsalicylic acid is an analgesic, anti-inflammatory, and anti-platelet drug that was first isolated from the bark of willow trees. The German pharmaceutical company Bayer began synthesizing the drug aspirin in the late 1800s. Since that time it has remained one of the most important and widely used drugs in medicine. Aspirin is a non-steroidal anti-inflammatory drug (NSAID) that irreversibly inhibits the enzyme cyclo-oxygenase (COX). COX has two isoforms COX-1 and COX-2 and aspirin is 170 times more potent at inhibiting COX-1 (Vane, Bakhle & Botting, 1998). The downstream effect of COX inhibition is decreased production of thromboxane A2, which leads to decreased platelet aggregation. Aspirin may also inhibit platelets through other mechanisms including inhibition of neutrophil-related platelet activation (Bolz & Pohl, 1997). The dose necessary for platelet inhibition in a given individual is debatable and it has been suggested that some patients are "aspirin resistant". In one study, doses as small as 37.5 mg per day decreased thromboxane A2 production by 98% 2-6 hours after the first dose (Perneby,

Wallen, Rooney, Fitzgerald & Hjemdahi, 2006). Aspirin is absorbed quickly in the upper gastrointestinal tract and platelets are affected as early as the portal circulation (Penderson & Fitzgerald, 1984). The plasma half-life of aspirin is approximately 20 minutes, but its effects are much longer because COX inhibition is irreversible. This essentially means that aspirin's effects last for the duration of the platelet lifespan or 7-10 days (Awtry & Loscalzo, 2000). When aspirin use is stopped platelet activity recovers approximately 10% per day as new platelets enter the circulation (Burch, Stanford & Majerus, 1979). The most common dosing regiments for platelet inhibition are 81 mg per day or 325 mg per day. Even with an 81 mg dose, the level of platelet inhibition is high and resistance is low and differences in measured platelet inhibition depend upon the assay and agonist used (Grubel, et al., 2007). One study suggested that the level of platelet inhibition from these doses is sex dependent with woman having greater residual platelet function for any given dose of aspirin (Qayyum, 2008).

Thienopyridines (Clopidogrel, Prasugrel, Ticagrelor)

Clopidogrel

Clopidogrel is a pro-drug whose active metabolite inhibits ADP-induced platelet aggregation by blocking the P2Y12 receptor. When added to aspirin, it has been shown to reduce mortality in acute coronary syndromes (Yusuf, et al., 2001)(Mehta, et al., 2001). It can also be used in place of aspirin for patients who have an aspirin allergy. Following an oral loading dose of 300 to 600 mg, maximum platelet inhibition occurs after 2-4 hours. The maintenance dose is then 75 mg per day. Without a loading dose, the time to peak platelet inhibition is 5-7 days (Hebert, et al., 1993).

Clopidogrel should be discontinued at least 5 days before elective surgery to ensure return of normal platelet function. Metabolism occurs primarily through the CYP2C19 hepatic enzyme system. Patients who are "poor-metabolizers" or have a "clopidogrel resistant" genotype may have a decreased response to clopidogrel because of a lower conversion of the pro-drug to its active form. For these reasons, the American College of Cardiology and American Heart Association recommend genotype testing in patients who are at moderate to high risk for adverse cardiovascular events (Holmes, et al., 2010).

Prasugrel

Prasugrel also inhibits the P2Y12 ADP receptor; however; compared to clopidogrel it reaches maximum platelet inhibition faster (30 minutes after a loading dose). It also has a higher percentage of maximum platelet inhibition compared to clopidogrel (80-85% vs 40-60%). Platelet aggregation returns to baseline 5-9 days after discontinuation and it is recommended to hold therapy for at least 7 days prior to elective cardiac surgery.

The oral loading dose of prasugrel is 60 mg followed by a daily maintenance dose of 10 mg per day. Prasugrel undergoes metabolism by esterase-mediated hydrolysis and CYP3A4 and CYP2B6 oxidation in the liver. The TRITON-TIMI 36 trial studied prasugrel compared to clopidogrel in patients with myocardial infarction and found net harm with prasugrel in patients with a history of transient ischemic attack or stroke (Wivott, et al., 2007). For STEMI patients, it was associated with a reduction in ischemic endpoints and a sustained mortality benefit. It was also associated with more CABG-related bleeding (Serebruany, 2010). When used in acute coronary syndromes, it is not recommended if future CABG is likely because of the increased bleeding risk.

Ticagrelor

Ticagrelor is a cyclopentyl-traizolopyrimidine drug that reversibly inhibits the P2Y12 receptor. It is not a prodrug and does not require metabolism for activation. It reaches maximum platelet inhibition 2 hours after a loading dose and achieves >90% inhibition of platelet aggregation, the highest of the thienopyridine drugs.

It is recommended to be held for 5 days prior to elective surgery. Recovery of platelet function is faster than with clopidogrel or prasugrel because its inhibition of the P2Y12 receptor is reversible. The dose of ticagrelor is a 180 mg oral loading dose followed by 90 mg twice per day. Ticagrelor is a CYP3A4 substrate and inhibitor so concurrent use of inhibitors or inducers should be avoided. It is also a weak inhibitor and substrate of P-glycoprotein. It primarily undergoes biliary excretion, but is also eliminated renally. Unfortunately, its use has not been evaluated in patients receiving intermittent hemodialysis or continuous renal replacement therapy.

The PLATO study compared ticagrelor to clopidogrel in acute coronary syndrome patients and found decreased vascular death, myocardial infarction, or stroke in patients receiving ticagrelor. There was an increase in non-CABG related bleeding, but no difference in CABG-related bleeding (Wallentin, et. al., 2009). Of note, the results favored ticagrelor in patients receiving an aspirin dose ≤100 mg. Therefore, an aspirin maintenance dose of 81 mg per day, rather than 325 mg per day, should be prescribed with ticagrelor.

Warfarin

Warfarin is named for the Wisconsin Alumni Research Foundation. The drug was discovered at the University of Wisconsin in the 1920s when spoiled sweet clover plants caused hemorrhagic deaths in cattle. Initially, it was used as a rat poison, but it is now the most commonly used oral anticoagulant in the world. Warfarin is a vitamin K antagonist that works by inhibiting the reduction of vitamin K to its active form. Structurally it is similar to vitamin K and it competes with it for Vitamin K reductase. This inhibits the production of vitamin K dependent clotting factors including factors: II, VII, IX, X, and proteins C and S.

It typically takes 3 to 5 days to achieve warfarin's full anticoagulant effects because of the differing half-lives of the various Vitamin K dependent factors. Dosing is individualized and based on several patient-specific factors including: age, nutritional status, concurrent medications, and hepatic function. Doses usually range from 2 to 10 mg per day and are adjusted based on the INR.

Warfarin is hepatically metabolized and is a major substrate of the CYP1A2 and CYP2C9 enzyme systems, which leads to important drug-drug interactions that may affect therapeutic response and require dose adjustments. Response is also altered by the vitamin K content of a patient's diet. Several genetic factors may increase patient sensitivity to warfarin, however the American College of Chest Physicians does not recommend routine pharmacogenomic testing (Guyatt, Akl, Crowther, Gutterman, & Schuunemann, 2012). The half-life of warfarin is highly variable and ranges from 20-60 hours. Warfarin is commonly used as a long-term anticoagulant in patients with mechanical heart valves. Table 1 shows the recommended INR based upon the type of valve.

Table 1. Target INR based upon type of heart valve (Stein et al., 2001)

Indication	*Target INR Range*
Mechanical aortic valve	2-3
Bileaflet or tilting disk mechanical mitral valve	2.5-3.5
Caged ball or caged disk mechanical mitral valve	2.5-3.5
Mechanical valves in both the aortic and mitral positions	2.5-3.5
Bioprosthetic mitral valve	2-3

Heparins (Unfractionated, Low-Molecular Weight Heparin, Fondaparinux)

Unfractionated Heparin

Heparin was discovered in 1916 by a Johns Hopkins University medical student (McLean, 1959). Today it is widely used as an anticoagulant for thrombotic diseases as well as anticoagulation for extracorporeal circulation including cardiopulmonary bypass. Its anticoagulant effects are dependent upon the enzyme antithrombin III, a critical endogenous anticoagulant. Unfractionated heparin contains heparin molecules of various sizes ranging from 3K to 30K daltons. Both bovine and porcine preparations have been used clinically. In order for heparin molecules to exert their anti-Xa activity a specific pentasaccharide unit must bind to antithrombin III (Bjork & Lindahal, 1982). Unfractionated heparin's anti-IIa activity occurs through a separate mechanism that is size dependent with larger molecules having greater anti-IIa activity. When large heparin molecules, anti-thrombin III, and factor IIa form a complex, factor IIa is rapidly inactivated. Ultimately, this leads to decreased conversion of fibrinogen to fibrin and a reduction in new clot formation (Hirsh & Levine, 1992). In some cases (including those of prolonged exposure to heparin), patients exhibit heparin resistance due to antithrombin III deficiency and this is manifested by an antithrombin III level of less than 80%.

Unfractionated heparin's action occurs immediately after intravenous administration and its elimination half-life is approximately 30-150 minutes. At low doses it is eliminated rapidly by non-renal mechanisms, but at high doses renal elimination appears to play a more significant role. Nevertheless, dose adjustment is unnecessary for patients with renal impairment (Hirsh, et. al., 2008).

Depending on the indication for anticoagulation and a patient's individual bleeding risk, a bolus dose of heparin may be given when an intravenous infusion is initiated in order to rapidly achieve a therapeutic aPTT. Maintenance infusion rates are weight based ranging from 10-18 units/kg/hour and titrated according to aPTT level or anti-Xa level. An aPTT of approximately 1.5-2.5 times normal or an anti-Xa level of 0.3-0.7 units/mL is considered therapeutic. Control aPTT values vary among hospitals, so target aPTT values will also differ somewhat. The aPTT can be measured every 6 hours until a therapeutic aPTT is achieved. At that point it can be measured less frequently in our experience. A number of dose-adjustment nomograms have been developed, however institution and indication-specific nomograms should be consulted (Cruickshank, Levine, Hirsh, Roberts & Siguenza, 1991)(Flaker, Barolozzi, Davis, McCabe & Cannon, 1994)(Raschke, Reilly, Guidry, Fontana, & Srinivas, 1993).

Low-Molecular Weight Heparin (LMWH)

Low-molecular weight heparins are derived from unfractionated porcine heparin that is benzylated and depolymerized. The average molecular weight of enoxaparin is 4.5K daltons, compared to an average of 16K daltons for unfractionated heparin. Low molecular weight heparin increases antithrombin III's activity against factor Xa, however it has little to no activity against factor IIa (Hirsh & Levine, 1992).

Low-molecular weight heparins are administered subcutaneously and have more predictable effects and a longer elimination half-life than unfractionated heparin. For treatment of thromboembolism, enoxaparin is typically dosed 1 mg/kg twice daily, or 1.5 mg/kg once daily. Anti-Xa activity can be measured in order to monitor the dose efficacy and make adjustments if needed, with a goal of 0.5-1 units/mL when dosing twice daily (Duplaga, Rivers & Nutescu, 2001). The peak effects of enoxaparin are seen 3-4 hours after injection and the half-life ranges from 4.5 to 7 hours. It is metabolized hepatically and eliminated renally, and therefore should be avoided in patients with renal failure or acute kidney injury (Farooq, et. al., 2004). Dose adjustments are typically required when the glomerular filtration rate is below 30 mL/min.

Fondaparinux

Fondaparinux is a synthetic polysaccharide that mimics the critical pentasaccharide sequence involved in increasing antithrombin III's activity against factor Xa. Like low molecular weight heparin, it has no activity against Factor IIa. Because fondaparinux is not derived from heparin and is a relatively small molecule, it can be used for anticoagulation in the setting of heparin induced thrombocytopenia (Blacker, Oertel & Valgus, 2008)(Harenberg, Jorg & Fenyvesi, 2004). Dosing is weight-based and administration is via subcutaneous injection. For treatment of thromboembolism, the dose is 5 mg per day for patients <50 kg, 7.5 mg per day for patients 50-100 kg, and 10 mg per day for patients >100 kg. Absorption is rapid after subcutaneous injection and the half-life is 17 to 21 hours. The half-life is prolonged in renal impairment, so use is not recommended in renal failure. When the glomerular filtration rate falls below 30 mL/min fondaparinux is contraindicated.

Direct Thrombin Inhibitors (Argatroban, Bivalirudin, Lepirudin, Dabigatran)

Argatroban

Argatroban reversibly binds thrombin inhibiting the conversion of fibrinogen to fibrin and feedback activation of factors V, VIII, XIII, and protein C. It also inhibits platelet aggregation through its effects on thrombin. It is administered as an intravenous infusion with a starting dose of 0.2-1 mcg/kg/min, and titrated to a dilute thrombin time or aPTT. We typically treat patients in the cardiac surgery intensive care unit with a starting dose of 0.5 mcg/kg/min and have observed few bleeding complications.

Argatroban is hepatically metabolized and partially eliminated in the urine. Its half-life is 39 to 51 minutes, but can be longer in patients with hepatic impairment. Critically ill patients with multiorgan dysfunction and post-cardiac surgery patients may have reduced drug clearance and a lower starting dose of 0.2 mcg/kg/min is recommended (Beiderlinden, Treschan, Gorlinger & Peters, 2007).

Bivalirudin

Bivalirudin is also a specific and reversible direct thrombin inhibitor. It is administered as an intravenous infusion with a starting dose of 0.03-0.15 mg/kg/hr. A lower starting rate of 0.03 mg/kg/hr is recommended for critically ill patients. Bivalirudin has an immediate onset of action and a half-life of approximately 25 minutes. It undergoes enzymatic metabolism by blood proteases (80%), but is also renally eliminated and may have a prolonged half-life in patients with significant renal impairment. In addition to its use as a treatment for thromboembolism, two multicenter trials (CHOOSE-ON and CHOOSE-OFF) demonstrated its safety and efficacy as an alternative to heparin in patients with heparin induced thrombocytopenia requiring on pump or off pump cardiac surgery (Koster et. al., 2007)(Dyke et. al., 2007). On-pump patients received a 1 mg/kg intravenous bolus followed by continuous infusion of 2.5 mg/kg/hour. A 50 mg bolus was also added to the priming solution of the cardiopulmonary bypass circuit. Off-pump patients received a 0.75 mg/kg bolus and a continuous infusion of 1.75 mg/kg/hour. When emergent reversal of bivalirudin anticoagulant effect is required renal replacement therapy or modified ultrafiltration can be performed.

Lepirudin

Lepirudin was the first direct thrombin inhibitor available. It is derived from hirudin which is an antithrombotic molecule produced by the salivary glands of medicinal leeches. Lepirudin is initiated with an intravenous bolus dose of 0.4 mg/kg followed by a continuous infusion of 0.15 mg/kg/hour. It undergoes renal elimination and therefore its dose should be reduced in patients with renal dysfunction. A recommended regimen for patients with a creatinine clearance less than 60 mL/min is a bolus dose of 0.2 mg/kg followed by an infusion rate of 0.0225-0.075 mg/kg/hour (Linkins, 2012). Its half-life can range from 10 minutes in healthy volunteers to 2 days in patients with marked renal impairment. Patients can also develop anti-hirudin antibodies while on treatment. These antibodies enhance the pharmacologic activity of the drug, and dose reductions may be required. Antibody formation typically does not occur until at least 5 days after starting therapy (Eichler, Friesen, Lubenow, Jaeger & Greinacher, 2000).

Dabigatran

Dabigatran is the first oral direct thrombin inhibitor. In 2010 it became FDA approved as an anticoagulant for non-valvular atrial fibrillation. Dabigatran is a prodrug whose active metabolite is a potent inhibitor of thrombin's active site. Currently, it is only available in a capsule formulation containing tartaric acid pellets, which prohibit its administration in enteral feeding tubes. The dose is 150 mg by mouth twice daily, but is reduced to 75 mg twice daily in patients with a creatinine clearance less than 30 mL/min. Its use is not recommended when creatinine clearance is less than 15 mL/min or in patients with end-stage renal disease. Dabigatran reaches peak plasma concentration 30 minutes to 2 hours after administration and steady state 3 days after initiating therapy. Absorption is delayed by ingestion of a high fat meal. Its half life is 12-17 hours and elimination is primarily renal. Dabigatran is a P-glycoprotein substrate and should be avoided with P-glycoprotein substrate inducers.

The RE-LY study compared dabigatran to warfarin in patients with non-valvular atrial fibrillation and found non-inferiority compared to warfarin. However dabigatran did have higher rates of GI bleeding (Connolly, 2009). The RE-ALIGN study evaluated dabigatran compared to warfarin in patients with mechanical heart valves. The trial was terminated early because of increased thrombosis and bleeding in patients receiving dabigatran. The authors postulate that warfarin may be more effective than dabigatran in preventing valvular thrombosis because it inhibits both the extrinsic and common pathways, whereas dabigatran exclusively inhibits thrombin in the common pathway. Based on the lack of benefit and increased risk demonstrated in this study, dabigatran should not be used for patients with mechanical heart valves (Eikelboom et. al., 2013).

Anti Xa Drugs (Rivaroxaban, Apixiban)

Rivaroxaban

Rivaroxaban is an oral, direct inhibitor of factor Xa. Through inhibition of Xa it decreases the conversion of prothrombin to thrombin and ultimately the conversion of fibrinogen to fibrin decreasing clot formation. For non-valvular atrial fibrillation, the dose of rivaroxaban is 20 mg per day. For patients with a creatinine clearance less than 50 mL/min, the dose is 15 mg per day. Its use is not recommended when creatinine clearance is below 15 mL/min or in patients with end stage renal disease. For venous thromboembolism prophylaxis, the approved dose is 10 mg per day. The time to peak anticoagulant activity is 2 to 4 hours. Rivaroxaban undergoes hydrolysis and CYP3A4 and 3A5 metabolism. It is primarily renally eliminated and its half-life is 5 to 9 hours.

In the ROCKET-AF study, rivaroxaban was non-inferior to warfarin when comparing rates of stroke and systemic embolism in patients with non-valvular atrial fibrillation. Rivaroxaban had less fatal and intracranial hemorrhages, but increased transfusion and gastrointestinal bleeds (Patel et. al., 2011). The ATLAS ACS 2-TIMI-52 studied the addition of rivaroxaban in acute coronary syndromes. This study observed a decrease in death from cardiovascular causes, but increased risk of bleeding in patients receiving rivaroxaban. Based on missing data, the FDA did not approve rivaroxaban for this indication (Mega, 2012). Rivaroxaban has also been studied for the treatment of venous thromboembolism. The EINSTEIN-DVT and EINSTEIN-PE studies both found rivaroxaban non-inferior to warfarin for treatment of deep vein thrombosis and pulmonary embolism (EINSTEIN investigators, 2010)(EINSTEIN-PE, 2012). An ongoing challenge for the new oral anticoagulants is the identification of a safe, rapid reversal strategy as there is not a specific reversal agent that has been validated. Both 3 and 4 factor prothrombin complexes have been used because they contain factor X, but the evidence for their use is limited.

Apixaban

Apixaban is also an orally administered factor Xa inhibitor. The dose for stroke prevention in patients with non-valvular atrial fibrillation is 5 mg twice per day and the dose for venous thromboemboliosm prophylaxis is 2.5 mg twice per day. There is no data for its use when creatinine clearance falls below 30 mL/min or in end stage renal disease. Apixaban reaches peak concentration one hour after oral administration and is metabolized hepatically by CYP3A4 and 3A5, with 27% renal elimination. It is also a P-glycoprotein substrate. It should be avoided with strong P-glycoprotein or CYP3A4 inducers or inhibitors. It has a half-life of 12 hours.

The ARISTOTLE study evaluated apixiaban in comparison to warfarin for patients with nonvalvular atrial fibrillation. The authors found that apixaban was superior to warfarin for the composite outcome of of stroke or systemic embolism (1.27% per year vs. 1.6% per year, HR 0.79), and also found less major and minor bleeding complications compared to warfarin (Granger et. al., 2011). Similar to rivaroxaban, apixaban did not demonstrate clinical benefit in patients with acute coronary syndromes and showed increased major bleeding events in the APPRAISE and APPRAISE-2 trials (APPRAISE, 2009)(APPRAISE-2, 2011). Anticoagulant doses, mechanisms, and pharmacokinetics are summarized in Table 2.

Therapeutic Drug Monitoring

Anti-Platelet Drugs

There are a variety of assays that can quantify platelet inhibition including aggregometry (impedance or light transmission), VerifyNow^R (Accumetrics, SanDiego, CA USA), PFA100 (Siemens USA, Cary, NC USA), and Plateletworks (Helena Labs, Beaumont, TX USA). Both thromboelastography (TEG) (Haemonetics, Braintree, MA USA) and thromboelastometry (ROTEM)(TEM USA, Research Triangle, NC USA) can also monitor platelet inhibition. Platelet mapping is used with TEG and "ROTEM platelet" is used for ROTEM. Despite the availability of these assays, routine anti-platelet drug monitoring has not gained widespread acceptance in clinical practice. The main reason for this is that it does not predict clinical events (Gachet & Aleil, 2008)(Breet et. al., 2010). Nevertheless select high-risk patients may require monitoring and for this reason the more commonly used clinical platelet assays will be described in greater detail.

VerifyNow^R

VerifyNow^R uses whole blood that is added to 4 wells with fibrinogen-activator coated beads. When blood enters the wells it is heated, mixed, and the activator pellets dissolve becoming suspended in the sample. The amount of platelet aggregation is estimated using light transmission through the sample. VerifyNow^R has both P2Y12 specific and aspirin specific tests (VeriftyNow^R PRU and VeriftyNow^R Aspirin). For the VerifyNow^R PRU, values less than 194 are highly specific for P2Y12 inhibition and for the VerifyNow Aspirin, ARU less than 550 indicates therapeutic inhibition. Unfortunately, there are not well-established therapeutic targets for either assay. Patients taking clopidogrel 75 mg per day commonly have PRU values below 250 and those taking aspirin 325 mg per day commonly have ARUs between 300 and 400 (Madsen, Saw, Kristensen, Schmidt & Pittendreigh, 2010).

PFA100

The PFA100 is a platelet function test that examines platelet function under high shear stress. Device membranes contain either collagen and epinephrine (coll-epi) or collagen and ADP (coll-adp) as an activator and the time to close a small aperture in the center is recorded as the closure time (CT). When platelet function is inhibited, the closure time becomes prolonged. Typically coll-epi is used first because it is sensitive to all platelet defects (drug induced and non-drug induced) and if the closure time is less than 180 seconds then platelet function is normal. If the closure time is longer than 180 seconds then the coll-adp assay is used to evaluate for aspirin effect. Coll-adp is relatively resistant to aspirin effect so if the coll-epi is abnormal and the coll-adp is normal (<120 seconds) this likely indicates aspirin effect. Unfortunately, the effects of P2Y12 inhibitors on CT for both assays are somewhat unpredictable.

Table 2. Anticoagulant medications

Medication	*Dose*	*Mechanism*	*Pharmacokinetics*
Antiplatelet drugs			
Aspirin	81-325 mg PO daily	COX inhibition	Metabolism: hepatic conjugation Half-life: 15-20 minutes Excretion: urine
Clopidogrel	Loading dose: 300-600 mg PO Maintenance: 75 mg PO daily	Blocks platelet P2Y12 (ADP) receptor	Metabolism: hepatic via CYP450 to active metabolite Half-life: 6 hours Excretion: urine (50%), feces (46%)
Prasugrel	Loading dose: 60 mg PO Maintenance dose: 10 mg daily	Blocks platelet P2Y12 (ADP) receptor	Metabolism: hepatic via CYP450 to active metabolite Half-life: 2-15 hours Excretion: urine (68%), feces (27%)
Ticagrelor	Loading dose: 180 mg PO Maintenance: 90 mg twice daily	Reversible antagonism of P2Y12 (ADP) receptor	Metabolism: hepatic via CYP450 Half-life: 7-9 hours Excretion: feces (58%), urine (26%)
Inhibitors of protein coagulant factors			
Warfarin	Starting dose 2-5 mg PO daily, adjusted to goal INR	Vitamin K antagonist	Metabolism: hepatic via CYP450 Half-life: 20-60 hours Excretion: urine
Unfractionated heparin	Starting infusion 10-18 units/kg/hour, adjusted to goal aPTT	Increases antithrombin III activity leading to IIa and Xa inhibition	Metabolism: hepatic Half-life: 1-2 hours Excretion: urine
Enoxaparin (LMWH)	1 mg/kg SQ twice daily or 1.5 mg/kg SQ daily	Increases antithrombin III activity leading to primarily Xa inhibition	Metabolism: hepatic Half-life: 17-21 hours (prolonged in renal impairment) Excretion: urine
Fondaparinux	<50 kg: 5 mg SQ daily 50-100 kg: 7.5 mg SQ daily >100 kg: 10 mg SQ daily	Increases antithrombin III-activity leading to selective Xa inhibition	Half-life: 17-21 hours (prolonged in renal impairment) Excretion: urine
Argatroban	Starting infusion 0.2-1 mcg/kg/min, adjusted to goal aPTT or DTT	Direct thrombin inhibitor	Metabolism: hepatic Half-life: 39-51 minutes (prolonged in hepatic impairment) Excretion: feces (65%), urine (22%)
Bivalirudin	Starting infusion 0.03-0.15 mg/kg/hour, adjusted to goal aPTT or DTT	Direct thrombin inhibitor	Metabolism: blood proteases Half-life: 25 minutes (prolonged in renal impairment) Excretion: urine (20%), proteolytic cleavage
Lepirudin	Starting infusion 0.0225-0.15 mg/kg/hour, adjusted to goal aPTT or DTT	Direct thrombin inhibitor	Metabolism: hydrolysis Half-life: 10 minutes (prolonged in renal impairment) Excretion: urine
Dabigatran	150 mg PO twice daily	Direct thrombin inhibitor	Metabolism: hepatic Half-life: 12-17 hours Excretion: urine
Rivaroxaban	10-20 mg PO daily	Factor Xa inhibitor	Metabolism: hepatic via CYP450 Half-life: 5-9 hours Excretion: urine (66%), feces (28%)
Apixaban	2.5-5 mg PO twice daily	Factor Xa inhibitor	Metabolism: hepatic via CYP450 Half-life: 12 hours Excretion: urine, feces

Plateletworks

Plateletworks estimates platelet function by comparing electronic impedance platelet counts in a control sample with a sample that is treated with an activator (collagen or ADP). The tubes containing agonist have a decrease in platelet count that is proportional to the degree of aggregation that occurs. Typically the result is reported as a total platelet count and then a functional count (which is equal to the total platelet count - remaining platelet count). Plateletworks has been shown to have poor discriminative power for detecting aspirin associated platelet inhibition in cardiac surgery patients (Lennon, Gibbs, Weightman, McGuire & Michalopoulos, 2004). Its discriminative power for detecting clopidogrel associated inhibition is slightly better (van Werkum et. al., 2010).

Unfractionated Heparin

There are a number of available assays for monitoring the anticoagulant effects of unfractionated heparin including the activated clotting time (ACT), activated partial thromboplastin time (aPTT), and the anti-Xa activity assay. The ACT has been used since the 1960s to monitor anticoagulation. The test uses a particulate activator of coagulation such as kaolin or celite and whole blood. When the activator comes in contact with whole blood the contact system (intrinsic pathway) is activated. ACT levels increase linearly as the level of heparin anticoagulation increases (Koerber et al., 1999). The aPTT is performed using platelet poor plasma (PPP), calcium (for citrated samples), and an activator, partial thromboplastin (phospholipid without tissue factor) to trigger clot formation. The time in seconds until a clot is formed is the aPTT.

The aPTT also correlates linearly with the plasma heparin concentration and its association is stronger than that of the ACT. Finally the anti-Xa assay is a chromogenic assay that measures the residual activity of factor Xa in samples treated with heparin. This assay is based on a standard curve that is estimated using standardized dilutions containing known amounts of heparin and Xa. When Xa is not inhibited, it releases the chromogenic substrate into solution allowing for light absorbance. A common substrate used is para-nitroaniline (pNA), which absorbs maximally at 405 nm. The amount of absorption is inversely related to the active Xa (or heparin) concentration in the solution. For unfractionated heparin the therapeutic range of anti-Xa activity is 0.3-0.7 units/mL. When unfractionated heparin is given intravenously all coagulation tests can be run within 5 minutes of drug administration.

Low Molecular Weight Heparin and Fondaparinux

Low molecular weight heparin and fondaparinux inhibit factor Xa through antithrombin III. These drugs do not require routine drug monitoring; however, in some cases (eg: extremes of body weight, abnormal renal function or prolonged therapy) it may be desirable to determine the drugs' anticoagulant activity. The anti-Xa assay is the most useful test and should be drawn approximately 3-4 hours after low molecular weight heparin administration (during peak activity). The recommended therapeutic range for low molecular weight heparin that is dosed once daily is 1-2 units/mL and for twice daily is 0.5-1 units/mL (Bates & Weitz, 2005). For fondaparinux the anti-Xa test should be drawn 3 hours after administration and the therapeutic range is 0.6-1.5 mg/L

Warfarin

Warfarin inhibits the vitamin K dependent synthesis of factors II, VII, IX, X, protein C, and protein S. Because it inhibits the synthesis of factor VII, which is in the extrinsic pathway, it prolongs the prothrombin time (PT) or international normalized ratio (INR) in a dose dependent manner. The PT is performed using platelet poor plasma, tissue factor, phospholipid, and calcium. The PT is reported in seconds until clot formation. The INR is a standardized ratio that is calculated against the international reference preparation (IRP). The INR is more commonly used for monitoring warfarin's anticoagulant effects than the PT because it is a standardized value and the PT is highly variable between labs.

Therapeutic drug monitoring for warfarin is important because it has a narrow therapeutic index and supratherapeutic levels increase the risk for major bleeding substantially. In elderly patients taking warfarin, the risk of a major bleeding is approximately 13 events per 100 patient years (Hylek, Evans-Molina, Shea, Henault & Regan, 2007). Warfarin's anticoagulant effects are also highly dependent upon genetic variations in hepatic microsomal enzymes and its clearance is altered by other common medications including amiodarone. Typically, the goal INR range for warfarin is 2 to 3; however, the INR is pushed up to 2.5 to 3.5 for some patients who have a high risk for thromboembolic events (eg: mechanical mitral valves).

Direct Thrombin Inhibitors

Either the aPTT or the dilute thrombin time (DTT) can be used to monitor the anticoagulant effects of direct thrombin inhibitors such as dabigatran, bivalirudin, and argatroban. The dilute thrombin time is performed by adding thrombin to platelet poor plasma diluted with normal plasma (4:1) and recording the number of seconds until clot forms. The therapeutic ranges for the various direct thrombin inhibitors are as follows: argatroban 60 to 100 seconds, bivalirudin 60 to 90 seconds, and lepirudin 60 to160 seconds (Love, Ferrell & Chandler, 2007). Dabigatran concentrations show a linear correlation with the dilute thrombin time (Avecilla, Ferrell, Chandler & Reyes 2012). The aPTT shows a curvilinear correlation with direct thrombin inhibitor levels (Fenyvesi, Jorg & Harenber, 2002). Other than for argatroban, the INR appears to be of limited utility in monitoring the anticoagulant effects of direct thrombin inhibitors (Gosselin et. al., 2004).

Dabigatran was approved as an anticoagulant therapy without the need for routine therapeutic drug monitoring, but dose adjustments are required when the creatinine clearance falls below 30 mL/min. In patients with acute kidney injury or recovering renal function therapeutic monitoring using either the aPTT or dilute thrombin time may be helpful. These tests may also be helpful in determining drug elimination prior to surgery.

Oral Xa-Inhibitors

Routine anticoagulation monitoring is not recommended for rivaroxaban or apixaban. Like dabigatran dose adjustment is required for patients with impaired renal function (<50mL/min with rivaroxaban and <30mL/min with apixaban). The anticoagulant activity of oral Xa-inhibitors can be monitored using chromogenic anti-Xa assays, the INR, or the aPTT (Samama et. al., 2010)(Hillarp et al., 2011) (Kubitza, Becka, Roth & Mueck 2008). Using the chromogenic anti-Xa assay, the blood concentration of rivaroxaban or apixaban can be estimated by plotting against a standardized curve. At present it is unclear which test is most accurate and cost efficient for monitoring anticoagulation with these drugs. Also the therapeutic ranges in terms of anti-Xa level, INR, and aPTT are not well described suggesting that routine monitoring is of limited utility at the present time.

Indications for Anticoagulation in the Cardiac Surgery ICU

Bioprosthetic Valve Replacement

Thrombosis of bioprosthetic heart valves is a rare occurrence and usually occurs early after implantation (Roudaut, Serri & Lafitte, 2007). In 2012, *Chest* published evidence-based guidelines for anticoagulation in patients with cardiac valve disease (Table 3)(Whitlock, Sun, Fremes, Rubens & Teoh, 2012). In these guidelines, aspirin mono-therapy (50mg to 100mg per day) is recommended for patients with a bioprosthetic valve replacement in any position except for the mitral valve for the first 3 months after surgery as long as there is no other indication for warfarin (eg: atrial fibrillation). For patients with a transcatheter stented bioprosthetic aortic valve dual anti-platelet therapy with aspirin (50mg to 100 mg per day) and clopidogrel (75 mg per day) is recommended for the first 3 months after surgery. For patients with a bioprosthetic mitral valve, warfarin therapy is recommended for 3 months after surgery with an INR goal of 2 to 3. After the first 3 months, mono-therapy with aspirin (50-100 mg per day) is recommended for all bioprosthetic heart valves if there is no other indication for warfarin. Aspirin is also recommended as initial therapy and long- term therapy for both mitral valve and aortic valve repairs.

Table 3. Chest anticoagulation guidelines after valve replacement

Type of valve and position	Anticoagulant drug	Target INR	Comments
Bioprosthetic mitral	Wafarin and ASA 50-100 mg/day for 3 months followed by ASA mono-therapy	2-3	Mitral valves require warfarin because they are at a higher risk for valvular thrombosis.
Bioprosthetic aortic	ASA 50-100 mg/day	N/A	For transcatheter AVR, ASA and clopidogrel x 3 months and then ASA alone after.
Bioprosthetic tricuspid or pulmonic	ASA 50-100 mg/day	N/A	Lower associated stroke risk than left sided heart valves.
Mechanical mitral	Warfarin	2.5-3.5	Some valves such as the On-X valve may have a lower thrombosis risk and require less anticoagulation. Oral DTIs are not recommended based on RE-ALIGN study. Add ASA for patients with low bleeding risk.
Mechanical aortic	Warfarin	2.0-3.0	Oral DTIs are not recommended based on RE-ALIGN study. Add ASA for patients with low bleeding risk.
Mitral valve repair	ASA 50-100 mg/day		Mitral valve repairs have a lower risk of valve thrombosis than bioprosthetic valves.

Mechanical Valve Replacement

Mechanical heart valves have a significantly higher risk for valvular thrombosis than bioprosthetic valves with estimates ranging from 0.3 to 1.3% per patient year (Horstkotte & Burckardt, 1995). Thromboembolic events also occur at a higher rate with estimates ranging from 0.7 to 6% per patient year. For mechanical valves the highest risk period is also in the first year after surgery with a decreasing risk after (Deviri, Sareli, Wisenbaugh & Cronje, 1991). The *Chest* recommendations for mechanical heart valve anticoagulation suggest initial postoperative therapy with heparin and bridging to warfarin as soon as possible for long-term therapy. For patients with mechanical aortic valves the recommended INR is 2 to 3 and for mechanical mitral valves it is 2.5 to 3.5. The guidelines also suggest adding anti-platelet therapy with aspirin (50 to 100mg per day) to warfarin for patients who are at low risk of bleeding complications.

Coronary Artery Bypass

The 1999 *Circulation* CABG guidelines recommended aspirin therapy to reduce the closure rate of saphenous vein grafts after CABG (Eagle et. al., 1999). These guidelines stated that aspirin doses from 100 mg per day to 1 g per day appeared to be "efficacious." There was no recommendation for dual anti-platelet therapy, but ticlopidine and clopidogrel were suggested as alternatives to aspirin mono-therapy in patients who could not take aspirin. In 2004 and 2011 updates were made to these guidelines that recommended aspirin mono-therapy for prevention of saphenous vein graft closure (Hillis, 2011). These updates emphasized that for aspirin's full benefit to be achieved it needs to be started within 48 hours of surgery. Clopidogrel was only recommended as an alternative mono-therapy in patients who could not take aspirin. In a previous randomized controlled trial comparing dual anti-platelet therapy after CABG to aspirin mono-therapy there was no benefit achieved with the addition of clopidogrel (Kulik, 2010).

Aortic Surgery

Endovascular stent grafting of aortic aneurysms is a new and rapidly growing field in medicine and unfortunately there are no good studies to guide anticoagulation practices after surgery. Clinically thromboembolic complications related to the graft appear to be uncommon with a rate less than 1% (Marin, Hollier, & Cha 2003). However, one study that performed CT imaging of recent intra-abdominal aortic stent grafts in 51 patients showed thrombotic material on 15% of grafts, an average of 9.8 months after surgery (Wu, et al., 2009). The main concern with any endovascular stent graft is that before the stent endothelializes it can develop thrombus that can embolize to organs such as the kidneys, brain, intestine, etc. In recent guidelines for endovascular abdominal aortic aneurysm repair, aspirin and clopidogrel were recommended postoperative therapies, but the guideline is vague with no duration of therapy mentioned (Walker et. al., 2010). Most current published recommendations are not based upon study data, but instead on extrapolation form the cardiology literature that relates to coronary artery stents. The major limitation of these recommendations is that large arteries have different flow dynamics than coronary arteries and thus the risk for thrombus is probably different.

In patients who have open surgical aortic replacement with a dacron graft (eg: gelweave) there is also little data to guide long term anti-platelet therapy. In our experience most patients are treated with aspirin monotherapy and clinical thromboembolic rates appear to be low.

To summarize, there is a paucity of data to guide anti-platelet therapy after aortic surgery (both endovascular and open replacement). Our recent pubmed search returned zero articles on the topic. In our opinion aspirin monotherapy is likely to be the safest and the most cost-efficient treatment at the present time and until future clinical studies are completed.

Heparin Induced Thrombocytopenia

Heparin induced thrombocytopenia (HIT) is a thrombophilic disorder that occurs when IgG antibodies bind to heparin platelet factor 4 complexes resulting in platelet activation through the CD32 receptor (Fc receptor) on platelet membranes. HIT leads to venous thromboembolism in approximately 50% of untreated patients and arterial thrombosis at a lower rate (Warkentin & Kelton, 1996). The overall mortality rate is approximately 25% (Wallis et al., 1999). In 2012 *Chest* published guidelines for HIT management that recommended initial anticoagulant therapy with argatroban, lepirudin, or the anti-Xa drug danaparoid in patients with normal renal function (Linkins et. al., 2012). In patients with significantly decreased renal function argatroban was recommended as first line therapy. In our experience, we use argatroban as first line therapy, typically starting with a dose of 0.5 mcg/kg/min. We use this lower dose in critically ill patients because of potentially altered hepatic function and an increased risk for bleeding complications.

The *Chest* guidelines recommend ultimate treatment with warfarin, but they recommend not starting it until the platelet count has recovered to at least 150x 10^9/Liter. The guideline also recommends 5 days of warfarin overlap with another non-heparin anticoagulant like argatroban. It remains unclear how long a patient should be anticoagulated for HIT. Typically by 3 months HIT antibodies are at very low levels so this would seem to be a reasonable duration of anticoagulant therapy (Kelton, 2002).

Atrial Fibrillation

New atrial fibrillation after cardiac surgery is common with incidence estimates between 10 and 65% (Alqahtani, 2010). The incidence increases with certain types of procedures such as combined CABG and valve procedures. Almost all new post-operative atrial fibrillation occurs in the first week after surgery (Aranki et. al., 1996). Approximately 90% of cases of new atrial fibrillation after cardiac surgery resolve by 6 to 8 weeks (Kowey et. al., 2001)(Landymore & Howell, 1991). The risk for clot formation in atrial fibrillation increases substantially after 48 hours of atrial fibrillation. For this reason the American College of Chest Physicians recommends 3 weeks of anticoagulation prior to elective cardioversion in persons who have had atrial fibrillation for greater than 48 hours (Singer et al., 2008). The mechanism for thrombus formation in atrial fibrillation is complex relating not only to stagnation of blood flow in the atrium, but also potentially to increases in clotting factors and atrial natriuretic peptide levels (Lip et. al., 1996)(Petersen, Kastrup, Willhelmsen & Schutten, 1988). Even when no clot is visualized before cardioversion, post procedure clot can form (Black, Hopkins, Lee & Walsh, 1993).

In cardiac surgery patients who have atrial fibrillation for greater than 48 hours and require urgent cardioversion our recommendation is to give heparin for anticoagulation immediately prior to the procedure as long as the risk for bleeding is minimal. Ideally trans-esophageal echocardiography should be performed prior to the procedure to rule out left atrial clot, but this is not always possible. Unfortunately, there is scant evidence to guide how long anticoagulation should be continued after cardioversion in this group of patients. In cardiology practice, patients with chronic atrial fibrillation are often anticoagulated for as long as 4 weeks after cardioversion; however, this is not our practice in cardiac surgery patients who we believe are at a higher risk for bleeding complications including delayed tamponade. We typically do not cardiovert patients in the cardiac surgery ICU who have been in atrial fibrillation for longer than 48 hours unless it will substantially improve their hemodynamics. In these cases when the patient is close to surgery, we only continue anticoagulation for 24 hours after the procedure.

For cardiac surgery patients who have hemodynamically stable atrial fibrillation lasting greater than 48 hours and a rate control strategy anticoagulation decisions should be based upon the $CHADS_2$ score (Gage et. al., 2001)(Table 4). This score allows for estimation of the annual stroke risk associated with chronic atrial fibrillation. It assigns points based upon the following risk factors: congestive heart failure, hypertension, age greater than 75, diabetes, and previous stroke. All risk factors are given 1 point except for stroke which is given 2 points. In our practice, patients with persistent atrial fibrillation and a $CHADS_2$ score greater than 2 receive chronic anticoagulation with warfarin. The target INR is typically 2 to 3. Because many patients have resolution of their atrial fibrillation warfarin can likely be stopped 2 to 3 months after surgery. In patients having the Cox-3 MAZE procedure for chronic atrial fibrillation we also typically give warfarin for 2-3 months.

Table adapted from Gage et. al., 2001. $CHADS_2$ score is calculated by giving 1 point for each of the following: congestive heart failure, hypertension, age of at least 75, and diabetes mellitus. 2 points is given for a prior stroke or transient ischemic attack.

Pulmonary Embolism and Deep Venous Thrombosis

Deep venous thrombosis occurs in approximately 13% of patients after heart surgery even in the setting of aggressive thromboprophylaxis (Schwann, Kistler, Engoren & Habib, 2010). The 2012 *Chest* venous thromboembolism prevention guidelines recommend mechanical prophylaxis only for cardiac surgery patients with an uncomplicated postoperative course (2C recommendation)(Gould, 2012). For patients with a prolonged postoperative course they recommend pharmacologic prophylaxis (2C recommendation). In our practice we treat patients who have no bleeding complications with subcutaneous heparin prophylaxis on the first postoperative day.

Pulmonary embolism is a rare, but potentially fatal complication after cardiac surgery occurring in approximately 3% of patients and carrying a mortality rate of approximately 20% (Josa et. al., 1993). When either a deep vein thrombosis or pulmonary embolism is high on the differential diagnosis hepa-

Table 4. $CHADS_2$ score

$CHADS_2$ score	**No of patients**	**No of strokes**	**Adjusted stroke rate per 100 patients years (95% CI)**
0	120	2	1.9 (1.2-3.0)
1	463	17	2.8 (2.0-3.8)
2	523	23	4.0 (3.1-5.1)
3	337	25	5.9 (4.6-7.3)
4	220	19	8.5 (6.3-11.1)
5	65	6	12.5 (8.2-17.5)
6	5	2	18.2 (10.5-27.4)

rin should be started immediately if there are no serious bleeding concerns. Due to increased bleeding risk post-operatively, we typically target a lower aPTT of 45-55 in most patients. Other centers target an anti-Xa level between 0.3 and 0.7 units/mL. Once the patient reaches a point where they are able to tolerate an oral drug and the risk for new procedures or bleeding is low he or she should be converted to an oral anti-coagulant. Warfarin is the most commonly used drug, but rivaroxaban is also an option in patients with thrombotic diseases and relatively normal renal function (Einstein investigators, 2010). Both apixaban and dabigatran are currently being compared to warfarin in the treatment of venous thromboembolism in the RECOVER-2 and AMPLIFY studies.

Duration of anticoagulation therapy for venous thromboembolism remains somewhat controversial. The *Chest* guidelines recommend 3 months of anticoagulation with warfarin and a target INR of 2 to 3 for a patient with a first time deep vein thrombosis (Guyatt, Akl, Crowther, Gutterman & Schunemann 2012). In patients with recurrent disease the recommendation is for longer therapy unless the patient has a high bleeding risk.

Risks of Anticoagulation in the Cardiac Surgery ICU

Cardiac surgery patients are at high risk for bleeding complications in the setting of anticoagulation for a number of reasons including thrombocytopenia, qualitative platelet dysfunction, and dilutional coagulopathy. The ICU physician caring for a cardiac surgery patient who requires anticoagulant therapy must always carefully assess the risk-benefit profile for an individual patient. Even when the risk for bleeding seems to have abated cardiac surgery patients are at risk for delayed tamponade when they receive anticoagulation (Ofori-Krakye et. al., 1991)(Malouf, Alam, Gharzeddine & Stefadouros, 1993). At present there is little data to help determine when patients can safely be therapeutically anticoagulated after cardiac surgery. This remains an important judgment call that the ICU physician must make given the patient's overall clinical picture.

FUTURE RESEARCH DIRECTIONS

A number of areas require further research to improve anticoagulant practices in post cardiac surgery patients including the role of novel oral anticoagulants in post cardiac surgery patients, optimal anticoagulation for extra-corporeal membrane oxygenation and ventricular assist devices, the duration of anticoagulation for heparin induced thrombocytopenia, the timing of thromboembolism prophylaxis in post cardiac surgery patients, and clarification of the risks associated with anticoagulation in post cardiac surgery patients. Because anticoagulant medications are commonly given to post cardiac surgery patients these studies are badly needed to guarantee best practice moving forward.

CONCLUSION

Anticoagulant medications are commonly used in post cardiac surgery patients for a number of indications. It is important for cardiac surgeons and ICU physicians to understand the basic pharmacology, contraindications, and complications associated with these drugs in order to limit the number of life threatening bleeding complications that occur. Today's physician is fortunate because a number of anticoagulant medications are available allowing for tailored use based upon an individual patient's medical history and comorbidities. When anticoagulant medications are properly selected, dosed, and monitored maximum benefit can be achieved with relatively minimal risk.

REFERENCES

Alexander, J. H., Lopes, R. D., James, S., Kilaru, R., He, Y., Mohan, P., & Wallentin, L. et al.APPRAISE-2 investigators. (2011). Apixaban with antiplatelet therapy after acute coronary syndrome. *The New England Journal of Medicine*, *365*(8), 699–708. doi:10.1056/NEJMoa1105819 PMID:21780946

Alqahtani, A. A. R. (2010). Atrial fibrillation post cardiac surgery trends towards management. *Heart Views*, *11*(2), 57–63. doi:10.4103/1995-705X.73212 PMID:21187998

APPRAISE Steering Committee and Investigators. (2009). Apixaban, an oral, direct, selective factor Xa inhibitor, in combination with antiplatelet therapy after acute coronary syndrome: Results of the Apixaban for Prevention of Acute Ischemic and Safety Events (APPRAISE) trial. *Circulation*, *119*(22), 2877–2885. doi:10.1161/CIRCULATIONAHA.108.832139 PMID:19470889

Aranki, S., Shaw, D., Adams, D., Rizzo, R., Couper, G., VanderVliet, M., & Burstin, H. R. et al. (1996). Predictors of Atrial Fibrillation After Coronary Artery Surgery: Current Trends and Impact on Hospital Resources. *Circulation*, *94*(3), 390–397. doi:10.1161/01.CIR.94.3.390 PMID:8759081

Avecilla, S. T., Ferrell, C., Chandler, W. L., & Reyes, M. (2012). Plasma diluted thrombin time to measure dabigatran etexilate therapy. *American Journal of Clinical Pathology*, *137*, 572–574. doi:10.1309/AJCPAU7OQM0SRPZQ PMID:22431533

Awtry, E. H., & Loscalzo, J. (2000). Aspirin. *Circulation*, *101*(10), 1206–1218. doi:10.1161/01.CIR.101.10.1206 PMID:10715270

Bates, S. M., & Weitz, J. I. (2005). Coagulation assays. *Circulation*, *112*(4), e53–e60. doi:10.1161/CIRCULATIONAHA.104.478222 PMID:16043649

Beiderlinden, M., Treschan, T. A., Gorlinger, K., & Peters, J. (2007). Argatroban anticoagulation in critically ill patients. *The Annals of Pharmacotherapy*, *41*(5), 749–754. doi:10.1345/aph.1H569 PMID:17440009

Bjork, I., & Lindahl, U. (1982). Mechanism of the anticoagulant action of heparin. *Molecular and Cellular Biology*, *48*(3), 161–182. PMID:6757715

Black, I. W., Hopkins, A. P., Lee, L. C. L., & Walsh, W. F. (1993). Evaluation of transoesophageal echocardiography before cardioversion of atrial fibrillation and flutter in nonanticoagulated patients. *American Heart Journal*, *126*(2), 375–381. doi:10.1016/0002-8703(93)91054-I PMID:8338008

Blacker, A. B., Oertel, M. D., & Valgus, J. M. (2008). Fondaparinux and the management of heparin-induced thrombocytopenia: The journey continues. *The Annals of Pharmacotherapy*, *43*(1), 1636–1646. PMID:19737996

Bolz, S. S., & Pohl, U. (1997). Indomethacin enhances endothelial NO release: Evidence for a role of PGI2 in the autocrine control of calcium-dependent autacoid production. *Cardiovascular Research*, *36*(3), 437–444. doi:10.1016/S0008-6363(97)00197-1 PMID:9534864

Breet, N. J., van Werkum, J. W., Bouman, H. J., Kelder, J. C., Ruven, H. J. T., Bal, E. T., & ten Berg, J. M. et al. (2010). Comparison of platelet function tests in predicting clinical outcomes in patients undergoing coronary stent implantation. *Journal of the American Medical Association*, *303*(8), 754–762. doi:10.1001/jama.2010.181 PMID:20179285

Burch, J. W., Stanford, N., & Majerus, P. W. (1979). Inhibition of platelet prostaglandin synthase by oral aspirin. *The Journal of Clinical Investigation*, *61*(2), 314–319. doi:10.1172/JCI108941 PMID:413839

Connolly, S. J., Ezekowitz, M. D., Yusuf, S., Eikelboom, J., Oldgren, J., Parekh, A., & Wallentin, L. et al. (2009). Dabigatran versus warfarin in patients with atrial fibrillation. *The New England Journal of Medicine*, *361*(12), 1139–1151. doi:10.1056/NEJMoa0905561 PMID:19717844

Cruickshank, M. K., Levine, M. N., Hirsh, J., Roberts, R., & Siguenza, M. (1991). A standard heparin nomogram for the management of heparin therapy. *Archives of Internal Medicine*, *151*(2), 333–337. doi:10.1001/archinte.1991.00400020085018 PMID:1789820

Deviri, E., Sareli, P., Wisenbaugh, T., & Cronje, S. L. (1991). Obstruction of mechanical heart valve prostheses: Clinical aspect and surgical management. *Journal of the American College of Cardiology*, *17*(3), 646–650. doi:10.1016/S0735-1097(10)80178-0 PMID:1993782

Duplaga, B. A., Rivers, C. W., & Nutescu, E. (2001). Dosing and monitoring of low-molecular-weight heparins in special populations. *Pharmacotherapy*, *21*(2), 218–234. doi:10.1592/phco.21.2.218.34112 PMID:11213859

Dyke, C. M., Aldea, G., Koster, A., Smedira, N., Avery, E., Aronson, S., & Lincoff, A. M. et al. (2007). Off-pump coronary artery bypass with bivalirudin for patients with heparin-induced thrombocytopenia or antiplatelet factor four/heparin antibodies. *The Annals of Thoracic Surgery*, *84*(3), 836–839. doi:10.1016/j.athoracsur.2007.04.007 PMID:17720385

Eagle, K. A., Guyton, R. A., Davidoff, R., Ewy, G., Fonger, J., Gardner, T. J., & Yusuf, S. et al. (1999). ACC/AHA guidelines for coronary artery bypass surgery: Executive summary and recommendations. *Circulation*, *100*, 1464–1480. doi:10.1161/01.CIR.100.13.1464 PMID:10500052

Eichler, P., Friesen, H. J., Lubenow, N., Jaeger, B., & Greinacher, A. (2000). Antihirudin antibodies in patients with heparin-induced thrombocytopenia treated with lepirudin: Incidence, effects on aPTT, and clinical relevance. *Blood*, *96*(7), 2373–2378. PMID:11001886

Eikelboom, J. W., Connolly, S. J., Brueckmann, M., Granger, C. B., Kappetein, A. P., Mack, M. J., & Van de Werf, F. et al. (2013). Dabigatran versus warfarin in patients with mechanical heart vales. *The New England Journal of Medicine*, *369*(13), 1206–1214. doi:10.1056/NEJMoa1300615 PMID:23991661

Fenyvesi, T., Jorg, I., & Harenber, J. (2002). Monitoring anticoagulant effects of direct thrombin inhibitors. *Seminars in Thrombosis and Hemostasis*, *28*(4), 361–368. doi:10.1055/s-2002-34305 PMID:12244483

Flaker, G. C., Barolozzi, J., Davis, V., McCabe, C., & Cannon, C. P. (1994). Use of a standardized heparin nomogram to achieve therapeutic anticoagulation after thrombolytic therapy in myocardial infarction. TIMI 4 investigators. *Archives of Internal Medicine*, *154*(13), 1492–1496. doi:10.1001/archinte.1994.00420130084011 PMID:8018004

Gachet, C., & Aleil, B. (2008). Testing antiplatelet therapy. *European Heart Journal Supplements*, *10*(suppl A), A28–A34. doi:10.1093/eurheartj/sum081

Gage, B., Waterman, A., Shannon, W., Boechler, M., Rich, M., & Radford, M. (2001). Validation of Clinical Classification Schemes for Predicting Stroke. *Journal of the American Medical Association*, *285*(22), 2864–2870. doi:10.1001/jama.285.22.2864 PMID:11401607

Gosselin, R. C., Dager, W. E., King, J. H., Janatpour, K., Mahackian, K., Larkin, E. C., & Owings, J. T. (2004). Effect of direct thrombin inhibitors, bivalirudin, lepirudin, and argatroban on prothrombin time and INR values. *American Journal of Clinical Pathology*, *121*(4), 593–599. doi:10.1309/D79K4YG-78NTNYY38 PMID:15080313

Gould, M. K., Garcia, D. A., Wren, S. M., Karnicolas, P. J., Arcelus, J. I., Heit, J. A., & Samama, C. M. (2012). Prevention of VTE in nonorthopedic surgical patients. *Chest*, *141*(2Suppl), e227s–e277s. PMID:22315263

Granger, C. B., Alexander, J. H., McMurray, J. J., Lopes, R. D., Hylek, E. M., Hanna, M., & Wallentin, L. et al. (2011). Apixaban versus warfarin in patients with atrial fibrillation. *The New England Journal of Medicine*, *365*(11), 981–992. doi:10.1056/NEJMoa1107039 PMID:21870978

Gurbel, P. A., Bliden, K. P., DiChiara, J., Newcomer, J., Weng, W., Neerchal, K., & Etherington, A. et al. (2007). Evaluation of dose related effects of aspirin on platelet function: Results from the aspirin induced platelet effect (ASPECT) study. *Circulation*, *115*(25), 3156–3164. doi:10.1161/CIRCULATIONAHA.106.675587 PMID:17562955

Guyatt, G. H., Akl, E. A., Crowther, M., Gutterman, D. D., & Schuunemann, H. J. (2012). Executive summary: Antithrombotic therapy and prevention of thrombosis, 9th ed: American College of Chest Physicians Evidence-Based Clinical Practice Guidelines. Chest. 141(2 Suppl), 7S-47S.

Harenberg, J., Jorg, I., & Fenyvesi, T. (2004). Treatment of heparin-induced thrombocytopenia with fondaparinux. *Haematologica*, *89*(8), 1017–1018. PMID:15339691

Herbert, J. M., Frehel, D., Vallee, E., Kieffer, G., Gouy, D., Berger, Y., & Maffrand, J. P. et al. (1993). Clopidogrel, a novel antiplatelet and antithrombotic agent. *Cardiovascular Drug Reviews*, *11*(2), 180–198. doi:10.1111/j.1527-3466.1993.tb00275.x

Hillarp, A., Baghhaei, F., Bagerber Blixter, I., Gustafsson, K. M., Stigendal, L., Sten-Linder, M., & Lindahl, T. L. et al. (2011). Effects of oral, direct factor Xa inhibitor rivaroxaban on commonly used coagulation assays. *Journal of Thrombosis and Haemostasis*, *9*(1), 133–139. doi:10.1111/j.1538-7836.2010.04098.x PMID:20946166

Hillis, D., Smith, P. K., Anderson, J. L., Bittl, J., Bridges, C. R., Byrne, J. G., & Winniford, M. D. et al. (2011). ACCF/AHA guideline for coronary artery bypass graft surgery: A report from the american college of cardiology foundation/American heart Association task force on practice guidelines. *Circulation*, *124*(23), e652–e735. doi:10.1161/CIR.0b013e31823c074e PMID:22064599

Hirsh, J., Bauer, K. A., Donati, M. B., Gould, M., Samama, M. M., & Weitz, J. I. (2008). Parenteral anticoagulants: American College of Chest Physicians Evidence-Based Clinical Practice Guidelines (8th edition). Chest, 133(6 Suppl), 141S-159S.

Hirsh, J., & Levine, M. N. (1992). Low molecular weight heparin. *Blood*, *79*(1), 1–17. PMID:1309422

Holmes, D. R. Jr, Dehmer, G. J., Kaul, S., Leifer, D., O'Gara, P. T., & Stein, M. (2010). ACCF/AHA clopidogrel clinical alert: approaches to the FDA "boxed warning": a report of the American College of Cardiology Foundation Task Force on clinical expert consensus documents and the American Heart Association endorsed by the Society for Cardiovascular Angiography and Interventions and the Society of Thoracic Surgeons. *Journal of the American College of Cardiology*, *65*(4), 321–341. doi:10.1016/j.jacc.2010.05.013 PMID:20633831

Horstkotte, D., & Burckardt, D. (1995). Prosthetic valve thrombosis. *The Journal of Heart Valve Disease*, *4*(2), 141–153. PMID:8556174

Hylek, E. M., Evans-Molina, C., Shea, C., Henault, L., & Regan, S. (2007). Major hemorrhage and tolerability of warfarin in the first year of therapy among elderly patients with atrial fibrillation. *Circulation*, *115*(21), 2689–2696. doi:10.1161/CIRCULATIONAHA.106.653048 PMID:17515465

Josa, M., Siouffi, S. Y., Silverman, A. B., Barsamian, E. M., Khuri, S. F., & Sharma, G. V. (1993). Pulmonary embolism after cardiac surgery. *Journal of the American College of Cardiology*, *21*(4), 990–996. doi:10.1016/0735-1097(93)90358-8 PMID:8450170

Kelton, J. G. (2002). Heparin induced thrombocytopenia: An overview. *Blood Reviews*, *16*(1), 77–80. doi:10.1054/blre.2001.0189 PMID:11914002

Koerber, J. M., Smythe, M. A., Begle, R. L., Mattson, J. C., Kershaw, B. P., & Westley, S. J. (1999). Correlation of activated clotting time and activated partial thromboplastin time to plasma heparin concentration. *Pharmacotherapy*, *19*(8), 922–931. doi:10.1592/phco.19.11.922.31573 PMID:10453963

Koster, A., Dyke, C. M., Aldea, G., Smedira, N. G., McCarthy, H. L. II, Aronson, S., & Lincoff, A. M. et al. (2007). Bivalirudin during cardiopulmonary bypass in patients with previous or acute heparin-induced thrombocytopenia and heparin antibodies: Results of the CHOOSE-ON trial. *The Annals of Thoracic Surgery*, *83*(2), 572–577. doi:10.1016/j.athoracsur.2006.09.038 PMID:17257990

Kowey, P., Stebbins, D., Igidbashian, L., Goldman, S., Sutter, F., Rials, S., & Marinchak, R. (2001). Clinical Outcome of Patients Who Develop PAF After CABG Surgery. *Pacing and Clinical Electrophysiology*, *24*(2), 191–193. doi:10.1046/j.1460-9592.2001.00191.x PMID:11270698

Kubitza, D., Becka, M., Roth, A., & Mueck, W. (2008). Dose-escalation study of the pharmacokinetics and pharmacodynamics of rivaroxaban in healthy elderly subjects. *Current Medical Research and Opinion*, *24*(10), 2757–2765. doi:10.1185/03007990802361499 PMID:18715524

Kulik, A., Le May, M. R., Voisine, P., Tardif, J. C., DeLarochelliere, R., Naidoo, S., & Ruel, M. et al. (2010). Aspirin plus clopidogrel versus aspirin alone after coronary artery bypass grafting. *Circulation*, *122*(25), 2680–2687. doi:10.1161/CIRCULATIONAHA.110.978007 PMID:21135365

Landymore, R. W., & Howell, F. (1991). Recurrent atrial arrhythmias following treatment for postoperative atrial fibrillation after coronary bypass operations. *European Journal of Cardio-Thoracic Surgery*, *5*(8), 436–439. doi:10.1016/1010-7940(91)90191-L PMID:1910852

Lennon, M. J., Gibbs, N. M., Weightman, W. M., McGuire, D., & Michalopoulos, N. (2004). A comparison of plateletworks and platelet aggregometry for the assessment of aspirin induced platelet dysfunction in cardiac surgical patients. *Journal of Cardiothoracic and Vascular Anesthesia*, *18*(2), 136–140. doi:10.1053/j.jvca.2004.01.015 PMID:15073699

Linkins, L. A., Dans, A. L., Moores, L. K., Bona, R., Davidson, B., Schulman, S., & Crowther, M. (2012). Treatment and prevention of heparin induced thrombocytopenia. *Chest*, *141*(2), e495s–e530s. PMID:22315270

Linkins, L. A., Dans, A. L., Moores, L. K., Bona, R., Davidson, B. L., Schulman, S., & Crowther, M. (2012). Treatment of prevention of heparin-induced thrombocytopenia: Antithrombotic therapy and prevention of thrombosis, 9th ed: American College of Chest Physicians Evidence-Based Clinical Practice Guidelines. Chest, 141(2 Suppl), e495S-530S.

Lip, G. Y. H., Lip, P. L., Zafaris, J., Watson, R. D., Bareford, D., Lowe, G. D., & Beevers, D. G. (1996). Fibrin D-dimer and B-thromboglobulin as markers of thrombogenesis and platelet activation in atrial fibrillation. Effects of introducing ultralow-dose warfarin and aspirin. *Circulation*, *94*(3), 425–431. doi:10.1161/01.CIR.94.3.425 PMID:8759084

Love, J. E., Ferrell, C., & Chandler, W. L. (2007). Monitoring direct thrombin inhibitors with a plasma diluted thrombin time. *Journal of Thrombosis and Haemostasis*, *98*(1), 234–242. PMID:17598018

Madsen, E. H., Saw, J., Kristensen, S. R., Schmidt, E. B., Pittendreigh, C., & Maurer-Spurej, E. (2010). Long term aspirin and clopidogrel response evaluated by light transmission aggregometry, verifynow, and thromboelastography in patients undergoing percutaneous coronary intervention. *Clinical Chemistry*, *56*(5), 839–847. doi:10.1373/clinchem.2009.137471 PMID:20224050

Malouf, J. F., Alam, S., Gharzeddine, W., & Stefadouros, M. A. (1993). The role of anticoagulation in the development of pericardial effusion and late tamponade after cardiac surgery. *European Heart Journal*, *14*(11), 1451–1457. doi:10.1093/eurheartj/14.11.1451 PMID:8299624

Marin, M., Hollier, L., & Cha, A. (2003). Endovascular stent graft repair of abdominal and thoracic aortic aneurysms. *Annals of Surgery*, *238*(4), 586–595. PMID:14530730

McLean, J. (1959). The discovery of heparin. *Circulation*, *19*(1), 75–78. doi:10.1161/01.CIR.19.1.75 PMID:13619023

Mega, J. L., Braunwald, E., Wiviott, S. D., Bassand, J. P., Bhatt, D. L., Bode, C., & Gibson, C. M. et al. (2012). Rivaroxaban in patients with a recent acute coronary syndrome. *The New England Journal of Medicine*, *366*(1), 9–19. doi:10.1056/NEJMoa1112277 PMID:22077192

Mehta, S. R., Yusuf, S., Peters, R. J., Bertrand, M. E., Lewis, B. S., Natarajan, M. K., & Fox, K. A. et al. (2001). Effects of pretreatment with clopidogrel and aspirin followed by long-term therapy in patients undergoing percutaneous coronary intervention: The PCI-CURE study. *Lancet*, *358*(9281), 527–533. doi:10.1016/S0140-6736(01)05701-4 PMID:11520521

Ofori-Krakye, S. K., Tyberg, T. I., Geha, A. S., Hammond, G. L., Cohen, L. S., & Langou, R. A. (1981). Late cardiac tamponade after open heart surgery: Incidence, role of anticoagulants in its pathogenesis and its relationship to the postcardiotomy syndrome. *Circulation*, *63*(6), 1323–1328. doi:10.1161/01.CIR.63.6.1323 PMID:7226478

Patel, M. R., Mahaffey, K. W., Garg, J., Pan, G., Singer, D. E., Werner, H., & Califf, R. M. et al. (2011). Rivaroxaban versus warfarin in nonvalvular atrial fibrillation. *The New England Journal of Medicine*, *365*(10), 883–891. doi:10.1056/NEJMoa1009638 PMID:21830957

Penderson, A. K., & Fitzgerald, G. A. (1984). Dose related kinetics of aspirin: Presystemic acetylation of platelet cyclooxygenase. *The New England Journal of Medicine*, *311*(19), 1206–1211. doi:10.1056/NEJM198411083111902 PMID:6436696

Perneby, C., Wallen, N. H., Rooney, C., Fitzgerald, D., & Hjemdahi, P. (2006). Dose and time-dependent antiplatelet effects of aspirin. *Journal of Thrombosis and Haemostasis*, *95*(4), 652–658. PMID:16601836

Petersen, P., Kastrup, J., Wilhelmsen, R., & Schutten, H. J. (1988). Atrial natriuretic peptide in atrial fibrillation before and after electrical cardioversion therapy. *European Heart Journal*, *9*, 639–641. PMID:2970387

Qayyum, R., Becker, D. M., Yanek, L. R., Moy, T. F., Becker, L. C., Faraday, N., & Vaidya, D. (2008). Platelet inhibition by 81 and 325 mg aspirin daily in men vs women without clinically apparent cardiovascular disease. *The American Journal of Cardiology*, *101*(9), 1359–1363. doi:10.1016/j.amjcard.2007.12.038 PMID:18435972

Raschke, R. A., Reilly, B. M., Guidry, J. R., Fontana, J. R., & Srinivas, S. (1993). The weight-based heparin dosing nomogram compared with a "standard care" nomogram. A randomized controlled trial. *Annals of Internal Medicine*, *119*(9), 874–881. doi:10.7326/0003-4819-119-9-199311010-00002 PMID:8214998

Roudaut, R., Serri, K., & Lafitte, S. (2007). Thrombosis of prosthetic heart valves: Diagnosis and therapeutic considerations. *Heart (British Cardiac Society)*, *93*(1), 137–142. doi:10.1136/hrt.2005.071183 PMID:17170355

Samama, M. M., Martinoli, J. L., LeFlem, L., Guinet, C., Plu-Bureau, G., Depasse, F., & Perzborn, E. (2010). Assessment of laboratory assays to measure rivaroxaban-an oral, direct factor Xa inhibitor. *Journal of Thrombosis and Haemostasis*, *103*(4), 815–825. doi:10.1160/TH09-03-0176 PMID:20135059

Schwann, T. A., Kistler, L., Engoren, M. C., & Habib, R. H. (2010). Incidence and predictors of postoperative deep vein thrombosis in cardiac surgery in the era of aggressive thromboprophylaxis. *The Annals of Thoracic Surgery*, *90*(3), 760–766. doi:10.1016/j.athoracsur.2010.03.117 PMID:20732491

Serebruany, V. L. (2010). Mortality in the TRITON trial: Update from the FDA prasugrel action package. *The American Journal of Cardiology*, *105*(9), 1356–1357. doi:10.1016/j.amjcard.2009.12.052 PMID:20403493

Singer, D. E., Albers, G. W., Dalen, J. E., Fang, M. C., & Go, A. Ss, Halperin J.L., Lip G.Y. & Manning WJ. (2008). Antithrombotic therapy in atrial fibrillation: American College of Chest Physicians Evidence-Based Clinical Practice Guidelines (8th Edition). Chest, 133(6 suppl), 546S-592S.

The EINSTEIN investigators. (2010). Oral rivaroxaban for symptomatic venous thromboembolism. *The New England Journal of Medicine*, *363*(26), 2499–2510. doi:10.1056/NEJMoa1007903 PMID:21128814

The EINSTEIN-PE Investigators. (2012). Oral rivaroxaban for the treatment of symptomatic pulmonary embolism. *The New England Journal of Medicine*, *366*(14), 1287–1297. doi:10.1056/NEJMoa1113572 PMID:22449293

Vane, J. R., Bakhle, Y. S., & Botting, R. M. (1998). Cyclooxygenases 1 and 2. *Annual Review of Pharmacology and Toxicology*, *38*(1), 97–120. doi:10.1146/annurev.pharmtox.38.1.97 PMID:9597150

vanWerkum, J., Kleibeuker, M., Postma, S., Bouman, H. J., Elsenberg, E. H., ten Berg, J. M., & Hackeng, C. M. (2010). A comparison between plateletworks assay and light transmittance aggregometry for monitoring the inhibitory effects of clopidogrel. *International Journal of Cardiology*, *140*(1), 123–126. doi:10.1016/j.ijcard.2008.10.046 PMID:19091430

Walker, T. G., Kalva, S. P., Yeddula, K., Wicky, S., Kundu, S., Drescher, P., & Cardella, J. F. et al. (2010). Clinical practice guideline for endovascular abdominal aortic aneurysm repair. *Journal of Vascular and Interventional Radiology*, *21*(11), 1632–1655. doi:10.1016/j.jvir.2010.07.008 PMID:20884242

Wallentin, L., Becker, R. C., Budaj, A., Cannon, C. P., Emanuelson, H., Held, C., & Harrington, R. A. et al. (2009). Ticagrelor versus clopidogrel in patients with acute coronary syndromes. *The New England Journal of Medicine*, *361*(11), 1045–1057. doi:10.1056/NEJMoa0904327 PMID:19717846

Wallis, D., Workman, D., Lewis, B., Steen, L., Pifarre, R., & Moran, J. (1999). Failure of early heparin cessation as treatment for heparin-induced thrombocytopenia. *The American Journal of Medicine*, *106*(6), 629–635. doi:10.1016/S0002-9343(99)00124-2 PMID:10378620

Warkentin, T. E., & Kelton, J. G. (1996). A 14 year study of heparin induced thrombocytopenia. *The American Journal of Medicine*, *101*(5), 502–507. doi:10.1016/S0002-9343(96)00258-6 PMID:8948273

Whitlock, R. P., Sun, J. C., Fremes, S. E., Rubens, F. D., & Teoh, K. H. (2012). Antithrombotic and thrombolytic therapy for valvular disease. *Chest*, *141*(2), e576s–e600s. PMID:22315272

Wiviott, S. D., Braunwald, E., McCabe, C. H., Montalescot, G., Ruzyllo, W., Gottlieb, S., & Antman, E. M. et al. (2007). Prasugrel versus clopidogrel in patients with acute coronary syndromes. *The New England Journal of Medicine*, *357*(20), 2001–2015. doi:10.1056/NEJMoa0706482 PMID:17982182

Wu, I., Liang, P., Huang, S., Chi, N., Lin, F., & Wang, S. (2009). The Significance of Endograft Geometry on the Incidence of Intraprosthetic Thrombus Deposits after Abdominal Endovascular Grafting. *European Journal of Vascular and Endovascular Surgery*, *38*(6), 741–747. doi:10.1016/j.ejvs.2009.09.004 PMID:19836272

Yusuf, S., Zhao, F., Mehta, S. R., Chrolavicius, S., Tognoni, G., & Fox, K. K. (2001). Effects of clopidogrel in addition to aspirin in patients with acute coronary syndromes without ST-segment elevation. *The New England Journal of Medicine*, *345*(7), 494–502. doi:10.1056/NEJMoa010746 PMID:11519503

KEY TERMS AND DEFINITIONS

Activated Partial Thromboplastin Time: Common laboratory coagulation assay that uses calcium, partial thromboplastin, and platelet poor plasma to measure the time until clot formation.

CHADS-2 Score: Scoring system for patients with chronic atrial fibrillation that predicts the annual stroke risk. Variables are congestive heart failure, hypertension, age >75, diabetes, and stroke.

Dilute Thrombin Time: Coagulation assay for direct thrombin inhibitors. Assay is performed by adding thrombin to diluted platelet poor plasma and measuring the time until clot formation.

Direct Thrombin Inhibitor: Class of medications including dabigatran, argatroban, lepirudin, and bivalirudin that directly inhibits factor IIa (thrombin).

Heparin Induced Thrombocytopenia: Thrombophilic disorder characterized by heparin-platelet factor IV complexes that lead to platelet activation, thrombocytopenia, and most commonly venous thrombosis.

Low Molecular Weight Heparin: Small chain heparin molecules with an average weight of around 4K Daltons. Anticoagulant effect occurs through enhancement of anti-thrombin III against Factor Xa.

Unfractionated Heparin: A glycosaminoglycan molecule that is highly sulfated and negatively charged. Unfractionated heparin is a mix of heparin molecules between 3 and 30K Daltons. Anticoagulant effect occurs through enhancement of anti-thrombin III activity against Factors Xa and IIa.

Warfarin: Vitamin K antagonist drug that inhibits the synthesis of Vitamin K dependent coagulation factors II, VII, IX, X, Protein C, and Protein S. Most commonly used oral anti-coagulant in the world.

Chapter 12
Sedation and Analgesia

Jordan Brand
San Francisco VA Medical Center, USA & University of California – San Francisco, USA

ABSTRACT

Patients in the cardiothoracic intensive care unit (CTICU) are subject to numerous physical and mental stresses. While most of these cannot be completely eliminated, intensivists have many tools in their armamentarium to alleviate patients' pain and suffering. This chapter will consider the importance of analgesia and sedation in the CTICU and the relevant consequences of over- or under-treatment. We will examine the tools available for monitoring and titrating analgesia and sedation in critically ill patients. The major classes of medications available will be reviewed, with particular attention to their clinical effects, metabolism and excretion, and hemodynamic characteristics. Lastly, experimental evidence will be assessed regarding the best strategies for treatment of pain and agitation in the CTICU, including use of non-pharmacologic adjuvants.

INTRODUCTION AND BACKGROUND

The experience of being in the intensive care unit (ICU) can present many stresses, both physical and psychological. Up to 77% of patients in the ICU suffer pain (Van Gulik et al., 2010) and 15% may go on to develop posttraumatic stress disorder (PTSD) (Girard et al., 2007). Many of the daily necessities of critical care, such as endotracheal intubation, mechanical ventilation, placement and maintenance of lines, and use of restraints, cause pain and distress, to say nothing of the discomfort that can come from surgical wounds and interventions. Through the use of judicious analgesia and sedation, intensivists are able to attenuate these stresses.

Inadequate sedation and analgesia have been associated with elevated catabolism, immunosuppression, hypercoagulability, and sympathetic overactivity (Consales, Chelazzi, Rinaldi, & De Gaudio, 2006). These effects are deleterious for patients in the perioperative period, even more so for those with cardiovascular disease, in whom they may precipitate arrhythmias and myocardial ischemia. Conversely, heavy sedation can lead to more time spent undergoing mechanical ventilation, longer ICU stays, and increased needs for imaging and other studies to evaluate patients' neurologic status, all of which put patients at risk for complications (Kress, Pohlman, O'Connor, & Hall, 2000).

DOI: 10.4018/978-1-4666-8603-8.ch012

As a result, it is critical to maintain a balance between providing adequate analgesia and sedation and limiting side effects. Several principles seem to logically follow from this:

1) Selection of medications should be tailored to the individual patient and situation.
2) There is growing evidence that the medications used in the ICU may impact long-term outcomes, so current best evidence and guidelines should be followed.
3) Titration of medications should be based on reproducible, validated measurements, and frequent reassessment is mandatory.
4) Use of non-pharmacologic measures should be optimized to reduce the need for medication.

While analgesics and sedatives can produce adverse effects, they have the potential to relieve suffering and improve patients' outcomes and quality of life. This is as true in the cardiothoracic population as in any other group of critically ill individuals. The goals of this chapter will be to discuss the assessment of pain and mental state in the cardiothoracic ICU (CTICU), review various options for providing analgesia and sedation, and provide a framework for evaluating the evidence and selecting the most appropriate agents and strategies for individual patients.

ASSESSMENT OF LEVEL OF ANALGESIA/SEDATION

Regardless of the sedative used, it is critical to monitor level of analgesia and sedation closely so as to avoid over- or under-dosing. For pain intensity, the gold standard is the patient's subjective report; when this is not available, clinicians are forced to estimate pain levels via observation of behavior. One simple and well-validated tool for measuring self-reported pain intensity is the Visual Analog Scale (VAS), which plots relative pain intensity along a line. An alternative is the Numerical Reporting Scale (NRS), which adds numerical increments to the VAS (Hawker, Mian, Kendzerska, & French, 2011).

When patients cannot report their pain intensity due to altered mental status or inability to communicate, an observational scale may be used, such as the Behavioral Pain Scale (BPS). The BPS relies on visual indicators of discomfort, assessed by a healthcare practitioner, and ranks pain intensity on a scale of 3 to 12 (see Table 1). This scale has been shown to have good reliability and validity in a broad population of critically ill patients (Cade, 2008). However, the BPS relies partially on increases in patient movement to indicate greater pain intensity, and some studies suggest that increased pain intensity is correlated with *decreased* movement, calling its results into question (Blenkham, Faughnan, & Morgan,

Table 1. The behavioral pain scale

Item	1 Point	2 Points	3 Points	4 Points
Facial Expression	Relaxed	Partially tightened	Fully tightened	Grimacing
Upper Limb Movements	No movement	Partially bent	Fully bent with finger extension	Permanently retracted
Compliance with Mechanical Ventilation	Tolerating movement	Coughing but tolerating ventilation for most of time	Fighting ventilator	Unable to control ventilation

(Adapted from Payen et al., 2001)

2002). When the BPS has been compared to self-reported measurements, it indeed has been found to underestimate pain intensity, especially at higher levels of discomfort. Therefore, it is appropriate to utilize patients' self-report of pain intensity whenever feasible (Ahlers et al., 2007).

Similarly, quantitative tests of level of sedation provide for more uniform assessment and trending of data over time. One of the most commonly used sedation assessment tools is the Ramsay Sedation Scale, which uses a series of numbers to identify levels of arousal ranging from severe agitation to coma (See Table 2). It exhibits good inter-rater reliability and has been used for many years, making it familiar to clinicians (Sessler, Grap, & Ramsay, 2009). The Ramsay scale, however, has several problems, one of which being that patients may fall under more than one of its levels at the same time if, for example, they are suffering from a mixed form of delirium. Additionally, the scale only has one score corresponding to agitation.

Another tool to assess sedation is the Richmond Agitation-Sedation Scale, or RASS (See Table 3). The RASS has the advantage of having a full range of responses quantifying both sedation and agitation, and has been found to have excellent inter-rater reliability (Sessler et al., 2002).

Table 2. The Ramsay Sedation Scale

Score	Definition
1	Anxious and agitated or restless or both
2	Cooperative, oriented, and tranquil
3	Responds to commands only
4	Brisk response to a light glabellar tap or loud auditory stimulus
5	Sluggish response to a light glabellar tap or loud auditory stimulus
6	No response to a light glabellar tap or loud auditory stimulus

(Adapted from Sessler, Grap, & Ramsay, 2009)

Table 3. The Richmond Agitation-Sedation Scale

Score	Term	Description
+4	Combative	Violent, immediate danger to staff
+3	Very Agitated	Pulls on or removes tube(s) or catheter(s) or has aggressive behavior towards staff
+2	Agitated	Frequent nonpurposeful movement or patient-ventilator dyssynchrony
+1	Restless	Anxious or apprehensive but movements not aggressive or vigorous
0	Alert and Calm	
-1	Drowsy	Not fully alert, but has sustained (more than 10 s) awakening, with eye contact, to voice
-2	Light Sedation	Briefly (less than 10 s) awakens with eye contact to voice
-3	Moderate Sedation	Any movement (but no eye contact) to voice
-4	Deep Sedation	No response to voice, but any movement to physical stimulation
-5	Unarousable	No response to voice or physical stimulation

(Adapted from Sessler, Grap, & Ramsay, 2009)

Since delirium is common in the ICU, it behooves clinicians to have an objective way of evaluating it and grading its severity. One of the most utilized tools for doing this is the Confusion Assessment Method for the Intensive Care Unit (CAM-ICU) (See Table 4). This instrument was the first developed to monitor for delirium in ICU patients receiving mechanical ventilation; it can also be used in patients who are not receiving ventilator support (Ely et al., 2001).

Unfortunately, visual observation and neurologic examination are not always adequate for evaluating a patient's level of sedation, especially if he or she is minimally responsive. An alternative method is to use physiologic variables, such as processed electroencephalography (EEG). The BIS monitor, a popular device used to assess depth of anesthesia in the operating room, analyzes the frequency spectrum of the EEG and produces an indexed value representing the patient's level of sedation. This device can assess states ranging from full alertness to deep anesthesia (Riker & Fraser, 2001). Unfortunately, the EEG signal can be degraded by artifact, especially in patients who are moving, but it can provide valuable information in those who appear to be deeply sedated or are receiving neuromuscular blockers.

ANALGESICS

Almost all patients in the CTICU will suffer from some degree of pain, whether it is due to surgical trauma or other sources. Risk factors for more severe postoperative pain include younger age, duration of surgery, and location of surgery; the thoracotomy incision is generally more painful than the median sternotomy

Table 4. Confusion assessment method for the intensive care unit (CAM-ICU)

Features and Descriptions	Absent	Present
1. Acute Onset or Fluctuating Course		
C. Is there evidence of an acute change in mental status from baseline? D. Did the abnormal behavior fluctuate during the past 24 hours as evidenced by fluctuations in the RASS or Glasgow Coma Scales?		
2. Inattention		
Did the patient have difficulty focusing attention (score of less than 8 on the visual or auditory components of the Attention Screening Examination)?		
3. Disorganized thinking		
Is there evidence of disorganized or incoherent thinking as evidenced by incorrect answers to 3 or more of the 4 questions and inability to follow commands? Questions: 5. Will a stone float on water? 6. Are there fish in the sea? 7. Does 1 pound weigh more than 2 pounds? 8. Can you use a hammer to pound a nail? Commands: 4. Are you having unclear thinking? 5. Hold up this many fingers. 6. Now do the same thing with the other hand.		
4. Altered level of consciousness		
Is the patient's level of consciousness anything other than alert, such as being vigilant or lethargic or in a stupor or coma?		
Overall CAM-ICU Assessment: Features 1 and 2 and either Feature 3 or 4		

(Adapted from Ely et al., 2001)

(Cogan, 2010). Analgesia is crucial for these patients for multiple reasons. Inadequate analgesia may result in hypertension, tachycardia, and other hemodynamic changes, increasing the risk of myocardial ischemia, arrhythmias, and bleeding (Rouby et al., 1981). It may also predispose patients to atelectasis and respiratory compromise. Likewise, while many analgesics have some sedative properties, it is difficult to achieve adequate sedation without sufficient analgesia. Therefore, it is prudent to ensure that a patient's pain is treated before adding additional sedatives to their regimen. It has also been suggested that inadequate analgesia may increase the risk of delirium, especially in the elderly (Morrison, 2003).

Numerous approaches to analgesia are available for CT surgery patients. Multiple approaches can be used simultaneously as "multimodal analgesia," potentially improving pain control and decreasing side effects. This strategy has been shown to be effective in both cardiac (Rafiq et al., 2014) and thoracic (Bottiger, Esper, & Stafford-Smith, 2014) surgical populations. The medications and techniques used to achieve pain control depend somewhat on the individual patient and surgery. In many cases, however, standardized perioperative analgesic algorithms can be developed to improve the efficacy and efficiency of perioperative analgesia.

OPIOIDS

Parenteral opioids are the mainstay of pain management for CT surgery patients. This approach offers flexibility, relative hemodynamic stability, and a manageable side effect profile. Some commonly used opioids include fentanyl, morphine, and hydromorphone (See Table 5). All opioids act through stimulation of opioid receptors in the central nervous system (CNS), which belong to the G-protein-coupled receptor family, causing multiple physiologic effects, including reliable dose-dependent analgesia. Other effects include miosis, pruritus, sedation, decreased gastrointestinal motility, and suppression of hypercarbic respiratory drive. Opioid analgesia appears to be mediated primarily by inhibition of pain signals via pathways involving the midbrain, medulla, and dorsal root ganglion of the spinal cord, as well as possibly at other sites (Basbaum & Fields, 2004). The most significant receptor subtype mediating analgesia for the majority of opioids is the μ-opioid receptor (Jordan & Devi, 1998).

The most severe toxicity of opioids is respiratory depression due to inhibition of the central response to hypercarbia. Up to 1% of patients receiving postoperative opioid analgesia may experience respiratory depression (Shapiro et al., 2005), and such events can result not just in morbidity and mortality, but also increased hospital length-of-stay and costs (Oderda et al., 2007). Patients receiving potent IV opioids

Table 5. Comparison of typical opioids used in the CTICU

Drug	Typical IV Bolus Dose	Onset	Duration of Action After Bolus	Metabolism	Active Metabolites?
Fentanyl	25-100 mcg	1-4 min	30-60 min	Hepatic	No
Morphine	2-5 mg	5-10 min	2-6 hrs	Hepatic	Yes
Hydromorphone	0.2-1 mg	5-10 min	3-5 hrs	Hepatic	No
Sufentanil	5-50 mcg	1-4 min	30-60 min	Hepatic	No
Remifentanil	0.5-1 mcg/kg	1 min	5-10 min	Plasma esterases	No

should be monitored closely for hypoxia and hypercarbia. The use of end-tidal CO2 (EtCO2) monitoring, "smart" infusion devices, and other interventions may mitigate such risks (Maddox, Oglesby, Williams, Fields, & Danello, 2006). Other opioid-related adverse effects include nausea, vomiting, pruritus, and constipation. Opioid administration is associated with development of tolerance and may necessitate dose escalation.

Some of these side effects can be treated with opioid antagonists. Naloxone, which is a non-selective opioid receptor antagonist, is useful in the management of respiratory depression. However, naloxone itself can induce rebound pain, tachycardia, and hypertension. It should therefore be administered in smaller, titrated doses (20-40 micrograms at a time) when the situation is less emergent. As an additional consideration, naloxone has an elimination half-life of roughly 30 minutes, so it may need to be redosed when used to counteract the effects of a long-acting opioid. Several new agents are being investigated to treat opioid-induced respiratory depression, such as serotonin agonists, ampakines, and minocycline, all of which help maintain respiratory drive via pathways that bypass opioid receptors (Dahan, Aarts, & Smith, 2010). While these agents are still being tested experimentally, they have the potential advantage of treating opioids' side effects without counteracting their analgesic effects. Nausea and vomiting may respond to 5HT-3 receptor antagonists and other antiemetics, and methylnaltrexone, a peripheral opioid antagonist, is useful in ameliorating adverse effects on gastrointestinal motility.

Hemodynamically, most opioids induce some degree of bradycardia and hypotension. This occurs due to a decrease in sympathetic and an increase in parasympathetic autonomic tone, mediated by the central nervous system (CNS). These changes can be potentiated by the use of other medications, like beta-blockers, that cause similar effects. Direct effects on cardiac contractility are variable between opioids but are probably relatively minor compared to other classes of sedative medications (Fukuda, 2010). Opioids may also exert protective effects against myocardial ischemia, although the clinical significance of this fact is unclear (Schultz, Hsu, & Gross, 1996).

Fentanyl

Fentanyl is a synthetic opioid that is highly lipophilic and has a relatively fast onset of action. It diffuses quickly in and out of the CNS. Fentanyl may be administered by bolus and can also be given via infusion at doses ranging from 25 to 200 mcg/hr. It is metabolized in the liver by CYP3A4 enzymes and has no active metabolites.

Although it has an elimination half-life of several hours, fentanyl's clinical effect is usually terminated via redistribution out of the CNS into other tissues, such as muscle and adipose tissue, rather than elimination. Therefore, it appears to have a shorter duration of action than would be expected based on its metabolism and elimination. However, fentanyl is notable in that its context-sensitive half-time increases substantially after 120-180 minutes of continuous infusion. At this point, non-CNS tissue compartments start to become saturated, and the drug's clinical effects will last much longer after discontinuing an infusion. Dosage may need to be adjusted accordingly (Hill, 2004). (See Figure 1)

Morphine

Morphine is the least lipophilic of the commonly used opioids. While morphine actually has a shorter elimination half-life than fentanyl, it diffuses more slowly out of the CNS once it has entered and thus appears to have a longer duration of action than fentanyl and other highly lipophilic opioids (Hug, Murphy,

Figure 1. Context-sensitive half-times of common analgesics/sedatives
(Adapted From Hughes, Glass, & Jacobs, 1992, and Egan et al., 1993)

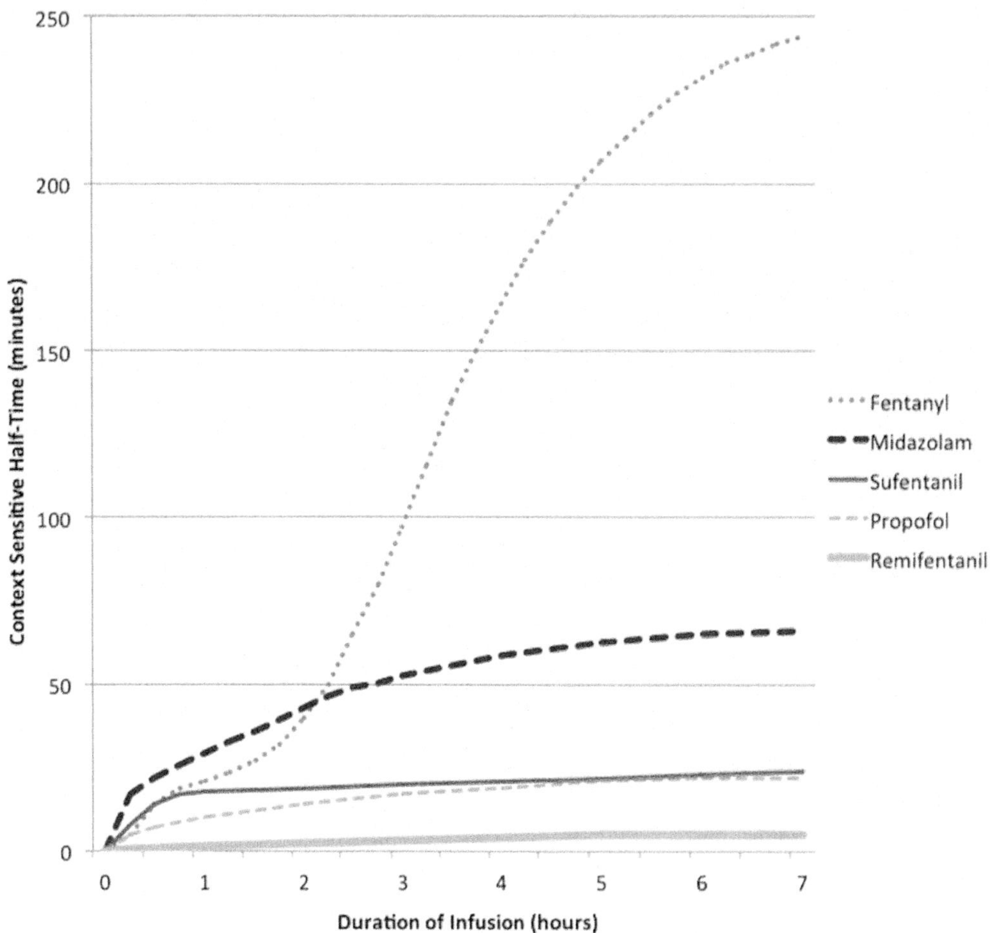

Rigel, & Olson, 1981). Morphine can cause prominent histamine release, particularly if given as a rapid bolus. Additionally, it is conjugated in the liver to morphine-3-glucuronide, which has neuroexcitatory properties, and morphine-6-glucuronide, which has properties similar to morphine itself (Christrup, 1997). Because these metabolites are partially excreted by the kidneys, repeated doses or prolonged infusion of morphine may have unpredictable effects in patients with renal insufficiency.

Hydromorphone

Hydromorphone, which has pharmacokinetic and dynamic properties similar to morphine, has a slightly more favorable side-effect profile. It appears to cause less histamine release and may have a more consistent duration of action; some pain specialists feel it may cause less nausea and constipation, although studies on this subject have produced mixed results (Felden et al., 2011; Wirz, Wartenberg, & Nadstawek, 2008). IV hydromorphone is roughly seven times as potent as IV morphine. Both morphine and hydromorphone are available in oral form although hydromorphone is less orally bioavailable than morphine.

Sufentanil

Sufentanil is a synthetic opioid that has similar properties to fentanyl but is 5-10 times more potent. It is commonly used intraoperatively during cardiac surgery and provides similar hemodynamic control to fentanyl (Thomson, Harding, & Hudson, 2000). However, sufentanil exhibits much less increase in context sensitive half-time than fentanyl with longer infusions (see Figure 2). Some studies have found that sufentanil consequently facilitates earlier emergence and more rapid extubation than other opioids, particularly when high doses of opioids are administered as adjuncts to general anesthesia (Sanford, Smith, Dec-Silver, & Harrison, 1986).

Remifentanil

Another potent and very short-acting synthetic opioid is remifentanil, which is particularly notable because it is metabolized by nonspecific plasma esterases instead of by hepatic enzymes. Therefore, remifentanil's duration of action is unaffected by hepatic or renal dysfunction. Its context sensitive half-time is the shortest of the opioids and is affected minimally by duration of infusion (see Figure 2). As a result, remifentanil is an ideal choice when patients may need frequent neurologic assessments or must undergo procedures that are short but painful (Ruggeri et al., 2011). Because remifentanil is so potent, it can cause pronounced bradycardia and hypotension, especially when bolused; it can instead be administered by infusion at doses of 0.05-2 mcg/kg/min. It can also easily induce apnea and should be dosed carefully when patients are breathing spontaneously.

While remifentanil has several practical advantages, it can also have adverse effects. When used intraoperatively, remifentanil can induce rapid opioid tolerance, which may result in higher postoperative narcotic requirements (Guignard et al., 2000) and even hyperalgesia (Angst, Koppert, Pahl, Clarke, & Schmelz, 2003). These effects may be particularly problematic in patients with chronic pain disorders and remifentanil should be used judiciously in this population.

KETAMINE

Ketamine is a phencyclidine derivative that can act as both an analgesic and a sedative/anesthetic. It acts primarily via antagonism of the *N*-methyl-D-aspartate (NMDA) receptor, but likely has numerous other targets, such as opioid receptors, monoaminergic receptors, muscarinic receptors, and ion channels (Hirota & Lambert, 1996). Higher doses of ketamine (1-2 mg/kg) will produce sedation and a "dissociative" state, which is characterized by an appearance of alertness although the patient will generally be amnestic and minimally responsive. Dense analgesia is also a prominent feature of this state. Ketamine has a fast onset (1-5 minutes after a bolus). It can also be administered by infusion as a sedative with doses in the range of 10-30 mcg/kg/min.

At lower, subanesthetic doses (4-5 mcg/kg/min), ketamine has relatively little sedative effect, but acts as an analgesic. A Cochrane review found that low-dose ketamine given postoperatively decreases opioid requirements and leads to less nausea and vomiting without substantial side effects (Bell, Dahl, Moore, & Kalso, 2006). It also seems to attenuate acute opioid tolerance (Kissin, Bright, & Bradley, 2000). This effect is particularly helpful in patients with high postoperative opioid requirements, either due to chronic opioid use or the magnitude of surgery itself.

Ketamine is metabolized in the liver, producing norketamine, a less potent active metabolite. Its clinical effect is terminated by redistribution, and it has an elimination half-life of 2 to 3 hours. Because of its active metabolite, the duration of action of ketamine may be prolonged in patients with liver or renal dysfunction or those who receive multiple doses.

Ketamine's major cardiovascular effect is stimulation of central sympathetic outflow. This results in increased heart rate, blood pressure, and cardiac output, as well as potentially increased pulmonary arterial pressures (Tweed, Minuck, & Mymin, 1972). These effects seem to be more prominent after bolus dosing than with infusions, and can be attenuated by premedication with benzodiazepines or other sedatives (Jackson, Dhadphale, & Callaghan, 1978). In some cases, this sympathetic stimulation may be beneficial, preserving hemodynamic stability. However, in critically ill patients, ketamine may occasionally cause hypotension, presumably due to its direct myocardial depressive effects, which are typically masked by increased sympathetic tone (Schwartz & Horwitz, 1975). Because of these diverse hemodynamic effects, use of ketamine in the CT surgery population requires careful monitoring.

An additional benefit of ketamine compared to opioids is its relatively benign respiratory profile. It has minimal effect on respiratory drive and airway reflexes, even with higher doses (Soliman, Brinale, & Kuster, 1975; Lanning & Harmel, 1975), and can act as a bronchodilator. However, ketamine can also cause an increase in salivation. Antisialogogues (such as glycopyrrolate) can be administered to avoid this effect.

Ketamine also has prominent neurologic effects. While it is sometimes cited as a proconvulsant and can induce epileptiform activity in deeper brain structures, it does not appear to induce generalized seizures (Myslobodsky, Golovchinsky, & Mintz, 1981). Likewise, while it was long thought to increase intracranial pressure (ICP), ketamine likely maintains or decreases ICP as long as ventilation is controlled and PaCO2 does not rise substantially (Mayberg, Lam, Matta, Domino, & Winn, 1995). Most prominently, ketamine can cause emergence delirium as its effect is wearing off. This state is characterized by hallucinations, vivid dreams, and confusion. Emergence delirium may occur in up to 30% of patients receiving higher-dose ketamine for anesthesia; risk factors include age > 15 years, female gender, total doses greater than 2 mg/kg, rapid administration, and a history of personality issues or frequent dreaming (White, Way, & Trevor, 1982). Premedication with GABA-ergic agents, particularly benzodiazepines, seems to lessen this effect, with midazolam being the preferred medication (Cartwright & Pingel, 2007). Interestingly, it seems that despite this effect, ketamine may not precipitate long-lasting delirium. In fact, low-dose ketamine administered intraoperatively may reduce delirium after cardiopulmonary bypass (CPB) via anti-inflammatory effects (Hudetz et al., 2009).

ADJUVANTS

Numerous other non-sedative medications may be used to augment the analgesic effect of opioids and ketamine. Ideally, this enables the reduction of a patient's analgesic dosage and thus reduces adverse effects. Multiple agents may be used together as part of a multimodal pain management strategy.

Non-Steroidal Anti-Inflammatory Drugs (NSAIDs)

NSAIDS act via inhibition of cyclooxygenase-1 (COX-1) and cyclooxygenase-2 (COX-2). These enzymes participate in the formation of mediators such as prostacyclin, prostaglandins, and thromboxane, causing fever, inflammation, and pain. While inflammation often serves an adaptive purpose, it can be counterproductive if it increases post-surgical pain and impedes recovery. Numerous NSAIDs have been used in the management of postoperative pain, such as diclofenac and ketorolac. Ketorolac is available in intravenous form, facilitating perioperative use.

NSAIDs exert potent analgesic and anti-inflammatory effects. They improve pain control after sternotomy and allow for decreases in opioid dosage, resulting in decreased rates of prolonged intubation, desaturation, and gastrointestinal side effects when compared to therapy with opioids alone (Fayaz et al., 2004). As an additional (and perhaps unintentional) benefit, use of ketorolac has been suggested to improve graft patency after coronary bypass grafting and possibly improve postoperative survival (Engoren, Hadaway, Schwann, & Habib, 2011). Ketorolac has been shown to have similar efficacy in relieving post-thoracotomy pain, resulting in improved respiratory parameters (Carretta et al., 1996). Thoracic surgical patients frequently have limited pulmonary reserve and may thus be unable to tolerate the respiratory depression that can result from high doses of systemic opioids.

Unfortunately, NSAIDs do have adverse effects that must be taken into account. All NSAIDs can induce some decrease in renal function, potentially resulting in fluid retention, hyperkalemia, and other abnormalities. These effects are particularly likely in individuals whose renal function is already impaired and are dependent on prostaglandin production to maintain renal blood flow and glomerular filtration rate (GFR). Interstitial nephritis is also possible but rare. Most of the decrease in GFR due to NSAIDs is reversible when the medication is discontinued (Whelton & Hamilton, 1991).

Because they decrease production of prostaglandins, NSAIDs can induce systemic hypertension. They are also known to cause gastropathy and upper gastrointestinal bleeding, due to decreased levels of prostaglandin-induced mucus and bicarbonate production. Older patients, those with a history of gastritis or peptic ulcers, and those taking steroids or anticoagulants are at higher risk (Hawkey, 2000). NSAIDs inhibit platelet function and may exacerbate postoperative bleeding, especially when combined with other antiplatelet agents or anticoagulants.

COX-2-specific NSAIDs may have some theoretical advantages over agents that inhibit both COX-1 and COX-2. COX-2 inhibitors induce lower rates of bleeding and gastropathy, which would seem to make them advantageous for perioperative use. However, concerns have been raised about whether these medications predispose patients to adverse cardiovascular events. (Some similar concerns exist for nonspecific NSAIDs as well.) In a study evaluating the use of valdecoxib and parecoxib, two COX-2 inhibitors, after coronary artery bypass grafting (CABG), it was found that use of these drugs vs. placebo resulted in higher rates of adverse cardiovascular events, such as myocardial infarction, stroke, and pulmonary embolism (Nussmeier et al., 2005). Such concerns have resulted in valdecoxib being withdrawn from the market, although parecoxib, its prodrug, remains available in some countries. In the aggregate, it appears that NSAIDs have a useful role in perioperative pain control, but should be used carefully, with close monitoring for side effects.

Acetaminophen

Acetaminophen is one of the most widely used pain medications in the world due to its perceived efficacy and benign side effect profile. Acetaminophen is typically administered orally or rectally; an intravenous formation is also available for perioperative use. It produces analgesic and antipyretic effects. The mechanisms of acetaminophen's effects remain poorly understood. While it has some inhibitory effects on the COX enzymes and inhibits prostacyclin production, it does not seem to strongly affect thromboxane, and thus has minimal effect on platelets (Trettin et al., 2014). It has been proposed that acetaminophen may act via activation of central serotonergic pathways and stimulation of the endocannabinoid system, as its effect seems more dependent on CNS concentration than systemic levels (Anderson, 2008).

While acetaminophen itself is a relatively weak analgesic, it exhibits synergistic effects with opioids and other analgesics. Administration of acetaminophen after major surgery reduces morphine consumption in a similar fashion as that found with NSAIDs. However, NSAIDs seem to have more benefit in reducing gastrointestinal side effects and may result in slightly less sedation (McDaid et al., 2010).

While acetaminophen confers minimal risk of postoperative bleeding or gastropathy, it does have notable adverse effects, the most significant of which is hepatotoxicity. Acetaminophen is metabolized by cytochrome enzymes in the liver to a reactive metabolite, *N*-acetyl-*p*-benzoquinone imine, which is usually bound and detoxified by glutathione. However, when large doses are given, glutathione is depleted and the metabolite binds to proteins. This results in oxidative stress, inflammation, and hepatic necrosis (Hinson, Roberts, & James, 2010). Certain patients, particularly those who habitually consume alcohol, are at higher risk, and total daily dosage may need to be limited. Theoretically, intravenous administration may be beneficial in these patients because it avoids first-pass metabolism in the liver.

REGIONAL ANALGESIA

While it requires some additional expertise, the use of regional techniques to provide analgesia after CT surgery has grown substantially. Use of regional analgesia can provide pain relief while avoiding some of the side effects of systemic medications.

Epidural Analgesia

Epidural analgesia involves the placement of a small flexible catheter in the space between the ligamentum flavum and the dura mater in the spinal canal. Medications, usually local anesthetics, opioids, or both in combination, are infused through the catheter. Pain is reduced via multiple mechanisms: local anesthetics block sodium channels on the spinal nerves in the paravertebral and intradural spaces, producing segmental analgesia that is proportional to the volume of medication administered (Bromage, 1975). Epidural opioids, in contrast, act on receptors both within the spinal cord and supraspinally. Supraspinal mechanisms seem to become more important when opioids are administered by infusion rather than bolus (George, 2006).

Thoracic epidural analgesia (TEA) has gained wide acceptance as the analgesic technique of choice for thoracotomy and, at some centers, video-assisted thoracic surgery (VATS). Typically, an epidural catheter is inserted in the mid-thoracic region, and a continuous infusion of medication is delivered, in some cases with additional bolus doses on demand via patient-controlled analgesia. When compared to systemic analgesics, TEA has been shown to reduce pain scores, time to extubation, ICU length of stay, consumption of rescue medication, and rates of postoperative arrhythmias, and seems to improve pulmonary measures such as functional residual capacity (FRC) (Guay, 2006). Other reviews have suggested that epidural analgesia reduces rates of pulmonary complications such as atelectasis and pneumonia (Ballantyne et al., 1998; Popping, Elia, Marret, Remy, & Tramer, 2008). On the other hand, these studies do not show an improvement in mortality with epidural analgesia. As an added benefit, some authors have concluded that use of TEA is associated with less chronic postthoracotomy pain, particularly if the epidural infusion is initiated preoperatively (Senturk et al., 2002). TEA can also be utilized in VATS, and has been shown to provide better analgesia than systemic analgesics (Yoshioka et al., 2006). However, it is not clear that this leads to fewer pulmonary complications after thoracoscopic surgery.

TEA has also been shown to have a role after cardiac surgery. Many of the same benefits posited in thoracic and abdominal surgery have been found in post-cardiac surgical patients. Several meta-analyses have found lower rates of arrhythmias and respiratory complications in cardiac patients who received epidural analgesia, as well as faster time to tracheal extubation (Liu, Block, & Wu, 2004; Svircevic et al., 2013). Notably, as with thoracic surgery, these investigators did not find any significant effect of TEA on rates of myocardial ischemia or mortality. The use of TEA in cardiac surgery has been limited by concerns over the risk of epidural hematoma, particularly when CPB requiring full heparinization is utilized. The risk of TEA-associated epidural hematoma after cardiac surgery has recently been estimated at roughly one in 5500, which is similar to the risk in the non-cardiac surgical population of one in 6600 (Hemmerling, Cyr, & Terrasini, 2013).

Besides the risk of hematoma formation, epidural analgesia has some other notable side effects. Epidural opioids can potentially cause any of the side effects of systemic opioids, although this is theoretically ameliorated by the lower total doses required. In particular, pruritus and urinary retention can be particularly severe (Ladak et al., 2009). Use of epidural local anesthetics substantially improves pain relief compared to epidural opioids alone and causes some degree of sympathectomy; while this may be beneficial in decreasing arrhythmias and myocardial oxygen demand, it can also lead to hypotension (Joshi, 2008). Hypotension may require reduction or temporary discontinuation of the epidural infusion.

Intrathecal Opioids

In some cases, intrathecal administration of opioids may be preferable to the epidural route. Because intrathecal injection is performed with a smaller needle than that used to place an epidural, it is theorized that the rate of spinal hematoma is lower with this technique. Additionally, because no catheter is left in place, there is no concern for how to accomplish catheter removal in patients who become coagulopathic or thrombocytopenic postoperatively or those who require postop anticoagulation. The rate of hematoma formation does seem to be somewhat lower with intrathecal injection, but such complications are extremely rare and thus rates vary widely across studies and between patient populations (Moen, Dahlgren, & Irestedt, 2004; Emazabel-Yunta et al., 2008).

Intrathecal opioids provide postop analgesia that is at least equivalent to that provided by intravenous narcotics. In cardiac surgery, they seem to reduce postoperative opioid requirements although they may also delay time to tracheal extubation (Chaney, Furry, Fluder, & Slogoff, 1997; Alhashemi, Sharpe, Harris, Sherman, & Boyd, 2000). Other data suggests an improvement in postoperative spirometric parameters and no change in time to extubation (Jacobsohn et al., 2005), but this has not been shown to translate into a decrease in complications, morbidity, or mortality. Studies examining patients undergoing thoracotomy also show decreased postop opioid requirements and improved respiratory function versus parenteral narcotics (Askar et al., 2007), although direct comparisons between epidural and intrathecal techniques are lacking.

One of the shortcomings of intrathecal injection is that because a catheter is generally not left in place, repeat doses of medication cannot be given, limiting the duration of analgesia. Intrathecal opioids can cause any of the side effects of systemic opioids, such as respiratory depression, nausea, vomiting, and pruritus. While this technique may be useful, it has not truly been shown to be superior to intravenous opioids, and since it is more expensive and effort-intensive, its appeal is likely to remain limited.

Paravertebral Infusion

Another regional technique that can enhance postoperative analgesia is continuous paravertebral infusion (CPI). In this technique, a catheter is inserted into the paravertebral space on the surgical side and local anesthetic is infused, anesthetizing the spinal nerves as they exit the intervertebral foramina and producing unilateral pain relief (Richardson, Lonnqvist, & Naja, 2011). No opioids are included in the infusion, and the sympathectomy induced is unilateral, providing improved hemodynamic stability. Meta-analyses have shown that CPI seems to result in equivalent analgesia after thoracotomy when compared to TEA, and may induce less urinary retention, nausea, and hypotension (Ding et al., 2014). In an intriguing study in breast cancer patients, CPI was even found to reduce rates of cancer recurrence and distant metastasis when compared to systemic opioid analgesia (Exadaktylos, Buggy, Moriarty, Mascha, & Sessler, 2006). However, because the benefits in this study were suggested to be due to attenuation of the stress response and decreased use of opioids (which can be immunomodulatory), it is worth noting that TEA may result in similar benefits. This is still a question in the early stages of investigation.

While it appears to have a good side-effect profile compared to epidural analgesia, CPI does have its own risks. Because it is still an invasive procedure close to the spinal cord, its use is limited in coagulopathic patients. It also has limited utility in pain relief after sternotomy, when unilateral analgesia may be inadequate. However, this technique seems likely to grow in popularity in the future.

SEDATIVES

While analgesia forms the basis of patient comfort, additional sedatives are sometimes necessary to ensure anxiolysis and ventilator synchrony. Numerous agents are available which may act through different pathways and thus can have divergent effects. The choice of agent is largely dependent on a patient's individual medical condition and needs.

BENZODIAZEPINES

Benzodiazepines (BZDs) have a long history as ICU sedatives. They interact with the Gamma aminobutyric acid type A (GABA-A) receptor and enhance the action of GABA, the primary inhibitory neurotransmitter in the CNS. This produces numerous effects including sedation, anxiolysis, muscle relaxation, and anterograde amnesia. The BZD binding site on the receptor is distinct from the binding sites for other GABA-ergic sedatives, such as barbiturates and ethanol, and BZDs' effects can be synergistic with these agents (Olsen, 1981). BZDs are metabolized by CYP450 enzymes in the liver, then undergo glucuronidation, and are finally excreted renally. Some have active metabolites. Three of the most commonly used benzodiazepines in critical care practice are midazolam, lorazepam, and diazepam (See Table 6).

BZDs have several advantages: they provide reliable anxiolysis and have a high specificity for inducing amnesia, which can be very useful for procedural sedation. This anterograde amnesia appears to be strongly related to the lipid solubility of the drug (Fox, Liu, & Kaye, 2011). BZDs are also useful for treating alcohol withdrawal and delirium tremens.

Another advantage to BZDs in patients with cardiovascular disease is their relatively benign hemodynamic profile. When given at clinically relevant doses, BZDs may cause mild vasodilation but only a slight drop in arterial blood pressure (Stoelting, 1981). They seem to have minimal effects on coronary blood flow (Marty, Nitenberg, Blanchet, Zouioueche, & Desmonts, 1986) and are generally well-tolerated even in patients that are hemodynamically unstable.

As with other sedatives, BZDs have several drawbacks. Because they are hepatically metabolized and renally cleared, they may have prolonged effects in patients with end-organ dysfunction. While BZDs modestly decrease respiratory drive and response to hypercapnea and hypoxia (Forster, Gardaz, Suter, & Gemperle, 1980), clinical experience indicates that they rarely cause respiratory failure when given in isolation (Gaudreault, 1991). Flumazenil, a competitive BZD receptor antagonist, is readily available to reverse BZD effects. However, it should be reserved for severe cases because of the relatively benign nature of BZD overdose and the risk of seizures and agitation with flumazenil administration, particularly if a patient has been taking BZDs chronically. When indicated, flumazenil is given in increments of 0.2 mg IV, up to 1 mg total.

More concerning for intensivists, BZDs have been implicated in increasing the risk of ICU delirium. Lorazepam, in particular, has been associated with the transition to delirium in critically ill patients. This relationship seems to be dose-dependent, with an increasing risk of delirium at doses from 0 to 20 mg/day and a plateau in risk after 20 mg/day (Pandharipande et al., 2006). Additionally, total lorazepam dose has been correlated with risk of post-traumatic stress disorder (PTSD) after intensive care (Girard et al., 2007). However, these relationships are strongest in cohort and case-control studies and thus may be affected by unmeasured biases. One possible mechanism by which BZDs may increase risk of PTSD is the very amnesia that leads many intensivists to use them: at least one study has indicated that patients who have delusional memories of their ICU stay, with no true memories, are actually at higher risk for PTSD than those with true memories of the ICU (Jones, Griffiths, Humphris, & Skirrow, 2001).

Midazolam

Midazolam is a fast-acting, water-soluble BZD that is very lipophilic. This results in a speedy onset of action and a high level of anterograde amnesia. It is available in IV, oral, and intranasal forms, although

Table 6. Comparison of benzodiazepines most commonly used in the CTICU

Drug	Typical IV Dose	Onset	Duration of Action After Bolus	Elimination Half-Life	Active Metabolites?
Midazolam	1-5 mg	1-5 min	20-60 min	2-6 hrs	No
Lorazepam	0.5-4 mg	2-5 min	1-4 hrs	12-18 hrs	No
Diazepam	2-10 mg	15-20 min	1-6 hrs	20-70 hrs	Yes

it has low oral bioavailability. Midazolam's clinical action is typically terminated by redistribution out of the CNS, and, like fentanyl, its context-sensitive half-time increases after a prolonged infusion (see Figure 2). When given as an infusion, doses for midazolam range from 1-10 mg/hr.

Lorazepam

Lorazepam has an onset of action that is similar to midazolam but has a longer duration of action. It also causes some anterograde amnesia. Because it undergoes direct glucuronidation without prior P450 metabolism and has no active metabolites, lorazepam's half-life is not substantially influenced by hepatic or renal dysfunction, making it an especially useful agent in critically ill patients (Olkkola & Ahonen, 2008). It can also be administered by continuous infusion at doses similar to midazolam. As previously mentioned, lorazepam has been associated with increased risk for delirium, but it is possible that this effect applies to all BZDs and lorazepam is simply the one most commonly used in the ICU setting.

Diazepam

Diazepam has a longer onset of action than midazolam or lorazepam. Because it has active metabolites (temazepam, oxazepam, and desmethyldiazepam), diazepam's apparent duration of action is much longer, and this effect is more pronounced in older patients or those with renal dysfunction. Indeed, it has been suggested that diazepam's half-life increases by 1 hour for every year of age after 40 (Griffin, Kaye, Bueno, & Kaye, 2013). Diazepam has prominent myorelaxant effects, especially at higher doses. Unlike midazolam and lorazepam, its IV formulation contains propylene glycol, which can cause injection pain and thrombophlebitis.

PROPOFOL

Propofol is a short-acting anesthetic that is chemically distinct from other sedatives. Because of its low solubility in aqueous solutions, it is prepared in a lipid emulsion containing soy and egg ingredients. Usual doses are 1-2.5 mg/kg for boluses and 1-5 mg/kg/hr for sedative infusions. Propofol has a very rapid onset (1-2 minutes) after bolus dosing and is cleared similarly quickly, with an initial redistribution half-life of 2-3 minutes and a longer elimination half-life of 34-56 minutes (Kanto & Gepts, 1989). Because the initial redistribution is what typically terminates the effect of propofol, its clinical effect usually dissipates in 5-10 minutes after a bolus. While propofol exhibits some increase in context-sensitive half-time with prolonged infusion, this effect is relatively mild compared to other sedatives (See Figure 2). In general, propofol induces a deeper state of unconsciousness than benzodiazepines or opioids, with more muscle relaxation (Dueck, Oberthuer, Wedekind, Paul, & Boerner, 2003). While this makes it useful for situations that demand heavy sedation, it also means that propofol must be given in a monitored environment and by clinicians experienced in its administration.

Propofol's metabolism is still a matter of some investigation. Very little propofol is excreted unchanged in the urine. While propofol undergoes hepatic metabolism, its rate of clearance seems to be greater than hepatic blood flow. The apparent explanation for this conundrum is that propofol is also metabolized in extrahepatic sites like the kidney and the lung. Experimental evidence suggests that 60% of propofol is metabolized in the liver and 33% in the kidney, with studies equivocal as to the lung's contribution (Hiraoka et al., 2005). Interestingly, propofol clearance does not seem to be affected significantly by cirrhosis or renal failure (Veroli et al., 1992; Morcos & Payne, 1985).

Hemodynamically, propofol is known to cause hypotension after an IV bolus. This effect is more pronounced than that induced by BZDs or opioids. Much of this decrease appears to be related to decreased systemic vascular resistance (SVR), although propofol may also have some myocardial depressant effects, especially if PaCO2 is maintained at normal values rather than allowed to rise (Searle & Sahab, 1993). Propofol can depress the baroreceptor response to hypotension, which can exacerbate these effects. It is notable that much acute hypotension from propofol may be related to the fast rise and equally fast drop-off in blood levels that follows a propofol bolus. When an administration protocol was used that was specifically designed to avoid overshoot of desired blood levels, researchers found that hypotension was minimal (Roberts, Dixon, Lewis, Tackley, & Prys-Roberts, 1988). Propofol seems to cause some decrease in coronary blood flow (likely due to decreased blood pressure) but also decreases myocardial oxygen consumption by a similar magnitude; these changes seem to reverse with stimulation (Stephan, Sonntag, Schenk, Kettler, & Khambatta, 1986). Overall, propofol is likely safe to use in all but the most unstable cardiac patients, but should be administered with caution, especially when given as a rapid bolus.

As previously stated, propofol acts as a respiratory depressant. When used at anesthetic doses, propofol depresses minute ventilation and shifts the CO2 response curve to the right (Allsop, Taylor, Grounds, & Morgan, 1988). It can cause periods of apnea after bolus administration. However, lower doses of propofol used to induce conscious sedation have not been shown to have a significant effect on respiratory variables (Rosa et al., 1992). Higher doses of propofol can also cause a decrease in airway muscle tone, which may induce or exacerbate airway obstruction (Mathru et al., 1996).

One complication of propofol administration that has more recently come to light is propofol infusion syndrome (PRIS), a severe metabolic disorder. This syndrome is characterized by bradycardia, arrhythmias, rhabdomyolysis, lactic acidosis, fatty liver, renal failure, and cardiovascular collapse if unchecked. While this syndrome is rare enough that its prevalence is difficult to measure, its severity and high risk of mortality (estimated around 60%) make it significant (Kam & Cardone, 2007). Risk factors that have been proposed include higher doses of propofol (> 10 mg/kg/hr), prolonged infusion, impaired nutritional status, critical illness, and younger age. The most likely mechanism for PRIS is that propofol interferes with fatty-acid oxidation and may affect the electron transport chain (Wolf, Weir, Segar, Stone, & Shield, 2001). In those who are malnourished and dependent on fatty acids for energy, this may result in global metabolic failure.

DEXMEDETOMIDINE

One of the newest sedatives to gain popularity is dexmedetomidine, which acts as an α-2 adrenergic receptor agonist. Dexmedetomidine produces anxiolysis, mild analgesia, and a sedative state that has been termed "calm responsiveness." Patients receiving this agent will frequently remain asleep until stimulated, at which point they awaken and can follow commands, but will return to sleep when the level of stimulation drops. Dexmedetomidine has very little effect on respiratory drive and as such, is increasingly seen as an ideal choice for sedating patients who are extubated and breathing spontaneously or those who may benefit from early extubation (Venn, Hell, & Grounds, 2000). On the other hand, these characteristics may make dexmedetomidine unsuitable for situations requiring deep sedation. It is typically administered via a bolus of 1 mg/kg over 15 minutes, followed by an infusion of 0.2-1 mcg/kg/hr.

Dexmedetomidine causes hemodynamic effects similar to other α-2 agonists such as clonidine: infusion of dexmedetomidine is associated with a decrease in heart rate and blood pressure, which may be quite profound in susceptible patients. Decreased blood pressure is primarily a result of reduced SVR, although cardiac output may decrease as well (Bloor, Ward, Belleville, & Maze, 1992). Bolus dosing can cause hypertension and bradycardia, which is thought to result from the increased α-1 agonist activity of the drug at higher concentrations, resulting in a temporary rise in SVR. In cardiac surgical patients, dexmedetomidine seems to decrease SVR and BP without significant effects on cardiac output, although mixed venous oxygen concentration has been noted to decrease (Ishikawa et al., 2006). It can blunt sympathetic responses to stimuli effectively but does not seem to have as significant an effect on baroreceptor response (Hogue et al, 2002).

Another advantage of dexmedetomidine is its fast onset and offset. Dexmedetomidine is metabolized both by the cytochrome P450 system and by direct glucuronidation and has no active metabolites. Like many other sedatives, it is redistributed extensively with an initial half-life of 6 minutes; its terminal elimination half-life is closer to 2 hours. Because dexmedetomidine has a high margin of cardiovascular and respiratory safety, it is usable in patients with hepatic impairment, although some dose adjustment may be necessary.

ANTIPSYCHOTICS

Antipsychotics are used both as a sedative and to treat delirium, a common problem in the CTICU. They produce varying degrees of sedation but have minimal effects on respiratory drive and thus can be advantageous in patients with compromised respiratory function (Tjia & Gitlin, 2010).

The two major categories of antipsychotics are typicals, such as haloperidol and thorazine, and atypicals, like olanzapine and quetiapine. Typical antipsychotics act primarily via dopaminergic (D2 receptor) antagonism and have a greater risk of associated extrapyramidal symptoms (EPS), such as Parkinsonism and tardive dyskinesia. Atypical antipsychotics modulate both dopaminergic and serotonergic systems and carry a lower risk of EPS, but have been associated with metabolic side effects such as weight gain and diabetes mellitus (Meltzer, 2012). Antipsychotics also have variable anticholinergic and α-adrenergic-blocking effects, which can potentially cause dry mouth, blurry vision, and hypotension (Guzman & Farinde, 2014). Lastly, but of substantial importance in the CTICU, is the risk of QTc interval prolongation with antipsychotics, which seems to be most prominent for haloperidol, droperidol, thioridazine, clozapine, and olanzapine, and can result in Torsades de Pointes in susceptible patients. Interestingly, low-dose quetiapine seems to have minimal effects on the QTc, while aripiprazole may actually shorten it (Goodnick, Jerry, & Parra, 2002). Careful ECG monitoring is essential in patients receiving these medications in the CTICU. In some studies of elderly dementia patients, antipsychotics (especially typicals) have been associated with increased overall mortality, but the relevance of this association with regard to shorter-term ICU therapy is unclear (Gill et al., 2007).

Antipsychotics, particularly haloperidol, have been shown to be efficacious in the treatment of acute delirium in the hospital setting (Lacasse, Perreault, & Williamson, 2006). However, this evidence has not always translated to the ICU, as other studies focusing specifically on critically ill patients have suggested no difference between groups receiving antipsychotics versus placebo in terms of days alive without delirium or coma (Girard et al., 2010). In contrast, Devlin et al. (2010) found that scheduled quetiapine combined with as-needed haloperidol produced faster resolution of delirium, reduced duration of delirium, and less agitation than haloperidol alone, as well as possibly better functional status at discharge, although quetiapine had a higher incidence of somnolence. Studies evaluating whether scheduled haloperidol can prevent the onset of delirium in the ICU have similarly produced mixed results (Page et al., 2013; Wang et al., 2012). Overall, while it seems the efficacy of antipsychotics in treating ICU delirium is not well established, these drugs may be useful in patients with or without delirium whose conditions warrant a sedative with minimal respiratory effects. Further research is necessary to compare the efficacy of antipsychotics to other sedatives and better delineate their best role as part of an overall sedative regimen.

TRENDS IN ANALGESIA AND SEDATION

Before assessing what are the best agents and strategies to apply to CTICU patients, it is instructive to see what patterns are most common in current practice and what approaches are recommended by professional societies. A recent summary of international surveys by Mehta, McCullagh, and Burry (2009) showed that while there is much variation across countries, several trends are evident. Lighter sedation is becoming more common, and propofol is being used progressively more than benzodiazepines. Shorter-acting opioids are also gaining in popularity, with fentanyl and remifentanil taking the place of morphine. At the time of this review, notably, dexmedetomidine was not a commonly used agent.

The most recent guidelines from the Society of Critical Care Medicine suggest how to further refine practice to fit the best evidence (Barr et al., 2013). This set of recommendations emphasized pain control and frequent reassessment of pain as a primary objective. Other evidence-based suggestions were to titrate agents to achieve light rather than deep sedation, to monitor patients closely for delirium, and to use early mobilization as a tool to prevent delirium. Epidural analgesia was suggested for certain types of procedures, although some uncertainty about its benefits was noted. Few recommendations were made for the use of individual pharmacologic agents.

CHOICE OF MEDICATIONS: IS THERE A "BEST AGENT?"

Many factors need to be considered in choosing an analgesic and sedative strategy for a given patient. It is instructive to lay out goals for the patient on daily rounds: is deep sedation required, due to hemodynamic instability or severe hypoxia, or would the patient benefit from lighter sedation and a greater focus on weaning from the ventilator? And are there any measures that can be taken to reduce the need for sedation and analgesia, such as instituting physical therapy, environmental modifications, or an improved sleep regimen?

An additional question to consider is how to minimize the adverse effects of the sedative regimen on the patient. One population that warrants specific concern is patients at greater risk for delirium, such as those with advanced age, sensory impairment, alcohol abuse, or electrolyte abnormalities (Elie, Cole, Primeau, & Bellavance, 1998). This is of particular importance as delirium has been associated with increased mortality and length of stay in critically ill patients (Ely et al., 2004), as well as increased

ICU and hospital costs (Milbrandt et al., 2004). In the cardiac surgery population, delirium may occur in more than 30% of patients. Risk factors include older age, medical comorbidities, decreased preoperative cognitive function, longer cardiopulmonary bypass time, and greater inflammatory response (Guenther et al., 2013). CT surgical patients who experience delirium have greater drops in postoperative cognition and are less likely to return to their preoperative baseline (Saczynski et al., 2012).

Other characteristics of the CT surgical population may impact choice of analgesics and sedatives. Hemodynamic instability may necessitate regimens that have less cardiovascular depressant effects. Organ failure may preclude the use of medications with long elimination half-lives or active metabolites. Patients with impaired pulmonary function may be unable to tolerate agents with prominent respiratory depressant effects. Considering these issues can help to tailor a patient's analgesic and sedative regimen to their needs.

A separate question is whether any one sedative regimen is better than another in terms of overall outcomes, and various studies have been undertaken to answer this question. As has been touched on before in this chapter, an important question is whether BZDs are associated with worse outcomes or more adverse events, particularly delirium. A meta-analysis examining BZD-based sedation vs. non-BZD-based sedation found that use of non-BZD regimens resulted in shorter ICU length of stay and shorter duration of mechanical ventilation but no significant difference in rates of delirium or mortality (Fraser et al., 2013). In a similar vein, another meta-analysis found that use of dexmedetomidine for ICU sedation was associated with a reduction in ICU length-of-stay and time to extubation, although this result was limited by high heterogeneity between studies (Pasin et al., 2013).

Several randomized studies have also been undertaken comparing specific sedatives in terms of efficacy and side effects. When midazolam and propofol have been compared, propofol seems to result in more time spent at target levels of sedation and earlier extubation than midazolam, especially after more prolonged infusions (Hall et al., 2001). This is intuitively sensible, since propofol has a substantially shorter context-sensitive half-time than midazolam. Even when the higher cost of propofol has been factored in, earlier weaning from mechanical ventilation seems to make propofol a more economically viable choice (Barrientos-Vega et al., 1997).

More recently, dexmedetomidine has grown in popularity and this is reflected in the literature. Pandharipande et al. (2007) conducted a randomized controlled trial (RCT) using lorazepam vs. dexmedetomidine for sedation in 106 mechanically ventilated medical and surgical patients. In this trial, patients receiving dexmedetomidine spent more time at their targeted level of sedation and also spent more days alive without delirium or coma. However, this latter composite outcome was driven primarily by more coma in the lorazepam group. There was a trend towards fewer days with delirium in the dexmedetomidine group but it did not reach significance. This study found no difference in mortality between groups.

A similar study was conducted in by Riker et al. (2009) comparing dexmedetomidine to midazolam for the sedation of critically ill, ventilated patients. In this instance, patients treated with dexmedetomidine spent less time on the ventilator, experienced less delirium, and were less likely to exhibit tachycardia and hypertension. Dexmedetomidine was, unsurprisingly, associated with more bradycardia, but the proportion of patients experiencing bradycardia that required treatment was much smaller. Notably, in this study, neither medication resulted in more time spent at the desired level of sedation.

Jakob et al. (2012) synthesized two multi-center Phase 3 RCTs, one comparing dexmedetomidine to midazolam and another comparing dexmedetomidine to propofol for sedation of mechanically ventilated ICU patients. This study found that all three agents were equivalent at maintaining desired levels of light to moderate sedation. Using dexmedetomidine seemed to lead to shorter duration of mechanical ventilation than midazolam and more ability to communicate with patients than either midazolam or propofol. However, dexmedetomidine caused more hypotension and bradycardia than either of the other sedatives used.

Results of trials conducted specifically in CT surgical patients have found similar results. When comparing an analgesic regimen based on morphine vs. one based on dexmedetomidine, with open-label propofol administered as needed for additional sedation in both groups, Shehabi et al. (2009) found that the dexmedetomidine-based regimen resulted in shorter duration of delirium, earlier extubation, and less vasopressor use than the morphine-based regimen, although it also produced more episodes of bradycardia. In this study, there was also a trend towards a lower incidence of delirium in the dexmedetomidine group, but it did not reach significance. In an open-label study, Maldonado et al. (2009) found that dexmedetomidine administered after valvular cardiac surgery resulted in less opioid use and substantially lower rates of delirium than midazolam or propofol. Notably, this study had a number-needed-to-treat to prevent delirium of just over 2, implying a large clinical effect; however, it was limited by its smaller size, its open-label structure, and a high dropout rate. In the aggregate, while it seems dexmedetomidine may have some distinct advantages as a sedative in critically ill CT surgery patients, the choice of medication regimen still needs to be tailored to the individual patient.

CHOICE OF SEDATIVE STRATEGY

Several approaches towards analgesic/sedative administration seem to be useful regardless of the specific drugs chosen. One of these is the use of daily sedation interruption (DSI), sometimes referred to as a "sedation vacation." In this technique, a period each day is designated wherein sedatives are withheld and patients are allowed to awaken. This allows assessment of the depth of sedation, facilitates neurologic examination, and can be an ideal opportunity to conduct spontaneous breathing trials. The foundational study on interruption of sedation by Kress, Pohlman, O'Connor, and Hall (2000) revealed that this approach leads to shorter duration of ventilation and ICU length-of-stay, as well as fewer diagnostic studies, than usual care, with no increase in complications like self-extubation.

One concern with this strategy is that withholding sedation may lead to more stress for patients, greater impact of traumatic experiences, and even more PTSD. However, the evidence does not suggest this. In fact, examining retrospective data, it seems that DSI is associated with unchanged rates of adverse psychological outcomes, as well as fewer symptoms of PTSD, and possibly lower eventual rates of PTSD (Kress et al., 2003). Most of the studies examining DSI have been in mixed medical-surgical populations, with few CT surgical patients included, but there is no reason to think such an approach would not be equally effective in CT patients as long as severe hemodynamic instability is not present.

Not all studies on sedation interruption, however, have found the same results. A Cochrane review by Burry et al. (2014), which examined 9 trials of DSI, found that the intervention reduced rates of tracheostomy but did not change duration of mechanical ventilation or ICU stay. The studies analyzed had significant heterogeneity, which may have affected the results. In a randomized trial, Mehta et al. (2013) studied 430 critically ill, ventilated patients who were being treated using a protocol designed to target light sedation. In this case, again, DSI did not change length of stay or duration of ventilation. Notably, the DSI group in this study received higher daily doses of analgesics and sedatives than the group that was treated via sedation protocol alone. It seems that some of the benefit from DSI may be related to light sedation and not the daily interruption itself. This is consistent with the results of the original study by Kress et al. (2000), in which the DSI group received significantly less sedatives and analgesics than the control group.

Another approach that has been evaluated is the use of analgesics with minimal or no sedation, even when patients are intubated. A trial by Strøm, Martinussen, and Toft (2010) randomized critically ill, mechanically ventilated patients to receive morphine boluses for analgesia with or without a concurrent propofol infusion. The group receiving propofol underwent daily interruption of sedation. Patients received haloperidol if they were felt to be delirious. Those in the morphine-only (or "no-sedation") group were assigned a dedicated caregiver to comfort and calm them if they were anxious or uncomfortable despite analgesics. If these measures failed repeatedly, patients in the "no-sedation" group could receive rescue sedatives by infusion. 18% of the patients in the "no-sedation" group eventually had to cross over and receive continuous sedatives. In the intent-to-treat analysis, this study found that the "no-sedation" group spent more time free from mechanical ventilation and had shorter LOS in the ICU and hospital. There was a trend towards lower ICU mortality in the "no-sedation" group but it was not significant. Conversely, the "no-sedation" group experienced more agitated delirium and received more haloperidol.

While this study creates interesting food for thought, it is not always feasible to forego sedation entirely, especially in patients who are unable to tolerate episodes of coughing, movement, or delirium. Again, while it seems prudent to limit any extraneous use of sedatives, a certain level may be necessary to avoid counterproductive stress responses. Intensivists must balance long-term outcome goals with the medical (and human) imperative to limit pain and anxiety when possible.

Another common strategy utilized in the CTICU is "fast-track" management. This term does not have a concrete definition, but involves various components of care in the intraoperative and postoperative periods that are designed to facilitate earlier ventilator weaning and extubation, shorter ICU stay, and improved recovery after CT surgery in appropriate patients. A meta-analysis of 25 trials by Zhu, Lee, and Chee (2012) evaluated two of the most common components of fast-track cardiac care, low-dose intraoperative opioids and early extubation protocols. They found that these 2 inverventions were associated with significantly shorter times until extubation and ICU length of stay; the fast-track patients had no increase in complications as a result. Other components not evaluated in this study include use of short-acting sedatives like remifentanil and dexmedetomidine and use of epidural analgesia. While fast-track recovery protocols do not clearly lead to shorter hospital stays or lower rates of complications, they appear safe and are consistent with the recognized goals of minimizing sedation and avoiding unnecessary interventions.

NON-PHARMACOLOGIC APPROACHES

While medications continue to be the mainstay of analgesia and sedation in the CTICU, other non-pharmacologic techniques may also prove useful. Physical therapy may facilitate early mobilization and can avoid painful stiffness and contractures, as well as potentially improve function and mood. Alternative therapies, such as acupuncture, massage, meditation, and visualization, may help to alleviate pain, although their use in the CTICU has not been well evaluated. Guided music therapy has been shown to decrease heart rate and myocardial oxygen demand and to improve sleep quality (Jacobi et al., 2002). As little of 20 minutes of music after cardiac surgery has been shown to significantly reduce anxiety and pain (Sendelbach, Halm, Doran, Miller, & Gaillard, 2006). Lastly, attention to sleep- frequently a rare commodity in the ICU- can potentially prevent delirium and help the healing process (Kamdar et al., 2013). Keeping the ICU quiet, turning down lights, and avoiding procedures overnight can all aid in this objective.

CONCLUSION/DIRECTIONS FOR FURTHER RESEARCH

Patients in the CTICU are at risk for pain and anxiety from many sources, many of which are unavoidable in the perioperative period. Through judicious use of medications and non-pharmacologic interventions, intensivists and surgeons can alleviate much of their distress. However, it is of paramount importance to avoid adverse effects that can result from analgesics and sedatives, such as hypotension, bradycardia, delirium, and prolonged mechanical ventilation. There are many ways to achieve these goals, and more research is needed to better delineate whether certain agents may confer benefits in terms of mortality, neurocognitive dysfunction, or other long-term outcomes. It is also less clear whether certain populations may benefit from different agents more than others. While inferences can be made about this possibility, little empirical evidence exists. Dexmedetomidine seems to hold great promise both as a sedative and an analgesic adjuvant, and it may be informative to evaluate its efficacy when combined with other agents such as ketamine for postoperative analgesia. Unfortunately, dexmedetomidine's use is limited by its relatively high cost, although some studies imply that this is outweighed by the shorter duration of ventilation associated with dexmedetomidine (Lachaine, 2012). While antipsychotics are frequently used in the CTICU, there is little data as to their efficacy as sedatives and how best to use them as part of a sedative strategy.

Regardless of which agents are used, sedation interruption, sedation protocols, and other approaches that limit deep sedation seem to hold potential benefits for patients. More research may help to predict which patients are the best candidates for "fast-track" management and whether specific sedative and analgesic protocols may improve outcomes in subsets of the population.

The role of non-pharmacologic techniques in alleviating pain and agitation in the CT surgical population is a field that is ripe for study. These techniques are particularly attractive because they may help limit adverse drug effects, although their relative efficacy needs to be tested in a more formalized way. It may be useful in the future to combine multiple types of analgesics, sedatives, and alternative approaches to establish clinical pathways and protocols based on best evidence. This will help standardize care and make the perioperative process more efficient and less traumatic.

REFERENCES

Ahlers, S. J. G. M., van Gulik, L., van der Veen, A. M., van Dongen, H. P. A., Bruins, P., Belitser, S. V., & Knibbe, C. A. J. et al. (2007). Comparison of different pain scoring systems in critically ill patients in a general ICU. *Critical Care (London, England)*, *12*(1), R15. doi:10.1186/cc6789 PMID:18279522

Alhashemi, J. A., Sharpe, M. D., Harris, C. L., Sherman, V., & Boyd, D. (2000). Effect of subarachnoid morphine administration on extubation time after coronary artery bypass graft surgery. *Journal of Cardiothoracic and Vascular Anesthesia*, *14*(6), 639–644. doi:10.1053/jcan.2000.18300 PMID:11139101

Allsop, P., Taylor, M. B., Grounds, R. M., & Morgan, M. (1988). Ventilatory effects of a propofol infusion using a method to rapidly achieve steady-state equilibrium. *European Journal of Anaesthesiology*, *5*, 293–303. PMID:3065083

Anderson, B. J. (2008). Paracetamol (acetaminophen): Mechanisms of action. *Paediatric Anaesthesia*, *18*(10), 915–921. doi:10.1111/j.1460-9592.2008.02764.x PMID:18811827

Angst, M. S., Koppert, W., Pahl, I., Clark, D. J., & Schmelz, M. (2003). Short-term infusion of the mu-opioid agonist remifentanil in humans causes hyperalgesia during withdrawal. *Pain*, *106*(1), 49–57. doi:10.1016/S0304-3959(03)00276-8 PMID:14581110

Askar, F. Z., Kocabas, S., Yucel, S., Samancilar, O., Cetin, H., & Uyar, M. (2007). The efficacy of intrathecal morphine in post-thoracotomy pain management. *The Journal of International Medical Research*, *35*(3), 314–322. doi:10.1177/147323000703500305 PMID:17593859

Ballantyne, J. C., Carr, D. B., deFerranti, S., Suarez, T., Lau, J., Chalmers, T. C., & Mosteller, F. et al. (1998). The comparative effects of postoperative analgesic therapies on pulmonary outcome: Cumulative meta-analyses of randomized, controlled trials. *Anesthesia and Analgesia*, *86*, 598–612. PMID:9495424

Barr, J., Fraser, G. L., Puntillo, K., Ely, E. W., Gelinas, C., Dasta, J. F., & Jaeschke, R. et al. (2013). Clinical practice guidelines for the management of pain, agitation and delirium in adult patients in the intensive care unit. *Critical Care Medicine*, *41*(1), 263–306. doi:10.1097/CCM.0b013e3182783b72 PMID:23269131

Barrientos-Vega, R., Mar Sanchez-Soria, M., Morales-Garcia, C., Robas-Gomez, A., Cuena-Boy, R., & Ayensa-Rincon, A. (1997). Prolonged sedation of critically ill patients with midazolam or propofol: Impact on weaning and costs. *Critical Care Medicine*, *25*(1), 33–40. doi:10.1097/00003246-199701000-00009 PMID:8989173

Basbaum, A. I., & Fields, H. L. (2004). Endogenous pain control mechanisms: Review and hypothesis. *Annals of Neurology*, *4*(5), 451–462. doi:10.1002/ana.410040511 PMID:216303

Bell, R. F., Dahl, J. B., Moore, R. A., & Kalso, E. (2006). Perioperative ketamine for acute postoperative pain. *Cochrane Database of Systematic Reviews*, *1*, 1–43. PMID:16437490

Blenkharn, A., Faughnan, S., & Morgan, A. (2002). Developing a pain assessment tool for use by nurses in an adult intensive care unit. *Intensive & Critical Care Nursing*, *1*(6), 332–341. doi:10.1016/S0964-3397(02)00071-X PMID:12526871

Bloor, B. C., Ward, D. S., Belleville, J. P., & Maze, M. (1992). Effects of intravenous dexmedetomidine in humans- II: Hemodynamic changes. *Anesthesiology*, *77*(6), 1134–1142. doi:10.1097/00000542-199212000-00014 PMID:1361311

Bottiger, B. A., Esper, S. A., & Stafford-Smith, M. (2014). Pain management strategies for thoracotomy and thoracic pain syndromes. *Seminars in Cardiothoracic and Vascular Anesthesia*, *18*(1), 45–56. doi:10.1177/1089253213514484 PMID:24336691

Bromage, P. R. (1975). Mechanism of action of extradural analgesia. *British Journal of Anaesthesia*, *47*, 199–211. PMID:1096918

Burry, L., Rose, L., McCullagh, I.J., Fergusson, D.A., Ferguson, N.D., & Mehta, S. (2014). Daily sedation interruption versus no daily sedation interruption for critically ill adult patients requiring invasive mechanical ventilation. *Cochrane Database of Systematic Reviews, Jul 9*, 7:CD009176.

Cade, C. H. (2008). Clinical tools for the assessment of pain in sedated critically ill adults. *Nursing in Critical Care, 13*(6), 288–297. doi:10.1111/j.1478-5153.2008.00294.x PMID:19128312

Carretta, A., Zannini, P., Chiesa, G., Altese, R., Melloni, G., & Grossi, A. (1996). Efficacy of ketorolac tromethamine and extrapleural intercostal nerve block on post-thoracotomy pain: A prospective, randomized study. *International Surgery, 81*, 224–228. PMID:9028977

Cartwright, P. D., & Pingel, S. M. (2007). Midazolam and diazepam in ketamine anesthesia. *Anaesthesia, 39*(5), 439–442. doi:10.1111/j.1365-2044.1984.tb07312.x PMID:6731772

Chaney, M. A., Furry, P. A., Fluder, E. M., & Slogoff, S. (1997). Intrathecal morphine for coronary artery bypass grafting and early extubation. *Anesthesia and Analgesia, 84*, 241–248. PMID:9024009

Christrup, L. L. (1997). Morphine metabolites. *Acta Anaesthesiologica Scandinavica, 41*(1), 116–122. doi:10.1111/j.1399-6576.1997.tb04625.x PMID:9061094

Cogan, J. (2010). Pain management after cardiac surgery. *Seminars in Cardiothoracic and Vascular Anesthesia, 14*(3), 201–204. doi:10.1177/1089253210378401 PMID:20705642

Consales, G., Chelazzi, C., Rinaldi, S., & De Gaudio, A. R. (2006). Bispectral index compared to Ramsay score for sedation monitoring in intensive care units. *Minerva Anestesiologica, 72*, 329–336. PMID:16675941

Dahan, A., Aarts, L., & Smith, T. W. (2010). Incidence, reversal, and prevention of opioid-induced respiratory depression. *Anesthesiology, 112*(1), 226–238. doi:10.1097/ALN.0b013e3181c38c25 PMID:20010421

Devlin, J. W., Roberts, R. J., Fong, J. J., Skrobik, Y., Riker, R. R., Hill, N. S., & Garpestad, E. et al. (2010). Efficacy and safety of quetiapine in critically ill patients with delirium: A prospective, multicenter, randomized, double-blind, placebo-controlled pilot study. *Critical Care Medicine, 38*(2), 419–427. doi:10.1097/CCM.0b013e3181b9e302 PMID:19915454

Ding, X., Jin, S., Niu, X., Ren, H., Fu, S., & Li, Q. (2014). A comparison of the analgesia efficacy and side effects of paravertebral compared with epidural blockade for thoracotomy: An updated meta-analysis. *PLoS ONE, 9*(5), e96233. doi:10.1371/journal.pone.0096233 PMID:24797238

Dueck, M. H., Oberthuer, A., Wedekind, C., Paul, M., & Boerner, U. (2003). Propofol impairs the central but not the peripheral part of the motor system. *Anesthesia and Analgesia, 96*, 449–455. PMID:12538195

Egan, T. D., Lemmens, H. J., Fiset, P., Hermann, D. J., Muir, K. T., Stanski, D. R., & Shafer, S. L. (1998). The pharmacokinetics of the new short-acting opioid remifentanil (GI87084B) in healthy adult male volunteers. *Anesthesiology, 79*(5), 881–892. doi:10.1097/00000542-199311000-00004 PMID:7902032

Elie, M., Cole, M. G., Primeau, F. J., & Bellavance, F. (1998). Delirium risk factors in elderly hospitalized patients. *Journal of General Internal Medicine, 13*(3), 204–212. doi:10.1046/j.1525-1497.1998.00047.x PMID:9541379

Ely, E. W., Margolin, R., Francis, J., May, L., Truman, B., Dittus, R., & Inouye, S. K. et al. (2001). Evaluation of delirium in critically ill patients: Validation of the Confusion Assessment Method for the Intensive Care Unit (CAM-ICU). *Critical Care Medicine*, *29*(7), 1370–1379. doi:10.1097/00003246-200107000-00012 PMID:11445689

Ely, E. W., Shintani, A., Truman, B., Speroff, T., Gordon, S. M., Harrell, F. E. Jr, & Dittus, R. S. et al. (2004). Delirium as a predictor of mortality in mechanically ventilated patients in the intensive care unit. *Journal of the American Medical Association*, *291*(14), 1753–1762. doi:10.1001/jama.291.14.1753 PMID:15082703

Emazabel-Yunta, I., Casado-Campo, I., Telletxea-Benguira, S., Torre-Mollinedo, F., Largo, L. F. O., & Maguregui, A. A. (2008). Subarachnoid hematoma following spinal anesthesia. *Ambulatory Surgery*, *14*, 49–52.

Engoren, M., Hadaway, J., Schwann, T. A., & Habib, R. H. (2011). Ketorolac improves graft patency after coronary artery bypass grafting: A propensity-matched analysis. *The Annals of Thoracic Surgery*, *92*(2), 603–609. doi:10.1016/j.athoracsur.2011.04.050 PMID:21801915

Exadaktylos, A. K., Buggy, D. J., Moriarty, D. C., Mascha, E., & Sessler, D. I. (2006). Can anesthetic technique for primary breast cancer surgery affect recurrence or metastasis? *Anesthesiology*, *105*(4), 660–664. doi:10.1097/00000542-200610000-00008 PMID:17006061

Fayaz, M. K., Abel, R. J., Pugh, S. C., Hall, J. E., Djaiani, G., & Mecklenburgh, J. S. (2004). Opioid-sparing effects of diclofenac and paracetamol lead to improved outcomes after cardiac surgery. *Journal of Cardiothoracic and Vascular Anesthesia*, *18*(6), 742–747. doi:10.1053/j.jvca.2004.08.012 PMID:15650984

Felden, L., Walter, C., Harder, S., Treede, R. D., Kayser, H., Drover, D., & Lotsch, J. et al. (2011). Comparative clinical effects of hydromorphone and morphine: A meta-analysis. *British Journal of Anaesthesia*, *107*(3), 319–328. doi:10.1093/bja/aer232 PMID:21841049

Forster, A., Gardaz, J. P., Suter, P. M., & Gemperle, M. (1980). Respiratory depression by midazolam and diazepam. *Anesthesiology*, *53*(6), 494–497. doi:10.1097/00000542-198012000-00010 PMID:7457966

Fox, C., Liu, H., & Kaye, A. D. (2011). Antianxiety agents. In Manchikanti, L., Trescot, A.M., and Christo, P.J. (Eds.), Clinical Aspects of Pain Medicine and Interventional Pain Management: A Comprehensive Review (pp. 543-552). Paducah, KY: ASIP Publishing.

Fraser, G. L., Devlin, J. W., Worby, C. P., Alhazzani, W., Barr, J., Dasta, J. F., & Spencer, F. A. et al. (2013). Benzodiazepine versus nonbenzodiazepine-based sedation for mechanically ventilated, critically ill adults: A systematic review and meta-analysis of randomized trials. *Critical Care Medicine*, *41*, S30–S38. doi:10.1097/CCM.0b013e3182a16898 PMID:23989093

Fukuda, K. (2010). Cardiovascular effects of opioids. In Miller's Anesthesia (7th ed.). Elsevier.

Gaudreault, P., Guay, J., Thivierge, R. L., & Verdy, I. (1991). Benzodiazepine poisoning: Clinical and pharmacological considerations and treatment. *Drug Safety*, *6*(4), 247–265. doi:10.2165/00002018-199106040-00003 PMID:1888441

George, M. J. (2006). The site of action of epidurally administered opioids and its relevance to postoperative pain management. *Anaesthesia*, *61*(7), 659–664. doi:10.1111/j.1365-2044.2006.04713.x PMID:16792611

Gill, S. S., Bronskill, S. E., Normand, S. L., Anderson, G. M., Sykora, K., Lam, K., & Rochon, P. A. et al. (2007). Antipsychotic drug use and mortality in older adults with dementia. *Annals of Internal Medicine*, *146*(11), 775–786. doi:10.7326/0003-4819-146-11-200706050-00006 PMID:17548409

Girard, T. D., Pandharipande, P. P., Carson, S. S., Schmidt, G. A., Wright, P. E., Canonico, A. E., & Ely, E. W. et al. (2010). Feasibility, efficacy, and safety of antipsychotics for intensive care unit delirium: The MIND randomized, placebo-controlled trial. *Critical Care Medicine*, *38*(2), 428–437. doi:10.1097/CCM.0b013e3181c58715 PMID:20095068

Girard, T. D., Shintani, A. K., Jackson, J. C., Gordon, S. M., Pun, B. T., Henderson, M. S., & Ely, E. W. et al. (2007). Risk factors for post-traumatic stress disorder symptoms following critical illness requiring mechanical ventilation: A prospective cohort study. *Critical Care (London, England)*, *11*(1), R28. doi:10.1186/cc5708 PMID:17316452

Goodnick, P. J., Jerry, J., & Parra, F. (2002). Psychotropic drugs and the ECG: Focus on the QTc interval. *Expert Opinion on Pharmacotherapy*, *3*(5), 479–498. doi:10.1517/14656566.3.5.479 PMID:11996627

Griffin, C. E. III, Kaye, A. M., Bueno, F. R., & Kaye, A. D. (2013). Benzodiazepine pharmacology and central nervous system-mediated effects. *Ochsner Journal*, *13*, 214–223. PMID:23789008

Guay, J. (2006). The benefits of adding epidural analgesia to general anesthesia: A metaanalysis. *Journal of Anesthesia*, *20*(4), 335–340. doi:10.1007/s00540-006-0423-8 PMID:17072704

Guenther, U., Theuerkauf, N., Frommann, I., Brimmers, K., Malik, R., Stori, S., & Popp, J. et al. (2013). Predisposing and precipitating factors of delirium after cardiac surgery: A prospective observational cohort study. *Annals of Surgery*, *257*(6), 1160–1167. doi:10.1097/SLA.0b013e318281b01c PMID:23426334

Guignard, B., Bossard, A. E., Coste, C., Sessler, D. I., Lebrault, C., Alfonsi, P., & Chauvin, M. et al. (2000). Acute opioid tolerance: Intraoperative remifentanil increases postoperative pain and morphine requirement. *Anesthesiology*, *93*(2), 409–417. doi:10.1097/00000542-200008000-00019 PMID:10910490

Guzman, F., & Farinde, A. (2014). *First-generation antipsychotics: an introduction.* Retrieved from http://psychopharmacologyinstitute.com/antipsychotics/first-generation-antipsychotics/

Hall, R. I., Sandham, D., Cardinal, P., Tweeddale, M., Moher, D., Wang, X., & Anis, A. H. (2001). Propofol vs midazolam for ICU sedation: A Canadian multicenter randomized trial. *Chest*, *119*(4), 1151–1159. doi:10.1378/chest.119.4.1151 PMID:11296183

Hawker, G. A., Mian, S., Kendzerska, T., & French, M. (2011). Measures of adult pain. *Arthritis Care and Research*, *63*(S11), S240–S252. doi:10.1002/acr.20543 PMID:22588748

Hawkey, C. J. (2000). Nonsteroidal anti-inflammatory drug gastropathy. *Gastroenterology*, *119*(2), 521–535. doi:10.1053/gast.2000.9561 PMID:10930388

Hemmerling, T. M., Cyr, S., & Terrasini, N. (2013). Epidural catheterization in cardiac surgery: The 2012 risk assessment. *Annals of Cardiac Anaesthesia*, *16*(3), 169–177. doi:10.4103/0971-9784.114237 PMID:23816670

Hill, S. A. (2004). Pharmacokinetics of drug infusions. *Continuing Education in Anaesthesia, Critical Care, and Pain*, *4*(3), 76–80. doi:10.1093/bjaceaccp/mkh021

Hinson, J. A., Roberts, D. W., & James, L. P. (2010). Mechanisms of acetaminophen-induced liver necrosis. *Handbook of Experimental Pharmacology*, *196*, 369–405. doi:10.1007/978-3-642-00663-0_12 PMID:20020268

Hiraoka, H., Yamamoto, K., Miyoshi, S., Morita, T., Nakamura, K., Kadoi, Y., & Horiuchi, R. et al. (2005). Kidneys contribute to the extrahepatic clearance of propofol in humans, but not lungs and brain. *British Journal of Clinical Pharmacology*, *60*(2), 176–182. doi:10.1111/j.1365-2125.2005.02393.x PMID:16042671

Hirota, K., & Lambert, D. G. (1996). Ketamine: Its mechanism(s) of action and unusual clinical uses. *British Journal of Anaesthesia*, *77*(4), 441–444. doi:10.1093/bja/77.4.441 PMID:8942324

Hogue, C. W. Jr, Talke, P., Stein, P. K., Richardson, C., Domitrovich, P. P., & Sessler, D. I. (2002). Autonomic nervous system responses during sedative infusions of dexmedetomidine. *Anesthesiology*, *97*(3), 592–598. doi:10.1097/00000542-200209000-00012 PMID:12218525

Hudetz, J. A., Patterson, K. M., Iqbal, Z., Gandhi, S. D., Byrne, A. J., Hudetz, A. G., & Pagel, P. S. et al. (2009). Ketamine attenuates delirium after cardiac surgery with cardiopulmonary bypass. *Journal of Cardiothoracic and Vascular Anesthesia*, *23*(5), 651–657. doi:10.1053/j.jvca.2008.12.021 PMID:19231245

Hug, C. C. Jr, Murphy, M. R., Rigel, E. P., & Olson, W. A. (1981). Pharmacokinetics of morphine injected intravenously into the anesthetized dog. *Anesthesiology*, *54*(1), 38–47. doi:10.1097/00000542-198101000-00008 PMID:7457981

Hughes, M. A., Glass, P. S. A., & Jacobs, J. R. (1992). Context-sensitive half-time in multicompartment pharmacokinetic models for intravenous anesthetic drugs. *Anesthesiology*, *76*(3), 334–341. doi:10.1097/00000542-199203000-00003 PMID:1539843

Ishikawa, S., Kugawa, S., Neya, K., Suzuki, Y., Kawasaki, A., Hayama, T., & Ueda, K. (2006). Hemodynamic effects of dexmedetomidine in patients after cardiac surgery. *Minerva Chirurgica*, *61*, 215–219. PMID:16858303

Jackson, A. P. F., Dhadphale, P. R., Callaghan, M. L., & Alseri, S. (1978). Haemodynamic studies during induction of anaesthesia for open-heart surgery using diazepam and ketamine. *British Journal of Anaesthesia*, *50*(4), 375–377. doi:10.1093/bja/50.4.375 PMID:656254

Jacobi, J., Fraser, G. L., Coursin, D. B., Riker, R. R., Fontaine, D., Wittbrodt, E. T., & Lumb, P. D. et al. (2002). …Lumb, P.D. (2002). Clinical practice guidelines for the sustained use of sedatives and analgesics in the critically ill adult: Sedation and Analgesia Task Force of the American College of Critical Care Medicine. *Critical Care Medicine*, *30*(1), 119–141. doi:10.1097/00003246-200201000-00020 PMID:11902253

Jacobsohn, E., Lee, T. W., Amadeo, R. J., Syslak, P. H., Debrouwere, R. G., Bell, D., & Avidan, M. et al. (2005). Low-dose intrathecal morphine does not delay early extubation after cardiac surgery. *Canadian Journal of Anaesthesia*, *52*, 848–857. PMID:16189338

Jakob, S. M., Ruokonen, E., Grounds, M., Sarapohja, T., Garratt, C., Pocock, S. J., & Takala, J. et al. (2012). Dexmedetomidine vs. midazolam of propofol for sedation during prolonged mechanical ventilation: Two randomized controlled trials. *Journal of the American Medical Association*, *307*(11), 1151–1160. doi:10.1001/jama.2012.304 PMID:22436955

Jones, C., Griffiths, R. D., Humphris, G., & Skirrow, P. M. (2001). Memory, delusions, and the development of acute posttraumatic stress disorder-related symptoms after intensive care. *Critical Care Medicine*, *29*(3), 573–580. doi:10.1097/00003246-200103000-00019 PMID:11373423

Jordan, B., & Devi, L. A. (1998). Molecular mechanisms of opioid receptor signal transduction. *British Journal of Anaesthesia*, *81*(1), 12–19. doi:10.1093/bja/81.1.12 PMID:9771268

Joshi, G. P., Bonnet, F., Shah, R., Wilkinson, R. C., Camu, F., Fischer, B., & Kehlet, H. et al. (2008). A systemic review of randomized trials evaluating regional techniques for postthoracotomy analgesia. *Anesthesia and Analgesia*, *107*(3), 1026–1040. doi:10.1213/01.ane.0000333274.63501.ff PMID:18713924

Kam, P. C. A., & Cardone, D. (2007). Propofol infusion syndrome. *Anaesthesia*, *62*(7), 690–701. doi:10.1111/j.1365-2044.2007.05055.x PMID:17567345

Kamdar, B. B., King, L. M., Collop, N. A., Sakamuri, S., Colantuoni, E., Neufeld, K. J., & Needham, D. M. et al. (2013). The effect of a quality improvement intervention on perceived sleep quality & cognition in a medical ICU. *Critical Care Medicine*, *41*(3), 800–809. doi:10.1097/CCM.0b013e3182746442 PMID:23314584

Kanto, J., & Gepts, E. (1989). Pharmacokinetic implications for the clinical use of propofol. *Clinical Pharmacokinetics*, *17*(5), 308–326. doi:10.2165/00003088-198917050-00002 PMID:2684471

Kissin, I., Bright, C. A., & Bradley, E. L. Jr. (2000). The effect of ketamine on opioid-induced acute tolerance: Can it explain reduction of opioid consumption with ketamine-opioid analgesic combinations? *Anesthesia and Analgesia*, *91*(6), 1483–1488. doi:10.1097/00000539-200012000-00035 PMID:11094005

Kress, J. P., Gehlbach, B., Lacy, M., Pliskin, N., Pohlman, A. S., & Hall, J. B. (2003). The long-term psychological effects of daily sedation interruption on critically ill patients. *American Journal of Respiratory and Critical Care Medicine*, *168*(12), 1457–1461. doi:10.1164/rccm.200303-455OC PMID:14525802

Kress, J. P., Pohlman, A. S., O'Connor, M. F., & Hall, J. B. (2000). Daily interruption of sedative infusions in critically ill patients undergoing mechanical ventilation. *The New England Journal of Medicine*, *342*(20), 1471–1477. doi:10.1056/NEJM200005183422002 PMID:10816184

Lacasse, H., Perreault, M. M., & Williamson, D. R. (2006). Systematic review of antipsychotics for the treatment of hospital-associated delirium in medically or surgically ill patients. *The Annals of Pharmacotherapy*, *40*(11), 1966–1973. doi:10.1345/aph.1H241 PMID:17047137

Lachaine, J., & Beauchemin, C. (2012). Economic evaluation of dexmedetomidine relative to midazolam for sedation in the intensive care unit. *The Canadian Journal of Hospital Pharmacy*, *65*(2), 103–110. doi:10.4212/cjhp.v65i2.1116 PMID:22529402

Ladak, S. S., Katznelson, R., Muscat, M., Sawhney, M., Beattie, W. S., & O'Leary, G. (2009). Incidence of urinary retention in patients with thoracic patient-controlled epidural analgesia (TPCEA) undergoing thoracotomy. *Pain Management Nursing*, *10*(2), 94–98. doi:10.1016/j.pmn.2008.08.001 PMID:19481048

Lanning, C. F., & Harmel, M. H. (1975). Ketamine anesthesia. *Annual Review of Medicine*, *26*(1), 137–141. doi:10.1146/annurev.me.26.020175.001033 PMID:1096753

Liu, S. S., Block, B. M., & Wu, C. L. (2004). Effects of perioperative central neuraxial analgesia on outcome after coronary artery bypass surgery. *Anesthesiology*, *101*(1), 153–161. doi:10.1097/00000542-200407000-00024 PMID:15220785

Maddox, R. R., Oglesby, H., Williams, C. K., Fields, M., & Danello, S. (2006). Continuous respiratory monitoring and a "smart" infusion system improve safety of patient-controlled analgesia in the postoperative. *American Journal of Health-System Pharmacy*, *63*, 157–164. doi:10.2146/ajhp050194 PMID:16390930

Maldonado, J. R., Wysong, A., van der Starre, P. J., Block, T., Miller, C., & Reitz, B. A. (2009). Dexmedetomidine and the reduction of postoperative delirium after cardiac surgery. *Psychosomatics*, *50*(3), 206–217. doi:10.1176/appi.psy.50.3.206 PMID:19567759

Marty, J., Nitenberg, A., Blanchet, F., Zouioueche, S., & Desmonts, J. M. (1986). Effects of midazolam on the coronary circulation in patients with coronary artery disease. *Anesthesiology*, *64*(2), 206–210. doi:10.1097/00000542-198602000-00013 PMID:2936281

Mathru, M., Esch, O., Lang, J., Herbert, M. E., Chaljub, G., Goodacre, B., & vanSonnenberg, E. (1996). Magnetic resonance imaging of the upper airway: Effects of propofol anesthesia and nasal continuous positive airway pressure in humans. *Anesthesiology*, *84*(2), 273–279. doi:10.1097/00000542-199602000-00004 PMID:8602656

Mayberg, T. S., Lam, A. M., Matta, B. F., Domino, K. B., & Winn, H. R. (1995). Ketamine does not increase cerebral blood flow velocity or intracranial pressure during isoflurane/nitrous oxide anesthesia in patients undergoing craniotomy. *Anesthesia and Analgesia*, *81*, 84–89. PMID:7598288

McDaid, C., Maund, E., Rice, S., Wright, K., Jenkins, B., & Woolacott, N. (2010). Paracetamol and selective and non-selective non-steroidal anti-inflammatory drugs (NSAIDs) for the reduction of morphine-related side effects after major surgery: A systematic review. *Health Technology Assessment*, *14*(17), 1–153. doi:10.3310/hta14170 PMID:20346263

Mehta, S., Burry, L., Cook, D., Fergusson, D., Steinberg, M., Granton, J., & Meade, M. et al. (2012). Daily sedation interruption in mechanically ventilated critically ill patients cared for with a sedation protocol: A randomized controlled trial. *Journal of the American Medical Association*, *308*(19), 1985–1992. doi:10.1001/jama.2012.13872 PMID:23180503

Mehta, S., McCullagh, I., & Burry, L. (2009). Current sedation practices: Lessons learned from international surveys. *Critical Care Clinics*, *25*(3), 471–488. doi:10.1016/j.ccc.2009.04.001 PMID:19576525

Meltzer, H. Y. (2012). Update on typical and atypical antipsychotic drugs. *Annual Review of Medicine*, *64*(1), 393–406. doi:10.1146/annurev-med-050911-161504 PMID:23020880

Milbrandt, E. B., Deppen, S., Harrison, P. L., Shintani, A. K., Speroff, T., Stiles, R. A., & Ely, E. W. et al. (2004). Costs associated with delirium in mechanically ventilated patients. *Critical Care Medicine*, *32*(4), 955–962. doi:10.1097/01.CCM.0000119429.16055.92 PMID:15071384

Moen, V., Dahlgren, N., & Irestedt, L. (2004). Severe neurological complications after central neuraxial blockades in Sweden, 1990-1999. *Anesthesiology*, *101*(4), 950–959. doi:10.1097/00000542-200410000-00021 PMID:15448529

Morcos, W. E., & Payne, J. P. (1985). The induction of anaesthesia with propofol compared in normal and renal failure patients. *Postgraduate Medical Journal*, *61*, 62–63. PMID:3877297

Morrison, R. S., Magaziner, J., Gilbert, M., Koval, K. J., McLaughlin, M. A., Orosz, G., & Siu, A. L. et al. (2003). Relationship between pain and opioid analgesics on the development of delirium following hip fracture. *The Journals of Gerontology. Series A, Biological Sciences and Medical Sciences*, *58*(1), 76–81. doi:10.1093/gerona/58.1.M76 PMID:12560416

Myslobodsky, M. S., Golovchinsky, V., & Mintz, M. (1981). Ketamine: Convulsant or anti-convulsant? *Pharmacology, Biochemistry, and Behavior*, *14*(1), 27–33. doi:10.1016/0091-3057(81)90099-X PMID:7465607

Nussmeier, N. A., Whelton, A. A., Brown, M. T., Langford, R. M., Hoeft, A., Parlow, J. L., & Verburg, K. M. et al. (2005). Complications of the COX-2 inhibitors parecoxib and valdecoxib after cardiac surgery. *The New England Journal of Medicine*, *352*(11), 1081–1091. doi:10.1056/NEJMoa050330 PMID:15713945

Oderda, G. M., Said, Q., Evans, R. S., Stoddard, G. J., Lloyd, J., Jackson, K., & Samore, M. H. et al. (2007). Opioid-related adverse drug events in surgical hospitalizations: Impact on costs and length of stay. *The Annals of Pharmacotherapy*, *41*(3), 400–406. doi:10.1345/aph.1H386 PMID:17341537

Olkkola, K. T., & Ahonen, J. (2008). Midazolam and other benzodiazepines. *Handbook of Experimental Pharmacology*, *182*, 335–360. doi:10.1007/978-3-540-74806-9_16 PMID:18175099

Olsen, R. W. (1981). GABA-benzodiazepine-barbiturate receptor interactions. *Journal of Neurochemistry*, *37*(1), 1–13. doi:10.1111/j.1471-4159.1981.tb05284.x PMID:6265597

Page, V. J., Ely, E. W., Gates, S., Zhao, X. B., Alce, T., Shintani, A., & McAuley, D. F. et al. (2013). Effect of intravenous haloperidol on the duration of delirium and coma in critically ill patients (Hope-ICU): A randomised, double-blind, placebo-controlled trial. *Lancet Respiratory Medicine*, *1*(7), 515–523. doi:10.1016/S2213-2600(13)70166-8 PMID:24461612

Pandharipande, P., Pun, B. T., Herr, D. L., Maze, M., Girard, T. D., Miller, R. R., & Ely, E. W. et al. (2007). Effect of sedation with dexmedetomidine vs. lorazepam on acute brain dysfunction in mechanically ventilated patients: The MENDS randomized controlled trial. *Journal of the American Medical Association*, *298*(22), 2644–2653. doi:10.1001/jama.298.22.2644 PMID:18073360

Pandharipande, P., Shintani, A., Peterson, J., Pun, B. T., Wilkinson, G. R., Dittus, R. S., & Ely, E. W. et al. (2006). Lorazepam is an independent risk factor for transitioning to delirium in intensive care unit patients. *Anesthesiology*, *104*(1), 21–26. doi:10.1097/00000542-200601000-00005 PMID:16394685

Pasin, L., Greco, T., Feltracco, P., Vittorio, A., Neto, C. N., Cabrini, L., & Zangrillo, A. et al. (2013). Dexmedetomidine as a sedative agent in critically ill patients: A meta-analysis of randomized controlled trials. *PLoS ONE*, *8*(12), e82913. doi:10.1371/journal.pone.0082913 PMID:24391726

Payen, J. F., Bru, O., Bosson, J. L., Lagrasta, A., Novel, E., Deschaux, I., & Jacquot, C. et al. (2001). Assessing pain in critically ill sedated patients by using a behavioral pain scale. *Critical Care Medicine*, *29*(12), 2258–2263. doi:10.1097/00003246-200112000-00004 PMID:11801819

Popping, D. M., Elia, N., Marret, E., Remy, C., & Tramer, M. R. (2008). Protective effects of epidural analgesia on pulmonary complications after abdominal and thoracic surgery: A meta-analysis. *Archives of Surgery*, *143*(10), 990–999. doi:10.1001/archsurg.143.10.990 PMID:18936379

Rafiq, S., Steinbrüchel, D. A., Wanscher, M. J., Andersen, L. W., Navne, A., Lilleoer, N. B., & Olsen, P. S. (2014). Multimodal analgesia versus traditional opiate based analgesia after cardiac surgery, a randomized controlled trial. *Journal of Cardiothoracic Surgery*, *9*(1), 52. doi:10.1186/1749-8090-9-52 PMID:24650125

Richardson, J., Lonnqvist, P. A., & Naja, Z. (2011). Bilateral thoracic paravertebral block: Potential and practice. *British Journal of Anaesthesia*, *106*(2), 164–171. doi:10.1093/bja/aeq378 PMID:21233114

Riker, R. R., & Fraser, G. L. (2001). Monitoring sedation, agitation, analgesia, neuromuscular blockade, and delirium in adult ICU patients. *Seminars in Respiratory and Critical Care Medicine*, *22*(02), 189–198. doi:10.1055/s-2001-13832 PMID:16088673

Riker, R. R., Shehabi, Y., Bokesch, P. M., Ceraso, D., Wisemandle, W., Koura, F., & Rocha, M. G. et al. (2009). Dexmedetomidine vs. midazolam for sedation of critically ill patients: A randomized trial. *Journal of the American Medical Association*, *301*, 489–499. doi:10.1001/jama.2009.56 PMID:19188334

Roberts, F. L., Dixon, J., Lewis, G. T., Tackley, R. M., & Prys-Roberts, C. (1988). Induction and maintenance of propofol anaesthesia. *Anaesthesia*, *43*(s1), 14–17. doi:10.1111/j.1365-2044.1988.tb09061.x PMID:3259089

Rosa, G., Conti, G., Orsi, P., D'Alessandro, F., La Rosa, I., DiGiugno, G., & Gasparetto, A. (1992). Effects of low-dose propofol administration on central respiratory drive, gas exchanges and respiratory pattern. *Acta Anaesthesiologica Scandinavica*, *36*(2), 128–131. doi:10.1111/j.1399-6576.1992.tb03438.x PMID:1549931

Rouby, J. J., Eurin, B., Glaser, P., Guillosson, J. J., Nafziger, J., Guesde, R., & Viars, P. (1981). Hemodynamic and metabolic effects of morphine in the critically ill. *Circulation*, *64*(1), 53–59. doi:10.1161/01.CIR.64.1.53 PMID:7237725

Ruggeri, L., Landoni, G., Guarrancino, F., Scolletta, S., Bignami, E., & Zangrillo, A. (2011). Remifentanil in critically ill cardiac patients. *Annals of Cardiac Anaesthesia*, *14*, 6–12. PMID:21196668

Saczynski, J. S., Marcantonio, E. R., Quach, L., Fong, T. G., Gross, A., Inouye, S. K., & Jones, R. N. (2012). Cognitive trajectories after postoperative delirium. *The New England Journal of Medicine, 367*(1), 30–39. doi:10.1056/NEJMoa1112923 PMID:22762316

Sanford, T. J. Jr, Smith, N. T., Dec-Silver, H., & Harrison, W. K. (1986). A comparison of morphine, fentanyl, and sufentanil anesthesia for cardiac surgery: Induction, emergence, and extubation. *Anesthesia and Analgesia, 65*(3), 259–266. doi:10.1213/00000539-198603000-00007 PMID:2937352

Schultz, J. E., Hsu, A. K., & Gross, G. J. (1996). Morphine mimics the cardioprotective effect of ischemic preconditioning via a glibenclamide-sensitive mechanism in the rat heart. *Circulation Research, 78*(6), 1100–1104. doi:10.1161/01.RES.78.6.1100 PMID:8635241

Schwartz, D. A., & Horwitz, L. D. (n.d.). Effects of ketamine on left ventricular performance. *The Journal of Pharmacology and Experimental Therapeutics, 194*, 410–414. PMID:1151766

Searle, N. R., & Sahab, P. (1993). Propofol in patients with cardiac disease. *Canadian Journal of Anesthesiology, 40*(8), 730–747. doi:10.1007/BF03009770 PMID:8403158

Sendelbach, S. E., Halm, M. A., Doran, K. A., Miller, E. H., & Gaillard, P. (2006). Effects of music therapy on physiological and psychological outcomes for patients undergoing cardiac surgery. *The Journal of Cardiovascular Nursing, 21*(3), 194–200. doi:10.1097/00005082-200605000-00007 PMID:16699359

Senturk, M., Ozcan, P. E., Talu, G. K., Kiyan, E., Camci, E., Ozyalcin, S., & Pembeci, K. et al. (2002). The effects of three different analgesia techniques on long-term postthoracotomy pain. *Anesthesia and Analgesia, 94*(1), 11–15. doi:10.1213/00000539-200201000-00003 PMID:11772793

Sessler, C. N., Gosnell, M. S., Grap, M. J., Brophy, G. M., O'Neal, P. V., Keane, K. A., & Elswick, R. K. et al. (2002). The Richmond agitation-sedation scale: Validity and reliability in adult intensive care unit patients. *American Journal of Respiratory and Critical Care Medicine, 166*(10), 1338–1344. doi:10.1164/rccm.2107138 PMID:12421743

Sessler, C. N., Grap, M. J., & Ramsay, M. A. E. (2009). Evaluating and monitoring analgesia and sedation in the intensive care unit. *Critical Care (London, England), 12*, 1–13. doi:10.1186/cc6147 PMID:18495053

Shapiro, A., Zohar, E., Zaslansky, R., Hoppenstein, D., Shabat, S., & Fredman, B. (2005). The frequency and timing of respiratory depression in 1524 postoperative patients treated with systemic or neuraxial morphine. *Journal of Clinical Anesthesia, 17*(7), 536–542. doi:10.1016/j.jclinane.2005.01.006 PMID:16297754

Shehabi, Y., Grant, P., Wolfenden, H., Hammond, N., Bass, F., Campbell, M., & Chen, J. (2009). Prevalence of delirium with dexmedetomidine compared with morphine based therapy after cardiac surgery: A randomized controlled trial (DEXmedetomidine COmpared to Morphine-DEXCOM Study). *Anesthesiology, 111*(5), 1075–1084. doi:10.1097/ALN.0b013e3181b6a783 PMID:19786862

Soliman, M. G., Brinale, G. F., & Kuster, G. (1975). Response to hypercapnia under ketamine anaesthesia. *Canadian Anaesthetists' Society Journal, 22*(4), 486–494. doi:10.1007/BF03004864 PMID:1139389

Stephan, H., Sonntag, H., Schenk, H. D., Kettler, D., & Khambatta, H. J. (1986). Effects of propofol on cardiovascular dynamics, myocardial blood flow and myocardial metabolism in patients with coronary artery disease. *British Journal of Anaesthesia*, *58*(9), 969–975. doi:10.1093/bja/58.9.969 PMID:3489478

Stoelting, R. K. (1981). Hemodynamic effects of barbiturates and benzodiazepines. *Cleveland Clinic Journal of Medicine*, *48*(1), 9–13. doi:10.3949/ccjm.48.1.9 PMID:7261393

Strøm, T., Martinussen, T., & Toft, P. (2010). A protocol of no sedation for critically ill patients receiving mechanical ventilation: A randomised trial. *Lancet*, *375*(9713), 475–480. doi:10.1016/S0140-6736(09)62072-9 PMID:20116842

Svircevic, V., Passier, M. M., Nierich, A. P., van Dijk, D., Kalkman, C. J., & van der Heijden, G. J. (2013). Epidural analgesia for cardiac surgery. *Cochrane Database of Systematic Reviews*, *6*, CD006715. PMID:23740694

Thomson, I. R., Harding, G., & Hudson, R. J. (2000). A comparison of fentanyl and sufentanil in patients undergoing coronary artery bypass surgery. *Journal of Cardiothoracic and Vascular Anesthesia*, *14*(6), 652–656. doi:10.1053/jcan.2000.18307 PMID:11139103

Tjia, M. W., & Gitlin, D. F. (2010). Use of antipsychotics in medically ill patients. In A. J. Rothschild (Ed.), *The evidence-based guide to antipsychotic medications* (pp. 215–243). Arlington, VA: American Psychiatric Publishing.

Trettin, A., Böhmer, A., Suchy, M. T., Probst, I., Staerk, U., & Stichtenoth, D. O. … Tsikas, D. (2014). Effects of paracetamol on NOS, COX, and CYP activity and on oxidative stress in healthy male subjects, rat hepatocytes, and recombinant NOS. *Oxidative Medicine and Cellular Longevity*. doi:10.1155/2014/212576 PMID:24799980

Tweed, W. A., Minuck, M., & Mymin, D. (1972). Circulatory responses to ketamine anesthesia. *Anesthesiology*, *37*(6), 613–619. doi:10.1097/00000542-197212000-00008 PMID:4652778

Van Gulik, L., Ahlers, S. J., Brkic, Z., Belitser, S. V., van Boven, W. J., van Dongen, E. P., & Bruins, P. et al. (2010). Improved analgesia after the realisation of a pain management programme in ICU patients after cardiac surgery. *European Journal of Anaesthesiology*, *27*(10), 900–905. doi:10.1097/EJA.0b013e32833d91c3 PMID:20848698

Venn, R. M., Hell, J., & Grounds, R. M. (2000). Respiratory effects of dexmedetomidine in the surgical patient requiring intensive care. *Critical Care (London, England)*, *4*(5), 302–308. doi:10.1186/cc712 PMID:11056756

Veroli, P., O'Kelly, B., Bertrand, F., Trouvin, J. H., Farinotti, R., & Ecoffey, C. (1992). Extrahepatic metabolism of propofol in man during the anhepatic phase of orthotopic liver transplantation. *British Journal of Anaesthesia*, *68*(2), 183–186. doi:10.1093/bja/68.2.183 PMID:1540462

Wang, W., Li, H., Wang, D., Zhu, X., Li, S., Yao, G., & Zhu, S. et al. (2012). Haloperidol prophylaxis decreases delirium incidence in elderly patients after noncardiac surgery: A randomized controlled trial. *Critical Care Medicine*, *40*(3), 731–739. doi:10.1097/CCM.0b013e3182376e4f PMID:22067628

Whelton, A., & Hamilton, C. W. (1991). Nonsteroidal anti-inflammatory drugs: Effects on kidney function. *Journal of Clinical Pharmacology*, *31*(7), 588–598. doi:10.1002/j.1552-4604.1991.tb03743.x PMID:1894754

White, P. F., Way, W. L., & Trevor, A. J. (1982). Ketamine- its pharmacology and therapeutic uses. *Anesthesiology*, *56*(2), 119–136. doi:10.1097/00000542-198202000-00007 PMID:6892475

Wirz, S., Wartenberg, H. C., & Nadstawek, J. (2008). Less nausea, emesis, and constipation comparing hydromorphone and morphine? A prospective open-labeled investigation on cancer pain. *Supportive Care in Cancer*, *16*(9), 999–1009. doi:10.1007/s00520-007-0368-y PMID:18095008

Wolf, A., Weir, P., Segar, P., Stone, J., & Shield, J. (2001). Impaired fatty acid oxidation in propofol infusion syndrome. *Lancet*, *357*(9256), 306–307. doi:10.1016/S0140-6736(00)04064-2 PMID:11558490

Yoshioka, M., Mori, T., Kobayashi, H., Iwatani, K., Yoshimoto, K., Terasaki, H., & Nomori, H. (2006). The efficacy of epidural analgesia after video-assisted thoracoscopic surgery: A randomized control study. *Annals of Thoracic and Cardiovascular Surgery*, *12*, 313–318. PMID:17095972

Zhu, F., Lee, A., & Chee, Y.E. (2012). Fast-track cardiac care for adult cardiac surgical patients. *Cochrane Database of Systematic Reviews, Oct 17*, 10:CD003587.

ADDITIONAL READING

Papadakos, P. J., & Compolo, F. (2011). Sedation in the ICU: Shifts and strategies. *Anesthesiology News*, *37*, 1–12.

Rowe, K., & Fletcher, S. (2008). Sedation in the intensive care unit. *Continuing Education in Anaesthesia, Critical Care, and Pain*, *8*(2), 50–55. doi:10.1093/bjaceaccp/mkn005

KEY TERMS AND DEFINITIONS

Analgesic: An agent or technique that provides relief from painful sensations.

Cardiothoracic: Of or pertaining to the heart, lungs, or other intrathoracic organs.

Cardiothoracic Intensive Care Unit: An ICU providing specialized preoperative and postoperative care for patients undergoing cardiothoracic surgery.

Context-Sensitive Half-Time: The time required for blood levels of a drug to drop by 50%, which may be due to redistribution, metabolism, or elimination, and which may vary after different durations of drug infusion.

Delirium: A multifactorial syndrome characterized by acute onset, a fluctuating course, as well as possible attentional deficits and an altered level of consciousness.

Elimination Half-Life: The time required for blood levels of a drug to drop by 50% due to elimination from the body.

Intensive Care Unit: Specialized hospital unit wherein patients are cared for who require support of vital organ functions, including those suffering from respiratory, circulatory, and renal failure.

Opioid: One of a class of analgesics related to naturally-derived opium.

Regional Analgesia: A technique by which analgesia is provided through blockade or modulation of afferent pain signals, not via systemic medications.

Sedative: A medication that induces a depressed level of consciousness.

Chapter 13
Vasodilating Agents

Shreyajit R. Kumar
Weill Cornell Medical College, USA

Andrew Sosa
Weill Cornell Medical College, USA

Ilan Margulis
Weill Cornell Medical College, USA

ABSTRACT

This chapter discusses the salient features of arterial and venous dilating agents commonplace in the management of the post-cardiotomy surgical patient. A keen understanding of the underlying cellular mechanism, pharmacology, indication, safety profile, and controversies of clinical utility of vasodilating agents is imperative for routine use. The evidenced-based examination of each therapeutic modality will strengthen the practitioner's fund of knowledge for management of each pathophysiological state.

INTRODUCTION

Vasodilating agents have a wide scope of therapeutic utility both intraoperatively and in the ICU setting. The rapid onset of vasodilators aide in treatment of aneurysm propagation, aneurysm dissection, and hypertensive crises. Pulmonary vasodilators are the crux of right-heart support with provision of inotropy, decreasing right ventricular preload, and decreasing pulmonary vascular resistance.

Intraoperatively, vasodilator-mediated hypotensive anesthetic technique preserves chief quality outcome measures. Bodies of evidence demonstrate 2-4 fold reduction of intraoperative blood loss(Sharrock, 1998), 50% reduction of in-hospital transfusion, decreased intraoperative time (Dolman, Bentley & Head, 2000).

Vasodilator drugs are classified based upon their site of activity. Dilation of the capacitance – venous – system will reduce preload, allowing an unloading of the myocardium. Decreased wall tension reduces myocardial oxygen demand, and optimizes overall Starling function. Dilation of the resistance – arteriole – system results in afterload reduction, improving effective myocardial contractility. The net result is augmentation of stroke volume and cardiac output.

DOI: 10.4018/978-1-4666-8603-8.ch013

MOLECULAR MECHANISMS: SMOOTH MUSCLE

Vascular smooth muscle constriction is dependent upon the translation of the synaptic action potential to muscle tension. Excitation-coupling describes the rise of intracellular calcium following receptor interaction with a neurotransmitter. Intracellular calcium rises trifold (see figure 1): (i) direct influx through voltage-gated calcium channels, (ii) g-protein ligand gated calcium channels, and (iii) IP3-phospholipase system. The latter, GTP binding protein – G Protein – is activated, and couples with phospholipase C to upregulate IP3 (inositol 1,4,5-triphosphate) production (Costanzo, 2014). The net effect is increased intracellular Calcium, liberated from the sarcoplasmic reticulum. Intracellular calcium-calmodulin complexes activate myosin cross-bridges, resulting in vasoconstriction. Increased systemic vascular resistance leads to a higher afterload and mean arterial pressure, and a parasympathetic bradycardic reflex. Alpha-receptor antagonism (*e.g.* phentolamine) perturbs intracellular calcium release, lowering overall systemic vascular resistance in a vasodilated state.

Figure 1. Trifold mechanism that increases intracellular smooth muscle calcium
This figure was published in Physiology, Fifth Edition. Costanzo, Linda. Figure 1-30 Mechanisms for increasing intracellular [Ca2+] in smooth muscle. Copyright Elsevier 2014.

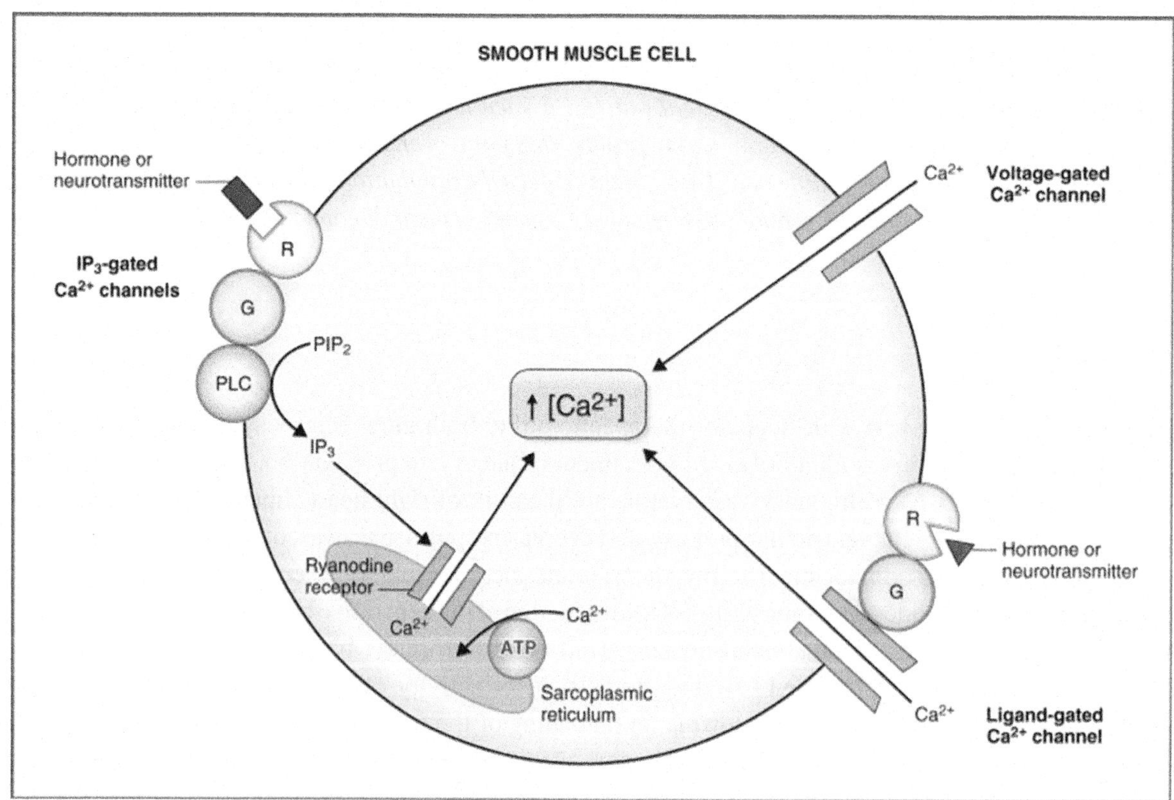

MOLECULAR MECHANISMS: MYOCARDIAL CONTRACTILITY AND AUTOMATICITY

Myocardial contractility is intimately dependent upon the excitation-coupling of cardiac action potential with intracellular calcium accumulation. Action potentials in the atrium, ventricular purkinje fibers, and sinoatrial nodes (Costanzo, 2014, see figure 2) involve four distinct phases of ion exchange (see table 1). Initial inward sodium flow results in rapid ventricular depolarization to +20mV. Long acting (L-type) calcium channels modulate a plateau phase and increased contractility. Myocardial tension is directly proportional to intracellular calcium concentrations. Repolarization to resting membrane potential is governed by potassium counterflow. Phase configuration varies in sinoatrial pacemaker cells, where a plateau – phase 2 – is absent, and the depolarization – phase 4 – dominates; this is the chief determinant of automaticity and heart rate.

Thus, L-channel calcium-channel blockade (*e.g.* diltiazem, verapamil) affect both myocyte arrhythmogenicity and vascular smooth muscle dilation.

MOLECULAR MECHANISMS: NITRIC OXIDE

Furchgott, Ignarro and Murad were jointly awarded the 1998 Nobel Prize in Medicine for their elucidation of nitric oxide (NO) mediated vasodilation in the late 1970s. The end-product of the NO system is upregulation of cyclic GMP (cGMP), which modulates smooth muscle vasodilation. Exogenous nitrates (nitroglycerin, isosorbide dinitrate) stimulate reduction of nitrate groups from S-nitrosothiol to form nitric oxide (NO). Endogenous NO is produced from the interaction of nitric oxide synthetase (NOS) and L-arginine at the smooth muscle endothelium. Two endothelial types of NOS exist – constitutive (cNOS) and inducible (iNOS). cNOS ("physiologic") represents a tonic response to shear forces from blood flow and vasoactive substances. iNOS ("pathologic") represents a phasic response from inflammation, endotoxin, and cytokine release (Klabunde, 2012, see figure 3). Septic states may increase NO

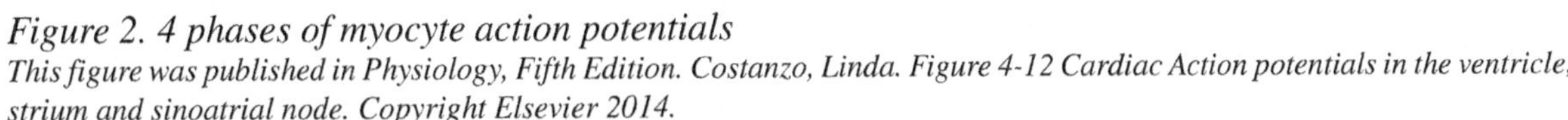

Figure 2. 4 phases of myocyte action potentials
This figure was published in Physiology, Fifth Edition. Costanzo, Linda. Figure 4-12 Cardiac Action potentials in the ventricle, strium and sinoatrial node. Copyright Elsevier 2014.

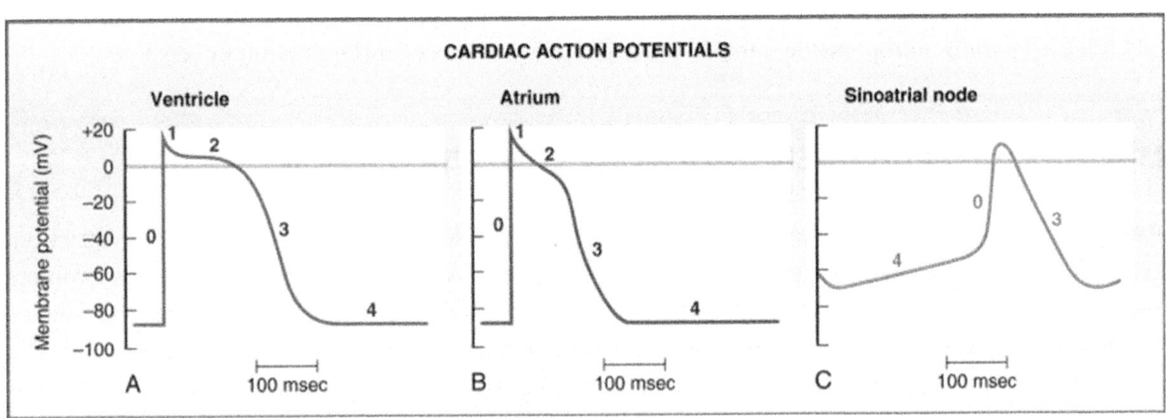

Table 1. 4 phases of myocyte action potentials

Phase	Activity	Dominant Current	Location
Phase 0	Upstroke	Na^+ influx	Ventricle, Atrium, SA node fibers
Phase 1	Initial Repolarization	K^+ efflux	Ventricle, Atrium fibers
Phase 2	Plateau	K^+ efflux = Ca^{2+} influx	Ventricle, Atrium Fibers
Phase 3	Repolarization	K^+ efflux	Ventricle, Atrium, SA node fibers
Phase 4	Resting membrane potential depolarization		Ventricle, Atrium, SA node fibers

Figure 3. Mechanism of NO-mediated cGMP upregulation
www.cvpharmacology.com, www.cvphysiology.com

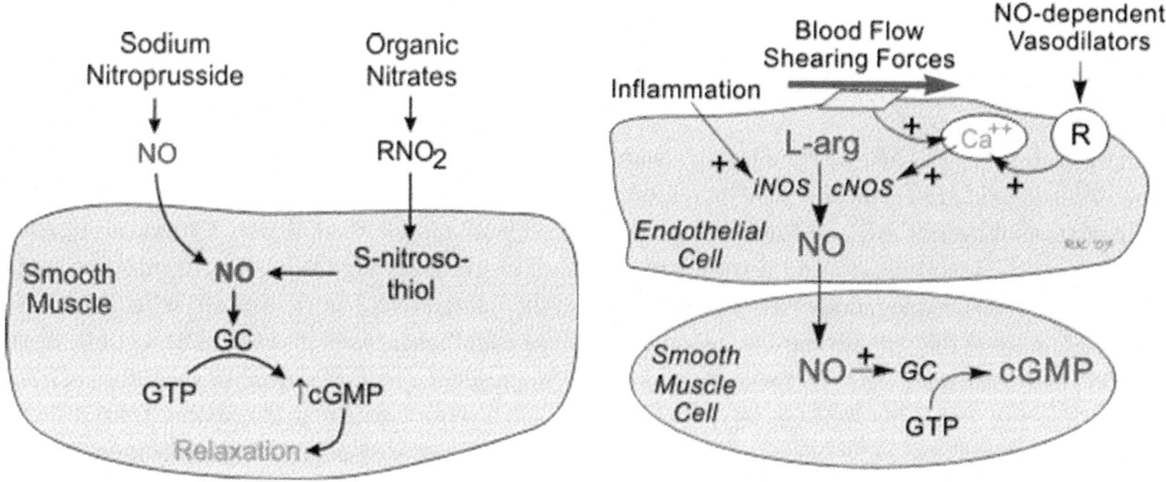

production from iNOS a thousand-fold, accounting for brisk decrease of systemic vascular resistance. Phosphodiesterase-5 will hydrolyze and inactivate cGMP. Thus, vasodilation may be maintained by PDE-5 inhibition (sildenafil, tadalafil), organic nitrates (nitroglycerin, isosorbide dinitrate), spontaneous NO release (sodium nitroprusside, inhaled nitric oxide), or states of inflammation or sepsis.

MOLECULAR MECHANISMS: PULMONARY HYPERTENSION

Panvasculopathy of pulmonary artery hypertension involves endothelial dysfunction, vasoconstriction, excess fibroproliferation and right ventricular dysfunction. Anatomically, these processes promote "onion-skinned", concentric thickened, intimal lesions; a net increase in pulmonary vascular resistance (Archer, Weir & Wilkins 2010). Pulmonary vascular modulation involves several distinct pathways. The vasodilator/antiproliferative pathway is regulated twofold: by cGMP (see figure 3) and cAMP. Prostacyclin promotes adenylate cyclase activity, cAMP production, and vascular relaxation. The Endothelin pathway causes potent vasoconstriction, via ET_A smooth muscle receptors. Working in an opposing fashion, ET_B receptors stimulate release of prostacyclin, NO, and vasodilation (Davies, 2008, see figure 4). PAH carries a 15% mortality rate, despite targeted vasodilatory and antiproliferative therapies. A keen understanding of these therapeutic agents augments the care of the post-cardiotomy patient.

Classification of Pulmonary Arterial Hypertension was recently modified during the 2013 Fifth World Symposium in Nice, France. The major consensus was to include the pediatric population, common with the adult classification (Galiè & Simonneau, 2013). The etiologies of pulmonary hypertension are: primary arterial hypertension, hypertension secondary to left heart disease, hypertension secondary to pulmonary disease, chronic thromboembolic pulmonary hypertension, and hypertension from unclear etiology (see Table 2).

NITROPRUSSIDE

Sodium nitroprusside directly dilates both arterial and venous vessels. Its complex molecular structure consists of a ferrous ion surrounded by a nitrosyl group and five cyanide moieties. Both venous and

Figure 4. Modulation of pulmonary vasculature
Davies, R, et al. "Molecular Mechanisms of Pulmonary Arterial Hypertension: Role of Mutations in the Bone Morphogenetic Protein Type II Receptor". Chest (2008) 134.6

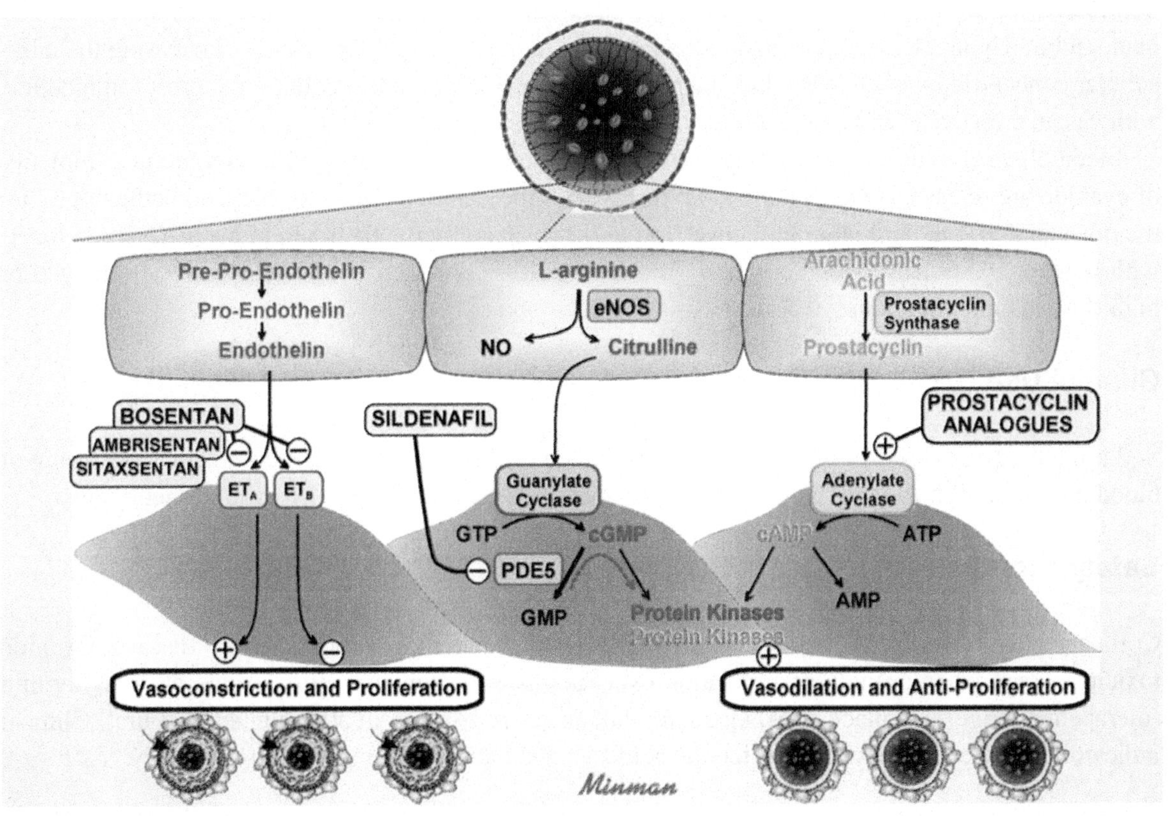

Table 2. WHO classification of pulmonary hypertension

WHO Classification	Pulmonary Hypertension Etiology	Example
I	Pulmonary arterial hypertension	Idiopathic, heritable, connective tissue disorder, HIV, schistosomiasis
II	Left heart Disease	LV dysfunction, valvular dysfunction, congenital cardiomyopathies
III	Lung disease/hypoxia	COPD, interstitial lung disease, OSA, high-altitude,
IV	Chronic Thromboembolic Pulmonary Hypertension	CTEPH
V	Multifactorial/unclear	Hematologic disorders, metabolic disorders: glycogen storage disease, Gaucher disease

Adapted from Galiè N, Simonneau G. (2013). Updated Clinical Classification of Pulmonary Hypertension. *J Am Coll Cardiol.* 62, 25_S

arterial vasculature are responsive to Nitroprusside, with a pronounced effect upon the arteriole system. Sodium Nitroprusside has a short half life and is only available in IV preparation, thus usually used as an infusion and titrated to effect.

Pharmacology

Sodium Nitroprusside binds to oxyhemoglobin in circulation to release nitric oxide, cyanide and met-hemoglobin. Upon release, nitric oxide activates smooth muscle guanylate cyclase, increasing the intra-cellular concentration of cGMP, which increases vascular smooth muscle dilation. Onset is immediate, with vascular recovery within 1-2 minutes of discontinuation.

Metabolism of sodium nitroprusside starts with the interaction of the drug with hemoglobin. 5 moieties of cyanide are released. One cyanide atom reacts with methemoglobin to form cyanomethemoglobin; the other moieties are available for conversion to thiocyanate by the liver and kidneys. Cyanide reacts with hepatic and renal rhodonase which facilitates its excretion as urinary thiocyanate. Prolonged or high-dose administration increase the risk of cyanide toxicity.

Clinical Use

Sodium Nitroprusside is commonly used in medical emergencies which require immediate lowering of blood pressure, such as acute hypertensive urgency/emergency and aortic dissections/aneurysms.

Safety Profile

Coronary steal phenomena may occur in patients with significant coronary artery disease. Cyanide toxicity occurs when cyanide accumulation overwhelms excretion. An infusion rate of 2mcg/kg/min (therapeutic range) will place an 80 kg adult adult at risk of toxicity in 500 minutes (8.3 hrs). Clinical indicators include tachyphylaxis, metabolic acidosis, and increased mixed venous oximetry.

Treatment of cyanide toxicity begins with administration of 100% oxygen. Amyl Nitrate and Sodium nitrate promotes cyanide binding to methhemoglobin, and excretion as cyanomethemoglobin. Thiosulfate and Hydroxycobalamin (vitamin B12) facilitates inactivation to urinary thiocyanate and cyanocobalamin, respectively.

Controversies

The misconcenception that cyanide toxicity is a frequent complication has been perpetuated in clinical practice. In 1987, 3,000 cases per year and 1,000 deaths per year of SNP cyanide toxicity in post-cardiac surgery patients were estimated (Sarvotham, 1987). A 2010 meta-analysis of 50 trials (approximately 4100 patients) reported an incidence of SNP-related adverse events of only 1.8%, and a scant mortality rate of 0.6% (Lockwood, Patka & Rabinovich, 2010).

Recent data has challenged the understanding that overwhelming a patients' rhodonase stores - and ability to create thiocyanate - results in cyanide toxicity. This toxic dose of SNP was based on measurements of cyanide and thiocyanate concentrations. Evidence now supports a second enzyme system (mercaptopyruvate sulfurtransferase), and several other chemical pathways that inactivate cyanide (Westley, Alder & Westley, 1983). Hence, patients have a more comprehensive ability to clear cyanide, than once believed.

Novel monitoring using lactate as a surrogate for cyanide toxicity, has been successfully reported. A prospective trial of 39 smoke-inhalation victims, lactate concentrations > 10 mmol/L had high sensitivity and specificity for cyanide intoxication (Baud, Borron, Mégarbane, 2002). Further literature supports base excess, in addition to lactate, as markers of acute cyanide toxicity; especially where resources limit the measurement of serum cyanide. Attention to tachyphylaxis, serum lactate levels, and development of a lactic acidosis, will all aide in safe use of sodium nitroprusside, as a first line agent in hypertensive emergencies.

Recently, Nitroprusside has been been implemented in many arenas not previously used in. It has been estimated that even after successful percutaneous coronary intervention, myocardial perfusion may remain compromised and regional myocardial dysfunction may still persist. A 781 patient meta-analysis investigated the use of intracoronary Nitroprusside injection in reducing the amount of no-reflow post intervention. This study demonstrated improved flow in the group of patients who received Nitroprusside, though did not find statistical significance, warranting further investigation. Interestingly, no adverse effects commonly described with nitroprusside use were reported in any of the studies examined (Zhao, Qi & Tian, 2014).

HYDRALAZINE

Hydralazine selectively dilates arterial blood vessels, in a fashion similar to organic nitrates.

Pharmacology

The exact mechanism by which hydralazine causes arterial vasodilation is poorly understood, aside from its effect upon activation of potassium-gated channels on vascular smooth muscle. Potassium efflux results in myocyte hyperpolarization and vasodilation. Other postulated effects include inhibition of intracellular calcium release, and nitric oxide-mediated cGMP vasodilation.

Clinical Use

Hydralazine is utilized in the treatment of arterial hypertension and congestive heart failure. Baroreceptor-induced reflex tachycardia precludes hydralazine use as a first-line antihypertensive agent. It is commonly used in conjunction with a beta-blocker to mitigate this effect. Hydralazine may also increase fluid retention by plasma renin upregulation. Thus, concominant diuretic use is prudent in the heart failure patient.

Fixed dose isosorbide dinitrate and hydralazine reduced heart failure mortality among black patients in the African-American Heart-Failure Trial (AHeFT). Hydralazine – a potent antioxidant – is postulated to decrease nitric oxide consumption by reactive oxygen species, which improves both vasorelaxation and remodeling. The AHeFT trial reported improved LV ejection fraction, and reduction of LV mass (Taylor, Ziesche & Yancy, 2004). Further investigation has hinted at functional improvements in diastolic dysfunction and exercise capacity is due to extracardiac effects, namely vasculature dilation.

Safety Profile

Common side effects include headache, drug-induced lupus and reflex tachycardia.

PHENTOLAMINE

Phentolamine is an alpha-1 and alpha-2 receptor antagonist. Its chief alpha-1 antagonism causes arterial vasodilation.

Pharmacology

Vascular smooth muscle is innervated by the autonomic nervous system – V1a, alpha and beta receptors. Alpha-1 receptor antagonism inhibits G-protein synthesis, IP3 signal transduction, and myosin chain activity. Smooth muscle contriction is prevented, resulting in arterial vasodilation.

Clinical Use

Phentolamine is commonly employed in cocaine-induced hemodynamic perturbations, when beta-blockade will cause unopposed alpha-mediated vasoconstriction. Patients with a pheochromocytoma benefit from phentolamine as a first-line anti-hypertensive agent. Phentolamine also will counteract the effects of extravasated vasopressor infusion, to prevent severe vasoconstriction.

Controversies

Preoperative control of hypertension has been long indoctrinated to decrease mortality in patients undergoing removal of a pheochromocytoma. A 48-year cohort of 108 patients established a 23-fold decrease of complications – 69% to 3% – from the use of antihypertensives (Goldstein, O'Neill & Holcomb, 1999). However, this timeframe encompasses a tremendous shift in surgical technique. After 1979, midline abdominal incision replaced a thoracoabdominal approach; since 1998, laparoscopic resection has become a mainstay practice. Recent literature has focused upon intraoperative, rather than preoperative, hemodynamic control. A 2009 study on 96 pheochromocytoma patients undergoing adrenalectomy, demonstrated preoperative hypertension was not predictive of intraoperative and postoperative hemodynamic instability (Lentschener, Gaujoux & Thillois, 2009). A retrospective practice evaluation deemed preoperative alpha-blockade redundant, emphasizing intraoperative control of hemodynamic instability. Plasma catecholamine release occurs during all phases of adrenalectomy – induction of general anesthesia, tracheal intubation, intrathoracic positive pressure administration, intraabdominal insufflation, and direct tumor manipulation. Optimal control of these hemodynamic perturbations should be achieved by increasing anesthetic depth, maintaining adequate muscle relaxation, intravascular fluid resuscitation, and judicious use of vasodilating agents. Systematic control of this hypertensive surgical response has replaced the prior emphasis on preoperative hemodynamic control.

Safety Profile

Headache, reflex tachycardia and orthostatic hypotension are common side effects. This effect is secondary to alpha 2 inhibition.

MINOXIDIL

Minoxidil is an arterial vasodilator which activated vascular smooth-muscle potassium channels. It is a second-line antihypertensive agent, and first-line treatment of alopecia; minoxidil will retard hair loss and promote follicular growth.

Pharmacology

Vascular smooth muscle is clad with potassium channels. Activation of these potassium channels leads to smooth muscle hyperpolarization, calcium channel closing, and decreased intracellular calcium concentration. Arterial vasodilation occurs from minimal myosin light chain activation.

Clinical Use

Due to its side effect profile, Minoxidil is not commonly employed as first line antihypertensive agents, utilized instead for refractory hypertension. Chronic use has been documented to result in positive cardiovascular changes – increases in end-diastolic volume and cardiac output. 2% - 5% Minoxidil solution was formulated to treat male pattern baldness and female baldness. Minoxidil also leads to hypertrichosis – an increased body hair pigmentation.

Safety Profile

Minoxidil can cause headaches, facial swelling and flushing. Patients commonly develop a reflex tachycardia secondary to a drop in blood pressure; this limits Minoxidil use in patients with coronary artery disease. Sodium and water retention may also occur, thus often prescribed with a loop diuretic. Oral Minoxidil has been linked to subendocardial papillary muscle necrosis, myocardial infarction and psueudoacromegaly (Nguyen & Marks, 2003). The alcohol and propylene glycol in topical formulations may result in dermatitis and dandruff. Case reports exist of pericardial effusions and tamponade physiology in patients taking mioxidil (Çilingiroğlu, Akkuş & Sethi, 2014). One such anecdote describes a patient treated supportively for a pericardial effusion, ultimately resolving upon minoxidil discontinuation.

CALCIUM CHANNEL BLOCKER – DIHYDROPRIDINE CLASS: AMLODIPINE, NICARDIPINE, NIFEDIPINE, NIMODIPINE

Calcium channels dispersed throughout vascular smooth muscle are targets for many pharmacological agents. These channels are also found on cardiac myocytes and nodal tissue. These drugs primarily affect arterial resistance vessels, with only minimal effects on venous capacitance vessels.

There are different classes of calcium channel blockers, which describe the relative selectivity of the agents for their target. Dihydropyridines target L-type calcium channels found on vascular smooth muscle and decrease mean arterial pressure. Other calcium channel blockers target cardiac myocytes and nodal tissue (Katz, 1996, see table 3).

Pharmacology

Calcium channels regulate the influx of calcium into the cell, regulating the state of vascular constriction. Calcium channel blockers block the influx of calcium into the cell. By blocking the influx of calcium into the cell, these agents lead to vascular smooth muscle dilation and a decrease in systemic vascular resistance.

Clinical Use

Amlodipine is long-acting dihydropyridine channel blocker, and is utilized in the management of hypertension and coronary artery disease.

Nicardipine is a dihydropyridine channel blocker, with a higher selectivity for coronary and cerebral vasculature. It is used in hypertension, stable angina, and Raynaud's phenomena.

Table 3. Diversity of calcium channel blockade

	Class	Heart Rate	Depression of AV/SA node conduction	Peripheral Vasodilation	Inotropic Effect	Coronary Artery Dilation
Verapamil	phenylalkylamine	-	++	+	Moderate negative	+
Diltiazem	benzothiazepine	-	+	+	Mild negative	+
Nifedipine	dihydropridine	+(rebound)	Minimal	++	None/minor negative	++
Nicardipine	dihydropridine	+(rebound)	None	++	None	+
Nimodipine	dihydropridine	None	None	0/+	None	None
Amlodipine	dihydropridine	None	None	++	Negative	+

Nifedipine primarily blocks L-type dihydropyridine channels. It is principally used in hypertensive emergencies, angina pectoris and Prinzmetal's angina, Raynaud's phenomena and tocolysis of premature labor.

Nimodipine is a dihydropyridine blocker. It is an antihypertensive, primarily used in prevention of cerebral vasospasm after subarachnoid hemorrhage

Safety Profile

Amlodipine is contraindicated in pregnancy. It is metabolized by the cytochrome p450 system, and should be used in caution in hepatic impairment, and with concominant use of any CYP4A-interacting agents. It causes peripheral edema, fatigue, flushing and palpitations. Less frequently, amlodipine may result in ginigival hyperplasia and gynecomastia.

Nicardipine may cause increased pedal edema, angina, tachycardia, postural hypotension. It should be used with caution in patients with an acute cerebral ischemia or hemorrhage, and in patients with hepatic impairment.

Nifedipine has caused reflex tachycardia, peripheral edema, dizziness, and should be used in caution with concominant use of any CYP4A-interacting agents.

Nimodipine has caused reflex tachycardia, peripheral edema and dizziness. It is contraindicated in unstable angina.

CALCIUM CHANNEL BLOCKER – BENZOTHIAZEPINE CLASS: DILTIAZEM

Diltizaem is a benzothiazepine, a calcium channel blocking agent of the non-dihydropyridine class. It is employed in both the management of chronic and acute conditions.

Pharmacology

Diltiazem has action at both the vascular smooth muscle and the cardiac myocytes. It is a class IV antiarrhythmic, hepatically metabolized by CYP34A. It causes a decrease in blood pressure with potent peripheral vasodilator and afterload reducing effects. Diltiazem depresses AV-nodal conduction, acting as a negative chronotrope. It is also a negative inotrope, decreasing overall contractility and myocardial oxygen consumption.

Clinical Use

Diltiazem is utilized in treatment of hypertension. It is effective in treatment supraventricular tachycardia, atrial fibrillation, and atrial flutter, owing its activity upon nodal tissue. Diltiazem is indicated in angina, causing coronary vasodilation.

Safety Profile

Diltazem may result in bradycardia, hypotension and flushing. It should not be used in patients with Wolf-Parkinson's White syndrome, from increased conduction via the accessory pathway – bundle of

Kent. Diltiazem must be avoided in patients with second or third-degree AV blockade, as it will further prolong AV nodal refractory periods. It should be used with caution in patients with hepatic insufficiency.

CALCIUM CHANNEL BLOCKER – PHENYLALKYLAMINE CLASS: VERAPAMIL

Verapamil is a calcium channel blocker which is most selective for cardiac myocytes, with minority activity at the vascular smooth muscle. This calcium channel blocker is unique in its ability to act selectively on cardiac receptors, exerting effect at the cardiac nodal tissue.

Pharmacology

Verapamil is a phenylalkylamine L-type calcium channel blocker. It is a class IV antiarrhythmic, decreasing impulse conduction through the sinoatrial and atrioventricular nodes. Calcium channel blockade in vascular smooth muscle causes a decrease in peripheral tone, vasodilation, and a cessation of vasospasm. Afterload reduction will result in an overall decrease of myocardial work and oxygen demand.

Clinical Use

Verapamil is utilized in treatment of atrial tachyarrhthmia, due to its ability to retard conduction through the atrioventricular node. It decreases systemic vascular resistance, effective as an antihypertensive agent. Reflex tachycardia and orthostatic hypotension are uncommon. Verapamil dilates the coronary system, and prevents coronary vasospasm, thus efficacious in the treatment for unstable and Prinzmetal's angina. Direct arterial injection in the surgical milieu will attenuate arterial vasospasm. Verapamil is also employed in treatment of cluster headaches.

Safety Profile

Verapamil should be avoided in patients with left ventricular dysfunction – ejection fraction less than 30%. A negative inotropic effect may exacerbate pulmonary edema or congestive heart failure. Patients with Wolf-Parkinson-White syndrome, have developed increased accessory pathway conduction with rapid ventricular response or fibrillation. Verapamil will also exacerbate any preexisting atrioventricular block, and should be utilized cautiously alongside other nodal blocking agents. It is metabolized by the CP450 system, and can result in a transaminitis. Additionally, Verapamil will raise serum concentrations and bioavailability of oral Dabigatran Exilate (Pradaxa), via p-glycoprotein transporter inhibition (Härtter, Sennewald, & Nehmiz, 2013).

NITRIC OXIDE (NO)

NO is a colorless, odorless gas first discovered as a vasodilator in 1987.

Pharmocology

NO rapidly diffuses across the alveoli into the pulmonary vasculature inducing guanylate cyclase to convert GTP to cGMP. Increased levels of cGMP inhibits calcium influx, inactivates calcium channels and decreases calcium release from the sarcoplasmic reticulum. This reduction in calcium enhances smooth muscle relaxation which decreases pulmonary vascular resistance. NO is rapidly metabolized in the blood stream by oxyhemoglobin to methemoglobin and nitrate. The rapid metabolism of NO prevents it from affecting the systemic vascular resistance.

NO also decreases shunt faction when administered to patients. As an inhaled medication, it will preferentially diffuse to ventilated alveoli and dilate the accompanying vasculature, thus decreasing the overall shunt fraction.

Clinical Use

NO can be administered via nasal cannula, face mask or endotracheal tube. Typical dose ranges from 1-20 parts per million (ppm). NO should be discontinued slowly, as abrupt discontinuation can lead to rebound pulmonary hypertension. By 1988, NO was quickly adopted for acute treatment of primary pulmonary hypertension. Utility in chronic treatment of this WHO Class I patient is currently under investigation.

Safety Profile

While NO is an effective for pulmonary vasodilator, it has several side effects. Part of its metabolism is the production of methemoglobin, which may accumulate as methemoglobinemia. Elevated levels of methemoglobin will lead to increased affinity of hemoglobin for oxygen, a left shift of the oxy-hemoglobin dissociation curve, and result in tissue hypoxia. NO is oxidized to nitrogen dioxide (NO2) in air, rapidly so when delivered in 100% oxygen. NO2 may increase airway reactivity, cause pulmonary edema, and diffuse airway inflammation.

Controversies

Initial practice of treating ARDS with NO was borne from a 1993 study of 10 patients with ARDS. This investigation hypothesized that pulmonary vasodilation improved cardiac function, oxygenation and reduced extravascular lung water; inhaled NO at 18 ppm resulted in an average increase of PaO2/FiO2 of 51mm HG (Rossaint, Falke & López, 1993). By 1998, a European survey confirmed 98.5% of practitioners deemed ARDS an indication for inhaled nitric oxide (Beloucif & Paven, 1998). However, six years later, a similar Canadian questionnaire demonstrated the majority of intensivists believed nitric oxide was possibly beneficial (45%) or had no net effect (28%) in treatment of acute lung injury (. This shift in practice was motivated by discouraging phase 3 trials; ARDS treatment with nitric oxide did not improve overall survival. A 2007 meta-analysis corroborated the lack of mortality benefit for nitric oxide in ALI or ARDS (Adhikari, Burns & Friedrich, 2007). Apprehension has been further supported by the extreme cost of nitric oxide administration, as well as tachyphylaxis and rebound pulmonary hypertension. Thus, the benefit of nitric oxide in ARDS remains dubious; its routine use in this patient population is not recommended.

PHOSPHODIESTERASE INHIBITORS

Phosophodiesterases (PDE) are populated throughout the pulmonary vasculature, and play a role in nitric oxide (NO) induced vasodilation. Endogenous nitric oxide is produced from L-arginine via nitric oxide synthase, which ultimately decreases pulmonary vasculature resistance (PVR). PDE-5 is responsible the specific metabolism of cGMP by hydrolysis of the phosphodiester bond. Decreased levels of cGMP lead to increased levels of intracellular calcium which induces pulmonary vasoconstriction. Phosphodiesterase inhibitors prevents the breakdown of cGMP and maintain pulmonary artery dilation. Increased cGMP levels in the corpus cavernosum lends to treatment for erectile dysfunction.

Sildenafil

Pharmacology

Sildenafil is a direct acting inhibitor of phosphodiesterase-5(PDE-5). Sildenafil is 96% protein bound with a peak onset time of 0.5-2 hours, and a half life of 4 hours. It is metabolized by the liver producing an active metabolite – N-desmethylsildenafil – excreted 80% through the GI tract and 13% by the kidneys. N-desmethylsildenafil is 50% as potent as sildenafil. Typical dosing needs to be adjusted for renal insufficiency.

Clinical Use

Sildenafil is a class I-a recommended treatment for PAH patients in WHO functional class II-III. Randomized control trials have shown sildenafil to improve exercise capacity, 6 minute walk test distance, decreased mean pulmonary artery pressure and increase cardiac index. The Sildenafil Use in Pulmonary Artery Hypertension (SUPER) study showed dose dependent improvement of 6 minute walk test, decrease in mean pulmonary artery pressure (MPAP) and increasing the cardiac index.

Safety Profile

Sildenafil is associated with priapism, headache, myalgia, flushing nausea, extremity pain, numbness, back pain, insomnia and hypotension.

Controversies

The use of sildenafil in an ICU setting for new-onset pulmonary hypertension from ARDS or acute lung injury has been reported, but not yet standard practice. Cases have reported successful treatment of massive pulmonary embolism with sildenafil. Reduction of mean pulmonary artery pressure and pulmonary vascular resistance, with increase in cardiac index and preserved mean arterial systemic pressure were achieved (Ganière, Feihl & Tagan, 2006). Similar positive reports have utilized sildenafil in conjunction with nitric oxide in a case of pulmonary embolism (Lewis, Bloch and Semigran, 2004). Large, randomized controlled studies are necessary to delineate the role of sildenafil in the critically ill patient. Synergy with nitric oxide is encouraging, and can be used routinely to bridge off inhaled nitric oxide therapy.

Tadalafil

Pharmacology

Similar to Sildenafil, Tadalafil is a PDE-5 inhibitor. Tadalafil is 94% protein bound with a peak onset time of 2-8 hours and a half-life of 15 hours. It is metabolized in the liver forming a weak metabolite, and is 61% excreted through the GI tract, and 36% is eliminated via the kidneys. It is given as a 40 mg tab once daily, which needs to be adjustment in renal insufficiency.

Clincial Use

Tadalafil a class I-b recommended medication for PAH patients with WHO functional class II-III. In the Pulmonary Arterial Hypertension and Response to Tadalafil (PHIRST) study, shown to improvement in 6 minute walk, and reduction in MPAP.

Safety Profile

Tadalafil is associated with priapism, headache, myalgia, flushing nausea, extremity pain, numbness, back pain, insomnia and hypotension.

PROSTANOIDS

Prostanoids are metabolites of arachidonic acid, and include prostaglandin I2(PGI2) and thromboxane A2 (TXA2). PGI2 and TXA2 work in opposing fashions in order to maintain pulmonary artery homeostasis. PGI2 is responsible for vasodilation, and prevention of platelet activation; TXA2 does the opposite.

Arachidonic acid is cleaved from membrane phospholipids via phospholipase a2 or phospholipase C. It is ultimately converted to prostaglandin I2, known as prostacyclin. Prostacyclin leads to increased levels of cAMP and cause venodilation and smooth muscle relaxation. Dysregulation of the prostacyclin formation has been demonstrated as an etiology of pulmonary artery hypertension.

Epoprostenol

Pharmacology

Epoprostenol is a prostacylin analogue, with a rapid onset of action, reaching steady state in the blood in 15 minutes. Epoprostenol must be delivered as a continuous infusion due to its short half life (3-6 minutes). It is unstable in solution, and rapidly metabolized via enzymatic hydrolysis in blood. Administration is challenging, as patients require a long term site for continuous infusion. Starting rate via central axis is 2ng/kg/min. It can be titrated up by 2ng/kg/min every 15 minutes until a decrease PAH symptoms are seen, usually seen between 20-40 ng/kg/min (Chaumais, Jobard & Huertas, 2010).

Clinical Use

Epoprostenol was the first developed prostanoid. It is a class Ia recommended medication for patients with WHO functional class III and IV pulmonary artery hypertension. It has been shown clinically to improve 6 minute walk test, quality of life, and cause significant reductions in mean pulmonary artery pressure. It is the only medication to be shown to improve survival in PAH patients.

Safety Profile

Centrally administered medications come with the risks of line infection as well as thrombosis formation. Epoprostenol has also been associated with flushing, headache, jaw pain, diarrhea, muscle pain, hyperglycemia and hyperthyroidism.

Treprostinil

Pharmacology

Treprostinil has a half life of 4.5 hours. A key difference of Treprostinil vs. its sibling epoprostenol is that it has a neutral pH. Central administration is not required, which mitigates the risk of thrombus formation and infection. The medication is also more stable, which allows it to be shipped in pre-made syringes without requiring daily reconstitution or use of ice pouches to maintain stability.

Treprostinil can be administered IV, subcutaneously or inhaled. Its initial infusion rate is 1.25 ng/kg/min which if well tolerated, can be increased by 1.25 ng/kg/min each week for the first 4 weeks. Initial inhalational dosing is 3 breaths (18ug) via an ultrasound pulsed delivery device every 4 hours while the patient is awake.

Clinical Use

Is a prostacyclin analogue with vasodilatory and antiplatelet effects. It is recommended in the treatment of WHO PAH class II-IV. It has been shown to improve 6 minute walk test performance, dyspnea fatigue rating, and overall pulmonary hemodynamics.

Safety Profile

Typical side effects include cough, headache, nausea, dizziness, flushing, throat irritation, diarrhea and phayngolaryngeal pain.

Iloprost

Pharmocology

Onset time of iloprost is almost immediate, however it has a short half life of only 20-25 minutes. It undergoes oxidation to form an inactive metabolite.

Inhaled Iloprost is started at a dosage of 2.5 ug/d and is increased up to 5ug/d. Iloprost has a longer half life than Epoprostenol and does not require a continuous infusion. It does, however, have to be administered 6-9 times daily via nebulization.

Clinical Use

Iloprost is a synthetic analogue of prostacyclin used for the treatment of WHO functional class III and IV PAH. It has been clinically shown to improve 6 minute walk test, mixed venous oxygen saturation, pulmonary vascular resistance, and mean pulmonary pressure.

Safety Profile

Iloprost is associated with jaw pain, headache, flushing, thrombosis and stroke.

ENDONTHELIN RECEPTOR ANTAGONISTS(ERA): BOSENTAN

ERAs work by antagonizing the binding of endothelin-1 to ETa, and ETb receptors. Endothelin-1 activation is responsible for vasoconstriction and proliferation of vascular smooth muscle. Increased expression of plasma and pulmonary endothelin-1 are demonstrated in patients with pulmonary hypertension. Bosentan has an increased affinity for the ETa receptor.

Pharmacology

Bosentan is hepatically metabolized and is excreted through the biliary tract. It has a half life of 5 hours. Bosentan is started at a dose of 62.5mg BID, after 4 weeks of this regimen it is increased to 125mg BID.

Safety Profile

Bosentan can cause severe hepatic dysfunction. Hepatic panel monitoring is necessary prior to initiating treatment, and then monthly. Other common side effects include headache, dizziness, abnormal hepatic function, flushing and syncope. Bosentan is teratogenic – pregnancy category X.

The BREATHE-1 trial confirmed the clinical benefit of Bosentan in WHO class III patients. An increase in 6 minute walk distance, improvement in Borg dyspnea index, and improvement in functional classification all reached statstical significance (Rubin, Badesch & Barst, 2002). Subsequent trials confirmed improved quality of life, increased survival, and improved right-ventricular metrics on echocardiography (Galiè, Hinderliter & Torbicki, 2003). BREATHE-4 and BREATH-5 confirmed utility of Bosentan in several PAH subgroups: HIV-infected patients (Sitbon, Gressin & Speich, 2004), and Eisenmenger syndrome, respectively.

There is a paucity of robust data examining Bosentan in several distinct arenas. Rationale exists for combination PAH therapy with agents affecting different pathways. Bosentan with epoprostenol was examined in BREATHE-2. While results trended towards improved functional response, and decreased adverse effects, the trial was underpowered, and did not meet statistical significance. The SERAPH (Sildenafil versus Endothelin Receptor Antagonist for Pulmonary Hypertension) trial is one of few studies comparing Bosentan with other specific agents for pulmonary hypertension. There was a significant improvement of 6 minute walk distance and cardiac index of the entire cohort, but no differences among the two treatment groups (Wilkins, Paul & Strange, 2005). Finally, the BENEFIT trial is the sole randomized, placebo-controlled, multicenter study examining Bosentan in inoperable WHO Class IV patients. No significant improvement of 6MWD, functional class, or time to clincal worsening was observed (Jaïs, D'Armini & Jansa, 2008). The 2008 World Symposium on PAH deemed more investigation is required in this patient subgroup.

International guidelines confirm specific subsets of patients clearly benefit from Bosentan as a safe, and well tolerated first-line therapy. However, further investigation needs to confirm its use in all classifications of PAH patients, combination therapy and superiority over other agents.

REFERENCES

Adhikari, N., Burns, K. E., Friedrich, J. O., Granton, J. T., Cook, D. J., & Meade, M. O. (2007). Effect of nitric oxide on oxygenation and mortality in acute lung injury: Systematic review and meta-analysis. *British Medical Journal*, *334*(7597), 779. doi:10.1136/bmj.39139.716794.55 PMID:17383982

Archer, S. L., Weir, E. K., & Wilkins, M. R. (2010). Basic Science of Pulmonary Arterial Hypertension for Clinicians. *Circulation*, *12*(18), 2045–2066. doi:10.1161/CIRCULATIONAHA.108.847707 PMID:20458021

Barst, R. J., Gibbs, J. S., Ghofrani, H. A., Hoeper, M. M., McLaughlin, V. V., Rubin, L. J., & Galiè, N. et al. (2009). Updated Evidence-Based Treatment Algorithm in Pulmonary Arterial Hypertension. *Journal of the American College of Cardiology*, *54*(1), S78–S84. doi:10.1016/j.jacc.2009.04.017 PMID:19555861

Baud, F. J., Barriot, P., Toffis, V., Riou, B., Vicaut, E., Lecarpentier, Y., & Bismuth, C. et al. (1991). Elevated blood CN concentrations in victims of smoke inhalation. *The New England Journal of Medicine*, *325*(25), 1761–1766. doi:10.1056/NEJM199112193252502 PMID:1944484

Baud, F. J., Borron, S. W., Mégarbane, B., Trout, H., Lapostolle, F., Vicaut, E., & Bismuth, C. et al. (2002). Value of lactic acidosis in the assessment of the severity of acute CN poisoning. *Critical Care Medicine*, *30*(9), 2044–2050. doi:10.1097/00003246-200209000-00015 PMID:12352039

Beloucif, S., & Paven, D. (1998). A European Survey of the use of inhaled nitric oxide in the ICU. Working group on inhaled NO in ICU of the European Society of Intensive Care Medicine. *Intensive Care Medicine*, *24*(8), 864–877. doi:10.1007/s001340050679 PMID:9757934

Benza, R., Tapson, V. F., Gomberg-Maitland, M., Poms, A., Barst, R. J., & McLaughlin, V. V. (2013). One-year Experience with Intravenous Treprostinil for Pulmonary Arterial Hypertension. *The Journal of Heart and Lung Transplantation*, *32*(9), 889–896. doi:10.1016/j.healun.2013.06.008 PMID:23953817

Channick, R. N., Voswinckel, R., Rubin, L. J., & Vultaggio, . (2012). Inhaled Treprostinil: A therapeutic review. *Drug Design. Development and Therapy*, *6*, 19–28. doi:10.2147/DDDT.S19281

Chaumais, M. C., Jobard, M., Huertas, A., Vignand-Courtin, C., Humbert, M., Sitbon, O., & Montani, D. et al. (2010). Pharmacokinetic Evaluation of Continuous Intravenous Epoprostenol. *Expert Opinion on Drug Metabolism & Toxicology*, *6*(12), 1587–1598. doi:10.1517/17425255.2010.534458 PMID:21077785

Choi, W. S., & Samman, N. (2008). Risks and benefits of deliberate hypotension in anesthesia: A systematic review. *International Journal of Oral and Maxillofacial Surgery*, *37*(8), 687–703. doi:10.1016/j.ijom.2008.03.011 PMID:18511238

Çilingiroğlu M, Akkuş N, Sethi S, Modi KA. (2014). Large pericardial effusion induced by minoxidil. *Türk Kardiyoloji Derneği arşivi: Türk Kardiyoloji Derneğinin yayın organıdı*, *40*(3), 255.

Costanzo, L. (2014). *Physiology* (5th ed.). Philadelphia: Saunders Elsevier.

Davies, R., & Morrell, N. W. (2008). Molecular Mechanisms of Pulmonary Arterial Hypertension: Role of Mutations in the Bone Morphogenetic Protein Type II Receptor. *Chest*, *134*(6), 1271–1277. doi:10.1378/chest.08-1341 PMID:19059957

Desmonts, J. M., & Marty, J. (1984). Anesthetic management of patients with pheochromocytoma. *British Journal of Anaesthesia*, *56*(7), 781–789. doi:10.1093/bja/56.7.781 PMID:6375708

Dolman, R. M., Bentley, K. C., Head, T. W., & English, M. (2000). The effect of hypotensive anesthesia on blood loss and operative time during Lefort 1 osteotomies. *Journal of Oral and Maxillofacial Surgery*, *58*(8), 834–839. doi:10.1053/joms.2000.8194 PMID:10935580

Fahmy, N. R. (1985). Nitroprusside vs a nitroprusside trimethaphan mixture for induced hypotension: Hemodynamic effects and CN release. *Clinical Pharmacology and Therapeutics*, *37*(3), 264–270. doi:10.1038/clpt.1985.38 PMID:3971651

Friederich, J. A., & Butterworth, J. F. (1995). Sodium Nitroprusside: Twenty years and counting. *Anesthesia and Analgesia*, *81*, 152–162. PMID:7598246

Galiè, N., Beghetti, M., Gatzoulis, M. A., Granton, J., Berger, R. M., & Lauer, A. et al.. (2006). Bosentan therapy in patients with Eisenmenger syndrome: A multicenter, double-blind, randomized, placebo-controlled study. *Circulation*, *114*(1), 48–54. doi:10.1161/CIRCULATIONAHA.106.630715 PMID:16801459

Galiè, N., Hinderliter, A. L., Torbicki, A., Fourme, T., Simonneau, G., Pulido, T., & Rubin, L. et al. (2003). Effects of the oral endothelin-receptorantagonist bosentan on echocardiographic and Doppler measures in patients with pulmonary arterial hypertension. *Journal of the American College of Cardiology*, *41*(8), 1380–1386. doi:10.1016/S0735-1097(03)00121-9 PMID:12706935

Galiè, N., Hoeper, M. M., Humbert, M., Torbicki, A., Vachiery, J. L., Barbera, J. A., & Simonneau, G. et al. (2009). Guidelines for the Diagnosis and Treatment of Pulmonary Hypertension. *The European Respiratory Journal*, *34*(6), 1219–1263. doi:10.1183/09031936.00139009 PMID:19749199

Galiè, N., & Simonneau, G. (2013). Updated Clinical Classification of Pulmonary Hypertension. [_S.]. *Journal of the American College of Cardiology*, *62*, 25. PMID:24355639

Ganière, V., Feihl, F., & Tagan, D. (2006). Dramatic beneficial effects of sildenafil in recurrent massive pulmonary embolism. *Intensive Care Medicine*, *32*(3), 452–454. doi:10.1007/s00134-005-0058-5 PMID:16450094

Goldstein, R., O'Neill, J. A. Jr, Holcomb, G. W. III, Morgan, W. M. III, Neblett, W. W. III, Oates, J. A., & Scott, H. W. Jr et al.. (1999). Clinical experience over 48 years with pheochromocytoma. *Annals of Surgery*, *229*(6), 755–764. doi:10.1097/00000658-199906000-00001 PMID:10363888

Hall, A. H., & Rumack, B. H. (1986). Clinical toxicology of CN. *Annals of Emergency Medicine*, *15*(9), 1067–1074. doi:10.1016/S0196-0644(86)80131-7 PMID:3526995

Härtter, S., Sennewald, R., Nehmiz, G., & Reilly, P. et al.. (2013). Oral bioavailability of dabigatran etexilate (Pradaxa®) after co-medication with verapamil in healthy subjects. *British Journal of Clinical Pharmacology*, *75*(4), 1053–1062. doi:10.1111/j.1365-2125.2012.04453.x PMID:22946890

Higenbottam, T., Pepke-Zaba, J., Scott, J., Woolman, P., Coutts, C., & Wallwork, J. (1988). Inhaled endothelial derived-relaxing factor (EDRF) in primary pulmonary hypertension (PPH). *The American Review of Respiratory Disease*, *137*, A107.

Hoette, S., O'Callaghan, D., Jardim, C., & Souza, R. (2010). Dual receptor blockade by bosentan: Clinical experience in treatment of pulmonary hypertension. *Journal of Receptor. Ligand and Channel Research*, *3*, 113–121.

Ichinose, F., Roberts, J. D., & Zapol, W. M. (2004). Inhaled Nitric Oxide: A Selective Pulmonary Vasodilator: Current Uses and Therapeutic Potential. *Circulation*, *109*(25), 3106–3111. doi:10.1161/01.CIR.0000134595.80170.62 PMID:15226227

Inhaled Nitric Oxide/INOpulse for Pulmonary Arterial Hypertension. (2015). In *ClinicalTrials.gov*. Retrieved from http://clinicaltrials.gov/ct2/show/record/NCT01457781

Ivankovich, A. D., Braverman, B., Stephens, T. S., Shulman, M., & Heyman, H. J. (1983). Sodium thiosulfate disposition in humans: Relation to sodium nitroprusside toxicity. *Anesthesiology*, *58*(1), 11–17. doi:10.1097/00000542-198301000-00003 PMID:6600205

Jaïs, X., D'Armini, A. M., Jansa, P., Torbicki, A., Delcroix, M., Ghofrani, H. A., & Rubin, L. J. et al. (2008). Bosentan for treatment of inoperable chronic thromboembolic pulmonary hypertension. *Journal of the American College of Cardiology*, *52*(25), 2127–2134. doi:10.1016/j.jacc.2008.08.059 PMID:19095129

Katz, A. M. (1996). Calcium channel diversity in the cardiovascular system. *Journal of the American College of Cardiology*, *28*(2), 522–529. doi:10.1016/0735-1097(96)00170-2 PMID:8800134

Klabunde, R. (2012). *Nitrodilators*. Retrieved from http://www.cvpharmacology.com/vasodilator/nitro.htm

Klabunde, R. (2012). *Nitric Oxide*. Retrieved from www.cvphysiology.com/bloodflow/BF011.htm

Lavoie, J. (2011). Blood transfusion risks and alternative strategies in pediatric patients. *Paediatric Anaesthesia*, *21*(1), 12–24. doi:10.1111/j.1460-9592.2010.03470.x PMID:21155923

Lentschener, C., Gaujoux, S., Tesniere, A., & Dousset, B. (2011). Point of Controversy: Perioperative care of patients undergoing pheochromocytoma removal – time for a reappraisal? *European Journal of Endocrinology*, *165*(3), 365–373. doi:10.1530/EJE-11-0162 PMID:21646289

Lentschener, C., Gaujoux, S., Thillois, J. M., Duboc, D., Bertherat, J., Ozier, Y., & Dousset, B. (2009). Increased arterial pressure is not predictive of haemodynamic instability in patients undergoing adrenalectomy for phaeochromocytoma. *Acta Anaesthesiologica Scandinavica*, *53*(4), 522–527. doi:10.1111/j.1399-6576.2008.01894.x PMID:19239408

Lewis, G. D., Bloch, K. D., & Semigran, M. J. (2004). Pulmonary thromboembolism superimposed on a congenital ventricular septal defect in a 50-year-old man inhaled nitric oxide and sildenafil to the rescue. *Cardiology in Review*, *12*(4), 188–190. doi:10.1097/01.crd.0000122635.12743.57 PMID:15191635

Lockwood, A., Patka, J., Rabinovich, M., Wyatt, K., & Abraham, P. (2010). Nitroprusside-associated cyanide toxicity in adult patients - fact or fiction? A critical review of the evidence and clinical relevance. *Open Access Journal of Clinical Trials*, *2*(133), 148.

Marino, P. (2007). *The ICU Book* (3rd ed.). Philadelphia: Lippincott Williams and Wilkins.

Meade, M., Jacka, M. J., Cook, D. J., Dodek, P., Griffith, L., & Guyatt, G. H. (2004). Survey of interventions for the prevention and treatment of acute respiratory distress syndrome. *Critical Care Medicine*, *32*(4), 946–954. doi:10.1097/01.CCM.0000120056.76356.AD PMID:15071383

Minoxidil. (2009). In *Official FDA Information, Side effects and Uses*. Retrieved from http://www.drugs.com/mtm/minoxidil.html

Nguyen, K., & Marks, J. G. Jr. (2003). Pseudoacromegaly induced by the long-term use of minoxidil. *Journal of the American Academy of Dermatology*, *48*(6), 962–965. doi:10.1067/mjd.2003.325 PMID:12789195

Pasala, K. K., Gujja, K., Prabhu, H., Vasavada, B., & Konka, S. et al.. (2012). Short-term Minoxidil Use Associated With Pericardial Effusion and Cardiac Tamponade: An Uncommon Presentation. *American Journal of Therapeutics*, *19*(6), e186–e188. doi:10.1097/MJT.0b013e3181f5371c PMID:21519225

Rossaint, R., Falke, K. J., López, F., Slama, K., Pison, U., & Zapol, W. M. (1993). Inhaled nitric oxide for the adult respiratory distress syndrome. *The New England Journal of Medicine*, *328*(6), 399–405. doi:10.1056/NEJM199302113280605 PMID:8357359

Rubin, L. J., Badesch, D. B., Barst, R. J., Galie, N., Black, C. M., Keogh, A., & Simonneau, G. et al. (2002). Bosentan therapy for pulmonary arterial hypertension. *The New England Journal of Medicine*, *346*(12), 896–903. doi:10.1056/NEJMoa012212 PMID:11907289

Sarvotham, S. S. (1987). Nitroprusside therapy in post-open heart hypertensives: A ritual tryst with CN death? *Chest*, *91*(5), 796. doi:10.1378/chest.91.5.796b PMID:3568793

Sastry, B. K., Narasimhan, C., Reddy, N. K., & Raju, B. S. (2004). Clinical Efficacy of Sildenafil in Primary Pulmonary Hypertension. *Journal of the American College of Cardiology*, *43*(7), 1149–1153. doi:10.1016/j.jacc.2003.10.056 PMID:15063421

Sharrock, N. E. (1998). Anesthesia. In The Adult Hip. Philadelphia: Lippincott - Raven Publishers.

Sitbon, O., Gressin, V., Speich, R., Macdonald, P. S., Opravil, M., Cooper, D. A., & Simonneau, G. et al. (2004). Bosentan for the treatment of human immunodeficiency virus-associated pulmonary arterial hypertension. *American Journal of Respiratory and Critical Care Medicine*, *170*(11), 1212–1217. doi:10.1164/rccm.200404-445OC PMID:15317666

Sitbon, O., McLaughlin, V., Badesch, D., Barst, R., Black, C., & Galie, N. et al.. (2005). Survival in patients with class III idiopathic pulmonary arterial hypertension treated with first line oral bosentan compared with an historical cohort of patients startedon intravenous epoprostenol. *Thorax*, *60*(12), 1025–1030. doi:10.1136/thx.2005.040618 PMID:16055621

Souza, R., Jardim, C., Martins, B., Cortopassi, F., Yaksic, M., Rabelo, R., & Bogossian, H. (2005). Effect of bosentan treatment on surrogate markers in pulmonary arterial hypertension. *Current Medical Research and Opinion*, *21*(6), 907–911. doi:10.1185/030079905X46232 PMID:15969891

Taylor, A. L., Ziesche, S., Yancy, C., Carson, P., D'Agostino, R. Jr, Ferdinand, K., & Cohn, J. N. et al. African-American Heart Failure Trial Investigators. (2004). Combination of isosorbide dinitrate and hydralazine in blacks with heart failure. *The New England Journal of Medicine*, *351*(20), 2049–2057. doi:10.1056/NEJMoa042934 PMID:15533851

Taylor, R. W., Zimmerman, J. L., Dellinger, R. P., Straube, R. C., Criner, G. J., & Davis, K. et al.. (2004). Low-dose inhaled nitric oxide in patients with acute lung injury: A randomized controlled trial. *Journal of the American Medical Association*, *291*, 1603–1609. doi:10.1001/jama.291.13.1603 PMID:15069048

Tsai, B., Turrentine, M. W., Sheridan, B. C., Wang, M., Fiore, A. C., Brown, J. W., & Meldrum, D. R. (2006). Differential Effects of Phosphodiesterase-5 Inhibitors on Hypoxic Pulmonary Vasoconstriction and Pulmonary Artery Cytokine Expression. *The Annals of Thoracic Surgery*, *81*(1), 272–278. doi:10.1016/j.athoracsur.2005.06.040 PMID:16368379

Verapamil. (2013). In *Official FDA Information, Side effects and Uses*. Retrieved from http://www.drugs.com/verapamil.html

Walshe, C., & Kevin, L. (2010). *Pulmonary Hypertension in ARDS: Is It Important and Should We Treat It? Evidence Based Practice of Critical Care*. Philadelphia: Saunders Elsevier. doi:10.1016/B978-1-4160-5476-4.00049-3

Weinberger, B., Laskin, D. L., Heck, D. E., & Laskin, J. D. (2001). The Toxicology of Inhaled Nitric Oxide. *Toxicological Sciences*, *59*(1), 5–16. doi:10.1093/toxsci/59.1.5 PMID:11134540

Westley, J. (1973). Rhodanese. *Advances in Enzymology and Related Areas of Molecular Biology*, *39*, 327–368. PMID:4583640

Westley, J., Adler, H., Westley, L., & Nishida, C. (1983). The sulfur transferases. *Fundamental and Applied Toxicology*, *3*(5), 377–382. doi:10.1016/S0272-0590(83)80008-6 PMID:6357923

Wilkins, M. R., Paul, G. A., Strange, J. W., Tunariu, N., Gin-Sing, W., Banya, W. A., & Gibbs, J. S. R. et al. (2005). Sildenafil versus endothelin receptor antagonist for pulmonary hypertension (SERAPH) study. *American Journal of Respiratory and Critical Care Medicine*, *171*(11), 1292–1297. doi:10.1164/rccm.200410-1411OC PMID:15750042

Wilson, R. M., De Silva, D. S., Sato, K., Izumiya, Y., & Sam, F. (2009). Effects of fixed-dose Isosorbide Dinitrate/Hydralazine on diastolic function and exercise capacity in hypertension-induced diastolic heart failure. *Hypertension*, *54*(3), 583–590. doi:10.1161/HYPERTENSIONAHA.109.134932 PMID:19620510

Zhao, S., Qi, G., Tian, W., Chen, L., & Sun, Y. (2014). Effect of Intracoronary Nitroprusside in Preventing No Reflow Phenomenon during Primary Percutaneous Coronary Intervention: A Meta-Analysis. *Journal of Interventional Cardiology*, *27*(4), 356–364. doi:10.1111/joic.12133 PMID:25041036

KEY TERMS AND DEFINITIONS

ALI: Acute Lung Injury. Spectrum of Widespread lung inflammation resulting in impaired oxygenation.

ARDS: Acute Respiratory Distress Syndrome. Widespread lung inflammation resulting in severe impairment of oxygenation.

Capacitance Vessels: Venous system vasculature.

cGMP: Cyclic GMP. Modulates smooth muscle vasodilation.

cNOS: Constitutive Nitric Oxide Synthetase.

CYP450: Cytochrome p450 hepatic enzyme system for drug metabolism.

ET_A: Endothelin-A receptor, results in pulmonary vasoconstriction and fibroproliferation.

ET_B: Endothelin-B receptor, results in pulmonary vasodilation and inhibits fibroproliferation.

iNOS: Inducible Nitric Oxide Synthetase.

IP_3: Inositol 1,4,5-triphosphate. Upregulated upon G-protein activation.

L-Type Calcium Channels: Long-acting calcium channels. Modulate plateau phase of myocardial action potential.

MPAP: Mean pulmonary arterial pressure.

NO: Nitric Oxide.

NOS: Nitric Oxide Synthetase.

PAH: Pulmonary Artery Hypertension.

PDE-5: Phosphodiesterase-5, hydrolyzes and inactivates cGMP.

PGI2: Prostaglandin I2. Arachadonic acid metabolite, results in pulmonary artery vasodilation and platelet inhibition.

PPM: Parts per million. Units of nitric oxide administration, varies from 0 – 20 ppm.

Resistance Vessels: Arteriole system vasculature.

SNP: Sodium Nitroprusside.

TXA2: Thromboxane A2. Arachadonic acid metabolite, results in pulmonary artery vasoconstriction and platelet activation.

Section 4

A Systematic Approach to Cardiothoracic Critical Care

Chapter 14
Neurologic Complications in the Cardiac Surgery Patient

Sheela Pai Cole
Stanford University, USA

Albert T. Cheung
Stanford University, USA

ABSTRACT

This chapter per the authors discusses the spectrum of complications that occur in the postoperative cardiac surgery patients. It evaluates the mechanistic role of cardiopulmonary bypass and the various cardiac surgical procedures in the development of cerebral injury. Furthermore, it evaluates the role of different intraoperative monitoring in early detection of cerebral injury in these patients. Finally, it provides evidence based practice guidelines for hemodynamic management as well as treatment of complications that are diagnosed in the cardiac surgical intensive care unit.

INTRODUCTION

Neurologic injuries have always been an important complication of cardiac operations. In a prospective study of patients undergoing open-heart operations published in 1970, 43% of patients were reported to suffer cerebral injury during operation with 15% of patients suffering permanent damage.(Tufo, Ostfeld, & Shekelle, 1970) In 1996, the rate of stroke in a multicenter study of patients undergoing elective coronary artery bypass (CABG) operations was reported as 3.1% and the rate of neurocognitive dysfunction reported as 3%.(Roach, Kanchuger, & Mora-Mangano, 1996) Perioperative neurologic injury as a consequence of cardiac operations have also been associated with increased mortality, increased morbidity, and decreased long-term survival.(Roach et al., 1996; Tarakji, 2011)

(Fortunately, contemporary studies indicate that the rate of stroke after CABG operations may be decreasing despite a cardiac surgical patient population with a greater risk profile for neurologic complications.(Tarakji, 2011)

DOI: 10.4018/978-1-4666-8603-8.ch014

Figure 1. Prevalence of perioperative stroke after coronary artery bypass graft surgery by year of operation, 1982-2010 modified from Tarakji et al (Tarakji, 2011)

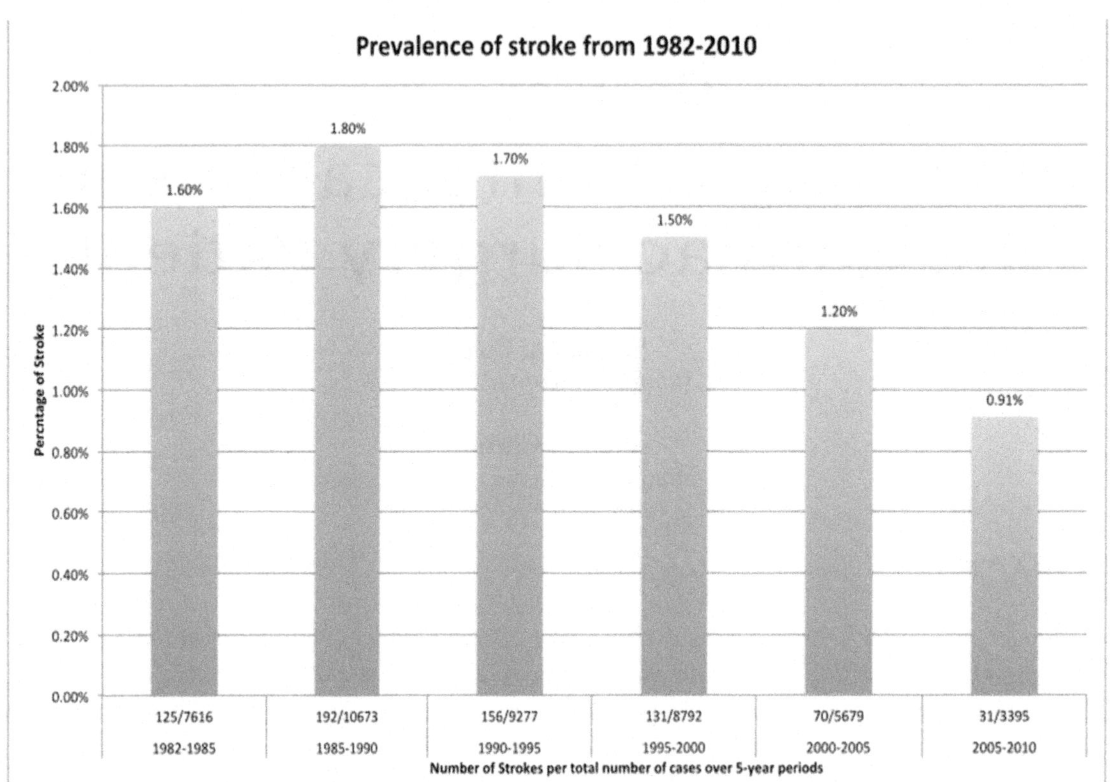

Major advances in understanding the causes of stroke and encephalopathy among cardiac surgical patients together with improvements in the anesthetic care and surgical techniques employed in the care of cardiac surgical patients to minimize the risk of neurologic complications may explain the progress that has been achieved over time.

Types of Perioperative Neurological Injury

Neurological complications of cardiac operations have generally been broadly classified as injuries as a consequence of stroke and injuries that are manifested by neurocognitive dysfunction or global encephalopathy without direct evidence of ischemic neurologic injury.(Roach et al., 1996) Stroke is caused by thromboembolism, cerebral hypoperfusion, or hemorrhage that may occur at any time in the perioperative period and produces ischemic neurologic injury associated with radiologic findings of cerebral infarction or hemorrhage. The precise etiology of neurocognitive dysfunction or encephalopathy has not been established, but is likely multifactorial. Subclinical ischemia, stroke, thromboembolism, or cerebral hypoperfusion may also be etiologic mechanisms that contribute to the development of perioperative neurocognitive dysfunction or global encephalopathy.

STROKE

Analysis of Society of Thoracic Surgeons (STS) database for Cerebrovascular Accident (CVA) after Coronary Artery Bypass Grafting (CABG) by year demonstrates that the rate of perioperative stroke has gradually decreased from a rate of 3% prior to 2000 to a rate of 1.8%, but has remained at approximately 1.2% since 2008. A meta-analysis examining 19 studies and about 2000 patients demonstrated that the risk of stroke after CABG was 1.2% compared to a risk of 0.34% after percutaneous coronary intervention (PCI). This finding suggested that procedural factors had a major role in the pathophysiology of perioperative stroke. The increased risk of stroke associated with complex open-heart procedures also supports the importance of procedural factors. The risk of stroke associated with mitral or aortic valve surgery averages 6%. The risk of stroke after combined CABG and valve operation can be as high as 7.9%(McKhann, Grega, Borowicz, Baumgartner, & Selnes, 2006). Patient factors that contribute to increased risk for stroke include advanced age, diabetes, hypertension, and a history of prior stroke or cerebrovascular accident.

The majority of perioperative strokes occur at the time of operation with 40% of all strokes diagnosed immediately upon emergence from general anesthesia.(Likosky et al., 2003) The risk of stroke is about 20% at 48 hours after operation and decreases further with each subsequent day after operation.(Likosky et al., 2003; McKhann et al., 2006) Serial neurologic examination in the first 3 days after cardiac operations has the greatest chance for detection of perioperative strokes.

Thromboembolism is believed to be the most common cause of perioperative stroke in the cardiac surgery patients

Figure 2. TEE image of left atrial appendage: Looking for cardiac source of emboli

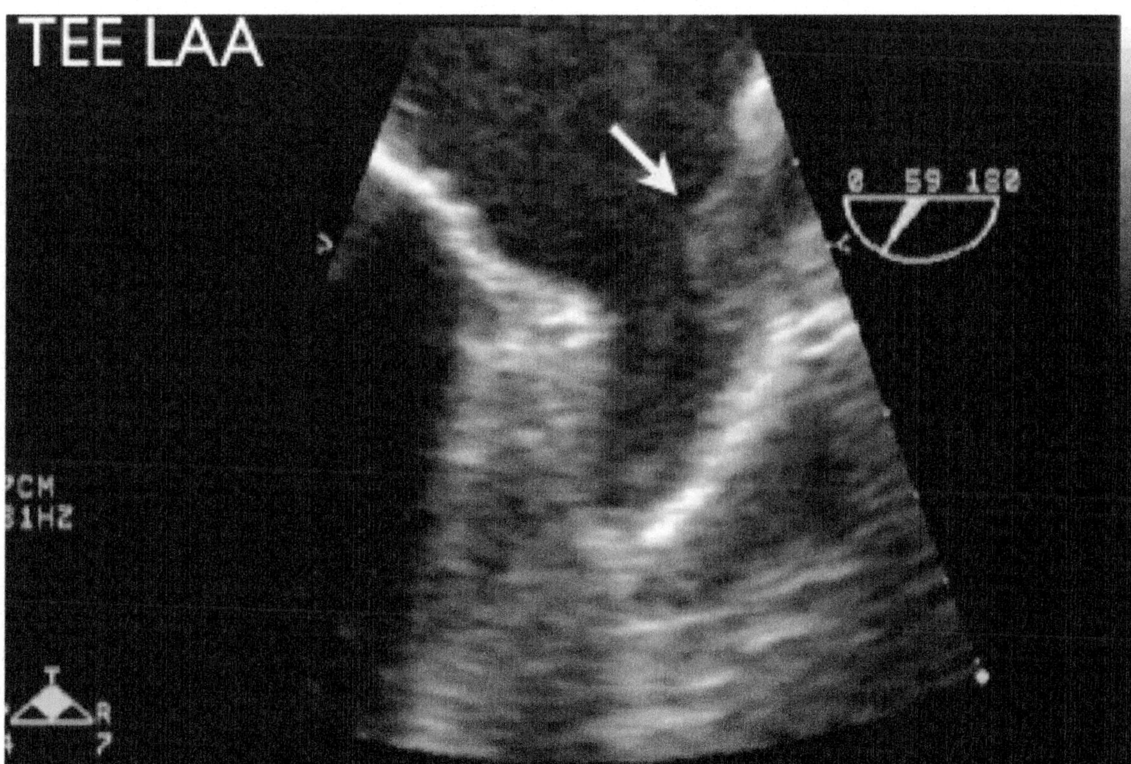

Neurologic examination and brain imaging studies in patients with thromboembolic stroke will reveal corresponding focal defects in the cerebrovascular territory that have been occluded. Sources of thromboembolism include atherosclerotic aortic plaque in the thoracic aorta, calcific debris, air, or thrombus. Thromboembolic strokes in the postoperative period may in part be explained by delayed embolism in patients with vulnerable atherosclerotic plaque that have been made unstable as a consequence of surgical instrumentation.(Gutsche et al., 2007)

Cerebral hypoperfusion will cause strokes in a watershed distribution of the brain at the margins of arterial supply that are most vulnerable to ischemia in response to hypotension (Gottesman et al., 2006).

Cerebral hypoperfusion can occur during cardiac operations as a consequence of hypotension, inadequate cardiac output, cardiopulmonary bypass, or elevated central venous pressure. Cerebral blood flow is normally maintained by autoregulation over a range of arterial pressures, but the autoregulatory threshold may be increased in chronic hypertension and maintaining "normal" mean arterial pressure throughout the operation may produce cerebral hypoperfusion in susceptible individuals.

Hemorrhagic strokes are the least common type of stroke in the perioperative period, but are typically catastrophic because of the need for systemic anticoagulation for cardiopulmonary bypass. Hemorrhagic strokes usually manifest as severe headache associated with progressive neurologic deficits. In the perioperative period, hemorrhagic strokes may occur as a consequence of mycotic aneurysm rupture in patients with endocarditis; hemorrhagic conversion of an acute embolic stroke involving a large vascular territory; or in patients with a recent ischemic stroke subjected to anticoagulation during cardiopulmonary bypass.

THE CLINICAL CONSEQUENCES OF PERIOPERATIVE STROKE

Stroke in the perioperative period has important short-term and long-term clinical consequences among cardiac surgical patients. One study showed a six-fold increase in mortality in patients with perioperative stroke, while another study demonstrated that the mortality in patients with strokes was 22% versus 6% in those without a stroke.(Bucerius, Gummert, & Borger, 2003; McKhann et al., 2006; Newman et al., 2006) The Northern New England Cardiovascular Disease Study Group compared survival in those with and without stroke after CABG and found lower survival rates at 1, 5 and 10 years after the injury. At 1 year the survival was 83% versus 94.1%, at 5 years 58.7% versus 83.3% and at 10 years 26.9% versus 61.9%, in patients with and without perioperative stroke, respectively. Cardiac surgical patients with perioperative stroke also had a 3-fold increase in 10-year mortality compared to patients without neurological complications.(Dacey et al., 2005) In a multicenter study, perioperative stroke was associated with a 10-fold increase in hospital mortality and increased intensive care unit length of stay, increased average hospital length of stay, and increased rate of discharge to skilled nursing facilities or rehabilitation centers.(Roach et al., 1996) Postoperative mortality and morbidity as a consequence of perioperative stroke is also much greater among elderly patients.

THE MANAGEMENT OF PERIOPERATIVE STROKE

Stroke is a neurologic emergency.(Jauch et al., 2013) Regardless of the mechanism of the stroke, the acute management of a stroke involves two principles. The first step is to perform a diagnostic evaluation to determine the anatomic location and extent of injury. The second step that can be implemented simultaneously is to intervene with the objective of preventing secondary injury.

Stroke should be suspected in patients who exhibit a delayed emergence from general anesthesia after operation or manifest focal neurologic deficits upon recovery from general anesthesia. Examples of early neurologic deficits may include a new facial droop or asymmetry, visual field deficits or gaze palsy, arm or leg weakness, speech impairments such as aphasia or dysarthria, extinction or inattention, decreased level of consciousness, or even seizures. The NIH stroke scale is a validated instrument that has been used to determine severity as well as serve as a prognosticator of acute ischemic stroke. Muir et al found NIHSS to be a valid instrument to predict severity and outcomes in stroke.(Muir, Weir, Murray, Povey, & Lees, 1996) A NIHSS score greater than 15 implies a severe stroke whereas a low score is prognostic of a good outcome both at 30 days as well as at 6 months.(Fonarow et al., 2012; Weimar et al., 2004)

If stroke is suspected, a neurology consultation for a full diagnostic evaluation should be requested immediately. Most centers have specialized stroke code teams that facilitate rapid mobilization of imaging and interventional teams. Early management should also include the administration of supplemental oxygen, treatment of cardiovascular disturbances, measurement of blood glucose levels, laboratory testing to assess coagulation function, and the discontinuation of medications that may impair the ability to perform a detailed neurologic examination.

The initial management of suspected stroke includes radiologic imaging performed concurrently to confirm the presence of ischemic stroke, localize the vascular territory at risk, and determine the

Figure 3. Acute ischemic stroke 30-day mortality rates by NIHSS. Standard error bars are displayed (Fonarow et al., 2012).

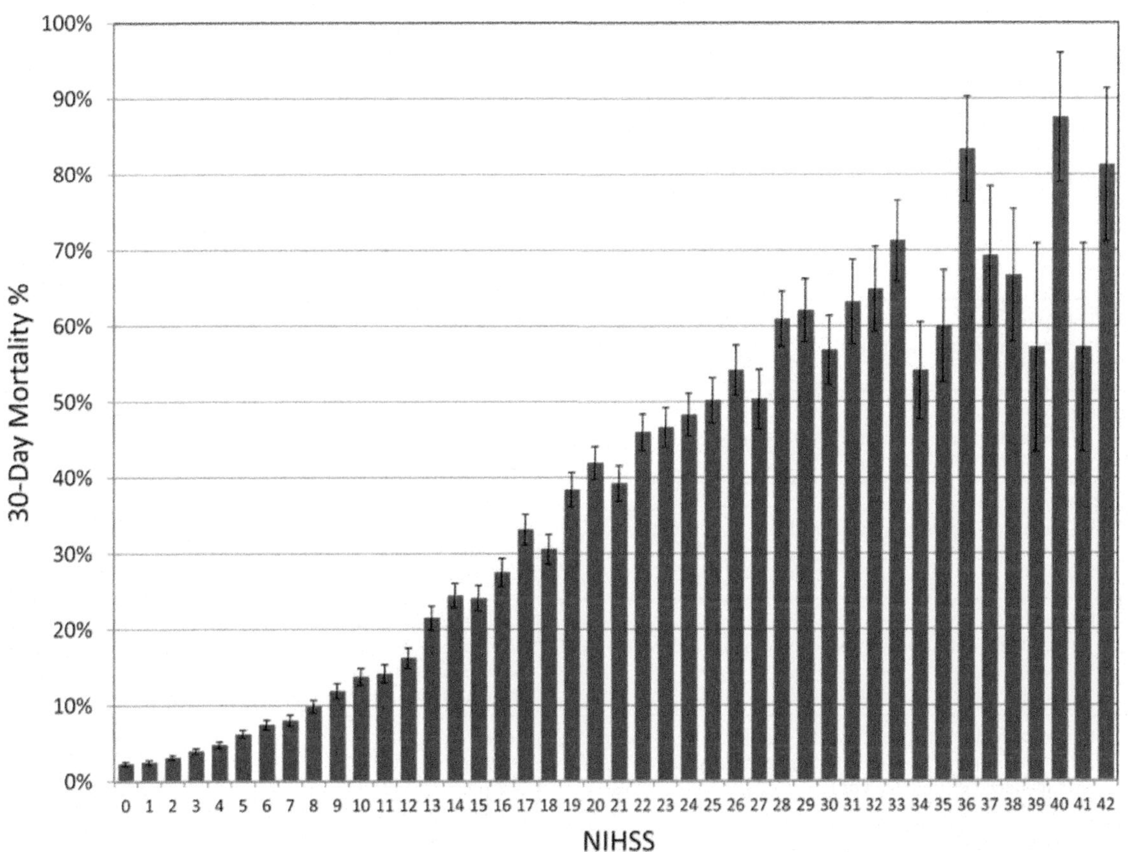

Table 1. NIHSS questionnaire used to determine stroke score

Category	Score/Description	Date/Time Initials
1a. Level of Consciousness (Alert, drowsy, etc.)	0=Alert 1=Drowsy 2=Stuporous 3=Coma	
1b. LOC Questions (Month, age)	0=Answers both correctly 1=Answers one correctly 2=Incorrect	
1c. LOC Commands (Open/close eyes, makes fist/let go)	0=Obeys both correctly 1=Obeys one correctly 2=Incorrect	
2. Best Gaze (Eyes open-patient follows examiners finger or face)	0=Normal 1=Partial gaze palsy 2=Forced deviation	
3. Visual fields (Introduce visual stimulus/threat to patient's visual field quadrants)	0=No visual loss 1=Partial hemianopia 2=Complete hemianopia 3=Bilateral hemianopia	
4. Facial Paresis (Show teeth, raise eyebrows and squeeze eyes shut)	0=Normal 1=Minor 2=Partial 3=Complete	
5a. Motor Arm- Left 5b. Motor Arm- Right (Elevate arm to 90 (sitting) 45 (supine))	0=No drift 1=Drift 2=Can't resist gravity 3=No effort against gravity 4=No movement X=Untestable	
6a. Motor leg- Left 6b. Motor leg- Right (Elevate leg to 30 if supine)	0=No drift 1=Drift 2=Can't resist gravity 3=No effort against gravity 4=No movement X=Untestable	
7. Limb Ataxia (Finger-nose, heel down shin)	0=No Ataxia 1=Present in one limb 2=Present in 2 limbs	
8. Sensory (Pin prick to face, arm, trunk and leg-compare side to side)	0=Normal 1=Partial loss 2=Severe loss	
9. Best language (Name item, describe a picture and	0=No aphasia 1=Mild to moderate aphasia 2=Severe aphasia 3=Mute	
10. Dysarthria (Evaluate speech clarity by patient repeating listed words)	0=Normal articulation 1=Mild to moderate slurring 2=Near unintelligible or worse X=intubated or other barrier	
11. Extinction and Inattention (Use information from prior testing to identify neglect or double simultaneous stimuli testing)	0=No neglect 1=Partial neglect 2=Complete neglect	

extent of the injury. Imaging also determines whether a patient is a candidate for endovascular stenting or thrombolytic therapy. The 2013 American Stroke Association consensus statement on the early management of acute ischemic stroke recommended non-contrast-enhanced computed tomographic (NECT) imaging of the brain and interpretation by an expert physician should be performed before initiating any specific therapy to treat acute ischemic stroke. Although magnetic resonance imaging (MRI) with diffusion weighted imaging (DWI) has emerged as the most sensitive and specific imaging technique to detect an acute infarct, these studies are rarely feasible for cardiac surgical patients in the early postoperative period because of the presence of indwelling epicardial pacing wires, pulmonary artery catheter, vasoactive drug infusions, and the need for mechanical ventilation or other life support systems.(Adams et al., 2007)

Once the diagnosis of ischemic stroke has been established, therapies should be focused on preventing secondary injury. Prevention of secondary injury involves providing supportive care, decreasing the risk of hemorrhagic conversion, minimizing cerebral edema, improving perfusion to the ischemic penumbra, and the treatment of acute complications. The ischemic penumbra is that region of the brain adjacent to the infarct and is most vulnerable to ischemia and infarction. A small number of patients may be candidates for intra-arterial thrombolytic therapy to revascularize a stroke caused by acute occlusion of the middle cerebral artery (MCA), but the risks and potential benefits of this therapy must be carefully considered among cardiac surgical patients immediately after operation.

AIRWAY AND VENTILATION

Hypoxia is common after acute stroke and may worsen cerebral injury in the setting of acute cerebral ischemia, but the efficacy of supplemental oxygen after stroke has yet to be established. Current recommendations for supplemental oxygen are to maintain oxygen saturation greater that 94% and to administer it in the least invasive method.(Jauch et al., 2013) Patients with stroke complicated by airway obstruction, hypoventilation, aspiration, pneumonia, or decreased consciousness may require tracheal intubation and mechanical ventilator support. The need for mechanical ventilation after an acute stroke is a bad prognostic sign and has an associated 50% 30-day mortality. Elective tracheal intubation and mechanical ventilator support may also be necessary for the management of patients with increased intracranial pressure or malignant brain edema after stroke. Frequent arterial blood gas measurement should be used to guide the management of mechanical ventilation. The autoregulation of cerebral blood flow is affected by arterial $PaCO_2$ and hypocarbia has the potential to decrease cerebral blood flow. Deliberate hyperventilation may be necessary to temporarily reduce intracranial pressure in the presence of life-threatening cerebral edema.

CIRCULATION

Extremes of blood pressure are associated with adverse outcome in acute ischemic stroke. Hypertension is common after stroke and may be explained by pre-existing hypertension or as a physiologic compensation for impaired cerebral perfusion. However, severe arterial hypertension may be harmful from the standpoint of hemorrhage, encephalopathy, cardiac complications, and end-organ dysfunction. For every 10-mmHg-increase above a systolic blood pressure of 180 mm Hg, the risk of neurological deterioration increased by 40% and the risk of poor outcome increased by 23%. In contrast, hypotension or over treatment hypertension is also associated with poor outcomes because it may exacerbate the ischemic injury. Castillo et al noted that the rates of neurological worsening, poor neurological outcomes, or death increased when the baseline systolic blood pressure was <100 mm Hg or the diastolic blood pressure was <70 mm Hg.(Castillo et al., 2004) For these reasons, guidelines suggest that arterial hypertension should only be treated only if it exceeds 185/110 mm Hg. Eligibility for reperfusion therapy has a similar arterial pressure threshold of 185/110 mm Hg. In the event that antihypertensive therapy is initiated in a patient with acute ischemic stroke, it should be titrated gradually with continuous arterial pressure monitoring to avoid hypotension and abrupt decreases in blood pressure. In patients with acute ischemic stroke who are not candidates for fibrinolytic or interventional therapies, mild induced hypertension may be beneficial for improving regional blood flow early after the onset of cerebral ischemia. The administration of vasopressor therapy can be justified in acute ischemic stroke to treat hypotension or to augment cerebral perfusion, but requires careful serial neurologic and cardiovascular assessment.

GLUCOSE CONTROL

As with arterial pressure, extremes of blood glucose concentration are also associated with worse outcomes after acute ischemic stroke. Hypoglycemia alters mental status and may mimic the symptoms of stroke. Hypoglycemia with blood glucose <60 mg/dl should be identified and treated immediately. Similarly, hyperglycemia with persistent glucose levels > 200 mg/dl in the first 24 after a stroke have also been a bad prognostic sign.(Baird et al., 2003) Secondary brain injury due to hyperglycemia may occur by two mechanisms. First, anaerobic glycolysis and lactic acidosis perpetuated by hyperglycemia may worsen tissue acidosis and increase free radical production. Second, the osmotic changes caused by glucose may worsen brain edema and increase the risk of hemorrhagic transformation. However, insulin infusion to control blood glucose concentration after acute stroke have yet to demonstrate effectiveness for improving outcomes after acute stroke. Because perioperative glucose control is routine in the management of cardiac surgery patients, normal clinical protocols can be followed in patients with acute ischemic stroke with attention to avoiding hypoglycemic episodes.

TEMPERATURE

Increased body temperature (fever) in the setting of acute ischemic stroke increases metabolic demands, enhances release of neurotransmitters and free radical production and is associated with worse neurologic outcomes. The negative effects of fever mandate that the source of fever be identified and treated. Additionally, preventing and treating fever with acetaminophen, aspirin, or cooling blankets may improve prognosis after a stroke. Although experimental evidence supports a beneficial action of deliberate hypothermia in conditions of brain ischemia, induced hypothermia has not been demonstrated to be effective for the treatment of acute ischemic stroke.

ROLE OF THROMBOLYTIC THERAPY

Thrombolytic therapy with the use of intravenous tissue plasminogen activator (t-PA) has been conclusively demonstrated to decreased mortality and morbidity after stroke to reopen the occluded vessel. Thrombolytic therapy is most effective when administered within 3 hours after onset of stroke, but may also provide benefit when administered up to 6 hours after stroke. However, major surgery or trauma within 14 days is a relative contraindication to treatment with thrombolytic therapy making most cardiac surgery patients ineligible because of a significant risk of hemorrhage. For this reason, intra-arterial t-PA is an alternative option that may decrease the risk of bleeding because the medication is delivered in high concentration to the area of blockage and it can be effective up to 6 six hours after stroke. Most studies using intra-arterial t-PA are small and demonstrate a benefit only when the stroke is in a large arterial distribution such as the middle cerebral artery (MCA). Rapid mobilization of the acute stroke team, interventional neuroradiology team, the cardiac surgical team, and assessment of the risks and benefits of the procedure are necessary to implement intra-arterial thrombolysis for stroke in a cardiac surgical patient. After thrombolysis, the patient should be observed in an intensive care unit to detect bleeding that may cause cardiac tamponade.

ANTICOAGULATION

Aspirin is routinely started immediately after operations in the majority of cardiac surgical patients and early administration of aspirin within 48 hours of stroke has been associated with improved outcomes and decreased mortality.(Adams et al., 2007) Aspirin should only be withheld in the presence of hemorrhagic complications or in patients receiving thrombolytic therapy. The available clinical evidence suggests that early administration of anticoagulants such as unfractionated heparin, low molecular weight heparin, or other antithrombotic agents were not effective for decreasing the severity of acute ischemic stroke or decreasing the risk of early recurrent stroke.(Jauch et al., 2013) The decision to initiate anticoagulation therapy should be based on other clinical conditions that justify systemic anticoagulation such as atrial fibrillation, mechanical prosthetic heart valve, or ventricular assist device and not specifically for the acute treatment of stroke.

ROLE OF SURGICAL AND ENDOVASCULAR PROCEDURES IN CARDIAC SURGICAL PATIENTS AT RISK FOR STROKE

Surgical procedures such as carotid endarterectomy (CEA) and percutaneous carotid stenting in combination with cardiac operations may be justified for patients who have concomitant coronary and carotid occlusive disease. Although considerable controversy exists concerning the timing of CEA in patients who require coronary artery bypass grafting (CABG), guidelines from the American Heart Association recommend CEA for symptomatic patients with 79% to 99% stenosis of the ipsilateral carotid artery or in asymptomatic patients with severe bilateral 79% to 99% carotid artery stenosis. For this reason, preoperative carotid artery Duplex imaging is warranted in cardiac surgical patients at risk for cerebral vascular disease.

INTRA-OPERATIVE STRATEGIES TO REDUCE THE RISK OF STROKE OR NEUROLOGIC INJURIES

Intraoperative stroke or neurologic injury can be caused by thromboembolic events, hypoperfusion, or adverse reaction to medications. Therapeutic strategies to minimize the risk of neurologic injury and to minimize the severity of injuries should they occur can be employed by both the surgical and anesthetic team during cardiac operations.

CARDIOPULMONARY BYPASS

Cardiopulmonary bypass or extracorporeal circulatory support has been implicated to increase the risk of stroke or neurologic injuries in cardiac operations. Mechanisms of injury as a consequence of cardiopulmonary bypass include hypoperfusion, non-pulsatile perfusion, blood interactions with non-biological surfaces, activation of the systemic inflammatory response, and microembolism. Procedures associated with the conduct of cardiopulmonary bypass such as cannulation of the aorta, venting of the left ventricle, and cross-clamping the ascending aorta increase the risk of atheroembolic events and arterial air embolism.

The ability to perform certain cardiac operations such as coronary artery bypass grafting without the use of cardiopulmonary bypass (off-pump CABG) has been advocated as a means to potentially decrease the risk of stroke associated with cardiac operations. Initial studies comparing on and off-pump CABG showed similar outcomes in both on and off pump groups when comparing stroke, renal and myocardial dysfunction. In centers that had a large volume of off-pump cases, there was decreased morbidity and end organ dysfunction(Moller, Penninga, Wetterslev, Steinbruchel, & Gluud, 2008; Nathoe, van Dijk, & Jansen, 2003; Sedrakyan, Wu, Parashar, Bass, & Treasure, 2006). However, based on the combined reports in over 30 years experience with off-pump CABG operations, the efficacy of this approach to reduce the risk of stroke remains controversial. A meta-analysis published in 2006 that included 3,996 patients in 41 randomized controlled trials spanning the period between 1980 and 2006 indicated a 50% risk reduction for stroke among patients undergoing off-pump CABG procedures compared to procedures performed with cardiopulmonary bypass.(Sedrakyan et al., 2006) In contrast, two other meta-analyses published at approximately the same time failed to detect a statistically significant reduction in the risk of stroke for off-pump versus on-pump CABG procedures.(Cheng, Bainbridge, & Martin, 2005; Takagi, Tanabashi, Kawai, & Umemoto, 2007) The decision to include trials that reported strokes that occurred more than 30 days after operation or trials with no event rates may explain differences in the conclusions based on meta-analysis. Furthermore, patients included in randomized controlled trials may represent a low risk group and underestimate the effectiveness of off-pump CBG for reducing the risk of stroke. Nevertherless, off-pump CABG, when feasible, may offer opportunities to decrease the risk of stroke among selected high risk patients.

The decisions to perform off-pump CABG in an effort to decrease the risk of stroke should also consider other potential risks of the procedure. For example, some studies have reported inferior graft patency in the off-pump group(Diegeler et al., 2013; Khan, 2004; Nathoe et al., 2003). In the Veterans Administration (VA) Randomized to on/off bypass (ROOBY) trial of 2,000 low-risk patients randomized to off-pump or on-pump CABG, the composite outcome which comprised of all-cause mortality, non-fatal myocardial infarction and need for repeat revascularization was higher in the off-pump group despite similar clinical outcomes at 30-day and at 1-year. Furthermore lower arterial and venous graft patency was documented as well both clinically as well as by coronary angiography(Hattler et al., 2012). In another study of 2,000 elderly patients randomized to on-pump vs. off-pump CABG, there was no difference in the composite end point of death, neurological injury or new renal replacement therapy at 30 days and again at 12 months.(Diegeler et al., 2013)

To investigate the effect of cardiac surgical techniques on the incidence and timing of perioperative strokes, Sabik and his group at the Cleveland clinic performed a retrospective chart review of 45,432 primary or redo CABG performed using four different techniques. The study found that postoperative stroke (postoperative day 2-5) was more common than intraoperative stroke. Among patients with intraoperative strokes, the incidence was greatest among operations performed using cardiopulmonary bypass together with aortic cross clamp along, and hypothermic circulatory arrest.(Tarakji, 2011)

AORTIC ATHEROMATOUS DISEASE AND RISK FACTORS FOR STROKE

Aortic atheromatous disease has been associated with a higher risk of stroke during cardiac surgery because patients with severe aortic atherosclerosis are independently at increased risk for cerebrovascular disease, stroke, and perioperative atheroembolic events. Studies have demonstrated an association between ascending aortic disease, carotid artery disease and atrial fibrillation as risk factors for stroke. Identifying patients with aortic atherosclerosis and grading the severity of pre-existing aortic atherosclerotic disease is useful for both risk assessment and operative planning. Initial. The routine use of TEE has helped improved the ability to characterized the severity of aortic atherosclerosis. The French Aortic Plaque in Stroke (FAPS) group first supported causality between aortic arch atheromas and stroke.(Amarenco, Cohen, & Tzouirio, 1994) In that study, it was also shown increased atheroma plaque thickness increased the risk of stroke. The odds ratio for stroke was 1.0 (no increased risk) in patients with plaques <1 mm in thickness, 3.9 for patients with plaques between 1.0 to 3.9-mm in thickness, and 13.8 in patient with plaques >4 mm in thickness. Mobile atheroma or atheromatous plaques with mobile elements represent the greatest risk for atheroemboli, especially in the setting of surgical instrumentation of the aorta. (Gutsche et al., 2007) The distribution of atheroma at specific locations within the ascending aorta may also affect stroke risk. Blood flow patterns in the thoracic aorta are not uniform with greatest flow velocities along the non-coronary cusp and along the lateral wall of the ascending aorta during systole in a counterclockwise spiral during systole(Laas, Kleine, & Hasenkam, 1999). This pattern of blood flow may explain the slightly higher risk of embolism when atheromatous plaques are located on the lateral wall of the ascending aorta.(Van der linden, Hadjinikolaou, & Bergman, 2001)

Identifying the location and severity of aortic atheromatous disease by CT scan or intraoperative TEE can influence the conduct of the cardiac operation in terms of the decision to perform off-pump CABG, the decision to use an aortic cross clamp, choosing the best position to cannulate the ascending aorta, or choosing alternative aortic cannulation sites. Although intraoperative TEE can detect and grade the severity of atherosclerosis in the descending thoracic aorta, it is less sensitive for the detection of disease in the distal ascending aorta and arch because the trachea partially obscures TEE ultrasound imaging in those segments. Nevertheless, the absence of severe atherosclerotic disease in the descending thoracic aorta by TEE imaging make it less likely that there is significant atherosclerotic disease involving the ascending aorta or arch. Intraoperative epiaortic ultrasound with a surface probe applied directly to the aorta through the open chest overcomes these limitations of TEE. Compared to TEE, epiaortic ultrasound provided high resolution imaging of the entire length of the ascending aorta to detect and characterize atheromatous plaques.(Ibrahim et al., 2008) (Suvarna et al., 2007) Studies have also demonstrated that epiaortic ultrasound was superior to surgical palpation of the aorta for detecting the presence and location of atherosclerotic plaques. (Royse, Royse, & Blake, 1998)]]

In a study examining the use of epiaortic ultrasound in 6,000 cardiac surgical patients, it was found that the use of epiaortic ultrasound changed surgical practice in about 4% of cases and influenced the decision to use alternative sites of aortic cannulation, alternative arterial cannulation strategies, and the decision to avoid the use of an aortic cross clamp(Rosenberger et al., 2008). Although the clinical application of epiaortic ultrasound is sensitive for detecting aortic atheroma, the routine application of this

Figure 4. TEE image of Aortic Atherosclerosis, a common source of embolic stroke after during cardiac surgery

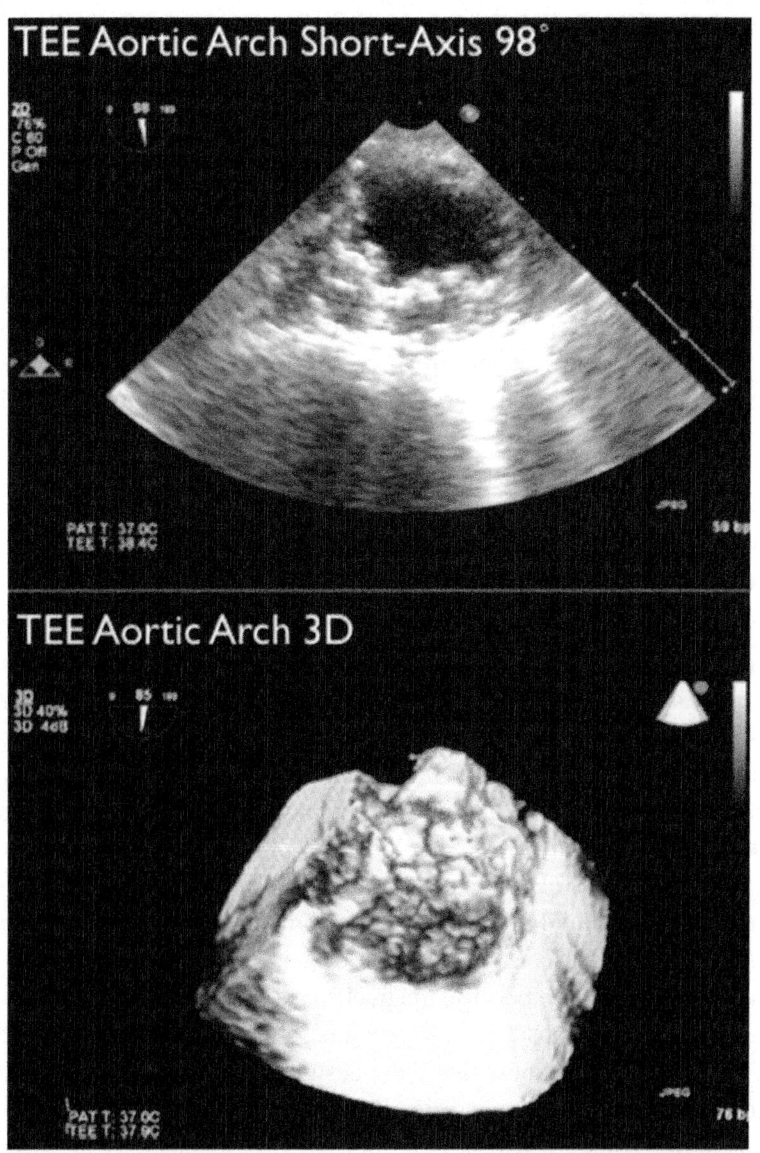

approach has yet to demonstrate efficacy for reducing the risk of stroke. In a study that employed both epiaortic ultrasound to identify aortic atheroma and transcranial ultrasound to detect cerebral emboli, the use of epiaortic imaging changed surgical practice in 30% of patients, but did not affect the number of embolic events that were detected by transcranial Doppler during cardiopulmonary bypass.(Djaiani et al., 2008) Despite its potential advantages, epiaortic ultrasound imaging is not universally performed for assessing the aorta prior to aortic manipulation for cannulation, cardioplegia device placement or aortic cross clamp placement. The reasons that may explain the limited adoption of epiaortic imaging include the limited availability of ultrasound imaging equipment for use in the operating room, reluctance by the operating the surgeon, and lack of data to support its efficacy(Suvarna et al., 2007).

In addition to ultrasound imaging, CT scanning, angiography, and MRI can be used for the preoperative assessment of aortic atherosclerosis. Cardiac gated computerized tomography with a multi-slice electrocardiographic-gated imaging cycled to respiration was found to be equivalent to TEE for evaluating atherosclerotic disease of the thoracic aorta(Hussain et al., 2008). In another study, CT angiography (CTA) was found to be less sensitive, but more specific than TEE in for detecting high-grade aortic atheromas(Barazangi et al., 2011). It should be noted that CT scan or CTA modalities have not been compared to epiaortic ultrasound imaging and may not be able to detect the presence of mobile atheroma. Diffusion weighted MRI has been used to identify white matter lesions and to provide a prognostic indicator for the risk of stroke, but there is limited data about its utility for the preoperative evaluation of thoracic aortic atherosclerosis.

Another clinical approach is to detect surrogates for aortic disease that predict the risk of perioperative stroke. It is well know that patients with a clinical history of prior stroke, transient ischemic attack, peripheral vascular disease, hypertension, diabetes mellitus, left ventricular dysfunction, atrial fibrillation, or tobacco use are at increased risk for perioperative stroke. Some studies suggest that increased carotid intimal thickness (CIMT) maybe a marker for significant aortic plaques. Harloff and colleagues showed an association between increased CIMT, worsening carotid stiffness or distensibilty and significant aortic plaques (plaques > 4mm) in acute ischemic strokes(Harloff et al., 2006). In another study, CIMT at the bifurcation of internal and external carotid arteries in asymptomatic patients was associated with the presence of atherosclerotic plaques in the aortic arch.(Tessitore et al., 2010)

SURGICAL STRATEGIES TO REDUCE THROMBOEMBOLIC EVENTS

Surgical manipulation or instrumentation of the ascending thoracic aorta and aortic arch can both cause atheroembolism or increase the subsequent risk for atheroembolism in susceptible patients with unstable plaque. Surgical techniques to minimize instrumentation of the ascending aorta include the use of off-pump CABG and the placement of a single aortic cross clamp for both cardiopulmonary bypass and the construction of the proximal coronary artery bypass grafts. If cardiopulmonary bypass must be employed, the axillary artery can be cannulated instead of the ascending aorta. Aortic cross clamping can sometimes be avoided in the absence of aortic regurgitation or by operating on the beating heart. Use of the internal mammary artery and branched arterial grafts can avoid the need to perform proximal aortic anastomosis for CABG procedures. Proximal arterial anastomotic devices that do not require aortic cross clamping have also been developed for CABG procedures.(Biancari, Catania, & D'Andrea, 2011; Thourani et al., 2014)

Clinical investigations employing the use of intra-aortic filters to capture atheroembolic debris during cardiac operations have been performed to both demonstrate the potential of surgical manipulations to cause thromboembolism and in an attempt to decrease the risk of cerebral embolization. In one study, the use of a parachute like device, which is integrated in the aortic cannula and expands after cannula placement (EmbolX Inc., Mountain View, CA, USA) was found to capture a large amount of debris during cardiopulmonary bypass, but did not affect the number of embolic events detected by transcranial Doppler monitoring(Eifert et al., 2003). Another study using this same device in 150 patients undergoing CABG procedures found no difference in cognitive outcomes at 3 months(Gerriets et al., 2010). It is possible that cerebral embolization that occurs at the time of aortic cannulation, aortic decannulation, or in the postoperative period may be a major source of stroke and devices that prevent cerebral embolization during cardiopulmonary bypass cannot prevent strokes that result from these events.

During cardiopulmonary bypass, blood is drained by the venous cannula into a venous reservoir and pumped through a heat exchanger and oxygenator before returning to the patient via the arterial cannula. The presence of cholesterol-laden plaque, microbubbles, and other microscopic debris that is generated during transit through the cardiopulmonary bypass circuit can be injected into the arterial circulation and cause cerebral embolization. The routine use of 25-micron in-line filters on arterial line of cardiopulmonary bypass circuit has helped reduce the presence of gaseous and other micro emboli, especially when bubble oxygenators were in use. The clinical benefit of arterial line filters was reported as early as 1988, but a subsequent study that compared 25-micron to 40-micron filters provided further support by demonstrating a decreased risk of neurocognitive injury. The use of 25-micron arterial filters has become an integral part of the modern cardiopulmonary bypass circuit.

During cardiopulmonary bypass, shed mediastinal blood is sometimes returned to the cardiopulmonary bypass reservoir via the cardiotomy suction device. Shed mediastinal blood may contain debris that may contribute to arterial embolization. Processing shed mediastinal blood through a red blood cell scavenging device can be employed to decrease the risk of arterial embolization from this source.

Aortic operations and valve operations that involve opening of the aorta and the left sided chambers of the heart are associated with an increased risk of stroke. In these open chamber cardiac operations, air can get trapped inside the heart and become a source for arterial embolization upon cardiac ejection. The routine use of TEE during cardiac surgery can be used to detect and assess the amount of air trapped within the left atrium and ventricle prior to cardiac ejection and to assist with during de-airing maneuvers. De-airing is typically performed after the aortic cross clamp is removed and prior to separation from CPB. Maneuvers that help to dislodge trapped intracavitary air include positive pressure breaths that expel air out of the pulmonary veins, Trendelenberg positioning to prevent air from going into the aortic arch, and the placement of a vent in the ascending aorta to aspirate residual air exiting the left ventricle. Systematic examination of non-dependent regions of the heart such as the anterior wall of the left atrium behind the aortic valve, the left atrial appendage, and along the interventricular septum in the left ventricle are common regions where intracardiac air can be trapped. Treatment of air embolism is mainly supportive. The administration of high-inspired oxygen concentration facilitates intravascular absorption and the administration of vasopressors to increase the arterial pressure improves arterial perfusion.

The insufflation of carbon dioxide into the surgical field will also reduce the risk of air embolization. Because solubility of carbon dioxide is greater than air, any gas trapped within the heart or aorta during open chamber procedures with carbon dioxide insufflation be rapidly absorbed by the blood. In 2003,

Kalpokas and colleagues conducted a small study comparing carbon dioxide insufflation to mechanical de-airing techniques and demonstrated a decrease in the amount of intra-cardiac air with carbon dioxide insufflation but the study was not powered to test for differences in neurocognitive outcomes. A subsequent study in 2008 by Martens et al found that decreasing the amount of intra-cardiac air with CO2 insufflation improved neurocognitive outcomes(Martens et al., 2008). Carbon dioxide insufflation has become a routine technique in cardiac surgery.

TECHNIQUES TO DECREASE THE SEVERITY OF NEUROLOGIC INJURY DURING CARDIAC OPERATIONS

Cardiopulmonary Bypass Machine Design

Interactions between blood components and the non-biologic surfaces of the cardiopulmonary bypass circuit causes the release of inflammatory mediators, activation of platelets, and destruction of blood cells that lead to a systemic inflammatory response. This inflammatory response has been implicated to contribute to many of the complications that are common among cardiac surgical patients in the immediate postoperative period that include neurocognitive dysfunction, as well as cardiac arrhythmias, acute renal injury, endothelial dysfunction, and multisystem organ failure. In addition, the volume required to prime the cardiopulmonary bypass circuit of the circuit causes hemodilution, that contributes further to the need for blood and blood component transfusions and their associated problems that include transfusion associated lung injury (TRALI) and transfusion associated circulatory overload (TACO). Efforts to decrease the physiologic impact of extracorporeal perfusion include minimizing the volume of the circuit and modifications to increase the biologic compatibility of the surfaces that are in contact with the blood. These changes limit the degree of hemodilution, decrease the total area of the blood-surface interface, and reduce the inflammatory response. This technology has led to the feasibility of providing long-term support for patients on extracorporeal membrane oxygenation (ECMO). Another example of this technology is the mini-extracorporeal circulation (MECC) that has a smaller volume circuit without a venous reservoir. These design modifications have been shown to reduce the level of markers of oxidative stress and inflammation, but have yet to demonstrate improved clinical outcomes. (Levy & Tanaka, 2003; Zeitani et al., 2013) (Immer et al., 2007) (Wiesenack, 2004)

Temperature Management on CPB

Deliberate hypothermia has a long history of use as a therapeutic intervention in cardiac operations to decrease the risk of ischemic injury to the brain and other organs during cardiopulmonary bypass and for cases that require temporary circulatory arrest. The original concept of employing hypothermia was based on the principle that decreasing body temperature would decrease the oxygen requirement of tissues thereby increasing the tolerance of organs to ischemic conditions. (Bigelow, Lindsay, & Greenwood, 1950) Subsequent studies have demonstrated that every 10 degree Celsius reduction in body temperature was associated with a 2.3-fold reduction in cerebral metabolic rate. (McCollough, Zhang, & Reich, 1999) Assuming the brain can tolerate a 5 minute duration of ischemia under normothermic conditions, the decrease in cerebral metabolism associated with hypothermia would predict that the brain could tolerate a 17 to 38 minute period of circulatory arrest at temperatures ranging between 15°C to 20°C. (McCollough et al., 1999) Existing clinical experience supports the effectiveness of deep hypothermia for protecting the brain from ischemic injury for a limited duration temporary circulatory arrest. (Appoo et al., 2006; Gaynor et al., 2005)

Contemporary studies have demonstrated that mild hypothermia was protective even when instituted after a period of ischemia due to cardiac arrest. (Bernard, Gray, & Buist, 2002; group, 2002) These studies suggest that the clinical benefits of deliberate hypothermia extend beyond its ability to decrease cerebral metabolic rate.

Despite the evidence supporting the beneficial actions of deliberate hypothermia for brain protection, considerable controversy remains regarding the direct application of deliberate hypothermia for cardiac operations. For example, the safe duration of deep hypothermic circulatory arrest, the optimal temperature for deep hypothermic circulatory arrest, and the best method for assessing brain temperature during deliberate hypothermia remain to be established. Furthermore, the clinical application of deliberate hypothermia has associated risks that must be considered in relation to its potential benefits. Deliberate hypothermia prolongs the duration of cardiopulmonary bypass, increases the risk for hyperthermia during rewarming, increases the risk for infection, and may contribute to postoperative coagulopathy.

Evidence suggests that hyperthermia during rewarming on CPB is detrimental and may contribute to mismatching of oxygen supply and demand during the period of reperfusion when the brain is most vulnerable to injury. Cerebral hyperthermia as a consequence of rapid rewarming or arterial inflow temperatures exceeding 37°C has been shown to be associated with worse neurologic and neurocognitive outcomes. (Alina M. Grigore et al., 2002; A. M. Grigore, Murray, Ramakrishna, & Djaiani, 2009; Sahu et al., 2009) Additional evidence to support an adverse effect of hyperthermia is the association between hyperthermia or fever and adverse neurologic outcomes among patients with stroke or brain injury.(Ginsberg & Busto, 1998)

There are no direct means to measure actual brain temperature when employing deliberate hypothermia. Temperature management during cooling and rewarming on cardiopulmonary bypass is guided by measurements using temperature probes in the nasopharynx, esophagus, tympanic membrane, bladder, rectum, arterial inflow, or venous return. The electroencephalogram (EEG) provides information on brain activity in response to deliberate hypothermia and the onset of electrocortical silence in the absence of anesthetic agents can be used as a physiologic surrogate for achieving satisfactory metabolic suppression produced and conditions deep hypothermic circulatory arrest.(Stecker, Cheung, & Pochettino, 2001)

Existing clinical evidence supports the use of deliberate hypothermia for the prevention of neurologic injury in patients undergoing cardiac operations. A review of the literature recommends the following approaches to the use of deliberate hypothermia in cardiac surgical patients. (A. M. Grigore et al., 2009)

1. Mild hypothermia is indicated for patients at low risk for neurologic injury by allowing the body temperature to drift to 34°C–35°C without active cooling and then slowly rewarming to temperatures not exceeding 37°C. (Newman et al., 2006)
2. Patients undergoing complex operation or who are at high risk for neurologic injury should be actively cooled to 28°C–30°C followed by slow rewarming to temperatures not exceeding 37°C. (Alina M. Grigore et al., 2002)
3. In patients at high risk for neurologic injury but relatively straightforward surgery: Active cooling to 32°C, gentle rewarming to 34°C–35°C, and weaning from CPB at 34°C–35°C may be preferred

to protect the brain in the OR as in the early postoperative period in the ICU(Sahu et al., 2009). Finally, hyperthermia is bad for the brain. Once the diagnosis of brain injury is made it is important to maintain normothermia i.e. <37 degree Celsius in the ICU.

Steroids and Pharmacologic Neuroprotection

Although anesthetic drugs that produce cerebral suppression, drugs that promote ischemic preconditioning, and anti-inflammatory agents all have theoretical potential to protect against ischemic neurologic injury, multiple studies have yet to definitively demonstrate clinical efficacy. (Chaney, 2002; Ho & Tan, 2009; Murphy, Whitlock, Gutsche, & Augoustides, 2013). Smaller studies have suggested that glucocorticoid administration may decrease ventilator dependence, atrial fibrillation(Halonen, 2007) and postoperative inotrope requirement.(Kilger et al., 2003; Murphy et al., 2013) The Dexamethasone for Cardiac Surgery Trial (DECS) published in 2012 failed to support a benefit of dexamethasone at a dose of 1 mg/kg on the incidence of major complications including stroke and atrial fibrillation after cardiac operations, but did show that patients receiving dexamethasone had a shorter hospital length of stay and a lower risk of delirium and infections. However a sub-study of the DECS trial employing neuropsychiatric testing at one and 12 months after operation failed to show a statistically significant benefit of dexamethasone on the incidence of postoperative cognitive decline.(Ottens, 2014) Despite the absence of definitive proof for the beneficial action of glucocorticoids, no adverse effect of steroids has been detected in any of the trials with respect to wound healing or infections. The Steroids in Cardiac Surgery (SIRS) trial is a multi center trial in progress with a planned enrollment of over 5,000 patients to further test role of steroids in cardiac surgery.

Role of Modified Ultrafiltration

Modified ultrafiltration can be performed during CPB to reduce the load of inflammatory mediators that have been implicated to contribute to the systemic inflammatory response. Although small studies have suggested that modified ultrafiltration may reduce the risk of lung injury and alveolar damage, the effect of modified ultrafiltration on neurologic outcomes have yet to be studied.

Hematocrit on CPB

Studies suggest that anemia and hemodilution as a consequence of cardiopulmonary bypass was a risk factor for neurologic morbidity. Karkouti et al. observed a 10% increased risk of stroke rate with each percent decrease in the nadir hematocrit(Karkouti et al., 2005; Karkouti et al., 2009). Newman et al. found a higher incidence of neurocognitive decline in elderly patients randomized to receive profound hemodilution (hematocrit of 15%–18%)(Newman et al., 2006). Furthermore the risk of developing acute renal failure or a significant increase in postoperative serum creatinine increased as hematocrit values decreased below 21%–24% on CPB(Ranucci, 2006). Despite the risks associated with anemia, the need for blood transfusion has also been linked to the risk of neurologic complications. (Koch et al., 2006) At present efforts to address the effects of anemia on adverse neurologic outcomes should be focused to techniques to both minimize hemodilution, blood loss, and transfusion requirements.

CEREBRAL HYPOPERFUSION

Early studies demonstrated that low arterial pressure during cardiopulmonary bypass was associated with cerebral damage. (Tufo et al., 1970) As a consequence, an effort is made to maintain a mean arterial pressure (MAP) of 50–60 mm Hg during CPB in the majority of adult patients undergoing cardiac operations. This practice is based on data supporting a MAP of 50 mm Hg as the lower limit of cerebral autoregulation(Murkin, Farrar, & Tweed, 1987). However, the lower limit of cerebral autoregulation may be increased in advanced age, chronic hypertension, cerebrovascular disease, peripheral vascular disease, increased pulse pressure, or diabetes mellitus. In these conditions, a higher MAP may be required to ensure adequate cerebral and end organ perfusion and may explain the reason for increased risk of stroke among patients with hypertension. A randomized controlled study comparing a target MAP of 50-60 mm Hg to a target MAP of 80-100 mm Hg during CPB showed a reduction in a composite cardiac and neurologic outcome in patients maintained at the greater MAP during elective CABG, but could not demonstrate a statistically significant decrease in the rate of stroke or postoperative cognitive decline. (Gold, Charlson, & Szatrowski, 1995) Another study has also supported the benefit of higher perfusion pressures on the risk of neurologic injuries among patients with severe aortic atherosclerosis. (Hartman, Yao, & Bruefach, 1996)

Because maintaining a high MAP during cardiac operations may not always be possible or desirable from the perspective of the need for vasopressor therapy, risk of bleeding, or optimizing cardiac performance, techniques such as near-infrared cerebral oximetry (NIRS) have been developed in an attempt to detect cerebral hypoperfusion during cardiac operations.

Commercially available NIRS cerebral oximeters estimate regional tissue oxygenation by transcutaneous measurement of oxygen saturation in the frontal cerebral cortex that may reflect the supply of substrate to vulnerable watershed regions of the rest of the brain. Near-infared cerebral oximetry (rSO2) utilizes 2 photo-detectors linked to a light source attached by adhesive pads to the forehead to selectively sample tissue at a specified depth beneath the skin. NIRS is not dependent on pulsatile flow making it feasible for used during CPB.

Because arterial blood cannot be distinguished from venous blood in the sample volume, the value for rSO2 that represents brain oxygenation consists of a weighted average that is approximately 75% venous and 25% arterial (Edmonds, 2002), but cerebral hypoperfusion would be expected to cause an decrease in both cerebral venous and arterial oxygen saturation(Kuroda, Houkin, & Abe, 1996). In theory, NIRS monitoring could provide an early warning for cerebral hypoperfusion. Interventions to respond to cerebral desaturation include augmenting the arterial pressure, augmenting CPB flow, increasing the arterial oxygen content, transfusion for anemia, normalizing arterial PaCO2, checking for evidence of arterial cannula malpositioning, and checking for venous outflow obstruction. (S. Conolly, Arrowsmith, & Klein, 2010; Edmonds, 2002; Kellermann & Jungwirth, 2010; Murkin, 2013) [78,]

Despite the physiologic rationale for NIRS monitoring, clinical evidence to support the clinical effectiveness of NIRS-guided interventions to treat cerebral hypoperfusion have yet to be definitively proven. A retrospective study of 2,297 patients who underwent cardiac surgery that compared the use of NIRS monitoring to conventional management found a nearly statistically significant decrease in stroke, duration of mechanical ventilation support, ICU length of stays and hospital.(Goldman, Sutter, Ferdinand, & Trace, 2004). A randomized controlled study by Murkin(Murkin, 2013) [78,] et al. Comparing the use of NIRS together with a NIRS-directed algorithm to optimize cerebral saturation to conventional management failed to demonstrate a decrease in adverse outcomes in the treatment group. The NIRS-directed

Figure 5. Operating principles of the use of near-infrared spectroscopy. On the screen, the large number indicates the ongoing brain oximetry values and the small number the baseline value obtained at the beginning of the recording from both the right (R) and the left (L) hemisphere usually obtained prior to induction of general anesthesia.

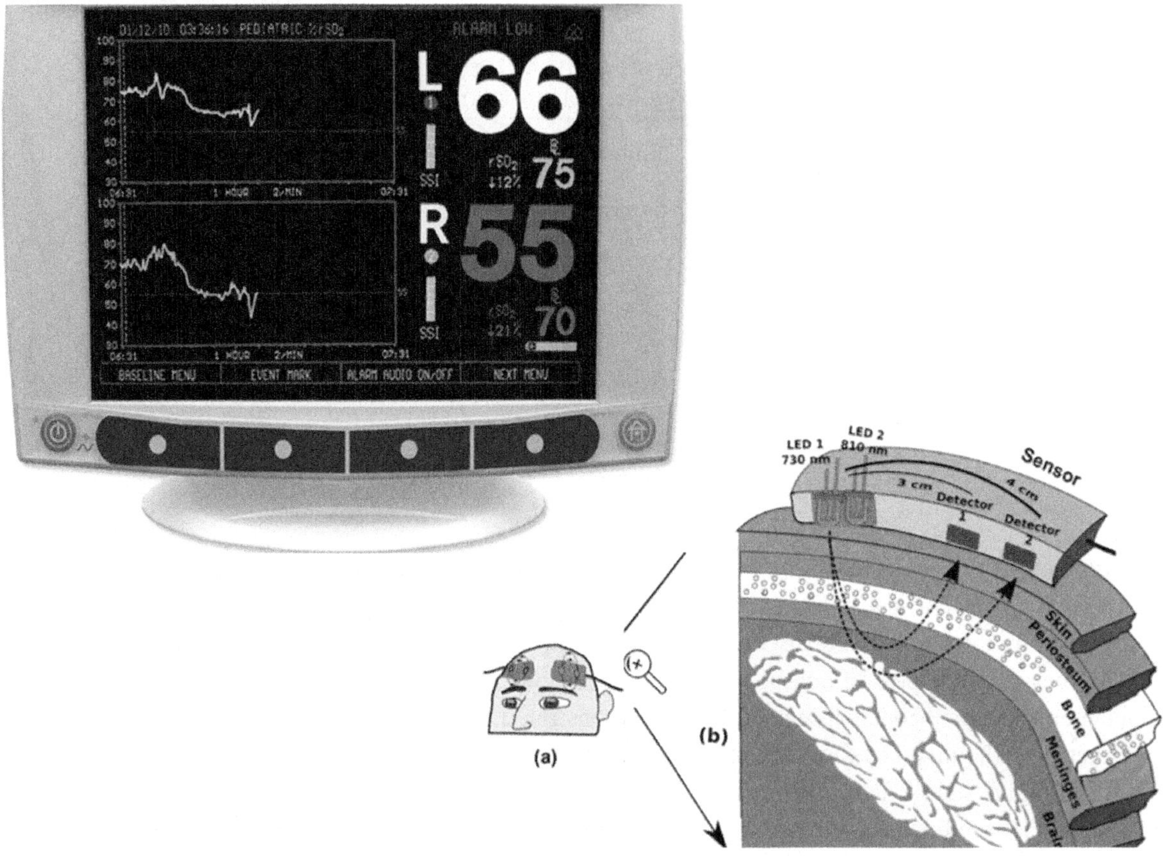

interventions included optimizing blood pressure or cardiac output, increasing PaCO2 to increase cerebral blood flow or blood transfusions to increase oxygen carrying capacity. However, the study demonstrated that interventions were effective in improving cerebral oxygen saturation and that lower baseline cerebral oxygen saturation or prolonged cerebral oxygen desaturations was associated with major organ morbidity and mortality. Another randomized trial of NIRS monitoring in elective CABG patients also failed to demonstrate the ability of NIRS to reduce the risk of postoperative cognitive decline, but did show that the duration and severity of cerebral desaturation during operation was associated with early postoperative decline and increased risk for prolonged hospitalization. (Slater et al., 2009) Additional studies also support the association between rSO2 values and postoperative morbidity and mortality. (Heringlake, 2011) Based on the existing evidence, NIRS monitoring of cerebral oxygen saturation is capable of identifying patients at risk for adverse outcomes but evidence to support the routine application of NIRS-guided interventions in cardiac surgical patients to decrease the incidence of adverse neurologic outcomes has yet to be established. Ongoing investigations employing NIRS technology to identify the cerebral autoregulatory threshold among individual patients may permit circulatory management to be individualized and yield additional clinical applications of NIRS. (Brady et al., 2010)

Figure 6. Stepwise approach to cerebral desaturation during cardiac surgery

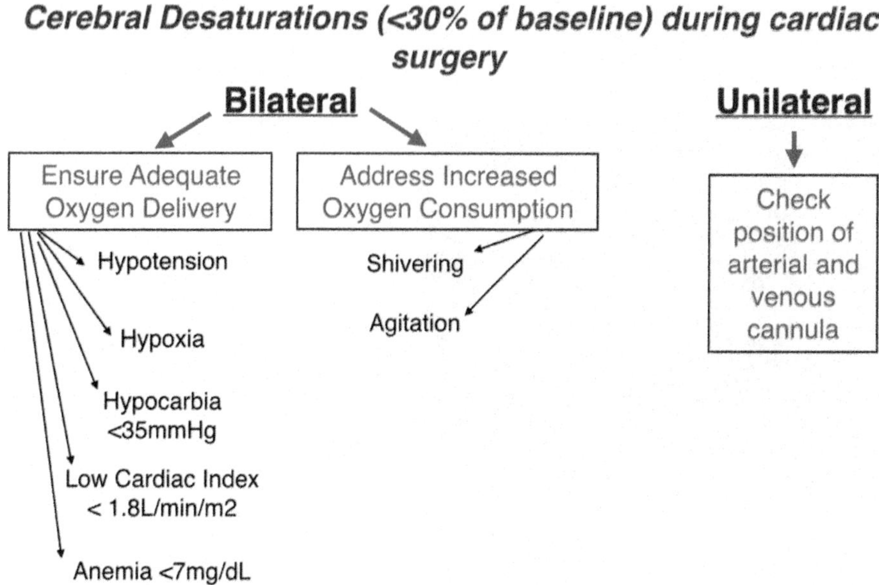

Attenuation of the electrical activity of the brain measured by electroencephalopathy (EEG) can also detect changes in cortical brain activity caused by hypoperfusion, hypothermia, or anesthetic drugs. Systems to monitor processed EEG signals such as the bispectral index (BIS) are commercially available to measure the depth of anesthesia during operations. Although these systems are not designed to detect cerebral perfusion, a recent study has demonstrated that cardiac surgical patients who had their anesthetic depth guided by the BIS values had a lower incidence of postoperative delirium compared to those whose anesthetic depth was targeted to the end-tidal anesthetic concentration. (E. L. Whitlock et al., 2014) This finding of an association between low anesthetic requirements and risk of postoperative delirium suggest that increased sensitivity to anesthetic agents may be a marker for patients at greater risk of adverse events and that intraoperative use of EEG or BIS to guide anesthetic management has the potential to decrease the risk of adverse neurologic complications.

PREVENTING POSTOPERATIVE THROMBOEMBOLIC COMPLICATIONS

In the immediate postoperative period after cardiac operations patients who had cardiac valve replacement with a prosthetic valve and patients who develop atrial fibrillation are at increased risk of stroke for thromboembolic stroke. Appropriate medical management of these two conditions has potential and may have contributed to the decreased incidence of postoperative stroke.

Atrial fibrillation occurs in approximately 27% to 40% of patients after cardiac operations. Most commonly, the onset of new postoperative atrial fibrillation occurs within the first 72 hours after cardiac surgery. As many as 40% of patients who develop postoperative atrial fibrillation will have a second episode within 2 days. Advanced age is a the single greatest risk factor for atrial fibrillation and for every 10-year increase in age beyond 70 years, the odds of development of atrial fibrillation increase by

75%.(Carrascal et al., 2014; Mathew, 2004; Mitchell, 2004) Treatment for postoperative atrial fibrillation involves ventricular rate control, restoration and maintenance of sinus rhythm and anticoagulation to decrease the risk of stroke. Ventricular rate control can be achieved with beta-blockers, amiodarone, digoxin, or diltiazem. Among these agents, beta-blockers and intravenous amiodarone are the most effective. Beta-blocker therapy should be resumed as soon as it is safe whether or not the patient had been on preoperative beta-blocker therapy. The only established contraindications for postoperative beta-blocker therapy are decompensated heart failure, hypotension, bradycardia, or heart block. For patients at risk for adverse effects of beta-blockade, the drug can be started with low doses and incrementally increased. Intravenous amiodarone can be administered alone or in combination with beta-blockers and is most commonly given as an intravenous infusion at 0.5 mg to 1.0 mg per minute followed by an intravenous loading dose of 2-5 mg/kg. Some patients will convert to sinus rhythm in response to pharmacologic treatment. Attempts to restore sinus with electrical cardioversion will also be more effective after beta-blocker or amiodarone therapy has been started. The treatment of postoperative pain, timely discontinuation of sympathomimetic drugs, and prevention of respiratory complications are also important adjuncts in the prevention and treatment of postoperative atrial fibrillation.

Current ACLS guidelines recommend that synchronized cardioversion for new onset atrial fibrillation is safe if the duration of atrial fibrillation has been less than 48 hours. After 48 hours it is recommended that transesophageal echocardiography be performed to determine the absence of a left atrial thrombus prior to performing electrical cardioversion. In 2005, the prophylactic amiodarone for prevention of atrial fibrillation in patients after revascularization, valve replacement or repair (PAPABEAR) study showed that a 13-day course of perioperative amiodarone was not only safe but also effective in decreasing the incidence of postoperative atrial fibrillation.

Scores based on clinical risk factors for stroke can be applied to guide the use of anticoagulation therapy for stroke prevention in patients with atrial fibrillation. A commonly used score assigns one point for a history of congestive heart failure, hypertension, age≥75 years, or diabetes mellitus and 2 points for prior stroke or transient ischemic attack (CHADS2).

A CHADS2 score of 2 indicates a high risk of stroke and a score of 0 indicates a low risk of stroke. The most recent American College of Chest Physicians (ACCP) guidelines for anticoagulation management of atrial fibrillation recommend that patients with a CHADS2 score of ≥1 will benefit from treatment

Table 2. CHADS2 scoring system used for the assessment of stroke risk in patients with AF. Patients receive 1 point for each risk factor and 2 points for the risk factor of previous stroke or TIA. Total scores range from 0 to 6.

Risk Factor	Score
Congestive Heart Failure	1
Hypertension	1
Age >75 years	1
Diabetes Mellitus	1
Prior CVA/TIA	2
Total Score	**0-6**

with aspirin combined with oral anticoagulation or antiplatelet therapy. (You et al., 2012) The decision to initiate anticoagulation or antiplatelet therapy in the early postoperative period must consider also the risk of bleeding and need for subsequent surgical procedures.

The risk of thromboembolic complications after valve replacement or repair is greatest immediately after operation because of exposed non-endothelialized surfaces and the prothrombotic state. (Cannegieter, Rosendaal, & Briet, 1994; Kulik et al., 2006) In the first six months after operation, the thromboembolic risk is up to seven times greater than in the following months and years. After aortic valve replacement, the risk of thromboembolic events decreases from 16 per 100 patient-years in the early postoperative period to 1.4 per 100 patient-years at 5 years. Similarly, after mitral valve replacement, the risk decreases over time from 21 per 100 patient-years to 2.5 per 100 patient-years.(Goldhaber, 2006; Kulik et al., 2006) The need for long-term oral anticoagulation with vitamin K antagonists (VKA) therapy in patients with mechanical prosthetic valves is well established. Aspirin therapy reduces the risk of thromboembolism from 4 to 8 per 100 patient-years to 2.2 per 100 patient-years and this risk is further reduced to 1 per 100 patient-years with oral VKA. Institution of anticoagulant therapy in the early postoperative period needs a multidisciplinary approach to assess the risks of bleeding and the benefits of achieving therapeutic anticoagulation. Typically, intravenous heparin is started as a bridge to oral anticoagulation in patients after mitral valve replacement where the risk of thrombosis is greatest while oral anticoagulation is administered alone to patients after aortic valve replacement that are at increased risk for postoperative bleeding.

The 2008 ACC/AHA guidelines for anticoagulation of patients with prosthetic heart valves recommended: (Bonow et al., 2008):

1. Older bileaflet mechanical or Medtronic Hall prostheses for AVR, in patients with no risk factors, VKA is indicated to achieve an INR of 2.0 to 3.0
2. Starr Edwards valves which have a higher risk of thrombosis need to be anticoagulated with VKA to an INR of 2.5-3.5
3. Any mechanical valve in the mitral position, VKA is indicated to achieve an INR of 2.5 to 3.5.

Table 3. Risk of stroke or systemic thromboembolism based on $CHADS_2$ score

$CHADS_2$ Score	Annual Stroke Rate, %(95% CI)	Thromboembolism
0	1.9 (1.2, 3.0)	1.24 (1.16, 1.33)
1	2.8 (2.0, 3.8)	3.56 (3.42, 3.7)
2	4.0 (3.1, 5.1)	5.4 (5.18, 5.63)
3	5.9 (4.6, 7.3)	9.89 (9.50, 10.31)
4	8.5 (6.3, 11.1)	13.70 (12.95, 14.48)
5	12.5 (8.2, 17.5)	12.57 (11.18, 14.14)
6	18.2 (10.5, 27.4)	17.17 (12.33, 23.92)
Low risk 0		1.24 (1.16, 1.33)
Intermediate risk 1		3.56 (3.42, 3.70)
High risk 2-6		7.97 (7.77, 8.17)

4. After AVR or MVR with a bioprosthetic valve and no risk factors, aspirin is indicated at 75 to 100 mg per day
5. After AVR or MVR with a bioprosthesis and risk factors; VKA is indicated to achieve an INR of 2.0 to 3.0.
6. For those patients who are unable to take warfarin after MVR or AVR, aspirin is indicated in a dose of 75 to 325 mg per day.

The 2012 ACCP guidelines for anticoagulation in patients after valve replacement or valve repair recommended:(R. P. Whitlock et al., 2012)

Bioprosthetic valves:

1. Bioprosthetic AVR with no additional risk factors for stroke: aspirin alone
2. Transcatheter AVR: dual antiplatelet therapy with aspirin and clopidogrel
3. Bioprosthetic MVR: VKA with INR goal of 2-3

Mechanical valves:

1. Bridging with heparin infusion or low molecular weight heparin until target INR is reached on VKA therapy.
2. Mechanical AVR: VKA INR goal 2-3
3. Mechanical MVR VKA INR goal 2.5-3.5
4. Mechanical AVR and MVR at low risk of bleeding, add aspirin to VKA.

Valve Repair:

1. Mitral valve repair: aspirin alone is sufficient
2. Aortic valve repair: aspirin alone is sufficient

SEIZURES

Seizures are reportedly less common after cardiac surgery with an incidence of approximately 0.5%. While convulsive seizures cause great concern to medical personnel and families, the nonconvulsive type of seizures are the ones that are frequently missed and not always benign. (Hunter & Young, 2011) The differential diagnosis of an obtunded patient includes both types of seizures; additionally seizures delay separation from mechanical ventilation as well as discharge from the ICU as well as hospital. While myoclonic jerks, shivering as well as shaking movements get mistaken for seizures, the three common types of seizures are generalized tonic clonic with generalized jerking movements of the entire body, focal convulsive or non convulsive.

Generalized tonic clonic seizures often witnessed by family members or nursing staff may appear as jerking rhythmic movements or as tonic stiffening followed by rhythmic jerking movements. Focal seizures may present as focal eye or head deviation or migrating seizure activity such as from face to hand. Nonconvulsive seizures are the most difficult to diagnose. There needs to be a high index of suspicion and is often a diagnosis made by continuous Electroencephalography (EEG) monitoring.

In the cardiac surgery patient, various etiologies including air emboli, micro emboli from cardiopulmonary bypass pump and blood pressure fluctuations have been implicated as causative agents of seizures. In cardiac surgery patients, given the increased risk of hemoorhagic complications, antifibrinolytics have been shown to decrease the incidence of bleeding in this patient population. Various agents have been used including aprotinin, aminocaproic acid and tranexamic acid (TXA). In the US, aprotinin has been withdrawn given the higher side effect profile, and the recent shortage of aminocaproic acid has resulted in patients receiving TXA. Furthermore, total dose used has varied (bolus plus continued infusion) from 60mg/kg to 260mg/kg. The recent resurgence in the use of antifibrinolytic agent tranexamic acid has been identified as epileptogenic in the postoperative period. (Manji et al., 2012; Martin, Wiesner, Breuer, Lange, & Tassani, 2008; Murkin et al., 2010)Manji et al conducted a retrospective study of about 6000 patients to evaluate the role of tranexamic acid in the causation of seizures. They looked at the use of tranexamic acid (TXA) as well as the dosages used in patients who developed seizures in the postoperative period. This study identified a higher incidence of seizures in patients that had received high-dose TXA during cardiac surgery. Furthermore, in 2010 Murkin et al described an increase in the seizure rate from 1.3% to 3.8% when higher doses of TXA were used in their study of 669 cardiac surgery cases.(Murkin et al., 2010) The BART trial, which established the safety of TXA in cardiac surgery patients, did not show an association between TXA and seizures, but the doses used in those patients were modest in comparison. (Fergusson et al., 2008) The incidence of seizures returned to baseline once lower doses of TXA were used. The mechanism behind TXA and seizures has been postulated to increased TXA bioavailability in the CSF. It is possible that the inflammatory response to cardiopulmonary bypass renders the blood-brain barrier more permeable to TXA. If TXA is required in cardiac surgery patients, it is best to limit its total dosage, as at lower doses the risk of seizures appears to be closer to baseline risk.

Seizures increase metabolic activity of the heart and brain and need to be stopped. Frequently, new-onset seizures in the cardiac surgery patient present within 24 hours of surgery occur while sedation is being weaned. First-line therapy includes benzodiazepines such as midazolam or lorazepam to stop followed by specific anti-epileptic medicines such as valproic acid, levetiracetam and phenytoin. Phenytoin has a narrow therapeutic index and causes bradycardia and hypotension in cardiac surgery patients and should be used cautiously. Levetiracetam and valproic acid are safe alternatives to phenytoin in the cardiac surgical ICU. Similar to stroke, rapid brain scanning should be performed to rule out an organic cause of seizures such as hemorrhage or infarction while additional diagnostic tests should be geared towards an inorganic cause of seizures such as infections and metabolic derangements. EEG monitoring is the gold standard in the diagnosis and management of seizures. While anesthetic drugs, benzodiazepines and barbiturates may appear to stop a seizure; an EEG is required to demonstrate cessation of seizure activity in the brain. Supportive therapy should include oxygen, blood pressure management and adequate management of the post-ictal state. Presence of prolonged seizures (>60 minutes) may require intubation and mechanical ventilation. The occurrence of status epilepticus while rare continues to be a poor prognosticator in the cardiac surgery patient.

ENCEPHALOPATHY

Encephalopathy is broad, nonspecific term, used to describe a syndrome of global brain dysfunction that can range in severity from neurocognitive deficits to coma. The syndrome is generally used to describe conditions of decreased level of consciousness or confusion without specific focal neurologic deficits.

Depending on the on the diagnostic criteria used to define encephalopathy, it may occur in approximately 10% of all cardiac surgery patients with an increased frequency among patients with a greater number of pre-existing medical conditions or among those undergoing more complex surgical procedures increases, so does the likelihood of developing encephalopathy(Bruggemans, 2013; Newman et al., 2006). A prospective study in 2002 found a 6% incidence of encephalopathy among 2,700 patients undergoing CABG operations. Patients with postoperative encephalopathy had a 7.5% increase in hospital mortality and a two-fold increase in hospital length of stay. In terms of quality of life markers, patients who with postoperative encephalopathy or stroke more likely to require rehabilitation and were less likely to discharged home after the hospitalization(McKhann, Grega, & BorowiczJr, 2002).

The diagnosis of encephalopathy does not refer to a specific etiology and should prompt a medical evaluation to search for underlying causes or conditions that may be contributing to global brain dysfunction. Although global brain injury caused by subclinical stroke, anoxia, or hypoferfusion combined with underlying predisposition to dementia may contribute to postoperative encephalopathy in cardiac surgical patients, treatment in the early postoperative period should be focused on identifying treatable conditions and supportive care. The recovery from sedatives and anesthetic agents administered during operations may also contribute to postoperative encephalopathy. A careful review of the anesthetic record will help to differentiate residual drug action from other causes of postoperative encephalopathy. Although high dose narcotic analgesics and benzodiazepines were commonly used for general anesthesia for cardiac operations, contemporary practice has evolved to using lower doses of narcotics in combination with anesthetic and sedative drugs that have short durations of action to promote early recovery from the effects of general anesthesia and faster liberation from mechanical ventilation as well decreasing the length of stay in the ICU. The Cochrane database review studied 25 trials in fast-track cardiac surgery and found that anesthetics that used low dose opioid techniques were associated with decreased ICU length of stay(Zhu, 2012). There is also evidence to suggest that opioid analgesics and benzodiazepines may contribute to postoperative delirium or cognitive decline in elderly patients. (Leung, Sands, Vaurio, & Wang, 2006)

Although the administration of narcotics and sedatives may contribute to postoperative encephalopathy, withdrawal from alcohol and other drugs during hospitalization may also cause encephalopathy. The two most common withdrawal syndromes in post-surgical patients are alcohol and benzodiazepines. The most manifestation of alcohol withdrawal is delirium tremens, which is characterized by hallucinations, agitation and signs of autonomic hyperactivity and typically occurs between 72-96 hours after cessation of drinking. However, both alcohol and benzodiazepine withdrawal may be manifested by confusion, agitation, and even seizures. Treatment for drug withdrawal is largely supportive with thiamine, beta-blockers and small doses of benzodiazepines, but drug treatment with benzodiazepines may also exacerbate the condition of there is other causes for the postoperative encephalopathy. A detailed medical and social history should be elicited whenever drug or alcohol withdrawal is suspected.

Postoperative renal or hepatic dysfunction may also contribute to postoperative encephalopathy. Up to 30% of cardiac surgery patients exhibit evidence of acute kidney injury and up to 1% may require renal replacement therapy. The causes of acute kidney in the cardiac surgery patient is likely multifactorial and contributing conditions such prolonged duration of CPB, hypoperfusion, or thromboembolism may also be factors in the etiology of postoperative encephalopathy. (Karkouti et al., 2005; Karkouti et al., 2009) Uremia associated with altered mentation or encephalopathy is a clinical indication for dialysis. Hepatic encephalopathy should be suspected in patients with a history of hepatic disease, abnormal liver function tests or hyperbilirubinemia. Pre-existing congestive hepatopathy, perioperative heart failure, hypoperfusion or venous congestion may be etiologic factors that can contribute to both hepatic dysfunction and brain injury manifested in the postoperative period. A Model for end-stage Liver disease (MELD) score greater than 13 at the time of operation has been shown to be a marker for post-surgical hepatic dysfunction(Suman, 2004). In patients with suspected hepatic encephalopathy, treatment with lactulose and rifaximin can be considered for eliminating ammonia from the gut to reduce the symptoms of encephalopathy(Bass, Mullen, & Sanyal, 2010).

Other medically treatable causes for postoperative encephalopathy in the cardiac surgery patient include electrolyte disorders, hypoglycemia, hypothyroidism, or adrenal dysfunction. These conditions can be diagnosed by standard laboratory testing. The risk for hypoglycemia may be increased among cardiac surgical patients where efforts to control blood glucose concentrations with insulin therapy is routine. Hyponatremia is common among patients with heart failure and hypernatremia is common after cardiac operations when sodium bicarbonate is used to treat metabolic acidosis. When the cause of postoperative encephalopathy cannot be determined, neurologic consultation and diagnostic brain imaging is a necessary part of the medical evaluation to assess for unusual or treatable causes of encephalopathy.

DELIRIUM

Delirium is an acute condition characterized by fluctuating attention, disorganized thinking, altered level of consciousness, disorientation, impaired memory, hallucinations, restlessness, and altered sleep. Delirium is one of the most common acute neurologic consequences of cardiac surgery and may affect approximately 5% to 80% of patients after operation. This wide variation in incidence is likely a consequence of differences used in the diagnostic criteria used to define this condition, efforts to identify patients with delirium, and reporting. In 2001, Ely and colleagues introduced the Confusion assessment method for the intensive care unit (CAM-ICU) to identify patients with delirium(Ely, Inouye, & Bernard, 2001; Soja et al., 2008). The routine clinical use of standardized tools for the assessment of delirium has improved reporting to characterize the incidence of postoperative delirium, identify factors that increase the risk of postoperative delirium and to develop improved strategies for preventing and managing delirium

The etiology and pathophysiology of delirium in the cardiac surgery patient is complex and multifactorial and includes many of the factors that contribute to postoperative encephalopathy. Low score on the mini-mental state examination, prior stroke or transient ischemic attack, depression, and malnutrition have been identified as preoperative risk factors for the development of delirium(Hudetz et al., 2011; Shadvar, Baastani, Mahmoodpoor, & Bilehjani, 2013; Stransky et al., 2011; Tomasi & von Dossow-Hanfstingl, 2014; E. L. Whitlock et al., 2014) In a study of patients undergoing CABG, or valve, or combined procedures with and without use of cardiopulmonary bypass, the risk of delirium quadrupled in the setting of increased risk factors.(Bilotta et al., 2011; Hudetz et al., 2011) Postoperative delirium as a distinct entity is associated with increased hospital and ICU length of stay, increased short

Recent attention has been directed to the role of anesthetic agents and sedative drugs administered during operation and in the intensive care in the development and duration of postoperative delirium. Because increased ICU length of stay and increased duration of pharmacologic sedation is associated with postoperative delirium, anesthetic regimens that promote early postoperative recovery and weaning from mechanical ventilator support show promise for decreasing the risk of postoperative delirium. Minimally invasive approaches to cardiac operations may also decrease the physiologic impact of cardiac surgery, reduce the duration of postoperative convalescence and reduce the risk of delirium.

Figure 7. Delirium assessment in the ICU using CAM-ICU scoring

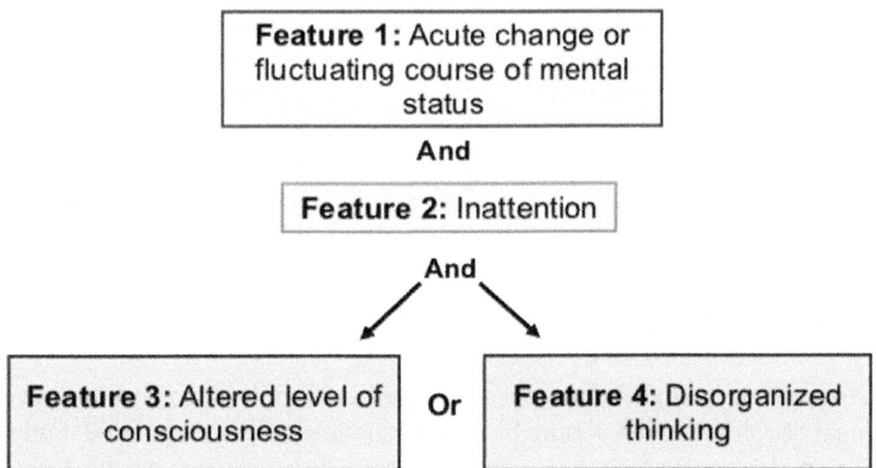

Studies have demonstrated that the incidence of delirium can be decreased along with a cost savings when dexmedetomidine was used instead of midazolam for sedation among ICU patients(McPherson et al., 2013; Pandharipande PP, 2005). Ongoing studies such as the PINOCCHIO trial is investigating the role of anesthetics that include propofol, sevoflurane and desflurane in the etiology of postoperative delirium. Preliminary data suggest that maintenance of general anesthesia with propofol instead of inhaled anesthetics may potentially decrease the incidence of postoperative delirium(Bilotta et al., 2011).

The treatment of postoperative delirium remains mostly supportive. Efforts to reestablish normal sleep-wake cycles, re-orient patients to their surroundings, manage postoperative pain, and physical rehabilitation can decrease the duration of delirium. Although physical restraints and drug therapy with agents such as haloperidol, quetiapine, or even sedative hypnotic drugs are sometimes necessary for the management of postoperative delirium, these interventions prolong recovery.

POST OPERATIVE COGNITIVE DECLINE

Postoperative cognitive decline (POCD) is a term used to describe a condition characterized by impaired memory, concentration, language comprehension, intellect, and social integration. In contrast to delirium, POCD normally refers to a condition that is manifest days to weeks after surgery and may become permanent.(Arrowsmith, Grocott, & Reves, 2000) (Bryson et al., 2011) Early postoperative cognitive decline has been associated with a risk of long-term cognitive deterioration at both 1 and 5 years after cardiac surgery(S. A. J. Conolly, klein AA, 2010; McKhann et al., 2002; Newman et al., 2006; Selnes, 2012). POCD may affect up to 40% of patients after cardiac operations, but its incidence varies widely according to how it is defined.(Selnes, 2012)

The risk factors for POCD after cardiac surgery are similar to those that that are believed to be associated with delirium. Older age, predisposition to dementia, low education level, diabetes, severe atherosclerotic disease, intraoperative hypotension, hypoxemia, medications, and infection have also been implicated in POCD. Existing evidence also suggest a genetic predisposition for POCD. Apolipoprotein E (APOE) is a component of plasma lipoprotein that is believed to play a central role in lipid transport and acetylcholine synthesis within the brain. Patients with the APO E4 allele Apolipoprotein E (APO E4) have been shown to be at risk for both Alzheimers disease and cardiovascular disease. Studies also support an association between the APO E4 allele and postoperative delirium and cognitive decline.

At present there no specific therapeutic interventions proven for the treatment of POCD. Management of POCD is directed at efforts to prevent or minimize the impact of anesthesia and surgery and facilitate early convalescence.

BRACHIAL PLEXUS INJURIES

Brachial plexus injuries and peripheral neuropathies after cardiac remain largely under investigated secondary to minimal discomfort and reporting by patients in the postoperative period. Early studies used somatosensory evoked potentials to estimate the role of sternal retractors especially during left internal mammary artery dissection in causing brachial plexopathy.(Vahl, Carl, Muller-Vahl, & Struck, 1991) Other studies have examined the role of arm positioning i.e. at the sides versus over the head during cardiac surgery in the incidence of nerve injuries.(Jellish, Blakeman, Warf, & Slogoff, 1997) Canbaz et al evaluated the role of pre-existing nerve injuries in the development of new postoperative peripheral nerve injuries, it appears that patients with history of a brachial plexopathy may have a relapse after cardiac surgery.(Canbaz et al., 2005) Kirsh et al showed increased width of sternal retraction was associated with brachial plexopathy. It appeared that 2 out of 5 patients had medial and lateral cord of the brachial plexus involved in injury.(Kirsh, Magee, Gago, Kahn, & Sloan, 1971) A study by Vander Salm et al, investigated the role of sternal retractors in patients with new onset peripheral neuropathy and discovered that sternal retractors in the 2nd intercostal space had higher incidence of first rib fractures and peripheral neuropathy versus retractors in the 4th intercostal space.(Vander Salm, Cereda, & Cutler, 1980) This was shown again by Baisden et al where they used retractors below the 4th intercostal space wherein there was a lower incidence of first rib fractures and brachial plexopathy.(Baisden, Greenwald, & Symbas, 1984) Another factor contributing to brachial plexus injury appears to be duration of cardiopulmonary bypass. Seyfer et al found that wider sternal retraction and prolonged duration of cardiopulmonary bypass were associated with increased incidence of injury.(Seyfer, Grammer, Bogumill, Provost, & Chandry, 1985) Asymmetric sternal retraction is used infrequently to harvest left internal mammary artery. Unlu et al investigated the role of asymmetric sternal retraction and found an increased incidence of brachial plexus injury in 571 CABG patients.(Unlu, Velioglu, Kocak, Becit, & Ceviz, 2007) Healey et al conducted a MEDLINE search to look at the incidence of nerve injury in an effort to develop a best practice paper. (Healey, O'Neill, Bilal, & Waterworth, 2013) The recommendations include caudally placed sternal retractors, minimizing width of sternal retraction and minimizing duration of cardiopulmonary bypass. Finally asymmetric chest retraction during LIMA harvest may predispose patients to brachial plexus injury in the postoperative period. In a small study, Ben-David et al showed that in contrast to non-cardiac surgery, brachial plexus injury after cardiac surgery, showed a sensory predominance with excellent recovery over 6-8 weeks. (Ben-David & Stahl, 1997) Physical rehabilitation, patient counseling and follow-up remain the cornerstone once the injury has occurred.

CONCLUSION

Neurologic complications ranging from stroke to postoperative cognitive decline remain an important complication of cardiac operations. Advances in anesthetic management, surgical techniques, and perfusion technology have shown promise in reducing the frequency and duration of this complication. At the same time, improved outcomes as a consequence of these advances in medical care have increased the number of patients with advanced disease and co-morbidities to undergo cardiac operations.

Important concepts for the prevention and treatment of neurologic complications include the early recognition of stroke and interventions to prevent secondary injury, decreasing the risk of thromboembolic events in the perioperative period, avoiding cerebral hypoperfusion, the application of deliberate hypothermia when temporary ischemia cannot be avoided, the judicious use of anesthetic and sedative drugs with greater safety profiles, and multidisciplinary approaches to facilitate early recovery and convalescence.

REFERENCES

Adams, H. P. Jr, del Zoppo, G., Alberts, M. J., Bhatt, D. L., Brass, L., Furlan, A., & Wijdicks, E. F. M. et al. (2007). Guidelines for the early management of adults with ischemic stroke: a guideline from the American Heart Association/American Stroke Association Stroke Council, Clinical Cardiology Council, Cardiovascular Radiology and Intervention Council, and the Atherosclerotic Peripheral Vascular Disease and Quality of Care Outcomes in Research Interdisciplinary Working Groups: The American Academy of Neurology affirms the value of this guideline as an educational tool for neurologists. *Circulation*, *115*(20), e478–e534. doi:10.1161/CIRCULATIONAHA.107.181486 PMID:17515473

Amarenco, P., Cohen, A., & Tzouirio, C. (1994). Atherosclerotic disease of the aortic arch and the risk of ischemic stroke. *The New England Journal of Medicine*, *331*(22), 1474–1479. doi:10.1056/NEJM199412013312202 PMID:7969297

Appoo, J. J., Augoustides, J. G., Pochettino, A., Savino, J. S., McGarvey, M. L., Cowie, D. C., & Bavaria, J. E. et al. (2006). Perioperative outcome in adults undergoing elective deep hypothermic circulatory arrest with retrograde cerebral perfusion in proximal aortic arch repair: Evaluation of protocol-based care. *Journal of Cardiothoracic and Vascular Anesthesia*, *20*(1), 3–7. doi:10.1053/j.jvca.2005.08.005 PMID:16458205

Arrowsmith, J. E., Grocott, H. P., Reves, J. G., & Newman, M. F. (2000). Central nervous system complications of cardiac surgery. *British Journal of Anaesthesia*, *84*(3), 378–393. doi:10.1093/oxfordjournals.bja.a013444 PMID:10793601

Baird, T. A., Parsons, M. W., Phan, T., Butcher, K. S., Desmond, P. M., Tress, B. M., & Davis, S. M. et al. (2003). Persistent poststroke hyperglycemia is independently associated with infarct expansion and worse clinical outcome. *Stroke*, *34*(9), 2208–2214. doi:10.1161/01.STR.0000085087.41330.FF PMID:12893952

Baisden, C. E., Greenwald, L. V., & Symbas, P. N. (1984). Occult rib fractures and brachial plexus injury following median sternotomy for open-heart operations. *The Annals of Thoracic Surgery*, *38*(3), 192–194. doi:10.1016/S0003-4975(10)62235-7 PMID:6332585

Barazangi, N., Wintermark, M., Lease, K., Rao, R., Smith, W., & Josephson, S. A. (2011). Comparison of computed tomography angiography and transesophageal echocardiography for evaluating aortic arch disease. *Journal of Stroke and Cerebrovascular Diseases*, *20*(5), 436–442. doi:10.1016/j.jstrokecerebrovasdis.2010.02.016 PMID:20813553

Bass, N. M., Mullen, K. D., Sanyal, A., Poordad, F., Neff, G., Leevy, C. B., & Forbes, W. P. et al. (2010). Rifaximin treatment in hepatic encephalopathy. *The New England Journal of Medicine*, *362*(12), 1071–1081. doi:10.1056/NEJMoa0907893 PMID:20335583

Ben-David, B., & Stahl, S. (1997). Prognosis of intraoperative brachial plexus injury: A review of 22 cases. *British Journal of Anaesthesia*, *79*(4), 440–445. doi:10.1093/bja/79.4.440 PMID:9389259

Bernard, S. A., Gray, T. W., Buist, M. D., Jones, B. M., Silvester, W., Gutteridge, G., & Smith, K. (2002). Treatment of comatose survivors of out-of-hospital cardiac arrest with induced hypothermia. *The New England Journal of Medicine*, *346*(8), 557–563. doi:10.1056/NEJMoa003289 PMID:11856794

Biancari, F., Catania, A., & D'Andrea, V. (2011). Elective endovascular vs. open repair for abdominal aortic aneurysm in patients aged 80 years and older: Systematic review and meta-analysis. *European Journal of Vascular and Endovascular Surgery*, *42*(5), 571–576. doi:10.1016/j.ejvs.2011.07.011 PMID:21820922

Bigelow, W. G., Lindsay, W. K., & Greenwood, W. F. (1950). Hypothermia It's possible role in cardiac surgery: An investigation of factors governing survival in dogs at low body temperatures. *Annals of Surgery*, *132*, 849–866. doi:10.1097/00000658-195011000-00001 PMID:14771796

Bilotta, F., Doronzio, A., Stazi, E., Titi, L., Zeppa, I. O., Cianchi, A., & Lumb, P. et al. (2011). Early postoperative cognitive dysfunction and postoperative delirium after anaesthesia with various hypnotics: Study protocol for a randomised controlled trial--the PINOCCHIO trial. *Trials*, *12*(1), 170. doi:10.1186/1745-6215-12-170 PMID:21733178

Bonow, R. O., Carabello, B. A., Chatterjee, K., de Leon, A. C. Jr, Faxon, D. P., & Freed, M. D. et al. American College of Cardiology/American Heart Association Task, F. (2008). (2008). Focused update incorporated into the ACC/AHA 2006 guidelines for the management of patients with valvular heart disease: a report of the American College of Cardiology/American Heart Association Task Force on Practice Guidelines (Writing Committee to Revise the 1998 Guidelines for the Management of Patients With Valvular Heart Disease): endorsed by the Society of Cardiovascular Anesthesiologists, Society for Cardiovascular Angiography and Interventions, and Society of Thoracic Surgeons. *Circulation*, *118*(15), e523–e661. doi:10.1161/CIRCULATIONAHA.108.190748 PMID:18820172

Brady, K., Joshi, B., Zweifel, C., Smielewski, P., Czosnyka, M., Easley, R. B., & Hogue, C. W. Jr. (2010). Real-time continuous monitoring of cerebral blood flow autoregulation using near-infrared spectroscopy in patients undergoing cardiopulmonary bypass. *Stroke*, *41*(9), 1951–1956. doi:10.1161/STROKEAHA.109.575159 PMID:20651274

Bruggemans, E. F. (2013). Cognitive dysfunction after cardiac surgery: Pathophysiological mechanisms and preventive strategies. *Netherlands Heart Journal; Monthly Journal of the Netherlands Society of Cardiology and the Netherlands Heart Foundation*, *21*(2), 70–73. doi:10.1007/s12471-012-0347-x PMID:23184600

Bryson, G. L., Wyand, A., Wozny, D., Rees, L., Taljaard, M., & Nathan, H. (2011). A prospective cohort study evaluating associations among delirium, postoperative cognitive dysfunction, and apolipoprotein E genotype following open aortic repair. *Canadian Journal of Anaesthesia*, *58*(3), 246–255. doi:10.1007/s12630-010-9446-6 PMID:21222188

Bucerius, J., Gummert, J. F., Borger, M. A., Walther, T., Doll, N., Onnasch, J. F., & Mohr, F. W. et al. (2003). Stroke after cardiac surgery: A risk factor analysis of 16,184 consecutive adult patients. *The Annals of Thoracic Surgery*, *75*(2), 472–478. doi:10.1016/S0003-4975(02)04370-9 PMID:12607656

Canbaz, S., Turgut, N., Halici, U., Sunar, H., Balci, K., & Duran, E. (2005). Brachial plexus injury during open heart surgery--controlled prospective study. *The Thoracic and Cardiovascular Surgeon*, *53*(5), 295–299. doi:10.1055/s-2005-865672 PMID:16208616

Cannegieter, S. C., Rosendaal, F. R., & Briet, E. (1994). Thromboembolic and bleeding complications in patients with mechanical heart valve prostheses. *Circulation*, *89*(2), 635–641. doi:10.1161/01.CIR.89.2.635 PMID:8313552

Carrascal, Y., Guerrero, A. L., Blanco, M., Valenzuela, H., Pareja, P., & Laguna, G. (2014). Postoperative stroke related to cardiac surgery in octogenarians. *Interactive Cardiovascular and Thoracic Surgery*, *18*(5), 596–601. doi:10.1093/icvts/ivu022 PMID:24556446

Castillo, J., Leira, R., Garcia, M. M., Serena, J., Blanco, M., & Davalos, A. (2004). Blood pressure decrease during the acute phase of ischemic stroke is associated with brain injury and poor stroke outcome. *Stroke*, *35*(2), 520–526. doi:10.1161/01.STR.0000109769.22917.B0 PMID:14726553

Chaney, M. A. (2002). Corticosteroids and cardiopulmonary bypass: A review of clinical investigations. *Chest*, *121*(3), 921–931. doi:10.1378/chest.121.3.921 PMID:11888978

Cheng, D. C., Bainbridge, D., Martin, J. E., & Novick, R. J. (2005). Does off-pump coronary artery bypass reduce mortality, morbidity, and resource utilization when compared with conventional coronary artery bypass? A meta-analysis of randomized trials. *Anesthesiology*, *102*(1), 188–203. doi:10.1097/00000542-200501000-00028 PMID:15618803

Conolly, S., Arrowsmith, J. E., & Klein, A. A. (2010). Deep hypothermic circulatory arrest. *Continuing Education in Anaesthesia. Critical Care & Pain*, *10*(5), 138–142. doi:10.1093/bjaceaccp/mkq024

Conolly, S. A. J., klein AA. (2010). Deep hypothermic circulatory arrest. *Continuing Education in Anaesthesia, Critical Care & Pain, 10*(5).

Dacey, L. J., Likosky, D. S., Leavitt, B. J., Lahey, S. J., Quinn, R. D., & Hernandez, F. Jr et al. Northern New England Cardiovascular Disease Study, G. (2005). Perioperative stroke and long-term survival after coronary bypass graft surgery. *The Annals of Thoracic Surgery*, *79*(2), 532–536, discussion 537. doi:10.1016/j.athoracsur.2004.07.027 PMID:15680829

Diegeler, A., Borgermann, J., Kappert, U., Breuer, M., Boning, A., Ursulescu, A., & Group, G. S. et al. (2013). Off-pump versus on-pump coronary-artery bypass grafting in elderly patients. *The New England Journal of Medicine*, *368*(13), 1189–1198. doi:10.1056/NEJMoa1211666 PMID:23477657

Djaiani, G., Ali, M., Borger, M. A., Woo, A., Carroll, J., Feindel, C., & Rakowski, H. et al. (2008). Epiaortic scanning modifies planned intraoperative surgical management but not cerebral embolic load during coronary artery bypass surgery. *Anesthesia and Analgesia*, *106*(6), 1611–1618. doi:10.1213/ane.0b013e318172b044 PMID:18499587

Edmonds, H. L. (2002). Multi-modality neurophysiologic monitoring for cardiac surgery. *The Heart Surgery Forum*, *5*, 225–228. PMID:12538134

Eifert, S., Reichenspurner, H., Pfefferkorn, T., Baur, B., von Schlippenbach, C., Mayer, T. E., & Reichart, B. et al. (2003). Neurological and neuropsychological examination and outcome after use of an intra-aortic filter device during cardiac surgery. *Perfusion*, *18*(1), 55–60. doi:10.1191/0267659103pf628oa PMID:12708766

Ely, E. W., Inouye, S. K., Bernard, G. R., Gordon, S., Francis, J., May, L., & Dittus, R. et al. (2001). Delirium in mechanically ventilated patients validity and reliabilty os the confusion assessment method for the intensive care unit. *Journal of the American Medical Association*, *286*(21), 2703–2710. doi:10.1001/jama.286.21.2703 PMID:11730446

Fergusson, D. A., Hebert, P. C., Mazer, C. D., Fremes, S. E., MacAdams, C., Murkin, J. M., & Pretorius, R. et al. (2008). A comparison of Aprotinin and Lysine analogues in high-risk cardiac surgery. *The New England Journal of Medicine*, *358*(22), 2319–2331. doi:10.1056/NEJMoa0802395 PMID:18480196

Fonarow, G. C., Saver, J. L., Smith, E. E., Broderick, J. P., Kleindorfer, D. O., Sacco, R. L., & Schwamm, L. H. et al. (2012). Relationship of national institutes of health stroke scale to 30-day mortality in medicare beneficiaries with acute ischemic stroke. *J Am Heart Assoc*, *1*(1), 42–50. doi:10.1161/JAHA.111.000034 PMID:23130117

Gaynor, J. W., Nicolson, S. C., Jarvik, G. P., Wernovsky, G., Montenegro, L. M., Burnham, N. B., & Clancy, R. R. et al. (2005). Increasing duration of deep hypothermic circulatory arrest is associated with an increased incidence of postoperative electroencephalographic seizures. *The Journal of Thoracic and Cardiovascular Surgery*, *130*(5), 1278–1286. doi:10.1016/j.jtcvs.2005.02.065 PMID:16256779

Gerriets, T., Schwarz, N., Sammer, G., Baehr, J., Stolz, E., Kaps, M., & Schonburg, M. et al. (2010). Protecting the brain from gaseous and solid micro-emboli during coronary artery bypass grafting: A randomized controlled trial. *European Heart Journal*, *31*(3), 360–368. doi:10.1093/eurheartj/ehp178 PMID:19541675

Ginsberg, M. D., & Busto, R. (1998). Combating hyperthermia in acute stroke. *Stroke*, *29*(2), 529–534. doi:10.1161/01.STR.29.2.529 PMID:9472901

Gold, J. P., Charlson, M. E., & Szatrowski, T. P. (1995). Improvement of outcomes after cardiac surgery. *The Journal of Thoracic and Cardiovascular Surgery*, *110*, 1302–1314. doi:10.1016/S0022-5223(95)70053-6 PMID:7475182

Goldhaber, S. Z. (2006). "Bridging" and mechanical heart valves: Perils, promises, and predictions. *Circulation*, *113*(4), 470–472. doi:10.1161/CIRCULATIONAHA.105.598268 PMID:16449725

Goldman, S., Sutter, F., Ferdinand, F., & Trace, C. (2004). Optimizing intraoperative cerebral oxygen delivery using noninvasive cerebral oximetry decreases the incidence of stroke for cardiac surgical patients. *The Heart Surgery Forum*, *7*(5), E376–E381. doi:10.1532/HSF98.20041062 PMID:15799908

Gottesman, R. F., Sherman, P. M., Grega, M. A., Yousem, D. M., Borowicz, L. M. Jr, Selnes, O. A., & McKhann, G. M. et al. (2006). Watershed strokes after cardiac surgery: Diagnosis, etiology, and outcome. *Stroke*, *37*(9), 2306–2311. doi:10.1161/01.STR.0000236024.68020.3a PMID:16857947

Grigore, A. M., Grocott, H. P., Mathew, J. P., Phillips-Bute, B., Stanley, T. O., Butler, A., & Newman, M. F. et al. (2002). The Rewarming Rate and Increased Peak Temperature Alter Neurocognitive Outcome After Cardiac Surgery. *Anesthesia and Analgesia*, *94*(1), 4–10. doi:10.1213/00000539-200201000-00002 PMID:11772792

Grigore, A. M., Murray, C. F., Ramakrishna, H., & Djaiani, G. (2009). A core review of temperature regimens and neuroprotection during cardiopulmonary bypass: Does rewarming rate matter? *Anesthesia and Analgesia*, *109*(6), 1741–1751. doi:10.1213/ANE.0b013e3181c04fea PMID:19923500

Group, T. h. a. c. s. (2002). Mild therapeutic hypothermia to improve the neurologic outcome after cardiac arrest. *N Engl J Med, 346*, 549-556.

Gutsche, J. T., Cheung, A. T., McGarvey, M. L., Moser, W. G., Szeto, W., Carpenter, J. P., & Bavaria, J. E. et al. (2007). Risk factors for perioperative stroke after thoracic endovascular aortic repair. *The Annals of Thoracic Surgery*, *84*(4), 1195–1200, discussion 1200. doi:10.1016/j.athoracsur.2007.04.128 PMID:17888969

Halonen, J. H. P., & Jarvinen, O. (2007). Corticosteroids for the prevention of atrial fibrillation after cardiac surgery. *Journal of the American Medical Association*, *297*(14), 1562–1567. doi:10.1001/jama.297.14.1562 PMID:17426275

Harloff, A., Strecker, C., Reinhard, M., Kollum, M., Handke, M., Olschewski, M., & Hetzel, A. et al. (2006). Combined measurement of carotid stiffness and intima-media thickness improves prediction of complex aortic plaques in patients with ischemic stroke. *Stroke*, *37*(11), 2708–2712. doi:10.1161/01.STR.0000244763.19013.dc PMID:17008632

Hartman, G. S., Yao, F. F., & Bruefach, M. (1996). Severity of aortic atheromatous disease diagnosed by transesophageal echocardiography predicts stroke and other outcomes associated with coronary artery surgery: A prospective study. *Anesthesia and Analgesia*, *83*, 701–708. PMID:8831306

Hattler, B., Messenger, J. C., Shroyer, A. L., Collins, J. F., Haugen, S. J., Garcia, J. A., & Grover, F. L. et al. (2012). Off-Pump coronary artery bypass surgery is associated with worse arterial and saphenous vein graft patency and less effective revascularization: Results from the Veterans Affairs Randomized On/Off Bypass (ROOBY) trial. *Circulation, 125*(23), 2827–2835. doi:10.1161/CIRCULATIONAHA.111.069260 PMID:22592900

Healey, S., O'Neill, B., Bilal, H., & Waterworth, P. (2013). Does retraction of the sternum during median sternotomy result in brachial plexus injuries? *Interactive Cardiovascular and Thoracic Surgery, 17*(1), 151–157. doi:10.1093/icvts/ivs565 PMID:23513004

Heringlake, M. G. C., & Kabler, J. H. (2011). Preoperative cerebral oxygen saturation and clinical outcomes in cardiac surgery. *Anesthesiology, 114*(1), 58–69. doi:10.1097/ALN.0b013e3181fef34e PMID:21178669

Ho, K. M., & Tan, J. A. (2009). Benefits and risks of corticosteroid prophylaxis in adult cardiac surgery: A dose-response meta-analysis. *Circulation, 119*(14), 1853–1866. doi:10.1161/CIRCULATIONAHA.108.848218 PMID:19332460

Hudetz, J. A., Iqbal, Z., Gandhi, S. D., Patterson, K. M., Byrne, A. J., & Pagel, P. S. (2011). Postoperative delirium and short-term cognitive dysfunction occur more frequently in patients undergoing valve surgery with or without coronary artery bypass graft surgery compared with coronary artery bypass graft surgery alone: Results of a pilot study. *Journal of Cardiothoracic and Vascular Anesthesia, 25*(5), 811–816. doi:10.1053/j.jvca.2010.05.003 PMID:20655248

Hunter, G. R., & Young, G. B. (2011). Seizures after cardiac surgery. *Journal of Cardiothoracic and Vascular Anesthesia, 25*(2), 299–305. doi:10.1053/j.jvca.2010.08.004 PMID:21036061

Hussain, S. I., Gilkeson, R. C., Suarez, J. I., Tarr, R., Schluchter, M., Landis, D. M., & Zaidat, O. O. (2008). Comparing multislice electrocardiogram-gated spiral computerized tomography and transesophageal echocardiography in evaluating aortic atheroma in patients with acute ischemic stroke. *Journal of Stroke and Cerebrovascular Diseases, 17*(3), 134–140. doi:10.1016/j.jstrokecerebrovasdis.2007.12.008 PMID:18436154

Ibrahim, K. S., Vitale, N., Tromsdal, A., Kirkeby-Garstad, I., Fraser, A. G., & Haaverstad, R. (2008). Enhanced intra-operative grading of ascending aorta atheroma by epiaortic ultrasound vs echocardiography. *International Journal of Cardiology, 128*(2), 218–223. doi:10.1016/j.ijcard.2007.05.035 PMID:17643531

Immer, F. F., Ackermann, A., Gygax, E., Stalder, M., Englberger, L., Eckstein, F. S., & Carrel, T. P. et al. (2007). Minimal extracorporeal circulation is a promising technique for coronary artery bypass grafting. *The Annals of Thoracic Surgery, 84*(5), 1515–1520, discussion 1521. doi:10.1016/j.athoracsur.2007.05.069 PMID:17954055

Jauch, E. C., Saver, J. L., Adams, H. P. Jr, Bruno, A., Connors, J. J., Demaerschalk, B. M., & Yonas, H. et al. (2013). Guidelines for the early management of patients with acute ischemic stroke: A guideline for healthcare professionals from the American Heart Association/American Stroke Association. *Stroke, 44*(3), 870–947. doi:10.1161/STR.0b013e318284056a PMID:23370205

Jellish, W. S., Blakeman, B., Warf, P., & Slogoff, S. (1997). Hands-up position during asymmetric sternal retraction for internal mammary artery harvest: A possible method to reduce brachialplexus injury. *Anesthesia and Analgesia*, *84*, 260. PMID:9024012

Karkouti, K., Djaiani, G., Borger, M. A., Beattie, W. S., Fedorko, L., Wijeysundera, D., & Karski, J. et al. (2005). Low hematocrit during cardiopulmonary bypass is associated with increased risk of perioperative stroke in cardiac surgery. *The Annals of Thoracic Surgery*, *80*(4), 1381–1387. doi:10.1016/j.athoracsur.2005.03.137 PMID:16181875

Karkouti, K., Wijeysundera, D. N., Yau, T. M., Callum, J. L., Cheng, D. C., Crowther, M., & Beattie, W. S. et al. (2009). Acute kidney injury after cardiac surgery: Focus on modifiable risk factors. *Circulation*, *119*(4), 495–502. doi:10.1161/CIRCULATIONAHA.108.786913 PMID:19153273

Kellermann, K., & Jungwirth, B. (2010). Avoiding stroke during cardiac surgery. *Seminars in Cardiothoracic and Vascular Anesthesia*, *14*(2), 95–101. doi:10.1177/1089253210370902 PMID:20478949

Khan, N. E. D., & Mister, R. (2004). A randomized comparison of Off-pump and On-pump multivessel coronary-artery bypass surgery. *2004, 350*, 21-28.

Kilger, E., Weis, F., Briegel, J., Frey, L., Goetz, A. E., Reuter, D., & Peter, K. et al. (2003). Stress doses of hydrocortisone reduce severe systemic inflammatory response syndrome and improve early outcome in a risk group of patients after cardiac surgery. *Critical Care Medicine*, *31*(4), 1068–1074. doi:10.1097/01.CCM.0000059646.89546.98 PMID:12682474

Kirsh, M. M., Magee, K. R., Gago, O., Kahn, D. R., & Sloan, H. (1971). Brachial plexus injury following median sternotomy incision. *The Annals of Thoracic Surgery*, *11*(4), 315–319. doi:10.1016/S0003-4975(10)65455-0 PMID:4927044

Koch, C. G., Li, L., Duncan, A. I., Mihaljevic, T., Cosgrove, D. M., Loop, F. D., & Blackstone, E. H. et al. (2006). Morbidity and mortality risk associated with red blood cell and blood-component transfusion in isolated coronary artery bypass grafting. *Critical Care Medicine*, *34*(6), 1608–1616. doi:10.1097/01.CCM.0000217920.48559.D8 PMID:16607235

Kulik, A., Rubens, F. D., Wells, P. S., Kearon, C., Mesana, T. G., van Berkom, J., & Lam, B. K. (2006). Early postoperative anticoagulation after mechanical valve replacement: A systematic review. *The Annals of Thoracic Surgery*, *81*(2), 770–781. doi:10.1016/j.athoracsur.2005.07.023 PMID:16427905

Kuroda, S., Houkin, K., Abe, H., Hoshi, Y., & Tamura, M. (1996). Near-infrared monitoring of carebral oxygenation state during carotid endarterectomy. *Surgical Neurology*, *45*(5), 450–458. doi:10.1016/0090-3019(95)00463-7 PMID:8629246

Laas, J., Kleine, P., Hasenkam, M. J., & Nygaard, H. (1999). Orientation of tilting disc and bileaflet aortic valve substitutes for optimal hemodynamics. *The Annals of Thoracic Surgery*, *68*(3), 1096–1099. doi:10.1016/S0003-4975(99)00780-8 PMID:10510028

Leung, J. M., Sands, L. P., Vaurio, L. E., & Wang, Y. (2006). Nitrous oxide does not change the incidence of postoperative delirium or cognitive decline in elderly surgical patients. *British Journal of Anaesthesia*, *96*(6), 754–760. doi:10.1093/bja/ael106 PMID:16670110

Levy, J. H., & Tanaka, K. A. (2003). Inflammatory response to cardiopulmonary bypass. *The Annals of Thoracic Surgery*, *75*(2), S715–S720. doi:10.1016/S0003-4975(02)04701-X PMID:12607717

Likosky, D. S., Marrin, C. A., Caplan, L. R., Baribeau, Y. R., Morton, J. R., Weintraub, R. M., & O'Connor, G. T. et al. (2003). Determination of etiologic mechanisms of strokes secondary to coronary artery bypass graft surgery. *Stroke*, *34*(12), 2830–2834. doi:10.1161/01.STR.0000098650.12386.B3 PMID:14605327

Manji, R. A., Grocott, H. P., Leake, J., Ariano, R. E., Manji, J. S., Menkis, A. H., & Jacobsohn, E. (2012). Seizures following cardiac surgery: The impact of tranexamic acid and other risk factors. *Canadian Journal of Anaesthesia*, *59*(1), 6–13. doi:10.1007/s12630-011-9618-z PMID:22065333

Martens, S., Neumann, K., Sodemann, C., Deschka, H., Wimmer-Greinecker, G., & Moritz, A. (2008). Carbon dioxide field flooding reduces neurologic impairment after open heart surgery. *The Annals of Thoracic Surgery*, *85*(2), 543–547. doi:10.1016/j.athoracsur.2007.08.047 PMID:18222261

Martin, K., Wiesner, G., Breuer, T., Lange, R., & Tassani, P. (2008). The risks of aprotinin and tranexamic acid in cardiac surgery: A one-year follow-up of 1188 consecutive patients. *Anesthesia and Analgesia*, *107*(6), 1783–1790. doi:10.1213/ane.0b013e318184bc20 PMID:19020118

Mathew, J. P. F. (2004). A multicenter risk index for atrial fibrillation after cardiac surgery. *Journal of the American Medical Association*, *291*(14), 1720–1729. doi:10.1001/jama.291.14.1720 PMID:15082699

McCollough, J. N., Zhang, N., & Reich, D. L. (1999). Cerebral metabolic suppression during hypothermic circulatory arrest in humans. *The Annals of Thoracic Surgery*, *67*(6), 1895–1899. doi:10.1016/S0003-4975(99)00441-5 PMID:10391334

McKhann, G. M., & Grega, M. A., & BorowiczJr, L. M. (2002). Encephalopathy and stroke after Coronary artery bypass grafting. *JAMA Neurology*, *59*, 1422–1428. PMID:12223028

McKhann, G. M., Grega, M. A., Borowicz, L. M. Jr, Baumgartner, W. A., & Selnes, O. A. (2006). Stroke and encephalopathy after cardiac surgery: An update. *Stroke*, *37*(2), 562–571. doi:10.1161/01.STR.0000199032.78782.6c PMID:16373636

McPherson, J. A., Wagner, C. E., Boehm, L. M., Hall, J. D., Johnson, D. C., Miller, L. R., & Pandharipande, P. P. et al. (2013). Delirium in the cardiovascular ICU: Exploring modifiable risk factors. *Critical Care Medicine*, *41*(2), 405–413. doi:10.1097/CCM.0b013e31826ab49b PMID:23263581

Mitchell, L. B. C., E.; Heilbron, B. (2004). Atrial fibrillation after cardiac surgery. *The Canadian Journal of Cardiology*, *21*(Suppl B), 45B–50B. PMID:16239988

Moller, C. H., Penninga, L., Wetterslev, J., Steinbruchel, D. A., & Gluud, C. (2008). Clinical outcomes in randomized trials of off- vs. on-pump coronary artery bypass surgery: Systematic review with meta-analyses and trial sequential analyses. *European Heart Journal*, *29*(21), 2601–2616. doi:10.1093/eurheartj/ehn335 PMID:18628261

Muir, K. W., Weir, C. J., Murray, G. D., Povey, C., & Lees, K. R. (1996). Comparison of neurological scales and scoring systems for acute stroke prognosis. *Stroke*, *27*(10), 1817–1820. doi:10.1161/01.STR.27.10.1817 PMID:8841337

Murkin, J. M. (2013). Is it better to shine a light, or rather to curse the darkness? Cerebral near-infrared spectroscopy and cardiac surgery. *European Journal of Cardio-Thoracic Surgery*, *43*(6), 1081–1083. doi:10.1093/ejcts/ezt186 PMID:23543201

Murkin, J. M., Falter, F., Granton, J., Young, B., Burt, C., & Chu, M. (2010). High-dose tranexamic Acid is associated with nonischemic clinical seizures in cardiac surgical patients. *Anesthesia and Analgesia*, *110*(2), 350–353. doi:10.1213/ANE.0b013e3181c92b23 PMID:19996135

Murkin, J. M., Farrar, J. K., Tweed, W. A., McKenzie, F. N., & Guiraudon, G. (1987). Cerebral autoregulation and flow/metabolism coupling during cardiopulmonary bypass: The influence of PaCO2. *Anesthesia and Analgesia*, *66*(9), 825–832. doi:10.1213/00000539-198709000-00003 PMID:3113288

Murphy, G. S., Whitlock, R. P., Gutsche, J. T., & Augoustides, J. G. (2013). Steroids for adult cardiac surgery with cardiopulmonary bypass: Update on dose and key randomized trials. *Journal of Cardiothoracic and Vascular Anesthesia*, *27*(5), 1053–1059. doi:10.1053/j.jvca.2013.04.022 PMID:24054192

Nathoe, H. M., van Dijk, D., Jansen, E. W. L., Suyker, W. J. L., Diephuis, J. C., van Boven, W.-J., & de Jaegere, P. P. T. et al. (2003). A comparison of On-pump and Off-pump coronary bypass surgery in low-risk patients. *The New England Journal of Medicine*, *348*(5), 394–402. doi:10.1056/NEJMoa021775 PMID:12556542

Newman, M. F., Mathew, J. P., Grocott, H. P., Mackensen, G. B., Monk, T., Welsh-Bohmer, K. A., & Mark, D. B. et al. (2006). Central nervous system injury associated with cardiac surgery. *Lancet*, *368*(9536), 694–703. doi:10.1016/S0140-6736(06)69254-4 PMID:16920475

Ottens, T. H. D., Dieleman, J. M., Sauër, A.-M. C., Peelen, L. M., Nierich, A. P., de Groot, W. J., & van Dijk, D. et al. (2014). Effects of dexamethasone on cognitive decline after cardiac surgery. *Anesthesiology*, *121*(3), 492–500. doi:10.1097/ALN.0000000000000336 PMID:25225745

Pandharipande, PP, J. J., Ely EW. (2005). Delirium: Acute cognitive dysfunction in the critically ill. *Current Opinion in Critical Care*, *11*, 360–368. PMID:16015117

Ranucci, M. B. B. (2006). Lowest hematocrit on cardiopulmonary bypass impairs the outcome in coronary surgery. *Texas Heart Institute Journal*, *33*, 300–305. PMID:17041685

Roach, G. W., Kanchuger, M., & Mora-Mangano, C. T. (1996). Adverse cerebral outcomes after coronary artery bypass surgery. *The New England Journal of Medicine*, *335*(25), 1857–1863. doi:10.1056/NEJM199612193352501 PMID:8948560

Rosenberger, P., Shernan, S. K., Loffler, M., Shekar, P. S., Fox, J. A., Tuli, J. K., & Eltzschig, H. K. et al. (2008). The influence of epiaortic ultrasonography on intraoperative surgical management in 6051 cardiac surgical patients. *The Annals of Thoracic Surgery*, *85*(2), 548–553. doi:10.1016/j.athoracsur.2007.08.061 PMID:18222262

Royse, C., Royse, A., & Blake, D. (1998). Screening the thoracic aorta for atheroma: A comparison of manual palpation, Transesophageal and epiaortic ultrasonography. *Annals of Thoracic and Cardiovascular Surgery*, *4*, 347–350. PMID:9914464

Sahu, B., Chauhan, S., Kiran, U., Bisoi, A., Lakshmy, R., Selvaraj, T., & Nehra, A. (2009). Neurocognitive function in patients undergoing coronary artery bypass graft surgery with cardiopulmonary bypass: The effect of two different rewarming strategies. *Journal of Cardiothoracic and Vascular Anesthesia*, *23*(1), 14–21. doi:10.1053/j.jvca.2008.07.010 PMID:18834816

Sedrakyan, A., Wu, A. W., Parashar, A., Bass, E. B., & Treasure, T. (2006). Off-pump surgery is associated with reduced occurrence of stroke and other morbidity as compared with traditional coronary artery bypass grafting: A meta-analysis of systematically reviewed trials. *Stroke*, *37*(11), 2759–2769. doi:10.1161/01.STR.0000245081.52877.f2 PMID:17008617

Selnes, O. A. G. R., & Grega, M. A. (2012). Cognitive and neurologic outcomes after Coronary artery bypass grafting. *The New England Journal of Medicine*, *366*(3), 250–257. doi:10.1056/NEJMra1100109 PMID:22256807

Seyfer, A. E., Grammer, N. Y., Bogumill, G. P., Provost, J. M., & Chandry, U. (1985). Upper extremity neuropathies after cardiac surgery. *The Journal of Hand Surgery*, *10*(1), 16–19. doi:10.1016/S0363-5023(85)80241-0 PMID:2981914

Shadvar, K., Baastani, F., Mahmoodpoor, A., & Bilehjani, E. (2013). Evaluation of the prevalence and risk factors of delirium in cardiac surgery ICU. *J Cardiovasc Thorac Res*, *5*(4), 157–161. doi:10.5681/jcvtr.2013.034 PMID:24404347

Slater, J. P., Guarino, T., Stack, J., Vinod, K., Bustami, R. T., Brown, J. M., 3rd, . . . Parr, G. V. (2009). Cerebral oxygen desaturation predicts cognitive decline and longer hospital stay after cardiac surgery. *Ann Thorac Surg, 87*(1), 36-44; discussion 44-35. doi: 10.1016/j.athoracsur.2008.08.070

Soja, S. L., Pandharipande, P. P., Fleming, S. B., Cotton, B. A., Miller, L. R., Weaver, S. G., & Ely, E. W. et al. (2008). Implementation, reliability testing, and compliance monitoring of the Confusion Assessment Method for the Intensive Care Unit in trauma patients. *Intensive Care Medicine*, *34*(7), 1263–1268. doi:10.1007/s00134-008-1031-x PMID:18297270

Stecker, M. M., Cheung, A. T., Pochettino, A., Kent, G. P., Patterson, T., Weiss, S. J., & Bavaria, J. E. (2001). Deep hypothermic circulatory arrest: 1. Effects of cooling on electroencephalogram and evoked potentials. *The Annals of Thoracic Surgery*, *71*(1), 14–21. doi:10.1016/S0003-4975(00)01592-7 PMID:11216734

Stransky, M., Schmidt, C., Ganslmeier, P., Grossmann, E., Haneya, A., Moritz, S., & Trabold, B. et al. (2011). Hypoactive delirium after cardiac surgery as an independent risk factor for prolonged mechanical ventilation. *Journal of Cardiothoracic and Vascular Anesthesia*, *25*(6), 968–974. doi:10.1053/j.jvca.2011.05.004 PMID:21741272

Suman, A. B., Barnes, D. S., Zein, N. N., Levinthal, G. N., Connor, J. T., & Carey, W. D. (2004). Predicting outcomes after cardiac surgery in patients with cirrhosis: A comparison of Child-Pugh and MELD scores. *Clinical Gastroenterology and Hepatology*, *2*(8), 719–723. doi:10.1016/S1542-3565(04)00296-4 PMID:15290666

Suvarna, S., Smith, A., Stygall, J., Kolvecar, S., Walesby, R., Harrison, M., & Newman, S. (2007). An intraoperative assessment of the ascending aorta: A comparison of digital palpation, transesophageal echocardiography, and epiaortic ultrasonography. *Journal of Cardiothoracic and Vascular Anesthesia*, *21*(6), 805–809. doi:10.1053/j.jvca.2007.05.014 PMID:18068056

Takagi, H., Tanabashi, T., Kawai, N., & Umemoto, T. (2007). Off-pump surgery does not reduce stroke, compared with results of on-pump coronary artery bypass grafting: A meta-analysis of randomized clinical trials. *The Journal of Thoracic and Cardiovascular Surgery*, *134*(4), 1059–1060. doi:10.1016/j.jtcvs.2007.07.006 PMID:17903537

Tarakji, K. G. S. (2011). Temporal Onset, risk factors and outcomes associated with stroke after coronary artery nypass grafting. *Journal of the American Medical Association*, *305*(4), 381–390. doi:10.1001/jama.2011.37 PMID:21266685

Tessitore, E., Rundek, T., Jin, Z., Homma, S., Sacco, R. L., & Di Tullio, M. R. (2010). Association between carotid intima-media thickness and aortic arch plaques. *Journal of the American Society of Echocardiography*, *23*(7), 772–777. doi:10.1016/j.echo.2010.04.012 PMID:20510582

Thourani, V. H., Razavi, S. A., Nguyen, T. C., Kilgo, P. D., Puskas, J. D., Guyton, R. A., & Halkos, M. E. et al. (2014). Incidence of postoperative stroke using the Heartstring device in 1,380 coronary artery bypass graft patients with mild to severe atherosclerosis of the ascending aorta. *The Annals of Thoracic Surgery*, *97*(6), 2066–2072, discussion 2072. doi:10.1016/j.athoracsur.2014.02.044 PMID:24726605

Tomasi, R., & von Dossow-Hanfstingl, V. (2014). Critical care strategies to improve neurocognitive outcome in thoracic surgery. *Current Opinion in Anaesthesiology*, *27*(1), 44–48. doi:10.1097/ACO.0000000000000026 PMID:24263687

Tufo, H. M., Ostfeld, A. M., & Shekelle, R. (1970). Central nervous system dysfunction following open-heart surgery. *Journal of the American Medical Association*, *212*(8), 1333–1340. doi:10.1001/jama.1970.03170210039006 PMID:5467674

Unlu, Y., Velioglu, Y., Kocak, H., Becit, N., & Ceviz, M. (2007). Brachial plexus injury following median sternotomy. *Interactive Cardiovascular and Thoracic Surgery*, *6*(2), 235–237. doi:10.1510/icvts.2006.137380 PMID:17669822

Vahl, C. F., Carl, I., Muller-Vahl, H., & Struck, E. (1991). Brachial plexus injury after cardiac surgery. The role of internal mammary artery preparation: A prospective study on 1000 consecutive patients. *The Journal of Thoracic and Cardiovascular Surgery*, *102*(5), 724–729. PMID:1682532

Van der linden, J., Hadjinikolaou, L., & Bergman, P. (2001). Postoperative stroke in cardiac surgery is related to the location and extent of atherosclerotic disease inthe ascending aorta. *J Am Coll Cardiol*, *38*(1), 131-135.

Vander Salm, T. J., Cereda, J. M., & Cutler, B. S. (1980). Brachial plexus injury following median sternotomy. *The Journal of Thoracic and Cardiovascular Surgery*, *80*(3), 447–452. PMID:7412350

Weimar, C., Konig, I. R., Kraywinkel, K., Ziegler, A., & Diener, H. C. (2004). Age and National Institutes of Health Stroke Scale Score within 6 hours after onset are accurate predictors of outcome after cerebral ischemia: Development and external validation of prognostic models. *Stroke*, *35*(1), 158–162. doi:10.1161/01.STR.0000106761.94985.8B PMID:14684776

Whitlock, E. L., Torres, B. A., Lin, N., Helsten, D. L., Nadelson, M. R., Mashour, G. A., & Avidan, M. S. (2014). Postoperative delirium in a substudy of cardiothoracic surgical patients in the BAG-RECALL clinical trial. *Anesthesia and Analgesia*, *118*(4), 809–817. doi:10.1213/ANE.0000000000000028 PMID:24413548

Whitlock, R. P., Sun, J. C., Fremes, S. E., Rubens, F. D., Teoh, K. H., & American College of Chest, P. (2012). Antithrombotic and thrombolytic therapy for valvular disease: Antithrombotic Therapy and Prevention of Thrombosis, 9th ed: American College of Chest Physicians Evidence-Based Clinical Practice Guidelines. *Chest, 141*(2 Suppl), e576S-600S. doi: 10.1378/chest.11-2305

Wiesenack, C. L. A., & Philipp, A. (2004). Four years' experience with a miniaturized extracorporeal circulation system and its influence on clinical outcomes. *Artificial Organs*, *28*(12), 1082–1088. doi:10.1111/j.1525-1594.2004.00030.x PMID:15554936

You, J. J., Singer, D. E., Howard, P. A., Lane, D. A., Eckman, M. H., Fang, M. C., ... American College of Chest, P. (2012). Antithrombotic therapy for atrial fibrillation: Antithrombotic Therapy and Prevention of Thrombosis, 9th ed: American College of Chest Physicians Evidence-Based Clinical Practice Guidelines. Chest, 141(2 Suppl), e531S-575S. doi:10.1378/chest.11-2304

Zeitani, J., Buccisano, F., Nardella, S., Flaminio, M., Prati, P., Chiariello, G., & Chiariello, L. et al. (2013). Mini-extracorporeal circulation minimizes coagulation abnormalities and ameliorates pulmonary outcome in coronary artery bypass grafting surgery. *Perfusion*, *28*(4), 298–305. doi:10.1177/0267659113478322 PMID:23411504

Zhu, F. L., A.; Chee, Y.E. (2012). Fast-track cardiac care for adult cardiac surgical patients. *The Cochrane Collaboration,* (10).

APPENDIX

Guidelines for anticoagulation and Antiplatelet therapy to decrease the risk of stroke in Patients with atrial fibrillation

1. CHADS2 =0, low risk of stroke, aspirin alone is adequate
2. CHADS2=1, intermediate risk of stroke, Aspirin plus clopidogrel is suggested
3. CHADS2 =2, high risk of stroke, Oral Dabigatran is preferred above Aspirin and clopidogrel
4. AF plus drug eluting coronary stents in first 12 months dual anti-platelet therapy is adequate, after 12 months, oral vitamin K antagonists (VKA, coumadin) are recommended with goal INR of 2-3
5. AF plus mitral stenosis, oral VKA with goal INR 2-3
6. AF plus stable CAD, oral VKA with goal INR 2-3

Chapter 15
Perioperative Respiratory Care and Complications

Peter Burrage
Harvard Medical School, USA

Zinaida Wadhwani
Kaiser Permanente, USA

Michael Nurok
Cedars Sinai Heart Institute, USA

ABSTRACT

Clinicians caring for patients with cardio-pulmonary disease invariably must manage the respiratory system. Doing so requires a basic understanding of physiology and the interaction of the heart and lung. The present chapter begins with rudimentary concepts of respiratory physiology, focusing on, gas exchange, pulmonary mechanics, and cardio-pulmonary interactions. These are used to develop an approach to mechanical ventilation and routine perioperative respiratory care of the patient having undergone a cardio-pulmonary procedure. The final section of this chapter addresses specific respiratory challenges encountered in caring for the critically ill cardiothoracic patient in addition to contemporary management strategies.

INTRODUCTION

The present chapter provides the reader with a systematic approach to the respiratory care of patients with cardio-pulmonary disease. The initial section focuses on physiology, specifically, gas exchange, respiratory mechanics, and cardio-pulmonary interactions. Basic understanding of these fundamentals creates a foundation for understanding respiratory pathophysiology.

A problem-oriented approach is provided in later sections of the chapter with a focus on routine mechanical ventilation and ventilator liberation following surgery. The final section of this chapter outlines specific management strategies for commonly encountered respiratory problems in the critical care unit.

DOI: 10.4018/978-1-4666-8603-8.ch015

Key words: Gas exchange, respiratory mechanics, cardio-pulmonary interaction, work of breathing, respiratory failure, mechanical ventilation, ventilator liberation, pulmonary edema, chronic obstructive pulmonary disease, pneumothorax, pleural effusion, acute respiratory distress syndrome.

BACKGROUND

The respiratory system's primary function is to exchange oxygen and carbon dioxide in support of metabolism. This is achieved by approximating blood and air over a large surface area. The heart and lungs move blood and air, permitting exchange of gas between alveoli, pulmonary capillaries, tissue, and eventually cells.

The respiratory system is made of two components, the lung and chest wall. Airways smaller than respiratory bronchioles contain alveoli that function as gas exchanging units. The chest wall includes the rib cage, abdomen, and diaphragm. Parietal and visceral pleura separate the chest wall from the lung with a potential pleural space between.

Respiratory Physiology and Pathophysiology

Gas Exchange

The most basic and essential action of the lung is the efficient exchange of gases between the blood and the external environment via the alveolus-blood interface. The movement of gases across this membrane is governed by passive diffusion, a process described by Fick's law of diffusion.

$$\dot{V}_{gas} \propto \frac{A}{T} \cdot D \cdot (P_1 - P_2)\; D \propto \frac{Sol}{\sqrt{MW}}$$

This law states that the rate of gas migration through a membrane is directly proportional to both the area of the membrane (A), and the difference in partial pressure of the gas on both sides of the membrane (P_1-P_2), and is inversely proportional to the thickness of the membrane (T). Given this relationship, the lung is structurally well suited for gas exchange with its large surface area (50-100 m^2) and thin alveolar walls (approximately 0.3 μm)(West, 2012). The transfer rate is also directly dependent on a diffusion constant (D) that is related to both the blood solubility (Sol) of the gas and its molecular weight (MW). The physiologic impact of the diffusion constant is illustrated by the fact that while CO_2 and O_2 have similar molecular weights and partial pressure differences, the relative solubility of CO_2 is much higher, allowing CO_2 transport to occur at 20-fold higher rates than O_2 transport.

Given the specific characteristics of a gas, its rate of transport can be classified as either diffusion limited or perfusion limited. Diffusion limitation occurs with gases that are very soluble in blood (e.g. – carbon monoxide), and therefore the partial pressure difference between the alveolus and blood is maintained throughout capillary transit, continually driving transport. In this situation, a large amount of gas can be absorbed into a relatively small volume of blood, and the amount of gas crossing the membrane is dependent on the rate of diffusion, not the volume of blood that traverses the capillary. Perfusion limitation is seen with gases that are less soluble in blood (e.g. – nitrous oxide), leading to partial pressure equilibration between both sides of the alveolar wall relatively early on in capillary transit. This causes the total amount of gas moving across the membrane to be dependent on the amount of blood flowing through the capillary bed, and to be minimally affected by the diffusion characteristics of the membrane.

In a normal patient in the resting state, the transit time of red blood cell (RBC) in the pulmonary capillary is approximately 0.75 second, and equilibration between alveolar P_{O2} and capillary P_{O2} is reached by 0.25 second(West, 2012). Even in exercise states with high cardiac outputs where the capillary transit time may approach 0.25 second, equilibration is usually still reached with no gradient in alveolar/end capillary P_{O2}. Therefore, oxygen transfer in the normal lung is largely perfusion limited. Similarly, in the normal lung, P_{CO2} equilibration occurs early on in capillary transit and is therefore perfusion limited. However, in certain pathologic states where the alveolar membrane is thickened (e.g. - pulmonary fibrosis, pulmonary edema), decreased in area (e.g. - COPD), or the diffusion characteristics of the capillary/alveolar membrane are otherwise abnormal (e.g. - pulmonary hypertension), the end capillary P_{O2} and P_{CO2} may not reach alveolar levels and therefore a component of diffusion limitation can also be introduced.

Respiratory Mechanics

The process of breathing requires the repetitive generation of pressure gradients, via changes in thoracic volume, to produce gas flow. In the spontaneously breathing patient, these changes are created by the actions of the muscles of inspiration and expiration, as well as the inherent structural mechanics of the chest wall and lung itself. In mechanically ventilated patients, the function of the inspiratory muscles is largely replaced with positive pressure, but the physical characteristics of the lung parenchyma still play a crucial role in the efficacy of ventilation.

Inspiration is an active process and the major muscle of inspiration is the diaphragm. This muscular sheet forms a dome shape at rest and travels as little as 1 cm with resting tidal breathing, to up to 10 cm with a vital capacity breath(West, 2012). Contraction of the diaphragm causes an increase in both the vertical dimension of the thoracic cavity, with movement of the abdominal contents downward and forward, as well as the transverse dimension, with lateral displacement of the ribs outward. Inspiration can also augmented by the external intercostal muscles that act to pull the ribs upwards and forwards in a "bucket handle" motion, with subsequent expansion of the thorax in the lateral and anteroposterior dimensions. Although used minimally in normal tidal breathing, the accessory muscles of inspiration, including the scalene and sternocleidomastoid muscles, can be active during exercise and periods of respiratory distress to help lift the first two ribs and the sternum, respectively. Notably, while paralysis of the diaphragm due to damage to the phrenic nerves can have a significant negative impact on ventilatory capacity, isolated paralysis of the external intercostal muscles secondary to intercostal nerve damage does not have a large effect as long as diaphragm function is maintained.

Expiration during tidal breathing is largely a passive process resulting from the elastic properties of the chest wall and lung counteracting the active expansion of these structures seen with inspiration. During exercise and other situations with active expiration, such as coughing or performing the Valsalva maneuver, the abdominal musculature plays the major role. The rectus abdominus, internal and external obliques, and transversus abdominus contract leading to increased intraabdominal pressure and subsequent elevation of the diaphragm. In addition, the internal intercostal muscles act to pull the ribs downward and inward leading to decreased thoracic volume.

It is the close juxtaposition of the visceral pleura covering the lung and the parietal pleura lining the inside of the thoracic cavity that allows the position changes of the chest wall made by the muscles of respiration to be efficiently transmitted to the lung. Although these two layers create a potential space, normally the intrapleural pressure is negative due to the combination of an air-tight thoracic cavity with the presence of pleural fluid that allows the layers to slide easily past each other while strongly resisting their separation(Jaeger & Blank, 2011). This relationship causes the chest wall and lung to move as a single unit, and disruption of this interaction by introducing air (pneumothorax), or fluid (hemothorax or empyema) into the pleural space can have significant effects on respiratory function.

The response of this unified chest wall/lung system to position changes is defined by the summation of the response of the individual components (see Fig. 1). While both the lung and chest wall are elastic structures, their equilibrium positions are different.

For example, although the lung is at equilibrium at residual volume (RV), which is roughly 20% of total lung capacity (TLC), the chest wall is at equilibrium at approximately 60% of TLC. Taken together, the equilibrium of the system as a whole, defined as the functional residual capacity (FRC), is approximately 40% of TLC. When the transpulmonary pressure, defined as the difference in pressure between inside the lung (alveoli) and outside the lung (intrapleural space), is increased by either expansion of the chest wall in spontaneous respiration, or introduction of positive pressure in mechanical ventilation, air flow occurs and the system increases in volume. The change in volume per unit change in pressure is known as the compliance and is expressed as the slope of the pressure-volume curve. While the isolated normal lung is easily distensible with a compliance of approximately 200 ml/cm H_2O, the compliance of the system

Figure 1. Static pressure volumes curves of the isolated chest wall (---), isolated lung parenchyma (--), and the unified respiratory system (-). RV – residual volume; FRC – functional residual capacity; TLC – total lung capacity. (Jaeger & Blank, 2011).

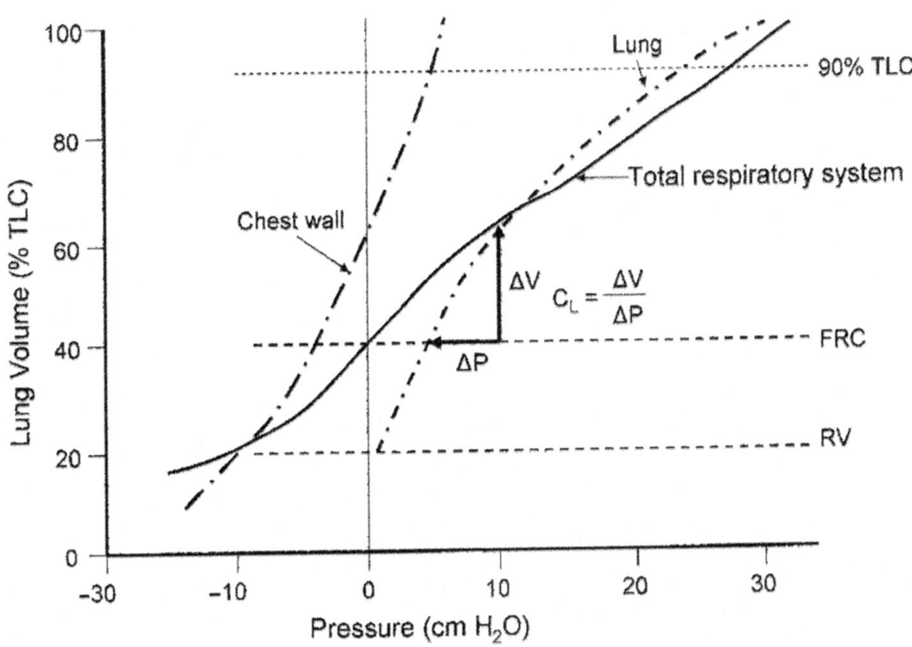

as a whole is in the range of 50-80 ml/cm H_2O due to the contribution of the significantly stiffer (i.e. – relatively noncompliant) chest wall(Jaeger & Blank, 2011; West, 2012). Decreases in compliance can be caused by increases in chest wall stiffness (e.g. - obesity, neuromuscular weakness, scoliosis, pectus excavatum, scleroderma), increases in lung stiffness (e.g. - pulmonary fibrosis, pulmonary edema, acute respiratory distress syndrome, tension pneumothorax, atelectasis), or both. Differentiating the etiology of decreased compliance (chest wall vs. lung) requires the measurement of intrapleural pressure. Esophageal pressure, as measured using an esophageal balloon, is thought to be the most accurate surrogate marker for intrapleural pressure in clinical use(Akoumianaki et al., 2014).

Cardio-Pulmonary Interaction

The unified goal of cardiac and pulmonary systems is to ensure adequate oxygen delivery to body tissues. There is significant interdependence between these two systems and disruption of function in either one can have adverse affects on the other, with negative downstream affects due to compromised oxygen distribution. There are two major reasons for the tight linkage of heart and lung function. First, they both share the thoracic cavity and therefore changes in pressure created by the function of one system act on the other. Second, they are essentially in series from a circulation standpoint with the lungs and pulmonary vasculature carrying flow from the right to the left-sided cardiac chambers. These anatomical relationships create a complex interaction where changes in respiratory function can have significant effects on the preload and afterload conditions for both the right and left heart.

Respiration affects preload of the right heart by altering the pressures in the thoracic cavity relative to extrathoracic compartments. The extrathoracic venous system has a low pressure, low resistance, high capacitance architecture, and venous return to the right heart is dependent on the pressure in the extrathoracic veins relative to the pressure in the right atrium (P_{RA}). The pressure in the extrathoracic venous reservoirs is thought to be equal to the mean circulatory filling pressure (P_{MCF}), which conceptually can be thought of as the elastic recoil potential stored in the circulatory system as the walls of the vasculature are distended with blood volume(Henderson, Griesdale, Walley, & Sheel, 2010). Changes in intrathoracic pressure during respiration are transmitted to the right atrium and because the pressure gradient driving venous return flow back to the right atrium is defined by P_{MCF} - P_{RA}, these changes also affect venous return. Increases in ITP, and therefore P_{RA}, such as those seen with positive pressure ventilation, can lead to decreased venous return and right heart preload.

The influence of respiration on right heart afterload is mediated through affects on the pulmonary vascular resistance (PVR) via both chemical and physical mechanisms. First, inadequate respiration can lead to respiratory acidosis and hypoxia, both of which cause vasoconstriction of the pulmonary vasculature. Second, respiration alters lung volumes which affect PVR in a biphasic pattern with PVR reaching its nadir at FRC and increasing as lung volumes decrease towards RV or increase towards TLC (see Fig. 2).

This relationship occurs because the pulmonary vascular bed contains both extra-alveolar vessels that lie in the interstitium and are exposed to intrapleural pressures, and alveolar vessels that run through the alveolar wall and are exposed to alveolar pressure. At lung volumes less than FRC, the radial traction on the extra-alveolar vessels provided by the interstitium begins to decrease, causing a fall in the cumula-

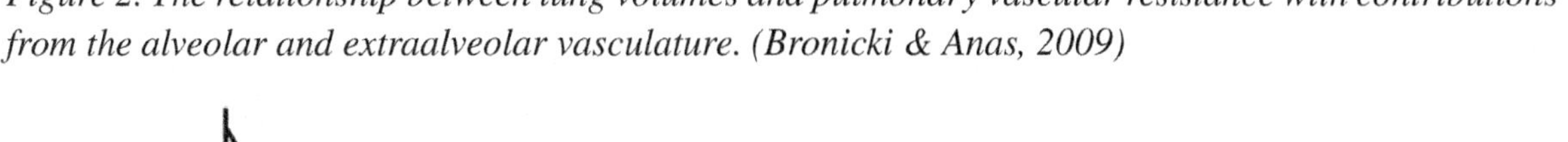

Figure 2. The relationship between lung volumes and pulmonary vascular resistance with contributions from the alveolar and extraalveolar vasculature. (Bronicki & Anas, 2009)

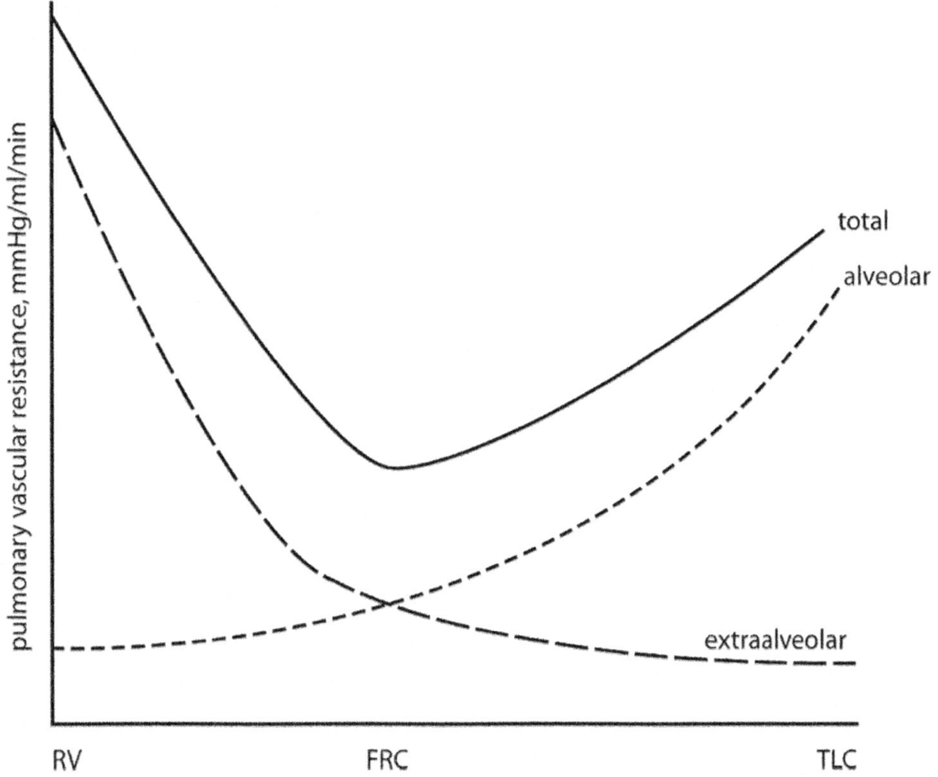

tive cross sectional area of these vessels, and therefore an increase in resistance. Further, decreasing lung volumes also cause atelectasis to develop with subsequent hypoxic vasoconstriction and increased vascular resistance in the collapsed lung tissue. Lung volumes greater than FRC also increase PVR because increased volume means increased distention of alveolar walls with subsequent compression of the vessels coursing through those walls, and increased resistance to flow.

Left heart preload can be altered by respiration mainly through effects on pulmonary venous return and right ventricular function. Increases in PVR lead to decreased volume transiting the pulmonary vasculature into the left heart, leading to decreased preload and cardiac output. In addition, as PVR increases, right ventricular diastolic pressures also rise causing a decrease in, and eventually reversal of, the pressure gradient across the interventricular septum. Reversal of the trans-septal gradient causes deformation of the septum towards the left ventricular cavity with decreased left ventricular volume and impaired filling in a phenomenon termed diastolic ventricular interdependence.

Changes in intrathoracic pressure with respiration can also have significant effects on left heart afterload, largely due to the effects on the transmural pressure (P_{TM}) of the left ventricle (LV) and intrathoracic arterial structures. The P_{TM} of the LV is equal to the aortic systolic blood pressure, which acts to impede blood flow out of the LV, minus the ITP, which acts to compress the LV and thereby assist in blood ejection. Given this concept, applying positive ITP would act to decrease the P_{TM}, and therefore the afterload, of the LV, while decreasing or creating negative ITP would lead to increased LV afterload. This effect is similar when applied to the arterial tree. Positive ITP compresses the intrathoracic arterial vessels, leading to decreased volumes and increased pressure relative to extrathoracic arteries. This gradient results in intrathoracic arterial blood being propelled into the extrathoracic vessels, allowing the LV to eject into a relatively volume depleted aorta against decreased afterload.

Understanding the effects of respiration on cardiac function is crucial to successfully caring for critically ill patients in whom optimization of oxygen delivery is an omnipresent goal. Careful consideration should be paid to the physiologic implications of changes in ITP because many of these patients are receiving mechanical ventilatory support. This is particularly important in patients who may have significant right and or left heart dysfunction.

Pulmonary Response to Cardiothoracic Surgery

Commonly after major cardiac surgery, especially that which employs extracorporeal circulation such as cardiopulmonary bypass (CPB), the body undergoes a significant inflammatory response characterized by increased capillary permeability, complement activation, leukocyte activation, and cytokine release. In addition to general surgical activators of the immune response including surgical tissue trauma, blood loss, transfusion and hypothermia, there are several mechanisms specific to CPB that are thought to be involved in the development of this inflammatory response. First, there is thought to be direct "contact activation" that occurs when the blood components of the immune system are exposed to the foreign materials of the CPB circuit. Second, after removal of the aortic cross clamp, there can be a component of ischemia-reperfusion injury to a number of major organs including the heart, lungs, kidneys, liver, and brain with subsequent immune system activation. Finally, the presence of endotoxemia post-CPB is also thought to play a role in the inflammatory cascade, although the etiology of these elevated endotoxin levels are still a matter of investigation(Laffey, Boylan, & Cheng, 2002). The cumulative effect of this robust immune response has important clinical ramifications as it can lead to a systemic inflammatory response syndrome (SIRS) that is commonly accompanied by organ dysfunction including myocardial depression, renal failure, acute lung injury, and multiple organ dysfunction syndrome (MODS). The development of MODS, which is thought to have an incidence of approximately 11% after CPB, carries a poor prognosis with mortality rates of approximately 41%(Laffey et al., 2002).

Isolated thoracic surgery may also lead to a vigorous inflammatory response. Postulated causes include lung manipulation, lung collapse (particularly in the setting of one lung ventilation), endothelial injury from changes in perfusion to lung regions with manipulation and from clamping and unclamping of pulmonary vasculature, oxidative stress from the need for elevated inspired oxygen concentration, ischemia reperfusion injury, and impaired lymphatic drainage from manipulation or resection of lymphatics(Jordan, Mitchell, Quinlan, Goldstraw, & Evans, 2000).

Positive Pressure Ventilation

During normal breathing, the lungs are expanded by the creation of negative intrapleural pressure through chest wall expansion. Air is then drawn into the alveoli down this pressure gradient. With positive pressure ventilation (PPV), air is mechanically propelled into the alveoli, and this nonphysiologic mechanism of lung expansion has a number of important effects on pulmonary and cardiac function.

In the upright, normal lung undergoing negative pressure ventilation, both ventilation and perfusion are highest in the dependent portions of the lung. The vertical variation in ventilation occurs due to a gradient in intrapleural pressure created by the weight of the lung. Due to the tendency of the lung to descend in the hemithorax, the intrapleural pressure surrounding the apices of the lung is more negative than the bases, leading to greater distention of these non-dependent alveoli at end expiration. With normal inspiration the dependent alveoli are more capable of expansion because their starting volume is smaller, so more ventilation is directed to these regions. The distribution of perfusion is debated, while there is a clear gravitational effect, with increased blood flow at the bases leading to optimal V/Q matching, perfusion also seems to be increased in the center of the thorax following the arborization of the cardiopulmonary tree(Glenny et al., 2000; Hakim, Lisbona, & Dean, 1987).

With the introduction of PPV, ventilation becomes more equally distributed throughout the lung thereby creating a dependent region of low V/Q with a relative overabundance of blood flow (i.e. – intrapulmonary shunt) and a non-dependent region of high V/Q with relatively increased ventilation (i.e.- alveolar dead space). This increased shunting can theoretically lead to decreased P_{aO2} while the increased dead space can lead to elevated P_{aCO2}. However, especially in patients with acute lung pathology, the negative effects of PPV on gas exchange are largely outweighed by the advantages of PEEP, a reduced work of breathing, and the maintenance of FRC(Buckley & Gillham, 2007; Hasan, 2010).

The use of positive pressure to expand alveoli also carries with it the risk of overdistention leading to potential barotrauma with the rupture of alveoli and respiratory bronchioles and creation of extrapulmonary air (e.g. – pneumothorax or pneumomediastinum). Importantly, it is an elevated transpulmonary pressure, defined as alveolar pressure – pleural pressure, that causes barotrauma, and not necessarily an isolated elevated peak airway pressure.

Conceptually, peak airway pressure is the pressure at end inspiration required to distend the lung and chest wall in addition to that required to overcome airway resistance. Plateau pressure is the pressure required to distend the lung and chest wall. It is measured in a paralyzed patient after end inspiration and approximates peak intra-alveolar pressure. In mechanically ventilated patients, the compliance of the respiratory system can be calculated by examining changes in volume in relationship to pressure. Dynamic compliance is measured while airflow is present and is calculated as Cdyn=Vt/(Ppeak-PEEP). Static compliance (Cstat=Vt/(Pplateau-PEEP) is measured after inspiration has ended and when airflow has terminated. Because dynamic compliance involves airflow, and therefore resistance, it is decreased in patients with elevated resistance, for e.g., bronchospasm. Resistance does not affect static compliance. As seen in Figure 3, the main risk for an elevated transpulmonary gradient is reduced lung compliance, despite the fact that reduced chest wall compliance and increased airway resistance can also lead to elevated peak pressures.

In addition to causing lung injury via barotrauma, PPV can also exacerbate existing lung injury secondary to inflammatory conditions, including systemic sepsis and pneumonia. Although multifactorial, the mechanisms behind ventilator induced lung injury are thought to involve overdistention ("volutrauma"), cyclic atelectasis, ("atelectotrauma"), contribution to existing inflammatory process by injuring lung tissue ("biotrauma"), and high oxygen concentrations leading to oxidative tissue damage(Pinhu, Whitehead, Evans, & Griffiths, 2003; Slutsky & Ranieri, 2013). These observations have led to the low

Figure 3. Transpulmonary pressure gradients in different pathologic states. Although peak airway pressures may be similarly elevated in these disease states, the transpulmonary pressures can be markedly different. (Buckley & Gillham, 2007).

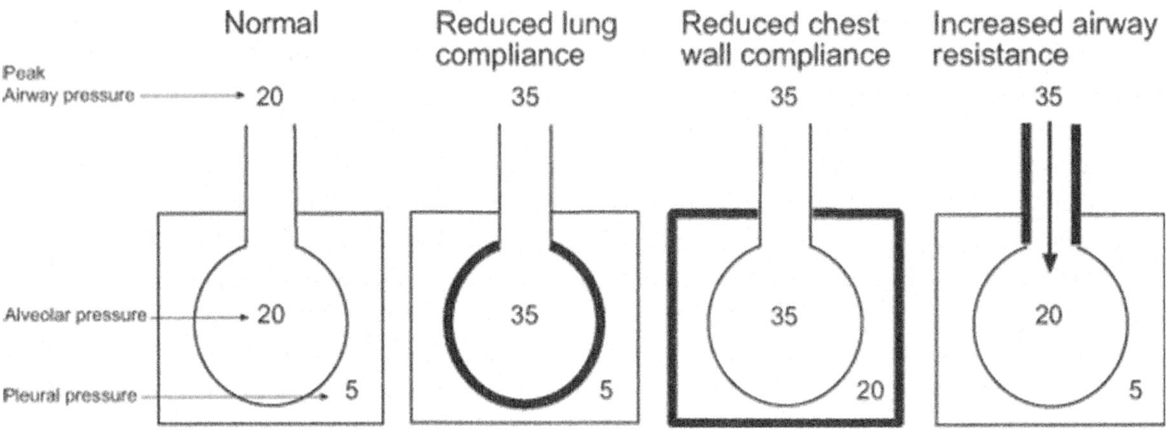

volume, high PEEP strategies currently recommended for patients with ARDS(2000), and more recently, transpulmonary pressure gradient-targeted ventilation strategies(Talmor et al., 2008), prone positioning (Guerin et al., 2013), and the use of extracorporeal support.

As discussed previously, respiration can have significant effects on cardiac function, specifically on the preload and afterload conditions for both sides of the heart. Due to the increases in ITP that are transmitted to the RA, the initiation of PPV can cause a marked reduction in right heart preload, especially in the setting of hypovolemia or high levels of PEEP. A portion of the elevated alveolar pressure generated by PPV is transmitted to the pulmonary capillaries, with greater pressure transmission occurring with more compliant lungs (i.e. – with alveoli more capable of distention). The increased pressure has several effects including greater right heart afterload due to increased PVR as well as increased left heart preload for the cardiac cycle immediately following the breath due to mobilization of blood volume already in the capillaries and pulmonary veins into the left atrium. With subsequent cardiac cycles, however, left heart preload is decreased due to the increased RV afterload. In the context of PPV, left heart afterload is also decreased due to both a decrease in P_{TM} of the LV, as well as a decreased intrathoracic aortic volume, which assists with LV ejection. Notably, the dynamic changes in arterial waveform variables seen with volume controlled mechanical ventilation including systolic pressure variation, stroke volume variation, and pulse pressure variation have been found to be accurate in identifying critically ill patients whose cardiac performance would be improved with fluid boluses. These associations, however, do not hold true for the spontaneously breathing or non-invasively ventilated patient(Marik, Cavallazzi, Vasu, & Hirani, 2009).

Mechanical Ventilation

Indications for Mechanical Ventilation

The reasons for invasive ventilation via tracheal intubation can be broken into two large categories: 1) airway control, and 2) respiratory failure. The need to secure a patient's airway can arise when the patient is at high risk for aspiration of gastric contents into the pulmonary tree or when the patency of the airway is threatened. These situations can be seen in patients with altered mental status, depressed airway reflexes, upper airway trauma, or the need for sedation during a procedure or lengthy imaging study where gaining control of the airway emergently may be complex (e.g. – patient obesity, distorted head and neck anatomy, minimal respiratory reserve in context of possible apneic periods).

The onset of acute respiratory failure (ARF) that would benefit from intubation and mechanical ventilation can be more insidious than indications for airway control, although ARF is commonly heralded by a sensation of dyspnea. This sensation may be more subtle in patients with underlying chronic lung disease, but a focused physical examination of the patient in potential respiratory failure should emphasize patient-reported shortness of breath, assessment of work of breathing, and mental status in addition to the standard vital sign and examination findings. Hypoxemia and respiratory acidosis can lead to depression of central nervous system and cardiovascular function that can manifest as confusion, agitation, systemic hypertension, angina, bradyarrhythmia, or evidence of myocardial ischemia.

A respiratory rate greater than 35 breaths/minute is consistent with an elevated WOB/respiratory distress and likely impending respiratory muscle failure. Although not routinely measured, the inability to generate a maximum inspiratory force of greater than -20 cm H_2O is suggestive of significant neuromuscular weakness and will likely result in inadequate ventilation. Critically decreased ventilatory capacity can also be identified by a forced expiratory volume in one second (FEV_1) of less than 10 mL/kg, and a forced vital capacity (FVC) of less than 15 mL/kg suggests an inability to mount an effective cough. Arterial blood gas analysis and chest radiography are helpful to assess of the degree and etiology of ARF(Chalaby M, 2010).

While these objective numerical thresholds have been established, in a given patient it is very important to follow the trends of these indicators, even when they are below the noted thresholds. This allows one to intervene before the clinical situation has markedly deteriorated, as the benefits of mechanical ventilation are consistently better when initiated electively instead of emergently(Hasan, 2010).

Respiratory Failure

Respiratory Failure may be defined as the inability to maintain normal blood gas partial pressure(Lumb & Nunn, 2005). It is variously defined as Type I "Hypoxemic" Respiratory Failure where PCO2 is normal or low and Type II "Hypercarbic" Respiratory Failure where PCO2 is elevated. Respiratory Failure is caused by Ventilatory Failure (failure to maintain normal alveolar gas partial pressure) and Venous Admixture due to a spectrum of ventilation and perfusion mismatch.

Hypoxemic Respiratory Failure

Conventionally hypoxemic respiratory failure is defined as a PaO_2 less than 60 mmHg with an FiO_2 of 0.5 or an alveolar-arterial gradient greater than 450 mmHg with an FiO_2 of 1.0, both of which are consistent with critically dysfunctional gas exchange in the lung. Arterial oxygen content is defined by the following relationship:

$$CaO2 = (1.31xHbxSaO2) + (0.003xPaO2)$$

CaO_2 is the oxygen content of arterial blood in mL/dL of blood, Hb is hemoglobin concentration in gm/dL, Sa O_2 is the oxygen saturation and PaO_2 is the partial pressure of oxygen in arterial blood. The constant 1.31 is the amount of oxygen bound per gram of hemoglobin (the theoretical limit yields a constant of 1.39 however, in vivo this has not been substantiated) and the constant 0.003 represents a multiplier to quantify the amount of oxygen dissolved in plasma. Evident from the equation above is the minimal contribution of dissolved oxygen relative to the hemoglobin-bound oxygen, thus arterial oxygen content depends mostly on hemoglobin concentration and oxygen saturation.

The mechanisms of hypoxemic respiratory failure include ventilation/perfusion (V/Q) mismatch, right-to-left intrapulmonary or intracardiac, atelectasis and hypoperfusion. The term shunt is often used ambiguously to refer to one of three scenarios: areas of pure shunt where V/Q=0 (i.e., there is no ventilation and just perfusion, areas of very low V/Q ratios, and to the solution to the shunt equation of venous admixture. There is a clear correlation between gas exchange impairment and the amount of alveolar collapse(Hedenstierna, Tokics, Strandberg, Lundquist, & Brismar, 1986). Atelectasis occurs regularly in dependent lung regions during general anesthesia in approximately 90% of patients and persists postoperatively potentiating hypoxemia (Lawrence et al., 1995; Lundquist, Hedenstierna, Strandberg, Tokics, & Brismar, 1995; Magnusson & Spahn, 2003). As a result, hypoxemia during the immediate perioperative period is most commonly due to low V/Q ratios, which results in pulmonary blood flow through edematous or poorly ventilated lung with inadequate absorption of O_2. Respiratory failure due to V/Q mismatching in this scenario, represents a spectrum between pure alveolar dead space ventilation (alveoli which lack perfusion but have ventilation) and pure shunt (alveoli not ventilated but perfused) plus different inhomogeneous V/Q ratios in between. Note that similar to shunt, the term "Dead Space" is variously used to define regions of pure dead space (V/Q= infinity, i.e. ventilation without perfusion), areas with high V/Q ratios, and the solution to the dead space equation. V/Q mismatching can often be corrected by supplemental oxygen, unlike pure shunt when a portion of cardiac output bypasses pulmonary capillary beds and is therefore refractory to increases of FiO_2.

Regional hypoxia in these areas (primarily low alveolar oxygen tension, and secondarily low mixed venous oxygen tension) stimulates hypoxic pulmonary vasoconstriction (HPV) resulting in improved V/Q matching. Understanding the effects of various physiologic conditions and drugs on HPV is complicated because of their multiple effects. For example, drugs that may directly inhibit HPV (inhalational anesthetics) may also decrease cardiac output, leading to increased oxygen extraction and lower mixed venous oxygen tension thereby increasing HPV with a net neutral effect(Lumb & Nunn, 2005). In general, HPV is inhibited by vasodilators and enhanced by vasoconstrictors. The effects of HPV by anesthetics and sedatives are controversial but it is generally thought that intravenous agents commonly used for sedation do not change HPV. (Benumof & Wahrenbrock, 1975; Reid, Slinger, & Lenis, 1996). In a patient with right ventricular failure administration of milrinone will decrease pulmonary vascular resistance (PVR) (along with nitroglycerin, sodium nitroprusside, and hydralazine) and potentially worsen PaO_2 by reducing HPV(Casthely, Lear, Cottrell, & Lear, 1982; Kato, Sato, & Nishino, 1998). Reduction of right ventricular afterload with inhaled PGI_2, inhaled NO, and sildenafil also has been shown to affect HPV in animal studies(Reichenberger et al., 2007; Weissmann et al., 2007). Current pharmacologic approaches to reverse ventricular remodeling in chronic heart failure using angiotensin II receptor blockers (ARBs) and angiotensin converting enzyme inhibitors (ACEi) recently have been shown to reduce PVR and in turn decrease HPV in acute hypoxia (Cargill & Lipworth, 1996; Kiely, Cargill, & Lipworth, 1996).

Hypoxemia can also present in patients with right-to-left intracardiac shunt that have mixing of deoxygenated blood from either the right atrium or ventricle with oxygenated blood from the left sided heart structures. Key to successful management of these patients is minimizing the shunt by reducing the pressure gradient across the lesion: either increasing the left sided pressure or decreasing the right sided pressures. As previously described, application of positive intrathoracic pressure or PEEP should be performed with caution because in a patient with patent foramen ovale (PFO) it can increase the shunt fraction and worsen hypoxemia(Cujec, Polasek, Mayers, & Johnson, 1993; Dewan, Gayasaddin, Angelillo, O'Donohue, & Mohiuddin, 1986).

Hypercarbic Respiratory Failure

Hypercarbic respiratory failure is defined as the inability to maintain a normal PaCO2. It occurs when alveolar ventilation falls behind CO2 production resulting in an increase of the arterial partial pressure of carbon dioxide. Acute versus chronic causes may be determined by the presence of an acute respiratory acidosis; in patients with chronic hypercarbia, acidosis is usually not present and plasma bicarbonate is slightly elevated. Hypercarbia is caused by increased CO2 production, hypoventilation, or increased dead space.

Excess CO2 production occurs most commonly in the setting of increased body temperature. Other causes include over-feeding with carbohydrates. ICU patients with marginal lung function may fail in either of these settings as CO2 production exceeds the ability to ventilate.

Hypoventilation is most commonly seen in the setting of airway obstruction however it can have several other etiologies including depression of the respiratory center secondary to sedative drugs or residual anesthesia, residual neuromuscular blockade, pre-existing neuromuscular disease affecting muscles of respiration and preexisting anatomic or surgical disruption of the chest wall. All result in inadequate minute ventilation with rising arterial CO_2 levels.

Hypercarbic respiratory failure from increased dead space (regions with high V/Q ratio) occur secondary to obstruction of pulmonary blood flow encountered with pulmonary embolus, pulmonary vascular disease, or decreased number of capillaries such as seen in emphysema. This is diagnosed in the setting of a normal minute ventilation with an elevated PCO2.

Risk Factors for Postoperative Respiratory Failure

Preoperative predictors associated with increased risk of postoperative respiratory dysfunction are the subject of debate. Multiple studies have looked at the incidence of postoperative pulmonary complications which include pneumonia, respiratory failure with prolonged mechanical ventilation, bronchospasm, atelectasis, and exacerbations of pre-existing chronic lung disease. None are conclusive and predicting which patients are at risk remains difficult. Patient risk factors can be grouped by history, physical examination, and laboratory measurements.

Age greater than 70, cardiac dysfunction, history of smoking, COPD, neuromuscular disease affecting respiratory muscles, myocardial dysfunction, diabetes, dyspnea at rest or with activities of daily living, and inability to climb one flight of stairs, and significant perioperative fluid administration have all been identified as risk factors(Arozullah, Daley, Henderson, & Khuri, 2000; Dales, Dionne, Leech, Lunau, & Schweitzer, 1993).

In patients with chronic obstructive pulmonary disease, incidence of postoperative pulmonary complications appears to be directly related to the severity of disease(Kroenke, Lawrence, Theroux, Tuley, & Hilsenbeck, 1993; Tarhan, Moffitt, Sessler, Douglas, & Taylor, 1973).

Risk factors that can be elicited by physical examination include, increased baseline work of breathing, preoperative wheezing not controlled by bronchodilators, signs of right ventricular dysfunction such as elevated JVP or lower extremity edema and cachexia. Concerning laboratory findings include a PaCO2 >45mmHg, room air PaO2<50mmHg, predicted post-operative FEV1<40% predicted, predicted post-operative DLCO<40% predicted, residual volume RV/total lung capacity TLC>30%, maximum oxygen consumption <15mL/kg/min, and elevated serum creatinine(Ramsay & Finley, 2011). Predicted post operative FEV1 after lung resection has been validated as the best predictor of requiring mechanical ventilation(Nakahara et al., 1988).

Ventilation Modes

In recent years, the complexity of modern ventilators has been steadily increasing with the ability to adjust nearly every attribute of the inspiratory cycle as well as microprocessor-based control systems that allow the ventilator to dynamically adjust support depending on patient effort and lung mechanics. Adding further to the intricacy is the fact that many of the new ventilator modes have different, manufacturer-specific names, despite functioning in the same way. Although there are significant distinctions between modes in terms of patient comfort, respiratory muscle unloading, and some surrogate physiologic variables, there is a dearth of data showing improved patient outcomes with any specific mode of ventilation(Baram & Richman, 2010; Branson & Johannigman, 2004). While an exhaustive description of existing ventilator modes is outside the scope of this chapter, an understanding of the basic principles underlying mechanical ventilation is essential to understand how changes in patient status/lung mechanics will alter the function of a particular mode and allow one to optimize settings for a given patient context (discussed in detail in the following section).

The parameters common to all modern ventilator modes are inspiratory flow control, cycling, trigger, positive end expiratory pressure (PEEP), and breath type. The pattern of inspiratory flow is set by the control variable, generally either volume control, or pressure control. In a volume control mode, the ventilator delivers a constant flow rate over the inspiratory time to achieve the set tidal volume. In this circumstance, while tidal volume is guaranteed, the airway pressure generated is variable, and fluctuations in lung compliance, specifically decreases in compliance, can lead to undesired elevated airway pressures. In a pressure control mode, the ventilator guarantees a pressure at which the breath is delivered, but both the flow rate and tidal volume delivered vary with the compliance of the lungs. In this mode, decreases in lung compliance can lead to decreases in delivered tidal volumes and potentially hypoventilation, while increases in lung compliance can lead to overdistention of lung tissue with potential volutrauma. With the drawbacks inherent in both volume control and pressure control modes, many newer ventilators also have what has been termed a "dual control" mode(Hasan, 2010). In this mode, the operator sets a guaranteed tidal volume but the flow control variable is pressure. Over a series of pressure control breaths, the ventilator can titrate the delivered pressure to achieve the set tidal volume. This allows the ventilator to dynamically adjust ventilation as lung mechanics change. This also allows the ventilator to adjust to changes in patient effort as it can decrease or increase the pressure delivered with each breath as the patient contributes more or less to the work of breathing.

Cycling defines how the ventilator switches from inspiration to expiration and is based on either time or flow characteristics. In mandatory breaths, cycling is time-based and is determined by the respiratory rate and time of inspiration or inspiration:expiration (I:E) ratio (approximately 1:2 in patients without lung pathology). In patients with significant obstructive disease, extended time for expiration is necessary to avoid dynamic hyperinflation that can lead to generation of autoPEEP and persistent elevated ITP with subsequent hemodynamic derangement. Alternatively, patients with hypoxemia due to V/Q mismatch (shunt) may benefit from relatively longer inspiratory times that may help recruit alveoli that are less compliant and require more time to fill. Flow-cycled ventilation is seen in supported ventilation, and the ventilator terminates inspiration when the flow rate falls below a percentage of the maximum flow rate seen earlier in the breath. This type of cycling is generally more comfortable for the spontaneously breathing patient and allows better synchrony with the ventilator. While cycling defines the transition from inspiration to expiration, triggering is the mechanism that ends expiration and begins inspiration. Similar to cycling, in mandatory breaths the initiation of inspiration is triggered by time. However, in an assisted breath, the ventilator can sense the patient initiate a respiratory effort through either a change in pressure or flow, and then support that breath. Flow triggering is thought to be more sensitive to a patient's respiratory effort and leads to improved synchrony and patient comfort(Tobin, 2001).

The PEEP setting determines ventilator behavior during end exhalation and it has been shown to prevent the collapse of alveoli and small airways and reduce lung water with subsequent increases in lung compliance and oxygenation(Buckley & Gillham, 2007). With decreasing lung compliance due to inflammatory injury or pulmonary edema, increasing levels of PEEP may be required to achieve these beneficial effects. It must be recognized that compliance is heterogeneous throughout the lung and that ideal PEEP in one zone may not be ideal in others. Increasing PEEP directly elevates ITP, which results in increased right heart afterload, decreased left heart preload, and can lead to hemodynamic perturbation. Therefore, PEEP should be titrated judiciously, especially in patients with compromised cardiac function. When there is uncertainty regarding the ideal level of PEEP in relation to cardiac function, consideration should be given for esophageal balloon guided optimization, although this approach may not maximize recruitable lung(Chiumello et al., 2014).

There are three types of breaths that can occur during mechanical ventilation, mandatory, supported/assisted, and unsupported/spontaneous. In a mandatory breath, the ventilator assumes all the WOB and delivers a breath independent of patient respiratory effort. A supported breath is initiated by the patient and contributed to by the ventilator, and therefore the ventilator is performing a portion of the WOB. Unsupported or spontaneous breaths are initiated and completed by the patient, who is responsible for all the WOB. Ventilator modes combine these breath types in different ways providing varying levels of support for the patient's WOB. For example, patients on assist control ventilation (ACV) receive a set number of mandatory breaths at a set tidal volume (volume control). If the patient makes a triggering respiratory effort, they receive a fully supported breath equal to the tidal volume of the mandatory breath, and this breath is counted towards the set respiratory rate. This type of mode guarantees a specific minute ventilation with minimal patient effort and allows for deep sedation or paralysis if necessary. However, at higher spontaneous respiratory rates, this can cause dynamic hyperinflation/autoPEEP. Additionally, if used for long periods of time, respiratory muscle deconditioning can occur due to the fact that every breath is fully volume supported.

Another example of a mode providing both mandatory and supported breaths is synchronized intermittent mandatory ventilation (SIMV), which is frequently combined with pressure support ventilation (PSV). In this mode, similar to ACV, there is a set number of mandatory breaths with a set tidal volume, but any patient-initiated efforts are only pressure-supported (generally with 5-10 cm H_2O) instead of the ventilator delivering the full mandatory breath volume. This theoretically allows the patient to maintain respiratory muscle activity while still ensuring a minimum minute ventilation. While theoretically advantageous, in practice, outcomes seem worse with SIMV and this mode is not recommended for routine use(Hess & MacIntyre, 2011). Alternatively, PSV alone sets only a level of pressure support (over PEEP) to be delivered when triggered by patient respiratory effort. This mode has no guaranteed minute ventilation but provides excellent synchrony and allows support to be easily titrated. While there are an ever-increasing number of ventilator modes, an understanding of the above variables in a given mode will assist in optimizing ventilator settings for a specific patient context.

Oxygen has adverse effects when delivered in non-physiologic inspired fractions (Martin & Grocott, 2013) and efforts should be made to keep FiO2 to the lowest levels necessary by optimizing ventilator settings. This may be done by the addition of PEEP, however the ideal settings are patient dependent and controversial. In a recent study, bedside positive end-expiratory pressure selection methods based on lung mechanics or absolute esophageal pressures provided positive end-expiratory pressure levels unrelated to lung recruitability and similar in mild, moderate, and severe acute respiratory distress syndrome, whereas a table-based method correlating PEEP levels to inspired oxygen concentration provided positive end-expiratory pressure levels related to lung recruitability progressively increasing from mild to moderate and severe acute respiratory distress syndrome(Chiumello et al., 2014). In an effort to minimize ventilator induced lung injury, contemporary ventilator strategies tend to result in hypercapnea which is labeled "permissive". There are not thought to be significant adverse effects associated with permissive hypercapnea and there is evidence for potential benefit in the setting of lung injury(O'Croinin, Ni Chonghaile, Higgins, & Laffey, 2005).

Patients with refractory hypoxemia despite optimal PEEP titration should be considered for inverse ratio ventilation strategies where the time spent in exhalation is less than the time spent in inspiration. Other modalities to improve ventilation and perfusion matching and limit mechanical ventilation induced lung injury include prone positioning(Guerin et al., 2013) and the use of extracorporeal support(Stewart, Jagelman, & Webster, 2011).

Discontinuing Mechanical Ventilation

Patients should be evaluated on a daily basis for the appropriateness of a spontaneous awakening (SAT) and then a spontaneous breathing trial (SBT(Girard et al., 2008; Medicine, 2013))(Girard et al., 2008; Group, 2013). Criteria to undergo a spontaneous awakening screen and then trial include the absence of seizures, substance withdrawal, and or agitation. Neuromuscular function must be intact and paralytic agents must not be in use. The SAT is conducted by stopping sedatives but continuing analgesics for active pain management while intensive care unit staff actively monitor the patient at the bedside. The SAT can be considered successful if the patient opens eyes to verbal stimulus and tolerates the interruption of sedation for a sustained period without exhibiting signs of sustained agitation, tachypnea, desaturation, dysrhythmia or respiratory distress. If any of these signs do develop, sedatives are restarted at a lower dose and titrated as needed with a goal of repeating the SAT the following day if no clear cause for failure can be identified.

After a successful SAT a Spontaneous Breathing Trial (SBT) should take place assuming the underlying pathology leading to the requirement for mechanical ventilation has improved. Guidelines for conducting an SBT include a PaO2/ FiO2 ratio of >200, adequate oxygen saturation, PEEP < 7.5 cm H_2O, FiO_2 < 50%, hemodynamic stability, and absence of myocardial ischemia.

The SBT is conducted using a spontaneous mode of ventilation and consideration should be given to using no PEEP as even low levels may sufficiently decrease the work of breathing to cause a patient to fail in its absence. The intensivist should assess the adequacy of gas exchange using an arterial blood gas, the condition of respiratory mechanics – for e.g., by calculating a "Rapid Shallow Breathing Index," (a low respiratory rate and high tidal volume with a ratio of <105 is reassuring)(Meade et al., 2001; Yang & Tobin, 1991) and the stability of hemodynamic parameters. In addition, consideration should be given to the degree of patient comfort, the predicted ability for the patient to protect their airway after extubation, and the difficulty of re-securing the airway should the patient require re-intubation. Patients satisfying these conditions can be extubated.

Patients who develop tachypnea, hypoxemia, hypotension, arrhythmias, changes in mental status, or other concerning signs should be provided with the minimum required ventilatory support to address these findings. The clinician should attempt to identify modifiable causes of respiratory failure and address these with a view to conducting a subsequent SBT. Patients failing an SBT and who are considered to be at risk for mechanical ventilation for more than 14 days may be evaluated for tracheostomy. This includes patients requiring high level of sedation to tolerate an endotracheal tube, those with marginal respiratory mechanics who may benefit from the lower resistance offered by a tracheostomy tube, patients who may derive psychological benefit from the ability to eat orally or communicate by speech, and those for who enhanced mobility may assist physical therapy efforts and improve functional outcomes. Additional benefits include improved pulmonary toilet, oral care, comfort, and having a secure airway (Freeman & Morris, 2012). Recent trials of early versus late tracheostomy have not yielded significant differences and this is likely due to the fact that physicians estimate poorly the ne(Henderson et al., 2010) ed for tracheostomy during the early period of respiratory failure(Terragni et al., 2010; Young, Harrison, Cuthbertson, Rowan, & TracMan, 2013)

Prolonged Mechanical Ventilation

In 2007 an international consensus group defined prolonged "weaning" as applying to a patient who fails at least three discontinuation attempts or requires more than 7 days of discontinuation attempts after the first attempt at ventilator liberation(Boles et al., 2007). Patients requiring prolonged weaning usually benefit from a gradual reduction of ventilator support in distinction to the majority of patients who can proceed directly to a spontaneous breathing trial and for whom the term "ventilator liberation" is preferred to "weaning".

Management strategies for patients requiring prolonged weaning should target the underlying cause for mechanical ventilation which may include inability to tolerate the work of breathing, cardiac load, neuromuscular weakness, neuropsychological states, metabolic impairments, nutritional deficits, and anemia(Boles et al., 2007). The elastic recoil of the lung and resistance to airflow are the principal influences of work of breathing. These may in turn be optimized by addressing poor lung compliance (e.g. pneumonia, pulmonary edema) and resistance to airflow (e.g. COPD, bronchospasm).

Patients requiring prolonged mechanical ventilation usually require tracheostomy. These can be placed in the operating room or percutaneously at the patient bedside by experienced intensivists. (Dennis, Eckert, Gunter, Morris, & May, 2013). In addition to the benefits discussed previously, tracheostomy in the setting of prolonged mechanical ventilation may facilitate weaning by decreasing turbulent airflow from a shorter and wider diameter tube than that used for translaryngeal intubation(Freeman & Morris, 2012).

Pain, Agitation, and Delirium in Mechanically Ventilated Patients

Mechanically ventilated patients in the ICU routinely experience pain with women reporting more pain than men after cardiac surgery(Milgrom et al., 2004; Yorke, Wallis, & McLean, 2004). Procedures performed in the ICU also contribute to pain. For these reasons, a standardized approach to assessing pain should be used and should incorporate metrics beyond simple vital signs.

A multi-modal approach to pain control with judicious use of non-opioid analgesics and non-pharmacologic measures may optimize respiratory function. The use of thoracic epidural, paravertebral and intercostal nerve block, as well as pump driven delivery of local anesthetic have also been shown to assist with post-thoracotomy pain for thoracic surgery. Regional anesthetic techniques and the use of epidural catheters must be balanced against the need for CPB, anticoagulants, and the risk of bleeding.

Once analgesic requirements have been adequately addressed, the need for sedation may be considered. Many patients may not require any sedation(Strom, Martinussen, & Toft, 2010). For those that do, available evidence supports using the lightest level of sedation required and this approach is associated with improved clinical outcomes(J. Barr et al., 2013).

Patients should be assessed for their level of sedation. The two most widely used and best-validated scales are the Richmond Agitation-Sedation Scale (RASS) and Sedation-Agitation Scale (SAS)(Medicine, 2013). Objective measures of brain function are not required unless clinically indicated for neurologic monitoring or for difficulty of subjectively quantifying level of sedation in patient requiring paralysis. Where sedatives are required, non-benzodiazepine medications should be used including dexmedetomidine or propofol(J. Barr et al., 2013).

Additional efforts should be made to optimize sleep for ICU patients. While non-pharmacologic strategies are preferred (controlling light and noise, clustering patient care activities, and decreasing stimuli at night to protect patients' sleep cycles) a sedative may be required(J. Barr et al., 2013).

Mechanically ventilated patients should be routinely monitored for delirium. The Confusion Assessment Method for the ICU (CAM-ICU) and the Intensive Care Delirium Screening Checklist (ICDSC) are the most valid and reliable delirium monitoring tools in adult ICU patients(J. Barr et al., 2013). The prevention and management of delirium are covered in detail in Chapter XX.

Early Extubation and "Fast Track" Considerations for Cardiac Surgery and Lung Resection

The use of "fast track" anesthetic and ICU protocols to achieve early extubation (usually defined as less than 6 hours of intubation after arrival in the ICU) in low to medium risk post-cardiac surgical patients is becoming more prevalent, especially in the current era of cost containment. In general, these protocols utilize lower doses of opioids and benzodiazepines intraoperatively, and short acting sedation regimens postoperatively(Myles & McIlroy, 2005). Early extubation reduces sedation requirements, decreases risk for pulmonary complications and facilitates accelerated mobilization. There is significant data confirming the safety and efficacy of early extubation in these patients, as well as decreases in overall cost likely due to shorter ICU stays, with a low risk for intraoperative awareness(Cheng et al., 1996; Dowd et al., 1998; Zhu, Lee, & Chee, 2012).

It is important to note that early extubation is a relative term compared to the prior widespread practice of keeping patients intubated and sedated overnight after cardiac surgery and does not decrease the importance of confirming hemodynamic stability, appropriate hemostasis, and achievement of normothermia prior to extubation. The disadvantages of early discontinuation of sedation and extubation should always be considered in the context of a given patient and include: 1) heightened sympathetic tone with associated hypertension, tachycardia and increased myocardial oxygen demand, 2) increased risk for bleeding with hypertension, and 3) possible respiratory compromise due to fluid overload and decreased analgesia leading to splinting, atelectasis, and hypoventilation. Risk models for predicting the need for longer term ventilation have been developed(Shroyer et al., 2003), and risk factors for failure of early extubation grouped into preoperative, intraoperative, and postoperative risk factors include:

Preoperative: Presence of pulmonary edema, cardiogenic shock, sepsis, urgent/emergent surgery, preoperative intubation, significant existing pulmonary or renal dysfunction

Intraoperative: Reoperations, cardiopulmonary bypass times greater than 4-6 hrs, use of deep hypothermic circulatory arrest, significant fluid or blood product administration, myocardial dysfunction requiring inotropic support or use of intraaortic balloon pump,

Postoperative: Significant chest tube output/mediastinal bleeding, requirement for blood products, stroke/altered mental status (Bojar, 2011)

Mechanical Ventilation in Specific Disease States

The intensivists should be mindful of the effects of positive pressure ventilation on the disease-state of a patient. This is particularly important when manipulating ventilator settings as changes in intrathoracic pressure have significant effects on the loading condition of the heart as described previously.

In patients having undergone pleurectomy or with intrapleural or mediastinal bleeding there is a theoretical advantage of using PEEP to approximate the lung to the chest wall and to tamponade bleeding structures. For patients having undergone lung resection and or anastomoses the ventilation strategy must minimize peak airway pressures to reduce the risk of a leak, fistulae, or anastomotic break down. PEEP must be used judiciously and titrated appropriately to FiO2. This often results in competing demands of minimizing airway pressure and minimizing the toxic effects of high inspired oxygen concentrations (particularly important in the setting of lung transplant) with PEEP titration. In practice, a compromise between the two demands is usually required.

Management of patients with a bronchopleural fistulae (BPF) resulting in inadequate ventilation or gross lung soilage requires immediate lung isolation and thoracostomy tube placement followed by surgical exploration(Baumann & Sahn, 1990). Thoracostomy tube size should permit the evacuation of the large volume of airflow that occurs across the defect. In mechanically ventilated patients without lung isolation, the ventilator will have a significant leak, although the leaked volume does appear to participate in gas exchange(Bishop, Benson, & Pierson, 1987).

Positive pressure ventilation is best avoided in patients with a BPF as airflow across the defects inhibits healing. For patients that require mechanical ventilation, strategies include minimizing airway pressures, decreasing minute ventilation and inspiratory time by increasing inspiratory flow, decreasing PEEP, decreasing chest tube suction as tolerated, and good pulmonary toilet. In resistant cases, the patient may be positioned with the BPF dependently to minimize ventilation to that lung, or differential ventilation through a double lumen tube may be attempted with two synchronized ventilators.

Short Term Perioperative Ventilatory Support

Patients deemed not appropriate for early extubation may require short-term ventilatory support as transient hemodynamic or pulmonary dysfunction is addressed. Acute postoperative respiratory insufficiency, defined as failure of oxygenation (PO2 < 60 mmHg on FiO2 of 0.5) or ventilation (PCO2 > 55 mmHg) while on mechanical ventilation, is seen in approximately 1% of patients undergoing surgery using CPB(Bojar, 2011). Most commonly this occurs after an acute systemic insult (e.g. - hypotension, sepsis) in the context of preexisting pulmonary dysfunction or for patients with risk factors reviewed above.

In the immediate postoperative period, difficulties with oxygenation generally outweigh ventilation (elimination of CO2) issues and an organized assessment of the patient can help identify the underlying etiology.

1. Ventilator/Breathing Circuit
    a. Confirm proper ventilator function and appropriate FiO2, tidal volume and minute ventilation
    b. Confirm endotracheal tube function (lack of kinking/mucous plugging, proper cuff inflation) and placement
2. Oxygen Delivery
    a. Confirm adequate cardiac output via pulmonary artery catheter, transesophageal echocardiography, or other method (stroke volume variation, pulse pressure variation, etc.)
    b. Assess for possible venous admixture due to low V/Q ratio or right-to-left shunt
    c. Confirm adequate hemoglobin levels
3. Intrinsic Pulmonary Pathology

Prevention of Pulmonary Complications

Although many pulmonary complications following surgery may not be preventable, attention to early mobilization and physical therapy, appropriate analgesia, and meticulous fluid management are good therapeutic strategies(Medicine, 2013).

In a widely cited study by Schweickert and colleagues, early physical and occupational therapy resulted in better functional outcomes at hospital discharge, a shorter duration of delirium, and more ventilator-free days compared to usual care(Schweickert et al., 2009). Therapy can be targeted to a patient's specific physical deficit and may include mobilization, chest physical therapy, incentive spirometry and deep breathing exercises. These aid in lung recruitment and may help with clearance of lung water.

Patients with marginal cardiac and pulmonary function are highly susceptible to excess intra and extravascular fluid. Meticulous attention to fluid balance and maintenance of euvolemia may decrease the risk of respiratory compromise. In a trial of patients with acute lung injury, a restrictive fluid management strategy did not change the primary outcome of sixty day mortality, but did result in improved lung function and shortened duration of mechanical ventilation and intensive care without increasing non-pulmonary organ failure(National Heart et al., 2006).

Non-Invasive Ventilation

Many patients with respiratory failure can be spared the complications of mechanical ventilation by receiving support from non-invasive positive pressure ventilation (NPPV). Since its earliest applications in COPD exacerbations and cardiogenic pulmonary edema, NPPV has become a widely accepted modality for *prevention* of mechanical ventilation in other patient populations. The indications for NPPV include, but are not limited to, cardiogenic pulmonary edema, hypoxemic respiratory failure, acute asthma, exacerbations of COPD, respiratory failure following lung resection and solid-organ transplants, and weaning from mechanical ventilation. There is good evidence demonstrating decreased risk of nosocomial infections in patients managed with NPPV(Girou et al., 2000; Nourdine et al., 1999) as compared to endotracheal intubation. In addition, NPPV reduces the risk of mortality, hospital stay, and endotracheal intubation in patients with COPD exacerbation and acute cardiogenic pulmonary edema(Hess & Fessler, 2007).

Careful patient selection should take place prior to initiation of NPPV as the positive pressure delivered to the oro- and nasopharynx will follow the path of least resistance and may result in distension (and possible rupture) of surfaces exposed to this pressure including the esophagus, stomach, lung resection sites, and or anastomoses. Contraindications to NPPV include uncooperative patient, facial trauma or anatomic abnormalities interfering with proper mask fit, copious secretions, compromised airway reflexes, cardiac or respiratory arrest, hemodynamic instability, and risk of rupture or leak of a site exposed to positive pressure(Mehta & Hill, 2001).

Application of NPPV allows for delivery of mechanical ventilation without an artificial airway and less invasive ICU management. An interface delivers gas from a positive-pressure ventilator to the patient's mouth or nose. The most common modalities are continuous positive airway pressure (CPAP) or bi-level positive airway pressure (BIPAP) where the ventilator cycles between a high and low airway pressure based on a patients respiratory effort. Many different interfaces are available. Nasal masks are usually triangular in shape with a soft silicone sealing surface. Full-face masks come in different sizes and fit over the nose and mouth. These, carry less risk of nasal bridge ulceration(Hill, 2013). Both interfaces demonstrate similar improvement rates for vital signs, dyspnea, and gas exchange in patients with acute respiratory failure, however because of the air leak through the mouth, the initial intolerance rate is higher in the nasal mask group(Kwok, McCormack, Cece, Houtchens, & Hill, 2003). Once a proper interface is chosen, it is connected to a specifically designed turbine ventilator for NPPV that provides pressure at set levels and that is able to compensate for leak, has adjustable trigger and cycle mechanism, inspiratory times and oxygen blenders. The most commonly encountered side-effects are patient discomfort and facial erythema. Flow related adverse effects involve nasal congestion, sinus pain, nasal or oral dryness and eye irritation.

Major complications occur in less than 5% of patients and include hypotension, aspiration pneumonia and pneumothorax(Mehta & Hill, 2001). Studies have shown increased mortality in patients who are unable to clear secretions, those requiring vasopressors, and who experience refractory hypoxemia. Patients should be evaluated carefully in the first one to two hours after initiation of NPPV to ensure stabilization and to allow for elective intubation if required(Confalonieri et al., 2005).

NPPV may be accepted by patients who have requested limitations on aggressive therapy. In one study, up to sixty percent of patients with "Do Not Resuscitate" orders had improvement of symptoms of respiratory distress following its application (Benhamou, Girault, Faure, Portier, & Muir, 1992).

Strategies for Managing Specific Perioperative Conditions

Pulmonary Hypertension

The diagnosis of pulmonary hypertension (PH) is generally defined as a mean pulmonary artery pressure (PAP) of $\geq$ 25 mm Hg as determined by the physiologic variables of left atrial pressure (LAP), cardiac output (CO), and PVR in the following relationship:

$$PAP = LAP + \frac{(CO + PVR)}{80}$$

Conceptually, PH can be divided into 1) pulmonary arterial hypertension (PAH), which is a pre-capillary phenomenon and requires an elevated PVR > 3 Woods units with a pulmonary capillary wedge pressure (PCWP) ≤ 15 mm Hg, and 2) pulmonary venous hypertension (PVH), which has a post-capillary mechanism and is characterized by a PCWP of > 15 mm Hg, consistent with an elevated LAP(Hoeper et al., 2013). There can be both dynamic (i.e. – reactive to inhaled 100% oxygen and nitric oxide) and fixed (i.e. – non-reactive) components to PH in a given patient. It is recommended that the initial diagnosis of PH be made based on direct pressure data from right heart catheterization, and not on RV systolic pressure (RSVP) estimations made by echocardiographic assessment of the tricuspid valve regurgitant jet, especially in patients with advanced lung disease(Arcasoy et al., 2003; Han, McLaughlin, Criner, & Martinez, 2007).

Accurate identification of patients with significant PH is important because of a body of literature demonstrating high postoperative morbidity and mortality rates of up to 25% in these patients after both cardiac and noncardiac surgeries (Kaw et al., 2011; Minai, Yared, Kaw, Subramaniam, & Hill, 2013; Reich et al., 1999; Roques et al., 1999). PH puts patients at higher risk for RV ischemia and *cor pulmonale* due to several mechanisms. In the context of PH, the RV will be subject to elevated afterload conditions, leading to increased oxygen demand. Further, the RV will hypertrophy to compensate for the elevated afterload creating additional myocardial mass requiring perfusion. While the RV normally receives perfusion during both systole and diastole, when PAP, and therefore RVSP, begins to approach systemic blood pressure, RV perfusion during systole declines thereby increasing the risk for ischemia. Additionally, as RV compliance decreases with continued hypertrophy and RV end diastolic filling pressure continues to rise, diastolic blood flow to the RV also decreases leading to worsening ischemia and RV failure. As discussed previously, due to ventricular interdependence, RV failure and dilatation also leads to changes in LV structure with resulting decreases in CO.

Clinically, PH has been classified by the World Health Organization (WHO) into 5 separate groups that are delineated based on the presumed etiology and pathology leading to the elevated PAP(Simonneau et al., 2013). Class I PH disorders are all specifically PAH and include idiopathic PAH, inheritable PAH, and PAH associated with HIV and with connective tissues disorders among others. These disorders are linked by a common mechanism of abnormal pulmonary endothelial and smooth muscle cell proliferation leading to progressive obstruction of the pulmonary vasculature. This causes an elevated PVR, and therefore PAP, in the context of a normal PCWP. WHO group II PH arises from elevated left-sided heart pressures, most commonly due to LV diastolic or systolic dysfunction, or left-sided heart valve pathology including stenosis or regurgitation of the mitral and/or aortic valves. The elevated LAP seen in these conditions is conducted in a retrograde manner to the pulmonary vasculature leading to an increased PCWP consistent with PVH. WHO group III is comprised of disorders causing PH due to intrinsic lung disease or recurrent hypoxia. This group includes COPD, interstitial lung disease, obstructive sleep apnea, and high altitude-induced hypoxia, and is unified by a mechanism of chronic hypoxia causing pulmonary artery smooth muscle cell hypertrophy and subsequently an elevated PVR. This is likely the most common subset seen postoperatively in the ICU, as between 40-50% of patients with advanced COPD or interstitial pulmonary fibrosis are thought to have PH(Han et al., 2007). Also know as chronic thromboembolic pulmonary hypertension (CTEPH), WHO group IV PH is associated with an elevated

PVR secondary to clot obstructing blood flow through the lungs. Finally, Group V PH is a mixed group of diseases with unclear or multifactorial mechanisms including hemolytic anemia, sarcoidosis, glycogen storage diseases, and fibrosing mediastinitis, among others.

In the perioperative setting, patients are exposed to a number of factors that increase their risk for PH exacerbation and potentially RV dysfunction and failure. First, it is essential to ensure that patients who are on chronic medical therapy for their PH continue to receive these medications or substitute agents to help avoid acute RV failure. Additionally, preoperative administration of anxiolytic medications such as benzodiazepines, especially in concert with opioids, can cause respiratory depression with resulting hypoxia, hypercarbia, and acute elevations in PAP. Increased sympathetic tone associated with noxious stimuli, including airway instrumentation, surgical stimulation, or postoperative pain also leads to increased PAP through autonomic reflex responses.

As discussed previously, the institution of PPV causes decreases in RV preload as well as increases in PVR, both factors that act to markedly decrease cardiac output from the RV. As many agents for the maintenance of general anesthesia are vasodilators, patients are at risk for decreased preload and subsequent episodes of hypotension, leading to increased risk for RV ischemia. Certain surgical procedures including lung resections, in which significant amounts of pulmonary vasculature are removed (e.g. - multiple lobectomy, pneumonectomy), hip replacements, during which pulmonary embolization of bone marrow, cement, and entrained air may occur, and laparoscopic procedures involving insufflation of the abdomen with CO_2 can involve substantial increases in PVR. Also, the SIRS response associated with CPB (discussed previously) also leads to acute increases in PVR as does the development of ALI OR ARDS. Large fluid shifts can be associated with major surgical procedures and while it is important to maintain RV preload in patients with PH, overzealous fluid replacement can worsen RV dilatation causing RV failure and decreased LV filling. With these considerations in mind, it is clear that optimal care of PH patients requires a significant level of vigilance, especially in the perioperative period.

Acute RV failure due to PH exacerbation in the postoperative period is likely due to an increase in the dynamic component of the patient's PH. Therefore, a good understanding of the mechanism driving a specific patient's PH can be essential to optimize interventions. Although support of systemic blood pressure to maintain RV perfusion and maintenance of a normal heart rate should be a main priority in all cases, if the patient has PAH, interventions should also be directed toward decreasing PVR, but if the patient has PVH, the focus should be on the reduction of LAP. In this situation, invasive arterial monitoring and a PA catheter may help direct management. In the case of hypotension with an appropriate CO, augmentation of SVR to restore adequate RV perfusion pressure with either a systemic vasoconstrictor such as vasopressin, or a combined inotrope-vasopressor such as norepinephrine, is commonly recommended(Minai et al., 2013). There is some data in non-human species that suggests vasopressin may have an SVR-selective vasconstrictive effect, but the existing data in humans is conflicting(Smith, Elliot, Kiely, & Channer, 2006). In contrast, norepinephrine has been shown to decrease the PAP/SBP ratio while maintaining cardiac output in patients with chronic PH(Kwak, Lee, Park, & Hong, 2002). More potent inotrope-chronotropes such as epinephrine and dopamine may be less desirable as they can lead to tachycardia and increase oxygen demand. Fluid can be administered to maintain adequate RV preload (CVP – 12-15), however this should be done cautiously as fluid overload can worsen RV failure.

If hypotension is accompanied by a decreased CO, an elevated RA pressure, and increased PVR, then following establishment of adequate systemic blood pressure, interventions should be made to reduce the PVR. Contributions to PVR from anxiety or pain should be judiciously addressed in the spontaneously breathing patient off ventilatory support, including the liberal use of regional anesthesia where appropriate. In the intubated patient, sedation should be deepened with possible paralysis to ensure comfort and avoid patient-ventilator dyssynchrony. FiO_2 and minute ventilation should be adjusted to avoid hypoxia, hypercarbia, and respiratory acidosis with avoidance of high airway pressures or high levels of PEEP. Ideally, tidal volumes should be set just above FRC as this will produce the lowest contribution to PVR (see Fig. 2).

Specific pharmacologic interventions to decrease PVR can also be initiated. Intravenous vasodilating agents such as nitroglycerin, nitroprusside and calcium channel blockers have been used effectively although they carry the risk of systemic vasodilation with associated decreases in blood pressure. Inhaled nitric oxide, although costly, allows selective pulmonary vasodilation with minimal effect on systemic blood pressure. Additionally, there are several classes of agents approved for treatment of Group I/PAH including the prostanoids (e.g. – Epoprostenol, Iloprost), endothelin receptor agonists (e.g. – Bosentan, Ambrisentan), and phosphodiesterase-5 (PDE-5) inhibitors (e.g. – sildenafil, tadalafil) however the use of the agents in acute RV failure has not been comprehensively studied. Notably, the use of Group I agents should likely be avoided in patients with Group II PH/PVH because of the development of pulmonary edema due to pulmonary vasculature vasodilation in the context of an elevated PCWP(D. L. Fox, Stream, & Bull, 2014). The PDE-3 antagonist milrinone is an ino-dilator and has been used successfully in intravenous form in patients with Group II PH after ventricular assist device placement and heart transplant, and inhaled form in patients undergoing mitral valve replacement(Eichhorn et al., 1987; Kihara et al., 2002; Wang, Gong, Zhou, & Dai, 2009). If these interventions are inadequate to maintain RV function, consideration should be given to mechanical support.

While no comprehensive guidelines currently exist for the perioperative management of patients with PH, a strong understanding of relevant physiology including vasoactive control of the pulmonary vasculature and cardiopulmonary interdependence is crucial to providing optimal care to these patients.

Acute Respiratory Distress Syndrome

Acute respiratory distress syndrome (ARDS) represents a continuum of acute hypoxemic respiratory failure. In 1994, the American-European Consensus Conference (AECC) proposed definitions for both ARDS and Acute Lung Injury (ALI). Both conditions were characterized by acute onset of severe hypoxemia, dyspnea, diffuse lung infiltrates and decreased compliance of the respiratory system. Criteria were based on a ratio of PaO2 to the fraction of inspired oxygen FiO2. ARDS was defined as a PaO2:FiO2 $\leq$200, and ALI as a PaO2:FiO2 was $\leq$300. In 2011, the current "Berlin" Definition for ARDS was developed with an emphasis on reliability and validity. The Berlin Definition establishes 3 categories of ARDS: mild (200mm Hg $<PaO_2/FiO_2\leq$300mm Hg), moderate (100mm Hg$<PaO_2/FiO_2\leq$200mm Hg), and severe ($PaO_2/FiO_2\leq$100mm Hg) with PEEP $\geq$ 5cm H_2O. The onset of hypoxemia must occur within 1 week of a known clinical insult or new or worsening respiratory symptoms. On chest X-ray or CT scan, bilateral opacities must be present, not fully explained by effusions, lobar collapse or nodules. Patients meet the new criteria for ARDS if their respiratory failure is not fully explained by fluid overload or cardiac failure, with some patients requiring echocardiography to exclude hydrostatic edema(Network, 2000).

The syndrome of ARDS has multiple causes, some of which may be treatable. These include infectious etiologies including pneumonia and sepsis. Other causes include pancreatitis, massive transfusion, chemical pneumonitis, and pulmonary contusion as a result of direct injury to the lung during surgery. ARDS is believed to occur following cardiopulmonary bypass in 1.3% of cases and patients over 60 years seem to be at higher risk(Messent, Sullivan, Keogh, Morgan, & Evans, 1992). The incidence approximates 3.9% following pulmonary resection with male patients and those undergoing resection for lung cancer were at higher risk.

The focus of treatment for ARDS remains supportive with the goal of minimizing mechanical ventilation induced trauma to the already damaged lung. It is important to recognize that ARDS represents a spectrum of disease with heterogeneous changes in lung compliance and ventilation and perfusion matching(Force et al., 2012). Strategies that are currently used to minimize ongoing lung injury include low tidal volume ventilation (6cc/kg) to avoid overdistention, high PEEP to avoid atelectotrauma, and recruitment maneuvers to inflate atelectatic lung. Additional therapies include optimizing fluid balance, paralysis in early severe ARDS(L. Papazian et al., 2010), and prone ventilation to optimize ventilation and perfusion matching, and the use of extra-corporeal support.

Pneumonia and Ventilator Associated Events

Pneumonia following thoracotomy is reported in between 2.2% and 6% of cases, with an incidence of 2-10% following cardiac surgery(Hortal et al., 2009; Wagnetz & de Perrot, 2011). Postoperative pneumonia has a mortality rate of 20-30% and has three pathogenic mechanisms: preoperative colonization with pathogenic bacteria, impaired host defenses secondary to critical illness and its therapies, and aspiration of contaminated secretions(Kollef, 1999). The most common culprit bacterial pathogens are the same as those found in community-acquired pneumonia- *Streptococcus* and *Haemophilus influenza*. The remainder of cases are caused by relatively high-grade pathogens such as methicillin-resistant *S. aureus (MRSA), Pseudomonas, Serratia and Enterobacter, Klebsiella pneumonia* (ESBL), *Acinetobacter* species especially in patients who have been in a hospital for ≥5 days or had prior nosocomial exposure. Ventilator-associated pneumonia (VAP) is a subgroup within postoperative pneumonia, and is defined as pneumonia occurring more than 48 hours following endotracheal intubation and initiation of mechanical ventilation, with a mortality rate between 20%-50% which can be even higher when infection is caused by high-risk pathogens(America, 2005; Chastre & Fagon, 2002).

Allou and colleagues identified five independent risk factors for postoperative pneumonia: age, presence of COPD, left ventricular ejection fraction, intraoperative RBC transfusion and duration of CPB. Scoring systems are available to assist in identifying patients at highest risk (Allou et al., 2014) The major risk factors for development of pneumonia following lung surgery are extent of pulmonary resection and COPD.

The diagnosis of pneumonia represents a clinical dilemma to the intensivist. The systemic signs of infection such as fever, tachycardia, and leukocytosis are nonspecific findings and can be caused by infectious and non-infectious process that releases cytokines. Pugin and colleagues developed a Critical Pulmonary Infectious Score (CPIS) as a tool for diagnosis of ventilator-associated pneumonia. It is a clinical score of 0-12 based on the following 6 variables: body temperature, leukocyte count, volume and character of tracheal secretion, arterial oxygenation, chest radiograph findings, Gram stain and tracheal aspirate culture results (Pugin et al., 1991). The score has been used in many subsequent studies. Using histologic examination of tissue (postmortem) as a gold standard for diagnosis, a CPIS score of 6 achieved specificity of 85% and sensitivity of 72% with an overall accuracy of 79% for the presence of VAP. Combination of the CPIS with quantitative culture resulted in an increase in specificity to 95% at the cost of diminished sensitivity of 67%(L Papazian et al., 1995). However, CPIS is over-inclusive in identifying patients with suspected VAP who need a prolonged course of antibiotics(Luyt, Chastre, & Fagon, 2004).

Sampling of lower respiratory tract mucosa with bronchoalveolar lavage (BAL) in patients with clinically suspected postoperative pneumonia remains critical to diagnosis. A quantitative culture analysis of the BAL with more than 10^4 cfu/mL (colony-forming units/mL) suggest a pneumonia.

Initial antibiotic coverage should be based on the prevalence of common microbes responsible for pneumonia at each institution and once microbiologic results become available, coverage should be tailored to the narrowest applicable spectrum of antibiotics. In patients at risk for multidrug resistant pathogens, initial empiric treatment should consist of combination antibiotic therapy covering MRSA (Vancomycin or Linezolid), antipseudomonal cephalosporin (Cefepime, Ceftazidime) or a carbapenem (Imipenem, Meropenem) or Piperacillin-Tazobactam. Other combinations consist of antipseudomonal fluoroquinolones (Ciprofloxacin, Levofloxacin) or aminoglycosides (Amikacin, Gentamicin) with Linezolid or Vancomycin (if high risk of MRSA) and Metronidazole. For patients with severe sepsis induced by pneumonia, consider double covering with two anti-pseudomonal agents until culture data are available. Immunocompromised patients should be additionally considered for anti-fungal coverage. An eight day course of antibiotic treatment is acceptable for most non-bacteremic patients with VAP(Chastre et al., 2003) but longer courses should be considered in the setting of an extended spectrum beta lactamase producing organism. Antibiotic therapy should be discontinued after 48-72 hours if cultures are negative or signs of infection have resolved(Micek, Ward, Fraser, & Kollef, 2004).

Since the establishment of the term ventilator associated pneumonia in 2002, this definition has been found to be neither sensitive nor specific. In 2014, a new term, *ventilator-associated event* (VAE) was established, which includes all the conditions that cause worsening oxygenation after a period of initial stability and require greater than 20% increase in the daily minimum FiO2 or an increase of at least 3cm in the daily minimum PEEP to maintain oxygenation(Raoof, Baumann, & Collaborative, 2014). Because VAE identifies broad range of events in patients on mechanical ventilation, it encompasses both infectious and non-infectious conditions, including complications occurring in this group of patients. Therefore, VAE definition has three tiers:

Tier 1: *Ventilator-associated condition* (VAC)- when the patient develops sustained hypoxemia of more than 2 days. The etiology of the hypoxemia is not taken into account.

Tier 2: *Infection-related ventilator-associated complication* (IVAC): hypoxemia in setting of infection or generalized inflammation (Temperature >38°C, <36°C, or WBC count ≥12,000 cells/mm^3 or ≤4,000 cells/mm^3) and a new antimicrobial agent is started and instituted for a minimum of 4 days.

Tier 3: *Probable or possible ventilator-associated pneumonia* (VAP): additional positive culture of sputum, endotracheal aspirate, BAL, lung tissue or protected specimen brushing, and/or purulent secretions (>25 neutrophils and <10 squamous epithelial cells per low power field (lpf, x100)). *Candida,* coagulase-negative *Staphylococcus,* and Enterococcus species are excluded from this criteria because they are not commonly regarded as true VAP pathogens.

VAE is not a clinical definition algorithm and is not intended for use in the management of patients, but instead serves as a surveillance tool to be implemented by the National Healthcare Safety Network (NHSN) for purposes of public reporting, inter-facility comparisons and pay-for-performance calculations. Additional guidance and tools are available on NHSN website http://www.cdc.gov/nhsn/acute-care-hospital/vae/index.html(Magill et al., 2013).

Pleural Effusion

Pleural effusions are common following cardiac surgery, and are seen in as many as 50% of patients, most commonly following violation of the pleural space(Light et al., 2002). Following cardiac surgery, pleural effusions result in blood from the mediastinum and serous fluid from the chest wall.

Pleural effusions may be classified as early (occurring within nine days following surgery) or late (more than fourteen days post-operatively)(Chiles et al., 1985; Judson, Handy, & Sahn, 1996, 1997). Early pleural effusions are usually exudative, bloody, and demonstrate a predominance of neutrophils. If early postoperative effusions decrease and the patient is making clinical progress, further workup is not indicated. For patients requiring further investigation, ultrasound and chest imaging can be used to assess size, location, and consistency of pleural effusion prior to thoracentesis. Late occurring pleural effusions should be investigated for chylothorax, empyema, pneumonia, or rejection in patients with lung or heart transplant.

Pneumo- and Hemothorax

Pneumothorax is defined as presence of air in the pleural space. The incidence of pneumothorax in mechanically ventilated ICU patients is anywhere between 4%-15%, with emphysematous lung disease and ARDS representing some of the risk factors(Strange, 1999). The three main mechanisms of air entry into pleural space are visceral pleural rupture allowing communication between the pleura and alveolar space, a communication between the pleural space and the atmosphere, and presence of gas-producing organisms within pleural space(Noppen & De Keukeleire, 2008).

Primary spontaneous pneumothoraces occur in subjects without underlying lung disease. Secondary spontaneous pneumothoraces arise in subjects with preexisting lung disease such as cystic fibrosis or emphysema(Haynes & Baumann, 2010). Iatrogenic pneumothoraces follow surgical violation of the pleural space during cardiac and thoracic surgery, and in the ICU after invasive procedures including thoracentesis, central line placement, or with positive pressure ventilation(Yarmus & Feller-Kopman, 2012).

Clinical signs and symptoms of pneumothorax in spontaneously breathing patient include sudden onset of respiratory distress, pleuritic chest pain, tachycardia, unilateral breath sounds and hypoxemia. An increase in airway pressure due to reduced chest compliance accompanies pneumothorax in mechanically ventilated subjects. Tension pneumothorax manifests with hypotension, cardiovascular collapse and a tracheal shift. While clinical features are helpful in diagnosis of pneumothorax, because of their nonspecific nature, imaging remains important in diagnosis with the exception of a hemodynamically significant tension pneumothorax which may need to be empirically managed by needle or tube drainage prior to radiologic confirmation.

Chest radiographic diagnosis of pneumothorax is confirmed by presence of a visceral pleural line seen without distal lung markings. Ultrasound is increasingly becoming the preferred diagnostic modality to exclude pneumothorax(Yarmus & Feller-Kopman, 2012). Computerized Tomography remains the gold standard for both sizing and diagnosis of pneumothorax(Kelly, Weldon, Tsang, & Graham, 2006).

Hemothorax is defined by the presence of blood in the pleural space. In post-thoracotomy patients, bleeding can result from slippage of ligatures around pulmonary vessels, bleeding from bronchial, intercostal arteries, the mediastinum, and raw pleural spaces. Postoperative bleeding is the most common indication for repeat thoracotomy after lung surgery(Sirbu et al., 1999). Following cardiac surgery, in patients with significant mediastinal bleeding, blood can drain into the opened pleural space and result in a hemothorax. Cardinal clinical findings in these patients consist of falling hematocrit and hemodynamic instability due to hypovolemia. Diagnosis of hemothorax can be established by continuous bloody chest tube output or CT scan of the chest.

The standard treatment of both pneumo- and hemothorax is tube thoracostomy, with the goal of complete drainage of either fluid or air to allow for full re-expansion of the lung and approximation of parietal and visceral pleura. There are three main chest tube types all containing a side and an end hole, in addition to a radio-opaque marker allowing for clear visualization of chest tube position on the chest X-ray. Serious complications can occur with chest tube insertion with inadvertent placement into major fissure or lung parenchyma(Campos & Parekh, 2011).

Disposable sterile dry suction chest drainage systems have replaced the traditional glass bottle systems. These newer systems are modeled on the three-bottle drainage system and also have three chambers; one for collection, a water seal chamber, and a suction control chamber. The collection chamber located on the left side of the system is connected directly to the chest tube allowing for drainage of blood or fluid in the pleural space. The middle chamber serves as a water seal and allows air to exit the pleural space on exhalation and prevents it from re-entering during inspiration. The suction-control chamber is located on the right side of the system; it is an automatic control valve that continuously balances the force of suction with the atmosphere allowing the delivery of accurate suction pressure. The water level in the water-seal chamber will rise with inhalation and return to baseline with exhalation, which is called tidaling (the reverse is true during mechanical ventilation). Other features included in the modern chest tube drainage system are: a suction control regulator, vacuum indicator, air leak monitor, suction monitor bellows, a manual high negativity vent and positive pressure release valve(Friedrich, 2012). The air leak monitor has numbered columns indicating the degree of air leak.

Because an air leak is a common concern following pulmonary resection, Cerfolio and colleagues developed an evidence-based approach for management of this complication. Air leaks occupying less than four of seven chambers are likely to decrease faster on water seal than on suction(Cerfolio, Bass, & Katholi, 2001). On postoperative day two and once air leaks have resolved chest tubes can be removed assuming no significant or expanding pneumothorax, subcutaneous emphysema, and drainage is less than 450 cc per day on water seal(Cerfolio & Bryant, 2008). Chest tube suction should be switched to -10cm H_2O from water seal if patients develop symptomatic enlarging pneumothorax or subcutaneous emphysema. Large air leaks and a pneumothorax >8cm in size predicts failure of simple water seal(Cerfolio, Bryant, Singh, Bass, & Bartolucci, 2005).

Pulmonary Edema

In ICU patients, the two most common forms of pulmonary edema result either from disruption of the alveolar-capillary membrane or increased net hydrostatic pressure across capillary beds. Movement of fluid across a capillary bed is described by the Starling equation:

$$Qf=Kf(Pv-Pint) - Kf(pV-pint)$$

Qf is net flow across the pulmonary capillary endothelium, *Kf* is the filtration coefficient of the microvascular endothelium, *Pv* and *Pint* represent the hydrostatic pressures in the capillary and interstitium respectively. *pV* and *pint* are plasma protein oncotic pressure and oncotic pressure of the interstitium(Meyer & Krishnamani, 2010).

Pulmonary edema can be classified as either cardiogenic or non-cardiogenic. Mechanistically, cardiogenic pulmonary edema results from increased pulmonary blood flow and pulmonary venous hypertension. Experimental models have shown that extravasation of intravascular fluid occurs once pulmonary capillary wedge pressure (PCWP) exceeds the plasma colloid osmotic pressure of 28 mmHg(Meyer & Krishnamani, 2010). With continued extravasation of fluid, the interstitial space will reach its maximum capacity (which is directly proportional to the functional capacity of the lymphatic system that drains interstitial fluid) and fluid will flood into the alveoli(Meyer & Krishnamani, 2010; Staub, Nagano, & Pearce, 1967). Upon injury of the alveolar-capillary membrane, proteins will leak from the capillary into the interstitium and result in impedance of capillary filtration(Meyer & Krishnamani, 2010).

Pulmonary causes of non-cardiogenic pulmonary edema that may be encountered in the cardiothoracic ICU include post-pneumonectomy pulmonary edema, re-expansion pulmonary edema following large volume thoracentesis, reperfusion injury following thromboendarterectomy, or lung transplantation. Non-pulmonary causes of non-cardiogenic pulmonary edema include transfusion related acute lung injury, systemic inflammation secondary to CPB, massive blood transfusion, sepsis, or neurogenic pulmonary edema. Clinical presentation is similar in all cases. Patients exhibit respiratory distress accompanied by hypoxemia, sometimes with wheezes and crackles. Specific signs of cardiogenic causes include a new heart murmur, S_3 or S_4 heart sound and elevated JVP. To distinguish between the mechanisms of pulmonary edema left ventricular function must be evaluated either by performing echocardiography or measuring PCWP with a pulmonary artery catheter (>18mmHg is indicative of increased hydrostatic pressure). In addition, a chest X-ray, electrocardiogram, and cardiac biomarkers such as troponin and B-type natriuretic peptide may be obtained, although the significance of the later in the perioperative setting and in critical illness is questionable(McGuinness & Sidebotham, 2007).

Management of pulmonary edema is aimed at treating the underlying cause. In cardiogenic pulmonary edema the goal is to decrease intrapulmonary fluid burden with diuretics, improve left ventricular function with inotropes and/or vasodilators (by decreasing preload and afterload), and reduce the pulmonary blood flow. Treatment of non-cardiogenic causes is generally supportive. In both cases, initiation of positive pressure ventilation improves shunt fraction, reduces work of breathing and improves oxygenation. In diuretic resistant patients or those with excess total body water with relative intravascular depletion, a combination of albumin and furosemide may increase plasma oncotic pressure and assist with diuresis and removal of lung water(Kitsios, Mascari, Ettunsi, & Gray, 2014).

Obstructive Airways Disease

The primary causes of airway obstruction encountered in the ICU are Chronic Obstructive Pulmonary Disease (COPD) and asthma. Both are characterized by increased airflow resistance and inflammation, however airflow resistance is largely reversible in asthma in contradistinction to COPD. COPD may be caused by emphysema or chronic bronchitis. A small portion of patients have a mixture of both COPD and asthma. Severe COPD is defined by an FEV1 less than 50% and FEV1/FVC ratio of less than 0.7. In these patients, postoperative bronchospasm can contribute to acute respiratory failure. The increase in airway resistance caused by bronchospasm increases work of breathing and leads to prolongation of expiration and auto-PEEP(Ramsay & Finley, 2011).

Preoperative preparation for patients with obstructive airways disease must focus on optimizing respiratory function. Chronic inflammation is central to the etiology of COPD. The inflammatory milieu in COPD is neutrophil and macrophage rich, where as in asthma there is eosinophil predominance. The presence of inflammatory cell types in sputum or BAL samples, specifically eosinophils, may predict steroid-responsiveness(Fujimoto, Kubo, Yamamoto, Yamaguchi, & Matsuzawa, 1999; Sutherland & Martin, 2003). In asthma, maintenance with inhaled corticosteroids reduces the inflammatory changes and incidence of exacerbations and improves lung mechanics. A combination therapy of inhaled corticosteroids and long-acting β_2 adrenergic agonists is required for a decrease in inflammation and disease control in severe COPD(Restrepo, 2009).

Clinical manifestation of bronchospasm includes wheezing, pulsus paradoxus, increased work of breathing with recession of intercostal spaces and supraclavicular fossae, paradoxical motion of the rib cage and the abdomen. In mechanically ventilated patients, an increase in peak inspiratory pressure, slow increase in expiratory capnograph waveform, and auto-PEEP are all suggestive of bronchospasm.

Non-invasive positive pressure ventilation (NPPV) may be used along with short acting inhaled beta$_2$-agonists for treatment of bronchospasm(Brochard et al., 1990; Kramer, Meyer, Meharg, Cece, & Hill, 1995). NPPV produces reductions in respiratory rate, patients' symptoms, increased tidal volumes and improved gas exchange(Brochard et al., 1990; Kramer et al., 1995). In COPD, most of the airflow obstruction is irreversible, however some patients do have a reversible component that can be treated with bronchodilator therapy. Inhaled β adrenergic agonists increase smooth muscle relaxation and bronchodilation by increasing intracellular levels of cyclic AMP. Short acting selective β_2 agonists such as albuterol or metaproterenol should be administered either by metered dose inhaler (MDI) 3-6 puffs every 30-60 minutes, or via nebulizer (0.5mL albuterol or 0.3mL metaproterenol in 2.5mL of normal saline). Alternatively, an inhaled cholinergic receptor antagonist, ipratropium can be given 3-10 puffs every 2-6 hours by MDI, or higher dose of 400mcg every 2 hours in intubated patients. Unlike stable disease, during COPD exacerbation, combination therapy of inhaled β_2 agonists with ipratropium does not result in better short-term bronchodilation than either agent alone(McCrory & Brown, 2002). The long-acting β_2 agonist salmeterol and nonselective phosphodiesterase inhibitor aminophylline, have failed to show any additional benefit during acute exacerbations of disease and should not be used during acute bronchospasm(R. G. Barr, Rowe, & Camargo, 2003). Through its alpha-adrenergic properties, racemic epinephrine may reduce respiratory mucosal edema. Administration of systemic adrenergic agonists (e.g. epinephrine) should be reserved for rescue therapy where selective β_2 agonists and corticosteroids are ineffective at relieving bronchospasm(Ramsay & Finley, 2011).

Administration, dosing and duration of corticosteroid therapy during COPD exacerbation remains controversial. Current guidelines advise 0.5-1 mg/kg of methylprednisolone every 6 hours, and duration of the steroid course should not exceed 14 days with transition to oral formulation after 72 hours of treatment (McCrory, Brown, Gelfand, & Bach, 2001). When compared to placebo, systemic corticosteroids improve airflow and decrease the risk of relapse. The lowest effective dose of corticosteroids and shortest duration of therapy should be provided(Woods, Wheeler, Finch, & Pinner, 2014).

The ICU patient with obstructive airways disease often has difficulty with secretions and these can be managed by judicious hydration, suctioning, humidification of inspired gases, mucolytics, and toilet bronchoscopy. Patients with severe, end-stage disease are highly sensitive to respiratory depressants and even small quantities of opioids or benzodiazepines may cause failure.

Ventilated patients with significant obstructive disease are at risk for "dynamic hyperinflation" where inspiration occurs before exhalation terminates. This results in increased intra-thoracic pressure as a result of auto-PEEP and hypotension that can cause cardiac arrest. Prevention of dynamic hyperinflation is achieved by the use of bronchodilators, a short I:E ratio (1:3 or more), low respiratory rates and tidal volumes, and the setting of PEEP levels to approximate a portion of a patient's auto-PEEP level. In the event of clinically significant hypotension, the patient should be disconnected from the ventilator and allowed to fully exhale while fluids are bolused.

Severe asthma may be treated with aggressive use of bronchodilators, oxygen, and epinephrine. Intravenous steroids should be administered recognizing that they will take several hours for their full effect to be realized. Helium oxygen mixtures, because of the lower density of helium compared to air, may be helpful in decreasing turbulent airflow in obstructive disease, however in practice, the relatively low FiO2 and high helium concentrations (70%) of these mixtures limits the usefulness of this approach. Intubation and mechanical ventilation may ultimately be required, and the intensivists should expect the need to ventilate at high peak airway pressure to overcome acute airflow resistance. For resistant disease, neuromuscular paralysis and administration of an inhalational anesthetic may be required. Cardiac dysfunction may contribute to acute respiratory failure from asthma as the catecholamine surge associated with the initiating asthmatic event may exacerbate valvular insufficiency resulting in excess lung water and worsening respiratory distress. In this setting, pharmacologically optimizing cardiac performance may reduce the severity of respiratory failure.

FUTURE RESEARCH DIRECTIONS

The practice of Critical Care Medicine is in continuous and rapid evolution. The systematic approach to respiratory care presented in this chapter relies on the state of knowledge at the time of publication, however this is in constant flux. Two areas of respiratory care that are likely to continue to see growth are innovation in ventilator technology and the turn towards extracorporeal support.

Ventilator technology and the understanding of the effects of mechanical ventilation are rapidly improving. New modes of ventilation attempt to gain better synchrony and optimization of ventilation. These include proportional assist ventilation (PAV) and neurally-adjusted ventilatory assist (NAVA) (Gilstrap & MacIntyre, 2013). PAV uses an algorithm to determine the additional support required by a ventilator to achieve a desired reduction in the work of breathing. NAVA uses an esophageal catheter with diaphragm EMG sensors to determine the onset, termination, and intensity of ventilatory effort and makes adjustments based on these. Like all new technologies, their application requires study of clinical effectiveness.

Despite improvements in ventilator technology, for patients requiring aggressive ventilator settings, the critical care community is increasingly turning towards more early application of extracorporeal support in hope of reducing ventilator induced lung injury(Slutsky & Ranieri, 2013). As experience is gained in using extracorporeal support, better understanding of the optimal indications and timing will emerge. Towards this end, a group recently used data from the Extracorporeal Life Support Organization (ELSO) to validate a score for predicting survival after ECMO(Schmidt et al., 2014).

The advent and application of novel technologies like ECMO occur by pushing limits of available care. This often means that patients don't individually benefit from the experimental studies in which they consent to participate, but that knowledge developed from these improves care for future patients and expands available therapies and their indications (R. e. C. Fox & Swazey, 2002).

Emerging technologies that fit this paradigm include improvements in ECMO devices, use of these in pre-hospital settings, and the advent of Extracorporeal Carbon Dioxide Removal (ECCOR)(Agerstrand, Bacchetta, & Brodie, 2014; Cove, Maclaren, Federspiel, & Kellum, 2012). These are all aimed at normalizing physiology during critical illness and preventing harm induced by mechanical ventilation at the non-physiologic settings often required for patients with severe respiratory disease.

CONCLUSION

The foundation of systematic respiratory care of the cardiothoracic intensive care unit patient is built on a clear understanding of respiratory physiology and a current understanding of the literature. The reader is encouraged to supplement the perspectives provided in this chapter with attention to new findings regularly published in current journals.

REFERENCES

Agerstrand, C. L., Bacchetta, M. D., & Brodie, D. (2014). ECMO for adult respiratory failure: Current use and evolving applications. *ASAIO Journal (American Society for Artificial Internal Organs)*, *60*(3), 255–262. doi:10.1097/MAT.0000000000000062 PMID:24625534

Akoumianaki, E., Maggiore, S. M., Valenza, F., Bellani, G., Jubran, A., Loring, S. H., & Brochard, L. et al. (2014). The application of esophageal pressure measurement in patients with respiratory failure. *American Journal of Respiratory and Critical Care Medicine*, *189*(5), 520–531. doi:10.1164/rccm.201312-2193CI PMID:24467647

Allou, N., Bronchard, R., Guglielminotti, J., Dilly, M. P., Provenchere, S., Lucet, J. C., & Montravers, P. et al. (2014). Risk factors for postoperative pneumonia after cardiac surgery and development of a preoperative risk score*. *Critical Care Medicine*, *42*(5), 1150–1156. doi:10.1097/CCM.0000000000000143 PMID:24351376

America, A. T. S. I. D. S. (2005). Guidelines for the management of adults with hospital-acquired, ventilator-associated, and healthcare-associated pneumonia. *American Journal of Respiratory and Critical Care Medicine*, *171*(4), 388–416. doi:10.1164/rccm.200405-644ST PMID:15699079

Arcasoy, S. M., Christie, J. D., Ferrari, V. A., Sutton, M. S., Zisman, D. A., Blumenthal, N. P., & Kotloff, R. M. et al. (2003). Echocardiographic assessment of pulmonary hypertension in patients with advanced lung disease. *American Journal of Respiratory and Critical Care Medicine*, *167*(5), 735–740. doi:10.1164/rccm.200210-1130OC PMID:12480614

Arozullah, A. M., Daley, J., Henderson, W. G., & Khuri, S. F. (2000). Multifactorial risk index for predicting postoperative respiratory failure in men after major noncardiac surgery. The National Veterans Administration Surgical Quality Improvement Program. *Annals of Surgery*, *232*(2), 242–253. doi:10.1097/00000658-200008000-00015 PMID:10903604

Baram, D., & Richman, P. (2010). Mechanical Ventilation in the Cardiac Care Unit. In A. Jeremias & D. L. Brown (Eds.), *Cardiac Intensive Care* (2nd ed., pp. 632–643). Philadelphia: Saunders Elsevier. doi:10.1016/B978-1-4160-3773-6.10050-3

Barr, J., Fraser, G. L., Puntillo, K., Ely, E. W., Gelinas, C., Dasta, J. F., & Jaeschke, R. et al. (2013). Clinical practice guidelines for the management of pain, agitation, and delirium in adult patients in the intensive care unit. *Critical Care Medicine*, *41*(1), 263–306. doi:10.1097/CCM.0b013e3182783b72 PMID:23269131

Barr, R. G., Rowe, B. H., & Camargo, C. A. (2003). Methylxanthines for exacerbations of chronic obstructive pulmonary disease. *Cochrane Database of Systematic Reviews,* (2), CD002168. doi: 10.1002/14651858.CD002168

Baumann, M. H., & Sahn, S. A. (1990). Medical management and therapy of bronchopleural fistulas in the mechanically ventilated patient. *Chest Journal*, *97*(3), 721–728. doi:10.1378/chest.97.3.721 PMID:2407455

Benhamou, D., Girault, C., Faure, C., Portier, F., & Muir, J. F. (1992). Nasal mask ventilation in acute respiratory failure. Experience in elderly patients. *Chest Journal*, *102*(3), 912–917. doi:10.1378/chest.102.3.912 PMID:1516421

Benumof, J. L., & Wahrenbrock, E. A. (1975). Local effects of anesthetics on regional hypoxic pulmonary vasoconstriction. *Anesthesiology*, *43*(5), 525–532. doi:10.1097/00000542-197511000-00008 PMID:1190522

Bishop, M. J., Benson, M. S., & Pierson, D. J. (1987). Carbon dioxide excretion via bronchopleural fistulas in adult respiratory distress syndrome. *Chest Journal*, *91*(3), 400–402. doi:10.1378/chest.91.3.400 PMID:3102170

Bojar, R. M. (2011). Respiratory Management. In R. M. Bojar (Ed.), Manual of perioperative care in adult cardiac surgery (5th ed.). Wiley-Blackwell.

Boles, J. M., Bion, J., Connors, A., Herridge, M., Marsh, B., Melot, C., & Welte, T. et al. (2007). Weaning from mechanical ventilation. *The European Respiratory Journal*, *29*(5), 1033–1056. doi:10.1183/09031936.00010206 PMID:17470624

Branson, R. D., & Johannigman, J. A. (2004). What is the evidence base for the newer ventilation modes? *Respiratory Care*, *49*(7), 742–760. PMID:15222907

Brochard, L., Isabey, D., Piquet, J., Amaro, P., Mancebo, J., Messadi, A. A., & Harf, A. et al. (1990). Reversal of acute exacerbations of chronic obstructive lung disease by inspiratory assistance with a face mask. *The New England Journal of Medicine*, *323*(22), 1523–1530. doi:10.1056/NEJM199011293232204 PMID:2122253

Bronicki, R. A., & Anas, N. G. (2009). Cardiopulmonary interaction. *Pediatric Critical Care Medicine*, *10*(3), 313–322. doi:10.1097/PCC.0b013e31819887f0 PMID:19307810

Buckley, D., & Gillham, M. (2007). Invasive Respiratory Support. In D. Sidebotham, A. McKee, M. Gillham, & J. H. Levy (Eds.), *Cardiothoracic Critical Care*. Philadelphia: Butterworth Heinemann Elsevier. doi:10.1016/B978-075067572-7.50032-1

Campos, J., & Parekh, K. R. (2011). Thoracic Imaging. In P. D. Slinger (Ed.), *Principles and practice of anesthesia for thoracic surgery* (pp. 35–48). New York: Elsevier. doi:10.1007/978-1-4419-0184-2_3

Cargill, R. I., & Lipworth, B. J. (1996). Lisinopril attenuates acute hypoxic pulmonary vasoconstriction in humans. *Chest Journal*, *109*(2), 424–429. doi:10.1378/chest.109.2.424 PMID:8620717

Casthely, P. A., Lear, S., Cottrell, J. E., & Lear, E. (1982). Intrapulmonary shunting during induced hypotension. *Anesthesia and Analgesia*, *61*(3), 231–235. doi:10.1213/00000539-198203000-00002 PMID:6802027

Cerfolio, R. J., Bass, C., & Katholi, C. R. (2001). Prospective randomized trial compares suction versus water seal for air leaks. *The Annals of Thoracic Surgery*, *71*(5), 1613–1617. doi:10.1016/S0003-4975(01)02474-2 PMID:11383809

Cerfolio, R. J., & Bryant, A. S. (2008). Results of a prospective algorithm to remove chest tubes after pulmonary resection with high output. *The Journal of Thoracic and Cardiovascular Surgery*, *135*(2), 269–273. doi:10.1016/j.jtcvs.2007.08.066 PMID:18242249

Cerfolio, R. J., Bryant, A. S., Singh, S., Bass, C. S., & Bartolucci, A. A. (2005). The management of chest tubes in patients with a pneumothorax and an air leak after pulmonary resection. *Chest Journal*, *128*(2), 816–820. doi:10.1378/chest.128.2.816 PMID:16100173

Chalaby, M. P. J. (2010). Acute Respiratory Failure. In A. Jeremias & D. L. Brown (Eds.), *Cardiac Intensive Care* (2nd ed., pp. 388–397). Philadelphia, PA: Saunders/Elsevier. doi:10.1016/B978-1-4160-3773-6.10031-X

Chastre, J., & Fagon, J.-Y. (2002). Ventilator-associated pneumonia. *American Journal of Respiratory and Critical Care Medicine*, *165*(7), 867–903. doi:10.1164/ajrccm.165.7.2105078 PMID:11934711

Chastre, J., Wolff, M., Fagon, J.-Y., Chevret, S., Thomas, F., Wermert, D., & Group, P. T. et al. (2003). Comparison of 8 vs 15 days of antibiotic therapy for ventilator-associated pneumonia in adults: A randomized trial. *Journal of the American Medical Association*, *290*(19), 2588–2598. doi:10.1001/jama.290.19.2588 PMID:14625336

Cheng, D. C., Karski, J., Peniston, C., Raveendran, G., Asokumar, B., Carroll, J., & Sandler, A. et al. (1996). Early tracheal extubation after coronary artery bypass graft surgery reduces costs and improves resource use. A prospective, randomized, controlled trial. *Anesthesiology*, *85*(6), 1300–1310. doi:10.1097/00000542-199612000-00011 PMID:8968177

Chiles, C., Guthaner, D. F., Jamieson, S. W., Stinson, E. B., Oyer, P. E., & Silverman, J. F. (1985). Heart-lung transplantation: The postoperative chest radiograph. *Radiology*, *154*(2), 299–304. doi:10.1148/radiology.154.2.3917571 PMID:3917571

Chiumello, D., Cressoni, M., Carlesso, E., Caspani, M. L., Marino, A., Gallazzi, E., & Gattinoni, L. et al. (2014). Bedside selection of positive end-expiratory pressure in mild, moderate, and severe acute respiratory distress syndrome. *Critical Care Medicine*, *42*(2), 252–264. doi:10.1097/CCM.0b013e3182a6384f PMID:24196193

Confalonieri, M., Garuti, G., Cattaruzza, M. S., Osborn, J. F., Antonelli, M., & Conti, G. et al.. (2005). A chart of failure risk for noninvasive ventilation in patients with COPD exacerbation. *The European Respiratory Journal*, *25*(2), 348–355. doi:10.1183/09031936.05.00085304 PMID:15684302

Cove, M. E., Maclaren, G., Federspiel, W. J., & Kellum, J. A. (2012). Bench to bedside review: Extracorporeal carbon dioxide removal, past present and future. *Critical Care (London, England)*, *16*(5), 232. doi:10.1186/cc11356 PMID:23014710

Cujec, B., Polasek, P., Mayers, I., & Johnson, D. (1993). Positive end-expiratory pressure increases the right-to-left shunt in mechanically ventilated patients with patent foramen ovale. *Annals of Internal Medicine*, *119*(9), 887–894. doi:10.7326/0003-4819-119-9-199311010-00004 PMID:8215000

Dales, R. E., Dionne, G., Leech, J. A., Lunau, M., & Schweitzer, I. (1993). Preoperative prediction of pulmonary complications following thoracic surgery. *Chest Journal*, *104*(1), 155–159. doi:10.1378/chest.104.1.155 PMID:8325061

Dennis, B. M., Eckert, M. J., Gunter, O. L., Morris, J. A., Jr., & May, A. K. (2013). Safety of bedside percutaneous tracheostomy in the critically ill: evaluation of more than 3,000 procedures.*Journal of American College of Surgeons, 216*(4), 858-865; discussion 865-857. doi: 10.1016/j.jamcollsurg.2012.12.017

Dewan, N. A., Gayasaddin, M., Angelillo, V. A., O'Donohue, W. J., & Mohiuddin, S. (1986). Persistent hypoxemia due to patent foramen ovale in a patient with adult respiratory distress syndrome. *Chest Journal*, *89*(4), 611–613. doi:10.1378/chest.89.4.611 PMID:3514169

Dowd, N. P., Cheng, D. C., Karski, J. M., Wong, D. T., Munro, J. A., & Sandler, A. N. (1998). Intraoperative awareness in fast-track cardiac anesthesia. *Anesthesiology, 89*(5), 1068-1073; discussion 1069A.

Eichhorn, E. J., Konstam, M. A., Weiland, D. S., Roberts, D. J., Martin, T. T., Stransky, N. B., & Salem, D. N. (1987). Differential effects of milrinone and dobutamine on right ventricular preload, afterload and systolic performance in congestive heart failure secondary to ischemic or idiopathic dilated cardiomyopathy. *The American Journal of Cardiology*, *60*(16), 1329–1333. doi:10.1016/0002-9149(87)90616-3 PMID:3687783

Force, A. D. T., Ranieri, V. M., Rubenfeld, G. D., Thompson, B. T., Ferguson, N. D., Caldwell, E., & Slutsky, A. S. et al. (2012). Acute respiratory distress syndrome: The Berlin Definition. *Journal of the American Medical Medical Association*, *307*(23), 2526–2533. doi:10.1001/jama.2012.5669 PMID:22797452

Fox, D. L., Stream, A. R., & Bull, T. (2014). Perioperative Management of the Patient With Pulmonary Hypertension. *Seminars in Cardiothoracic and Vascular Anesthesia*, *18*(4), 310–318. doi:10.1177/1089253214534780 PMID:24828282

Fox, R. C., & Swazey, J. P. (2002). The courage to fail: a social view of organ transplants and dialysis (New ed.). New Brunswick, NJ: Transaction Publishers.

Freeman, B. D., & Morris, P. E. (2012). Tracheostomy practice in adults with acute respiratory failure. *Critical Care Medicine*, *40*(10), 2890–2896. doi:10.1097/CCM.0b013e31825bc948 PMID:22824938

Friedrich, A. (2012). Management of common complications following thoracic surgery. In P. M. Hartigan (Ed.), *Practical Handbook of Thoracic Anesthesia* (pp. 291–310). New York: Springer. doi:10.1007/978-0-387-88493-6_17

Fujimoto, K., Kubo, K., Yamamoto, H., Yamaguchi, S., & Matsuzawa, Y. (1999). Eosinophilic inflammation in the airway is related to glucocorticoid reversibility in patients with pulmonary emphysema. *Chest. Journal, 115*(3), 697–702. PMID:10084478

Gilstrap, D., & MacIntyre, N.Implications for Clinical Management. (2013). Patient-ventilator interactions. Implications for clinical management. *American Journal of Respiratory and Critical Care Medicine, 188*(9), 1058–1068. doi:10.1164/rccm.201212-2214CI PMID:24070493

Girard, T. D., Kress, J. P., Fuchs, B. D., Thomason, J. W., Schweickert, W. D., Pun, B. T., & Ely, E. W. et al. (2008). Efficacy and safety of a paired sedation and ventilator weaning protocol for mechanically ventilated patients in intensive care (Awakening and Breathing Controlled trial): A randomised controlled trial. *Lancet, 371*(9607), 126–134. doi:10.1016/S0140-6736(08)60105-1 PMID:18191684

Girou, E., Schortgen, F., Delclaux, C., Brun-Buisson, C., Blot, F., Lefort, Y., & Brochard, L. et al. (2000). Association of noninvasive ventilation with nosocomial infections and survival in critically ill patients. *Journal of the American Medical Association, 284*(18), 2361–2367. doi:10.1001/jama.284.18.2361 PMID:11066187

Glenny, R. W., Lamm, W. J., Bernard, S. L., An, D., Chornuk, M., Pool, S. L., . . . Robertson, H. T. (2000). Selected contribution: redistribution of pulmonary perfusion during weightlessness and increased gravity. *Journal of Applied Physiology (1985), 89*(3), 1239-1248.

Group, I. D. a. C. I. S. (2013). *Awakening and Breathing Coordination*. Retrieved June 5, 2014, from http://www.icudelirium.org/medicalprofessionals.html

Guerin, C., Reignier, J., Richard, J. C., Beuret, P., Gacouin, A., Boulain, T., . . . Group, P. S. (2013). Prone positioning in severe acute respiratory distress syndrome. *N Engl J Med, 368*(23), 2159-2168.

Hakim, T. S., Lisbona, R., & Dean, G. W. (1987). Gravity-independent inequality in pulmonary blood flow in humans. *Journal of Applied Physiology (1985), 63*(3), 1114-1121.

Han, M. K., McLaughlin, V. V., Criner, G. J., & Martinez, F. J. (2007). Pulmonary diseases and the heart. *Circulation, 116*(25), 2992–3005. doi:10.1161/CIRCULATIONAHA.106.685206 PMID:18086941

Hasan, A. (2010). *Understanding Mechanical Ventilation: A Practical Handbook* (2nd ed.). Dordrecht: Springer. doi:10.1007/978-1-84882-869-8

Haynes, D., & Baumann, M. H. (2010). Management of pneumothorax. *Seminars in Respiratory and Critical Care Medicine, 31*(6), 769–780. doi:10.1055/s-0030-1269837 PMID:21213209

Hedenstierna, G., Tokics, L., Strandberg, A., Lundquist, H., & Brismar, B. (1986). Correlation of gas exchange impairment to development of atelectasis during anaesthesia and muscle paralysis. *Acta Anaesthesiologica Scandinavica, 30*(2), 183–191. doi:10.1111/j.1399-6576.1986.tb02393.x PMID:3085429

Henderson, W. R., Griesdale, D. E., Walley, K. R., & Sheel, A. W. (2010). Clinical review: Guyton--the role of mean circulatory filling pressure and right atrial pressure in controlling cardiac output. *Critical Care (London, England), 14*(6), 243. doi:10.1186/cc9247 PMID:21144008

Hess, D. R., & Fessler, H. E. (2007). Respiratory controversies in the critical care setting. Should noninvasive positive-pressure ventilation be used in all forms of acute respiratory failure? *Respiratory Care*, *52*(5), 568–578, discussion 578–581. PMID:17484789

Hess, D. R., & MacIntyre, N. R. (2011). Ventilator discontinuation: Why are we still weaning? *American Journal of Respiratory and Critical Care Medicine*, *184*(4), 392–394. doi:10.1164/rccm.201105-0894ED PMID:21844511

Hill, N. (2013). Noninvasive Positive-Pressure Ventilation. In M. J. Tobin (Ed.), *Principles and practice of mechanical ventilation* (3rd ed.). New York: McGraw-Hill Medical.

Hoeper, M. M., Bogaard, H. J., Condliffe, R., Frantz, R., Khanna, D., Kurzyna, M., & Badesch, D. B. et al. (2013). Definitions and diagnosis of pulmonary hypertension. *Journal of the American College of Cardiology*, *62*(25Suppl), D42–D50. doi:10.1016/j.jacc.2013.10.032 PMID:24355641

Hortal, J., Giannella, M., Perez, M. J., Barrio, J. M., Desco, M., Bouza, E., & Munoz, P. (2009). Incidence and risk factors for ventilator-associated pneumonia after major heart surgery. *Intensive Care Medicine*, *35*(9), 1518–1525. doi:10.1007/s00134-009-1523-3 PMID:19557389

Jaeger, J. M., & Blank, R. S. (2011). Essential Anatomy and Physiology of the Respiratory System and the Pulmonary Circulation. In P. D. Slinger (Ed.), *Principles and Practice of Anesthesia for Thoracic Surgery* (pp. 51–69). New York: Springer. doi:10.1007/978-1-4419-0184-2_4

Jordan, S., Mitchell, J. A., Quinlan, G. J., Goldstraw, P., & Evans, T. W. (2000). The pathogenesis of lung injury following pulmonary resection. *The European Respiratory Journal*, *15*(4), 790–799. doi:10.1034/j.1399-3003.2000.15d26.x PMID:10780775

Judson, M. A., Handy, J. R., & Sahn, S. A. (1996). Pleural effusions following lung transplantation. Time course, characteristics, and clinical implications. *Chest Journal*, *109*(5), 1190–1194. doi:10.1378/chest.109.5.1190 PMID:8625665

Judson, M. A., Handy, J. R., & Sahn, S. A. (1997). Pleural effusion from acute lung rejection. *Chest Journal*, *111*(4), 1128–1130. doi:10.1378/chest.111.4.1128 PMID:9106602

Kato, R., Sato, J., & Nishino, T. (1998). Milrinone decreases both pulmonary arterial and venous resistances in the hypoxic dog. *British Journal of Anaesthesia*, *81*(6), 920–924. doi:10.1093/bja/81.6.920 PMID:10211020

Kaw, R., Pasupuleti, V., Deshpande, A., Hamieh, T., Walker, E., & Minai, O. A. (2011). Pulmonary hypertension: An important predictor of outcomes in patients undergoing non-cardiac surgery. *Respiratory Medicine*, *105*(4), 619–624. doi:10.1016/j.rmed.2010.12.006 PMID:21195595

Kelly, A. M., Weldon, D., Tsang, A. Y., & Graham, C. A. (2006). Comparison between two methods for estimating pneumothorax size from chest X-rays. *Respiratory Medicine*, *100*(8), 1356–1359. doi:10.1016/j.rmed.2005.11.022 PMID:16406560

Kiely, D. G., Cargill, R. I., & Lipworth, B. J. (1996). Angiotensin II receptor blockade and effects on pulmonary hemodynamics and hypoxic pulmonary vasoconstriction in humans. *Chest Journal*, *110*(3), 698–703. doi:10.1378/chest.110.3.698 PMID:8797414

Kihara, S., Kawai, A., Fukuda, T., Yamamoto, N., Aomi, S., Nishida, H., & Koyanagi, H. et al. (2002). Effects of milrinone for right ventricular failure after left ventricular assist device implantation. *Heart and Vessels*, *16*(2), 69–71. doi:10.1007/s380-002-8320-z PMID:11833845

Kitsios, G. D., Mascari, P., Ettunsi, R., & Gray, A. W. (2014). Co-administration of furosemide with albumin for overcoming diuretic resistance in patients with hypoalbuminemia: A meta-analysis. *Journal of Critical Care*, *29*(2), 253–259. doi:10.1016/j.jcrc.2013.10.004 PMID:24268626

Kollef, M. H. (1999). Epidemiology and risk factors for nosocomial pneumonia. Emphasis on prevention. *Clinics in Chest Medicine*, *20*(3), 653–670. doi:10.1016/S0272-5231(05)70242-2 PMID:10516910

Kramer, N., Meyer, T. J., Meharg, J., Cece, R. D., & Hill, N. S. (1995). Randomized, prospective trial of noninvasive positive pressure ventilation in acute respiratory failure. *American Journal of Respiratory and Critical Care Medicine*, *151*(6), 1799–1806. doi:10.1164/ajrccm.151.6.7767523 PMID:7767523

Kroenke, K., Lawrence, V. A., Theroux, J. F., Tuley, M. R., & Hilsenbeck, S. (1993). Postoperative complications after thoracic and major abdominal surgery in patients with and without obstructive lung disease. *Chest Journal*, *104*(5), 1445–1451. doi:10.1378/chest.104.5.1445 PMID:8222804

Kwak, Y. L., Lee, C. S., Park, Y. H., & Hong, Y. W. (2002). The effect of phenylephrine and norepinephrine in patients with chronic pulmonary hypertension*. *Anaesthesia*, *57*(1), 9–14. doi:10.1046/j.1365-2044.2002.02324.x PMID:11843735

Kwok, H., McCormack, J., Cece, R., Houtchens, J., & Hill, N. S. (2003). Controlled trial of oronasal versus nasal mask ventilation in the treatment of acute respiratory failure. *Critical Care Medicine*, *31*(2), 468–473. doi:10.1097/01.CCM.0000045563.64187.20 PMID:12576953

Laffey, J. G., Boylan, J. F., & Cheng, D. C. (2002). The systemic inflammatory response to cardiac surgery: Implications for the anesthesiologist. *Anesthesiology*, *97*(1), 215–252. doi:10.1097/00000542-200207000-00030 PMID:12131125

Lawrence, V. A., Hilsenbeck, S. G., Mulrow, C. D., Dhanda, R., Sapp, J., & Page, C. P. (1995). Incidence and hospital stay for cardiac and pulmonary complications after abdominal surgery. *Journal of General Internal Medicine*, *10*(12), 671–678. doi:10.1007/BF02602761 PMID:8770719

Light, R. W., Rogers, J. T., Moyers, J. P., Lee, Y. C., Rodriguez, R. M., Alford, W. C. Jr, & Tedder, M. et al. (2002). Prevalence and clinical course of pleural effusions at 30 days after coronary artery and cardiac surgery. *American Journal of Respiratory and Critical Care Medicine*, *166*(12 Pt 1), 1567–1571. doi:10.1164/rccm.200203-184OC PMID:12406850

Lumb, A. B., & Nunn, J. F. (2005). *Nunn's applied respiratory physiology* (6th ed.). Edinburgh, Philadelphia: Elsevier Butterworth Heinemann.

Lundquist, H., Hedenstierna, G., Strandberg, A., Tokics, L., & Brismar, B. (1995). CT-assessment of dependent lung densities in man during general anaesthesia. *Acta Radiologica*, *36*(6), 626–632. doi:10.3109/02841859509176761 PMID:8519574

Luyt, C.-E., Chastre, J., & Fagon, J.-Y. (2004). Value of the clinical pulmonary infection score for the identification and management of ventilator-associated pneumonia. *Intensive Care Medicine*, *30*(5), 844–852. doi:10.1007/s00134-003-2125-0 PMID:15127196

Magill, S. S., Klompas, M., Balk, R., Burns, S. M., Deutschman, C. S., Diekema, D., & Lipsett, P. et al. (2013). Developing a new, national approach to surveillance for ventilator-associated events. *American Journal of Critical Care*, *22*(6), 469–473. doi:10.4037/ajcc2013893 PMID:24186816

Magnusson, L., & Spahn, D. R. (2003). New concepts of atelectasis during general anaesthesia. *British Journal of Anaesthesia*, *91*(1), 61–72. doi:10.1093/bja/aeg085 PMID:12821566

Marik, P. E., Cavallazzi, R., Vasu, T., & Hirani, A. (2009). Dynamic changes in arterial waveform derived variables and fluid responsiveness in mechanically ventilated patients: A systematic review of the literature. *Critical Care Medicine*, *37*(9), 2642–2647. doi:10.1097/CCM.0b013e3181a590da PMID:19602972

Martin, D. S., & Grocott, M. P. (2013). Oxygen therapy in critical illness: Precise control of arterial oxygenation and permissive hypoxemia. *Critical Care Medicine*, *41*(2), 423–432. doi:10.1097/CCM.0b013e31826a44f6 PMID:23263574

McCrory, D. C., Brown, C., Gelfand, S. E., & Bach, P. B. (2001). Management of acute exacerbations of COPD: A summary and appraisal of published evidence. *Chest Journal*, *119*(4), 1190–1209. doi:10.1378/chest.119.4.1190 PMID:11296189

McCrory, D. C., & Brown, C. D. (2002). Anti-cholinergic bronchodilators versus beta2-sympathomimetic agents for acute exacerbations of chronic obstructive pulmonary disease. *Cochrane Database of Systematic Reviews*, (4): CD003900. doi:10.1002/14651858.CD003900 PMID:12519615

McGuinness, S., & Sidebotham, D. (2007). Specific Causes of Respiratory Failure. In D. Sidebotham, A. McKee, M. Gillham, & J. H. Levy (Eds.), *Cardiothoracic Critical Care*. Philadelphia: Butterworth Heinemann Elsevier. doi:10.1016/B978-075067572-7.50030-8

Meade, M., Guyatt, G., Cook, D., Griffith, L., Sinuff, T., Kergl, C., & Epstein, S. et al. (2001). Predicting success in weaning from mechanical ventilation. *Chest Journal*, *120*(6Suppl), 400S–424S. doi:10.1378/chest.120.6_suppl.400S PMID:11742961

Medicine, S. C. C. (2013). *Guidelines*. Retrieved June 5, 2014, from http://www.iculiberation.org/Guidelines/Pages/default.aspx

Mehta, S., & Hill, N. S. (2001). Noninvasive ventilation. *American Journal of Respiratory and Critical Care Medicine*, *163*(2), 540–577. doi:10.1164/ajrccm.163.2.9906116 PMID:11179136

Messent, M., Sullivan, K., Keogh, B. F., Morgan, C. J., & Evans, T. W. (1992). Adult respiratory distress syndrome following cardiopulmonary bypass: Incidence and prediction. *Anaesthesia*, *47*(3), 267–268. doi:10.1111/j.1365-2044.1992.tb02134.x PMID:1566999

Meyer, T., & Krishnamani, R. (2010). Acute heart failure and pulmonary edema. In A. Jeremias & D. L. Brown (Eds.), *Cardiac Intensive Care* (pp. 291–308). Philadelphia: Saunders. doi:10.1016/B978-1-4160-3773-6.10024-2

Micek, S. T., Ward, S., Fraser, V. J., & Kollef, M. H. (2004). A randomized controlled trial of an antibiotic discontinuation policy for clinically suspected ventilator-associated pneumonia. *Chest Journal*, *125*(5), 1791–1799. doi:10.1378/chest.125.5.1791 PMID:15136392

Milgrom, L. B., Brooks, J. A., Qi, R., Bunnell, K., Wuestfeld, S., & Beckman, D. (2004). Pain levels experienced with activities after cardiac surgery. *American Journal of Critical Care*, *13*(2), 116–125. PMID:15043239

Minai, O. A., Yared, J. P., Kaw, R., Subramaniam, K., & Hill, N. S. (2013). Perioperative risk and management in patients with pulmonary hypertension. *Chest Journal*, *144*(1), 329–340. doi:10.1378/chest.12-1752 PMID:23880683

Myles, P. S., & McIlroy, D. (2005). Fast-track cardiac anesthesia: Choice of anesthetic agents and techniques. *Seminars in Cardiothoracic and Vascular Anesthesia*, *9*(1), 5–16. doi:10.1177/108925320500900102 PMID:15735840

Nakahara, K., Ohno, K., Hashimoto, J., Miyoshi, S., Maeda, H., Matsumura, A., & Kawashima, Y. et al. (1988). Prediction of postoperative respiratory failure in patients undergoing lung resection for lung cancer. *The Annals of Thoracic Surgery*, *46*(5), 549–552. doi:10.1016/S0003-4975(10)64694-2 PMID:3190329

National Heart. (2006). Comparison of two fluid-management strategies in acute lung injury. *The New England Journal of Medicine*, *354*(24), 2564–2575. doi:10.1056/NEJMoa062200 PMID:16714767

Network, T. A. R. D. S. (2000). Ventilation with lower tidal volumes as compared with traditional tidal volumes for acute lung injury and the acute respiratory distress syndrome. The Acute Respiratory Distress Syndrome Network. *The New England Journal of Medicine*, *342*(18), 1301–1308. doi:10.1056/NEJM200005043421801 PMID:10793162

Noppen, M., & De Keukeleire, T. (2008). Pneumothorax. *Respiration*, *76*(2), 121–127. doi:10.1159/000135932 PMID:18708734

Nourdine, K., Combes, P., Carton, M. J., Beuret, P., Cannamela, A., & Ducreux, J. C. (1999). Does non-invasive ventilation reduce the ICU nosocomial infection risk? A prospective clinical survey. *Intensive Care Medicine*, *25*(6), 567–573. doi:10.1007/s001340050904 PMID:10416907

O'Croinin, D., Ni Chonghaile, M., Higgins, B., & Laffey, J. G. (2005). Bench-to-bedside review: Permissive hypercapnia. *Critical Care (London, England)*, *9*(1), 51–59. doi:10.1186/cc2918 PMID:15693984

Papazian, L., Forel, J. M., Gacouin, A., Penot-Ragon, C., Perrin, G., Loundou, A., & Investigators, A. S. et al. (2010). Neuromuscular blockers in early acute respiratory distress syndrome. *The New England Journal of Medicine*, *363*(12), 1107–1116. doi:10.1056/NEJMoa1005372 PMID:20843245

Papazian, L., Thomas, P., Garbe, L., Guignon, I., Thirion, X., Charrel, J., & Gouin, F. et al. (1995). Bronchoscopic or blind sampling techniques for the diagnosis of ventilator-associated pneumonia. *American Journal of Respiratory and Critical Care Medicine*, *152*(6 Pt 1), 1982–1991. doi:10.1164/ajrccm.152.6.8520766 PMID:8520766

Pinhu, L., Whitehead, T., Evans, T., & Griffiths, M. (2003). Ventilator-associated lung injury. *Lancet*, *361*(9354), 332–340. doi:10.1016/S0140-6736(03)12329-X PMID:12559881

Pugin, J., Auckenthaler, R., Mili, N., Janssens, J. P., Lew, P. D., & Suter, P. M. (1991). Diagnosis of ventilator-associated pneumonia by bacteriologic analysis of bronchoscopic and nonbronchoscopic "blind" bronchoalveolar lavage fluid. *The American Review of Respiratory Disease*, *143*(5 Pt 1), 1121–1129. doi:10.1164/ajrccm/143.5_Pt_1.1121 PMID:2024824

Ramsay, J., & Finley, A. (2011). Postoperative Respiratory Failure and Treatment. In P. D. Slinger (Ed.), *Principles and Practice of Anesthesia for Thoracic Surgery* (pp. 609–633). New York: Springer. doi:10.1007/978-1-4419-0184-2_42

Raoof, S., Baumann, M. H., & Collaborative, C. C. S. (2014). An official multi-society statement: ventilator-associated events: the new definition. *Critical Care Medicine*, *42*(1), 228–229. doi:10.1097/CCM.0000000000000191 PMID:24346542

Reich, D. L., Bodian, C. A., Krol, M., Kuroda, M., Osinski, T., & Thys, D. M. (1999). Intraoperative hemodynamic predictors of mortality, stroke, and myocardial infarction after coronary artery bypass surgery. *Anesthesia and Analgesia*, *89*(4), 814–822. PMID:10512249

Reichenberger, F., Kohstall, M. G., Seeger, T., Olschewski, H., Grimminger, F., Seeger, W., & Ghofrani, H. A. (2007). Effect of sildenafil on hypoxia-induced changes in pulmonary circulation and right ventricular function. *Respiratory Physiology & Neurobiology*, *159*(2), 196–201. doi:10.1016/j.resp.2007.07.005 PMID:17851140

Reid, C. W., Slinger, P. D., & Lenis, S. (1996). A comparison of the effects of propofol-alfentanil versus isoflurane anesthesia on arterial oxygenation during one-lung ventilation. *Journal of Cardiothoracic and Vascular Anesthesia*, *10*(7), 860–863. doi:10.1016/S1053-0770(96)80046-2 PMID:8969391

Restrepo, R. D. (2009). A stepwise approach to management of stable COPD with inhaled pharmacotherapy: A review. *Respiratory Care*, *54*(8), 1058–1081. PMID:19650947

Roques, F., Nashef, S. A., Michel, P., Gauducheau, E., de Vincentiis, C., Baudet, E., . . . Thulin, L. (1999). Risk factors and outcome in European cardiac surgery: analysis of the EuroSCORE multinational database of 19030 patients. *European Journal of Cardiothoracic Surgery, 15*(6), 816-822; discussion 822-813.

Schmidt, M., Bailey, M., Sheldrake, J., Hodgson, C., Aubron, C., Rycus, P. T., & Pilcher, D. et al. (2014). Predicting Survival after Extracorporeal Membrane Oxygenation for Severe Acute Respiratory Failure. The Respiratory Extracorporeal Membrane Oxygenation Survival Prediction (RESP) Score. *American Journal of Respiratory and Critical Care Medicine*, *189*(11), 1374–1382. doi:10.1164/rccm.201311-2023OC PMID:24693864

Schweickert, W. D., Pohlman, M. C., Pohlman, A. S., Nigos, C., Pawlik, A. J., Esbrook, C. L., & Kress, J. P. et al. (2009). Early physical and occupational therapy in mechanically ventilated, critically ill patients: A randomised controlled trial. *Lancet*, *373*(9678), 1874–1882. doi:10.1016/S0140-6736(09)60658-9 PMID:19446324

Shroyer, A. L., Coombs, L. P., Peterson, E. D., Eiken, M. C., DeLong, E. R., Chen, A., . . . Edwards, F. H. (2003). The Society of Thoracic Surgeons: 30-day operative mortality and morbidity risk models. *Annals of Thoracic Surgery, 75*(6), 1856-1864; discussion 1864-1855.

Simonneau, G., Gatzoulis, M. A., Adatia, I., Celermajer, D., Denton, C., Ghofrani, A., & Souza, R. et al. (2013). Updated clinical classification of pulmonary hypertension. *Journal of the American College of Cardiology*, *62*(25Suppl), D34–D41. doi:10.1016/j.jacc.2013.10.029 PMID:24355639

Sirbu, H., Busch, T., Aleksic, I., Lotfi, S., Ruschewski, W., & Dalichau, H. (1999). Chest re-exploration for complications after lung surgery. *The Thoracic and Cardiovascular Surgeon*, *47*(2), 73–76. doi:10.1055/s-2007-1013114 PMID:10363604

Slutsky, A. S., & Ranieri, V. M. (2013). Ventilator-induced lung injury. *The New England Journal of Medicine*, *369*(22), 2126–2136. doi:10.1056/NEJMra1208707 PMID:24283226

Smith, A. M., Elliot, C. M., Kiely, D. G., & Channer, K. S. (2006). The role of vasopressin in cardiorespiratory arrest and pulmonary hypertension. *Open Journal of Medicine*, *99*(3), 127–133. doi:10.1093/qjmed/hcl009 PMID:16467356

Staub, N. C., Nagano, H., & Pearce, M. L. (1967). Pulmonary edema in dogs, especially the sequence of fluid accumulation in lungs. *Journal of Applied Physiology*, *22*(2), 227–240. PMID:6017888

Stewart, N. I., Jagelman, T. A., & Webster, N. R. (2011). Emerging modes of ventilation in the intensive care unit. *British Journal of Anaesthesia*, *107*(1), 74–82. doi:10.1093/bja/aer114 PMID:21613281

Strange, C. (1999). Pleural complications in the intensive care unit. *Clinics in Chest Medicine*, *20*(2), 317–327. doi:10.1016/S0272-5231(05)70144-1 PMID:10386259

Strom, T., Martinussen, T., & Toft, P. (2010). A protocol of no sedation for critically ill patients receiving mechanical ventilation: A randomised trial. *Lancet*, *375*(9713), 475–480. doi:10.1016/S0140-6736(09)62072-9 PMID:20116842

Sutherland, E. R., & Martin, R. J. (2003). Airway inflammation in chronic obstructive pulmonary disease: Comparisons with asthma. *The Journal of Allergy and Clinical Immunology*, *112*(5), 819–827, quiz 828. doi:10.1016/S0091-6749(03)02011-6 PMID:14610463

Talmor, D., Sarge, T., Malhotra, A., O'Donnell, C. R., Ritz, R., Lisbon, A., & Loring, S. H. et al. (2008). Mechanical ventilation guided by esophageal pressure in acute lung injury. *The New England Journal of Medicine*, *359*(20), 2095–2104. doi:10.1056/NEJMoa0708638 PMID:19001507

Tarhan, S., Moffitt, E. A., Sessler, A. D., Douglas, W. W., & Taylor, W. F. (1973). Risk of anesthesia and surgery in patients with chronic bronchitis and chronic obstructive pulmonary disease. *Surgery*, *74*(5), 720–726. PMID:4742756

Terragni, P. P., Antonelli, M., Fumagalli, R., Faggiano, C., Berardino, M., Pallavicini, F. B., & Ranieri, V. M. et al. (2010). Early vs late tracheotomy for prevention of pneumonia in mechanically ventilated adult ICU patients: A randomized controlled trial. *Journal of the American Medical Association*, *303*(15), 1483–1489. doi:10.1001/jama.2010.447 PMID:20407057

Tobin, M. J. (2001). Advances in mechanical ventilation. *The New England Journal of Medicine*, *344*(26), 1986–1996. doi:10.1056/NEJM200106283442606 PMID:11430329

Wagnetz, D., & de Perrot, M. (2011). Postthoracotomy surgical management and complications. In P. D. Slinger (Ed.), *Principles and Practice of Anesthesia for Thoracic Surgery* (pp. 661–673). New York: Springer. doi:10.1007/978-1-4419-0184-2_45

Wang, H., Gong, M., Zhou, B., & Dai, A. (2009). Comparison of inhaled and intravenous milrinone in patients with pulmonary hypertension undergoing mitral valve surgery. *Advances in Therapy*, *26*(4), 462–468. doi:10.1007/s12325-009-0019-4 PMID:19381522

Weissmann, N., Gerigk, B., Kocer, O., Nollen, M., Hackemack, S., Ghofrani, H. A., & Grimminger, F. et al. (2007). Hypoxia-induced pulmonary hypertension: Different impact of iloprost, sildenafil, and nitric oxide. *Respiratory Medicine*, *101*(10), 2125–2132. doi:10.1016/j.rmed.2007.05.025 PMID:17643279

West, J. B. (2012). *Respiratory physiology: the essentials* (9th ed.). Philadelphia: Wolters Kluwer Health/ Lippincott Williams & Wilkins.

Woods, J. A., Wheeler, J. S., Finch, C. K., & Pinner, N. A. (2014). Corticosteroids in the treatment of acute exacerbations of chronic obstructive pulmonary disease. *International Journal of Chronic Obstructive Pulmonary Disease*, *9*, 421–430. doi:10.2147/COPD.S51012 PMID:24833897

Yang, K. L., & Tobin, M. J. (1991). A prospective study of indexes predicting the outcome of trials of weaning from mechanical ventilation. *The New England Journal of Medicine*, *324*(21), 1445–1450. doi:10.1056/NEJM199105233242101 PMID:2023603

Yarmus, L., & Feller-Kopman, D. (2012). Pneumothorax in the critically ill patient. *Chest Journal*, *141*(4), 1098–1105. doi:10.1378/chest.11-1691 PMID:22474153

Yorke, J., Wallis, M., & McLean, B. (2004). Patients' perceptions of pain management after cardiac surgery in an Australian critical care unit. *Heart and Lung: The Journal of Acute and Critical Care*, *33*(1), 33–41. doi:10.1016/j.hrtlng.2003.09.002 PMID:14983137

Young, D., Harrison, D. A., Cuthbertson, B. H., Rowan, K., & TracMan Collaborators, . (2013). Effect of early vs late tracheostomy placement on survival in patients receiving mechanical ventilation: The TracMan randomized trial. *Journal of the American Medical Association*, *309*(20), 2121–2129. doi:10.1001/jama.2013.5154 PMID:23695482

Zhu, F., Lee, A., & Chee, Y. E. (2012). Fast-track cardiac care for adult cardiac surgical patients. *Cochrane Database of Systematic Reviews*, *10*, Cd003587. doi:10.1002/14651858.CD003587.pub2 PMID:23076899

ADDITIONAL READING

Akoumianaki, E., Maggiore, S. M., Valenza, F., Bellani, G., Jubran, A., Loring, S. H., & Brochard, L. et al. (2014). The application of esophageal pressure measurement in patients with respiratory failure. *American Journal of Critical Care Medicine*, *189*(5), 520–531. doi:10.1164/rccm.201312-2193CI PMID:24467647

Barr, J., Fraser, G. L., Puntillo, K., Ely, E. W., Gelinas, C., Dasta, J. F., & Jaeschke, R. et al. (2013). Clinical practice guidelines for the management of pain, agitation, and delirium in adult patients in the intensive care unit. *Critical Care Medicine*, *41*(1), 263–306. doi:10.1097/CCM.0b013e3182783b72 PMID:23269131

Buckley, D., & Gillham, M. (2007). Invasive Respiratory Support. In D. Sidebotham, A. McKee, M. Gillham, & J. H. Levy (Eds.), *Cardiothoracic Critical Care*. Philadelphia: Butterworth Heinemann Elsevier. doi:10.1016/B978-075067572-7.50032-1

Gilstrap, D., & MacIntyre, N. Implications for Clinical Management. (2013). Patient-ventilator interactions. Implications for clinical management. *American Journal of Respiratory and Critical Care Medicine*, *188*(9), 1058–1068. doi:10.1164/rccm.201212-2214CI PMID:24070493

Guerin, C., Reignier, J., Richard, J. C., Beuret, P., Gacouin, A., Boulain, T., & Group, P. S. et al. (2013). Prone positioning in severe acute respiratory distress syndrome. *The New England Journal of Medicine*, *368*(23), 2159–2168. doi:10.1056/NEJMoa1214103 PMID:23688302

Hasan, A. (2010). *Understanding Mechanical Ventilation: A Practical Handbook* (2nd ed.). Dordrecht: Springer. doi:10.1007/978-1-84882-869-8

Henderson, W. R., Griesdale, D. E., Walley, K. R., & Sheel, A. W. (2010). Clinical review: Guyton--the role of mean circulatory filling pressure and right atrial pressure in controlling cardiac output. *Critical Care (London, England)*, *14*(6), 243. doi:10.1186/cc9247 PMID:21144008

Hess, D. R., & Fessler, H. E. (2007). Respiratory controversies in the critical care setting. Should noninvasive positive-pressure ventilation be used in all forms of acute respiratory failure? *Respiratory Care*, *52*(5), 568–578, discussion 578–581. PMID:17484789

Hill, N. (2013). Noninvasive Positive-Pressure Ventilation. In M. J. Tobin (Ed.), *Principles and practice of mechanical ventilation* (3rd ed.). New York: McGraw-Hill Medical.

Jaeger, J. M., & Blank, R. S. (2011). Essential Anatomy and Physiology of the Respiratory System and the Pulmonary Circulation. In P. D. Slinger (Ed.), *Principles and Practice of Anesthesia for Thoracic Surgery* (pp. 51–69). New York: Springer. doi:10.1007/978-1-4419-0184-2_4

Kutlu, C. A., Williams, E. A., Evans, T. W., Pastorino, U., & Goldstraw, P. (2000). Acute lung injury and acute respiratory distress syndrome after pulmonary resection. *The Annals of Thoracic Surgery*, *69*(2), 376–380. doi:10.1016/S0003-4975(99)01090-5 PMID:10735666

Laffey, J. G., Boylan, J. F., & Cheng, D. C. (2002). The systemic inflammatory response to cardiac surgery: Implications for the anesthesiologist. *Anesthesiology*, *97*(1), 215–252. doi:10.1097/00000542-200207000-00030 PMID:12131125

Lumb, A. B., & Nunn, J. F. (2005). *Nunn's applied respiratory physiology* (6th ed.). Edinburgh, Philadelphia: Elsevier Butterworth Heinemann.

Martin, D. S., & Grocott, M. P. (2013). Oxygen therapy in critical illness: Precise control of arterial oxygenation and permissive hypoxemia. *Critical Care Medicine*, *41*(2), 423–432. doi:10.1097/CCM.0b013e31826a44f6 PMID:23263574

Meyer, T., & Krishnamani, R. (2010). Acute heart failure and pulmonary edema. In A. Jeremias & D. L. Brown (Eds.), *Cardiac Intensive Care* (pp. 291–308). Philadelphia: Saunders. doi:10.1016/B978-1-4160-3773-6.10024-2

Minai, O. A., Yared, J. P., Kaw, R., Subramaniam, K., & Hill, N. S. (2013). Perioperative risk and management in patients with pulmonary hypertension. *Chest Journal*, *144*(1), 329–340. doi:10.1378/chest.12-1752 PMID:23880683

Myles, P. S., & McIlroy, D. (2005). Fast-track cardiac anesthesia: Choice of anesthetic agents and techniques. *Seminars in Cardiothoracic and Vascular Anesthesia*, *9*(1), 5–16. doi:10.1177/108925320500900102 PMID:15735840

Simonneau, G., Gatzoulis, M. A., Adatia, I., Celermajer, D., Denton, C., Ghofrani, A., & Souza, R. et al. (2013). Updated clinical classification of pulmonary hypertension. *Journal of the American College of Cardiology*, *62*(25Suppl), D34–D41. doi:10.1016/j.jacc.2013.10.029 PMID:24355639

Slutsky, A. S., & Ranieri, V. M. (2013). Ventilator-induced lung injury. *The New England Journal of Medicine*, *369*(22), 2126–2136. doi:10.1056/NEJMra1208707 PMID:24283226

The Acute Respiratory Distress Syndrome Network. (2000). Ventilation with lower tidal volumes as compared with traditional tidal volumes for acute lung injury and the acute respiratory distress syndrome. The Acute Respiratory Distress Syndrome Network. *The New England Journal of Medicine*, *342*(18), 1301–1308. doi:10.1056/NEJM200005043421801 PMID:10793162

Wagnetz, D., & De Perrot, M. (2011). Postthoracotomy surgical management and complications. In P. D. Slinger (Ed.), *Principles and Practice of Anesthesia for Thoracic Surgery* (pp. 661–673). New York: Springer. doi:10.1007/978-1-4419-0184-2_45

West, J. B. (2012). *Respiratory physiology: the essentials* (9th ed.). Philadelphia: Wolters Kluwer Health/Lippincott Williams & Wilkins. Mechanical Ventilation.

Zhu, F., Lee, A., & Chee, Y. E. (2012). Fast-track cardiac care for adult cardiac surgical patients. *Cochrane Database of Systematic Reviews*, *10*, Cd003587. doi:10.1002/14651858.CD003587.pub2 PMID:23076899

KEY TERMS AND DEFINITIONS

Acute Respiratory Distress Syndrome (ARDS): A syndrome of lung injury from multiple etiologies characterized by hypoxemia of varying degrees quantified by the PaO2/ FiO2 ratio. This syndrome develops within one week of a known clinical insult with new or worsening respiratory symptoms not explained by fluid overload or cardiac failure. The current definition requires bilateral opacities that are not fully explained by effusions, lobar collapse or nodules.

Acute Respiratory Failure: The acute inability to maintain normal blood gas partial pressures of oxygen and/or carbon dioxide. Acute Respiratory Failure is caused by ventilatory failure (failure to maintain normal alveolar gas partial pressure) or venous admixture due to a spectrum of ventilation and perfusion mismatch.

Compliance: A quantification of the change in volume caused by a given change in pressure. In mechanically ventilated patients, "Dynamic Compliance" is measured while airflow is present and is calculated as Cdyn=Vt/(Ppeak-PEEP). Static compliance (Cstat=Vt/(Pplateau-PEEP) is measured after inspiration has ended and when airflow has terminated. Dynamic Compliance is decreased with increased airflow resistance whereas Static Compliance is not affected.

Dead Space: Variously refers to lung regions of pure dead space (V/Q= infinity, i.e. ventilation without perfusion), areas with high V/Q ratios, and the solution to the dead space equation.

Positive End Expiratory Pressure (PEEP): The pressure in alveoli above atmospheric pressure at end expiration. Extrinsic PEEP is delivered by a mechanical ventilator and by convention is referred to as Continuous Positive Airway Pressure (CPAP) in non-intubated patients. Intrinsic or "Auto" PEEP occurs because of incomplete expiration due to obstructive lung pathology and "air trapping".

Pulmonary Vascular Resistance (PVR): The resistance that must be overcome by the right ventricle to create forward flow in the pulmonary vasculature. Calculated as the difference between mean PA pressure and LAP divided by the cardiac output.

Shunt: Variously refers to lung regions of pure shunt where V/Q=0 (i.e., perfusion without ventilation), areas of very low V/Q ratios, and to the solution to the shunt equation for venous admixture.

Spontaneous Awakening Trial (SAT): The first step in ventilator liberation where sedatives are stopped but active analgesics are maintained. The goal of the SAT is to determine the patient's appropriateness for a Spontaneous Breathing Trial, and usually requires that the patient opens their eyes to verbal stimulus and tolerates the interruption of sedation for a sustained period without exhibiting signs of sustained agitation, tachypnea, desaturation, dysrhythmia or respiratory distress.

Spontaneous Breathing Trial (SBT): A trial of spontaneous ventilation following a successful Spontaneous Awakening Trial to evaluate the patient's appropriateness for ventilator liberation. The intensivist should assess for the adequacy of gas exchange, respiratory mechanics, and hemodynamic stability. In addition, prior to extubation, consideration should be given to the degree of patient comfort, the predicted ability for the patient to protect their airway after extubation, and the difficulty of re-securing the airway should the patient require re-intubation. An SBT should be conducted daily in intubated patients.

Transpulmonary Pressure: The pressure across the lung parenchyma (also referred to as transmural pressure) and defined as alveolar pressure, the pressure inside the lung, minus pleural pressure. During mechanical ventilation the change in pleural pressure required for a given volume change is dominated by chest wall mechanics and is positive during lung inflation. Unlike pleural pressure, the change in transpulmonary pressure across the lung required for a given volume change is the same during both spontaneous and mechanical ventilation.

Chapter 16
Cardiovascular System

Wolf Benjamin Kratzert
UCLA, USA

Eva Katherine Boyd
UCLA, USA

ABSTRACT

This chapter addresses underlying physiology, diagnostics, and management of common cardiovascular abnormalities in the patient after cardiac surgery. The goal is to provide insights into daily management, areas of controversy, and future directions in the field. After reviewing basic physiologic principles of cardiac output and circulation; problems affecting the postoperative hemodynamic state will be addressed individually. Specific topics include the low cardiac output syndrome, right ventricular failure, myocardial ischemia, diastolic dysfunction, vasodilatory syndrome, rhythm disturbances, pericardial tamponade, and cardiac arrest. Patients with postoperative open chests, or after orthotopic heart transplantation are also discussed.

INTRODUCTION

Postoperative care of the patient undergoing cardiac surgery presents with unique challenges in the field of critical care medicine. Management of the cardiovascular system plays an essential role, as it addresses the fundamental pathophysiologic state of these patients. Abnormalities in hemodynamics often lead to malfunction of other organs such as the central nervous system, lungs, liver, and kidneys, and achievement of adequate cardiovascular performance is key to recovery. Aberrations in cardiovascular physiology are frequently related to the initial underlying disease state, preexisting comorbidities, surgical procedure performed, and intraoperative events and management. A precise understanding of the preoperative pathophysiology and intraoperative course aids in postoperative management. Additionally, certain physiologic patterns are recognizable during specific phases of the postoperative period. Hemodynamic changes are often predictable to the experienced cardiothoracic intensivist, and subtle deviations from these patterns are detected to prevent adverse events.

This chapter reviews the basic concepts of cardiovascular physiology and pathophysiology specific to the post cardiac surgery patient. After a brief review of basic cardiac physiology, specific changes

DOI: 10.4018/978-1-4666-8603-8.ch016

in hemodynamics, and cardiac rhythm disturbances, the pathogenesis, diagnosis, and management of postoperative complications are systematically discussed. The goal of this chapter is to give insights and guidance into prediction, evaluation, and management of acute cardiovascular changes in the post cardiothoracic surgery patient, and offer insights into current controversies in the field.

BASIC PHYSIOLOGIC PRINCIPLES

Achieving adequate oxygen delivery to meet tissue metabolic demands is the primary objective to ensure smooth recovery from cardiac surgery. As systemic blood pressure does not always equal satisfactory organ perfusion, it is imperative to understand the physiologic principles of hemodynamics and tissue oxygenation.

Mean systemic blood pressure (MAP) is the product of cardiac output (CO) and systemic vascular resistance (SVR) added to the central venous pressure (CVP). As CVP is normally low, it is commonly omitted when using the formula for clinical purposes. Cardiac output equals stroke volume (SV) times heart rate (HR). The stroke volume is determined by preload, contractility, and afterload, which themselves are affected by ventricular compliance, interventricular dependence, and cardiac rhythm, among other components (see FIGURE 1). Rhythm disturbances, intrinsic and extrinsic metabolic factors, and postoperative pacing affect heart rate. The cardiac index (CI) is calculated to adjust for the individual patient, and can be derived by dividing CO by the body surface area (BSA). The normal values of the hemodynamic parameters mentioned are seen in Figure 2.

Figure 1. Components determining mean arterial pressure (MAP). Qt = cardiac output, SVR = systemic vascular resistance; SV = stroke volume; HR = heart rate; AVC = arterial vascular compliance

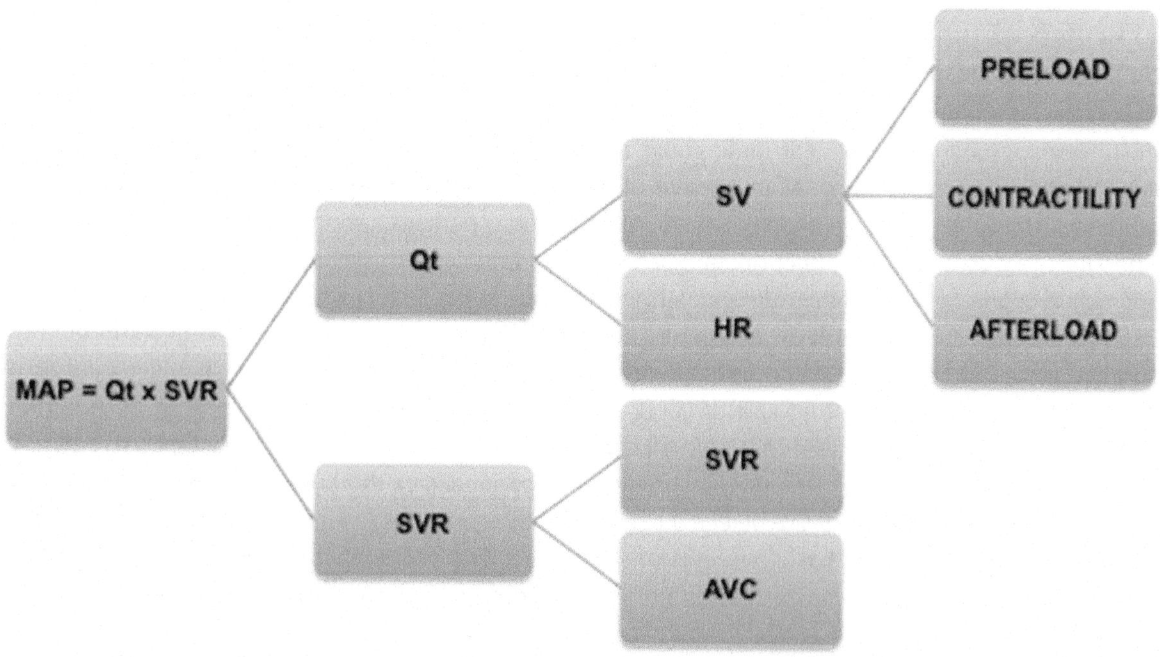

Figure 2. Hemodynamic formulas and normal values. CVP = central venous pressure; Pra = right atrial pressure

PARAMETER	FORMULA	NORMAL VALUES
HEART RATE (HR)		60 – 90 bpm
STROKE VOLUME (SV)		60 – 90 ml
CARDIAC OUTPUT (Qt)	CO = SV x HR	4 – 6 L/min
CARDIAC INDEX (CI)	CI = Qt / BSA	2.5 – 3 L/min/m^2
SYSTEMIC VACULAR RESISTANCE (SVR)	SVR = (MAP – Pra / Qt) x 80	800 – 1200 dyne x s/cm^5
PULMONARY VASCULAR RESISTANCE (PVR)	PVR = (PAPsys – PAOP / Qt) x80	120 – 200 dyne x s/cm^5
MEAN ARTERIAL PRESSURE (MAP)	MAP = Qt x SVR	70 – 100 mmHg
SYSTEMIC SYSTOLIC PRESSURE (SBP)		100 – 140 mmHg
PULMONARY SYSTOLIC PRESSURES (PAPsys)		15 – 25 mmHg
PULMONARY DIASTOLIC PRESSURES (PAPdiast)		5 – 12 mmHg
PULMONARY MEAN PRESSURES (PAPmean)		8 – 15 mmHg
PULMONARY ARTERY OCCLUSION PRESSURE (PAOP)		5 – 12 mmHg
CENTRAL VENOUS PRESSURE (CVP)		2 – 8 mmHg
OXYGEN DELIVERY (DO_2)	DO_2 = Qt x CaO_2	1000 ml/min
ARTERIAL OXYGEN CONTENT (CaO_2)	CaO_2 = 1.39 x Hgb x SaO_2 + 0.003 x PaO_2	200 ml/min
OXYGEN CONSUMPTION (VO_2)	VO_2 = Qt (CaO_2 – CvO_2)	250 ml/min
MIXED VENOUS OXYGEN SATURATION (SVO_2)		65 – 75 %

Preload

Preload refers to the degree of myocardial fiber stretch at end-diastole, and is commonly expressed by left ventricular (LV) end-diastolic volume (LVEDV). As it not only affects the CO by changes in SV, but also alters the force of contraction based on the Frank starling mechanism, preload is one of the most significant factors of alteration in CO (see FIGURE 3). Besides venous return, left ventricular preload can be affected by heart rate and rhythm. Tachycardia and irregular atrial contractions causing shortening or loss of diastolic filling time, especially in patients with decreased LV compliance, can significantly decrease LV preload. In addition, states of RV overload or dysfunction can lead to compromised LV filling secondary to displacement or dysfunction of the interventricular septum.

Left atrial filling pressures are commonly used as a surrogate for LVEDV. Direct left atrial pressures (LAP), pulmonary artery occlusion pressures (PAOP), or pulmonary artery diastolic pressures (PAD) measurements can be used to estimate LVEDV. In patients without preexisting pulmonary hypertension or intrinsic pulmonary disease the PAD is usually 2 – 4 mmHg higher than PAOP. When using filling pressures as surrogate for LVEDV in order to optimize cardiac preload, it is important to notice the effect

Figure 3. Frank-Starling-Curve: Relationship of preload and contractility. Normal ventricular function, increased contractility, and decreased contractility.

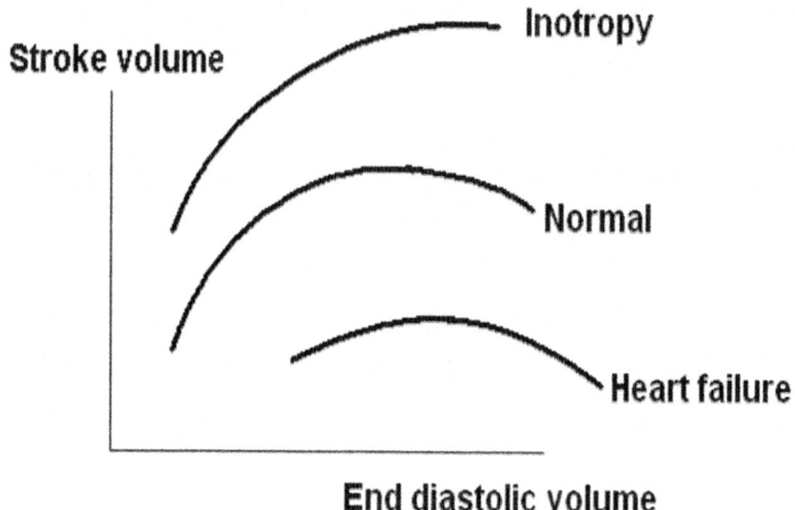

of ventricular compliance on filling pressures. Left ventricular compliance can be decreased by multiple disease states, such as chronic hypertension, aortic stenosis, ischemic or non-ischemic cardiomyopathy, diastolic dysfunction, and post cardiopulmonary bypass (CPB). With decreased compliance, higher filling pressures are needed to achieve adequate ventricular filling. CVP has shown to be a poor marker for preload assessment due to differences in ventricular compliance of the left and right atria, tricuspid regurgitation, and biventricular dysfunction post cardiac surgery (Marik, Baram, & Vahid, 2008; Marik, Monnet, & Teboul, 2011). Direct measurement of left atrial pressures via LAP lines, more common in pediatric cardiac surgery, is gradually disappearing from adult cardiac surgery as the risk of bleeding outweighs the benefits in most situations. In recent years, direct left ventricular volume measurement by echocardiography has become more common. Echocardiography has the advantage of providing a more complete assessment of filling and functional status of the left and right heart simultaneously.

Contractility

Contractility is the intrinsic strength of myocardial contraction independent of preload and afterload, and reflects ventricular systolic function. As seen in FIGURE 3, changes in contractility will result in different stroke volumes at certain preload conditions, and thereby alter cardiac output. In addition, contractility of myocardial fibers can be affected by heart rate (Bowditch reflex) and rhythm, as tachycardia or irregular rhythm interfere with the timing and efficiency of fiber contraction.

As the cardiothoracic patient often has compromised systolic ventricular function, assessment and management of ventricular contractility is a constant component of perioperative care. In the clinical setting, contractility can be quantified by ejection fraction (EF) with echocardiography, or indirectly by changes in CO when filling pressures and SVR remain constant. As the postoperative period is very dynamic, determination of ventricular function is complex and incorporation of many hemodynamic devices is necessary. Utilization of CO measurements by pulmonary artery catheter (PAC) to infer information about myocardial function has the advantage of continuous monitoring and real-time correlation to intervention. However, it is important to keep in mind that the PAC-derived CO reflects the right-sided myocardial function and thereby only indirectly gives information about the left ventricular systolic function. PAC-derived CO is also preload, afterload, heart rate, and rhythm dependent, and can give inaccurate results in patients with valvular pathologies, such as tricuspid regurgitation (see SECTION 6). In this situation, echocardiography again has shown to be a useful tool, as actual contraction of the myocardium can be visualized in addition to filling status and coexisting valvular pathologies.

Afterload

Afterload is defined as left ventricular wall stress during systole, and can be calculated by using the Laplace law: wall stress (σ) = ventricular pressure (P) x ventricular radius (r) / wall thickness (h). Clinically, this equation is infrequently used, as the components of the formula are not readily available. Instead, systemic vascular resistance (SVR) is used as surrogate for wall stress. It is important to notice that SVR, as measured clinically by PAC, only reflects the non-pulsatile component of impedance to left ventricular ejection, and does not incorporate compliance of the arterial tree.

In the postoperative cardiac patient, changes in SVR are most often associated with the post cardiopulmonary bypass vasodilatory state. States with increased SVR, often seen in patients with chronic HTN or aortic stenosis after valve replacement, can impair CO significantly. Therefore, hemodynamic management directed towards alterations of SVR, should incorporate systemic BP, CO, and biomarkers for end-organ perfusion.

Tissue Oxygenation

Tissue oxygenation depends on the adequate balance of oxygen delivery (DO2) and oxygen consumption (VO2). As seen in FIGURE 4, the four components determining tissue oxygenation are CO, hemoglobin (Hgb), arterial oxygen saturation (SaO2), and tissue oxygen consumption. All of these components are modifiable, and the basis of perioperative cardiovascular optimization. The mixed venous oxygen saturation (SvO2) measured from the pulmonary artery, is used clinically to reflect adequacy and changes in tissue oxygenation. The goal is an SvO2 of greater than 60% in most patients.

Oxygen delivery is the sum of CO and arterial oxygen content (CaO2). CaO2 incorporates the majority of oxygen bound to Hgb (1.34 x Hgb x SaO2) and a small, unbound part dissolved in plasma (PaO2 x 0.003). The equation emphasizes the importance CO and Hgb have in oxygen delivery as compared to PaO2, and helps to explain mechanisms of compensation. When PaO2 values increase above 60 mmHg, hemoglobin-bound oxygen levels remain relatively unchanged, and further increases in FiO2 have nominal effect on arterial oxygen content and global oxygen delivery. Given a normal oxygen-hemoglobin dissociation curve, the goal arterial oxygen tension is 60 – 90 mmHg to minimize side effects of hyperoxemia.

The optimal Hgb level for patients post cardiac surgery has been point of debate for decades. More recent guidelines suggest that lower levels of Hgb in the range of 7 – 8 g/dl are not harmful in this patient population, and having higher thresholds for transfusion can avoid complications associated with blood product administration (Society of Thoracic Surgeons Blood Conservation Guideline Task Force et al., 2007).

Tissue oxygen consumption is dependent on the oxygen extraction and utilization. Oxygen extraction of most organs varies with the amount of oxygen delivery. Different pathophysiologic states alter

Figure 4. Components affecting tissue oxygenation. Tissue oxygenation is determined by the four major components of cardiac output, hemoglobin, oxygenation, and oxygen consumption. VO2 = oxygen consumption; DO2 = oxygen delivery; Qt = cardiac output; CaO2 = arterial oxygen content; Hgb = Hemoglobin; SaO2 = arterial oxygen saturation; PaO2 = arterial oxygen content; SV = stroke volume; HR = heart rate

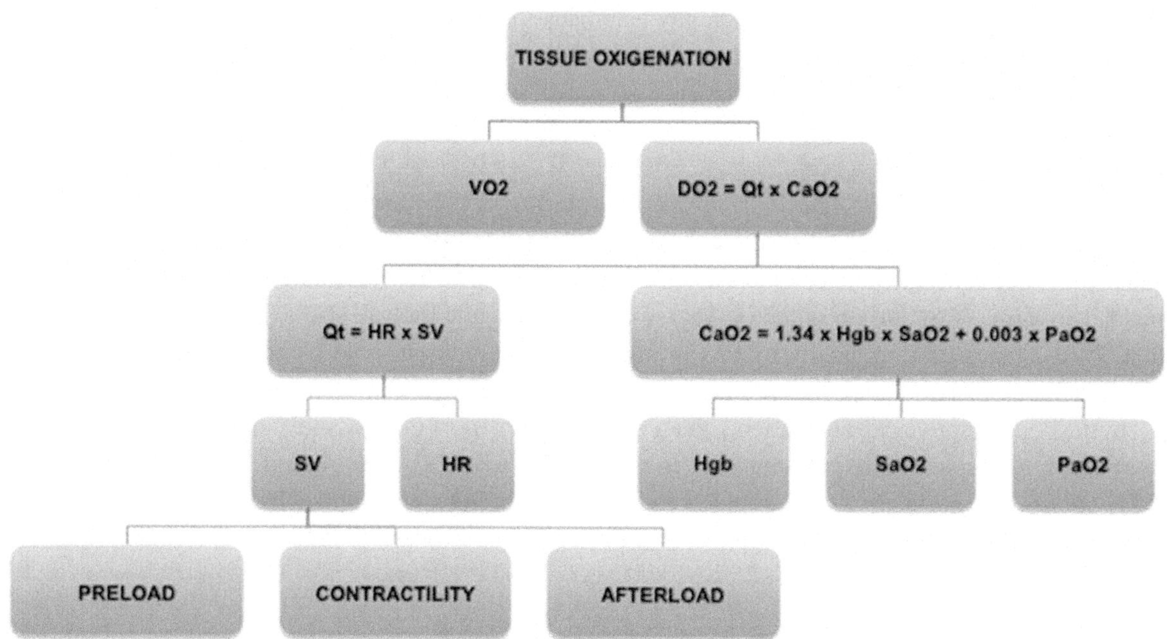

this balance, which is reflected by changes of SVO2 levels. SvO2 in cardiogenic, hypovolemic, and obstructive shock is decreased, due to decreased O2 delivery and compensatory increased extraction. In distributive shock states, like sepsis, SvO2 can be significantly elevated secondary to increase in CO, arteriovenous shunting, and impaired mitochondrial oxygen utilization. VO2 is altered by perioperative components of sedation, body temperature, perfusion, and paralysis. During the initial postoperative hours, oxygen consumption increases over time due to normalization of the cardiovascular physiology.

Oxygen supply and demand in the myocardium differs from the rest of the body. As myocardial oxygen demand (mvO2) is 20 times higher than in skeletal muscles, the body adjusts by increasing coronary blood flow and maximizing O2 extraction. Further increase in O2 demand can only be met by increasing coronary blood flow. When coronary blood flow is compromised due to coronary artery disease or ventricular hypertrophy, increases in mvO2 can result in myocardial ischemia. The fine balance of myocardial oxygen supply and demand is easily disrupted, and minimizing factors that can increase myocardial oxygen consumption is of vital importance.

Clinical Assessment of Circulation

Assessment of circulation can be difficult in the first couple of hours postoperatively, and systematic evaluation following the basic principles of hemodynamics as described above, is the best approach to differentiate etiologies. Despite utilization of physical examination, cardiovascular monitors for CO and tissue perfusion, specific imaging modalities, and laboratory values reflecting tissue perfusion, alteration of normal body physiology often impairs the assessment of hemodynamics. CPB, hypothermia, surgical stress, mechanical ventilation, and medications have significant effects on physiologic homeostasis. Polyuria is often seen despite inadequate intravascular volume status and delayed rewarming can cause cool extremities despite adequate CO. Even without ongoing hypoperfusion, high catecholamine levels or inadequate hepatic and renal clearance can affect biomarker such as lactate levels. Hyperlactatemia can have rare and unexpected causes such as reperfusion injury in the setting of mechanical assist devices or from persistent localized ischemia of limbs or splanchnic vasculature.

POSTOPERATIVE PHYSIOLOGY

The postoperative course after cardiac surgery is highly dependent on preoperative pathology, comorbidities, and intraoperative course. Surgical technique, type of graft used, post-procedural pathologies, length of CPB, effectiveness of myocardial protection, and temperature management all contribute to outcome and recovery time. Details of specific pathologies and their postoperative implications can be found in Section 5 of this book.

Within the first 6 – 12 hours after surgery, cardiovascular changes are very dynamic. Persistent bleeding, fluid loss from capillary leak, myocardial stunning, and vasodilatory states result in combinations of cardiogenic, hypovolemic, and vasodilatory shock states. This contributes significantly to the challenges in diagnosis and management of these complex and critically ill patients. The equilibration of normothermia after cardiopulmonary bypass amplifies these challenges. The initial rewarming on CPB is often followed by a drop in temperature due to ongoing resuscitation and difficulty in maintaining normothermia in the OR and during patient transport (Ramsay, Ralley, Whalley, DelliColli, & Wynands, 1985). After arrival in the ICU, the patient will become normothermic over time, but time to normalization can vary greatly. Rewarming is associated with an increase in O2 consumption, CO2 production, and vasodilation, and the slope of the rewarming curve correlates with dynamic fluctuations during this period (see FIGURE 5) (Ramsay et al., 1985). Following this initial period, the subsequent 24 hours are usually the period when cardiovascular support is weaned, fast-track patients moved to less acute care, and complex patients declare themselves in the direction of further recovery.

Hemodynamic goals in the postoperative period should be based on the individual patient, taking into account their specific pathology and comorbidities. Figure 6 shows hemodynamic and echocardiographic findings in different shock states, which can aid diagnosis and management of critical ill patients. The CI and SvO2 as indicators for myocardial function and adequate organ perfusion should be maintained at a normal range (CI > 2.2 $l/min/m^2$ and SvO2 > 60%). In deciding if the patient benefits from high- or low-normal values, the intensivist must consider the baseline myocardial function, as well as preexisting end-organ dysfunction. The same applies to blood pressure targets, as certain patients may require higher MAP's due to higher preexisting autoregulation curves or lower targets in consideration of surgical anastomoses. Also, cardiomyopathy patients may require lower than normal SVR and preload, to maintain adequate CO and avoid congestive heart failure (CHF).

Figure 5. Equilibrium of normothermia after CPB in the ICU. Initial post-CPB afterdrop in temperature associated with increase in systemic vascular resistance (SVR), decrease in oxygen consumption (VO2), and dioxide production (VCO2), is followed by a period of rewarming in the ICU, during which SVR vasodilation occurs, and VO2 and VCO2 increases. This period is the time of maximum hemodynamic instability and increased risk for hemodynamic or respiratory compromise, due to rapid changes in metabolism to which the intensivist has to adjust to. Extent of hemodynamic instability depends on slope and duration of the rewarming phase. OR = operating room; CPB = cardiopulmonary bypass; ICU = intensive care unit (Adopted from: Slade RN: Management of the adult cardiac patient in the intensive care unit. In Ream AK, Fogdall RP: Acute Cardiovascular Management: Anesthesia and Intensive Care. Philadelphia, LB Lippincott, 1982, p 495).

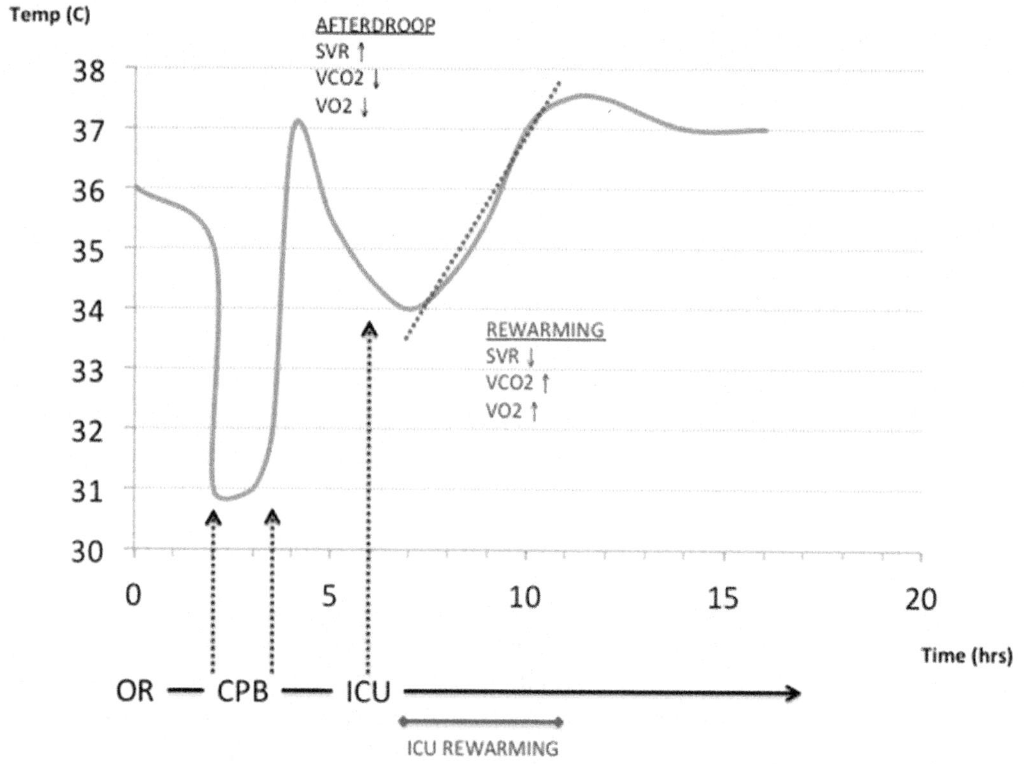

Low Cardiac Output State

Low CO post cardiac surgery can have multiple etiologies, including decreased preload, myocardial dysfunction, increased afterload, and rhythm disturbances (Figure 7). Bleeding, increased capillary leakage, and post CPB polyuria can decrease intravascular volume and thereby venous return to the heart. When active bleeding is source of hypovolemia, surgical bleeding needs to be ruled out. Aggressive resuscitation has to be performed while bearing in mind the potential for dilutional coagulopathy leading to further exacerbation of bleeding, right ventricular compromise, and complications from blood trans-

Figure 6. Hemodynamic and echocardiographic findings in different shock states. "Kissing papillary muscles", as seen in hypovolemic shock, is described as collapse of the LV chamber during ventricular systole. "Equalization of pressures" in tamponade of diastolic pressures is often masked by inotropic and vasopressor support. Abnormal IVS motion can be differentiated into diastolic and systolic motion of the IVS into the LV depending on RV-volume vs RV-pressure overload. IVS = interventricular septum; RA = right atrium; RV = right ventricle; PE = pulmonary embolus; TR = tricuspid regurgitation

	HEMODYNAMICS				ECHOCARDIOGRAPHY				
SHOCK	**CO**	**PAP**	**PAOP**	**CVP**	**CONTRACTILITY**	**LVEDV**	**LVESV**	**IVC DIAMETER**	**OTHER**
HYPOVOLEMIC	↓	↓	↓	↓	*hyperdynamic*	↓	↓	↓	***"kissing papillary muscles"***
DISTRIBUTIVE	↑	N/↓	N/↓	N/↓	*hyperdynamic*	N/↓	↓	N/↓	
CARDIOGENIC *LV*	↓	↑	↑	↑	*depressed LV*	↑	↑	↑	
CARDIOGENIC *RV*	↓	↓	N/↓	↑	*depressed RV*	N/↓	N/↓	↑	***RV dilation + abnormal IVS motion +/- significant TR***
OBSTRUCTIVE *TAMPONADE*	↓	↓	↑	↑	*hyperdynamic*	↓	↓	↑	***Pericardial effusion +/- clot + RA/RV collapse +/- "Equalization of pressures"***
OBSTRUCTIVE *PE*	↓	↓	↓	↑	*hyperdynamic*	↓	↓	↑	***+/- RV dilation & dysfunction***

fusions. Less common etiologies for decreased preload are tamponade, intra-abdominal hypertension, pulmonary embolus, right ventricular failure, and arrhythmias. Hemodynamic effects from low preload states are frequently exacerbated by positive pressure ventilation (Luecke & Pelosi, 2005; Michard & Teboul, 2000), and ventilator settings need to be adjusted in these situations. Factors that increase intra-thoracic pressures, such as PEEP, mainstem endotracheal intubation, patient-ventilator dyssynchrony, pulmonary obstructive disease, pulmonary edema, significant pleural effusion, or pneumothorax need to be addressed. Occasionally, deepening of sedation or even paralysis is needed to stabilize the hemodynamically unstable patient in the setting of patient-ventilator dyssynchrony. Because of the variety of etiologies affecting preload and thereby CO, it is important to differentiate between right- and left-ventricular preload, and management should consider each side in isolation, in order to improve left ventricular stroke volume and CO.

Reduced CO due to an increase in afterload can have multiple causes in the postoperative period (see Figure 8). Sympathetic activation resulting in increased SVR occurs with pain, shivering, and emergence from anesthesia. Abnormalities in intravascular volume status and acid-base homeostasis cause endogenous activation of the renin-angiotensin system and neurohumeral reflexes. As previously

Figure 7. Common and uncommon etiologies of low cardiac output states and its management post cardiac surgery. SVR = systemic vascular resistance; RV = right ventricle; CM = cardiomyopathy

	ETIOLOGY		MANAGEMENT
COMMON	HYPOVOLEMIA	- Polyuria - Bleeding	*volume resuscitation*
COMMON	PATIENT-VENT-DYSYNCHRONY		*optimize ventilation* *↑ sedation +/- paralysis*
COMMON	HIGH SVR		*treat etiology of ↑ SVR* *arterial vasodilator*
COMMON	MYOCARDIAL DYSFUNCTION	- Myocardial stunning - Acute myocardial ischemia - LV diastolic dysfunction - RV dysfunction - Stress-induced CM (Takotsubo)	*inotropic support*
COMMON	ARRHYTHMIAS		*control heart rate and rhythm* *cardiac pacing*
UNCOMMON	DYNAMIC LVOT OBSTRUCTION		*↑ ventricular pre- and afterload*
UNCOMMON	VALVULAR PATHOLOGY		*supportive +/- surgical or interventional treatment*
UNCOMMON	CARDIAC TAMPONADE		*volume* *inotropic support*
UNCOMMON	PULMONARY EMBOLUS		*supportive +/- systemic anticoagulation*
UNCOMMON	TENSION PNEUMOTHORAX		*Needle thoracotomy followed by thoracotomy tube*

discussed, residual hypothermia causes peripheral vasoconstriction. In addition, increased PVR secondary to PHTN, increased intrathoracic pressure, and pulmonary edema can lead to right ventricular low CO, especially if RV dysfunction exists preoperatively. Management is directed at balancing SVR and PVR by the use of specific arterial vasodilators to optimize biventricular CO and end-organ perfusion. If ventricular function is normal, frequently used vasodilators are nicardipine, sodium nitroprusside and nitroglycerine. When myocardial function is depressed, inodilators such as dobutamine or milrinone can add inotropy in addition to afterload reduction.

While acute and ongoing myocardial ischemia is infrequent and will be discussed later, temporary myocardial dysfunction in the setting of myocardial stunning and low cardiac output syndrome (LCOS) is common after cardiac surgery. Myocardial stunning following ischemic episodes, reperfusion injury, long cardiopulmonary bypass times, and electrical cardioversion or defibrillation, can be significant depending on the intraoperative course and effectiveness of myocardial protection. Myocardial stunning is associated with an initial decrease in myocardial function, which typically recovers within the first 24 hours, but can persist up to a week postoperatively (Licker et al., 2012).

LCOS is defined as post CPB need for inotropic or mechanical hemodynamic support for over 30 min in the operating room (OR) or intensive care unit (ICU), despite normalization of preload, afterload, rhythm, and electrolyte variables. The prevalence ranges from 2 – 9%, depending on the surgical procedure, and is associated with increased morbidity and mortality. Preoperative risk factors include age,

Figure 8. Common and uncommon etiologies of increased systemic vascular resistance post cardiac surgery

	ETIOLOGY
COMMON	PAIN
	EMERGENCE FROMM ANESTHESIA
	SHIVERING
	INAPPROPRIATE VASOPRESSOR THERAPY
	HYPOTHERMIA
	HYPERCARBIA
UNCOMMON	RENAL DISEASE
	PROSTHETIC VALVE DYSFUNCTION
	INTRACRANIAL PATHOLOGY

female gender, EF less than 40%, congestive heart failure (CHF), stroke, and renal failure. Intraoperative risk factors have been identified as redo- or emergent surgery, cardiogenic shock, poor myocardial protection, and prolonged CPB (greater than 90 minutes) and aortic cross-clamp times. Over the last two decades, prevalence of preoperative risk factors for left ventricular dysfunction and reoperation has increased. While incidence has decreased during this time, mortality of LCOS continues to increase, making preoperative patient selection and risk assessment of significant importance (Algarni, Elhenawy, Maganti, Collins, & Yau, 2012; Algarni, Maganti, & Yau, 2011; Maganti, Rao, Borger, Ivanov, & David, 2005; Maganti et al., 2010).

Whereas many etiologies of low CO can be easily reversed, LCOS and postoperative myocardial stunning may rely on temporary supportive management with inotropes and afterload reduction, until the myocardium has regained its systolic function. Preoperative evaluation for risk factors of LCOS often allows for more precise management during the intraoperative and early postoperative period. Figure 9 shows a common approach to management of post CPB low CO. Optimization of heart rate by external temporary pacing is commonly the first choice to improve CO, but additional inotropic support is often required. Inotropic support is available in the form of pharmacologic agents and mechanical devices. Inotropes can be differentiated into inopressors like epinephrine or dopamine, and inodilators such as dobutamine and milrinone. When used, careful choice of individual pharmacologic intervention and consideration of drug-specific mechanisms is pertinent for optimal hemodynamic management. Mechanical support can range from IABP to VA-ECMO and ventricular assist devices (VADs). With continuous advancement in device technology and increasing experience in their placement and management, utilization is growing in large cardiovascular centers with high acuity patient population. The indication

Figure 9. Algorithm for hemodynamic management in the post cardiac surgery period

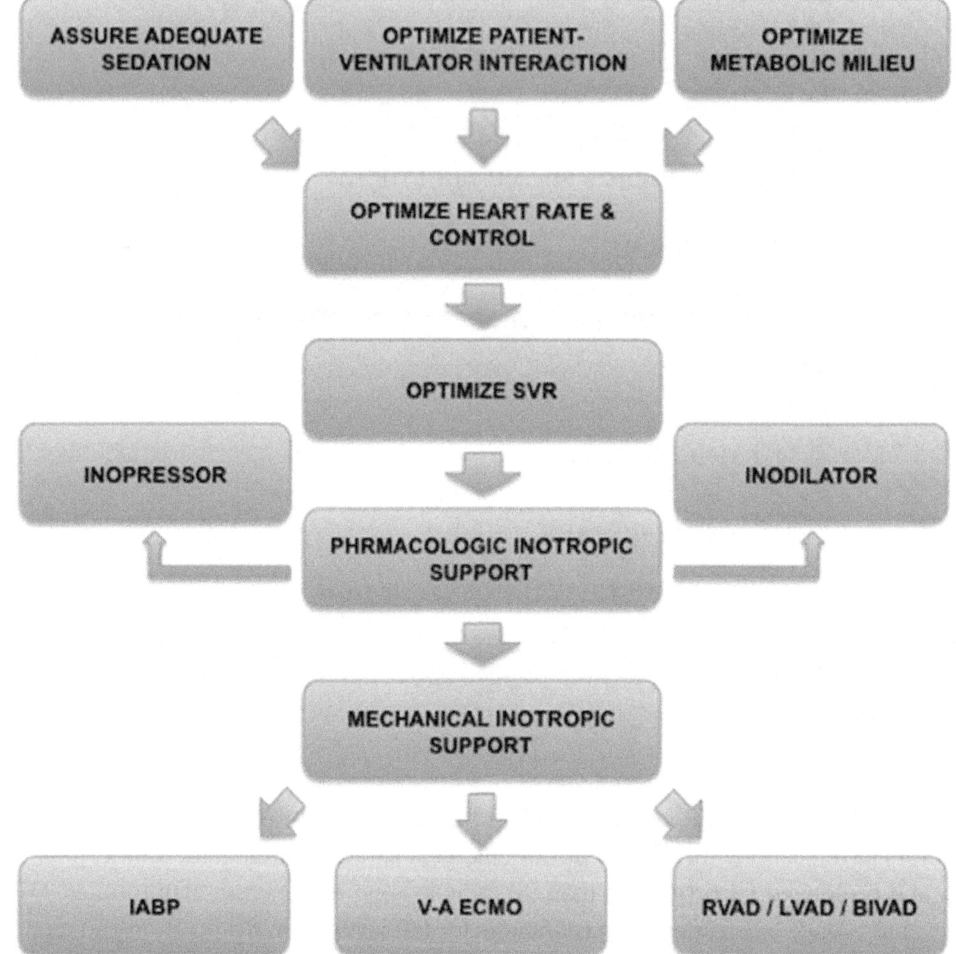

for and timing of placement is a continuously evolving and controversial subject. Further details of these devices and their management would exceed the scope of this chapter and will be discussed separately in chapter 29 of this book.

Right Ventricular Failure

Right ventricular (RV) systolic failure plays a significant role in global low CO state and inadequate perfusion, and carries significant mortality after cardiac surgery. Preexisting PHTN, as a significant risk factor for RV failure, has been included in perioperative risk scores for cardiac surgery (Euroscore and Parsonnet score). In addition, certain procedures such as heart transplantation and left ventricular assist devices carry high prevalence of acute postoperative RV failure. As awareness of its significance has increased over the years, understanding of pathophysiology and specific management has improved (Haddad, Couture, Tousignant, & Denault, 2009).

Low CO states should always be evaluated for right ventricular failure, especially in the high-risk patient populations mentioned above. Where CVP by itself is a poor indicator for RV function, the concomitant use of PAC and CVP monitoring can indicate worsening RV dysfunction [illegible] narrowing PA to RA pressure gradients, and the new onset of TR (V-waves) on CVP tracing. Echocardiography can support diagnosis and management, and can help in differentiating isolated RV failure from [illegible]induced right-sided compromise. Other more indirect indicators for right-sided failure are jugular vein distention and hepatic congestion with serum markers indicating liver dysfunction.

Specific treatment must be directed at the underlying etiology. Temporary improvement of RV function can be achieved by decreasing right-sided afterload with non-specific or specific vasodilators, such as nitroglycerin or inhaled nitric oxide (iNO), and by increasing RV contractility with inotropic support such as milrinone, dobutamine, and epinephrine. Specific pulmonary vascular dilators, such as inhaled nitric oxide or inhaled epoprostenol are now commonly used in significant RV failure due to their localized vasodilatory effect on the pulmonary vasculature without systemic vasodilation.

When utilizing inotropes and vasoconstrictors, attention must be paid to individual pulmonary vasoconstrictive effects of each drug. For this reason, milrinone and vasopressin, as nonsympathomimetic drugs with minimal pulmonary vasoconstrictive attributes, have been advocated. Utilization of newer drugs like inhaled milrinone or levosimendan, a calcium sensitizer, are under investigation, and possibly present additional medications for the management of RV failure (L. C. Price, Wort, Finney, Marino, & Brett, 2010). The use of a temporary right mechanical assist device (RVAD) may be warranted in situations where the patient is at high risk of significant RV compromise, due to a preexisting left mechanical assist device (LVAD).

One of the most important and controversial, but often neglected aspects in acute RV failure remains volume optimization (Cecconi, Johnston, & Rhodes, 2006; Mebazaa, Karpati, Renaud, & Algotsson, 2004). In normal physiologic states, the right ventricle has better compliance when compared to the LV, and allows for larger changes in venous return. Simultaneously, with a relatively small muscle mass, acute increases in RV afterload are not as well tolerated. When RV compliance is impaired in chronic RV dysfunction, post CPB, or in the setting of myocardial ischemia, the RV functions on a very narrow position of the Frank Starling curve, and even small volume changes can cause acute RV decompensation. Whereas, during the initial acute hypotensive phase of RV failure, a fluid challenge may temporarily increase right-sided CO and, thereby, improve hemodynamics for a short period of time, continuous fluid administration is detrimental to the failing ventricle. With inadequate RV forward flow and frequently concomitant tricuspid valve regurgitation, the RV is almost always volume overloaded, and functions on the descending slope of the Frank-Starling curve. The RV enters a vicious cycle of worsening failure as seen in Figure 10, and any further increase in volume promotes the downward spiral. Therefore, especially when persistent postoperative bleeding occurs, prompt measures should be taken to minimize the need for continuous volume resuscitation. Temporary inotropic support and afterload reduction, in addition to aggressive fluid removal by diuresis or continuous venous-venous hemofiltration (CVVH), is often the only option to optimize RV size to the point that RV function recovers and supportive measures can be weaned (L. C. Price et al., 2010).

A deviation from this pathophysiology exists in the pediatric and adult congenital heart disease, where RV function can be reduced to a passive conductor state. But this is rarely the case in the general adult cardiac population, and should not prompt adoption of very specific fluid management in this setting to the regular cardiac patient.

Figure 1 physiology of right ventricular failure. RV = right ventricle; LV = left ventricle; TR = tricuspi regurgitation; CO = cardiac output; RV WT = right ventricular wall tension; MAP = mean a pressures; IVS = intraventricular septum.

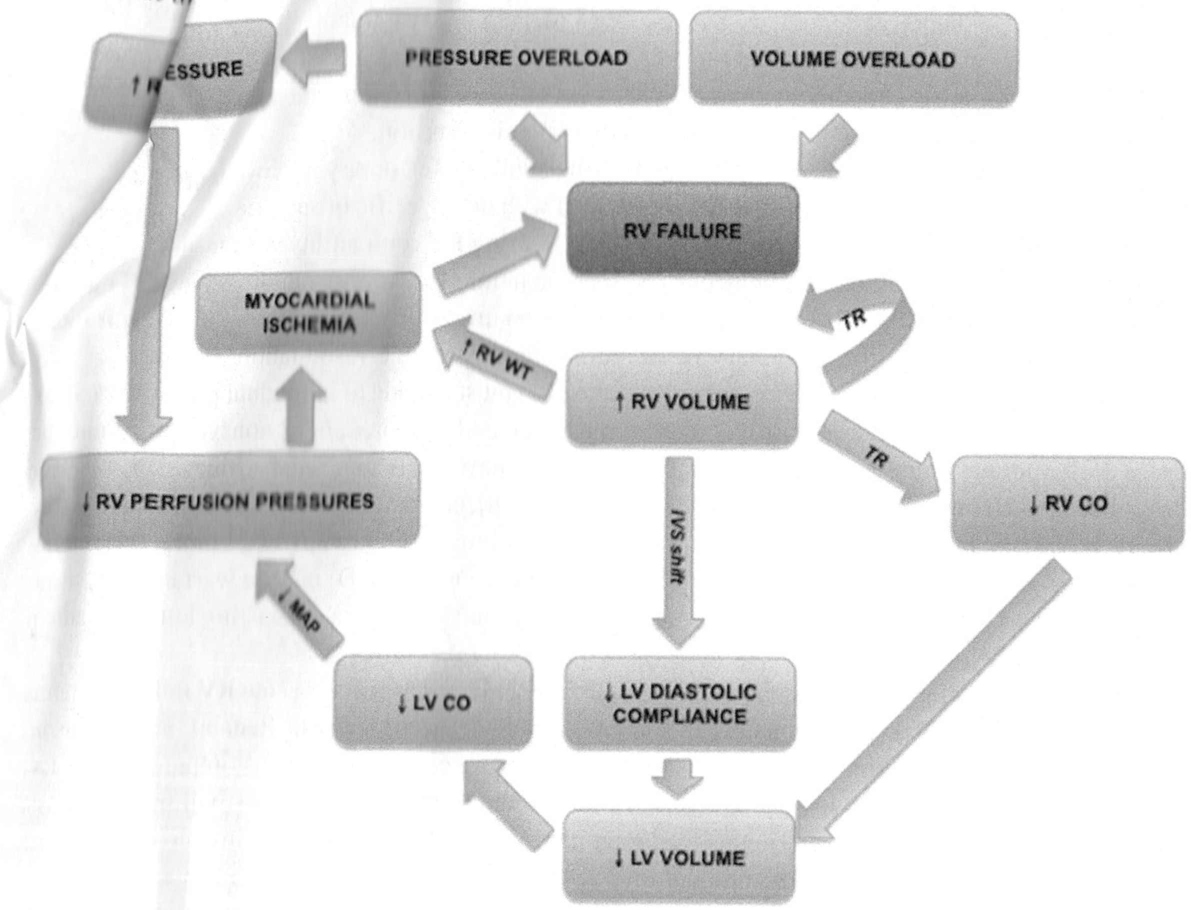

Myocardial Ischemia

Acute myocardial infarction (MI) during or after revascularization therapy can be caused by intraoperative myocardial injury, coronary dissection, failure of reperfusion, or graft thrombosis. A rare event in the post cardiac surgery period, a MI requires emergent recognition and management, and is associated with high mortality (Rasmussen et al., 1997).

More commonly, myocardial ischemia occurs secondary imbalance in to oxygen demand and supply, and should be considered when new ECG changes appear. At high risk are patients with generalized CAD, patients in danger of subendocardial hypoperfusion due to ventricular hypertrophy or increased wall tension, and patients with suboptimal vascular targets and revascularization. Other perioperative etiologies include coronary vasospasm, air emboli, or mechanical compromise from kinking or compression.

Besides ECG changes, cardiac biomarkers are part of the initial diagnostic evaluation for MI. Elevated myocardial enzymes troponin (Tn) and creatinine kinase (CK-MB) have been associated with increased short- and long-term mortality after cardiac surgery (Domanski et al., 2011; Lurati Buse et al., 2010;

Petäjä, Salmenperä, Pulkki, & Pettilä, 2009). Timing and degree of elevation have been shown to play a prognostic role, and even though exact cut-off values have not been identified, most studies agree that the greater the elevation in biomarker, the greater the risk of adverse outcome. Current consensus of several international cardiovascular societies suggests that a rise in Tn greater than 10 times the upper limit of normal in patients with preoperative normal baseline levels, plus new pathological Q-waves or new LBBB and/or angiographic or echocardiographic evidence of new myocardial ischemia, is suggestive of acute MI after cardiac surgery (Moussa et al., 2013; Thygesen et al., 2012).

In general, acute ST changes in the postoperative period, especially when associated with hemodynamic instability or signs of low cardiac output, should trigger prompt evaluation and diagnosis. Significant ST elevation or new myocardial dysfunction in vascular graft territory should trigger immediate involvement of the interventional cardiologist and cardiothoracic surgeon, for possible percutaneous or open re-revascularization. Initial stabilization in the ICU should focus on optimizing myocardial oxygen supply and demand. Augmentation of diastolic perfusion pressures and coronary vasodilation can be achieved with vasopressors and nitroglycerine, and by avoiding tachycardia, hypoxemia, hypercarbia, shivering, and pain. Administration of red blood cells may additionally be warranted in profoundly anemic patients to optimize oxygen delivery.

Coronary vasospasm is difficult to diagnose in the postoperative period, as it is a diagnosis of exclusion at the bedside. ECG and echocardiographic changes can suggest the diagnosis when other causes of myocardial hypoperfusion are ruled out, while definitive diagnosis is made by angiography. When suspected, treatment involves vasodilators such as nitroglycerine or calcium channel blockers.

Air embolus, causing transient blockage of coronary vessels, often presents with new conduction abnormalities, such as atrio-ventricular conduction delay or blocks and RV dysfunction. Involvement of the RCA territory is more common due to anatomical takeoff of the coronary vasculature. Immediate treatment is aimed at distal advancement of the embolus by coronary vasodilators and increasing coronary perfusion pressures, as well as supportive management of symptomatic bradyarrhythmias and myocardial dysfunction.

Diastolic Heart Failure

In diastolic heart failure, the systolic ventricular function and EF is preserved, but the early relaxation and late filling phase of ventricular diastole is impaired. Diastolic dysfunction is commonly caused by ventricular hypertrophy and increased wall stiffness, as seen in patients with chronic systemic HTN, aortic stenosis, CAD, cardiomyopathy, and advanced age. It results in increased left ventricular end-diastolic pressures (LVEDP) and left atrial pressures (LAP), and subsequent increased risk of pulmonary congestion and CHF.

The presence of diastolic dysfunction preoperatively has been linked to increased risk of postoperative systolic dysfunction in patients undergoing cardiac surgery (Apostolakis, Baikoussis, Parissis, Siminelakis, & Papadopoulos, 2009; Licker et al., 2010). New or worsening diastolic dysfunction post CPB is common, but usually recovers to baseline within 24 - 48 hrs. Clinically, SV and CO associated with increased filling pressures are suggestive of diastolic dysfunction, but other conditions causing reduction in diastolic function such as RV volume overload, pericardial tamponade, or tachyarrhythmia's, must be ruled out. Definite diagnosis is best made with echocardiography.

Patients with diastolic dysfunction often show fragile postoperative hemodynamics. When underfilled, inadequate SV causes low CO and significant hypotension. Arrhythmias resulting in loss of atrial contraction, such as supraventricular tachyarrhythmias or premature atrial contractions (PAC's), can lead to significant compromise in LV loading and subsequent hemodynamic instability. Therefore adequate volume loading to often higher than normal filling pressures, especially in patients with long standing diastolic dysfunction, is pertinent in the perioperative period.

Vasodilatory Syndrome

Postoperative vasodilatory state and distributive shock is common after cardiac surgery. Persistent hypotension, low SVR, and normal or high cardiac output which responds poorly to volume resuscitation and requires significant vasopressor support, has been described as vasoplegic or vasodilatory syndrome. Whereas temporary low SVR occurs in 20 - 40% of patients after cardiac surgery, the incidence of vasoplegic syndrome has been described as 5 - 10% and is associated with increased mortality and morbidity. An even higher prevalence is seen in patients with end-stage heart failure requiring LVAD support. In addition to sepsis and systemic inflammatory response, preoperative ACE inhibitors, ca-channel blockers, and intravenous Heparin are recognized as risk factors of vasodilatory syndrome. Early and persistent intraoperative hypotension during CPB acts as intraoperative indicator for postoperative manifestation (Shanmugam, 2005; Sidebotham, McKee, Gillham, Levy, 2007).

Management focuses on adequate intravascular volume resuscitation and vasoconstriction with potent vasopressors such as norepinephrine and vasopressin. Caution is advised in patients with depressed myocardial function, as overt arterial vasoconstriction can further exacerbate poor ventricular function and decrease CO. In extreme vasoplegic shock, the use of methylene blue has been reported, but should be avoided in patients with significant pulmonary hypertension, as its function is directed at competitive inhibition of nitric oxide, a potent pulmonary vasodilator (Shanmugam, 2005; Sidebotham et al., 2007).

Heart Rate and Arrhythmias

Heart rate can significantly contribute to improving or worsening the hemodynamic profile after cardiac surgery. Sinus bradycardia can decrease CO, especially in patients with advanced age or low myocardial function. At the same time, excessive sinus tachycardia can compromise CO, especially when ventricular diastolic dysfunction exists and ventricular filling is impaired. Many factors, including sympathetic tone, pain, sedation and agitation, and certain medications, affect the heart rate postoperatively, and have to be optimized in order to avoid adverse effects. Utilization of temporary atrial pacing can often help considerably to improve hemodynamics, and heart rates between 80 – 100 bpm are the goal for most situations.

Rhythm disturbances are common after cardiac surgery. In the postoperative course, they not only have diagnostic value and can herald ongoing cardiac dysfunction, but they can also have significant effect on hemodynamic performance, especially in patients with already compromised cardiac function. The most common are atrial tachyarrhythmias, with an incidence reported between 10 - 65% depending on the surgical procedure. Ventricular arrhythmias are less common and are mostly associated with electrolyte abnormalities, reperfusion syndromes, or ongoing ischemia. Conduction abnormalities and bradyarrhythmias have an incidence ranging between 1 - 30%, depending on the procedure and type of arrhythmia, but can have significant long-term implications by requiring permanent pacing (Chung, 2000; Echahidi, Pibarot, O'Hara, & Mathieu, 2008; Peretto, Durante, Limite, & Cianflone, 2014). In addition, the post cardiac surgery period carries the risk of pharmacologically induced arrhythmias or arrhythmias in the setting of dysfunctional temporary pacing.

Multiple risk factors for arrhythmias in the perioperative period have been described. The etiology is frequently multifactorial, and the significance of each individual component has not been clearly defined. Patient related predisposing factors are age, structural heart disease such as atrial enlargement, and non-cardiac diseases such as obesity and chronic obstructive pulmonary disease. Proarrhythmic factors related to the perioperative course are more complex. Cardiac trauma and inflammation can lead to subclinical or symptomatic pericarditis with increased cardiac irritability. Increased sympathetic tone and catecholamines contribute to the incidence of tachyarrhythmias. Electrolyte abnormalities, especially hypokalemia and hypomagnesemia, have been associated with rhythm disturbances ranging from premature atrial or ventricular beats and atrial tachyarrhythmias to ventricular tachyarrhythmias and torsades de pointes (TdP). Furthermore, ongoing ischemic injury or reperfusion injury post procedure commonly presents with significant ventricular ectopies. Certain procedures, such as aortic valvular surgery and heart transplantation, have an increased risk for bradyarrhythmias after surgery, and medications with nodal-blocking attributes, such as amiodarone, are frequently used in the postoperative period.

Atrial tachycardias can be divided into categories by their regularity and origin of rhythm (see figure 11). Of these, postoperative atrial fibrillation (POAF) is the most common, and it carries an increased morbidity and mortality. The highest incidence is seen on postoperative (POD) day 2 and 3, while 70% of POAF has developed by POD 4, and only 6% occurs after POD 6 (Echahidi et al., 2008; Maisel, Rawn, & Stevenson, 2001; Peretto et al., 2014). It is associated with increased risk for thromboembolic events, hemodynamic compromise, ventricular tachycardias, and complications from the treatment of POAF.

The goal of perioperative management of POAF is identification of the high-risk patient for prophylactic treatment, management of acute episodes, and prevention of subsequent complications. In recent years the use of protocols for POAF prophylaxis has become more established in order to weight risk and benefits of prophylactic management in individual patients undergoing cardiac surgery. Current recom-

Figure 11. Common arrhythmias post cardiac surgery. Tachyarrhythmias and bradyarrhythmias are differentiated, as well as supraventricular from ventricular origin. VT = ventricular tachycardia; TdP = torsades de pointes; V-fib = ventricular fibrillation; SA = sinoatrial; AV = atrioventricular; AVNRT = atrioventricular nodal reentry tachycardia.

SUPRAVENTRICULAR TACHYARRHYTHMIAS	VENTRICULAR TACHYARRHYTHMIAS	BRADYARRHYTMIAS
Sinus tachycardia	Monomorphic VT	Sinus bradycardia
Atrial fibrillation (A-fib)	Polymorphic VT (including TdP)	Sick sinus syndrome
Atrial flutter	Ventricular fibrillation (V-fib)	SA nodal block
Accelerated junctional rhythm	Accelerated ventricular rhythm	AV nodal block
AVNRT / accessory pathways		Slow A-fib
Ectopic atrial tachycardia		Ventricular escape rhythms

mendations to minimize the risk for POAF consist of resumption of preoperatively prescribed beta blocker as soon as possible, initiation of temporary beta-blocker or amiodarone therapy in patients at increased risk, and by optimizing postoperative risk factors (Echahidi et al., 2008). Most prophylactic protocols recommend initiation of prophylaxis on POD 0 or 1 and continuing for 2 to 6 weeks postoperatively, as seen in Figure 12. Given the variety of perioperative prevention strategies described in the literature, controversy remains about their significance in regards to clinical outcome, length of hospital stay, and hospital costs. More novel approaches looking at the use of anti-inflammatory medications like colchicine, ketorolac, steroids, statins, and N3-polyunsaturated fatty acids, as well as temporary postoperative atrial pacing have been suggested, but the evidence is still scare (Bradley et al., 2005; Fuster et al., 2006).

The management of acute episodes of atrial tachyarrhythmias is divided into rate versus rhythm control, and possible anticoagulation for persistent atrial fibrillation or flutter (see Figure 13). Initially, the decision has to be made whether a patient's hemodynamics are compromised enough by the arrhythmia to warrant immediate synchronized cardioversion. If time allows, preceding electrical cardioversion

Figure 12. Example of an atrial fibrillation prophylaxis protocol for patients with increased risk of POAF. Shown is the protocol used in the cardiothoracic ICU at UCLA. Patient with increased risk receive either a beta blocker, amiodarone, or a bata blocker plus amiodarone starting on POD 0 to 1. Amiodarone is continued for two weeks postoperatively.

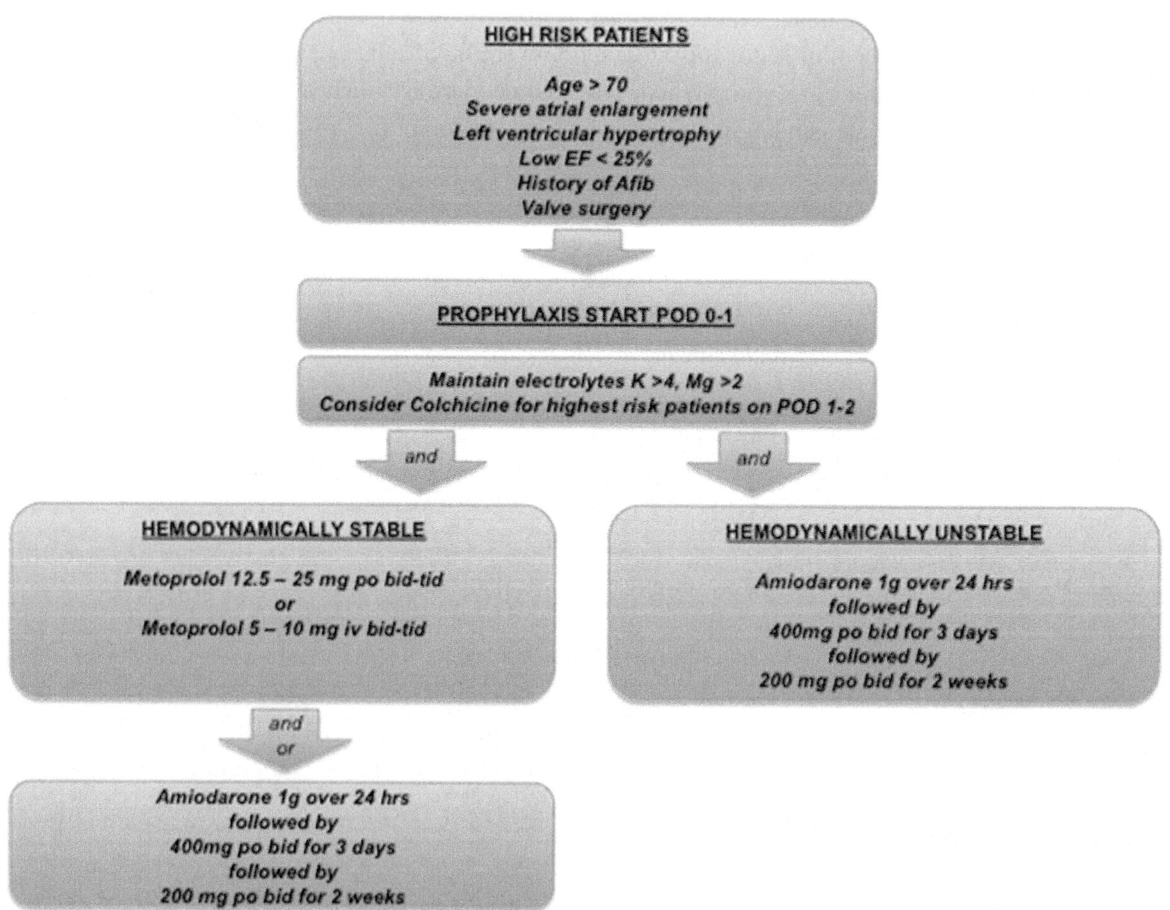

Figure 13. A-fib management in the post cardiac surgery patient. DCCV = synchronized direct current cardioversion.

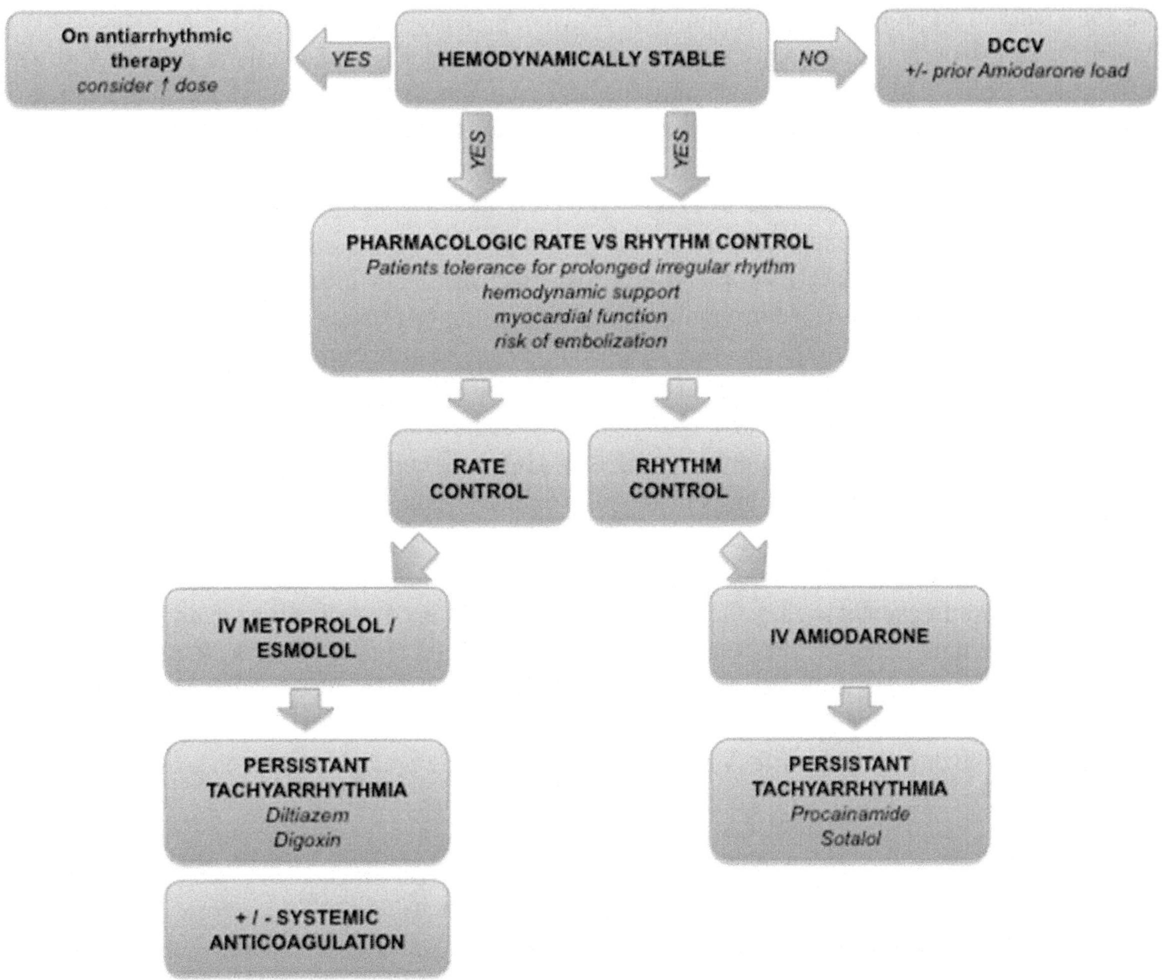

by an amiodarone bolus can have a positive effect on the success of cardioversion and maintenance of sinus rhythm. If the patient is hemodynamically stable, the intensivist can decide between rate control versus chemical rhythm control. This depends on the patient's comorbidities and the ability to tolerate prolonged loss of atrial contraction. In the majority of cases POAF is transient, and not every patient needs cardioversion. Especially when the risk of for intracardiac thrombus is high, the need for cardioversion, whether chemically or electrically, should be carefully considered, and prior echocardiographic assessment for thrombus is warranted. Patients on beta-blocker therapy preoperatively should resume this as early as possible in the postoperative period. Beta-blockers are also the first line recommendation in patients who do not require immediate cardioversion, and do not have significant myocardial dysfunction or hemodynamic compromise. Given the impact of adrenergic stimulation on the etiology of POAF perioperatively, and the relatively benign pharmacologic profile of beta blockers, they are preferred over other rate-controlling agents like calcium-channel blockers or digoxin in the postoperative period. In patients with depressed ventricular function, amiodarone is considered a safer choice due less hemodynamic compromise. Amiodarone is also the drug of choice in the ICU, if chemical cardioversion is warranted. In comparison to other agents such as Sotalol, propafenone, or ibutilide, amiodarone has safer side-effect profile. However, amiodarone, as other antiarrhythmic agents, can induce TdP in patients with QT prolongation. Also, some clinicians hesitate to use amiodarone in patients with significant pulmonary pathology or after lung transplantation, due to the rare but major complication of pulmonary fibrosis with long-term administration (Fuster et al., 2006). When available, temporary atrial or ventricular pacing at higher rates can be attempted to improve CO by providing a regularly paced rhythm. In addition, when functional atrial wires are present, conversion to SR can be accomplished in patients with atrial flutter by rapid atrial overdrive pacing.

Ventricular premature beats (PVC's) and ventricular tachycardia (VT) are most often due to electrolyte, acid-base, or oxygenation abnormalities. In patients with pre-existing atrioventricular conduction abnormalities, atrial tachycardia with aberrancy should be in the differential diagnosis to VT, but most wide complex tachycardias are ventricular in origin (see figure 11). Intermittent PVC's and non-sustained VT's have not been shown to impact short or long-term outcomes, but complex and prolonged ventricular arrhythmias in patients with ventricular dysfunction are associated with increased morbidity and mortality (Chung, 2000). When persistent and associated with hemodynamic instability, evaluation for underlying graft dysfunction, ongoing myocardial ischemia, or reperfusion injury should be performed. When TdP occur in the postoperative period, QT-prolonging medications need to be considered as triggering agents as they are frequently used in the ICU. Some commonly used medications include amiodarone, atypical antipsychotics, haloperidol, sotalol, metoclopramide, and high doses of ondansetron. Another mechanism of ventricular tachycardia or ventricular fibrillation (VF) post cardiac surgery has been described as the R-on-T phenomenon. Caused by malfunction of a temporary pacemaker, an electrical stimulus delivered during the ventricular repolarization phase can precipitate sudden arrhythmias. Even though extremely rare, given the high frequency of postoperative temporary pacing, awareness of the phenomenon and appropriate management of temporary pacing is imperative. Due to myocardial tissue swelling and mechanical irritation, dysfunction of temporary pacemaker leads with loss of atrial or ventricular sensing is common in the early postoperative period. Therefore, daily testing of pacemaker sensing and pacing thresholds to avoid ventricular undersensing, and avoidance of asynchronous pacing or atrial pacing in the absence of an atrial lead is recommended (Schulman, Stecker, & Rozner, 2012).

Acute treatment of any ventricular arrhythmia is guided by the hemodynamic profile of the patient and the complexity and duration of the arrhythmia. Asymptomatic ventricular ectopies or tachycardia, especially when non-sustained, do not routinely need intervention, and will often resolve by optimizing electrolyte and acid-base homeostasis. Sustained ventricular tachycardia can be treated with lidocaine or amiodarone as first-line agents. Other drugs that can be utilized are procainamide and bretylium. TdP are best treated by immediate withdrawal of offending medications, normalization of hypokalemia if present, and administration of magnesium. If unresponsive, mexelitine can be used as an antiarrhythmic medication as lidocaine normally has little effect in TdP. For any VT or VF, atrial or ventricular overdrive pacing can be attempted when rates are slow enough, but electrical cardioversion or defibrillation following ACLS algorithms is the treatment of choice when the patient is in extremis or unresponsive to pharmacologic management.

Bradyarrhythmias and conduction abnormalities (see figure 11) during the postoperative period are often temporary. They are commonly caused by intraoperative ischemia and cold injury to the conduction system, adjacent tissue swelling, and nodal-blocking medications administered in the perioperative period. Certain procedures carry an increased incidence of postprocedural conduction abnormalities.

Aortic valve replacement is associated with hemorrhage, edema, and suture-induced injury of the atrioventricular node and bundle of His. Mitral valve surgery, especially when performed by transseptal approach, can interrupt the sinoatrial node. In addition, newer procedures, such as transcatheter aortic valve replacement (TAVR), are associated with increased risk of temporary and permanent AV-block and long-term pacemaker necessity due to mechanical irritation of the adjacent conduction system. Pharmacologically induced bradycardia is often due to sedatives like dexmedetomidine, beta-blocker therapy, or antiarrhythmic agents affecting the AV node such as amiodarone. Conversion to NSR can be followed by bradyarrhythias, especially when patients are treated aggressively with nodal-blocking agents in the setting of POAF. In situations with pre-existing conduction abnormalities, treatment of POAF can be particularly difficult, as tachy-brady arrhythmias can occur with pharmacologic management.

Management of bradyarrhythmias in the postoperative period is based on temporary pacing, and the majority of patients undergoing heart surgery have ventricular and/or atrial temporary pacing wires placed. Daily testing of pacemaker thresholds is part of routine pacemaker management, to assure appropriate function if arrhythmias occur. Temporary pacing in cardiac surgery patients is common, and as temporary pacing can add significant hemodynamic support, every intensivist should become familiar with the appropriate management of these mechanical devices. Most common pacing modes are atrial pacing in AAI, ventricular pacing in VVI, or dual-chamber pacing in DDD mode. When atrial leads are present and AV conduction is appropriate, atrial pacing is preferred, as atrial systole is maintained. Ventricular pacing does not depend on AV conduction, but loss of atrial contraction can cause profound hypotension in patients with diastolic dysfunction. Once out of the operating room, asynchronous pacing should be avoided as it can induce ventricular tachyarrhythmias. Prolonged presence of conduction abnormalities is suggestive of permanent structural damage, and when pacer-dependence exists, consultation with an electrophysiologist is warranted. Evaluation for permanent pacemaker necessity is usually warranted when heart block persists over 7 days postoperatively.

Pericardial Effusion and Tamponade

Cardiac tamponade after open-heart surgery is a rare but potentially life-threatening complication. While small residual pericardial effusions are common, hemodynamically compromising tamponade occurs in only up to 6% of cases (S. Price, Prout, Jaggar, Gibson, & Pepper, 2004). Development of unexplained low CO post cardiac surgery is suggestive of tamponade, especially when preceded by sudden cessation of significant initial postoperative mediastinal chest tube output. Clinical presentation of post cardiac surgery tamponade can differ from tamponade of other medical etiologies. As patients are often on hemodynamic support, and fluid collection can present as loculated effusions or clot in unusual locations, clinical signs may be subtle. Hypotension, significant SV-variation on arterial line tracing, equalization of intracardiac pressures, and signs of low CO with low SvO2 and end-organ hypoperfusion, are common indicators of cardiac tamponade. The diagnosis of tamponade is a clinical one, and only pericardial effusion with hemodynamic compromise meets the criteria. For diagnosis and further evaluation of the pericardial effusion and clot, echocardiography is the modality of choice. A complete echocardiographic examination includes assessment for compression of right atrial or ventricular chambers, changes in ventricular inflow suggestive of tamponade physiology, and looking for loculated clot or fluid collections in unusual locations.

Management depends on extent and acuity of hemodynamic compromise. Small effusions can cause tamponade physiology in the volume-depleted heart or in patients with baseline marginal myocardial function; whereas patients with normal ventricular function and adequate volume status may not show any signs of cardiovascular compromise. Initial temporizing management consists of aggressive fluid resuscitation and inotropic support. The decision for definitive treatment by surgical re-exploration should be made quickly, as re-exploration, especially when delayed, has been associated with increased length of hospital stay and morbidity (Čanádyová, Zmeko, & Mokráček, 2012). The extent of hemodynamic compromise, significance of tamponade physiology on existing low CO-state, and expected improvement with chest opening, guides the decision-making when evaluating the need for re-exploration.

Delayed tamponade has been described up to three months postoperatively. Risk factors include postoperative anticoagulation and overdose of anticoagulation, and post-pericardiotomy syndrome. Therefore, even in the seemingly stable patient with protracted time after cardiac surgery, signs of low CO should trigger suspicion and evaluation for cardiac tamponade.

Circulatory Arrest

The incidence of cardiac arrest after cardiac surgery ranges between 0.7 – 2.9%, with a survival-to-discharge rate described in 17 – 79%. The reason for good survival outcomes in this patient population is the high incidence of reversible etiologies of cardiac arrest, and the prompt identification and treatment of these in the cardiac ICU. The two most common etiologies are ventricular fibrillation and cardiac tamponade (Dimopoulou, Anthi, Michalis, & Tzelepis, 2001; Dunning et al., 2009). Therefore, unexplained cardiac arrest should always be thought of as tamponade until proven otherwise.

General management of cardiac arrest with BLS and ACLS has been extensively described and details would exceed the scope of this chapter (Neumar et al., 2010). However, with the unique etiologies of cardiac arrest in post cardiac surgery patients and the change in provider background specialty in the cardiac ICU's over the recent years, developments of specific cardiac advance life support (CALS) protocols have been advocated (see FIGURE 14) (Dunning et al., 2009; 2006). The goal is to optimize the management of cardiopulmonary resuscitation (CPR) specifically in regards to the post cardiac surgery patient, and train personnel without cardiac surgery background to be able to perform more invasive intervention and avoid delays in appropriate care, when needed.

Specific emphasis in cardiac advance life support is targeted at early defibrillation, adequate fluid resuscitation, cautious use of epinephrine, and emergent resternotomy for release of cardiac tamponade and for internal cardiac massage. Caution in the use of epinephrine is based on the common etiology of cardiac arrests in this specific patient population and the potential adverse effects of epinephrine with inappropriate use. As specific management of cardiac arrest from tamponade or arrhythmias rapidly restores CO, excessive epinephrine use results hypertension, tachycardia, and tachyarrhythmias. Early resternotomy and internal cardiac massage, both have shown to improve outcomes in cardiac arrest after cardiac surgery (Vanden Hoek et al., 2010). When performing CPR while an intraaortic balloon pump (IABP) is in place, recommendations are to change the trigger to pressure trigger mode, and to an asynchronous internal rate when no cardiac massage is performed for a prolonged time.

The utilization of extracorporeal membrane oxygenator (ECMO) for cardiovascular life support has shown improved survival in children. In recent years increased interest has been in the use of ECMO to support CPR (E-CPR) in the adult population, especially in patients with refractory cardiogenic shock or post cardiac surgery. Small studies and case reports show encouraging results, and increased application is seen in medical centers with significant experience in ECMO technology and its use, but further

Figure 14. Cardiac advanced life support (CALS) algorithm. VF = ventricular fibrillation; VT = ventricular tachycardia; PEA = pulseless electrical activity; CPR = cardiopulmonary resuscitation; DC SCHOCK = direct current defibrillation. (Adopted from: Dunning J, et al. EACTS guidelines of a patient who arrests after cardiac surgery. Eur J cardiothorac Surg (2009). Oxford University Press. doi:10.1016/j.ejcts.2009.01.033

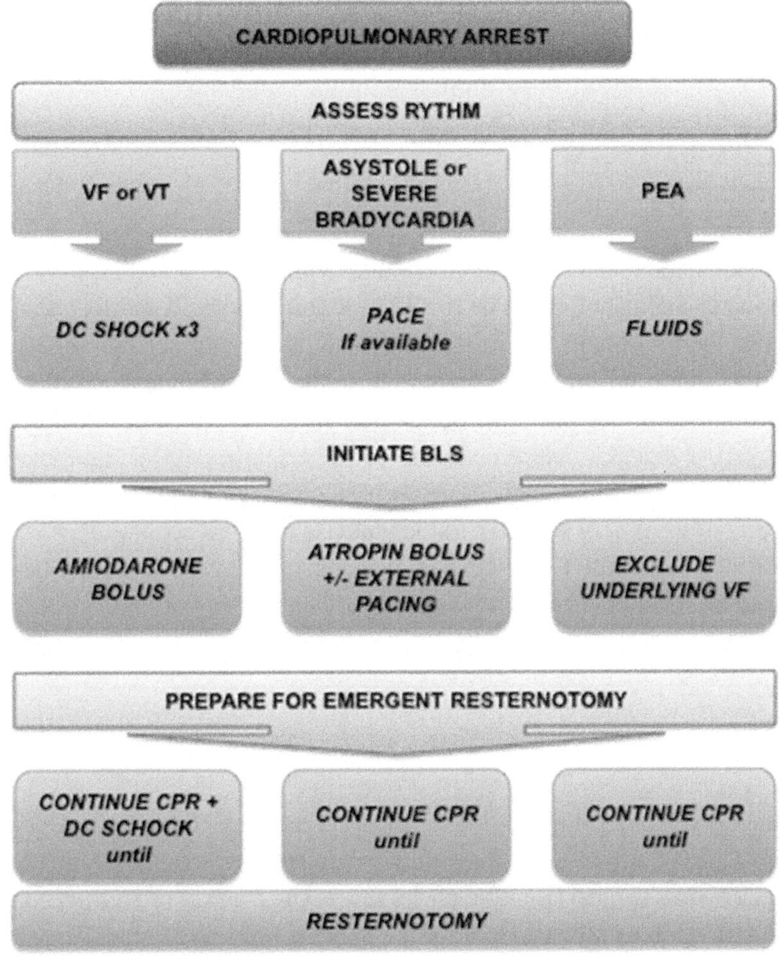

studies are warranted (Cardarelli, Young, & Griffith, 2009; Hsu et al., 2010; Thiagarajan et al., 2009). As ECMO carries significant risks for neurologic or bleeding complications, risk-benefit assessment, patient selection, and long-term outcomes need to be further evaluated before ECPR should be recommended on a broader scale.

Postoperative Open Chest

Postoperative open chest management (OCM) with delayed sternal closure (DSC) has been described for patients with significant postcardiotomy shock, mediastinal edema, and post orthotopic heart transplantation heart failure. More common in pediatric cardiac surgery, the incidence of OCM in the adult population is around 1.7%. Retrospective analyses have ameliorated initial concerns about increased morbidity and mortality due to increased sternal wound infections, and sternal closure usually occurs by POD 2 - 3.

Specific considerations for the management of OCM in the ICU focus on the hemodynamic optimization in anticipation of chest closure once cardiac swelling has improved. Sedation and analgesia, adjustment to ventilator strategies, hemodynamic stabilization, gentle diuresis for optimization of tissue edema, and prevention of infections directs the daily management. Many clinicians recommend broad-spectrum antibiotic coverage during open chest, and for the first 5 days post chest closure (Anderson et al., 2002; Takayama, Leone, & Aldea, 2006).

Heart Transplantation

Aside from the general hemodynamic management that applies to all post cardiac surgery patients, post heart transplantation management focuses on low CO secondary to bradycardia and on right ventricular graft dysfunction. As the transplanted heart is denervated, relative or absolute bradycardia is common and can significantly compromise left and right ventricular CO. Maintenance of heart rates between 90-110 is accomplished with temporary pacing or pharmacologic pacing, as needed. Pre heart transplantation, chronic left ventricular failure results in chronic changes of the pulmonary vasculature, and pulmonary hypertension is not uncommon. A newly transplanted RV, previously unexposed to elevated pulmonary artery pressures, is very sensitive to the increase in afterload as well as volume overload. As hemodynamics improve within the first couple of days postoperatively and mobilization of interstitial fluid occurs, the patient must be carefully evaluated for changes in volume status. Fluid management with maintenance of low cardiac filling pressures is pertinent to avoid graft failure during this time.

REFERENCES

Algarni, K. D., Elhenawy, A. M., Maganti, M., Collins, S., & Yau, T. M. (2012). Decreasing prevalence but increasing importance of left ventricular dysfunction and reoperative surgery in prediction of mortality in coronary artery bypass surgery: trends over 18 years. *The Journal of Thoracic and Cardiovascular Surgery, 144*(2), 340–6– 346.e1. doi:10.1016/j.jtcvs.2011.06.043

Algarni, K. D., Maganti, M., & Yau, T. M. (2011). Predictors of Low Cardiac Output Syndrome After Isolated Coronary Artery Bypass Surgery: Trends Over 20 Years. *Ats, 92*(5), 1678–1684. doi:10.1016/j.athoracsur.2011.06.017 PMID:21939957

Anderson, C. A., Filsoufi, F., Aklog, L., Farivar, R. S., Byrne, J. G., & Adams, D. H. (2002). Liberal use of delayed sternal closure for postcardiotomy hemodynamic instability. *Ats, 73*(5), 1484–1488. PMID:12022537

Apostolakis, E. E., Baikoussis, N. G., Parissis, H., Siminelakis, S. N., & Papadopoulos, G. S. (2009). Left ventricular diastolic dysfunction of the cardiac surgery patient; a point of view for the cardiac surgeon and cardio-anesthesiologist. *Journal of Cardiothoracic Surgery, 4*(1), 67. doi:10.1186/1749-8090-4-67 PMID:19930694

Bradley, D., Creswell, L. L., Hogue, C. W., Epstein, A. E., Prystowsky, E. N., & Daoud, E. G.American College of Chest Physicians. (2005). Pharmacologic prophylaxis: American College of Chest Physicians guidelines for the prevention and management of postoperative atrial fibrillation after cardiac surgery. *Chest, 128*(2Suppl), 39S–47S. doi:10.1378/chest.128.2_suppl.39S PMID:16167664

Čanádyová, J., Zmeko, D., & Mokráček, A. (2012). Re-exploration for bleeding or tamponade after cardiac operation. *Interactive Cardiovascular and Thoracic Surgery, 14*(6), 704–707. doi:10.1093/icvts/ivs087 PMID:22434857

Cardarelli, M. G., Young, A. J., & Griffith, B. (2009). Use of extracorporeal membrane oxygenation for adults in cardiac arrest (E-CPR): a meta-analysis of observational studies. *ASAIO Journal (American Society for Artificial Internal Organs: 1992), 55*(6), 581–586. doi:10.1097/MAT.0b013e3181bad907

Cecconi, M., Johnston, E., & Rhodes, A. (2006). What role does the right side of the heart play in circulation? *Critical Care (London, England), 10 Suppl 3*(Suppl 3), S5. doi:10.1186/cc4832

Chung, M. K. (2000). Cardiac surgery: Postoperative arrhythmias. *Critical Care Medicine, 28*(10Suppl), N136–N144. doi:10.1097/00003246-200010001-00005 PMID:11055682

Dimopoulou, I., Anthi, A., Michalis, A., & Tzelepis, G. E. (2001). Functional status and quality of life in long-term survivors of cardiac arrest after cardiac surgery. *Critical Care Medicine, 29*(7), 1408–1411. doi:10.1097/00003246-200107000-00018 PMID:11445698

Domanski, M. J., Mahaffey, K., Hasselblad, V., Brener, S. J., Smith, P. K., & Hillis, G. et al.. (2011). Association of myocardial enzyme elevation and survival following coronary artery bypass graft surgery. *Journal of the American Medical Association, 305*(6), 585–591. doi:10.1001/jama.2011.99 PMID:21304084

Dunning, J., Fabbri, A., Kolh, P. H., Levine, A., Lockowandt, U., Mackay, J., et al. (2009, July). Guideline for resuscitation in cardiac arrest after cardiac surgery. *European Journal of Cardio-Thoracic Surgery: Official Journal of the European Association for Cardio-Thoracic Surgery*. Oxford University Press. doi:10.1016/j.ejcts.2009.01.033

Dunning, J., Nandi, J., Ariffin, S., Jerstice, J., Danitsch, D., & Levine, A. (2006). The Cardiac Surgery Advanced Life Support Course (CALS): Delivering significant improvements in emergency cardiothoracic care. *The Annals of Thoracic Surgery, 81*(5), 1767–1772. doi:10.1016/j.athoracsur.2005.12.012 PMID:16631670

Echahidi, N., Pibarot, P., O'Hara, G., & Mathieu, P. (2008). Mechanisms, prevention, and treatment of atrial fibrillation after cardiac surgery. *Journal of the American College of Cardiology, 51*(8), 793–801. doi:10.1016/j.jacc.2007.10.043 PMID:18294562

Fuster, V., Rydén, L. E., Cannom, D. S., Crijns, H. J., Curtis, A. B., & Ellenbogen, K. A. et al.. (2006). ACC/AHA/ESC 2006 Guidelines for the Management of Patients With Atrial Fibrillation--Executive Summary. *Circulation, 114*(7), 700–752. doi:10.1161/CIRCULATIONAHA.106.177031 PMID:16908781

Haddad, F., Couture, P., Tousignant, C., & Denault, A. Y. (2009). The right ventricle in cardiac surgery, a perioperative perspective: II. Pathophysiology, clinical importance, and management. *Anesthesia and Analgesia, 108*(2), 422–433. doi:10.1213/ane.0b013e31818d8b92 PMID:19151265

Hsu, P.-S., Chen, J.-L., Hong, G.-J., Tsai, Y.-T., Lin, C.-Y., & Lee, C.-Y. et al.. (2010). Extracorporeal membrane oxygenation for refractory cardiogenic shock after cardiac surgery: Predictors of early mortality and outcome from 51 adult patients. *European Journal of Cardio-Thoracic Surgery: Official Journal of the European Association for Cardio-Thoracic Surgery*, *37*(2), 328–333. doi:10.1016/j.ejcts.2009.07.033 PMID:19748279

Licker, M., Cikirikcioglu, M., Inan, C., Cartier, V., Kalangos, A., Theologou, T., & Diaper, J. et al. (2010). Preoperative diastolic function predicts the onset of left ventricular dysfunction following aortic valve replacement in high-risk patients with aortic stenosis. *Critical Care (London, England)*, *14*(3), R101. doi:10.1186/cc9040 PMID:20525242

Licker, M., Diaper, J., Cartier, V., Ellenberger, C., Cikirikcioglu, M., Kalangos, A., & Bendjelid, K. et al. (2012). Clinical review: Management of weaning from cardiopulmonary bypass after cardiac surgery. *Annals of Cardiac Anaesthesia*, *15*(3), 206–223. doi:10.4103/0971-9784.97977 PMID:22772515

Luecke, T., & Pelosi, P. (2005). Clinical review: Positive end-expiratory pressure and cardiac output. *Critical Care (London, England)*, *9*(6), 607–621. doi:10.1186/cc3877 PMID:16356246

Lurati Buse, G. A., Koller, M. T., Grapow, M., Bolliger, D., Seeberger, M., & Filipovic, M. (2010). The prognostic value of troponin release after adult cardiac surgery - a meta-analysis. *European Journal of Cardio-Thoracic Surgery: Official Journal of the European Association for Cardio-Thoracic Surgery*, *37*(2), 399–406. doi:10.1016/j.ejcts.2009.05.054 PMID:19699102

Maganti, M., Badiwala, M., Sheikh, A., Scully, H., Feindel, C., David, T. E., & Rao, V. (2010). Predictors of low cardiac output syndrome after isolated mitral valve surgery. *The Journal of Thoracic and Cardiovascular Surgery*, *140*(4), 790–796. doi:10.1016/j.jtcvs.2009.11.022 PMID:20152992

Maganti, M. D., Rao, V., Borger, M. A., Ivanov, J., & David, T. E. (2005). Predictors of low cardiac output syndrome after isolated aortic valve surgery. *Circulation*, *112*(9Suppl), I448–I452. doi:10.1161/CIRCULATIONAHA.104.526087 PMID:16159861

Maisel, W. H., Rawn, J. D., & Stevenson, W. G. (2001). Atrial fibrillation after cardiac surgery. *Annals of Internal Medicine*, *135*(12), 1061–1073. doi:10.7326/0003-4819-135-12-200112180-00010 PMID:11747385

Marik, P. E., Baram, M., & Vahid, B. (2008). Does central venous pressure predict fluid responsiveness? A systematic review of the literature and the tale of seven mares. *Chest*, *134*(1), 172–178. doi:10.1378/chest.07-2331 PMID:18628220

Marik, P. E., Monnet, X., & Teboul, J.-L. (2011). Hemodynamic parameters to guide fluid therapy. *Annals of Intensive Care*, *1*(1), 1. doi:10.1186/2110-5820-1-1 PMID:21906322

Mebazaa, A., Karpati, P., Renaud, E., & Algotsson, L. (2004). Acute right ventricular failure--from pathophysiology to new treatments. *Intensive Care Medicine*, *30*(2), 185–196. doi:10.1007/s00134-003-2025-3 PMID:14618229

Michard, F., & Teboul, J. L. (2000). Using heart-lung interactions to assess fluid responsiveness during mechanical ventilation. *Critical Care (London, England)*, *4*(5), 282–289. doi:10.1186/cc710 PMID:11094507

Moussa, I. D., Klein, L. W., Shah, B., Mehran, R., Mack, M. J., Brilakis, E. S., ... (2013). Consideration of a new definition of clinically relevant myocardial infarction after coronary revascularization: an expert consensus document from the Society for Cardiovascular Angiography and Interventions (SCAI). (Vol. 62, pp. 1563–1570). doi:10.1016/j.jacc.2013.08.720

Neumar, R. W., Otto, C. W., Link, M. S., Kronick, S. L., Shuster, M., Callaway, C. W., & Morrison, L. J. et al. (2010). Part 8: adult advanced cardiovascular life support: 2010 American Heart Association Guidelines for Cardiopulmonary Resuscitation and Emergency Cardiovascular Care. *Circulation*, *122*(18Suppl 3), S729–S767. doi:10.1161/CIRCULATIONAHA.110.970988 PMID:20956224

Peretto, G., Durante, A., Limite, L. R., & Cianflone, D. (2014). Postoperative arrhythmias after cardiac surgery: Incidence, risk factors, and therapeutic management. *Cardiology Research and Practice*, (3): 615987–15. doi:10.1155/2014/615987 PMID:24511410

Petäjä, L., Salmenperä, M., Pulkki, K., & Pettilä, V. (2009). Biochemical injury markers and mortality after coronary artery bypass grafting: A systematic review. *The Annals of Thoracic Surgery*, *87*(6), 1981–1992. doi:10.1016/j.athoracsur.2008.12.063 PMID:19463650

Price, L. C., Wort, S. J., Finney, S. J., Marino, P. S., & Brett, S. J. (2010). Pulmonary vascular and right ventricular dysfunction in adult critical care: current and emerging options for management: a systematic literature review. *Critical Care (London, England)*, *14*(5), R169. doi:10.1186/cc9264 PMID:20858239

Price, S., Prout, J., Jaggar, S. I., Gibson, D. G., & Pepper, J. R. (2004). "Tamponade" following cardiac surgery: Terminology and echocardiography may both mislead. *European Journal of Cardio-Thoracic Surgery: Official Journal of the European Association for Cardio-Thoracic Surgery*, *26*(6), 1156–1160. doi:10.1016/j.ejcts.2004.08.020 PMID:15541977

Ramsay, J. G., Ralley, F. E., Whalley, D. G., DelliColli, P., & Wynands, J. E. (1985). Site of temperature monitoring and prediction of afterdrop after open heart surgery. *Canadian Anaesthetists' Society Journal*, *32*(6), 607–612. doi:10.1007/BF03011406 PMID:3878219

Rasmussen, C., Thiis, J. J., Clemmensen, P., Efsen, F., Arendrup, H. C., & Saunamäki, K. et al.. (1997). Significance and management of early graft failure after coronary artery bypass grafting: Feasibility and results of acute angiography and re-re-vascularization. *European Journal of Cardio-Thoracic Surgery: Official Journal of the European Association for Cardio-Thoracic Surgery*, *12*(6), 847–852. doi:10.1016/S1010-7940(97)00268-6 PMID:9489868

Schulman, P. M., Stecker, E. C., & Rozner, M. A. (2012). R-on-T and cardiac arrest from dual-chamber pacing without an atrial lead. *Heart Rhythm: the Official Journal of the Heart Rhythm Society*, *9*(6), 970–973. doi:10.1016/j.hrthm.2012.01.023 PMID:22300663

Shanmugam, G. (2005). Vasoplegic syndrome--the role of methylene blue. *European Journal of Cardio-Thoracic Surgery: Official Journal of the European Association for Cardio-Thoracic Surgery*, *28*(5), 705–710. doi:10.1016/j.ejcts.2005.07.011 PMID:16143539

Sidebotham, McKee, Gillham, & Levy. (2007). *Cardiothoracic Critical Care*. Elsevier Health Sciences.

Society of Thoracic Surgeons Blood Conservation Guideline Task Force, Ferraris, V. A., Ferraris, S. P., Saha, S. P., Hessel, E. A., Haan, C. K., et al. (2007, May). Perioperative blood transfusion and blood conservation in cardiac surgery: The Society of Thoracic Surgeons and The Society of Cardiovascular Anesthesiologists clinical practice guideline. *The Annals of Thoracic Surgery*. doi:10.1016/j.athoracsur.2007.02.099

Takayama, H., Leone, R. J., & Aldea, G. S. (2006). *Open-chest management after heart transplantation*. Texas Heart Institute.

Thiagarajan, R. R., Brogan, T. V., Scheurer, M. A., Laussen, P. C., Rycus, P. T., & Bratton, S. L. (2009). Extracorporeal membrane oxygenation to support cardiopulmonary resuscitation in adults. *The Annals of Thoracic Surgery*, *87*(3), 778–785. doi:10.1016/j.athoracsur.2008.12.079 PMID:19231388

Thygesen, K., Alpert, J. S., Jaffe, A. S., Simoons, M. L., Chaitman, B. R., White, H. D., ... (2012). Third universal definition of myocardial infarction. (Vol. 126, pp. 2020–2035). doi:10.1161/CIR.0b013e31826e1058

Vanden Hoek, T. L., Morrison, L. J., Shuster, M., Donnino, M., Sinz, E., Lavonas, E. J., & Gabrielli, A. et al. (2010). Part 12: cardiac arrest in special situations: 2010 American Heart Association Guidelines for Cardiopulmonary Resuscitation and Emergency Cardiovascular Care. *Circulation*, *122*(18Suppl 3), S829–S861. doi:10.1161/CIRCULATIONAHA.110.971069 PMID:20956228

Chapter 17
Acute Kidney Injury following Cardiac Surgery

Bryan Romito
University of Texas Southwestern Medical Center, USA

Joseph Meltzer
David Geffen School of Medicine at UCLA, USA

ABSTRACT

The primary goal of this chapter is to provide the reader with an overview of basic renal physiology and function and to review the identification, pathogenesis, and treatment of acute kidney injury following cardiac surgery. Particular focus will be directed toward the diagnostic criteria for acute kidney injury, short- and long-term impacts on patient outcomes, role of novel biomarkers, mechanisms of acute renal injury, general management principles, preventative strategies, and the influence of anesthetic and surgical techniques on its development. The content of this chapter will serve to underscore a particularly harmful but likely underappreciated problem affecting patients in the cardiothoracic critical care setting.

INTRODUCTION

Fundamental critical care principles include early recognition, stabilization, and prevention of secondary injury. Especially given the aging cardiac surgical population and the heavy burden of coexisting disease this cohort carries, following these tenants is essential to avoid poor outcomes. Consequently this chapter will primarily focus on the early diagnosis, anticipation, and management of acute kidney injury following cardiac surgery. The specific aim is to highlight established prevention strategies and draw attention to emerging diagnostic tools and therapeutic agents.

BACKGROUND

The development of acute kidney injury following cardiac surgery is common and contributes to considerable patient morbidity, mortality, and resource utilization. Given the increasing number of cardiac

DOI: 10.4018/978-1-4666-8603-8.ch017

surgical procedures performed and the substantial burden of comorbid disease in this patient population, the search for early markers of injury, specific prevention practices, new pharmacologic therapies, and timely management methods is essential. In line with ongoing research efforts, the future of disease management lies in the avoidance of medications, physiologic states, and iatrogenic procedures that promote renal injury in the perioperative period. Furthermore, the investigation into innovative therapies to prevent injury at the cellular and molecular levels represents the next phase of treatment.

RENAL ANATOMY AND PHYSIOLOGY

The Nephron

The kidney has a number of important physiologic functions including balancing electrolytes to maintain cardiovascular stability and prevention of dysrhythmias; preserving volume status through the regulation of salt and water; maintaining pH by regulating acid-base status for the appropriate functioning of medications, enzymes, and cells; eliminating drug metabolites and toxins; and production of renin, erythropoietin, and calcitriol.

The nephron is the functional unit of the kidney, and each kidney contains approximately 1 million nephrons. The proximal end of the nephron consists of Bowman's capsule surrounding a glomerulus, a network of capillaries supplied by an afferent arteriole and drained by an efferent arteriole. Collectively, this unit is known as the renal corpuscle. The basement membranes of the glomerular endothelial cells form a filter that prevents charged molecules, large proteins, and cells from entering the nephron while allowing ions, amino acids, and water to freely pass. Fluid is initially absorbed from the glomerulus into Bowman's capsule and then subsequently flows through the proximal tubule, loop of Henle, distal tubule, and finally to the collecting duct (see Figure 1). In the proximal tubule, as sodium and water are reabsorbed, organic anions and cations are secreted. Other molecules and ions transported here include glucose, proteins, amino acids, bicarbonate, chloride, potassium, magnesium, calcium, and lactate. Next fluid travels to the loop of Henle where it becomes concentrated, creating a gradient that allows for additional fluid reabsorption via osmosis further down the nephron. Also in the loop of Henle, sodium, chloride, potassium, calcium, and magnesium are reabsorbed. The initial segment of the distal tubule, called the macula densa, functions primarily to monitor the chloride concentration of the passing fluid. Based on this concentration, the macula densa alters afferent arteriolar tone and renin release to regulate changes in the glomerular filtration rate (GFR). The distal tubule also reabsorbs and secretes electrolytes and regulates acid-base status by adjusting the fluid's hydrogen ion and bicarbonate concentration. Finally as the fluid enters the collecting duct, the concentration gradient created by the loop of Henle allows for further water reabsorption and the formation of hypertonic urine (Loutzenhiser, Griffin, Williamson, & Bidani, 2006).

Renal Blood Flow

The combined blood flow through the kidneys consists of approximately 25% of the total cardiac output.

Each kidney typically receives its blood supply from a single renal artery, a branch off the aorta and is drained by a single renal vein which empties into the inferior vena cava. The difference in pressure between the renal artery and renal vein creates a transrenal pressure gradient, which drives the perfusion

Figure 1. Structure of the nephron.
Adapted with permission from: Melican, K., Sandoval, R. M., Kader, A., Josefsson, L., Tanner, G. A., Molitoris, B. A., & Richter-Dahlfors, A. (2011). Uropathogenic Escherichia coli P and Type 1 Fimbriae Act in Synergy in a Living Host to Facilitate Renal Colonization Leading to Nephron Obstruction. PLoS Pathogens, 7(2), e1001298.

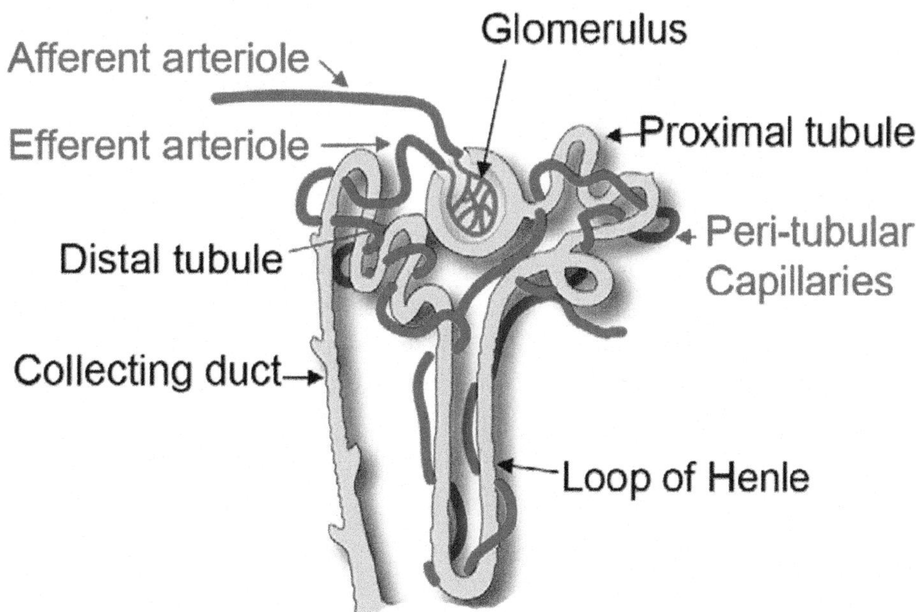

of the kidney. Approximately 90% of the total renal blood flow (RBF) perfuses the renal cortex and the cortical nephrons, while only 10% of the RBF perfuses the renal medulla and the juxtamedullary nephrons. This anatomic arrangement makes the renal medulla relatively vulnerable to ischemic injury in times of decreased perfusion. Autoregulation of RBF is accomplished by intrinsic fluctuations in the resistance of the afferent glomerular arterioles in response to arterial pressure changes. This autoregulatory mechanism acts to maintain kidney perfusion when mean arterial blood pressure (MAP) ranges from approximately 50 -150 mmHg in normotensive individuals (Loutzenhiser et al., 2006).

Glomerular Filtration Rate

The glomerular filtration rate is defined as the rate of fluid filtration from the glomerulus into Bowman's capsule, and it is the most commonly used measurement of renal function. GFR is ideally measured from the renal clearance of inulin, which is freely filtered but not reabsorbed or secreted by the renal tubule. It is more practical to estimate GFR using creatinine clearance; however, this measurement is somewhat less accurate as there is some secretion of creatinine by renal tubules and a number of physiologic factors influence creatinine levels. For this reason, the commonly used equations to estimate GFR incorporate serum creatinine concentration along with other characteristics including age, gender, weight, and race (National Kidney Foundation, 2014).

The normal value of GFR is reported as 120 mL/min in men and 100 mL/min in women, but body surface area and age can also affect this value. Typically the greater the body surface area, the greater the kidney size, function, and GFR. GFR decreases with increasing age at a rate of approximately 1% with each decade after age 20, thought secondary to age-related loss of native kidney function. Additionally it must be noted that with advancing age, there are also likely significant comorbidities present that negatively affect kidney function, such as atherosclerosis and diabetes (National Kidney Foundation, 2014).

Normally afferent arteriolar dilation or efferent arteriolar constriction will increase GFR. If renal blood flow is compromised, then autoregulation of the afferent and efferent arteriolar tone will attempt to maintain GFR. The afferent arterioles contain juxtaglomerular cells that produce renin, which increases afferent arteriolar pressure to maintain renal blood flow. As a result, if a decrease in systemic blood pressure results in decreased renal blood flow, then renin production will be stimulated. Ultimately, renin is released in response to β-adrenergic stimulation, decreases in afferent arteriolar pressure, or decreases in chloride flow past the macula densa. Once released, renin cleaves angiotensinogen to angiotensin I, which is subsequently converted by angiotensin converting enzyme (ACE) to angiotensin II in the lungs. Angiotensin II acts to increase water intake, vasoconstriction, and sodium and water retention, thus increasing blood pressure, renal perfusion, and GFR. It is important to note that when MAP falls below the lower limit of autoregulation (typically 50 mmHg), GFR can cease (National Kidney Foundation, 2014).

ACUTE KIDNEY INJURY

Incidence and Disease Burden

Following sepsis, the use of cardiopulmonary bypass (CPB) for cardiac surgery is the second most common cause of acute kidney injury in the intensive care unit (ICU) (Vives, Wijeysundera, & Rao, 2014). Depending on the definition used and specific population studied, acute kidney injury (AKI) occurs in 2-40% of patients undergoing cardiac surgical procedures (Lenihan, Montez-Rath, Mora Mangano, Chertow, & Winkelmayer, 2013; Dardashti, Ederoth, Algotsson, Bronden, & Bjursten, 2013).

For patients who develop severe forms of AKI, the reported mortality incidence varies widely but can range from 35-83%. By comparison, the reported mortality for post-coronary artery bypass graft (CABG) patients who do not develop AKI is less than 3% (Dasta, Kane-Gill, Durtschi, Pathak, & Kellum, 2008). When the AKI is severe enough to require renal replacement therapy (RRT), the mortality can reach as high as 90% (Lenihan et al., 2013; Dasta et al., 2008). Furthermore, patients who require RRT postoperatively may experience doubling of their postoperative costs and tripling of their ICU costs (Mariscalco, Lorusso, Dominici, Renzulli, & Sala, 2011). Analyzing statistics from the Nationwide Inpatient Sample (a random sample of roughly 20% of all community hospitals in the United States that participate in the Healthcare Cost and Utilization Project) for the years 1999 to 2008 revealed that the inpatient mortality of cardiac surgery-associated AKI (CSA-AKI) was 12.8% and CSA-AKI requiring dialysis was 35.3% (Lenihan et al., 2013).

Perhaps even more concerning than the rate of mortality in this population is the fact that the rate of postoperative AKI has increased over the period of 1999 to 2008. Whether this is the result of better diagnostic tools, a greater degree of awareness, a higher risk of patient selection, or a trend toward performing more complex surgical procedures, the presence of postoperative AKI following cardiac surgery remains a significant problem (Lenihan et al., 2013). The presence of CSA-AKI is also associated with increases in sternal wound infections, postoperative arrhythmias, length of stay, total cost, and both short- and long-term mortality (Billings et al., 2012). Even small, transient impairments in renal function are associated with increased mortality. In these patients the risk of death may remain increased for up to 10 years, even if the serum creatinine returns to baseline by the time of hospital discharge. Finally, both the severity (as measured by peak serum creatinine concentration) and duration of AKI following cardiac surgery directly reduce mortality (Brown, Kramer, Coca, & Parikh, 2010). Specifically it has been independently associated with an eight-fold increase in the odds of death at 30 days (Billings et al., 2012).

Defining Acute Kidney Injury

There are a number of classification systems used for defining and quantifying the degree of AKI. Presently, the most commonly used definitions are the Risk/Injury/Failure/Loss/End-Stage (RIFLE) criteria and the AKI Network (AKIN) classification (see Figure 2) (Bastin et al., 2013). The RIFLE criteria was developed by the Acute Dialysis Quality Initiative (ADQI) group and includes three progressive stages of injury (Risk, Injury, Failure) and two outcome categories (Loss, End Stage Renal Disease). The three stages are defined on the basis of either urine output or changes in the serum creatinine, whichever is worse. The two outcome categories are defined by the duration of the loss of renal function (KDIGO, 2012). Patients should be staged according to whichever criterion gives them the highest stage. The RIFLE criteria are widely used and have been validated as a tool for diagnosing the development of AKI following cardiac surgery.

The AKIN classification is a simplified version of the RIFLE definition that has recently emerged as an alternative to the established RIFLE criteria (Stafford-Smith, Shaw, & Swaminathan, 2009). Multiple studies have shown that both the RIFLE and AKIN classifications are valid tools that can be

Figure 2. RIFLE and AKIN classifications.
Reproduced with permission from: Cruz, D. N., Ricci, Z., & Ronco, C. (2009). Clinical review: RIFLE and AKIN – time for reappraisal. Critical Care, 13(3), 211.

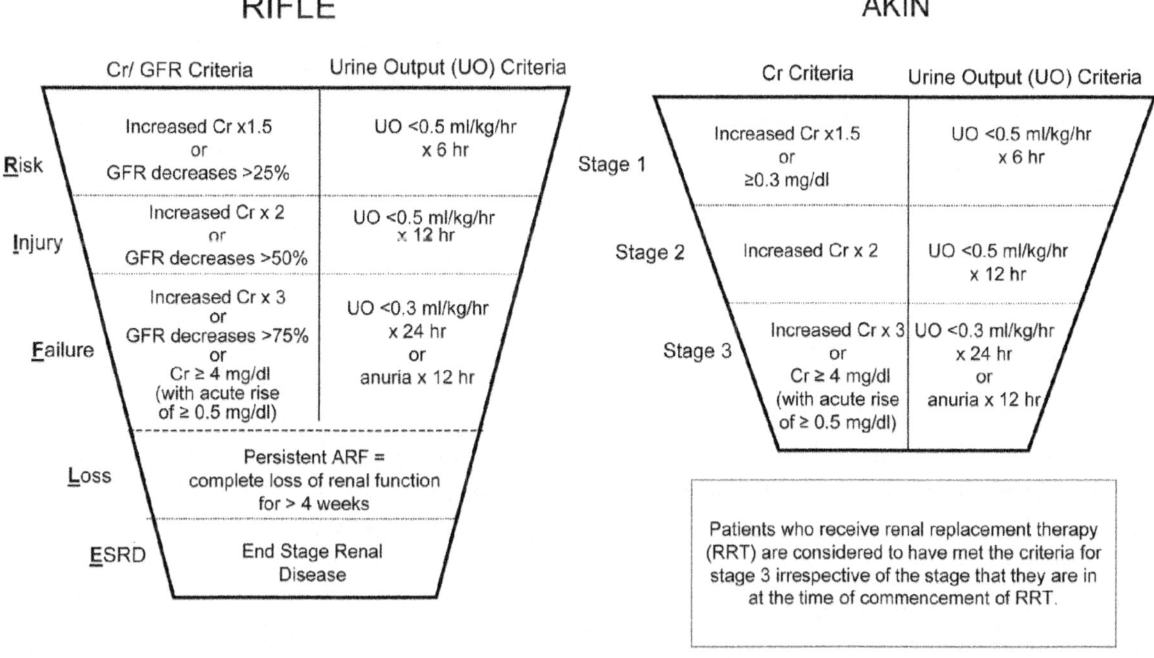

used to identify patients with AKI after cardiac surgery, with one offering little advantage over the other (Bastin et al., 2013). In the hopes of creating one universal classification scheme, the Kidney Disease: Improving Global Outcomes (KDIGO) initiative formulated the KDIGO classification in 2012, which is a combination of the RIFLE and AKIN criteria (KDIGO, 2012). In a recently published single center cohort study of post-cardiac surgery patients comparing the use of the KDIGO classification with the AKIN and RIFLE criteria, the authors found no difference in patient classification when using either the KDIGO or AKIN criteria. In this study however, the AKIN criteria correlated better with hospital mortality than the RIFLE classification (KDIGO, 2012). Both the RIFLE and AKIN criteria have been examined extensively and independently validated, and to date despite considerable research, there is no consensus as to which of these schemes should be routinely employed. Further studies are needed to evaluate whether the KDIGO classification is superior to these two established diagnostic standards.

BIOMARKERS OF RENAL INJURY

Given the substantial disease burden, there has been much interest in the search for biomarkers that may lead to the early identification of patients with CSA-AKI. Theoretically the ideal biomarker should be easy to measure noninvasively, highly-sensitive and specific for the early detection of CSA-AKI, readily quantifiable, and able to guide risk stratification (Wyckoff & Augoustides, 2012). While a number of potential candidates have been studied, the search for the biomarker that fulfills all of the above criteria remains ongoing. This section will review some of the markers that have shown promise in this setting.

Serum Creatinine

As previously mentioned, creatinine clearance is often used as an estimate of GFR; however levels are influenced by factors other than renal function, such as muscle mass, age, weight, and gender (Wyckoff & Augoustides, 2012). Although easily measured and often a component of routine electrolyte panels, creatinine has low sensitivity and specificity for the diagnosis of AKI. As such the use of serum creatinine alone as a biomarker for CSA-AKI will likely delay the diagnosis at least 24 hours or more following the initial period of renal injury (Wyckoff & Augoustides, 2012). Finally, increases in creatinine may be detected only after a substantial reduction in GFR. In this manner creatinine often reflects renal injury that has already occurred, rather than that which is ongoing (Haase et al., 2009).

Neutrophil Gelatinase-Associated Lipocalin (NGAL)

NGAL is a molecule that has been identified in neutrophils and is readily released by renal tubular cells in response to injury (Wyckoff & Augoustides, 2012; McIlroy, Wagener, & Lee, 2010). Of all of the biomarkers studied in CSA-AKI, NGAL seems to show the most promise. It is easily detected in the blood or urine as it undergoes little degradation (Wyckoff & Augoustides, 2012). Additionally, changes in NGAL levels occur rapidly, confirming its utility as a dynamic marker of the pattern of renal injury (Haase et al., 2009). There is evidence that even in the absence of serum creatinine elevations NGAL levels can detect subclinical AKI. In adults undergoing cardiac surgery, both elevated plasma and urinary NGAL levels significantly correlated with the risk of death, need for RRT, and prolonged ICU and hospital stays (Wyckoff & Augoustides, 2012). It has been reported that an acute elevation in urinary

NGAL can accurately diagnose ongoing AKI within 2-8 hours of cardiac surgery (McIlroy et al., 2010). However like many trials involving biomarkers, conflicting results have been reported. More recent studies have suggested that elevations in urinary NGAL levels are only able to accurately identify CSA-AKI in patients with normal baseline renal function (estimated GFR 90 -120 mL/min). Future trials are needed to clarify the impact of baseline renal dysfunction on the predictive value of urinary NGAL in this patient population (McIlroy et al., 2010).

Cystatin C

Cystatin C is a cysteine protease inhibitor that is normally synthesized by all nucleated cells. It is freely filtered by the glomerulus and released into the blood following renal injury (Wald et al., 2010). Like creatinine, plasma cystatin C levels can be affected by age and gender. Following cardiac surgery, cystatin C may be a better reflection of chronic kidney impairment rather than acute renal dysfunction (Haase et al., 2009). Although inferior to NGAL in terms of early identification of injury, plasma cystatin C has also been shown to independently predict the severity and duration of CSA-AKI within 24 hours of injury (Wyckoff & Augoustides, 2012). Note that combining cystatin C and NGAL increases their predictive value in this setting, although not enough to reach statistical significance (Haase et al., 2009).

Kidney Injury Molecule-1 (KIM-1)

KIM-1 is a transmembrane protein that becomes markedly elevated in renal proximal tubular cells after injury. Urinary values of KIM-1 have proven to be an early diagnostic marker for AKI (Liang et al., 2010). A recent meta-analysis evaluating the utility of urinary KIM-1 following cardiac surgery showed it to be a valid diagnostic marker, especially between 2-12 hours after CPB. The authors noted that, versus children, the accuracy of KIM-1 was lower in adults (Shao et al., 2014). One possible explanation for this finding is the notion that a number of comorbid diseases commonly found in adults undergoing cardiac surgery (hypertension, diabetes, and atherosclerosis) may influence the interpretation of KIM-1 levels (Shao et al., 2014). This feature may limit its usefulness as a diagnostic tool in high risk populations.

Interleukin-18 (IL-18)

IL-18 is a pro-inflammatory cytokine that is produced by macrophages and released into the urine following kidney injury. Multiple studies have shown that IL-18 levels may have useful prognostic value in the setting of CSA-AKI. Urinary IL-18 levels significantly predicted the risk of CSA-AKI and reached peak values within 6 hours after surgery. IL-18 was also found to correlate with risk of death, need for RRT, and prolonged ICU and hospital stay (Wyckoff & Augoustides, 2012). However as elevations in IL-18 are not specific for kidney injury, this biomarker may not be particularly reliable as the sole diagnostic test.

MECHANISMS OF INJURY IN CSA-AKI

The development of renal dysfunction following cardiac surgery likely involves the interplay between multiple pathologic injury mechanisms. A few of the most important contributors will be discussed in this section.

Immunologic

Immunologic pathways implicated include oxidative stress, systemic inflammatory response activation, endotoxin release, ischemia-reperfusion injury, and neurohormonal pathway activation (Moss & Lamarche, 2012; Haase, Bellomo, & Hasse-Fielitz, 2010). Some of these pathways are better defined than others. In particular, the foreign CPB circuit induces a global inflammatory response that results in renal interstitial inflammation with the subsequent development of tubular injury (Mariscalco et al., 2011). The institution of CPB may decrease renal perfusion by up to 30% via alterations in vasomotor tone (Vives et al., 2014). As AKI also occurs in the absence of CPB, there is little doubt that other mechanisms play important roles in the pathogenesis.

There is evidence to suggest that increased levels of oxidative stress may play a role in the development of AKI following cardiac surgery, as evidenced by increased intraoperative plasma concentrations of F2-isoprostanes, markers of systemic lipid peroxidation and oxidative injury (Billings et al., 2012). In experimental models, these compounds impair renal perfusion and promote cellular injury. They may also have diagnostic utility. When measured intraoperatively, elevated plasma levels of F2-isoprostanes may predict AKI after cardiac surgery; however, further studies are needed to explore the value of serum F2-isoprostane concentration as an early biomarker for oxidative stress or kidney injury (Billings et al., 2012).

Microemboli

CPB-induced microembolism release may also represent an important contribution to the development of CSA-AKI. Such embolic events have been diagnosed using transcranial Doppler techniques and have been found to be independently associated with postoperative AKI (Mariscalco et al., 2011; Moss & Lamarche, 2012). These emboli are often heterogeneous in composition and may be composed of fibrin and platelet collections, fat particles, cellular debris, and air (Vives et al., 2014). Due to their small size, they may not be effectively filtered by the CPB system. If present, they can directly injury the renal capillary beds and play a role in causing renal dysfunction.

Oxygen Supply-Demand Mismatch

Imbalances between renal oxygen supply and demand also contribute to the development of AKI following cardiac surgery. Reductions in cardiac output during the transition to and from CPB likely represent a time of renal hypoperfusion with the possibility for tubular ischemia (Hasse et al., 2010). Often encountered in the setting of cardiac surgery, anemia also reduces global tissue oxygen delivery. The renal medulla represents a particularly vulnerable area as the normal partial pressure of oxygen is very low in this region. In the setting of acute anemia from blood loss, dilutional effects, or reductions in cardiac output, this area may experience ischemic injury (Karkouti et al., 2009). This unique anatomical feature, coupled with the commonly associated perioperative conditions of renal vasoconstriction, hemodilution, and loss of pulsatile flow during CPB help to account for the high incidence of AKI following cardiac surgery (Moss & Lamarche, 2012; Mariscalco et al., 2011).

Hemolysis

The CPB circuit exposes red blood cells (RBCs) to excessive shear forces, promoting cell lysis. The resultant release of free hemoglobin and free labile iron molecules into the systemic circulation may directly injure tubular cells (Hasse et al., 2010; Mariscalco et al., 2011). Free labile iron has specifically been implicated in altering renal tubular function by inducing protein oxidation and free radical formation (Hasse et al., 2010). Normally when combined with haptoglobin, hemoglobin will be transferred to the liver to undergo metabolism. However in the presence of free radicals released during widespread systemic inflammatory responses or times of profound hemolysis, free labile iron will be released by hemoglobin into the circulation, where it can then directly induce kidney injury. In light of this mechanism, it has been shown that haptoglobin administration may have beneficial effects on hemolysis-induced renal injury. Furthermore, there is data from animal studies stating that the use of deferoxamine, an iron chelation agent, may provide some amelioration from iron-induced nephropathy in this setting (Hasse et al., 2010). Trials evaluating the effectiveness of deferoxamine for the prevention of AKI are ongoing.

Rhabdomyolysis

In a similar mechanism to RBC hemolysis, rhabdomyolysis-induced myoglobinemia following CPB may play a role in the development of postoperative AKI following cardiac surgery. Myoglobin is released following muscle injury and is rapidly cleared by the kidneys. Excessive myoglobinemia may further exacerbate ischemic injury to the proximal and distal tubules (Benedetto et al., 2010). Furthermore, the associated hypovolemia and acidemia that often accompany cardiac surgery only serve to magnify the negative effects of myoglobin on tubular cells. More studies are needed to explore the practical impact of rhabdomyolysis on postoperative renal function following cardiac surgery.

It is believed that these various mechanisms of injury together induce prerenal azotemia, adenosine triphosphate (ATP) depletion, free radical generation, complement cascade activation, renal medullary congestion with inflammatory cells, and ultimately renal tubular dysfunction (Moss & Lamarche, 2012; Mariscalco et al., 2011).

RISK FACTORS FOR CSA-AKI

Multiple risk factors for the development of CSA-AKI have been identified, and Table 1 highlights a number of these important perioperative considerations. Some of the potentially modifiable risk factors will be discussed in this section.

Anemia

The development of anemia in cardiac surgery is multifactorial, resulting from hemodilution from CPB priming solutions, intravenous fluid-associated dilution, coagulopathy, and surgical bleeding (Linden et al., 2011). Anemia reduces global oxygen delivery and can predispose to tubular ischemia. Despite the presence of normal serum creatinine values, many anemic patients have subclinical kidney dysfunction

Table 1. Perioperative CSA-AKI Risk factors

Preoperative	Intraoperative	Postoperative
Anemia	Anemia	Acute myocardial infarction
CHF	Aortic cross clamp duration	Anemia
CKD	Aortic dissection	Hypotension
COPD	Aprotinin	Hypovolemia
Depressed LV function	CPB duration	IABP
Female gender	Emergency surgery	Inotropes
Genetic predisposition	Hemodilution	Low cardiac output state
IABP	Hypothermic CPB	Nephrotoxic medications
IDDM	IABP	Packed red blood cells
Increasing age	Inotropes	Presence of an open chest
Inotropes	Microembolism	Rhabdomyolysis
Nephrotoxic medications	Need to restart CPB	Vasoconstrictors
Peripheral arterial disease	Nephrotoxic medications	
Tobacco use	Non-pulsatile flow on CPB	
	Oliguria	
	Packed red blood cells	
	Recent contrast exposure	
	Revision surgery	
	SBP hypotension	
	Surgery duration	
	Valvular or combined surgery	

CHF, congestive heart failure; *CKD*, chronic kidney disease; *COPD*, chronic obstructive pulmonary disease; *CPB*, cardiopulmonary bypass; *IABP*, intra-aortic balloon pump; *IDDM*, insulin-dependent diabetes mellitus; *LV*, left ventricular; *SBP*, systolic blood pressure.

and increased levels of oxidative stress (Karkouti, 2012). It has been reported that the nadir hematocrit during CPB is associated with postoperative renal injury, elevated serum creatinine values, and reductions in estimated GFR (Linden et al., 2011; Loor et al., 2012).

RBC Transfusion

As previously mentioned, while impaired oxygen delivery from anemia can lead to acute renal injury, so may the transfusion of packed RBCs for the correction of anemia. While the intent of RBC transfusion is to improve oxygen supply-demand ratios, the inherent characteristics of the red blood cells may contribute to the development of AKI (Moss & Lamarche, 2012). As their storage time increases, RBCs become depleted of ATP and 2, 3-diphosphoglycerate (2, 3-DPG), cellular energy sources necessary for proper function. During this time, red blood cells also accumulate both pro-inflammatory mediators and free iron molecules. Transfusion of these mediators may induce a systemic inflammatory response, increase the level of oxidative stress, and further exacerbate the effects of impaired oxygen delivery from the underlying anemia (Moss & Lamarche, 2012).

Systolic Blood Pressure Hypotension

Intraoperative isolated systolic blood pressure reductions below that of baseline values have been independently associated with the development of AKI following CABG as measured by elevations in postoperative serum creatinine concentrations (Aronson et al., 2013). This finding may suggest that, when feasible, intraoperative maintenance goals for both systolic and mean arterial pressure should be considered.

Timing of Surgery after Cardiac Catheterization

If the urgency of the procedure allows, it may be beneficial to avoid contrast administration (such as during cardiac catheterization) in close proximity to cardiac surgery, as these agents may induce renal medullary ischemia and glomerular cell injury (Mariscalco et al., 2011). Although there has been some conflicting data, cardiac surgery within 5 days of cardiac catheterization may increase the odds of developing AKI (Vives et al., 2014). The most recent (2011) update of the American College of Cardiology/American Heart Association guideline for CABG surgery recommends delaying surgery following coronary angiography in patients with baseline renal insufficiency (Ozkaynak et al., 2014; Hillis et al., 2011).

CPB Time

The duration of time spent on CPB is likely proportional to the complexity of the surgical procedure. An increased duration of CPB has been found to be an independent predictor of mortality and risk factor for the development of AKI following cardiac surgery. Although a threshold time beyond which complications are more likely to occur has not been clearly identified, results suggest that durations greater than 115 minutes may increase the risk CSA-AKI (Kumar, Suneja, Bayman, Weide, & Tarasi, 2012; Salis et al., 2008).

On Versus Off-Pump Procedures

The off-pump CABG (OPCAB) technique will avoid exposure to the extracorporeal CPB circuit, theoretically reducing the level of systemic inflammatory response. This practice may reduce the incidence of AKI, although the non-use of standardized definitions of AKI has made this outcome difficult to measure by meta-analysis (Bansal, 2012). As such there is conflicting data on the effectiveness of this technique on postoperative renal outcomes. At this time, its widespread adoption cannot be recommended, but it may be an option to consider in patients who are at particularly high risk of developing postoperative renal dysfunction (Vives et al., 2014).

IMPACT OF PHARMACOLOGIC AGENTS

Given the high degree of comorbid disease, potential for hemodynamic instability, and procedural complexity, patients undergoing cardiac surgery typically receive a number of pharmacologic agents in the perioperative setting. Not surprisingly, many of these medications can influence the development of postoperative AKI.

Angiotensin Converting Enzyme Inhibitors/ Angiotensin Receptor Blockers (ACEi/ARBs)

The preoperative use of these medications is associated with postoperative increases in serum creatinine levels following cardiac surgery (Coca et al., 2013). This may be a result of prolonged intraoperative hypotension induced by their negative effects on angiotensin II and also by the development of glomerular hypofiltration via angiotensin II inhibition of efferent arteriolar vasoconstriction. The use of these agents in the preoperative setting however, was not associated with the increase in four biomarkers that have become widely accepted as validated markers of structural kidney injury (urine NGAL, urine IL-18, urine KIM-1, urine L-FABP), nor a number of other outcomes such as length of ICU stay, length of hospital stay, or duration of mechanical ventilation (Coca et al., 2013). Despite the somewhat conflicting results, it may be prudent to withhold these medications preoperatively prior to cardiac surgery in order to decrease the risk of AKI, especially in higher risk patients. The risk of withdrawal of these medications must also be carefully considered, as they have been proven to provide long-term reductions in mortality in a number of patients.

Furosemide

In general, diuretics are not recommended for the prevention or treatment of AKI, with a possible exception being in the management of accompanying volume overload (KDIGO, 2012). In theory, use of the loop diuretic furosemide may decrease oxygen consumption in the loop of Henle and medullary tubular segments, thus reducing the magnitude of ischemic insults. Furthermore, loop diuretics may decrease recovery time in AKI by promoting the expulsion of debris that may obstruct renal tubules. Despite these theoretical benefits, there is evidence of harm associated with the administration of loop diuretics to prevent or treat AKI, and their use is not routinely recommended (Vives et al., 2014).

Mannitol

Mannitol is an osmotic diuretic that may increase renal blood flow, yet there is no conclusive evidence that it confers any benefit in the setting of AKI (Vives et al., 2014). In many centers, mannitol is added to the priming fluid of the CPB circuit in order to prevent postoperative renal dysfunction; however the results of this practice are not consistent as mannitol in this setting has not been proven to have any beneficial effects on any marker of renal function (Vives et al., 2014).

Dopamine

Low dose dopamine (at doses between 1-3 mcg/kg/min) will induce renal vasodilation and increase urine output; however, the use of dopamine has consistently failed to confer any renoprotection (KDIGO, 2012). There is convincing evidence that in the setting of AKI, dopamine offers no benefit, and may even be harmful, increasing renal vascular resistance, inducing tachyarrhythmias, and increasing the possibility for myocardial ischemia (KDIGO, 2012). Especially in the immediate post-cardiac surgery period, the development of tachyarrhythmias may be particularly concerning given the already increased incidence of atrial fibrillation in this patient population. For these reasons, low dose dopamine is not recommended either for the prevention or treatment of AKI.

Fenoldopam

Fenoldopam is a selective dopamine 1 receptor agonist that reduces systemic vascular resistance and increases renal blood flow (Zangrillo et al., 2012). There is evidence that receipt of a 24-hour infusion of fenoldopam may prevent AKI in patients at high risk for developing renal dysfunction. Fenoldopam may also confer protective anti-inflammatory effects independent of its vasodilatory action (Vives et al., 2014). A meta-analysis examining the effects of fenoldopam on AKI after cardiac surgery revealed that fenoldopam significantly reduced the risk of AKI; however, it was associated with a higher rate of hypotensive episodes and/or the use of vasopressors. Furthermore, it was found to have no effect on the use of RRT, hospital or ICU length of stay, or overall survival. Despite some inconsistency in the reported benefits, during cardiac surgery fenoldopam has been found to decrease the risk of AKI (Zangrillo et al., 2012). Given its propensity to induce hypotension it may have a limited role in the post-cardiac surgery population, where hemodynamic instability is not uncommon. Finally, there has not been consistent data from highly-powered multicenter trials to recommend its routine use for either the prevention or treatment of AKI (Vives et al., 2014).

Statins

Despite their reported reductions in inflammation and oxidative stress, statins have failed to consistently display any renal protection when given preoperatively to patients undergoing cardiac surgery using CPB. There may be a reduction in AKI rates in patients in which these medications are restarted early in the postoperative period (versus those patients in which they are withdrawn), although more studies are needed to clarify the potential benefit of statins in this setting (Bolesta, Uhrin, & Guzek, 2011).

N-Acetylcysteine

N-acetylcysteine (NAC) is a thiol-based compound that has been shown to reduce oxygen free radical production. It has shown promise as a beneficial therapeutic agent in both the setting of prevention of contrast-induced nephropathy and reduction of AKI rates following CPB in rat models. There is conflicting data, although multiple meta-analyses have shown that NAC is likely not beneficial for the prevention of post-cardiac surgery AKI. It is also not likely useful in reducing the need for RRT, ICU length of stay, or hospital length of stay. As such, its routine use is not recommended (Adabag, Ishani, Bloomfield, Ngo, & Wilt, 2009).

Sodium Bicarbonate

The use of sodium bicarbonate is controversial. It has been shown to be a scavenger of free radicals and may increase urine output. Furthermore, the urinary alkalinization associated with sodium bicarbonate administration may protect against some of the inflammatory mechanisms of injury implicated in CSA-AKI (Hasse et al., 2010). It has shown some benefit in this setting, as the perioperative use of a bicarbonate infusion reduced the incidence of AKI versus placebo; however, the pooled data do not support its routine use in the prevention of CSA-AKI (Stafford-Smith et al., 2009; Vives et al., 2014).

Nesiritide

Nesiritide is a recombinant form of brain natriuretic peptide that has been approved by the Food and Drug Administration (FDA) for the use of acute decompensated heart failure (KDIGO, 2012; Brown et al., 2008). It may improve both urine output and estimated GFR and may decrease the rise in serum creatinine, especially in patients with baseline renal insufficiency. Nesiritide may also have benefits in reducing hospital length of stay, the need for RRT, and both in-hospital and 30-day mortality. In a pilot trial examining its effects on patients undergoing cardiac surgery, nesiritide infusion during and after CPB improved serum creatinine values in a subset of patients with left ventricular dysfunction (KDIGO, 2012). Although there is potential therapeutic benefit to the use of nesiritide in cardiac surgery, to date the results are based on small studies, and further investigation is needed. Nesiritide is also not FDA-approved for this indication, so its use is not recommended.

Erythropoietin

Erythropoietin is a glycoprotein that is normally produced in the kidney that acts to control red blood cell production in the bone marrow. It may also have actions as an anti-inflammatory and anti-oxidant (Bock & Gottlieb, 2010). As reported in a recently published randomized control trial, when administered after cardiac surgery, erythropoietin did not significantly improve the incidence of AKI, urinary NGAL concentration, inflammatory cytokine levels, hospital stay, or mortality (Endre et al., 2010). However when given prophylactically prior to cardiac surgery for three days and at induction of anesthesia, compared to placebo, intravenous erythropoietin significantly reduced the incidence of cardiac-surgery associated AKI, mean ICU stay, and mean hospital stay (Tasanarong, Duangchana, Sumransurp, Homvises, & Satdhabudha, 2013). It also reduced postoperative increases in serum creatinine and decreases in estimated GFR. Finally, urinary NGAL levels were significantly lower than placebo at multiple early time points (Tasanarong et al., 2013).

There seems to be no evidence that the administration of erythropoietin following the development of AKI offers any protection from further injury or promotes earlier resolution of the injury already incurred, but it may have benefit when given early prior to cardiac surgery (Tasanarong et al., 2013). Given these results, further investigation into the proper timing of erythropoietin administration in cardiac surgery may provide valuable insight.

IMPACT OF ANESTHETIC AND SURGICAL MANAGEMENT

Although perhaps not classically considered risk factors for the development of AKI, there is emerging evidence that both the anesthetic and surgical technique can impact the degree of postoperative renal dysfunction following cardiac surgery.

Anesthetic Maintenance

Propofol binds to the gamma-aminobutyric acid (GABA) receptor in the central nervous system and is a widely used anesthetic agent. It possesses anti-inflammatory, anti-oxidant, and immune-modulating properties and has long been the subject of considerable research given these characteristics. Experimental studies have shown that propofol may be effective in reducing the incidence of AKI following ischemia-reperfusion injury (Yoo, Shim, Song, Yang, & Kwak, 2014). In patients undergoing valvular heart surgery under CPB, versus sevoflurane, anesthetic maintenance with propofol significantly reduced the incidence of postoperative AKI as measured by the AKIN criteria. Furthermore when AKI did develop, it did so to a less severe degree in the propofol group versus the sevoflurane group. The use of propofol was also associated with a smaller elevation in inflammatory mediators (interleukin-6, C-reactive protein) and cystatin C (Yoo et al., 2014). While previous studies of propofol in this setting failed to demonstrate a significant benefit, these recent results may be attributed to a higher target plasma concentration of propofol. These findings are particularly exciting given that CSA-AKI has few modifiable, anesthesia-specific risk factors.

Glycemic Management

Independent of the cause, hyperglycemia portends a poor prognosis in cardiac surgical patients. It can intensify the magnitude of ischemia-reperfusion injury, increase the oxidative stress response, promote endothelial dysfunction, and induce kidney injury (Song, Shim, Yoo, Oh, & Kwak, 2013). The use of CPB may further induce hyperglycemia by triggering insulin resistance and invoking a global systemic inflammatory response. Additionally, many of the cardioplegia solutions used during CPB contain high amounts of dextrose, which will only exacerbate intraoperative hyperglycemia (Song et al., 2013).

The precise range for optimal glycemic control in the setting of critical illness has not been clearly defined. Published in 2009, the landmark NICE-SUGAR study found that critically ill patients managed according to an intensive glucose target of 81-108 mg/dL had higher 90-day mortality than those patients managed according to a conventional glucose target of < 180 mg/dL, thought secondary to the development of hypoglycemia (NICE-SUGAR, 2009). Despite the known complications associated with hyperglycemia, in a study of patients undergoing OPCAB, the achievement of intensive intraoperative normoglycemia (< 110 mg/dL) was not associated with any reduction in the risk of renal dysfunction postoperatively (Song et al., 2013). While recommendations vary, in light of the current evidence authorities have suggested more liberal target glucose ranges of 110-149 mg/dL or 140-180 mg/dL (KDIGO, 2012; Bilotta & Rosa, 2012).

Transcatheter vs. Surgical Approach

As patients presenting for cardiac surgery have an increasing number of medical comorbidities, operative management of these high risk individuals has evolved. As such, transcatheter aortic valve replacement (TAVR) has emerged as an alternative to the classical surgical aortic valve replacement (SAVR). The transcatheter technique, while less invasive than its surgical counterpart, does require the administration of contrast dye, which is a known risk factor for the development of AKI (Nguyen et al., 2013).

When the degrees of postoperative renal dysfunction following these two techniques were compared, the patients who underwent the transcatheter approach had a greater increase in their postoperative glomerular filtration rate versus patients who underwent the surgical approach. In this study, the administration of contrast material during TAVR was not associated with increased rates of AKI or the need for RRT. Furthermore, postoperative renal dysfunction was associated with increased short-term and long-term mortality, hospital length of stay, and ICU length of stay in SAVR patients but not in patients undergoing TAVR (Nguyen et al., 2013). It is important to note that other results indicate that both the development of postoperative AKI and the need for RRT following TAVR seem to depend on the amount of contrast agent administered intraoperatively (Linden et al., 2011). The findings of these studies suggest that TAVR may be an especially attractive alternative to SAVR for the management of aortic valve disease in patients at a high risk for developing postoperative renal injury.

Off-Pump Coronary Artery Bypass

As mentioned previously, there has been a considerable amount of interest in the impact of OPCAB on postoperative renal function, as this technique eliminates the need for need for CPB. While the data has been inconsistent, the results of some studies suggest that the OPCAB procedure is a protective factor for AKI. The results of one particular observational study by Massoudy et al. (2008) reveal that not only did significantly fewer OPCAB patients develop AKI, but they also had lower peak serum creatinine values postoperatively. Although not significant, there was also a trend toward a reduced need for RRT versus those patients who underwent CABG on CPB (Massoudy et al., 2008).

Conversely, despite its theoretical benefits a number of studies of the OPCAB technique have not demonstrated a consistent renoprotective effect. Some authors argue that one possible reason for the large disparity among trials is that prior studies have included mostly patients with normal baseline renal function while patients with chronic kidney disease (those whom are likely to benefit most) constitute only a fraction of the study population (Chawla et al., 2012). In a large retrospective cohort study of patients with chronic kidney disease by Chawla et al. (2012), the OPCAB technique was associated with a reduction in a composite outcome of in-hospital mortality or the need for RRT. In this group of patients, the benefit derived from the OPCAB technique was inversely proportional to the baseline renal function. The results of this study suggest that OPCAB may be an attractive alternative to conventional CABG in patients with underlying renal insufficiency (Chawla et al., 2012).

PREVENTION AND TREATMENT OF CSA-AKI

Despite the long list of risk factors, unfortunately only a small number of these are modifiable from a management prospective (Karkouti et al., 2009). Additionally, there are no drugs that have consistently been shown to offer renal protection in this setting (Vives et al., 2014). Essential principles include avoidance of hemodynamic instability, minimization of CPB duration, early correction of anemia, prevention of unnecessary blood transfusion, avoidance of nephrotoxic medications, and possible postponement of surgery following contrast administration. As specific management options are somewhat limited, this section will primarily focus on strategies to reduce the development of CSA-AKI.

Perioperative Anemia Management

Like in other settings, the risks of tolerating a lower hematocrit have to be weighed against the risks of erythrocyte transfusion. Low intraoperative nadir hematocrit may be an independent risk factor for the development of AKI. Although the cut-off value has been a point of some debate, expert societies have recommended maintaining a hematocrit of at least 21% during CPB (Mariscalco et al., 2011; Karkouti,

2012; Vives et al., 2014). As preoperative anemia is an important risk factor for the development of low nadir hematocrits intraoperatively, interventions to correct anemia prior to surgery may ultimately decrease both the risk of developing postoperative AKI and those associated with red cell transfusion (Linden et al., 2011).

Preoperative approaches to help reduce the rate of intraoperative RBC transfusion may include early treatment with erythropoietin and iron, although there is conflicting data to support this (Karkouti et al., 2009; Vives et al., 2014). Prophylactically transfusing anemic patients 1-2 days before surgery may allow time for the kidneys to recover from the effects of the transfusion prior to being subjected to the negative effects of CPB (Karkouti, 2012). Intuitively, it is also likely beneficial to discontinue or avoid the use of any drug that may impair coagulation mechanisms (Karkouti et al., 2009). Other strategies include the minimization of hemodilution via careful volume replacement along with the administration of fibrinolysis inhibitors to minimize blood transfusions.

If possible, only administering blood products that have been stored for short durations may help to mitigate some of the negative effects of transfusion. During prolonged storage periods, red blood cells undergo a number of irreversible changes, including depletion of both ATP and 2, 3-DPG, which acts to alter the oxygen binding affinity of hemoglobin. Extended storage times also induce changes in the RBC membrane leading to accumulation of pro-inflammatory cytokines, reduced deformability, and the promotion of hemolysis. Another strategy for reducing transfusion-associated AKI includes washing of blood products to remove inflammatory mediators and free hemoglobin that may have accumulated during prolonged storage times (Karkouti, 2012).

Intraoperative Strategies

Maintaining stable hemodynamics, by preventing hypotension and achieving adequate global perfusion, is required to prevent end-organ ischemia. The use of positive inotropes may be needed to maintain cardiac output, especially given the high incidence of valvulopathy and impaired myocardial function in this patient population. If CPB is used, maintaining flows > $3L/min/m^2$ may help to prevent the development of AKI (Mariscalco et al., 2011). Avoidance of CPB or the use of pulsatile techniques can be beneficial as they may improve tissue oxygen delivery and creatinine clearance (Karkouti, 2012; Vives et al., 2014). As previously discussed, it may be prudent to advocate for an OPCAB technique in a patient who is at a high risk of developing postoperative AKI based on their degree of preoperative comorbidities and risk factors. Other intraoperative strategies include minimizing hemodilution from excessive crystalloid administration, the use of cell salvage techniques, and initial priming of the CPB circuit with autologous blood.

Postoperative Care

In general, the treatment of patients with AKI in this setting is primarily supportive (Lenihan et al., 2013; Dirkes & Hodge, 2007). Optimizing hemodynamics, correcting metabolic and electrolyte aberrations, ensuring proper intravascular fluid balance, and avoiding nephrotoxic agents are important management strategies in preventing further renal injury. Practically speaking, achieving these goals may involve beginning inotropic or vasopressor support, administering a fluid bolus, frequently treating abnormal serum chemistry values, changing antibiotic regimens, or initiating renal replacement therapy.

RENAL REPLACEMENT THERAPY

Background

In the setting of severe renal dysfunction, RRT should be initiated to avoid ongoing kidney injury and to maintain fluid, acid-base, and electrolyte homeostasis (KDIGO, 2012; Hall & Fox, 2006). During times of failure, the kidneys are no longer able to perform their normal functions of toxin excretion, solute balance, and maintenance of intravascular volume status. As such, the decision to begin RRT is usually based on clinical and laboratory features of volume overload, azotemia, severe acidosis, or life-threatening metabolic derangements (KDIGO, 2012; Moss & Lamarche, 2012; Hall & Fox, 2006). A detailed description of the subtypes of renal replacement therapy is beyond the scope of this chapter. In general, the modes of RRT commonly employed in the critical care setting include intermittent hemodialysis (IHD) and continuous renal replacement therapy (CRRT). Each of these methods has its own specific advantages and disadvantages, but neither mode provides mortality benefits over the other (Moss & Lamarche, 2012; Hall & Fox, 2006).

Intermittent hemodialysis rapidly removes solutes and volume via diffusion across a semi-permeable membrane. It is the most efficient mode of renal replacement; however the development of hypotension may preclude its use in critically ill patients already requiring inotropes or vasopressors. Furthermore, as treatments are episodic, the control of volume status and uremia can be inconsistent between dialysis sessions. IHD is considerably less expensive than CRRT and requires less of a staffing commitment (Dirkes & Hodge, 2007; Hall & Fox, 2006).

CRRT is a newer form of renal replacement therapy that can be considered a slower, more controlled variation of IHD. As its name states it allows for continuous solute, fluid, and electrolyte balance. This mode offers greater hemodynamic stability versus IHD as the rate of solute and volume clearance is reduced. CRRT requires a significant staffing presence and is more expensive than IHD. There are a number of subtypes of CRRT based on the mechanism of clearance, including continuous venovenous hemofiltration (CVVH), continuous venovenous hemodialysis (CVVHD), continuous venovenous hemodiafiltration (CVVHDF), and slow continuous ultrafiltration (SCUF) (Dirkes & Hodge, 2007; Hall & Fox, 2006). The general design of a CVVHD circuit is shown in Figure 3.

Renal Replacement Therapy in CSA-AKI

Kidney injury severe enough to require RRT develops in roughly 1-5% of patients, and as previously stated, the mortality can range from 50-90% (Lenihan et al., 2013; Dasta et al., 2008; Srivastava, D'Silva, Tang, Sogliani, & Ngaage, 2012; Muralidhar et al., 2013). This substantial risk of death is not transient, as patients who require dialysis in this setting have significant increases in both 1-year and 10-year mortality rates compared with those patients who do not develop AKI (Vives et al., 2014). Specifically 5-year survival rates can range from 27%-62%, depending on the baseline degree of renal dysfunction (Srivastava et al., 2012). While the mortality in this subset of patients is extremely high, it is unlikely that those with normal or even moderately-elevated baseline serum creatinine levels will require RRT upon discharge from the hospital following the development of AKI after cardiac surgery (Steinthorsdottir, Kandler, Windelov, & Steinbruchel, 2013).

There is controversy surrounding the timing of renal replacement therapy in critically ill patients. While conflicting data exists, earlier initiation of RRT following the development of AKI may offer survival

Figure 3. General design of a CVVHD circuit.
Adapted with permission from: Bellomo, R., Ronco, C. (2000). Continuous haemofiltration in the intensive care unit. Critical Care, 4, 339-345.

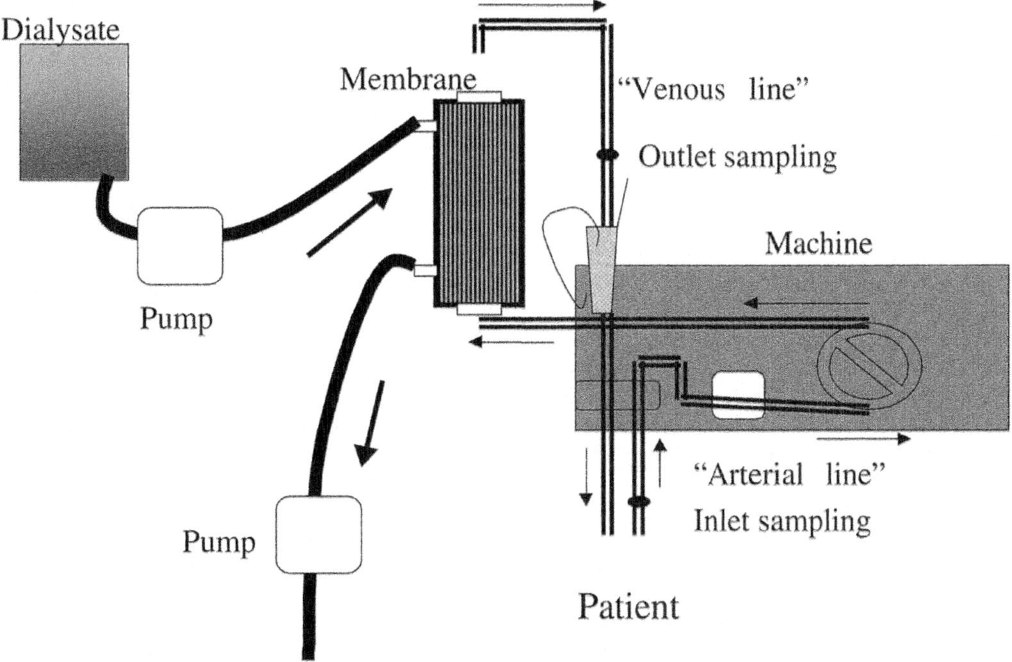

benefits, however no definitive treatment recommendations regarding the timing of RRT in this setting are available (Karvellas et al., 2011; Elahi, Asopa, Pflueger, Hakim, & Matata, 2009). In the absence of formal guidelines, a number of authors have proposed treatment algorithms to help guide management, and an example is shown in Figure 4.

FUTURE RESEARCH DIRECTIONS

Cyclin-Dependent Kinase Inhibitors

Cyclin-dependent kinases (Cdks) help to govern cell cycle progression between different phases and thus regulate cell growth, proliferation, and destruction. As such, Cdks have been the target of a number of anti-proliferative agents in cancer therapy (Fry et al., 2004; DiRocco et al., 2014). Progression through certain stages is dependent on the phosphorylation of specific proteins by different Cdks. PD 0332991 is a potent small molecule inhibitor of Cdk4/6 which, in animal studies, induces cell cycle arrest in renal epithelial cells and may offer protection from apoptosis, reducing further kidney damage following AKI. While PD 0332991 reduced inflammatory markers and macrophage infiltration into injured kidney tissue 72 hours after surgery in experimental settings, future studies are needed before such agents can be adopted into clinical practice (Fry et al., 2004; DiRocco et al., 2014).

Figure 4. A proposed algorithm for the initiation of RRT in adults.
Reproduced with permission from: Bagshaw, S. M., Cruz, D. N., Gibney, R. N., & Ronco, C. (2009). A proposed algorithm for initiation of renal replacement therapy in adult critically ill patients. Critical Care, 13(6), 317.

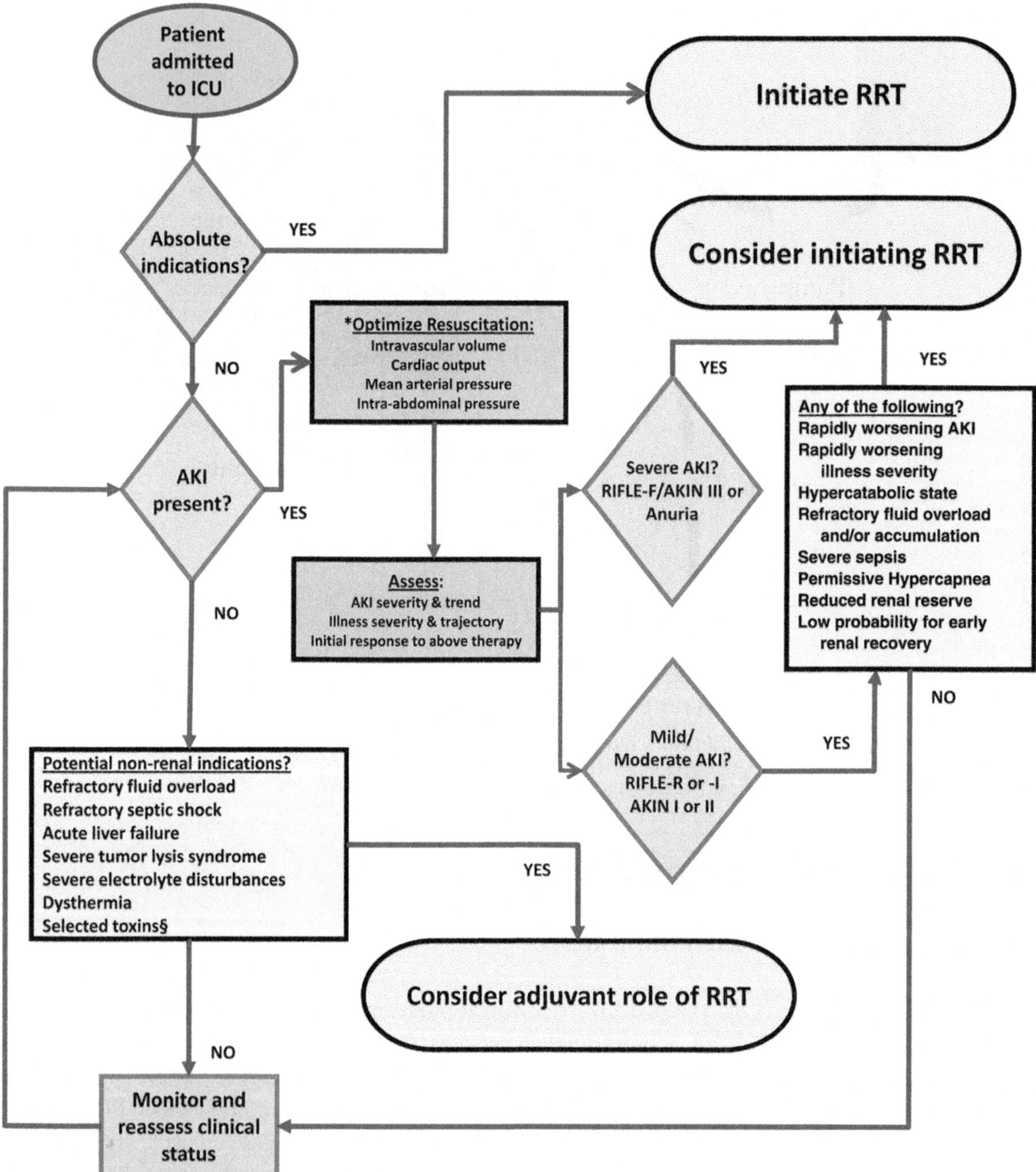

Phosphodiesterase Inhibitors

Phosphodiesterase (PDE) inhibitors prevent the breakdown of cyclic GMP (cGMP) and augment endogenous nitric oxide (NO) pathways. Preserved NO bioavailability may be renoprotective, promoting vasodilation and protecting against oxidative injury. In a post-CPB porcine model, intravenous administration of sildenafil, a phosphodiesterase-5 (PDE-5) inhibitor, prevented endothelial dysfunction, inflammation, and renal tubular alterations. In this study, sildenafil reduced post-CPB AKI as measured by creatinine clearance and the urinary biomarker IL-18 (Patel et al., 2011). Given these promising results, a safety and tolerability study evaluating the use of sildenafil for the prevention of post-cardiac surgery AKI in humans is presently ongoing.

Remote Ischemic Preconditioning

Remote ischemic preconditioning is a phenomenon whereby brief periods of distal limb ischemia and reperfusion confer systemic protection against periods of prolonged ischemia. Found in experimental studies to protect against myocardial ischemia, the precise mechanism of how this cascade works has not been conclusively identified but may involve a combination of neuronal, humoral, and anti-inflammatory pathways. Given its means of systemic attenuation of the inflammatory response, there are theoretical benefits in the prevention and treatment of AKI. Unfortunately, the results of a recently published randomized trial evaluating the effects of lower limb ischemic preconditioning on the development of AKI following complex valvular heart surgery failed to show any benefits in terms of reducing the

Figure 5. Potential mediators of remote ischemic preconditioning.
Adapted with permission from: Lim, S. Y., & Hausenloy, D. J. (2012). Remote Ischemic Conditioning: From Bench to Bedside. Frontiers in Physiology, 3, doi:10.3389/fphys.2012.00027.

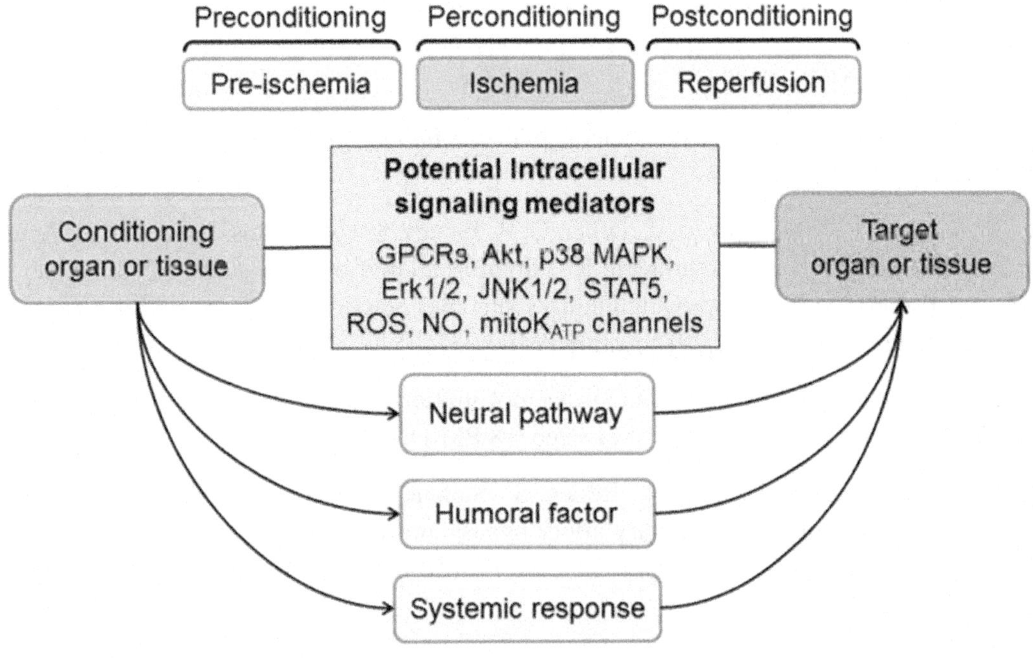

increase in NGAL and cystatin C levels (Choi et al., 2011). Despite these results, previous trials have demonstrated beneficial effects of remote ischemic preconditioning in this setting, and additional studies re-evaluating its utility may prove valuable. A diagram depicting the potential mediators of remote ischemic preconditioning is shown in Figure 5.

CONCLUSION

Despite considerable research effort, the development of acute kidney injury following cardiac surgery remains a frequently-occurring, highly-morbid complication. Following its development, patients also suffer increases in both short- and long-term mortality rates. Promising advances in markers of earlier detection and new prevention strategies, coupled with an increased level of awareness among practitioners, will allow for continued outcome improvement. Ultimately further investigation into novel therapies for acute kidney injury in this setting represents the next chapter of future management.

REFERENCES

Adabag, A. S., Ishani, A., Bloomfield, H. E., Ngo, A. K., & Wilt, T. J. (2009). Efficacy of N-acetylcysteine in preventing renal injury after heart surgery: A systematic review of randomized trials. *European Heart Journal, 30*(15), 1910–1917. doi:10.1093/eurheartj/ehp053 PMID:19282300

Aronson, S., Phillips-Bute, B., Stafford-Smith, M., Fontes, M., Gaca, J., Mathew, J. P., & Newman, M. F. (2013). The Association of Postcardiac Surgery Acute Kidney Injury with Intraoperative Systolic Blood Pressure Hypotension. *Anesthesiology Research and Practice, 2013*, 1–7. doi:10.1155/2013/174091 PMID:24324489

Bagshaw, S. M., Cruz, D. N., Gibney, R. N., & Ronco, C. (2009). A proposed algorithm for initiation of renal replacement therapy in adult critically ill patients. *Critical Care (London, England), 13*(6), 317. doi:10.1186/cc8037 PMID:19909493

Bansal, S. (2012). Post-surgical acute kidney injury. *Clinical Queries: Nephrology, 1*(1), 50–57. doi:10.1016/S2211-9477(11)70008-5

Bastin, A. J., Ostermann, M., Slack, A. J., Diller, G. P., Finney, S. J., & Evans, T. W. (2013). Acute kidney injury after cardiac surgery according to Risk/Injury/Failure/Loss/End-stage, Acute Kidney Injury Network, and Kidney Disease: Improving Global Outcomes classifications. *Journal of Critical Care, 28*(4), 389–396. doi:10.1016/j.jcrc.2012.12.008 PMID:23743540

Bellomo, R., & Ronco, C. (2000). Continuous haemofiltration in the intensive care unit. *Critical Care (London, England), 4*(6), 339–345. doi:10.1186/cc718 PMID:11123877

Benedetto, U., Angeloni, E., Luciani, R., Refice, S., Stefanelli, M., Comito, C., & Sinatra, R. et al. (2010). Acute kidney injury after coronary artery bypass grafting: Does rhabdomyolysis play a role? *The Journal of Thoracic and Cardiovascular Surgery, 140*(2), 464–470. doi:10.1016/j.jtcvs.2010.03.028 PMID:20416892

Billings, F. T., Pretorius, M., Schildcrout, J. S., Mercaldo, N. D., Byrne, J. G., Ikizler, T. A., & Brown, N. J. (2012). Obesity and Oxidative Stress Predict AKI after Cardiac Surgery. *Journal of the American Society of Nephrology*, *23*(7), 1221–1228. doi:10.1681/ASN.2011090940 PMID:22626819

Bilotta, F., & Rosa, G. (2012). Glycemia management in critical care patients. *World Journal of Diabetes*, *3*(7), 130–134. doi:10.4239/wjd.v3.i7.130 PMID:22816025

Bock, J. S., & Gottlieb, S. S. (2010). Cardiorenal Syndrome: New Perspectives. *Circulation*, *121*(23), 2592–2600. doi:10.1161/CIRCULATIONAHA.109.886473 PMID:20547939

Bolesta, S., Uhrin, L. M., & Guzek, J. R. (2011). Preoperative Statins and Acute Kidney Injury After Cardiac Surgery: Utilization of a Consensus Definition of Acute Kidney Injury. *The Annals of Pharmacotherapy*, *45*(1), 23–30. doi:10.1345/aph.1P384 PMID:21205946

Brown, J. R., Cochran, R. P., Mackenzie, T. A., Furnary, A. P., Kunzelman, K. S., Ross, C. S., & O'Connor, G. T. et al. (2008). Long-Term Survival After Cardiac Surgery is Predicted by Estimated Glomerular Filtration Rate. *The Annals of Thoracic Surgery*, *86*(1), 4–11. doi:10.1016/j.athoracsur.2008.03.006 PMID:18573389

Brown, J. R., Kramer, R. S., Coca, S. G., & Parikh, C. R. (2010). Duration of Acute Kidney Injury Impacts Long-Term Survival After Cardiac Surgery. *The Annals of Thoracic Surgery*, *90*(4), 1142–1148. doi:10.1016/j.athoracsur.2010.04.039 PMID:20868804

Chawla, L. S., Zhao, Y., Lough, F. C., Schroeder, E., Seneff, M. G., & Brennan, J. M. (2012). Off-Pump versus On-Pump Coronary Artery Bypass Grafting Outcomes Stratified by Preoperative Renal Function. *Journal of the American Society of Nephrology*, *23*(8), 1389–1397. doi:10.1681/ASN.2012020122 PMID:22595302

Choi, Y. S., Shim, J. K., Kim, J. C., Kang, K., Seo, Y. H., Ahn, K., & Kwak, Y. L. (2011). Effect of remote ischemic preconditioning on renal dysfunction after complex valvular heart surgery: A randomized controlled trial. *The Journal of Thoracic and Cardiovascular Surgery*, *142*(1), 148–154. doi:10.1016/j.jtcvs.2010.11.018 PMID:21272897

Coca, S. G., Garg, A. X., Swaminathan, M., Garwood, S., Hong, K., Thiessen-Philbrook, H., & Parikh, C. R. et al.TRIBE-AKI Consortium. (2013). Preoperative angiotensin-converting enzyme inhibitors and angiotensin receptor blocker use and acute kidney injury in patients undergoing cardiac surgery. *Nephrology, Dialysis, Transplantation*, *28*(11), 2787–2799. PMID:24081864

Cruz, D. N., Ricci, Z., & Ronco, C. (2009). Clinical review: RIFLE and AKIN – time for reappraisal. *Critical Care (London, England)*, *13*(3), 211. doi:10.1186/cc7759 PMID:19638179

Dardashti, A., Ederoth, P., Algotsson, L., Brondén, B., & Bjursten, H. (2013). Incidence, dynamics, and prognostic value of acute kidney injury for death after cardiac surgery. *The Journal of Thoracic and Cardiovascular Surgery*, *147*(2), 800–807. doi:10.1016/j.jtcvs.2013.07.073 PMID:24100099

Dasta, J. F., Kane-Gill, S. L., Durtschi, A. J., Pathak, D. S., & Kellum, J. A. (2008). Costs and outcomes of acute kidney injury (AKI) following cardiac surgery. *Nephrology, Dialysis, Transplantation*, *23*(6), 1970–1974. doi:10.1093/ndt/gfm908 PMID:18178605

Dirkes, S., & Hodge, K. (2007). Continuous Renal Replacement Therapy in the Adult Intensive Care Unit. *Critical Care Nurse*, *27*(2), 61–80. PMID:17389414

Dirocco, D. P., Bisi, J., Roberts, P., Strum, J., Wong, K., Sharpless, N., & Humphreys, B. D. (2014). CDK4/6 inhibition induces epithelial cell cycle arrest and ameliorates acute kidney injury. *AJP: Renal Physiology*, *306*(4), F379–F388. PMID:24338822

Elahi, M., Asopa, S., Pflueger, A., Hakim, N., & Matata, B. (2009). Acute kidney injury following cardiac surgery: Impact of early versus late haemofiltration on morbidity and mortality. *European Journal of Cardio-Thoracic Surgery*, *35*(5), 854–863. doi:10.1016/j.ejcts.2008.12.019 PMID:19216088

Endre, Z. H., Walker, R. J., Pickering, J. W., Shaw, G. M., Frampton, C. M., Henderson, S. J., & George, P. M. et al. (2010). Early intervention with erythropoietin does not affect the outcome of acute kidney injury (the EARLYARF trial). *Kidney International*, *77*(11), 1020–1030. doi:10.1038/ki.2010.25 PMID:20164823

Fry, D. W., Harvey, P. J., Keller, P. R., Elliott, W. L., Meade, M., Trachet, E., & Toogood, P. L. et al. (2004). Specific inhibition of cyclin-dependent kinase 4/6 by PD 0332991 and associated antitumor activity in human tumor xenografts. *Molecular Cancer Therapeutics*, *3*(11), 1427–1438. PMID:15542782

Haase, M., Bellomo, R., Devarajan, P., Ma, Q., Bennett, M. R., Möckel, M., & Haase-Fielitz, A. et al. (2009). Novel Biomarkers Early Predict the Severity of Acute Kidney Injury After Cardiac Surgery in Adults. *The Annals of Thoracic Surgery*, *88*(1), 124–130. doi:10.1016/j.athoracsur.2009.04.023 PMID:19559209

Haase, M., Bellomo, R., & Haase-Fielitz, A. (2010). Novel Biomarkers, Oxidative Stress, and the Role of Labile Iron Toxicity in Cardiopulmonary Bypass-Associated Acute Kidney Injury. *Journal of the American College of Cardiology*, *55*(19), 2024–2033. doi:10.1016/j.jacc.2009.12.046 PMID:20447525

Hall, N. A., & Fox, A. J. (2006). Renal replacement therapies in critical care. *Continuing Education in Anaesthesia. Critical Care & Pain*, *6*(5), 197–202.

Hillis, L. D., Smith, P. K., Anderson, J. L., Bittl, J. A., Bridges, C. R., Byrne, J. G., & Winniford, M. D. et al. (2011). 2011 ACCF/AHA Guideline for Coronary Artery Bypass Graft Surgery: A Report of the American College of Cardiology Foundation/American Heart Association Task Force on Practice Guidelines. *Circulation*, *124*(23), e652–e735. doi:10.1161/CIR.0b013e31823c074e PMID:22064599

Karkouti, K. (2012). Transfusion and risk of acute kidney injury in cardiac surgery. *British Journal of Anaesthesia*, *109*(suppl 1), i29–i38. doi:10.1093/bja/aes422 PMID:23242748

Karkouti, K., Sawchuk, C., Dupuis, J., Crowther, M., Cheng, D. C., Callum, J. L., & Beattie, W. S. et al. (2009). Acute Kidney Injury After Cardiac Surgery: Focus on Modifiable Risk Factors. *Circulation*, *119*(4), 495–502. doi:10.1161/CIRCULATIONAHA.108.786913 PMID:19153273

Karvellas, C. J., Farhat, M. R., Sajjad, I., Mogensen, S. S., Leung, A. A., Wald, R., & Bagshaw, S. M. (2011). A comparison of early versus late initiation of renal replacement therapy in critically ill patients with acute kidney injury: A systematic review and meta-analysis. *Critical Care (London, England)*, *15*(1), R72. PMID:21352532

Kidney Disease; Improving Global Outcomes (KDIGO) Acute Kidney Injury Work Group. (2012). KDIGO Clinical Practice Guideline for Acute Kidney Injury. *Kidney International. Supplement*, *2*(1), 1–138.

Kumar, A. B., Suneja, M., Bayman, E. O., Weide, G. D., & Tarasi, M. (2012). Association Between Postoperative Acute Kidney Injury and Duration of Cardiopulmonary Bypass: A Meta-Analysis. *Journal of Cardiothoracic and Vascular Anesthesia*, *26*(1), 64–69. doi:10.1053/j.jvca.2011.07.007 PMID:21924633

Lenihan, C. R., Montez-Rath, M. E., Mangano, C. T., Chertow, G. M., & Winkelmayer, W. C. (2013). Trends in Acute Kidney Injury, Associated Use of Dialysis, and Mortality After Cardiac Surgery, 1999 to 2008. *The Annals of Thoracic Surgery*, *95*(1), 20–28. doi:10.1016/j.athoracsur.2012.05.131 PMID:23272825

Liang, X., Liu, S., Chen, Y., Yan, L., Li, H., Xuan, H., & Shi, W. et al. (2010). Combination of urinary kidney injury molecule-1 and interleukin-18 as early biomarker for the diagnosis and progressive assessment of acute kidney injury following cardiopulmonary bypass surgery: A prospective nested case–control study. *Biomarkers*, *15*(4), 332–339. doi:10.3109/13547501003706558 PMID:20233133

Lim, S. Y., & Hausenloy, D. J. (2012). Remote Ischemic Conditioning: From Bench to Bedside. *Frontiers in Physics*, *3*. doi: doi:10.3389/fphys.2012.00027 PMID:22363297

Linden, A. V., Kempfert, J., Rastan, A. J., Holzhey, D., Blumenstein, J., Schuler, G., & Walther, T. et al. (2011). Risk of acute kidney injury after minimally invasive transapical aortic valve implantation in 270 patients. *European Journal of Cardio-Thoracic Surgery*, *39*(6), 835–843. doi:10.1016/j.ejcts.2010.11.034 PMID:21186126

Loor, G., Li, L., Sabik, J. F. III, Rajeswaran, J., Blackstone, E. H., & Koch, C. G. (2012). Nadir hematocrit during cardiopulmonary bypass: End-organ dysfunction and mortality. *The Journal of Thoracic and Cardiovascular Surgery*, *144*(3), 654–662.e4. doi:10.1016/j.jtcvs.2012.03.058 PMID:22507841

Loutzenhiser, R., Griffin, K., Williamson, G., & Bidani, A. (2006). Renal autoregulation: new perspectives regarding the protective and regulatory roles of the underlying mechanisms. *AJP: Regulatory. Integrative and Comparative Physiology*, *290*(5), R1153–R1167. doi:10.1152/ajpregu.00402.2005

Mariscalco, G., Lorusso, R., Dominici, C., Renzulli, A., & Sala, A. (2011). Acute Kidney Injury: A Relevant Complication After Cardiac Surgery. *The Annals of Thoracic Surgery*, *92*(4), 1539–1547. doi:10.1016/j.athoracsur.2011.04.123 PMID:21872837

Massoudy, P., Wagner, S., Thielmann, M., Herold, U., Kottenberg-Assenmacher, E., Marggraf, G., & Herget-Rosenthal, S. et al. (2008). Coronary artery bypass surgery and acute kidney injury--impact of the off-pump technique. *Nephrology, Dialysis, Transplantation*, *23*(9), 2853–2860. doi:10.1093/ndt/gfn153 PMID:18388121

Mcilroy, D. R., Wagener, G., & Lee, H. T. (2010). Neutrophil Gelatinase-Associated Lipocalin and Acute Kidney Injury after Cardiac Surgery: The Effect of Baseline Renal Function on Diagnostic Performance. *Clinical Journal of the American Society of Nephrology; CJASN*, *5*(2), 211–219. doi:10.2215/CJN.04240609 PMID:20056755

Melican, K., Sandoval, R. M., Kader, A., Josefsson, L., Tanner, G. A., Molitoris, B. A., & Richter-Dahlfors, A. (2011). Uropathogenic *Escherichia coli* P and Type 1 Fimbriae Act in Synergy in a Living Host to Facilitate Renal Colonization Leading to Nephron Obstruction. *PLoS Pathogens*, *7*(2), e1001298. doi:10.1371/journal.ppat.1001298 PMID:21383970

Moss, E., & Lamarche, Y. (2012). Acute Kidney Injury Following Cardiac Surgery: Prevention, Diagnosis, and Management. In M. Polenakovic (Ed.), Renal Failure: The Facts (pp. 129–156). Rijeka, Croatia: InTech; Retrieved from http://www.intechopen.com/books/renal-failure-the-facts/acute-kidney-injury-following-cardiac-surgery-prevention-diagnosis-and-treatment, doi:10.5772/37434

Muralidhar, K., Bhagyashri, K., Guptha, R., Hegde, N., Ahmed, I., & Vincent, L. (2013). Determinants of renal replacement therapy after adult cardiac surgery. *Asian Cardiovascular & Thoracic Annals*, *21*(5), 533–538. doi:10.1177/0218492312461638 PMID:24570554

National Kidney Foundation. (2014). *Frequently asked questions about GFR estimates*. Retrieved from http://www.kidney.org/professionals

Nguyen, T. C., Babaliaros, V. C., Razavi, S. A., Kilgo, P. D., Guyton, R. A., Devireddy, C. M., & Thourani, V. H. et al. (2013). Impact of varying degrees of renal dysfunction on transcatheter and surgical aortic valve replacement. *The Journal of Thoracic and Cardiovascular Surgery*, *146*(6), 1399–1407. doi:10.1016/j.jtcvs.2013.07.065 PMID:24075566

NICE-SUGAR Study Investigators. (2009). Intensive Versus Conventional Glucose Control In Critically Ill Patients. *The New England Journal of Medicine*, *360*(13), 1283–1297. doi:10.1056/NEJMoa0810625 PMID:19318384

Ozkaynak, B., Kayalar, N., Gümüs, F., Yücel, C., Mert, B., Boyacioğlu, K., & Erentuğ, V. (2014). *Time from cardiac catheterization to cardiac surgery: a risk factor for acute kidney injury? Interactive Cardiovascular and Thoracic Surgery*. Retrieved from; doi:10.1093/icvts/ivu023

Patel, N. N., Lin, H., Toth, T., Jones, C., Ray, P., Welsh, G. I., & Murphy, G. J. et al. (2011). Phosphodiesterase-5 Inhibition Prevents Postcardiopulmonary Bypass Acute Kidney Injury in Swine. *The Annals of Thoracic Surgery*, *92*(6), 2168–2176. doi:10.1016/j.athoracsur.2011.07.002 PMID:21983073

Salis, S., Mazzanti, V. V., Merli, G., Salvi, L., Tedesco, C. C., Veglia, F., & Sisillo, E. (2008). Cardiopulmonary Bypass Duration Is an Independent Predictor of Morbidity and Mortality After Cardiac Surgery. *Journal of Cardiothoracic and Vascular Anesthesia*, *22*(6), 814–822. doi:10.1053/j.jvca.2008.08.004 PMID:18948034

Shao, X., Tian, L., Xu, W., Zhang, Z., Wang, C., Qi, C., & Mou, S. et al. (2014). Diagnostic Value of Urinary Kidney Injury Molecule 1 for Acute Kidney Injury: A Meta-Analysis. *PLoS ONE*, *9*(1), e84131. doi:10.1371/journal.pone.0084131 PMID:24404151

Song, J. W., Shim, J. K., Yoo, K. J., Oh, S. Y., & Kwak, Y. L. (2013). Impact of intraoperative hyperglycaemia on renal dysfunction after off-pump coronary artery bypass. *Interactive Cardiovascular and Thoracic Surgery*, *17*(3), 473–478. doi:10.1093/icvts/ivt209 PMID:23690431

Srivastava, V., D'silva, C., Tang, A., Sogliani, F., & Ngaage, D. L. (2012). The impact of major perioperative renal insult on long-term renal function and survival after cardiac surgery. *Interactive Cardiovascular and Thoracic Surgery*, *15*(1), 14–17. doi:10.1093/icvts/ivs106 PMID:22473666

Stafford-Smith, M., Shaw, A., & Swaminathan, M. (2009). Cardiac surgery and acute kidney injury: Emerging concepts. *Current Opinion in Critical Care*, *15*(6), 498–502. doi:10.1097/MCC.0b013e328332f753 PMID:19812485

Steinthorsdottir, K. J., Kandler, K., Agerlin Windeløv, N. A., & Steinbrüchel, D. A. (2013). Renal replacement therapy after cardiac surgery; renal function recovers. *Scandinavian Cardiovascular Journal*, *47*(5), 303–306. doi:10.3109/14017431.2013.821625 PMID:23915029

Tasanarong, A., Duangchana, S., Sumransurp, S., Homvises, B., & Satdhabudha, O. (2013). Prophylaxis with Erythropoietin versus Placebo Reduces Acute Kidney Injury and Neutrophil Gelatinase-Associated Lipocalin in Patients Undergoing Cardiac Surgery: A Randomized, Double-Blind Controlled Trial. *BMC Nephrology*, *14*(1), 136. doi:10.1186/1471-2369-14-136 PMID:23829828

Vives, M., Wijeysundera, D., & Rao, V. (2014). Cardiac surgery-associated acute kidney injury. *Interactive Cardiovascular and Thoracic Surgery*, 1–9. doi: doi:10.1093/icvts/ivu014 PMID:24535092

Wald, R., Liangos, O., Perianayagam, M. C., Kolyada, A., Herget-Rosenthal, S., Mazer, C. D., & Jaber, B. L. (2010). Plasma Cystatin C and Acute Kidney Injury after Cardiopulmonary Bypass. *Clinical Journal of the American Society of Nephrology; CJASN*, *5*(8), 1373–1379. doi:10.2215/CJN.06350909 PMID:20522534

Wyckoff, T., & Augoustides, J. G. (2012). Advances in Acute Kidney Injury Associated with Cardiac Surgery: The Unfolding Revolution in Early Detection. *Journal of Cardiothoracic and Vascular Anesthesia*, *26*(2), 340–345. doi:10.1053/j.jvca.2012.01.001 PMID:22405191

Yoo, Y., Shim, J., Song, Y., Yang, S., & Kwak, Y. (2014). Anesthetics influence the incidence of acute kidney injury following valvular heart surgery. *Kidney International*, *86*(2), 414–422. doi:10.1038/ki.2013.532 PMID:24429400

Zangrillo, A., Biondi-Zoccai, G. G., Frati, E., Covello, R. D., Cabrini, L., Guarracino, F., & Landoni, G. et al. (2012). Fenoldopam and Acute Renal Failure in Cardiac Surgery: A Meta-Analysis of Randomized Placebo-Controlled Trials. *Journal of Cardiothoracic and Vascular Anesthesia*, *26*(3), 407–413. doi:10.1053/j.jvca.2012.01.038 PMID:22459931

ADDITIONAL READING

Abraham, V. S., & Swain, J. A. (2000). Cardio-pulmonary bypass and the kidney. In G. P. Gravlee, R. F. Davis, M. Kurusz, & J. R. Utley (Eds.), *Cardio-pulmonary bypass: Principles and practice* (2nd ed., pp. 382–391). Philadelphia, PA: Lippincott Williams & Wilkins.

Arora, P., Kolli, H., Nainani, N., Nader, N., & Lohr, J. (2012). Preventable risk factors for acute kidney injury in patients undergoing cardiac surgery. *Journal of Cardiothoracic and Vascular Anesthesia*, *26*(4), 687–697. doi:10.1053/j.jvca.2012.03.001 PMID:22516466

Bellomo, R., Auriemma, S., Fabbri, A., D'Onofrio, A., Katz, N., McCullough, P. A., & Ronco, C. et al. (2008). The pathophysiology of cardiac surgery-associated acute kidney injury (CSA-AKI). *The International Journal of Artificial Organs*, *31*(2), 166–178. PMID:18311733

Bingol, H., Akay, H. T., Iyem, H., Bolcal, C., Oz, K., Sirin, G., & Tatar, H. et al. (2007). Prophylactic dialysis in elderly patients undergoing coronary bypass surgery. *Therapeutic Apheresis and Dialysis*, *11*(1), 30–35. doi:10.1111/j.1744-9987.2007.00452.x PMID:17309572

Durmaz, I., Yagdi, T., Calkavur, T., Mahmudov, R., Apaydin, A. Z., Posacioglu, H., & Engin, C. et al. (2003). Prophylactic dialysis in patients with renal dysfunction undergoing on-pump coronary artery bypass surgery. *The Annals of Thoracic Surgery*, *75*(3), 859–864. doi:10.1016/S0003-4975(02)04635-0 PMID:12645707

Garcia-Fernandez, N., Perez-Valdivieso, J. R., Bes-Rastrollo, M., Vives, M., Lavilla, J., Herreros, J., & Monedero, P. (2011). Timing of renal replacement therapy after cardiac surgery: A retrospective multicenter Spanish cohort study. *Blood Purification*, *32*(2), 104–111. doi:10.1159/000324195 PMID:21372568

Goebel, U., Siepe, M., Schwer, C. I., Schibilsky, D., Foerster, K., Neumann, J., & Loop, T. et al. (2010). Inhaled carbon monoxide prevents acute kidney injury in pigs after cardiopulmonary bypass by inducing a heat shock response. *Anesthesia and Analgesia*, *111*(1), 29–37. PMID:20519418

Haase, M., Haase-Fielitz, A., Bagshaw, S. M., Ronco, C., & Bellomo, R. (2007). Cardiopulmonary bypass-associated acute kidney injury: A pigment nephropathy? *Contributions to Nephrology*, *156*, 340–353. doi:10.1159/000102125 PMID:17464145

Haase, M., Haase-Fielitz, A., & Bellomo, R. (2010). Cardiopulmonary bypass, hemolysis, free iron, acute kidney injury and the impact of bicarbonate. *Contributions to Nephrology*, *165*, 28–32. doi:10.1159/000313741 PMID:20427952

Hingorani, S., Molitoris, B. A., & Himmelfarb, J. (2009). Ironing out the pathogenesis of acute kidney injury. *American Journal of Kidney Diseases*, *53*(4), 569–571. doi:10.1053/j.ajkd.2009.01.002 PMID:19324244

Ho, J., Lucy, M., Krokhin, O., Hayglass, K., Pascoe, E., Darroch, G., & Reslerova, M. et al. (2009). Mass spectrometry-based proteomic analysis of urine in acute kidney injury following cardiopulmonary bypass: A nested case-control study. *American Journal of Kidney Diseases*, *53*(4), 584–595. doi:10.1053/j.ajkd.2008.10.037 PMID:19070948

Ishani, A., Nelson, D., Clothier, B., Schult, T., Nugent, S., Greer, N., & Ensrud, K. E. et al. (2011). The magnitude of acute serum creatinine increase after cardiac surgery and the risk of chronic kidney disease, progression of kidney disease, and death. *Archives of Internal Medicine*, *171*(3), 226–233. doi:10.1001/archinternmed.2010.514 PMID:21325112

Ji, Q., Mei, Y., Wang, X., Feng, J., Cai, J., Zhou, Y., & Hu, D. et al. (2011). Timing of continuous veno-venous hemodialysis in the treatment of acute renal failure following cardiac surgery. *Heart and Vessels*, *26*(2), 183–189. doi:10.1007/s00380-010-0045-9 PMID:21063880

Landoni, G., Bove, T., Székely, A., Comis, M., Rodseth, R. N., Pasero, D., & Bellomo, R. et al. (2013). Reducing mortality in acute kidney injury patients. systematic review and international web-based survey. *Journal of Cardiothoracic and Vascular Anesthesia*, *27*(6), 1384–1398. doi:10.1053/j.jvca.2013.06.028 PMID:24103711

Lu, J. C., Coca, S. G., Patel, U. D., Cantley, L., & Parikh, C. R.Translational Research Investigating Biomarkers and Endpoints for Acute Kidney Injury (TRIBE-AKI) Consortium. (2009). Searching for genes that matter in acute kidney injury: A systematic review. *Clinical Journal of the American Society of Nephrology; CJASN*, *4*(6), 1020–1031. doi:10.2215/CJN.05411008 PMID:19443624

Mann, B., Doig, C. J., Lee, H., Dean, S., Tonelli, M., Johnson, D., & Donaldson, C. (2003). Cost of acute renal failure requiring dialysis in the intensive care unit: Clinical and resource implications of renal recovery. *Critical Care Medicine*, *31*(2), 449–455. doi:10.1097/01.CCM.0000045182.90302.B3 PMID:12576950

Metnitz, P. G., Krenn, C. G., Steltzer, H., Lang, T., Ploder, J., Lenz, K., & Druml, W. et al. (2002). Effect of acute renal failure requiring renal replacement therapy on outcome in critically ill patients. *Critical Care Medicine*, *30*(9), 2051–2058. doi:10.1097/00003246-200209000-00016 PMID:12352040

Mishra, J., Mori, K., Ma, Q., Kelly, C., Yang, J., Mitsnefes, M., & Devarajan, P. et al. (2004). Amelioration of ischemic acute renal injury by neutrophil gelatinase-associated lipocalin. *Journal of the American Society of Nephrology*, *15*(12), 3073–3082. doi:10.1097/01.ASN.0000145013.44578.45 PMID:15579510

Pannu, N., Klarenbach, S., Wiebe, N., Manns, B., Tonelli, M., & Alberta Kidney Disease Network, . (2008). Renal replacement therapy in patients with acute renal failure: A systematic review. *Journal of the American Medical Association*, *299*(7), 793–805. doi:10.1001/jama.299.7.793 PMID:18285591

Pannu, N., & Noel Gibney, R. T. (2005). Renal replacement therapy in the intensive care unit. *Therapeutics and Clinical Risk Management*, *1*(2), 141–150. doi:10.2147/tcrm.1.2.141.62908 PMID:18360553

Parikh, C. R., Coca, S. G., Thiessen-Philbrook, H., Shlipak, M. G., Koyner, J. L., Wang, Z., & Garg, A. X. et al.Translational Research Investigating Biomarkers and Endpoints for Acute Kidney Injury (TRIBE-AKI) Consortium. (2011). Postoperative biomarkers predict acute kidney injury and poor outcomes after adult cardiac surgery. *Journal of the American Society of Nephrology*, *22*(9), 1748–1757. doi:10.1681/ASN.2010121302 PMID:21836143

Parikh, C. R., Devarajan, P., Zappitelli, M., Sint, K., Thiessen-Philbrook, H., Li, S., & Krawczeski, C. D. et al.Translational Research Investigating Biomarkers and Endpoints for Acute Kidney Injury (TRIBE-AKI) Consortium. (2011). Postoperative biomarkers predict acute kidney injury and poor outcomes after pediatric cardiac surgery. *Journal of the American Society of Nephrology*, *22*(9), 1737–1747. doi:10.1681/ASN.2010111163 PMID:21836147

Portilla, D., Dent, C., Sugaya, T., Nagothu, K. K., Kundi, I., Moore, P., & Devarajan, P. et al. (2008). Liver fatty acid-binding protein as a biomarker of acute kidney injury after cardiac surgery. *Kidney International*, *73*(4), 465–472. doi:10.1038/sj.ki.5002721 PMID:18094680

Shaw, A., Swaminathan, M., & Stafford-Smith, M. (2008). Cardiac surgery-associated acute kidney injury: Putting together the pieces of the puzzle. *Nephron. Physiology*, *109*(4), 55–60. doi:10.1159/000142937 PMID:18802376

Shroyer, A. L., Grover, F. L., Hattler, B., Collins, J. F., McDonald, G. O., Kozora, E., & Novitzky, D. et al.Veterans Affairs Randomized On/Off Bypass (ROOBY) Study Group. (2009). On-pump versus off-pump coronary artery bypass surgery. *The New England Journal of Medicine*, *361*(19), 1827–1837. doi:10.1056/NEJMoa0902905 PMID:19890125

Slocum, J. L., Heung, M., & Pennathur, S. (2012). Marking renal injury: Can we move beyond serum creatinine? *Translational Research; the Journal of Laboratory and Clinical Medicine*, *159*(4), 277–289. doi:10.1016/j.trsl.2012.01.014 PMID:22424431

Sreeram, G. M., Grocott, H. P., White, W. D., Newman, M. F., & Stafford-Smith, M. (2004). Transcranial Doppler emboli count predicts rise in creatinine after coronary artery bypass graft surgery. *Journal of Cardiothoracic and Vascular Anesthesia*, *18*(5), 548–551. doi:10.1053/j.jvca.2004.07.010 PMID:15578463

Swaminathan, M., Shaw, A. D., Phillips-Bute, B. G., McGugan-Clark, P. L., Archer, L. E., Talbert, S., & Stafford-Smith, M. et al. (2007). Trends in acute renal failure associated with coronary artery bypass graft surgery in the United States. *Critical Care Medicine*, *35*(10), 2286–2292. doi:10.1097/01.CCM.0000282079.05994.57 PMID:17944016

von Heymann, C., Sander, M., Foer, A., Heinemann, A., Spiess, B., Braun, J., & Spies, C. et al. (2006). The impact of an hematocrit of 20% during normothermic cardiopulmonary bypass for elective low risk coronary artery bypass graft surgery on oxygen delivery and clinical outcome—a randomized controlled study. *Critical Care (London, England)*, *10*(2), R58. doi:10.1186/cc4891 PMID:16606474

Zimmerman, R. F., Ezeanuna, P. U., Kane, J. C., Cleland, C. D., Kempananjappa, T. J., Lucas, F. L., & Kramer, R. S. (2011). Ischemic preconditioning at a remote site prevents acute kidney injury in patients following cardiac surgery. *Kidney International*, *80*(8), 861–867. doi:10.1038/ki.2011.156 PMID:21677633

KEY TERMS AND DEFINITIONS

Afferent: Conducting toward a specific structure or area.

Azotemia: A condition characterized by abnormally high blood levels of nitrogenous compounds.

Efferent: Conducting away from a specific structure or area.

Hemodilution: An increase in the fluid content of blood which results in a reduced concentration of cells.

Hemolysis: Red blood cell destruction with the subsequent release of intracellular components.

Normotensive: Indicating normal arterial blood pressure, approximately 120/80 mmHg.

Renal Cortex: The outer portion of the kidney. Its functions include ultrafiltration and erythropoietin production.

Renal Medulla: The inner portion of the kidney. It functions to maintain salt and water balance.

Rhabdomyolysis: Muscle breakdown with the subsequent release of muscle fiber contents.

Chapter 18
Gastrointestinal Issues in the Cardiothoracic ICU

Carrie Harvey
University of Michigan Health System, USA

Katherine Klein
University of Michigan Health System, USA

Michael Maile
University of Michigan Health System, USA

ABSTRACT

A thorough understanding of gastrointestinal issues in critical illness is necessary to optimize management of the cardiothoracic patient. Post-operatively, these patients are at increased risk of GI complications due a combination of underlying vascular disease, cardiopulmonary bypass, and low cardiac output, all of which lead to splanchnic hypoperfusion and subsequent damage to the gut mucosa. While GI complications are uncommon, they are associated with a disproportionately high rate of morbidity and mortality. Presence of unexplained fever, leukocytosis, bacteremia, hemodynamic compromise or abdominal pain or distention are concerning and require prompt assessment. Other GI management issues include delivery of adequate nutrition to counteract catabolism and promote wound healing and stress ulcer prophylaxis in patients with risk factors for upper gastrointestinal bleeding.

INTRODUCTION

Gastrointestinal management is an important component in the systems-based care of the critically ill patient. Although GI issues may appear minor when compared to the cardiorespiratory derangements encountered in the cardiothoracic ICU, certain complications can be catastrophic. Additionally, the best practices regarding nutrition and stress ulcer prophylaxis can be confusing due to differing interpretations of the literature. This chapter will therefore present an evidence-based foundation of four major topics: the differential diagnosis of abdominal pain, specific gastrointestinal complications, nutrition in the critically ill patient, and stress ulcer prophylaxis.

DOI: 10.4018/978-1-4666-8603-8.ch018

BACKGROUND

Gastrointestinal (GI) complications develop in 1-2% of cardiac surgery patients, but with mortality rates reaching 30% (Rodriguez et al., 2010). This excessively high rate is felt due to both delay in diagnosis, due to non-specific signs and symptoms, and the types of complications, such as GI bleeding and mesenteric ischemia, which already carry a poor prognosis.

Cardiac surgery with or without cardiopulmonary bypass (CPB) increases tissue oxygen demands while also causing a profound reduction in splanchnic perfusion (Fiore et al., 2006; Velissaris et al., 2003). This effect is further exacerbated by low cardiac output and the use of vasoconstrictors (Ohri & Velissaris, 2006). The resultant tissue hypoxia leads to breakdown of typical mucosal functions and potential for atrophy, ulceration, bacterial translocation, the systemic inflammatory response syndrome, and eventually, multi-system organ failure. Risk factors for the development of GI complications are listed in Table 1 (D'Ancona et al., 2003; Filsoufi et al., 2007; Mangi et al., 2005; McSweeney et al., 2004; Rodriguez et al., 2010).

Typical signs of an acute abdominal process, such as fever, leukocytosis, and hemodynamic changes are not specific and common in critical illness. As many patients are sedated, physical exam is unreliable. Diagnostic studies, such as CT scan, can be logistically difficult if the patient is unstable. Therefore, deviation from the normal post-operative course should prompt workup for an acute abdominal process to avoid delays in diagnosis.

Figure 1 outlines the incidence of various GI complications as determined from a review of over 150,000 cardiac surgery patients. Other considerations in the differential diagnosis include: small bowel obstruction, *Clostridium difficile* colitis, abdominal compartment syndrome, retroperitoneal hemorrhage, and urinary tract infection.

Evaluation requires review of the patient's medical and surgical history, serial abdominal exams, relevant laboratory tests (e.g. serum lactate, transaminases, lipase, stool *C. difficile* toxin PCR), and appropriate diagnostic imaging. For the majority of acute abdominal processes, CT abdomen with contrast remains the best initial study. An upright (or lateral) abdominal radiograph can evaluate for intra-peritoneal free air. If biliary pathology is suspected, upper abdominal ultrasound is the best initial study, with follow-up HIDA scan in select cases. Plain abdominal radiograph can be used to evaluate for bowel obstruction, but is far less sensitive and specific than CT scan and is of limited utility. Consultation with general surgery early is recommended, not only to help guide diagnosis, but also because early surgical exploration may reduce morbidity and mortality (Hackert et al., 2003). In general, patients have improved cardiac function post-operatively and are able to withstand anesthesia and an abdominal operation if necessary (Rodriguez et al., 2010).

Table 1. Risk factors for the development of GI complications following cardiac surgery

Pre-Operative	Operative	Post-Operative
Age >70 years	Emergent procedure	Use of vasoconstrictors
Poor left ventricular function	Duration of CPB	Use of intra-aortic balloon pump
Peripheral vascular disease	Multiple blood transfusions	Multiple blood transfusions
Chronic renal failure		Surgical re-exploration
Anticoagulant use		Dysrhythmias

Adapted from: Rodriguez et al., Journal of Cardiac Surgery, 2010

Figure 1. Incidence of GI complications following cardiac surgery
Adapted from: Rodriguez et al., Journal of Cardiac Surgery, 2010

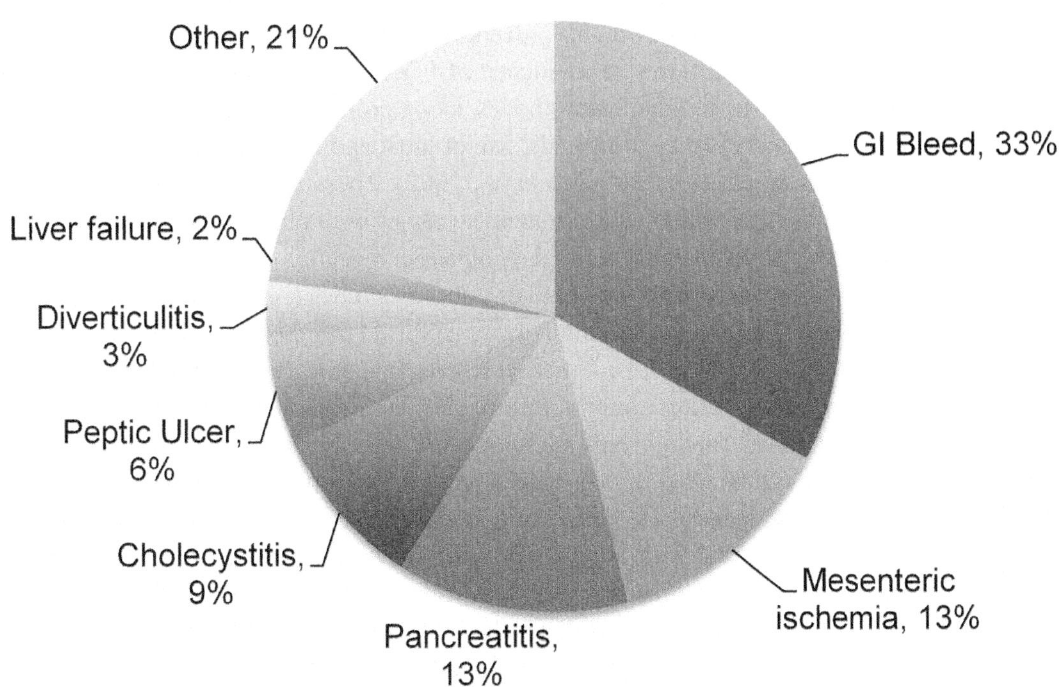

SPECIFIC GASTROINTENSTINAL COMPLICATIONS

Post-Operative Nausea and Vomiting

Post-operative nausea and vomiting (PONV) is a common issue amongst surgical patients. Without pharmacological antiemetic treatment, the PONV rate is approximately 30% in the general population and as high as 70% in patients at high risk (Gan et al., 2003). Risk factors for PONV include female gender, nonsmoker status, history of PONV or motion sickness, post operative opioid use, increased duration of surgery, and intra-abdominal, orthopedic or major gynecologic surgeries (Gan et al., 2003). Given the common occurrence of PONV and the impact it has on the medical system following surgery, many guidelines have been published focusing on risk stratification, minimization of PONV, and customized, multimodal pharmacological approaches.

Prevention

A common causative agent for PONV is the use of opioids in the post-operative setting. While cardiothoracic surgery often requires the use of opioid therapy early in the post- operative course, minimization of dosages and frequency has been found to reduce the incidence of PONV (Williams et al., 2007). The use of regional anesthesia, as well as a combination of intravenous and regional anesthesia, has also decreased PONV. Further risk reduction strategies include adequate patient hydration, preferential use of total intravenous and/ or regional anesthesia, and minimization of intraoperative neostigmine and nitrous oxide (Williams et al., 2007).

Routine Prophylaxis

There is no true consensus or "gold standard" for preventing PONV, but several studies have identified opportunities in patient care to minimize the incidence of PONV. These studies report a multimodal approach, including the avoidance of volatile anesthetics, using propofol as the "induction" and "maintenance" anesthetic of choice, avoidance of opioids, use of local and regional anesthesia, and routine, low-dose administration of antiemetics (Williams et al., 2007). There are many pathways and receptors involved in PONV, which allow for multiple areas to target with pharmacological therapy. Most common treatments utilize phenothiazines (block dopaminergic receptors in the chemoreceptor trigger zone), butyrophenones (dopamine receptor antagonists), antihistamines (act on the vomiting center and vestibular pathways), benzamides (block dopaminergic receptors at the chemoreceptor trigger zone and also have peripheral antiemetic properties), anticholinergics (antagonize muscarinic and histaminic receptors in the vestibular and vomiting centers), dexamethasone, serotonin receptor antagonists, and/or aprepitant (selectively binds and antagonizes the substance P/neurokinin-1 receptor) (Williams et al., 2007). With the number of pharmacological options available, many combinations exist to best suit each patient. Many institutions have focused on the use of a serotonin receptor antagonist with the addition of dexamethasone and/or droperidol with good clinical efficacy. Patients who received preoperative anxiolysis (midazolam), prophylactic antiemetics on induction and at the end of surgery, induction and maintenance anesthesia with propofol, and local anesthetic with ketorolac at the end of the case had a complete response rate with no reported PONV of 80% (Gan et al., 2014).

Treatment

PONV can still occur despite appropriate prophylaxis approaches. In this situation, the antiemetic choice should be of a different receptor class than was used for prophylaxis (Jokinen et al., 2012). Combinations of antiemetics that have an immediate onset of action like serotonin receptor antagonists or low dose droperidol with antiemetics that have a long half-life like dexamethasone, scopolamine, or NK1 receptor antagonists have shown to help with recurrence of PONV (Jokinen et al., 2012). In refractory cases of PONV, further causes should be investigated, including pain, hypotension, hypoxia, drug interactions, gastrointestinal abnormalities, nasogastric tube position, mobilization, or increased eye pressure (Jokinen et al., 2012). If PONV is still present, other options for treatment include low-dose propofol infusions, acupressure and/or acupuncture, alpha 2 antagonists, mirtazapine, gabapentin, intravenous fluid hydration, low-dose naloxone, or midazolam (Gan et al., 2014; Jokinen et al., 2012; Williams et al., 2007).

Summary

PONV is a major concern in surgical patients and can account for post operative complications such as disruption of suture lines, esophageal tissue damage, metabolic problems, dehydration, delayed hospital discharge, aspiration pneumonia, and decreased patient satisfaction (Gan et al., 2014). A multimodal approach to prophylaxis and treatment of PONV has been shown to be most effective. A better understanding of the mechanism of drug activity as well as combination therapy can help standardize the approach to PONV. Further research in this area has focused on the early identification of patients at risk for PONV, implementation of a standardized approach to PONV, and minimizing the side effects associated with many of the pharmacologic agents used in treatment algorithm.

Ileus and Obstruction

As mentioned previously, low cardiac output following cardiothoracic surgery places patients at increased risk for gastrointestinal complications postoperatively (Viana et al., 2013). In addition, use of postoperative inotropes, narcotics, and the inflammatory process of the cardiopulmonary circuit further increases the risk for ileus, obstruction or pseudo-obstruction (Tenofsky, Beamer, & Smith, 2000).

Diagnosis

Postoperative ileus or obstruction can increase patient discomfort and prolong hospital stays; therefore, prompt identification and treatment can positively influence patient care. Postoperative ileus has been defined as decreased gastrointestinal motility after surgery associated with abdominal distention, accumulation of gas and fluids in the bowel, delayed passage of flatus or defecation, and a lack or decrease in bowel sounds (Kehlet & Holte, 2001). Ileus is extremely common in postoperative patients and is thought to be a result of sympathetic activation of the intestines causing inhibition of motility of the gastrointestinal tract (Kehlet & Holte, 2001). Diagnosis is confirmed with the use of plain radiographic films of the abdomen showing distended, air-filled bowel with no clear sign of obstruction. Colonic pseudo-obstruction can also appear similar to an ileus state, but is limited to colonic dilatation. Bowel obstructions can also commonly occur in postsurgical patients and presents with abdominal pain, distention, constipation or obstipation, and dilated bowel loops on plain radiographic films with a transition point. Diagnosis for bowel obstructions often include CT scans of the abdomen and pelvis to further evaluate the location of the transition point, bowel wall thickening, mesenteric venous congestion, mesenteric fluid, ascites, concern for bowel wall ischemia, and/or unusual course of the mesenteric vasculature (Maung et al., 2012).

Treatment

Prevention strategies to reduce ileus include limiting intravenous fluid to reduce intestinal edema, nasogastric decompression if the patient is at risk for aspiration, early ambulation, early enteral feeding, gum chewing, use of epidural anesthesia, and opioid-sparing analgesia (Tu et al., 2014). When it occurs despite these measures, conventional treatments focus on nasogastric decompression, early mobilization, limiting opioid pain relief, prokinetics, early enteral feeding, and use of epidural anesthesia for pain control. However, further investigation has shown nasogastric decompression may actually prolong ileus and cause atelectasis and fever in early postoperative patient populations (Kehlet & Holte, 2001). In patients that suffer from colonic pseudo-obstruction (Ogilvie's Syndrome) treatment is based on cecal diameter measured with either a plain abdominal radiograph or CT of the abdomen and pelvis. If the patient's cecum measures less than 13 cm in diameter, conservative treatment can be considered and consists of bowel rest, nasogastric decompression, enemas, fluid resuscitation, prokinetic agents, and/or possible neostigmine. However, if the cecum measures greater than 13cm in diameter, or the patient fails conservative therapy, then colonoscopic decompression is recommended (Tenofsky et al., 2000). Further failure of colonoscopic decompression should lead to operative management with a right hemicolectomy or cecostomy. Mortality also increases significantly if the patient does not respond to medical interventions and requires surgical correction, with mortality rates as high as 50% (Tenofsky et al., 2000).

The treatment of bowel obstructions is also classified as operative versus non-operative. Operative management should be considered in patients who have concern for bowel ischemia, fever, leukocytosis, tachycardia, continuous pain, metabolic acidosis, peritonitis, are sepsis. Operative management in both partial and complete obstructions have shown reduction in recurrence rates and longer disease-free interval (Maung et al., 2012). Non-operative management for bowel obstructions includes serial abdominal exams, bowel rest, nasogastric decompression, and CT examination with water-soluble contrast for obstructions that do no resolve within 48 hours. There have been many discussions based on the timing of operative exploration in patients who have not resolved with conservative management. Most recent evidence-based practices point to waiting no longer than 3-5 days for operative exploration in bowel obstructions without clinical signs of deterioration or concern of ischemia (Sperry & Cohen, 2014). In patients who have undergone a laparotomy within the past 30 days, it is recommended to wait 6-14 days prior to operative exploration as surgery can be extremely difficult due to adhesion formation (Sperry & Cohen, 2014).

Summary

Early recognition and treatment of post-operative ileus and obstruction can greatly decrease patient discomfort, morbidity, hospital costs, and length of hospital stay. Early operative intervention is required in any patient who is acutely decompensating or has signs of ischemic bowel. Focusing on early enteral feeding, early mobility, and limiting opioid analgesia has shown direct benefit in reducing post-operative ileus and bowel obstruction. New areas of research have focused on μ-opioid receptor antagonists to reduce length of patient recovery from ileus and can be used in conjunction with the other approaches (Tu et al., 2014).

Diarrhea

Although considered a common symptom among critically ill patients, the incidence of diarrhea is unknown, primarily because no standardized definition exists. The most widely accepted definition is frequent (≥3 to 5 per day) and soft stools (≥250 ml/day) (Whelan et al., 2004). It can result from a variety of mechanisms, all of which lead to increased fecal water content. A useful distinction is differentiating between infectious and non-infectious causes, as summarized in Table 2 (Wiesen, Van Gossum, & Preiser, 2006). Determination of the etiology requires a standardized approach so that more serious causes are recognized and treated appropriately.

Table 2. Common causes of diarrhea in the critically ill

Infectious	Non-Infectious
Clostridium difficile	Gut hypermotility
Viral enteritis/colitis	Gut ischemia
Other bacterial causes	Drug-associated (e.g. sorbitol, magnesium)
	Hypoalbuminemia

Adapated from: Wiesen et al., Current Opinion in Critical Care, 2006

Infectious Diarrhea

A multitude of bacteria and viruses can lead to diarrhea, although these are rarely tested for specifically as they often resolve spontaneously and are treated conservatively. The exception is *Clostridium difficile*, an anaerobic Gram-positive bacillus that produces a toxin that leads to mucosal necrosis, and in severe cases, colonic dilation and perforation. Diagnosis is made by the presence of the toxin antigen in stool and should be suspected in the setting of diarrhea, fever, leukocytosis, and/or abdominal pain or distention. Sigmoidoscopy, if performed, will demonstrate pseudomembranes, which manifest as raised yellow or white plaques. Abdominal computed tomography will show marked colonic thickening. Contact precautions with non-permeable gown and gloves should be used in suspected or confirmed cases of *C. difficile* colitis (Zilberberg & Shorr, 2013).

An epidemiologic study from 2005 found that up to 30% of all hospitalized patients are asymptomatically colonized with *C. difficile,* however, colitis does not occur until there is significant overgrowth (Modena et al., 2005). Consequently, a large amount of research has resulted to determine what risk factors exist for developing C. difficile infection (CDI).

It is well-accepted that the use of quinolones and cepholosporins are associated with increased risk of CDI, therefore, judicious use of these agents is warranted based on the patient's clinical context and local antibiotic resistance patterns (Modena et al., 2005; Yip et al., 2001). Early observational studies found an association between proton pump inhibitor (PPI) use and CDI, but only one study has specifically evaluated this relationship in the ICU setting (Buendgens et al., 2014). The authors identified stress ulcer prophylaxis with PPIs as an independent risk factor for development of CDI in medical patients (odds ratio [OR] = 3.1), but this was a single-center retrospective study. Additionally, underlying disease severity is also a known risk factor (Kyne et al., 2002). Since the sickest patients are frequently on stress ulcer prophylaxis, it is possible that the development of CDI is due more to disease severity than the PPI itself (Novak et al., 2014).

Treatment of CDI depends on severity but should always include discontinuation of any offending antibiotics. The classification by severity and corresponding treatment recommendation per the Infectious Disease Society of America is summarized in Table 3 (Cohen et al., 2010). Recurrent disease generally warrants tapered or pulsed vancomycin therapy and should be done in consultation with an Infectious Disease specialist. Fulminant colitis requires consultation with General Surgery for subtotal colectomy or other surgical management (Carchman et al., 2012). It should be noted that 20% of patients with fulminant colitis will not have diarrhea, due to associated colonic dilation and ileus (Adams & Mercer, 2007).

Non-Infectious Diarrhea

Once CDI has been excluded as a cause of diarrhea, non-infectious etiologies can be considered. The exception is mesenteric ischemia, which is associated with several risk factors seen in cardiothoracic patients, including older age, underlying vascular disease, and cardiopulmonary bypass. Due to its high mortality, mesenteric ischemia should always be considered in the differential diagnosis of diarrhea. This topic is covered in detail later in this chapter.

Diarrhea is frequently seen in the context of enteral nutrition, which is thought to be due to formula osmolality and mode of administration (Chang & Huang, 2013; Wiesen et al., 2006). There is no difference in the incidence of diarrhea between gastric and jejunal feeding (Juan C Montejo et al., 2002). Contrary to popular belief, there are no large studies that demonstrate less diarrhea using continuous

Table 3. Classification of initial C. difficile infection

Severity	Clinical data	Treatment
Mild to moderate	Leukocytosis with WBC <15,000 cells/ μL **AND** serum creatinine <1.5 times baseline level	Metronidazole 500 mg by mouth 3 times per day for 10-14 days
Severe	Leukocytosis with WBC >15,000 cells/ μL **OR** serum creatinine ≥1.5 times baseline level	Vancomycin 125 mg by mouth 4 times per day for 10-14 days
Complicated	Hypotension/shock, ileus, megacolon	Vancomycin 500 mg by mouth 4 times per day, plus metronidazole 500 mg intravenously every 8 hours. Add vancomycin enema 500 mg every 6 hours if ileus

Adapted from: Cohen et al., Infection Control and Hospital Epidemiology, 2009

feeds rather than intermittent boluses, although continuous infusions are more practical from a nursing perspective (MacLeod et al., 2007; Serpa et al., 2003). Although intuitive, the addition of fiber has not been proven to be of benefit in critically ill patients receiving enteral feeding (Yang et al., 2005). Finally, the use probiotics remains controversial and are not currently recommended by any major society guidelines (Morrow, 2009; Theodorakopoulou et al., 2013).

Certain medications are well known to cause osmotic diarrhea. Those most frequently implicated in the critical care setting are listed in Table 4. Different formulations of many of these medications are available for substitution (Dickerson & Melnik, 1988).

If diarrhea persists, is not due to infection of ischemia, and is contributing to hypovolemia, skin breakdown, or patient discomfort, an anti-peristaltic agent (e.g. loperamide) can be used to decrease frequency of stools. It is important to remember that anti-peristaltic agents should never be used as part of the treatment regimen for CDI, as this can predispose to development of toxic megacolon (Cohen et al., 2010).

Summary

Diarrhea is frequently encountered in the critical care setting. The two most serious causes of diarrhea are ischemic colitis and *C. difficile* infection. CDI must be considered in critically ill patients with diarrhea,

Table 4. Common hyperosmolar medications used in the ICU

Medication
Acetaminophen elixir, 65 mg/mL
Cimetidine solution, 60 mg/mL
Dexamethasone solution, 1 mg/mL
Docusate sodium syrup, 3.3 mg/mL
Ferrous sulfate liquid, 60 mg/mL
Multivitamin liquid
Potassium chloride liquid, 10%
Sodium phosphate liquid, 0.5 g/mL

Adapted from: Dickerson and Melnick, American Journal of Hospital Pharmacy, 1988 particularly in the setting of abdominal pain or distention, unexplained fever or leukocytosis, or recent or current antibiotic use, particularly quinolones and cephalosporins. Further prospective studies regarding CDI risk with PPI use and potential benefit with probiotics are warranted, given current conflicting data.

Gastrointestinal Bleeding

With the advent of cardiopulmonary bypass for cardiac surgery, many patients experience an increase incident of gastrointestinal bleeding. Gastrointestinal organs are at increased risk for ischemic injury during cardiac surgery given the frequent use of the cardiopulmonary bypass circuit. The circuit creates an environment of non-pulsatile blood flow, reduced blood pressure, and oxygen shunting resulting in distal hypoxia at the intestinal villi (D'Ancona et al., 2003), placing patients at increased risk for postoperative gastrointestinal complications. Many cardiothoracic patients post operatively require anticoagulation and thus are at a higher risk for bleeding and more specifically gastrointestinal bleeding. Further advances in surgical management of cardiac disease including mechanical valves, ventricular assist devices, total artificial heart implantation, stent placement, and the need for cardiopulmonary bypass places this patient population at higher rates of bleeding associated with heparin use, antiplatelet therapy, and long-term anticoagulants (Bunte et al., 2013; Mathias et al., 2012; Mudd & Gelow, 2013). Particularly gastrointestinal bleeding affects approximately 1.5% of patients and has a mortality rate up to 39% (Bhat et al., 2012).

Prevention

As gastrointestinal bleeding is not an uncommon post operative complication in cardiac patients there have been several studies looking for risk factors to help better characterize patients prior to surgery. Several risk factors include age above 75 years, New York Heart Association classification IV, history of peptic ulcer disease, low cardiac output postoperatively, and prolonged ventilation duration >48 hours (Dong et al., 2012). However, gastrointestinal bleeding can be from various sources and should be further identified. Common causes of gastrointestinal bleeding are from peptic ulceration, duodenal ulceration, and/or ischemic sloughing from the bowel related to hypoperfusion (Egleston et al., 1993). Gastrointestinal bleeding can present with coffee ground emesis, hematochezia, melena, and/or hematemesis. These symptoms often present approximately 10 days after surgery and can lead to the need for transfusions of blood products, endoscopic therapy, and even definitive surgical management (Bhat et al., 2012). Given this concern, many institutions have protocolized gastrointestinal prophylaxis with H-2 receptor antagonists or proton-pump inhibitors post operatively for all patients after cardiac surgery. Further discussion of the topic of gastrointestinal prophylaxis will be addressed later in this chapter.

Treatment

Many of the patients who develop the complication of gastrointestinal bleeding are the most critically ill and cannot be moved for further diagnostic evaluation of their anemia. Common methods for diagnosis include placement of a nasogastric tube for lavage and decompression of stomach contents for further localization of gastrointestinal bleeding. In addition, use of endoscopic therapies have also allowed for diagnostic and therapeutic interventions in gastric and duodenal ulcers and bleeding. Initial therapy for gastrointestinal bleeding should be supportive care with transfusions as needed, strict monitoring of anticoagulation levels, and avoiding hypoperfusion when possible. However, the need for an operation may be necessary in patients with worsening clinical conditions, episodes of re-bleeding, or continued bleeding (Egleston et al., 1993).

Summary

While gastrointestinal bleeding following cardiac surgery is uncommon, it is associated with a significant mortality. Therefore, careful attention should be paid to identifying patients who are at risk for gastrointestinal bleeding postoperatively, appropriate prophylaxis, and quick institution of therapy when evidence of gastrointestinal bleeding is present. Further areas of study include new modalities for anticoagulation and antiplatelet therapy following cardiac surgery, combination therapy for GI prophylaxis, and new endoscopic therapy approaches to bleeding peptic and duodenal ulcers.

Mesenteric Ischemia

Cardiac surgery often requires the use of the cardiopulmonary bypass machine and can place patients at increased risk for mesenteric ischemia. While abdominal complications are uncommon following cardiopulmonary bypass (0.4%-2.9%), acute mesenteric ischemia (AMI) represents 10%-67% of these complications (Eris et al., 2013). Additionally, AMI does carry a high mortality risk between 70% and 100% (Eris et al., 2013; Kiessling et al., 2014). Presentation and diagnosis is often delayed given the intubated and sedated status of many of these patients.

Diagnosis

Clinical presentation can often be delayed and diagnosis often requires invasive testing. Therefore, risk factors for postoperative ischemia should be acknowledged such as arterial hypotension, postoperative heart failure, renal insufficiency, age >70 years, hypovolemia, extended cardiopulmonary bypass time >150 minutes, New York Heart Association class III-IV, active smoker, sepsis, intra-aortic balloon pump support, vasopressor use, and preexisting atherosclerotic lesions (Eris et al., 2013). Biological markers, clinical findings and radiological studies can help diagnose acute mesenteric ischemia when evaluated as a whole. Biological markers including leukocytosis, creatinine elevation, metabolic acidosis, transaminase elevation, PT <40%, lipase elevation, LDH elevation and CPK elevation can be suggestive of mesenteric ischemia, but are not definitive tests when used individually (Abboud et al., 2008). Clinical findings include hypotension, prolonged ileus, abdominal pain, abdominal guarding, abdominal distention, melena, hematochezia, cyanosis and/or fever. Radiologic studies can also be used to help diagnose mesenteric ischemia including plain films of the abdomen, abdominal ultrasound with doppler of mesenteric vessels, abdominal CT scan, rectosigmoidoscopy, and/or angiography. However, if clinical suspicion is high, prompt surgical intervention has shown to reduce mortality associated with AMI (Abboud et al., 2008).

Treatment

Treatment for mesenteric ischemia focuses on early detection of signs and symptoms and prompt surgical evaluation if concern for a correctable ischemic event occurred. Patients who have isolated, local ischemic effects are best suited for surgical correction and improved mortality rates. There has also been an association with patients who undergo cardiac surgery without the use of the cardiopulmonary circuit, routine epiaortic ultrasonography to identify and avoid debris in the aorta, active screening and treatment for heparin induced thrombocytopenia, avoidance of clamping the aorta, close monitoring of patients postoperatively with fast-track extubation plans, and minimal sedation that have helped reduce mesenteric ischemia events (Mangi et al., 2005).

Summary

Correctly identifying patients pre-operatively and performing selective angiography prior to cardiac surgery for those who are at increased risk for mesenteric ischemia may help to decrease mortality associated with such events postoperatively. Further work is focusing on early identification of ischemic events and the use of catheter directed treatment with thrombolytics, stent placements, or surgical revascularization versus the need for early surgical resection of infarcted bowel (Abboud et al., 2008).

Abdominal Compartment Syndrome

Intra-abdominal hypertension (IAH) and ACS have been increasingly recognized in a wide variety of critically ill patients, including those without any acute abdominal insult (Malbrain et al., 2004). Additionally, the diagnosis has been shown to be an independent predictor of mortality (Malbrain et al., 2005; Vidal et al., 2008). Consequently, it is imperative that critical care providers are familiar with the prevention, diagnosis, and treatment of IAH and ACS.

Definition

The World Society of Abdominal Compartment Syndrome (WSACS) has defined IAH as an intra-abdominal pressure ≥12 mm Hg and ACS as an intra-abdominal pressure ≥25 mm Hg that is associated with new organ dysfunction or failure (Cheatham et al., 2007). ACS is also classified as either primary, due to an acute intra-abdominal or retroperitoneal insult, or secondary, from massive fluid resuscitation and subsequent bowel edema or ascites. Measurements should be taken at end-expiration in the supine position, with the zero point at the mid-axillary line (Cheatham et al., 2007).

Pathophysiology

The development of ACS is similar to other compartment syndromes in that the underlying process leads to increased pressure within a non-expandable space, which causes decreased microvascular perfusion. At IAP of approximately 20 mm Hg, tissue ischemia ensues, which causes release of inflammatory mediators, capillary leak, and worsening tissue edema, which perpetuates the cycle (An & West, 2008).

Increasing IAP also leads to decreased blood flow to the other abdominal organs, causing liver failure, renal failure, and oliguira (Handschin, Weber, Renner, & Clavien, 2005; Shear & Rosner, 2006). The expansion of the abdominal cavity forces the diaphragm up into the chest, which leads to a decrease in pulmonary compliance and subsequent increase in airway pressures to deliver the same tidal volume (Pelosi, Quintel, & Malbrain, 2007). Compression of the inferior vena cava and subsequent decreased venous return will decrease cardiac output and eventually progress to obstructive shock.

Risk Factors

Risk factors outlined by the WSACS include diminished abdominal wall compliance, increased intra-luminal contents, increased abdominal contents, and capillary leak (Cheatham et al., 2007; Holodinsky et al., 2013). The most common risk factor is massive fluid resuscitation, defined by WSACS as >5 liters of intravenous fluid within 24 hours. A small prospective trial of 188 patients found that ≥3 liters of crystalloid administered in the Emergency Department led to odds ratio of 23 in development of ACS, although this study was specific to trauma patients (Zsolt Balogh et al., 2003). It is recommended that at risk patients have a baseline measurement of IAP at admission to the ICU and at least every 8 hours thereafter (Cheatham et al., 2007).

No studies to date have evaluated the cardiothoracic surgical population specifically, but it can be presumed that many of the same risk factors apply, such as large volume resuscitation and sepsis. A recent meta-analysis examining ACS after endovascular repair of ruptured abdominal aortic aneurysm may be of interest for those providers that also care for vascular surgery patients and can be found in the additional reading section.

Diagnosis

Diagnosis requires an understanding of the risk factors so that those patients can be assessed for IAH. Although several methods exist, the most widely accepted is via bladder pressure. The technique involves instillation of 25 mL of sterile saline into the bladder via a Foley catheter, clamping of the catheter tubing, insertion of a needle into the specimen collection port, and connection to a pressure transducer (Cheatham et al., 2007). As mentioned above, the transducer must be zeroed appropriately and the patient supine and at end-expiration for an accurate measurement. This can be done intermittently or continuously (Z Balogh, Jones, D'Amours, Parr, & Sugrue, 2004).

Clinically, the triad of tense abdomen, increasing peak airway pressures, and oliguria is extremely non-specific and cannot be relied upon for diagnosis. CT findings such as bowel wall thickening with edema can alert the clinician to the possibility of IAH and/or ACS (Al-Bahrani et al., 2007).

Treatment

Ideally, ACS is "treated" by prevention, which involves screening of at-risk patients and correction of any insults before ACS develops. This, in part, relies on an accurate end-points of resuscitation to avoid excess fluid administration. Currently, the most accepted measures of adequate resuscitation remain the normalization of central venous pressure, lactate, mixed venous oxygen saturation, and base deficit (Englehart & Schreiber, 2006).

Once ACS develops, consultation with a general surgeon for possible decompressive laparotomy is indicated. Although decompression will lead to rapid and dramatic improvements in hypotension, oliguria, and airway pressures, secondary issues such as ischemic-reperfusion injury, open abdominal wound complications, and unsuccessful closure are unfortunately common. Consequently, non-surgical options should also be considered (Table 5) (An & West, 2008). Risks and benefits of each must be weighed within the patient's clinical context and done in consultation with a general surgeon.

Table 5. Non-surgical treatment options for IAH/ACS

Gastric decompression (gastric tube to suction)
Prokinetic agents (e.g. erythromycin, metoclopramide)
Rectal decompression (enemas, rectal tube)
Patient positioning (reverse Trendelenburg)
Sedation
Neuromuscular blockade
Diuretics
Ultrafiltration
Paracentesis

Adapted from: An and West, Critical Care Medicine, 2008

Summary

IAH and ACS carry a high risk of morbidity and mortality and require aggressive screening of at-risk patients for diagnosis due to non-specific signs and symptoms. There are no studies specifically evaluating the cardiothoracic surgical patient, but among mixed ICU patients, certain presenting diagnoses, the presence of shock or metabolic derangement, and the volume of crystalloids used in the initial resuscitation are important risk factors. Successful treatment requires prompt diagnosis and consultation with a general surgeon for non-operative versus operative intervention. Further research, including prospective evaluation of new risk factors derived from a recent meta-analysis and validating a single-center screening tool, is warranted (Holodinsky et al., 2013; Iyer et al., 2014).

Acute Hepatic Failure

Acute liver failure following cardiac surgery is a rare event occurring in approximately 1% of all cases (Raman et al., 2002). However, the mortality associated with such an event is close to 65%. Given the rarity of such failure, little research has been done on this topic. It is well known that patients with preoperative liver disease and associated cirrhosis are poor candidates for cardiac surgery, but very few studies have evaluated the impact of acute onset liver failure after surgery (Hein et al., 2006). Previously hypothesized theories report acute liver failure is a result of a low flow state associated with cardiopulmonary bypass and decreased cardiac output (Raman et al., 2002). Secondarily, acute liver failure can also be a result of congestion from right heart failure leading to obstruction of the intrahepatic small biliary tract (Kumon et al., 1986).

Prevention

There are multiple factors that place a patient at higher risk for acute liver failure after a cardiac procedure, including prolonged cardiopulmonary bypass time, low cardiac output state, vasopressor and/or inotropic support postoperatively, and high filling pressures (Raman et al., 2002). Additionally, combined coronary artery bypass and valve operations, a history of cardiac failure, diabetes, hypertension, and female gender placed patients at increased risk for post-operative liver failure (Raman et al., 2002; Yilmaz et al., 1996).

Diagnosis/Treatment

Diagnosis of acute liver failure often relies on liver function assays including bilirubin, alkaline phosphatase, alanine transaminase (ALT), and lactate dehydrogenase. Previous studies have shown consistency with a ten-fold increase in ALT levels within 48 hours after surgery, and a concurrent increase in lactate dehydrogenase in acute liver failure patients (Raman et al., 2002). The lactate typically returns to normal levels 2-3 days after surgery and the ALT returns to normal levels 5-7 days after surgery. Histological diagnosis, though obtained rarely, reveals centrilobular hepatic necrosis, which is characteristic of acute ischemia. Treatment of acute liver failure is focused on correcting the underlying hypo-perfusion, right heart failure, and/or hypovolemia (Polson & Lee, 2005; Strassburg, 2003). Liver transplantation in this patient population is rarely required (Polson & Lee, 2005). Supportive care becomes of utmost importance in correcting any underlying lactic acidosis, coagulation abnormalities, and monitoring cardiac output (Strassburg, 2003).

Summary

Acute liver failure is a rare but deadly event following cardiac surgery. Quick identification and aggressive correction of underlying causes for liver ischemia are necessary to avoid the need for liver transplantation. Future areas of study have focused on identifying particular hepatic cells responsible in ischemia, including Kupffer cells and hepatocytes, to modulate their activity with TNF-alpha following surgery.

Pancreatitis

Postoperative pancreatitis occurs in 0.01% to 19% of all cardiac patients. This postoperative complication has been noted to increase hospital stay and increase mortality (Chung et al., 2013). Patients who progress to infected pancreatic necrosis have had associated mortality of 15%-30% (Kambhampati et al., 2014). There is a range of pancreatic injury from very mild abdominal complaints, to elevations in laboratory findings, to hemorrhagic or necrotizing pancreatitis.

Prevention/Diagnosis

The diagnosis of pancreatitis often presents with vague symptoms including abdominal pain, inability to tolerate oral intake, nausea, abdominal distention, ileus, fever, and/or elevation in lipase and amylase (Haas & Massachusetts, 1985). Some studies suggest that elevation in lipase is more specific for the diagnosis of pancreatitis postoperatively as hyperamylasemia may result from increased production in pancreatic tissue or due to salivary gland secretion, but typical studies have used the presence of hyperamylasemia for diagnosis (Fernandez-del Castillo et al., 1991). Pancreatitis often presents with a range of symptoms and associated severity. Definitions on tissue biopsy or autopsy have mild pancreatitis defined as scattered focal parenchymal necrosis and fat necrosis (Feiner, 1976). Moderate pancreatitis is similar parenchymal changes seen in mild pancreatitis with more areas affected. Severe pancreatitis has been defined as confluent zones of necrosis. Given most patients do no undergo pancreatic biopsy postoperatively, the clinician is often left with determining severity based on clinical symptoms and imaging with CT scan of the abdomen with IV contrast.

Similar to many abdominal complications following cardiothoracic surgery, acute pancreatitis is considered a result of splanchnic hypoperfusion and ischemic injury to acinar cells. Given the mortality associated with pancreatitis, several studies have tried to identify risk factors. The population most sensitive to develop postoperative acute pancreatitis had hypertension, renal disease, biliary disease, or a history of pancreatitis preoperatively (Chung et al., 2013). Intra-operative risk factors include the use of a non-pulsatile cardiopulmonary bypass circuit, hypothermia, atheromatous or cholesterol emboli, and the presence of venous sludging related to extracorporeal circulation. Furthermore, patients who progress to fatal pancreatitis had continued, significant postoperative hypotension for periods greater than 24 hours after surgery. Severe pancreatitis was also associated with hypercalcemia and increased administration of calcium chloride postoperatively (Fernandez-del Castillo et al., 1991).

Treatment

Given the spectrum of severity of pancreatitis after cardiothoracic surgery, there are multiple approaches to treatment. In mild cases of pancreatitis, a supportive care model is often sufficient with pancreatic tissue healing with no sequelae, or mild areas of pancreatic fibrosis. Supportive measures should focus on fluid resuscitation, bowel rest, pain control, nutritional support, and antibiotics when necessary (Kambhampati et al., 2014). More severe cases can progress to necrotizing pancreatitis or hemorrhagic pancreatitis. Prompt and early operative drainage and debridement in patients that develop hemodynamic compromise is imperative to reduce mortality (Tsiotos et al., 1994). Many studies have also evaluated the use of new medications to help reduce mortality or lessen symptom severity. Such medications include anti-secretory agents, protease inhibitors, immunomodulators, and anti-oxidants. However, these medications still lack adequately powered, reproducible clinical trials associated with their findings (Kambhampati et al., 2014).

Summary

Acute pancreatitis has a wide range of severity from minimal discomfort to requiring emergent surgery and possible death. Early diagnosis is often delayed given the intubated, sedated status of many of the patients and vague laboratory disturbances in many cases of pancreatitis. However, prolonged delay in diagnosis can lead to significant morbidity and even mortality. Future areas of study have focused on new medications to help treat pancreatitis when diagnosed as well as identifying patients at increased risk for development of pancreatitis and providing medications to prevent irreversible damage.

NUTRITION IN THE CRITICALLY ILL

It is well-accepted that critically ill patients enter a catabolic state secondary to underlying systemic inflammatory processes. The ensuing energy deficit leads to breakdown of lean tissue for gluconeogenesis, resulting in severe weakness, difficulty weaning from mechanical ventilation, need for rehabilitation, and increased mortality (De Jonghe et al., 2007; Singer et al., 2009). Yet, the seemingly simple task of providing calories to counteract these complications is anything but straightforward. Over the last decade, a substantial increase in the number of randomized, controlled trials investigating the optimal amount, timing, and route of nutrition has led to a new debate over nutritional practice in the ICU.

Oral Diet

In patients able to eat volitionally, a specialty cardiac diet low in sodium and cholesterol is recommended for the majority of patients in the cardiothoracic ICU setting. Adequate nutrition is necessary for wound healing, so control of post-operative nausea with anti-emetics and supplementation with high-calorie shakes (e.g. Boost) should be encouraged. Maintenance intravenous fluids should be stopped when patients are tolerating a diet.

Pharyngeal Dysfunction

Dysphagia has been noted in up to 50% of cardiac surgery patients who are intubated more than 48 hours (Barke et al., 2009). Predisposing factors include older age, diabetes, COPD, stroke, heart failure, and sepsis. Studies have also shown increased risk in patients who undergo intra-operative TEE (Hogue et al., 1995; Rousou et al., 2000). Thus, bedside swallow or modified barium swallow testing should occur in all patients in accordance with institutional guidelines. Interventions include speech therapy consultation, modified diet, and in some cases, initiation of enteral nutrition.

Initiation of Enteral Nutrition

Enteral nutrition (EN) remains the preferred route of nutrition due to a trophic effect on gut mucosa, although there have been no large, high-quality studies that show an outcomes benefit using this approach (Casaer & Van den Berghe, 2014; Doig et al., 2009). Both the American Society of Parenteral and Enteral Nutrition (ASPEN) and European Society of Parenteral and Enteral Nutrition (ESPEN) recommend initiation of EN within 24-48 hours of admission to the ICU (grade C). ASPEN bases this recommendation on one meta-analysis from 2001 that showed a significant reduction in infectious morbidity and hospital length of stay when compared to delayed feedings (Marik & Zaloga, 2001; Martindale et al., 2009). In comparison, ESPEN guidelines argue that after reviewing methodology of the various trials, there is no definitive data showing improvement using early EN (Kreymann et al., 2006).

Contrary to popular thought, the presence of bowel sounds or passage of flatus or stool is not required for the initiation of enteral feeding (grade B) (Kozar et al., 2002; Martindale et al., 2009). Additionally, in the setting of hemodynamic instability, EN may be provided with caution to patients requiring stable and low doses, although "low" remains subjective. EN should be discontinued if there is an escalating vasopressor requirement, signs of intolerance to feeding (abdominal distention, increasing nasogastric tube output), and/or worsening metabolic acidosis or base deficit (Kozar et al., 2002; Zaloga, Roberts, & Marik, 2003).

Optimal Energy Requirements

Indirect calorimetry remains the most accurate way to determine energy needs, but it is difficult to perform and rarely done in critically ill patients (Frankenfield & Ashcraft, 2011). Hundreds of equations exist to predict energy needs, although most experts caution dependence on any given formula, given the complexity of critically ill patients. Age, previous nutritional status, and ongoing disease processes all contribute to individual energy needs.

ASPEN makes no specific recommendations on how to determine energy requirements, but does advocate advancing to goal within 48-72 hours, or providing at least 50-65% of prescribed nutrition during the first week. ESPEN has a simpler recommendation of 20-25 kcal/kg/day during the acute phase of illness. Overfeeding has been associated with adverse outcomes and can inadvertently occur in elderly patients due to sarcopenia, which reduces energy needs (Raynaud-Simon, Revel-Delhom, & Hébuterne, 2011). Conversely, in obese patients (BMI >30), hypocaloric feeding with 60-70% of target energy requirements, or 11-14 kcal per kg actual body weight per day, is recommended (Martindale et al., 2009). For severely undernourished patients, 25-30 kcal/kg/day is recommended (Kreymann et al., 2006). The Tight Calorie Control Study (TICACOS) randomized patients to receive EN with an energy target determined by indirect calorimetry or according to 25 kcal/kg/day (Singer et al., 2011). This single-center pilot study found a non-significant trend towards decreased mortality in those patients with more individualized energy targets. Large randomized trials are needed to determine if a true mortality benefit exists.

Since malnutrition is associated with worse outcomes, it is intuitive that meeting energy targets would be beneficial, particularly in patients with an anticipated longer duration of mechanical ventilation (e.g. acute respiratory distress syndrome). The Trophic vs. Full-Energy Enteral Nutrition in Mechanically Ventilated Patients with Acute Lung Injury (EDEN) trial randomized 1000 patients to receive either trophic EN (10-20 ml/hr) or full EN (calculated as 25-30 kcal/kg/day) for 6 days, with the primary endpoint of ventilator free days. Despite the trophic EN cohort developing a much larger energy deficit, there were no differences between groups in ventilator-free days, 60 day mortality, or infectious complications (Needham et al., 2013; Rice et al., 2012). These results may lead to changes in the next society guideline updates.

Selection of Formula

The majority of critically ill patients can be given a standard isotonic, high-protein formula, which will provide all macronutrients, free water, electrolytes, trace minerals, and vitamins. Initial concerns that whole proteins could not be adequately digested in critical illness led to a handful of trials comparing whole protein with peptide-based formulas, with no clear advantage and no current recommendation for use (Kreymann et al., 2006; Martindale et al., 2009). Concentrated formulas are available if fluid restriction is necessary. Soluble fiber can be added if diarrhea develops.

In patients with renal injury, standard enteral formulations are considered safe, however, if significant electrolyte abnormalities exist or develop, a renal specific formula can be considered (grade E). Patients receiving continuous renal replacement therapy lose approximately 10-15 g amino acids per day and should consequently receive more protein, between 1.5-2.5 g/kg/day (grade C) (Martindale et al., 2009). Standard formulas are also safe for use in patients with hepatic failure. Feeding in pancreatitis remains a controversial topic and is reviewed separately in this chapter.

Adjunctive Treatment

Recent enthusiasm for glutamine supplementation has diminished due to several recent trials, although society guidelines published prior to these studies recommend enteral glutamine to burn and trauma patients, with conflicting opinions for mixed ICU patients (grade B recommendation per ASPEN, not recommended per ESPEN). Glutamine, a non-essential amino acid synthesized in skeletal muscle, was hypothesized to be "conditionally essential" during critical illness, due to loss of muscle mass and presumed decrease in synthesis (Casaer & Van den Berghe, 2014). A 2002 meta-analysis of early studies showed decreased mortality, ICU length of stay, and infectious risk in those patients that received glutamine supplementation (Novak et al., 2002). However, the recent Scottish Intensive Care Glutamine or Selenium Evaluative Trial (SIGNET) showed no benefit with parenteral glutamine and the Reducing Deaths Due to Oxidative Stress (REDOXS) trial showed an absolute increase in the rate of death of 6.5% at 6 months in those that received enteral glutamine (Andrews et al., 2011; D. Heyland et al., 2013).

Similarly, no high-quality evidence exists to support the routine use of omega-3 fatty acids, which have anti-inflammatory properties and therefore thought to be of benefit in critically ill patients, particularly those with adult respiratory distress syndrome. Again, society guidelines lag behind current evidence, as the most recent ASPEN guidelines from 2009 assign a grade A recommendation for omega-3 supplementation in acute lung injury (Martindale et al., 2009). However, the 2011 OMEGA trial was stopped for futility, as omega-3 fatty acid supplementation did not improve the primary end point of ventilator-free days or other clinical outcomes in patients with acute lung injury (Rice et al., 2011). More recently, a multicenter study of 300 patients compared immune-modulating high-protein (IMHP) nutrition containing glutamine, omega-3 fatty acids, selenium, and antioxidants with standard EN in mechanically ventilated adult patients. IMHP did not improve infectious complications or other clinical end points with possible harm as suggested by increased mortality at 6 months (van Zanten et al., 2014). Thus, expert opinion based on the most recent literature does not support routine glutamine or omega-3 fatty acid supplementation (Casaer & Van den Berghe, 2014; Marik & Zaloga, 2008).

Gastric vs. Small Bowel Feeding

Gastrointestinal dysfunction develops during critical illness, leading to large gastric residual volumes (GRV) with EN and a subsequent longstanding concern for increased risk of aspiration pneumonia. The GRV that can be safely tolerated has been controversial, prompting several studies comparing rates of ventilator associated pneumonia (VAP) between the two routes.

Based on more than 12 randomized trials and 3 meta-analyses, changing the level of infusion of EN from the stomach to the small bowel does reduce the incidence of regurgitation and aspiration, but this has not resulted in a significant decrease in the rate of VAP or mortality (Heyland et al., 2002; Ho, Dobb, & Webb, 2006; Marik & Zaloga, 2003). Since that time, two more large randomized, controlled trials have been published. The Gastric Residual Volume during Enteral Nutrition in ICU Patients (REGANE) trial found that GRVs of 500 mL were not associated with increased pneumonia, duration of mechanical ventilation, or gastrointestinal complications (Montejo et al., 2010). Similiarly, the Effect of Not Monitoring Residual Gastric Volume on the Risk of Ventilator-Associated Pneumonia in Adults Receiving Mechanical Ventilation and Early Enteral Feeding (NUTRIREA-1) trial randomized 449 patients and found that omitting routine GRV did not increase the risk of developing VAP (Reignier et al., 2013).

Per both ASPEN and ESPEN guidelines, either route of feeding is acceptable. Small bowel feeding should only be initiated if the patient is deemed high risk for aspiration or has demonstrated intolerance to gastric feeding (grade C) (Martindale et al., 2009). Risk factors include previous intolerance to gastric feeding, known gastric outlet obstruction, prone positioning, vomiting, and significant opioid requirement. Intolerance is defined as complaints of pain or distention, concerning physical exam findings, lack of flatus or stool, and/or abdominal radiograph findings suggestive of ileus. Holding EN for GRV <500 mL in the absence of any of these findings should be avoided (grade B). Persistent GRV between 250-500 mL should, however, lead to implementation of measures to reduce the risk of aspiration, including head of bed elevation to 30-45 degrees, continuous rather than intermittent delivery, and/or addition of prokinetic motility agents (Martindale et al., 2009). Addition of intravenous metoclopramide or erythromycin can improve gastric emptying, leading to better tolerance of EN, although no studies have shown a significant change in clinical outcomes (Berne et al., 2002; Yavagal, Karnad, & Oak, 2000). Metoclopramide, a dopamine and serotonin receptor antagonist, should be avoided in patients with Parkinson's Disease or those taking other neuroleptic drugs (e.g. typical antipsychotics and phenothiazines) due to risk of extrapyramidal symptoms. Erythromycin can cause QT prolongation and caution should therefore be taken in cardiac surgery patients.

Role of Parenteral Nutrition

As stated above, EN is the preferred route of feeding in the critically ill. By nature of their operation and post-operative course, cardiothoracic surgery patients are less likely to require parenteral nutrition (PN). However, if and when supplemental PN should be initiated is a controversial topic and worth reviewing, with focus on three recent trials.

In well-nourished patients, ASPEN guidelines recommend hypocaloric EN (or no nutrition, if EN is not feasible) for up to 1 week before considering PN (grade C) (Martindale et al., 2009). In contrast, ESPEN recommends initiation of PN within 48 hours of ICU admission to minimize any energy deficit (grade C) (Kreymann et al., 2006). The difference is based on a variety of complications (e.g. liver function abnormalities, infections) observed in older studies (Braunschweig et al., 2001; Grau et al., 2007; Peter, Moran, & Phillips-Hughes, 2005). These studies were performed before the era of glucose control (see *Glucose Control* below) and the worse outcomes with PN are now thought to be secondary to significant hyperglycemia, rather than PN itself.

The Early Parenteral Nutrition in Adult Critically Ill Patients (EPaNIC) trial was a multi-center randomized study of over 4600 patients that directly compared the American and European recommendations (Casaer et al., 2011). It is also the only large study of clinical nutrition with a predominance of cardiac surgery patients. All patients received early initiation of EN with tight glycemic control (80-110 mg/dL), followed by early PN (within 48 hours) or late PN (after day 7). Those patients who received late PN had less infectious complications and decreased duration of mechanical ventilation, but there was no significant difference in mortality between groups.

In the Early Parenteral Nutrition study, 1372 patients with a temporary contraindication to EN received either no nutrition or PN initiated on day one (Gordon S Doig et al., 2013). The early PN group had significantly fewer days of mechanical ventilation, but no difference in the primary endpoint of 60 day mortality. As compared to the EPaNIC trial, the early PN group did not have more infectious complications.

The Supplemental Parenteral Nutrition on Infection Rate, Duration of Mechanical Ventilation, and Rehabilitation in ICU Patients (SPN) trial investigated patients who were eligible to receive EN, but did not meet their targeted energy requirement after 3 days (Heidegger et al., 2013). 305 patients were enrolled, all of whom were receiving less than 60% of their target goal, as determined by indirect calorimetry. Patients were then randomized to receive supplemental PN or continue with EN alone from days 4-8, with primary outcome of nosocomial infection during days 4-28. Those in the supplemental

PN group received a greater number of calories, however, the rate of infection was unchanged. Although this study showed no increased rate of bacteremia with PN, it also showed no clinical benefit (Casaer, Wilmer, & Van den Berghe, 2013).

The three aforementioned trials have yet to incorporated into updated society guidelines. In the interim, clinical judgment regarding early versus late PN in a well-nourished patient should be exercised. The exception is the malnourished patient in whom EN is not feasible, in which PN can be initiated as soon as the patient is stabilized (grade C) (Martindale et al., 2009). Serial efforts to initiate EN should be made in patients receiving solely PN. Once 60% or more of energy requirements are met with EN, PN can be terminated (grade E) (Martindale et al., 2009).

Glucose Control

Critical illness and its associated stress response lead to hyperglycemia in most patients. A landmark study in 2001 showed decreased morbidity and mortality in patients randomized to tight glucose control of 80-110 mg/dL, as compared to standard care of <215 mg/dL (van den Berghe et al., 2001). Although this initially caused a shift in clinical practice, subsequent studies failed to consistently find a mortality benefit. In 2009, the Normoglycemia in Intensive Care Evaluation-Survival Using Glucose Algorithm Regulation (NICE-SUGAR) trial found increased mortality in the tight glycemic group when compared to modest blood sugar control of 140-180 mg/dL, which is now the current standard of care (Finfer et al., 2009). Glucose control and application in the cardiothoracic surgery population is described in further detail in the Endocrine and Metabolic Management chapter.

Summary

In critically ill patients, enteral nutrition is the preferred route of feeding and should be initiated within 24-48 hours of admission to the ICU. Various methods exist to estimate total energy needs, with 20-25 kcal/kg/day a simple and validated option. Patients can be safely fed by either gastric or small bowel feeding. When enteral nutrition alone cannot meet energy targets, supplemental parenteral nutrition should be considered. Use of protocols to avoid overfeeding is strongly recommended (Doig et al., 2008). Controversy exists regarding the use immune-modulating nutrition, such as glutamine and omega-3 fatty acids. Despite a resurgence of research in nutrition, no studies to date have shown a decrease in mortality. Data regarding best nutritional practices specific to the cardiothoracic surgery population is very limited.

STRESS ULCER PROPHYLAXIS

Stress ulceration was first described over 40 years ago and refers to the acute erosive insult to the upper gastrointestinal tract associated with critical illness (Peura, 1986). The disease process is described as a spectrum ranging from asymptomatic stress-related mucosal damage to life-threatening bleeding. A large, prospective study of medical and surgical ICU patients published by the Canadian Critical Care Trials Group in 1994 provided the definitions, prevalence, and risk factors most widely accepted today. Overt bleeding is defined as the presence of hematemesis, bloody gastrointestinal aspirate or melena. Clinically significant bleeding is overt bleeding that leads to hemodynamic instability or the need for blood transfusion (Cook et al., 1994).

Prevalence

Based on endoscopic data, between 75-100% of critically ill patients develop stress-related mucosal damage within 24 hours of admission (Mutlu, Mutlu, & Factor, 2001). However, the prevalence of clinically significant bleeding in all critically ill patients is only 1.5%, and negligible (0.45%) in cardiac surgery patients (Shin & Abah, 2012). Independent risk factors identified include mechanical ventilation >48 hours (odds ratio [OR] = 15.6, p<0.001) and coagulopathy (OR = 9.5, p<0.001). Other identified risk factors include traumatic brain injury, injury severity score of >15, acute renal failure, and high-dose steroid use (Cook et al., 1994).

A subsequent study by the same group found that although rare, clinically significant bleeding led to a relative risk of ICU mortality of 1-4 and in those that survived, an increased ICU stay of 4-8 days (Cook et al., 2001). Despite a myriad of research on this topic, no trials have shown a survival benefit despite various prophylactic regimens (Marik et al., 2010).

Mechanism

Critical illness leads to splanchnic vasoconstriction (Maynard et al., 1993). Associated hypovolemia and/or decreased cardiac output lead to hypoperfusion of the gastric mucosa and subsequent alterations in the protective mucus barrier. Cardiothoracic ICU patients with significant underlying vascular disease may be especially susceptible, although this has not been formally studied.

Pharmacology

Prevention of stress ulceration has been attempted by either cytoprotection or acid suppression. The most widely studied agents include sucralfate, histamine-2 receptor antagonists (H2RA), and proton pump inhibitors (PPI).

Sucralfate act a physical barrier by adhering to gastric epithelial cells, which protects the mucosa from the effects of acid. When compared to H2RA, different studies report conflicting evidence regarding superiority of either agent and rates of associated pneumonia (Cook et al., 1998; Huang, Cao, Liao, Wu, & Gao, 2010). Sucralfate has been shown to impair absorption of enteral feeds and medications (Daley, Rebuck, Welage, & Rogers, 2004). For this reason, as well as ease of administration of other IV agents, it is rarely used first-line anymore.

H2RAs block histamine binding to gastric parietal cell receptors, with a resultant decrease in acid secretion. Many early studies regarding stress ulcer prophylaxis used H2RA, which has been proven to reduce clinically significant bleeding when compared to placebo (Cook, Witt, Cook, & Guyatt, 1991). Use is associated with tachyphylaxis, leading to concerns about long-term efficacy (Plummer, Blaser, & Deane, 2014).

PPIs inhibit the hydrogen/potassium ATPase enzyme of gastric parietal cells, which prevents the secretion of hydrogen ions into the gastric lumen. No randomized controlled trials have ever compared PPIs to placebo, however, a recent meta-analysis comparing PPIs to H2RA found a decreased risk of overt and clinically significant bleeding with PPIs (relative risk [RR] = 0.35) (Alhazzani et al., 2013). However, another meta-analysis found H2RA to be superior in reducing clinically significant bleeding in those patients not receiving enteral nutrition (Marik et al., 2010). Both admit that the statistical analyses were limited by trial methodology and sparse data. Interestingly, the Surviving Sepsis guidelines "suggest" PPI use over H2RA, despite only grade 2C evidence (Dellinger et al., 2013).

Additionally, although intravenous PPIs are the overwhelming choice among American ICUs, there is evidence that PPI suspension can consistently raise gastric pH and prevent clinically significant bleeding (Barletta & Sclar, 2014; Phillips et al., 1996). No studies have directly compared intravenous versus suspension formulations in terms of efficacy and/or cost.

Proton pump inhibitor therapy has also been associated with an increase in infectious complications such as pneumonia and *Clostridium difficile* diarrhea, although this association was not seen in a recent meta-analysis (Alhazzani et al., 2013; Barletta et al., 2013; Herzig, Howell, Ngo, & Marcantonio, 2009; Howell et al., 2010).

A small number of older studies have evaluated whether any stress ulcer prophylaxis is necessary, but these were not randomized controlled trials and were performed primarily in the medical ICU population (Faisy et al., 2003; Zandstra & Stoutenbeek, 1994). A recent meta-analysis of cardiac surgery patients concluded that routine prophylaxis is still warranted (Shin & Abah, 2012).

The protective effect of enteral feeding is also controversial. Although it has been demonstrated that enteral feeding does not significantly raise gastric pH, there are no studies directly comparing enteral feeding to placebo or other pharmacologic agent (Gurman et al., 1990) Again, there is not sufficient evidence to recommend discontinuation of prophylaxis in patients receiving enteral nutrition.

The optimal timing and duration of therapy has not been extensively studied in prospective trials. The majority of society guidelines recommend initiation at the onset of risk factors and continued for the duration of critical illness (Plummer et al., 2014).

Summary

Currently, stress ulcer prophylaxis is recommended in critically ill patients with risk factors, despite a general consensus that the quality of existing data is low (Krag et al., 2014). These recommendations are based on data from over 20 years ago, during which the management of critically ill patients has changed drastically. Importantly, no studies to date have shown a mortality benefit with stress ulcer prophylaxis.

FUTURE RESEARCH

While significant progress has been made in the management of GI issues in critical illness, many more clinical questions have arisen. In mesenteric ischemia, one of the most lethal GI complications, outcomes data comparing endovascular to conventional surgical management is pending. The addition of novel anticoagulant and antiplatelet agents means that further research is needed to determine the optimal post-operative regimen for those patients who require anticoagulation. Prospective studies regarding *Clostridium difficile* infection risk with PPI use and potential benefit with probiotics are warranted, given conflicting data. Similarly, large randomized clinical trials to revisit if and when stress ulcer prophylaxis is necessary are also justified. Continued research regarding the optimal timing, route, and nitrogen content of nutritional support is ongoing (Brisard et al., 2014).

CONCLUSION

As described above, it is imperative that clinicians appreciate and understand the multitude of gastrointestinal issues that can arise during critical illness. Development of an acute abdomen carries a very high mortality rate and thus requires prompt diagnosis and intervention. Nutrition in the critically ill patient is a controversial topic with varying recommendations regarding optimal nutritional practices. Stress ulcer prophylaxis remains a quality measure for hospitals and should be given to patients receiving mechanical ventilation or with an existing coagulopathy. Consultation with speech therapy, nutrition services, gastroenterology or general surgery may be warranted.

REFERENCES

Abboud, B., Daher, R., Sleilaty, G., Madi-Jebara, S., El Asmar, B., Achouch, R., & Jebara, V. (2008). Is prompt exploratory laparotomy the best attitude for mesenteric ischemia after cardiac surgery? *Interactive Cardiovascular and Thoracic Surgery*, *7*(6), 1079–1083. doi:10.1510/icvts.2008.176271 PMID:18815161

Adams, S. D., & Mercer, D. W. (2007). Fulminant Clostridium difficile colitis. *Current Opinion in Critical Care*, *13*(4), 450–455. doi:10.1097/MCC.0b013e3282638879 PMID:17599017

Al-Bahrani, A. Z., Abid, G. H., Sahgal, E., O'shea, S., Lee, S., & Ammori, B. J. (2007). A prospective evaluation of CT features predictive of intra-abdominal hypertension and abdominal compartment syndrome in critically ill surgical patients. *Clinical Radiology*, *62*(7), 676–682. doi:10.1016/j.crad.2006.11.006 PMID:17556037

Alhazzani, W., Alenezi, F., Jaeschke, R. Z., Moayyedi, P., & Cook, D. J. (2013). Proton pump inhibitors versus histamine 2 receptor antagonists for stress ulcer prophylaxis in critically ill patients: A systematic review and meta-analysis. *Critical Care Medicine*, *41*(3), 693–705. doi:10.1097/CCM.0b013e3182758734 PMID:23318494

An, G., & West, M. A. (2008). Abdominal compartment syndrome: A concise clinical review. *Critical Care Medicine*, *36*(4), 1304–1310. doi:10.1097/CCM.0b013e31816929f4 PMID:18379259

Andrews, P. J. D., Avenell, A., Noble, D. W., Campbell, M. K., Croal, B. L., Simpson, W. G., … Cook, J. A. (2011). Randomised trial of glutamine, selenium, or both, to supplement parenteral nutrition for critically ill patients. *British Medical Journal*, *342*, d1542.

Balogh, Z., Jones, F., D'Amours, S., Parr, M., & Sugrue, M. (2004). Continuous intra-abdominal pressure measurement technique. *American Journal of Surgery*, *188*(6), 679–684. doi:10.1016/j.amjsurg.2004.08.052 PMID:15619483

Balogh, Z., McKinley, B. A., Holcomb, J. B., Miller, C. C., Cocanour, C. S., Kozar, R. A., & Moore, F. A. et al. (2003). Both primary and secondary abdominal compartment syndrome can be predicted early and are harbingers of multiple organ failure. *The Journal of Trauma*, *54*(5), 848–859. doi:10.1097/01.TA.0000070166.29649.F3 PMID:12777898

Barker, J., Martino, R., Reichardt, B., Hickey, E. J., & Ralph-Edwards, A. (2009). Incidence and impact of dysphagia in patients receiving prolonged endotracheal intubation after cardiac surgery. *Canadian Journal of Surgery*, *52*(2), 119–124. PMID:19399206

Barletta, J. F., El-Ibiary, S. Y., Davis, L. E., Nguyen, B., & Raney, C. R. (2013). Proton pump inhibitors and the risk for hospital-acquired Clostridium difficile infection. *Mayo Clinic Proceedings*, *88*(10), 1085–1090. doi:10.1016/j.mayocp.2013.07.004 PMID:24012413

Barletta, J. F., & Sclar, D. A. (2014). Use of proton pump inhibitors for the provision of stress ulcer prophylaxis: Clinical and economic consequences. *PharmacoEconomics*, *32*(1), 5–13. doi:10.1007/s40273-013-0119-5 PMID:24271943

Berne, J. D., Norwood, S. H., McAuley, C. E., Vallina, V. L., Villareal, D., Weston, J., & McClarty, J. (2002). Erythromycin reduces delayed gastric emptying in critically ill trauma patients: A randomized, controlled trial. *The Journal of Trauma*, *53*(3), 422–425. doi:10.1097/00005373-200209000-00004 PMID:12352474

Bhat, M., Larocque, M., Amorim, M., Herba, K., Martel, M., De Varennes, B., & Barkun, A. (2012). Prediction and prevention of upper gastrointestinal bleeding after cardiac surgery: A case control study. *Chinese Journal of Gastroenterology and Hepatology*, *26*(6), 340–344. PMID:22720275

Braunschweig, C. L., Levy, P., Sheean, P. M., & Wang, X. (2001). Enteral compared with parenteral nutrition: A meta-analysis. *The American Journal of Clinical Nutrition*, *74*(4), 534–542. PMID:11566654

Brisard, L., Le Gouge, A., Lascarrou, J.-B., Dupont, H., Asfar, P., Sirodot, M., & Reignier, J. et al. (2014). Impact of early enteral versus parenteral nutrition on mortality in patients requiring mechanical ventilation and catecholamines: Study protocol for a randomized controlled trial (NUTRIREA-2). *Trials*, *15*(1), 507. doi:10.1186/1745-6215-15-507 PMID:25539571

Buendgens, L., Bruensing, J., Matthes, M., Dückers, H., Luedde, T., Trautwein, C., & Koch, A. et al. (2014). Administration of proton pump inhibitors in critically ill medical patients is associated with increased risk of developing Clostridium difficile-associated diarrhea. *Journal of Critical Care*, *29*(4), 696.e11–696.e15. doi:10.1016/j.jcrc.2014.03.002 PMID:24674763

Bunte, M. C., Blackstone, E. H., Thuita, L., Fowler, J., Joseph, L., Ozaki, A., & Mountis, M. M. et al. (2013). Major bleeding during heartmate II support. *Journal of the American College of Cardiology*, *62*(23), 2188–2196. doi:10.1016/j.jacc.2013.05.089 PMID:23994419

Carchman, E. H., Peitzman, A. B., Simmons, R. L., & Zuckerbraun, B. S. (2012). The role of acute care surgery in the treatment of severe, complicated Clostridium difficile-associated disease. *Journal of Trauma and Acute Care Surgery*, *73*(4), 789–800. doi:10.1097/TA.0b013e318265d19f PMID:23026914

Casaer, M. P., Mesotten, D., Hermans, G., Wouters, P. J., Schetz, M., Meyfroidt, G., & Van den Berghe, G. et al. (2011). Early versus late parenteral nutrition in critically ill adults. *The New England Journal of Medicine*, *365*(6), 506–517. doi:10.1056/NEJMoa1102662 PMID:21714640

Casaer, M. P., & Van den Berghe, G. (2014). Nutrition in the Acute Phase of Critical Illness. *The New England Journal of Medicine*, *370*(13), 1227–1236. doi:10.1056/NEJMra1304623 PMID:24670169

Casaer, M. P., Wilmer, A., & Van den Berghe, G. (2013). Supplemental parenteral nutrition in critically ill patients. *Lancet*, *381*(9879), 1715. doi:10.1016/S0140-6736(13)61068-5 PMID:23683628

Chang, S.-J., & Huang, H.-H. (2013). Diarrhea in enterally fed patients: Blame the diet? *Current Opinion in Clinical Nutrition and Metabolic Care*, *16*(5), 588–594. doi:10.1097/MCO.0b013e328363bcaf PMID:23799327

Cheatham, M. L., Malbrain, M. L. N. G., Kirkpatrick, A., Sugrue, M., Parr, M., De Waele, J., & Wilmer, A. et al. (2007). Results from the international conference of experts on intra-abdominal hypertension and abdominal compartment syndrome. II. *Recommendations. Intensive Care Med*, *33*(6), 951–962. doi:10.1007/s00134-007-0592-4 PMID:17377769

Chung, J. W., Ryu, S. H., Jo, J. H., Park, J. Y., Lee, S., Park, S. W., & Chung, J. B. et al.J.W. (2013). Clinical implications and risk factors of acute pancreatitis after cardiac valve surgery. *Yonsei Medical Journal*, *54*(1), 154–159. doi:10.3349/ymj.2013.54.1.154 PMID:23225812

Cohen, S. H., Gerding, D. N., Johnson, S., Kelly, C. P., Loo, V. G., McDonald, L. C., & Wilcox, M. H. et al. (2010). Clinical practice guidelines for Clostridium difficile infection in adults: 2010 update by the society for healthcare epidemiology of America (SHEA) and the infectious diseases society of America (IDSA). *Infection Control and Hospital Epidemiology*, *31*(5), 431–455. doi:10.1086/651706 PMID:20307191

Cook, D., Guyatt, G., Marshall, J., Leasa, D., Fuller, H., Hall, R., & Kirby, A. et al. (1998). A comparison of sucralfate and ranitidine for the prevention of upper gastrointestinal bleeding in patients requiring mechanical ventilation. Canadian Critical Care Trials Group. *The New England Journal of Medicine*, *338*(12), 791–797. doi:10.1056/NEJM199803193381203 PMID:9504939

Cook, D. J., Fuller, H. D., Guyatt, G. H., Marshall, J. C., Leasa, D., Hall, R., & Willan, A. et al. (1994). Risk factors for gastrointestinal bleeding in critically ill patients. Canadian Critical Care Trials Group. *The New England Journal of Medicine*, *330*(6), 377–381. doi:10.1056/NEJM199402103300601 PMID:8284001

Cook, D. J., Griffith, L. E., Walter, S. D., Guyatt, G. H., Meade, M. O., Heyland, D. K., & Tryba, M. et al. (2001). The attributable mortality and length of intensive care unit stay of clinically important gastrointestinal bleeding in critically ill patients. *Critical Care (London, England)*, *5*(6), 368–375. doi:10.1186/cc1071 PMID:11737927

Cook, D. J., Witt, L. G., Cook, R. J., & Guyatt, G. H. (1991). Stress ulcer prophylaxis in the critically ill: A meta-analysis. *The American Journal of Medicine*, *91*(5), 519–527. doi:10.1016/0002-9343(91)90189-5 PMID:1835294

D'Ancona, G., Baillot, R., Poirier, B., Dagenais, F., de Ibarra, J. I. S., Bauset, R., & Doyle, D. et al. (2003a). Determinants of gastrointestinal complications in cardiac surgery. *Texas Heart Institute Journal*, *30*(4), 280–285. PMID:14677737

D'Ancona, G., Baillot, R., Poirier, B., Dagenais, F., de Ibarra, J. I. S., Bauset, R., & Doyle, D. et al. (2003b). Determinants of gastrointestinal complications in cardiac surgery. *Texas Heart Institute Journal*, *30*(4), 280–285. PMID:14677737

Daley, R. J., Rebuck, J. A., Welage, L. S., & Rogers, F. B. (2004). Prevention of stress ulceration: Current trends in critical care. *Critical Care Medicine*, *32*(10), 2008–2013. doi:10.1097/01.CCM.0000142398.73762.20 PMID:15483408

De Jonghe, B., Bastuji-Garin, S., Durand, M.-C., Malissin, I., Rodrigues, P., Cerf, C., & Sharshar, T. et al. (2007). Respiratory weakness is associated with limb weakness and delayed weaning in critical illness. *Critical Care Medicine*, *35*(9), 2007–2015. doi:10.1097/01.ccm.0000281450.01881.d8 PMID:17855814

Dellinger, R. P., Levy, M. M., Rhodes, A., Annane, D., Gerlach, H., Opal, S. M., & Moreno, R. et al. (2013). Surviving sepsis campaign: international guidelines for management of severe sepsis and septic shock: 2012. *Critical Care Medicine*, *41*(2), 580–637. doi:10.1097/CCM.0b013e31827e83af PMID:23353941

Dickerson, R. N., & Melnik, G. (1988). Osmolality of oral drug solutions and suspensions. *American Journal of Health-System Pharmacy*, *45*(4), 832–834. PMID:3376967

Doig, G. S., Heighes, P. T., Simpson, F., Sweetman, E. A., & Davies, A. R. (2009). Early enteral nutrition, provided within 24 h of injury or intensive care unit admission, significantly reduces mortality in critically ill patients: A meta-analysis of randomised controlled trials. *Intensive Care Medicine*, *35*(12), 2018–2027. doi:10.1007/s00134-009-1664-4 PMID:19777207

Doig, G. S., Simpson, F., Finfer, S., Delaney, A., Davies, A. R., Mitchell, I., & Dobb, G. (2008). Effect of evidence-based feeding guidelines on mortality of critically ill adults: A cluster randomized controlled trial. *Journal of the American Medical Association*, *300*(23), 2731–2741. doi:10.1001/jama.2008.826 PMID:19088351

Doig, G. S., Simpson, F., & Sweetman, E. (2013). Early parenteral nutrition in critically ill patients with short-term relative contraindications to early enteral nutrition: A randomized controlled trial. *Journal of the American Medical Association*, *309*(20), 2130–2138. doi:10.1001/jama.2013.5124 PMID:23689848

Dong, G., Liu, C., Xu, B., Jing, H., Li, D., & Wu, H. (2012). Postoperative abdominal complications after cardiopulmonary bypass. *Journal of Cardiothoracic Surgery*, *7*(1), 108. doi:10.1186/1749-8090-7-108 PMID:23046511

Egleston, C. V, Wood, a E., Gorey, T. F., & McGovern, E. M. (1993). Gastrointestinal complications after cardiac surgery. *Annals of the Royal College of Surgeons of England*, *75*(1), 52–56. PMID:8422146

Englehart, M. S., & Schreiber, M. A. (2006). Measurement of acid-base resuscitation endpoints: Lactate, base deficit, bicarbonate or what? *Current Opinion in Critical Care*, *12*(6), 569–574. doi:10.1097/MCC.0b013e328010ba4f PMID:17077689

Eris, C., Yavuz, S., Yalcinkaya, S., Gucu, A., Toktas, F., & Yumun, G. (2013). … Ozyazıcıoglu, A. (2013). Acute mesenteric ischemia after cardiac surgery: An analysis of 52 patients. *TheScientificWorldJournal*, 631534. PMID:24288499

Faisy, C., Guerot, E., Diehl, J. L., Iftimovici, E., & Fagon, J. Y. (2003). Clinically significant gastrointestinal bleeding in critically ill patients with and without stress-ulcer prophylaxis. *Intensive Care Medicine*, *29*(8), 1306–1313. doi:10.1007/s00134-003-1863-3 PMID:12830375

Feiner, H. (1976). Pancreatitis after cardiac surgery. *American Journal of Surgery*, *131*(6), 684–688. doi:10.1016/0002-9610(76)90178-1 PMID:937646

Fernandez-del Castillo, C., Harringer, W., Warshaw, A., Vlahakes, G. J., Koski, G., Zaslavsky, A. M., & Rattner, D. W. (1991). Risk factors for pancreatic cellular injury after cardiopulmonary bypass. *The New England Journal of Medicine*, *325*(6), 382–387. doi:10.1056/NEJM199108083250602 PMID:1712076

Filsoufi, F., Rahmanian, P. B., Castillo, J. G., Scurlock, C., Legnani, P. E., & Adams, D. H. (2007). Predictors and outcome of gastrointestinal complications in patients undergoing cardiac surgery. *Annals of Surgery*, *246*(2), 323–329. doi:10.1097/SLA.0b013e3180603010 PMID:17667513

Finfer, S., Chittock, D. R., Su, S. Y.-S., Blair, D., Foster, D., Dhingra, V., & Ronco, J. J. et al. (2009). Intensive versus conventional glucose control in critically ill patients. *The New England Journal of Medicine*, *360*(13), 1283–1297. doi:10.1056/NEJMoa0810625 PMID:19318384

Fiore, G., Brienza, N., Cicala, P., Tunzi, P., Marraudino, N., Schinosa, L., & Fiore, T. (2006). Superior mesenteric artery blood flow modifications during off-pump coronary surgery. *The Annals of Thoracic Surgery*, *82*(1), 62–67. doi:10.1016/j.athoracsur.2006.02.012 PMID:16798189

Frankenfield, D. C., & Ashcraft, C. M. (2011). Estimating energy needs in nutrition support patients. *Journal of Parenteral and Enteral Nutrition*, *35*(5), 563–570. doi:10.1177/0148607111415859 PMID:21832143

Fredriksson, P., Jaakkola, N., & Jaakkola, J. J. K. (2007). Management and outcomes of small bowel obstruction in older adult patients: A prospective cohort study. *Canadian Journal of Surgery*, *57*(6), 1–7.

Gan, T. J., Diemunsch, P., Habib, A. S., Kovac, A., Kranke, P., Meyer, T., & Tramèr, M. R. et al. (2014). Consensus guidelines for the management of postoperative nausea and vomiting. *Anesthesia and Analgesia*, *118*(1), 85–113. doi:10.1213/ANE.0000000000000002 PMID:24356162

Gan, T. J., Meyer, T., Apfel, C. C., Chung, F., Davis, P. J., Eubanks, S., & Watcha, M. et al. (2003). Consensus guidelines for managing postoperative nausea and vomiting. *Anesthesia and Analgesia*, *97*(5), 62–71. doi:10.1213/01.ANE.0000068580.00245.95 PMID:12818945

Grau, T., Bonet, A., Rubio, M., Mateo, D., Farré, M., Acosta, J. A., & Mesejo, A. et al. (2007). Liver dysfunction associated with artificial nutrition in critically ill patients. *Critical Care (London, England)*, *11*(1), R10. doi:10.1186/cc5670 PMID:17254321

Gurman, G., Samri, M., Sarov, B., Bearman, J. E., & Heilig, I. (1990). The rate of gastrointestinal bleeding in a general ICU population: A retrospective study. *Intensive Care Medicine*, *16*(1), 44–49. doi:10.1007/BF01706324 PMID:2107235

Haas, G. S., & Massachusetts, B. (1985). Acute Pancreatitis After Cardiopulrnonary Bypass. *American Journal of Surgery*, *149*(4), 508–515. doi:10.1016/S0002-9610(85)80048-9 PMID:2580453

Hackert, T., Kienle, P., Weitz, J., Werner, J., Szabo, G., Hagl, S., & Schmidt, J. et al. (2003). Accuracy of diagnostic laparoscopy for early diagnosis of abdominal complications after cardiac surgery. *Surgical Endoscopy*, *17*(10), 1671–1674. doi:10.1007/s00464-003-9004-1 PMID:12915977

Handschin, A. E., Weber, M., Renner, E., & Clavien, P.-A. (2005). Abdominal compartment syndrome after liver transplantation. *Liver Transplantation*, *11*(1), 98–100. doi:10.1002/lt.20295 PMID:15690542

Heidegger, C. P., Berger, M. M., Graf, S., Zingg, W., Darmon, P., Costanza, M. C., & Pichard, C. et al. (2013). Optimisation of energy provision with supplemental parenteral nutrition in critically ill patients: A randomised controlled clinical trial. *Lancet*, *381*(9864), 385–393. doi:10.1016/S0140-6736(12)61351-8 PMID:23218813

Hein, O. V., Birnbaum, J., Wernecke, K., England, M., Konertz, W., & Spies, C. (2006). Prolonged intensive care unit stay in cardiac surgery: Risk factors and long-term-survival. *The Annals of Thoracic Surgery*, *81*(3), 880–885. doi:10.1016/j.athoracsur.2005.09.077 PMID:16488688

Herzig, S. J., Howell, M. D., Ngo, L. H., & Marcantonio, E. R. (2009). Acid-suppressive medication use and the risk for hospital-acquired pneumonia. *Journal of the American Medical Association*, *301*(20), 2120–2128. doi:10.1001/jama.2009.722 PMID:19470989

Heyland, D., Muscedere, J., Wischmeyer, P. E., Cook, D., Jones, G., Albert, M., & Day, A. G. et al. (2013). A randomized trial of glutamine and antioxidants in critically ill patients. *The New England Journal of Medicine*, *368*(16), 1489–1497. doi:10.1056/NEJMoa1212722 PMID:23594003

Heyland, D. K., Drover, J. W., Dhaliwal, R., & Greenwood, J. (2002). Optimizing the benefits and minimizing the risks of enteral nutrition in the critically ill: Role of small bowel feeding. *Journal of Parenteral and Enteral Nutrition*, *26*(6Suppl), S51–S55. doi:10.1177/014860710202600608 PMID:12405623

Ho, K. M., Dobb, G. J., & Webb, S. A. R. (2006). A comparison of early gastric and post-pyloric feeding in critically ill patients: A meta-analysis. *Intensive Care Medicine*, *32*(5), 639–649. doi:10.1007/s00134-006-0128-3 PMID:16570149

Hogue, C. W. Jr, Lappas, G. D., Creswell, L. L., Ferguson, T. B. Jr, Sample, M., Pugh, D., & Lappas, D. G. et al. (1995). Swallowing dysfunction after cardiac operations. Associated adverse outcomes and risk factors including intraoperative transesophageal echocardiography. *The Journal of Thoracic and Cardiovascular Surgery*, *110*(2), 517–522. doi:10.1016/S0022-5223(95)70249-0 PMID:7637370

Holodinsky, J. K., Roberts, D. J., Ball, C. G., Reintam Blaser, A., Starkopf, J., & Zygun, D. (2013). Risk factors for intra-abdominal hypertension and abdominal compartment syndrome among adult intensive care unit patients: A systematic review and meta-analysis. *Critical Care (London, England)*, *17*(5), R249. doi:10.1186/cc13075 PMID:24144138

Howell, M. D., Novack, V., Grgurich, P., Soulliard, D., Novack, L., Pencina, M., & Talmor, D. (2010). Iatrogenic gastric acid suppression and the risk of nosocomial Clostridium difficile infection. *Archives of Internal Medicine*, *170*(9), 784–790. doi:10.1001/archinternmed.2010.89 PMID:20458086

Huang, J., Cao, Y., Liao, C., Wu, L., & Gao, F. (2010). Effect of histamine-2-receptor antagonists versus sucralfate on stress ulcer prophylaxis in mechanically ventilated patients: A meta-analysis of 10 randomized controlled trials. *Critical Care (London, England)*, *14*(5), R194. doi:10.1186/cc9312 PMID:21034484

Imrie, C. W., McKay, A. J., Benjamin, I. S., & Blumgart, L. H. (1978). Secondary acute pancreatitis: Aetiology, prevention, diagnosis and management. *British Journal of Surgery*, *65*(6), 399–402. doi:10.1002/bjs.1800650609 PMID:656756

Iyer, D., Rastogi, P., Åneman, A., & D'Amours, S. (2014). Early screening to identify patients at risk of developing intra-abdominal hypertension and abdominal compartment syndrome. *Acta Anaesthesiologica Scandinavica*, *58*(10), 1267–1275. doi:10.1111/aas.12409 PMID:25307712

Jokinen, J., Smith, A. F., Roewer, N., Eberhart, L. H. J., & Kranke, P. (2012). Management of Postoperative Nausea and Vomiting. How to Deal with Refractory PONV. *Anesthesiology Clinics*, *30*(3), 481–493. doi:10.1016/j.anclin.2012.07.003 PMID:22989590

Kambhampati, S., Park, W., Habtezion, A., Kambhampati, S., Park, W., & Habtezion, A. (2014). Pharmacologic therapy for acute pancreatitis. *World Journal of Gastroenterology*, *20*(45), 16868–16880. doi:10.3748/wjg.v20.i45.16868 PMID:25493000

Kehlet, H., & Holte, K. (2001). Review of postoperative ileus. *American Journal Surgery, 182*(5A Suppl), 3S–10S.

Kiessling, A., Reyher, C., Philipp, M., Beiras-fernandez, A., & Moritz, A. (2015). Real-Time Measurement of Rectal Mucosal Microcirculation During Cardiopulmonary Bypass. *Journal of Cardiothoracic and Vascular Anesthesia*, *29*(1), 89–94. doi:10.1053/j.jvca.2014.07.003 PMID:25440640

Kozar, R. A., McQuiggan, M. M., Moore, E. E., Kudsk, K. A., Jurkovich, G. J., & Moore, F. A. (2002). Postinjury enteral tolerance is reliably achieved by a standardized protocol. *The Journal of Surgical Research*, *104*(1), 70–75. doi:10.1006/jsre.2002.6409 PMID:11971680

Krag, M., Perner, A., Wetterslev, J., Wise, M. P., & Hylander Møller, M. (2014). Stress ulcer prophylaxis versus placebo or no prophylaxis in critically ill patients: A systematic review of randomised clinical trials with meta-analysis and trial sequential analysis. *Intensive Care Medicine*, *40*(1), 11–22. doi:10.1007/s00134-013-3125-3 PMID:24141808

Kreymann, K. G., Berger, M. M., Deutz, N. E. P., Hiesmayr, M., Jolliet, P., Kazandjiev, G., & Spies, C. et al. (2006). ESPEN Guidelines on Enteral Nutrition: Intensive care. *Clinical Nutrition (Edinburgh, Lothian)*, *25*(2), 210–223. doi:10.1016/j.clnu.2006.01.021 PMID:16697087

Kumon, K., Tanaka, K., Hirata, T., Naito, Y., & Fujita, T. (1986). Organ failures due to low cardiac output syndrome following open heart surgery. *Japanese Circulation Journal*, *50*(4), 329–335. doi:10.1253/jcj.50.329 PMID:3489109

Kyne, L., Sougioultzis, S., McFarland, L. V., & Kelly, C. P. (2002). Underlying disease severity as a major risk factor for nosocomial Clostridium difficile diarrhea. *Infection Control and Hospital Epidemiology*, *23*(11), 653–659. doi:10.1086/501989 PMID:12452292

MacLeod, J. B. A., Lefton, J., Houghton, D., Roland, C., Doherty, J., Cohn, S. M., & Barquist, E. S. (2007). Prospective randomized control trial of intermittent versus continuous gastric feeds for critically ill trauma patients. *The Journal of Trauma*, *63*(1), 57–61. doi:10.1097/01.ta.0000249294.58703.11 PMID:17622869

Malbrain, M. L. N. G., Chiumello, D., Pelosi, P., Bihari, D., Innes, R., Ranieri, V. M., & Gattinoni, L. et al. (2005). Incidence and prognosis of intraabdominal hypertension in a mixed population of critically ill patients: A multiple-center epidemiological study. *Critical Care Medicine*, *33*(2), 315–322. doi:10.1097/01.CCM.0000153408.09806.1B PMID:15699833

Malbrain, M. L. N. G., Chiumello, D., Pelosi, P., Wilmer, A., Brienza, N., Malcangi, V., & Gattinoni, L. et al. (2004). Prevalence of intra-abdominal hypertension in critically ill patients: A multicentre epidemiological study. *Intensive Care Medicine*, *30*(5), 822–829. doi:10.1007/s00134-004-2169-9 PMID:14758472

Mangi, A. A., Christison-Lagay, E. R., Torchiana, D. F., Warshaw, A. L., & Berger, D. L. (2005). Gastrointestinal complications in patients undergoing heart operation: An analysis of 8709 consecutive cardiac surgical patients. *Annals of Surgery*, *241*(6), 895–901. doi:10.1097/01.sla.0000164173.05762.32 PMID:15912039

Marik, P. E., Vasu, T., Hirani, A., & Pachinburavan, M. (2010). Stress ulcer prophylaxis in the new millennium: A systematic review and meta-analysis. *Critical Care Medicine*, *38*(11), 2222–2228. doi:10.1097/CCM.0b013e3181f17adf PMID:20711074

Marik, P. E., & Zaloga, G. P. (2001). Early enteral nutrition in acutely ill patients: A systematic review. *Critical Care Medicine*, *29*(12), 2264–2270. doi:10.1097/00003246-200112000-00005 PMID:11801821

Marik, P. E., & Zaloga, G. P. (2003). Gastric versus post-pyloric feeding: A systematic review. *Critical Care (London, England)*, *7*(3), R46–R51. doi:10.1186/cc2190 PMID:12793890

Marik, P. E., & Zaloga, G. P. (2008). Immunonutrition in critically ill patients: A systematic review and analysis of the literature. *Intensive Care Medicine*, *34*(11), 1980–1990. doi:10.1007/s00134-008-1213-6 PMID:18626628

Martindale, R. G., McClave, S. A., Vanek, V. W., McCarthy, M., Roberts, P., Taylor, B., & Cresci, G. et al. (2009). Guidelines for the provision and assessment of nutrition support therapy in the adult critically ill patient: Society of Critical Care Medicine and American Society for Parenteral and Enteral Nutrition: Executive Summary. *Critical Care Medicine*, *37*(5), 1757–1761. doi:10.1097/CCM.0b013e3181a40116 PMID:19373044

Mathias, J., Mathias, E., Jausset, F., Oliver, A., Sellal, C., Laurent, V., & Regent, D. (2012). Aorto-enteric fistulas: A physiopathological approach and computed tomography diagnosis. *Diagnostic and Interventional Imaging*, *93*(11), 840–851. doi:10.1016/j.diii.2012.07.003 PMID:23092721

Maung, A., Johnson, D. C., Piper, G. L., Barbosa, R. R., Rowell, S. E., Bokhari, F., & Kerwin, A. J. et al. (2012). Evaluation and management of small-bowel obstruction. *Journal of Trauma and Acute Care Surgery*, *73*(5), S362–S369. doi:10.1097/TA.0b013e31827019de PMID:23114494

Maynard, N., Bihari, D., Beale, R., Smithies, M., Baldock, G., Mason, R., & McColl, I. (1993). Assessment of splanchnic oxygenation by gastric tonometry in patients with acute circulatory failure. *Journal of the American Medical Association*, *270*(10), 1203–1210. doi:10.1001/jama.1993.03510100053032 PMID:8355382

McSweeney, M. E., Garwood, S., Levin, J., Marino, M. R., Wang, S. X., Kardatzke, D., & Wolman, R. L. et al. (2004). Adverse gastrointestinal complications after cardiopulmonary bypass: Can outcome be predicted from preoperative risk factors? *Anesthesia and Analgesia*, *98*(6), 1610–1617. doi:10.1213/01.ANE.0000113556.40345.2E PMID:15155313

Modena, S., Bearelly, D., Swartz, K., & Friedenberg, F. K. (2005). Clostridium difficile among hospitalized patients receiving antibiotics: A case-control study. *Infection Control and Hospital Epidemiology*, *26*(8), 685–690. doi:10.1086/502603 PMID:16156324

Montejo, J. C., Grau, T., Acosta, J., Ruiz-Santana, S., Planas, M., García-De-Lorenzo, A., & López-Martínez, J. et al. (2002). Multicenter, prospective, randomized, single-blind study comparing the efficacy and gastrointestinal complications of early jejunal feeding with early gastric feeding in critically ill patients. *Critical Care Medicine*, *30*(4), 796–800. doi:10.1097/00003246-200204000-00013 PMID:11940748

Montejo, J. C., Miñambres, E., Bordejé, L., Mesejo, A., Acosta, J., Heras, A., & Manzanedo, R. et al. (2010). Gastric residual volume during enteral nutrition in ICU patients: The REGANE study. *Intensive Care Medicine*, *36*(8), 1386–1393. doi:10.1007/s00134-010-1856-y PMID:20232036

Morrow, L. E. (2009). Probiotics in the intensive care unit. *Current Opinion in Critical Care*, *15*(2), 144–148. doi:10.1097/MCC.0b013e3283252d2d PMID:19300087

Mudd, J. O., & Gelow, J. M. (2013). Bleeding after heartmate II implantation: A cloud in the silver lining. *Journal of the American College of Cardiology*, *62*(23), 2197–2198. doi:10.1016/j.jacc.2013.08.696 PMID:23994418

Mutlu, G. M., Mutlu, E. A., & Factor, P. (2001). GI complications in patients receiving mechanical ventilation. *Chest*, *119*(4), 1222–1241. doi:10.1378/chest.119.4.1222 PMID:11296191

Needham, D. M., Dinglas, V. D., Morris, P. E., Jackson, J. C., Hough, C. L., Mendez-Tellez, P. A., & Hopkins, R. O. et al. (2013). Physical and cognitive performance of patients with acute lung injury 1 year after initial trophic versus full enteral feeding EDEN Trial follow-up. *American Journal of Respiratory and Critical Care Medicine*, *188*(5), 567–576. doi:10.1164/rccm.201304-0651OC PMID:23805899

Novak, F., Heyland, D. K., Avenell, A., Drover, J. W., & Su, X. (2002). Glutamine supplementation in serious illness: A systematic review of the evidence. *Critical Care Medicine*, *30*(9), 2022–2029. doi:10.1097/00003246-200209000-00011 PMID:12352035

Ohri, S. K., & Velissaris, T. (2006). Gastrointestinal dysfunction following cardiac surgery. *Perfusion*, *21*(4), 215–223. doi:10.1191/0267659106pf871oa PMID:16939115

Pelosi, P., Quintel, M., & Malbrain, M. L. N. G. (2007). Effect of intra-abdominal pressure on respiratory mechanics. *Acta Clinica Belgica*, *62*(Suppl 1), 78–88. doi:10.1179/acb.2007.62.s1.011 PMID:24881704

Peter, J. V., Moran, J. L., & Phillips-Hughes, J. (2005). A meta-analysis of treatment outcomes of early enteral versus early parenteral nutrition in hospitalized patients. *Critical Care Medicine*, *33*(1), 213–220. doi:10.1097/01.CCM.0000150960.36228.C0 PMID:15644672

Peura, D. A. (1986). Stress-related mucosal damage. *Clinical Therapeutics*, *8*(Suppl A), 14–23. PMID:2878727

Phillips, J. O., Metzler, M. H., Palmieri, M. T., Huckfeldt, R. E., & Dahl, N. G. (1996). A prospective study of simplified omeprazole suspension for the prophylaxis of stress-related mucosal damage. *Critical Care Medicine*, *24*(11), 1793–1800. doi:10.1097/00003246-199611000-00006 PMID:8917027

Plummer, M. P., Blaser, A. R., & Deane, A. M. (2014). Stress ulceration: prevalence, pathology and association with adverse outcomes. *Critical Care, 18*(2), 213.

Polson, J., & Lee, W. M. (2005). AASLD position paper: The management of acute liver failure. *Hepatology (Baltimore, Md.), 41*(5), 1179–1197. doi:10.1002/hep.20703 PMID:15841455

Raman, J. S., Kochi, K., Morimatsu, H., Buxton, B., & Bellomo, R. (2002). Severe ischemic early liver injury after cardiac surgery. *The Annals of Thoracic Surgery, 74*(5), 1601–1606. doi:10.1016/S0003-4975(02)03877-8 PMID:12440615

Raynaud-Simon, A., Revel-Delhom, C., & Hébuterne, X. (2011). Clinical practice guidelines from the French health high authority: Nutritional support strategy in protein-energy malnutrition in the elderly. *Clinical Nutrition (Edinburgh, Lothian), 30*(3), 312–319. doi:10.1016/j.clnu.2010.12.003 PMID:21251732

Reignier, J., Mercier, E., Le Gouge, A., Boulain, T., Desachy, A., Bellec, F., & Lascarrou, J.-B. et al. (2013). Effect of not monitoring residual gastric volume on risk of ventilator-associated pneumonia in adults receiving mechanical ventilation and early enteral feeding: A randomized controlled trial. *Journal of the American Medical Association, 309*(3), 249–256. doi:10.1001/jama.2012.196377 PMID:23321763

Rice, T. W., Wheeler, A. P., Thompson, B. T., DeBoisblanc, B. P., Steingrub, J., & Rock, P. (2011). Enteral omega-3 fatty acid, gamma-linolenic acid, and antioxidant supplementation in acute lung injury. *Journal of the American Medical Association, 306*(14), 1574–1581. doi:10.1001/jama.2011.1435 PMID:21976613

Rice, T. W., Wheeler, A. P., Thompson, B. T., Steingrub, J., Hite, R. D., Moss, M., & Rock, P. et al. (2012). Initial trophic vs full enteral feeding in patients with acute lung injury. *Journal of the American Medical Association, 307*(8), 795–803. doi:10.1001/jama.2012.137 PMID:22307571

Rodriguez, R., Robich, M. P., Plate, J. F., Trooskin, S. Z., & Sellke, F. W. (2010). Gastrointestinal complications following cardiac surgery: A comprehensive review. *Journal of Cardiac Surgery, 25*(2), 188–197. doi:10.1111/j.1540-8191.2009.00985.x PMID:20149010

Rousou, J. A., Tighe, D. A., Garb, J. L., Krasner, H., Engelman, R. M., Flack, J. E. III, & Deaton, D. W. (2000). Risk of dysphagia after transesophageal echocardiography during cardiac operations. *The Annals of Thoracic Surgery, 69*(2), 486–489. doi:10.1016/S0003-4975(99)01086-3 PMID:10735685

Shear, W., & Rosner, M. H. (2006). Acute kidney dysfunction secondary to the abdominal compartment syndrome. *Journal of Nephrology, 19*(5), 556–565. PMID:17136682

Shin, J.-S., & Abah, U. (2012). Is routine stress ulcer prophylaxis of benefit for patients undergoing cardiac surgery? *Interactive Cardiovascular and Thoracic Surgery, 14*(5), 622–628. doi:10.1093/icvts/ivs019 PMID:22345061

Singer, P., Anbar, R., Cohen, J., Shapiro, H., Shalita-Chesner, M., Lev, S., & Madar, Z. et al. (2011). The tight calorie control study (TICACOS): A prospective, randomized, controlled pilot study of nutritional support in critically ill patients. *Intensive Care Medicine, 37*(4), 601–609. doi:10.1007/s00134-011-2146-z PMID:21340655

Singer, P., Berger, M. M., Van den Berghe, G., Biolo, G., Calder, P., Forbes, A., & Pichard, C. et al. (2009). ESPEN Guidelines on Parenteral Nutrition: Intensive care. *Clinical Nutrition (Edinburgh, Lothian)*, *28*(4), 387–400. doi:10.1016/j.clnu.2009.04.024 PMID:19505748

Sperry, J., & Cohen, M. J. (2014). Acute Obstruction. *The Surgical Clinics of North America*, *94*(1), 77–96. doi:10.1016/j.suc.2013.10.001 PMID:24267500

Strassburg, C. P. (2003). Shock liver. *Best Practice & Research. Clinical Gastroenterology*, *17*(3), 369–381. doi:10.1016/S1521-6918(03)00025-8 PMID:12763502

Tenofsky, P. L., Beamer, L., & Smith, R. S. (2000). Ogilvie syndrome as a postoperative complication. *Archives of Surgery*, *135*(6), 682–687. doi:10.1001/archsurg.135.6.682 PMID:10843364

Theodorakopoulou, M., Perros, E., Giamarellos-Bourboulis, E. J., & Dimopoulos, G. (2013). Controversies in the management of the critically ill: The role of probiotics. *International Journal of Antimicrobial Agents*, *42*(Suppl), S41–S44. doi:10.1016/j.ijantimicag.2013.04.010 PMID:23664676

Tsiotos, G. G., Mullany, C. J., Zietlow, S., & van Heerden, J. (1994). Abdominal complications following cardiac surgery. *American Journal of Surgery*, *167*(6), 553–557. doi:10.1016/0002-9610(94)90096-5 PMID:8209926

Tu, C. P., Tsai, C. H., Tsai, C. C., Huang, T. S., Cheng, S. P., & Liu, T. P. (2014). Postoperative ileus in the elderly. *International Journal of Gerontology*, *8*(1), 1–5. doi:10.1016/j.ijge.2013.08.002

Van den Berghe, G., Wouters, P., Weekers, F., Verwaest, C., Bruyninckx, F., Schetz, M., & Bouillon, R. et al. (2001). Intensive insulin therapy in critically ill patients. *The New England Journal of Medicine*, *345*(19), 1359–1367. doi:10.1056/NEJMoa011300 PMID:11794168

Van Zanten, A. R. H., Sztark, F., Kaisers, U. X., Zielmann, S., Felbinger, T. W., Sablotzki, A. R., & Hofman, Z. et al. (2014). High-protein enteral nutrition enriched with immune-modulating nutrients vs standard high-protein enteral nutrition and nosocomial infections in the ICU: A randomized clinical trial. *Journal of the American Medical Association*, *312*(5), 514–524. doi:10.1001/jama.2014.7698 PMID:25096691

Velissaris, T., Tang, A., Murray, M., El-Minshawy, A., Hett, D., & Ohri, S. (2003). A prospective randomized study to evaluate splanchnic hypoxia during beating-heart and conventional coronary revascularization. *European Journal of Cardio-Thoracic Surgery*, *23*(6), 917–924. doi:10.1016/S1010-7940(03)00167-2 PMID:12829067

Viana, F. F., Chen, Y., Almeida, A., Baxter, H. D., Cochrane, A. D., & Smith, J. (2013). Gastrointestinal complications after cardiac surgery: 10-year experience of a single australian centre. *ANZ Journal of Surgery*, *83*(9), 651–656. doi:10.1111/ans.12134 PMID:23530720

Vidal, M. G., Ruiz Weisser, J., Gonzalez, F., Toro, M. A., Loudet, C., Balasini, C., & Estenssoro, E. et al. (2008). Incidence and clinical effects of intra-abdominal hypertension in critically ill patients. *Critical Care Medicine*, *36*(6), 1823–1831. doi:10.1097/CCM.0b013e31817c7a4d PMID:18520642

Whelan, K., Judd, P. A., Preedy, V. R., & Taylor, M. A. (2004). Enteral feeding: The effect on faecal output, the faecal microflora and SCFA concentrations. *The Proceedings of the Nutrition Society*, *63*(1), 105–113. doi:10.1079/PNS2003317 PMID:15099408

Wiesen, P., Van Gossum, A., & Preiser, J.-C. (2006). Diarrhoea in the critically ill. *Current Opinion in Critical Care*, *12*(2), 149–154. doi:10.1097/01.ccx.0000216583.64804.46 PMID:16543792

Williams, B. a, Kentor, M. L., Skledar, S. J., Orebaugh, S. L., & Vallejo, M. C. (. (2007). Eliminating postoperative nausea and vomiting in outpatient surgery with multimodal strategies including low doses of nonsedating, off-patent antiemetics: Is "zero tolerance" achievable? *TheScientificWorldJournal*, *7*, 978–986. doi:10.1100/tsw.2007.132 PMID:17619779

Yang, G., Wu, X.-T., Zhou, Y., & Wang, Y.-L. (2005). Application of dietary fiber in clinical enteral nutrition: A meta-analysis of randomized controlled trials. *World Journal of Gastroenterology*, *11*(25), 3935–3938. PMID:15991297

Yavagal, D. R., Karnad, D. R., & Oak, J. L. (2000). Metoclopramide for preventing pneumonia in critically ill patients receiving enteral tube feeding: A randomized controlled trial. *Critical Care Medicine*, *28*(5), 1408–1411. doi:10.1097/00003246-200005000-00025 PMID:10834687

Yilmaz, T., Arslan, M., Demirkilç, U., Ozal, E., Kuralay, E., Bingöl, H., … Oztürk, O. Y. (1996). Gastrointestinal complications after cardiac surgery. *European Journal of Cardiothoracic Surgery, 10*(9), 763–7.

Yip, C., Loeb, M., Salama, S., Moss, L., & Olde, J. (2001). Quinolone use as a risk factor for nosocomial Clostridium difficile-associated diarrhea. *Infection Control and Hospital Epidemiology*, *22*(9), 572–575. doi:10.1086/501954 PMID:11732787

Zaloga, G. P., Roberts, P. R., & Marik, P. (2003). Feeding the hemodynamically unstable patient: A critical evaluation of the evidence. *Nutrition in Clinical Practice*, *18*(4), 285–293. doi:10.1177/0115426503018004285 PMID:16215052

Zandstra, D. F., & Stoutenbeek, C. P. (1994). The virtual absence of stress-ulceration related bleeding in ICU patients receiving prolonged mechanical ventilation without any prophylaxis. A prospective cohort study. *Intensive Care Medicine*, *20*(5), 335–340. doi:10.1007/BF01720905 PMID:7930027

Zilberberg, M. D., & Shorr, A. F. (2013). Preventing Clostridium Difficile Infection in the Intensive Care Unit. *Critical Care Clinics*, *29*(1), 11–18. doi:10.1016/j.ccc.2012.10.006 PMID:23182524

ADDITIONAL READING

Alberda, C., Gramlich, L., Jones, N., Jeejeebhoy, K., Day, A. G., Dhaliwal, R., & Heyland, D. K. (2009). The relationship between nutritional intake and clinical outcomes in critically ill patients: Results of an international multicenter observational study. *Intensive Care Medicine*, *35*(10), 1728–1737. doi:10.1007/s00134-009-1567-4 PMID:19572118

Bojar, R. M. (2011). Post-ICU Care and Other Complications. Manual of Perioperative Care in Adult Cardiac Surgery, Fifth Edition (pp. 694–705).

Casaer, M. P., Wilmer, A., Hermans, G., Wouters, P. J., Mesotten, D., & Van Den Berghe, G. (2013). Role of disease and macronutrient dose in the randomized controlled epanic trial a post hoc analysis. *American Journal of Respiratory and Critical Care Medicine*, *187*(3), 247–255. doi:10.1164/rccm.201206-0999OC PMID:23204255

Fredriksson, P., Jaakkola, N., & Jaakkola, J. J. K. (2007). Management and outcomes of small bowel obstruction in older adult patients: A prospective cohort study. *Canadian Journal of Surgery*, *57*(6), 1–7.

Harvey, S. E., Parrott, F., Harrison, D. A., Bear, D. E., Segaran, E., Beale, R., & Rowan, K. M. et al. (2014). Trial of the Route of Early Nutritional Support in Critically Ill Adults. *The New England Journal of Medicine*, *371*(18), 1673–1684. doi:10.1056/NEJMoa1409860 PMID:25271389

Imrie, C. W., McKay, A. J., Benjamin, I. S., & Blumgart, L. H. (1978). Secondary acute pancreatitis: Aetiology, prevention, diagnosis and management. *British Journal of Surgery*, *65*(6), 399–402. doi:10.1002/bjs.1800650609 PMID:656756

Johnson, W. C., & Nabseth, D. C. (1974). Visceral Infarction Following Aortic Surgery. *Annals of Surgery*, *180*(3), 312–318. doi:10.1097/00000658-197409000-00010 PMID:4277757

Karkos, C. D., Menexes, G. C., Patelis, N., Kalogirou, T. E., Giagtzidis, I. T., & Harkin, D. W. (2014). A systematic review and meta-analysis of abdominal compartment syndrome after endovascular repair of ruptured abdominal aortic aneurysms. *Journal of Vascular Surgery*, *59*(3), 829–842. doi:10.1016/j.jvs.2013.11.085 PMID:24439324

Koretz, R. L. (2009). Enteral nutrition: A hard look at some soft evidence. *Nutrition in Clinical Practice*, *24*(3), 316–324. doi:10.1177/0884533609335378 PMID:19483061

Kron, I. L., Harman, P. K., & Nolan, S. P. (1984). The measurement of intra-abdominal pressure as a criterion for abdominal re-exploration. *Annals of Surgery*, *199*(1), 28–30. doi:10.1097/00000658-198401000-00005 PMID:6691728

Losser, M.-R., Damoisel, C., & Payen, D. (2010). Bench-to-bedside review: Glucose and stress conditions in the intensive care unit. *Critical Care (London, England)*, *14*(4), 231. doi:10.1186/cc9100 PMID:20727232

Manzanares, W., Langlois, P. L., & Hardy, G. (2013). Update on antioxidant micronutrients in the critically ill. *Current Opinion in Clinical Nutrition and Metabolic Care*, *16*(6), 719–725. doi:10.1097/MCO.0b013e32836599e5 PMID:24100672

Mowatt-Larssen, C. A., Brown, R. O., Wojtysiak, S. L., & Kudsk, K. A. (1992). Comparison of tolerance and nutritional outcome between a peptide and a standard enteral formula in critically ill, hypoalbuminemic patients. *Journal of Parenteral and Enteral Nutrition*, *16*(1), 20–24. doi:10.1177/014860719201600120 PMID:1738214

Novack, L., Kogan, S., Gimpelevich, L., Howell, M., Borer, A., Kelly, C. P., & Novack, V. et al. (2014). Acid suppression therapy does not predispose to Clostridium difficile infection: The case of the potential bias. *PLoS ONE*, *9*(10), e110790. doi:10.1371/journal.pone.0110790 PMID:25343667

Serpa, L. F., Kimura, M., Faintuch, J., & Ceconello, I. (2003). Effects of continuous versus bolus infusion of enteral nutrition in critical patients. *Revista Do Hospital Das Clinicas. Faculdade de Medicina Da Universidade de Sao Paulo*, *58*(1), 9–14.

Singer, P., Hiesmayr, M., Biolo, G., Felbinger, T. W., Berger, M. M., Goeters, C., & Pichard, C. et al. (2014). Pragmatic approach to nutrition in the ICU: Expert opinion regarding which calorie protein target. *Clinical Nutrition (Edinburgh, Lothian)*, *33*(2), 246–251. PMID:24434033

Skillman, J. J., Bushnell, L. S., Goldman, H., & Silen, W. (1969). Respiratory failure, hypotension, sepsis, and jaundice. A clinical syndrome associated with lethal hemorrhage from acute stress ulceration of the stomach. *American Journal of Surgery*, *117*(4), 523–530. doi:10.1016/0002-9610(69)90011-7 PMID:5771525

Vanderheyden, S., Casaer, M. P., Kesteloot, K., Simoens, S., De Rijdt, T., Peers, G., & Mesotten, D. et al. (2012). Early versus late parenteral nutrition in ICU patients: Cost analysis of the EPaNIC trial. *Critical Care (London, England)*, *16*(3), R96. doi:10.1186/cc11361 PMID:22632574

KEY TERMS AND DEFINITIONS

Bacterial Translocation: Migration of bacterial organisms from the intestinal lumen to normally sterile tissues, due to breakdown of mucosal barrier functions from inflammation or necrosis of gut epithelial cells.

Indirect Calorimetry: Measurement of oxygen consumption and carbon dioxide production to determine metabolic rate, considered gold-standard for determining a patient's individual energy requirements.

Ogilvie's Syndrome: A pseudo-obstruction of the colon, essentially acute colonic dilation without associated mechanical obstruction.

Splanchnic Circulation: Vasculature that originates from the celiac, superior mesenteric, and inferior mesenteric arteries and supplies the majority of intra-abdominal organs.

Stress-Related Clinically Significant Bleeding: Overt bleeding that leads to hemodynamic changes or drop in hemoglobin > 2 mg/dL.

Stress-Related Mucosal Disease: Diffuse, superficial, upper gastrointestinal mucosal damage.

Stress-Related Overt Bleeding: Hematemesis, bloody or coffee-ground nasogastric aspirate, melena, or hematochezia.

Stress-Related Ulceration: Discrete lesion that extends into the gastric submucosa.

Trophic Feeds: A volume of enteral nutrition that is too low to meet full nutritional needs but has some presumed gastrointestinal benefit (i.e. prevents gut mucosal atrophy).

Chapter 19
Infection and Immune System

Peter von Homeyer
University of Washington, USA

ABSTRACT

Infections are a major cause of mortality in intensive care unit (ICU) patients and the most common non-cardiac complications after cardiac surgery. Commonly encountered infections in the cardiothoracic ICU include pneumonia, bloodstream infections, and surgical site infections. At the beginning of this chapter, general measures of infection control and prevention are introduced. Those can help reduce infections and are best implemented in a bundled care fashion. Specifically for ICU patients, care bundles aimed at ventilator-associated pneumonia and central line-associated bloodstream infection have been successfully implemented, studied, and revised. In the next section, antibiotic treatment principles are described. Treatment with antibiotic drugs is an important part of therapy for infectious complications and is under continuous revision given the changing and diverse spectrum of microorganisms and the emergence of multidrug-resistance. In the central part of the chapter, specific infections are discussed in detail with regards to etiology, incidence, diagnosis, and therapy. Finally, the concept of systemic inflammatory response is described which is a common clinical problem after cardiac surgery, particularly with the use of cardiopulmonary bypass. Several immunologic mechanisms have been found to be associated with this and the clinical picture can be confused with sepsis.

INTRODUCTION

Infections remain a major cause of mortality in patients admitted to the intensive care unit (ICU). Most infections encountered following cardiothoracic surgery are hospital-acquired or nosocomial with an incidence of around 5% (Gelijns et al., 2014; Michalopoulos, Geroulanos, Rosmarakis, & Falagas, 2006). The majority of infectious complications concern the lungs, the blood stream, or the surgical site.

Systemic inflammatory response and interaction with the immune system play an important role after cardiac surgery, particularly with the use of cardiopulmonary bypass (CPB) (Larmann & Theilmeier, 2004; Paparella, Yau, & Young, 2002). While the pathophysiology is somewhat different, the clinical picture can resemble that of sepsis or septic shock.

DOI: 10.4018/978-1-4666-8603-8.ch019

In this chapter, we will first discuss measures to control and prevent infections in the ICU environment and basic concepts of antibiotic therapy. The second focus will be on the epidemiology, pathophysiology, diagnosis, and clinical management of common infections in the cardiothoracic surgical population. Lastly, the incidence, pathophysiology, and management of systemic inflammation as a non-specific host response with or without evidence of infection will be addressed.

BACKGROUND

Postoperative care on the ICU has improved significantly over the last decade, particularly with the advent of protocols and checklists guiding early extubation, glucose control, and blood conservation, to mention a few. Major healthcare-acquired infections, however, remain an important factor, as they do significantly contribute to morbidity, mortality, and cost (Stone et al., 2014).

The overall rate of infections following cardiac surgery has also improved over the years (Kollef et al., 1997), but the incidence now remains constant at around 5% (Michalopoulos et al., 2006). Unfortunately, studies looking at overall infection rates are rare, so epidemiologic data in this population is limited. More commonly, studies focus on specific infections and subgroups of patients, and clinical risk factors for acquiring major infections after cardiac surgery have been described (Fowler et al., 2005; Lola et al., 2011). One reason for a stable infection rate despite more aggressive measures to prevent infection is the fact that the population of patients undergoing major cardiothoracic surgery today is older and shows more comorbidities than ten years ago. Surgical practice also underwent a significant shift with a decrease in so-called routine operations and an exponential increase in complexity, i.e. surgery for adult congenital heart disease and end-stage heart failure.

Antibiotic drugs are a mainstay of therapy for infections and are more commonly used in the ICU than in other patient populations. Adequate perioperative prophylaxis using antibiotics is a well-accepted practice and drug choice and duration of prophylaxis is outlined in the respective guidelines put forward by the Society of Thoracic Surgeons (Edwards, Engelman, Houck, Shahian, & Bridges, 2006; Engelman et al., 2007). Conversely, overuse and uncritical initiation of therapy has significantly increased resistance to antibiotic drugs in the last 20 years (Livermore, 2005; Fournier et al., 2013). Multi-resistant bacteria are more and more present, and there are very few therapeutic options to treat infections caused by those highly pathogenic organisms. Absence of an indication for antibiotic therapy and wrong drug choices increase selection and promote development of resistant bacteria. It is therefore of utmost importance to limit and rationalize the use of antibiotic drugs to reduce further selection and maintain therapeutic options for the treatment of the most severe infections for our patients and the entire population. Most likely, there will not be any new antibiotic drug development in the near future particularly for the treatment of gram-negative bacteria, so preserving the effectiveness of existing drugs is an important principle. In addition to overuse, inadequate dose and duration of therapy, using the same antibiotic drug for the same indication over a long period of time can also increase selection.

In addition to the inappropriate use of antibiotics, other factors like indwelling catheters, immunosuppression, uncontrolled hyperglycemia, and non-adherence to infection control measures predispose the patient in the ICU to healthcare-acquired or nosocomial infections. Aside from perioperative antibiotic prophylaxis, interventions to prevent nosocomial infections include strict and adequate hand hygiene and the use of gloves and other protective accessories like gowns and masks when indicated (Pincock, Bernstein, Warthman, & Holst, 2012). Patient isolation may become necessary when colonization or infection with a resistant and contagious organism is suspected or in cases when patients are particularly susceptible to infections, i.e. after transplant surgery. A hospital infection surveillance program is an important quality measure to gain a better understanding of infection types and rates as well as the frequency of resistant organisms causing infections within an institution (Jarvis, 2003; Gastmeier et al., 2006).

Infection can result in an inflammatory response syndrome, which can be further categorized into sepsis, severe sepsis, and septic shock. Some common nosocomial infections in the cardiac surgical patient on the ICU frequently show clinical features of sepsis, particularly ventilator-associated pneumonia (VAP). However, sepsis is not a common clinical syndrome in postoperative cardiothoracic surgical patients, and other mechanisms of systemic inflammation have to be taken into consideration when treating a patient presenting with vasodilatory shock. A variety of pathophysiologic processes have been described in the systemic inflammatory response syndrome following cardiac surgery including surgical trauma, exposure to an extracorporeal circulation and duration of CPB, hypothermia, blood transfusion, and ischemia-reperfusion injury.

GENERAL MEASURES OF INFECTION CONTROL AND PREVENTION

Nosocomial infections are the most common complications for hospitalized patients and prevention and infection control have been identified as important measures of patient safety (Burke, 2003). Several risk factors have been identified that makes ICU patients particularly prone to nosocomial infections. Skin integrity is compromised by indwelling catheters and surgical wounds and immunosuppression is often present, be it secondary to drugs, related to underlying conditions such as diabetes, or due to critical illness per se. Modifiable risk factors include health care personnel and the hospital environment.

Hand Hygiene

Hand hygiene is regarded the most important measure of preventing healthcare-associated infections (Allegranzi & Pittet, 2009). Decontaminative hand hygiene should be performed before and after every patient care contact, before any clean or aseptic procedure, after exposure to bodily fluids, and after contact with a patient's surroundings (Pittet, Allegranzi, & Boyce, 2009). It is also important that hand hygiene is done after performing a task with a non-sterile glove. Non-sterile gloves should be worn whenever direct contact with the patient's bodily fluids is possible. Whenever splash or spray of bodily fluids is expected, gown, mask, and eye protection should be added for personal protection. Alcohol-based hand rubs are first choice and widely accepted as optimal for hand hygiene in the healthcare environment (Widmer, 2000; Girou, Loyeau, Legrand, Oppein, & Brun-Buisson, 2002). There is some debate whether the use alcohol-based hand rubs has increased the spread of Clostridium difficile, however studies could not prove this association (Boyce, Ligi, Kohan, Dumigan, & Havill, 2006). In case of suspected or proven Clostridium difficile colonization or infection, mechanical friction while hand washing with an antiseptic soap reduces the amount of spores on the skin more effectively than alcohol-based solutions (Jabbar et al., 2010). While reports have questioned the direct effect of hand hygiene on the reduction of healthcare-associated infections (Backman, Zoutman, & Marck, 2008), its widespread implementation and support by various government organizations has made it become standard of practice. It is conceivable that the reduction in healthcare-associated infections observed over the years is due to improved measures of infection prevention and the introduction of preventive care bundles, of which the promotion of hand hygiene is one part (Pincock, et al., 2012). It seems that regular staff education, behavioral reinforcement and accountability, and reliable point-of-care access to hand hygiene resources are critically important pieces in the successful implementation of a hand hygiene program (Kendall, Landers, Kirk, & Young, 2012).

Hospital Environment

Inadequate hand hygiene can lead to spread of organisms from colonized hands of healthcare personnel to surfaces and structures in patients' and other hospital rooms (Duckro, Blom, Lyle, Weinstein, & Hayden, 2005). Patient rooms can potentially harbor clinically significant microorganisms for quite some time (Huang, Datta, & Platt, 2006). This has led to enhanced room cleaning methods including the use of UV light to make previously marked areas of contamination visible (Carling, Parry, & Von Beheren, 2008). Along with continuing education for environmental staff, water and air filtration systems should be closely monitored.

Patient isolation measures may be necessary for certain patients colonized or infected with multi-resistant microorganisms which pose a risk to other patients in an ICU setting. This procedure is commonly referred to as source isolation and patients should be cared for in a single room. If airborne pathogens are of concern, the patient room should be a negative-pressure environment. Protective gowns are now standard in addition to gloves when caring for patients with methicillin-resistant Staphylococcus aureus (MRSA) (Jernigan, Titus, Gröschel, Getchell-White, & Farr, 1996) or vancomycin-resistant enterococci (VRE) (Srinivasan et al., 2002). If transmission by droplet is a potential problem, masks and eye protection should be part of personal protection. Protective isolation is another form of isolation, which separates patients at higher risk for infections from the remaining patients on the unit. This method is routinely used after heart or lung transplantation and in patients who are otherwise heavily immunosuppressed. A clear sign on the door indicating the type of precaution is needed to inform staff and visitors before entering the patient room. Personal protective gear should be discarded before leaving the room.

Healthcare Personnel

Continuing staff education is an integral part of a culture change towards infection prevention and increased patient safety. Studies show that periodic educational interventions can lead to a decrease of hospital-acquired infections (Zack et al., 2002; Warren et al., 2004). At the same time, adequate ICU staffing is an essential part of infection control, and variation in nursing staffing and different levels of training have an impact on infection rates (Hugonnet, Chevrolet, & Pittet, 2007).

Screening and Surveillance

It is widely recognized that resistant microorganisms are on the rise, and therefore it is extremely important to find ways to contain and eradicate those organisms. Colonized patients admitted to an ICU, while not infected themselves, pose a serious risk for other potentially immunosuppressed patients. Obtaining surveillance cultures to detect for example MRSA or VRE has been implemented on many ICU resulting in decreased colonization and infection rates (Perencevich et al., 2004; Gastmeier et al., 2006; Huang et al., 2006). The practice of obtaining cultures to detect certain resistant organisms is usually referred to as active surveillance. On the other hand, passive surveillance describes a general daily infection checklist when rounding on an ICU patient, including assessing for signs of infection, analysis of certain laboratory parameters, sending culture samples when infection is suspected, and checking indwelling lines for potential removal. While active surveillance as described above has become common practice for ICU admissions, the usefulness of routine surveillance cultures for any general hospital admission remains unclear. Studies have shown different results (Harbarth et al., 2008; Robiscek et al., 2008) and risk factors for MRSA or VRE colonization should be taken into account when culturing a patient newly admitted to the hospital.

Other Preventive Measures

Hyperglycemia and malnutrition have been identified as patient risk factors for hospital-acquired infections. Given the suppressive effects of hyperglycemia on immune function, it is conceivable that this can lead to an increased infection rate in these patients (Blondet & Beilman, 2007). An association between inadequate blood glucose control and an increased rate of postoperative wound infections has been described for diabetic patients after cardiac surgery (Latham, Lancaster, Covington, Pirolo, & Thomas Jr., 2001). This has led to various interventions around blood glucose control for perioperative cardiothoracic surgical patients. Similar to hyperglycemia, poor nutritional status affects immune function (Keusch, 2003). A low albumin level correlates with and increased risk of postoperative infection in cardiac surgery patients (Rapp-Kesek, Ståhle, & Karlsson, 2004). In some patients, supplemental nutrition is indicated. Enteral feeding has consistently been shown to superior to parenteral nutrition (Radrizzani et al., 2006).

GENERAL PRINCIPLES OF ANTIBIOTIC THERAPY

Therapeutic Strategies

The two major principles of antibiotic therapy are targeted and empiric therapy. Targeted therapy requires culture acquisition and diagnosis with speciation of the causing organism. This is followed by a highly specific drug choice, and this is generally the most effective and rational method of antibiotic therapy. After initial sample acquisition, empiric therapy should be started promptly since an immediate start of antibiotic therapy can be life saving and must not be delayed. One study found that in septic patients mortality increases by 7.6% for every hour without effective antibiotic therapy (Kumar et al., 2006). "The Tarragona Strategy" defined some of the principles for early empiric treatment of severe infections in the ICU (Sandiumenge, Diaz, Bodi, & Rello, 2003); these include: "Look at your patient" (clinical presentation and comorbidities), "Hit hard and early" (adequate drug choice and dosage), and "Listen to your hospital" (knowledge of the local antibiogram).

In addition to those overarching principles, one should consider all aspects of antibiotic drug pharmacology, including tissue penetration, patient's organ dysfunction, side effects, and drug interactions (Udy, Roberts, & Lipman, 2013) (Table 1).

Table 1. Principles of antibiotic drug choice

Organism	Patient	Antibiotic Drug
Spectrum - Community-acquired - Healthcare-acquired - Nosocomial	Clinical presentation and risk factors	Spectrum
Antibiogram and local resistance	Predisposing comorbidities	Side effects
	Antibiotic "history"	Tissue penetration
	Organ dysfunction	Pharmacology
	Allergies, age, pregnancy	

Antibiotic Drug Choice

It is important to understand the differences in the spectrum of organisms when treating community-acquired versus nosocomial infections. Community-acquired infections are relatively easy to predict. It becomes more problematic with healthcare-acquired infections in patients that are transferred from long-term care facilities, dialysis units, or nursing homes. Finally, nosocomial infections are hardest to predict in terms of the causing organism and multi-resistant bacteria are more common. The effectiveness of antibiotic drugs is highly dependent on the local resistance situation.

There is no antibiotic drug that covers all bacteria, some are only against gram-positive bacteria, others only against gram-negative bacteria, some against aerobic and others against anaerobic bacteria, or they have varying stability against bacterial beta-lactamase. For example, newer generation cephalosporins are more stable when exposed to bacterial beta-lactamase than first and second-generation cephalosporins. Another example is that certain antibiotics have no therapeutic effect on certain bacteria, i.e. cephalosporins are not effective against enterococci. Most common antibiotics are not effective against Pseudomonas aeruginosa, as this particular bacterium has very small pores, which most antibiotic molecules cannot penetrate.

Important for effective antibiotic therapy is to achieve an adequate tissue concentration at the site of the infection. This has an impact on antibiotic drug choice. As a general principle, in well-perfused organs such as the lungs or the bladder, most antibiotics will reach adequate tissue concentrations. Less-perfused organs such as bones or the central nervous system and meninges, certain antibiotics will not penetrate due to molecule size. For example, vancomycin is a large molecule and does not penetrate well into the cerebrospinal fluid. Other antibiotics tend to accumulate in certain tissues, i.e. clindamycin in bones. The worst penetration is seen in poorly perfused areas such as abscesses or necrotic tissue, i.e. diabetic gangrene foot or necrotizing fasciitis. In these cases, source control becomes more important than antibiotic therapy.

Some antibiotics are bactericidal, some are bacteriostatic, and in some the effect depends on the organism present. Bactericidal antibiotics kill almost all targeted bacteria in a matter of about 24 hours. Bacteriostatic antibiotics mainly inhibit bacterial growth, but can also reduce the amount of the bacteria slowly over time. Antibiotic drugs targeting the cell wall are generally bactericidal, drugs interfering with the protein synthesis usually act bacteriostatic. Some antibiotics are bactericidal against some bacteria, but bacteriostatic against others, i.e. linezolid is bactericidal against streptococci, but only bacteriostatic against staphylococci and enterococci (Tables 2 and 3).

The minimum inhibitory concentration (MIC) is the lowest concentration of an antibiotic that will inhibit the visible growth of an isolated microorganism after overnight incubation (18-24 hours). The minimum bactericidal concentration (MBC) is the lowest concentration of a bactericidal antibiotic required to kill a particular microorganism. A bacterium is sensitive to a certain antibiotic if the MIC is such that an adequate tissue concentration can be achieved without administering toxic doses of the drug.

Particularly in the ICU setting where we treat critically ill patients that frequently have comorbidities, antibiotic therapy must be tailored considering all relevant patients factors that may interfere with the drug chosen. The severity of the infectious illness is an important factor impacting drug choice as well as predisposing factors such as immunodeficiency or diabetes. Drug allergies, recent exposure to antibiotic drugs, and pregnancy also play an important role. Certain antibiotics should not be used in children, as their effect on growth is not completely understood (fluoroquinolones, tetracyclin). The most common acute patient factors influencing antibiotic drug choice and dosage in the ICU are organ dysfunction, especially renal and hepatic dysfunction. As most antibiotics are metabolized via hepatic or biliary excretion or renal clearance, doses and/or dosing interval have to be adjusted accordingly if these organs are dysfunctional due to critical illness. Ideally, patients with renal insufficiency should not receive nephrotoxic antibiotics, i.e. vancomycin or aminoglycosides.

When combining different antibiotic drugs to treat a severe infection, it makes sense to combine different types of antibiotics, for example a bactericidal and a bacteriostatic drug, i.e. cephalosporin and fluoroquinolone. The two main reasons for combination therapy in the critically ill patient are broadening of the spectrum of organisms and antibiotic synergy. The addition of beta-lactamase inhibitors to penicillins is a means to broaden the spectrum of the penicillin, which would have otherwise been inactivated by bacterial beta-lactamase. On the other hand, the combination of antibiotics with the same mechanism of action is generally not helpful and can in fact promote the development of resistance, i.e. carbapenem therapy can induce the production of specific beta-lactamases that make the bacteria resistant to penicillins and cephalosporins.

As a general principle, any antibiotic therapy should be reevaluated after two to four days of therapy. If the patient continues to have fevers or otherwise does not show clinical improvement, antibiotic therapy should be changed or broadened after careful review of culture results. The antibiotic drug may not be effective, but other reasons for ineffective therapy include the development of secondary resistance or

Table 2. Types of antibiotic drugs

Bactericidal	Dependent on Organism	Bacteriostatic
Penicillins Cephalosporins Carbapenems Aminoglycosides Fluoroquinolones Rifampicin Vancomycin Daptomycin	Linezolid Chloramphenicol Erythromycin Azithromycin Clindamycin	Chloramphenicol Sulfonamides Tetracycline Clindamycin Linezolid Tigecycline Macrolides

Table 3. Antibiotic drugs commonly used in the intensive care unit and their characteristics

Drug	Spectrum	Comments
Aztreonam	Gram-negative including Pseudomonas aeruginosa	Inactivated by ESBL, safe in patients with penicillin allergy
1st Generation cephalosporins (i.e. cefazolin)	Gram-positive (methicillin-susceptible) Few gram-negative	
2nd Generation cephalosporins (i.e. cefuroxime)	Less gram-positive than 1st generation More gram-negative than 1st generation	
3rd Generation cephalosporins (i.e. ceftazidime)	Few gram-positive Broad gram-negative coverage including Pseudomonas aeruginosa (some)	Penetrate the central nervous system
4th Generation cephalosporins (i.e. cefepime)	Coverage like 3rd generation, but greater resistance against beta-lactamases	
Clindamycin	Gram-positive cocci (including some MRSA) Anaerobes	High incidence of Clostridium difficile-associated diarrhea
Colistin	Gram-negative rods including multi-resistant pseudomonas, acinetobacter, and klebsiella	Nephrotoxic, old drug which fell out of favor Often last resort for multi-resistant gram-negative rods
Daptomycin	Gram-positive cocci including MRSA	Severe skin and soft tissue infections and endocarditis
Macrolides (i.e. azithromycin)	Gram-positive cocci Haemophilus influenzae	Usually for treatment of mild infections
Aminoglycosides (i.e. gentamicin)	Gram-negative rods Synergy against some Gram-positive cocci	Nephrotoxic and ototoxic
Carbapenems (i.e. meropenem)	Ultra-broad coverage	Imipenem can cause seizures
Linezolid	Gram-positive cocci including MRSA and VRE	Last resort antibiotic for severe gram-positive infections
Metronidazole	Anaerobes Entameba hystolitica Clostridium difficile	
Penicillins	Mostly Gram-positive cocci Some penicillins cover Gram-negative rods as well, i.e. piperacillin/tazobactam	Decreasing efficacy due to beta-lactamase producing bacteria Increased efficacy with beta-lactamase inhibitors, i.e. tazobactam
Fluoroquinolone (i.e. ciprofloxacin)	Gram-negative rods Some Gram-positive cocci (streptococcus usually resistant)	Only ciprofloxacin has sufficient pseudomonas coverage Moxifloxacin provides no coverage for urinary tract infections
Vancomycin	Gram-positive cocci including MRSA Clostridium difficile (only oral administration)	Nephrotoxic and ototoxic Can cause significant allergic reactions with whole-body rash and hypotension (red-man syndrome) Need loading dose and adequate trough serum tissue levels to avoid development of resistance
Tigecyclin	Gram-positive cocci including MRSA Some Gram-negative rods (not pseudomonas)	Last resort antibiotic for severe gram-positive infections
ESBL = extended-spectrum beta-lactamase, MRSA = methicillin-resistant Staphylococcus aureus, VRE = vancomycin-resistant enterococci		

growth of a second organism. It is important to recognize the difference between colonization and infection. The mere finding of an organism in a culture is no proof of clinically relevant infection. So again, the patient's clinical presentation has to correlate with the culture findings to justify antibiotic therapy.

Multi-Resistant Organisms

Multi-resistant organisms are an increasing problem in the ICU and therapeutic options are limited. One important principle is early detection of a multi-resistant bacterium and subsequent placement of the patient in isolation to avoid spread of the organism.

MRSA is now a common cause for nosocomial and healthcare-acquired infections. The reservoir for the organism is often the nose, throat, or skin of personnel or visitors. They are usually colonized and not ill. When transferred to a critically ill patient, the organism often causes infection. Spread of the organism can only be avoided if the patient is properly isolated and personnel is compliant with hand hygiene measures. Antibiotic therapy for MRSA is only indicated if there is proven infection (Boucher, Miller, & Razonable, 2010). In the ICU, these are most commonly pneumonia and wound infections. Colonized individuals are treated with topical antibiotics and decontaminants. Enterococci are enteric pathogens that have a natural resistance against many common antibiotics. More recently, some Enterococcus faecium species have developed resistance against vancomycin, which was traditionally an antibiotic for the most severe infections in the ICU. An important factor for the rise of VRE is the uncritical use of vancomycin. VRE infections are usually endogenous infections, most commonly urinary tract infections (UTI) and peritonitis (Table 4).

Many enterobacteria species have the ability to produce beta-lactamases that can inactivate some of the beta-lactam antibiotics. More recently, extended-spectrum beta-lactamase (ESBL) producing enterobacteria have been found to be resistant to all available penicillins including piperacillin-tazobactam and fourth-generation cephalosporins such as cefepime. The only effective beta-lactam remaining are the carbapenems. Similar to MRSA or VRE, patients with proven ESBL enterobacterial infections must be isolated and strict hygienic measures must be applied. Most recently, there have been reports about carbapenem-resistant enterobacteria, particularly klebsiella, which is another significant threat with very few therapeutic options left.

Non-lactose fermenting Gram-negative rods are relevant nosocomial organism that are modest and often reside in wet areas of the hospital. The best-known bacterium is Pseudomonas aeruginosa. Pseudomonas

Table 4. Treatment options for multi-resistant gram-positive bacteria

Antibiotic	MRSA	VRE
Vancomycin	++	0
Linezolid	++	++
Fosfomycin	++	0
Rifampicin	++*	+*
Tigecyclin	++	++
Daptomycin	++	?
MRSA = methicillin-resistant Staphylococcus aureus, VRE = vancomycin-resistant enterococci, ++ = good effect, + = fair effect, 0 = no effect, * = combination therapy only		

and similar bacteria tend to develop secondary resistance under antibiotic therapy. A combination therapy is usually indicated, and at times the only option are potentially toxic antibiotic drugs such as colistin.

Selection and "Collateral Damage"

Antibiotic drugs do not only attack pathogenic organisms, but also affect physiological flora, i.e. in the colon. If antibiotic therapy is unidirectional and not frequently changed or rotated, there will be selection of certain organisms, i.e. enterobacteria when cephalosporins are used. These can then colonize the patient in other areas of the body and potentially cause infection. Strategies to address this phenomenon include antibiotic combination and antibiotic cycling or rotation (Martinez et al., 2006).

Diarrhea during antibiotic therapy is multifactorial, but in about 30% of the cases this is due to Clostridium difficile. Some individuals have Clostridium difficile in their gut, but when undergoing antibiotic therapy, subsequent damage of the physiological flora of the gut can cause this microorganism to grow in an uncontrollable fashion. Depending on the severity this can cause Clostridium difficile-associated diarrhea or Clostridium difficile colitis. Some antibiotic drugs are more prone to causing diarrhea (Table 5). Clostridium difficile colitis can cause very severe disease in the ICU and often goes along with high fevers and a substantial increase in white blood cell count. Therapy should always be per os vancomycin, metronidazole is rarely indicated (Surawicz et al., 2013).

Strategies to Optimize Antibiotic Therapy

Interdisciplinary workgroups, guideline-driven therapy, and antibiotic stewardship programs are more recent developments to address the increasing complexity around antibiotic therapy in the hospital. Inadequate diagnosis may lead to poor antibiotic drug choices and subsequently impairs therapeutic success and patient outcomes. This is most impactful on the ICU where the most severe infections are treated (Kumar, 2009, Kaki et al., 2011).

SPECIFIC INFECTIONS

Pneumonia

Background

VAP is also the most commonly encountered infection in ventilated ICU patients and is linked to increased length of stay, cost, and mortality (Safdar, Dezfoulian, Collard, & Saint, 2005). It is defined as a pneumonia that occurs 48-72 hours (or later) following endotracheal intubation, characterized by

Table 5. Antibiotic drugs and risk of causing Clostridium difficile-associated diarrhea

High Risk	Medium Risk	Low Risk
Clindamycin	Cotrimoxazole	Fluoroquinolones
Aminopenicillins	Carbapenems	Macrolides
Cephalosporins	Tetracyclin	Aminoglycosides

signs of systemic infection, a new or progressive lung infiltrate on chest radiograph, and the detection of a causative agent (Kalanuria, Zai, & Mirski, 2014). A distinction is made between early-onset and late-onset VAP (more than four days of mechanical ventilation). This has therapeutic implications, as late-onset VAP is more likely to be caused by multidrug resistant (MDR) bacteria.

Pneumonia is also the most common infectious complication after heart surgery and bears a significant morbidity and mortality (Fitch & Whitman, 2014) and has a negative impact on long-term survival (Ibañez et al., 2014). In a recent meta-analysis, the mean prevalence of VAP was reported to be 6.4% for all patients and 35.2% for patients who are ventilated for more than 48 hours (He et al., 2014). Risk factors for VAP after cardiac surgery have been described in a number of studies. Conclusively, age > 70, underlying chronic lung disease, emergency surgery, perioperative blood transfusions, reintubation, and days of mechanical ventilation seemed to be the most important independent risk factors for developing VAP after cardiac surgery (El Solh, Bhora, Pineda, & Dhillon, 2006; Hortal et al., 2009, Sheng et al., 2014). Those findings have led to the development of preoperative risk scores (Allou et al., 2014).

The presence of an endotracheal tube and the need for mechanical ventilation are probably the most important risk factors leading up to a VAP infection. Bacteria grow and form a biofilm on the inside of the endotracheal tube, secretions can pool above and trickle down around the endotracheal tube cuff, and the absence of a functioning mucociliary clearance mechanism can help infectious microorganisms access the lower respiratory tract. Sources for these infectious microorganisms include the pharynx, sinuses, and the stomach, where normal flora is replaced by pathogenic material. One aggravating factor in the pathogenesis of VAP may be the suppressed immune response of critically ill patients. In addition to the systemic impairment, local dysregulation of the pulmonary compartment with deactivation and reduction of alveolar macrophages has been demonstrated in patients following cardiac surgery (Chalk et al., 2013).

Community-Acquired Pneumonia

Community-acquired pneumonia (CAP) is a rare cause of respiratory disease in the cardiac ICU. However, patients may have been exposed to pathogens in the community or in the immediate family, especially when young children are around. These patients are often asymptomatic going into the hospital and into surgery, and a subclinical bacterial or even viral infection may exacerbate in the context of systemic inflammation following surgery and CPB (McFarlane, MacDonald, Collins, Molyneaux, & Carman, 2009). Another study showed that one out of five patients had a positive gram stain on a preoperatively obtained tracheal aspirate, which led to a five-fold increase in the incidence of postoperative pneumonia (Carrel, Eisinger, Vogt, & Turina, 2001). With an aging surgical population and an increase in comorbidities, postoperative exacerbation of community-acquired infections may become more prevalent and needs consideration when treating these patients.

Healthcare-Associated Pneumonia

The concept of healthcare-associated pneumonia (HAP) was introduced by the American Thoracic Society in 2005 to describe an entity that occurs in non-hospitalized patients with recent or chronic contact with the healthcare system (Ewig, Welte, & Torres, 2012). The definition further specified that patients had to be nursing home residents, had been hospitalized for more than two days in the preceding 90 days, were on home infusion therapy or wound care, or were receiving care in an outpatient hemodialysis center (Poch & Ost, 2009). The clinical course and especially the spectrum of organisms resembled a nosocomial rather than a CAP, thus HAP required a more aggressive initial empiric antibiotic regimen.

The HAP concept is subject to substantial debate, as it appears that the incidence of multi-resistant pathogens is lower than initially suspected and mortality has not improved despite more aggressive treatment (Dobler & Waterer, 2013). A recent meta-analysis came to the conclusion that the excess mortality associated with HAP is primarily due to age and comorbidities rather than multi-resistant bacteria causing pneumonia and not covered by antibiotic therapy (Chalmers, Rother, Salih, & Ewig, 2014). It is suggested that broad-spectrum antibiotic therapy should be applied on the basis of individual risk assessment rather than HAP guidelines in order to prevent antibiotic overuse and potential increase in multi-resistant organisms.

Diagnosis

VAP is often diagnosed primarily based on clinical and radiographic findings and there is currently no commonly accepted gold standard for the diagnosis of VAP (Rea-Neto et al., 2008; Grgurich, Hudcova, Lei, Sarwar, & Craven, 2013) (Table 6). The clinical findings are signs of systemic infection, including fever, deteriorating gas exchange, altered mental status, abnormal white blood cell count, and purulent secretions. The classic radiographic finding is a new or progressive infiltrate. Since often only a few of those signs are present, scoring systems have been suggested (Pugin et al., 1991), but have not found widespread clinical use due to limited sensitivity and specificity (Schurink et al., 2004; Croce et al., 2006, Parks et al., 2012). The presence or absence of a pulmonary infiltrate may help to differentiate between pneumonia from tracheobronchitis, but the clinical significance of this is unclear (Craven, Lei, Ruthazer, Sarwar, & Hudcova, 2013).

If pneumonia is suspected, a sputum sample should be obtained prior to the initial dose of antibiotics. The sputum sample can be obtained as an endotracheal aspirate, a bronchoalveolar lavage (BAL), or from a protected specimen brush (PSB) from the lower airways. The sample is then analyzed in a quantitative or semi-quantitative fashion for gram stain and culture. Gram stains will quickly detect pus and the presence of bacteria, while cultures help identify specific bacteria and their antibiotic sensitivity. For BAL or PSB, the diagnostic threshold is 10^3 and 10^4 colony-forming units (CFU)/mL, respectively. Sometimes culture results are reported semi-quantitatively with a positive result being moderate (+++) or heavy (++++) agar growth. It is important to understand that the mere presence of microorganisms in tracheal secretions is not an indication for antibiotic therapy. Positive cultures have to be at least semi-quantitative and also have to be correlated with the clinical presentation as mentioned above. Common organisms isolated that rarely cause infections include Streptococcus viridans, Neisseria species, Candida species, and coagulase-negative staphylococci. Most cases of VAP after cardiac surgery are caused by Gram-negative bacteria, particularly Pseudomonas aeruginosa (Table 7).

Prevention

Early on, VAP was identified as a potentially preventable nosocomial infection. Several preventive strategies have been described (Muscedere et al., 2008). Subsequently, the Institute for Healthcare Improvement (IHI) recommended the implementation of a ventilator care bundle in 2004 (Resar et al., 2005). The updated 5-element IHI ventilator bundle includes: head of bed elevation, oral care with chlorhexidine, stress ulcer prophylaxis, deep venous thrombosis prophylaxis, and daily sedation vacation with spontaneous breathing trials. The implementation of this care bundle has led to impressive reductions in VAP rates (Blamoun et al., 2009), however the quality of the evidence has been questioned

Table 6. Clinical diagnosis of ventilator-associated pneumonia (VAP)

Johanson Criteria	At least 2 of the following: fever > 38°C; leukocytosis or leukopenia; purulent secretions		
	PLUS		
	A new or progressive chest radiographic infiltrate		
Clinical Pulmonary Infection Score (CPIS)	Temperature (°C): 36.5-38.4: 0 points; 38.5-38.9: 1 point; <36 or >39: 2 points	Oxygenation (P_aO_2/F_iO_2): >240 or ARDS: 0 points; ≤240 and no ARDS: 2 points	Tracheal secretions: absence of secretions: 0 points; non-purulent secretions: 1 point; purulent secretions: 2 points
	Blood leukocytes (cells/μl): 4,000-11,000: 0 points; <4000 or >11,000: 1 point; ≥50% bands: 2 points	Pulmonary radiograph: no infiltrate: 0 points; radiographic progression (CHF and ARDS excluded): 2 points	Endotracheal aspirate: minimal or no growth: 0 points; moderate or heavy growth: 1 point; same bacteria seen on Gram stain: add 1 point
Total score >6 consistent with VAP CHF = congestive heart failure, ARDS = acute respiratory distress syndrome			
Clinical Diagnostic Approach	At least 2 of the following: 1) temperature: >38°C; 2) WBC: >12,000/μl, or <4,000/μl; 3) purulent sputum[a]; hypoxia[b]	New and persistent infiltrate	BAL ≥10^4 cfu/ml; PSB ≥10^3 cfu/ml; endotracheal aspirate: semi-quantitative moderate (+++) to heavy (++++) growth or quantitative ≥10^{5-6} cfu/ml
[a]Purulent sputum defined as at least 25 neutrophils and less than or equal to 10 squamous epithelial cells per low-power field [b]Hypoxia defined as increase in inspired oxygen of at least 0.2 or an increase in positive end-expiratory pressure of greater than 3 cm H_2O WBC = white blood cells, BAL = bronchoalveolar lavage, PSB = protected specimen brush, cfu = colony forming units			

From: Grgurich et al., Current Opinion in Infectious Diseases, 2013

Table 7. Common microorganisms causing ventilator-associated pneumonia (VAP) after cardiac surgery

Microorganism	Mean Frequency (%)
Gram-positive	
• Staphylococcus aureus	20.2
• MSSA	13.1
• MRSA	14.1
Gram-negative	
• Pseudomonas aeruginosa	23.2
• Klebsiella pneumonia	9.5
• Acinetobacter baumanii	10.7
• Escherichia coli	10.2
• Stenotrophomonas maltophilia	4.8
• Haemophilus influenza	19.5
• Proteus vulgaris	2.4
Fungus	
• Candida albicans	7.2
MSSA = methicillin-sensitive Staphylococcus aureus, MRSA = methicillin-resistant Staphylococcus aureus	

From: He et al., Journal of Thoracic and Cardiovascular Surgery, 2014

(Zilberberg, Shorr, & Kollef, 2009; Klompas, 2010). A major drawback is the lack of a gold standard for the diagnosis of VAP making the interpretation of VAP incidence and the reduction thereof difficult (Klompas, 2007; Wip & Napolitano, 2009). The second point of criticism is the fact that VAP rates are used as an indicator of quality of care and has been implemented by many hospitals as a patient safety goal. Redistribution of reimbursement money from the "outliers" to the high performance institutions has increased the pressure to minimize or even abolish VAP (Mietto, Pinciroli, Patel, & Berra, 2013). The potential flaw here is under-reporting of VAP rates. The Centers for Disease Control and Prevention (CDC) recently published new guidelines for surveillance with the general aim to increase objectivity and improve comparability (Magill et al., 2013; Klompas 2013).

Since the implementation of the ventilator bundle, additional preventive strategies have been studied and some of those proven effective (Klompas et al., 2014). This has led to several modifications of the original bundle with the advantage of further improving VAP prevention, but with the disadvantage of significant variation across institutions (Eom et al., 2014) (Table 8).

Table 8. Recommendations for preventing ventilator-associated pneumonia (VAP)

Recommendation	Rationale	Intervention
Basic practices	Good evidence that the intervention decreases the average duration of mechanical ventilation, length of stay, mortality, and/or cost; benefits likely outweigh risks	• Use non-invasive positive pressure ventilation in selected populations • Manage patients without sedation whenever possible • Interrupt sedation daily • Assess readiness to extubate daily • Perform spontaneous breathing trials with sedatives turned off • Facilitate early mobility • Utilize endotracheal tubes with subglottic secretion drainage ports for patients expected to require more than 48-72 hours of mechanical ventilation • Change the ventilator circuit only if visibly soiled or malfunctioning • Elevate head of bed to 30-45°
Special approaches	Good evidence that the intervention improves outcomes but insufficient data available on possible risks May lower VAP rates but insufficient data to determine impact on duration of mechanical ventilation, length of stay, or mortality	• Selective oral or digestive decontamination • Regular oral care with chlorhexidine • Prophylactic probiotics in selected populations • Ultrathin polyurethane endotracheal tube cuffs • Automated control of endotracheal cuff pressure • Saline instillation before tracheal suctioning • Mechanical toothbrushing
Generally not recommended	Lowers VAP rate but ample data suggests no impact on duration of mechanical ventilation, length of stay, or mortality No impact on VAP rates, average duration of mechanical ventilation, length of stay, or mortality	• Silver-coated endotracheal tubes • Kinetic beds • Prone positioning • Stress ulcer prophylaxis • Early tracheostomy • Monitoring residual gastric volumes • Early parenteral nutrition • Closed endotracheal suctioning

From: Klompas et al., Infection Control and Hospital Epidemiology, 2014

Avoiding Intubation and Minimizing Sedation

Avoiding prolonged intubation is one of the general principles of modern ICU care and the benefit of non-invasive ventilation (NIV) has been well established in the setting of respiratory failure from chronic obstructive pulmonary disease or cardiogenic pulmonary edema (Hess, 2005). One has to be cautious about the timing of NIV, as it can be ineffective and potentially harmful in patients with altered mental status from more severe hypercapnia or severe hypoxemia. The largest study so far in cardiac surgery patients showed a reduction of pulmonary complications including pneumonia with the use of prophylactic NIV (Zarbock et al., 2009). The results of a few other studies on this topic are promising, but overall data is limited in this specific patient population (Cabrini et al., 2013).

Minimizing sedation has become standard practice in most ICU settings, and this concept should also apply to patient after CT surgery. Whenever possible, patients should be managed without continuous sedation or if necessary with agents other than benzodiazepines, i.e. propofol or dexmedetomidine (Barr et al., 2013). If sedation is required, daily interruption is recommended (Kress, Pohlman, O'Connor, & Hall, 2000; Mehta et al., 2012) and spontaneous awakening trials should be paired with spontaneous breathing trials to assess readiness for extubation (Girard et al., 2008). This should ideally be part of a daily protocol and even be done on patients without the plan for an early extubation, i.e. in the postoperative setting of an open chest or short-term mechanical circulatory support. In summary, the application of weaning protocols and the daily assessment of readiness for extubation should be the core of VAP prevention on the ICU, as studies have consistently shown that these measures decrease ventilator days and ICU length of stay and possibly mortality.

Improving Physical and Pulmonary Condition

Physiotherapy and early mobility protocols are now widely applied in various ICU settings (McWilliams et al., 2014). This approach may also include specific respiratory therapy in the perioperative period, such as deep breathing and coughing exercises and incentive spirometry. While the general usefulness of prophylactic respiratory physiotherapy has been subject to debate (Pasquina, Tramèr, & Walder, 2003), inspiratory muscle training has been shown to be effective in reducing atelectasis and pneumonia, particularly when applied preoperatively (Hulzebos et al., 2006).

Minimizing Pooling of Subglottic Tracheal Secretions

In a recent meta-analysis, endotracheal tubes that were equipped to provide continuous aspiration of subglottic secretions (CASS) were associated with a 55% decrease in VAP rate, however length of stay and mortality were unchanged (Lacherade et al., 2010; Muscedere et al., 2011). The effectiveness of CASS in reducing VAP in patients ventilated for more than 48 hours was also demonstrated in patients after cardiac surgery. In addition to that, CASS led to a reduction in time on mechanical ventilation and the use of antimicrobial agents in these patients (Bouza et al., 2008). Identifying patients that will require more than 48-72 hours of intubation and mechanical ventilation preoperatively could prove a clinical challenge.

Elevating the Head of the Bed

Head of bed elevation has been part of the initial VAP bundle and has become a widespread practice on the ICU, however the evidence is based on three randomized trials with only one showing a reduction in VAP rates. A meta-analysis has confirmed the beneficial effect and given the simplicity of this preventive measure, it should remain standard practice (Alexiou, Ierodiakonou, Dimopoulos, & Falagas, 2009). Prolonged postoperative hemodynamic instability sometimes encountered after cardiac surgery could make this intervention challenging or impossible.

Decontaminating the Oropharynx and Digestive Tract

Selective decontamination of the oropharynx and digestive tract has been widely adopted in Europe largely based on a meta-analysis and a more recent large randomized trial demonstrating a reduction of VAP rates and mortality (Silvestri, van Saene, Casarin, Berlot, & Gullo 2008; De Smet et al., 2009). This practice is still subject to debate. The main trials were conducted in the Netherlands, and there is concern in the US that it might increase the incidence of MDR bacterial infections and Clostridium difficile infections, particularly in institutions with a high baseline rate of MDR bacteria (Oostdijk et al., 2014).

Performing Oral Care with Chlorhexidine

Antiseptic oral care to reduce the incidence of VAP has been studied extensively. There is evidence that the application of chlorhexidine either as a mouth rinse or gel can reduce VAP rates by up to 40%, but no mortality has been shown (Chlebicki & Safdar, 2007; Shi et al., 2013; Klompas, Speck, Howell, Greene, & Berenholtz, 2014). The concept of antiseptic oral care seems to be most effective in patients after cardiac surgery, as demonstrated in a large trial (Segers, Speekenbrink, Ubbink, van Ogtrop, & de Mol 2006).

Using Endotracheal Tubes with Ultrathin Polyurethane Cuffs

Ultrathin polyurethane (PU) cuff membranes seal more effectively against the tracheal wall than traditional polyvinyl chloride (PVC) cuffs. Secretions accumulating in the subglottic space can leak around the endotracheal tube cuff, contaminate the lower airways and promote colonization and potentially infection. The use of endotracheal tubes with PU cuffs resulted in a lower incidence of early (Poelaert et al., 2008) as well as late-onset VAP (Lorente, Lecuona, Jimenez, Mora, & Sierra, 2007). Similar to the dilemma with endotracheal tubes with CASS capacity, it is challenging to decide in advance which patients would benefit from the more expensive PU cuff tube. A recent trial in cardiac surgery patients found the cutoff for an increased risk of VAP at about 16 hours of mechanical ventilation (Poelaert, Haentjens, & Blot, 2014).

Other Measures to Prevent VAP

Silver-coated endotracheal tubes were found to be effective in reducing VAP but in one randomized trial (Kollef et al., 2008) and its use is not generally recommended. Administration of probiotics has been discussed, but one should be cautious in immunocompromised patients, as the risk of gut translocation and subsequent infection can increase.

Treatment

VAP has a good prognosis if treatment is initiated without delay. Studies suggest that a delay in antimicrobial therapy is associated with prolonged mechanical ventilation and increased mortality (Iregui,

Ward, Sherman, Fraser, & Kollef, 2002; Luna et al., 2006; Mariya Joseph et al., 2012). Therefore, empiric antibiotic therapy should be initiated within the first 24 hours after onset of symptoms and clinical suspicion of VAP. In postoperative pneumonia, the choice of antibiotic is determined by the onset of symptoms. Early-onset VAP have a lower incidence of MDR bacteria, so treatment is more in line with the therapy of CAP or HAP. On the other hand, late-onset VAP after cardiac surgery is often caused by Pseudomonas aeruginosa (He et al., 2014), so empiric antibiotic therapy has to be adjusted accordingly.

For CAP, HAP, or early-onset VAP without further risk factors, an aminopenicillin with beta-lactamase inhibitor (i.e. ampicillin/sulbactam) or a basic third-generation cephalosporin (i.e. ceftriaxone or cefotaxime) plus a macrolide (i.e. azithromycin) is a sufficient empiric therapy, which should be continued for a total of 7-8 days. Alternatively, a basic fluoroquinolone (i.e. moxifloxacine or levofloxacine) can be used.

For HAP or VAP with risk factors for MDR bacteria, initial empiric therapy comprises of an ureidopenicilline with beta-lactamase inhibitor (i.e. piperacillin/tazobactam), an antipseudomonal third-generation cephalosporin (i.e. cefepime or ceftazidime), or a carbapenem (i.e. imipenem or meropenem). In addition to this, a glycopeptide (i.e. vancomycin) or an oxazolidinone (i.e. linezolid) should be given, particularly if MRSA is a concern within the institution. The typical therapy duration is 7-8 days, when pseudomonas or MRSA infection is proven, therapy should continue for a total of 10-14 days.

Combination therapy for VAP with risk factors (cefepime, piperacillin/tazobactam, or meropenem plus ciprofloxacine or an aminoglycoside) has traditionally been suggested (Eggimann & Revelly, 2006; Heyland, Dodek, Muscedere, Day, & Cook, 2008) and is also recommended in current guideline documents (American Thoracic Society & Infectious Disease Society of America, 2005). Conversely, a meta-analysis showed that the combination of drugs had no benefit over adequate monotherapy (Aarts, Hancock, Heyland, McLeod, & Marshall, 2008). The guidelines aside, it is paramount to consider patient risk factors and clinical presentation when treating for VAP and suspecting MDR microorganisms (Kett et al., 2011).

Since empiric therapy and inadequate de-escalation has been linked to increased antibiotic resistance within institutions, it is important to reevaluate therapy every 24 hours after initiation for the purpose of either de-escalating or increasing coverage. Total treatment days for VAP should be limited to 7-8 days, unless additional risk factors or proven MDR infection exist (Dimopoulos et al., 2013). Aerosolized administration of antibiotics has traditionally been reserved for patients with chronic pulmonary disease such as cystic fibrosis colonized with MDR bacteria. There is some beginning evidence that in VAP caused by MDR microorganisms such as pseudomonas or acinetobacter, the addition of inhaled antibiotics (i.e. colistin) can facilitate eradication, decrease resistance, and reduce the use and side effects of systemic agents, for example the significant nephrotoxicity of systemic colistin (Abu-Salah & Dhand, 2011; Palmer & Smaldone, 2014). For MRSA pneumonia, there is some evidence that linezolid has outcome advantages over vancomycin (Wunderink et al., 2012), but mortality was not affected by drug choice, and a meta-analysis showed no superiority of linezolid over glycopeptide antibiotics (Walkey, O'Donnell, & Wiener, 2011).

Surgical Site Infections

Background

Sternal Wound Infections

Surgical sites prone to postoperative infections include the sternal wound, the sternum itself, the mediastinum, the pleural space, and wounds related to vein or artery harvest and cutdown or cannulation sites. Sternal wound complications can be further differentiated in superficial wound infections and deep sternal wound infections (DSWI). DSWI carries considerable morbidity and increased mortality after cardiac surgery, both immediately postoperatively (Kubota et al., 2013) and long-term (Toumpoulis, Anagnostopoulos, DeRose, & Swistel, 2005). In a study including more than 1,000 postoperative cardiac surgery patients, the incidence of superficial wound infections was 3.3%, while 2.5% of patients developed DSWI (Heilmann et al., 2013). Several studies aimed at identifying risk factors for DSWI have been conducted. In the majority of studies, diabetes mellitus, morbid obesity, chronic obstructive pulmonary disease, redo surgery, blood transfusion, and the use of bilateral mammary arteries as coronary grafts were described as carrying an increased risk (Diez et al., 2007; Filsoufi et al., 2009, Risnes, Abdelnoor, Almdahl, & Svennevig, 2010; Floros et al., 2011) (Table 9).

Pleural Space Infections

Pleural effusions are a common complication after cardiothoracic surgical procedures. Most of them are of transsudative nature and resolve after drainage, diuresis, or treatment of the underlying condition, i.e. post-pericardiotomy syndrome. On the other hand, patients with primary pleural space infections may present to the cardiothoracic ICU in the setting before or immediately after thoracic exploration for diagnosis and treatment of an effusion or empyema. Complicated exsudative pleural effusions and empyema are a result of bacterial invasion of the pleural space (Brims, Lansley, Waterer, & Lee, 2010). Aside from a postoperative infection, pneumonia is the leading cause of a complicated effusion or empyema, commonly referred to as a parapneumonic effusion. Complicated effusions and empyema carry a significant mortality, so early treatment is critical (Davies, Kearney, Gleeson, & Davies, 1999).

Table 9. Risk factors for the development of deep sternal wound infections after cardiac surgery

Preoperative	Intraoperative
• Diabetes mellitus • Hemodynamic instability • Blood transfusion • Active smoking or history of COPD • Obesity • Type of operation	• Use of bilateral mammary arteries • Emergency surgery • Re-exploration for bleeding • Redo surgery • Operative time • Blood transfusion • Prolonged ventilation
MSSA = methicillin-sensitive Staphylococcus aureus, MRSA = methicillin-resistant Staphylococcus aureus	

From: Mauermann et al., Best Practice & Research in Clinical Anaesthesiology, 2008

Device-Related Infections

Device-related infections have come into the focus of cardiothoracic surgeons with the increasing prevalence of heart failure and use of ventricular assist devices (VAD). The International Society for Heart and Lung Transplantation has recently presented consensus guidelines describing the diagnosis and therapy of device-related infections (Hannan et al., 2011). Driveline exit site infections are a major cause of morbidity and occur in approximately 19% of continuous-flow VAD patients after 12 months of support (Goldstein et al., 2012). The presence of an infected driveline often leads to and increased length of stay and readmissions in this patient population. Longer duration of support appears to be the most important factor for the development of driveline infection (Sharma et al., 2012).

Diagnosis

Sternal Wound Infections

The majority of bacteria isolated from sternal wounds remain Gram-positive microorganisms. In North America and Europe, Staphylococcus aureus and coagulase-negative staphylococci are the leading bacteria causing sternal wound infections (Mauermann, Sampathkumar, & Thompson, 2008). Sternal wound infections generally present with localized cellulitis, swelling, warmth, tenderness, and potentially purulent discharge. Sternal instability can be an indicator of deep infection. Wounds swabs and blood cultures should be sent for Gram-stain and culture before the initial dose of empiric antibiotics. If a deeper infection or mediastinitis is suspected, imaging studies, such as computed tomography (CT) of the chest, can help confirm the diagnosis. Often times, the diagnosis is eventually made upon surgical re-exploration.

Pleural Space Infections

Patients with empyema often have significant clinical symptoms such as fever, malaise, and respiratory distress. A chest radiograph may or may not detect an effusion, as those fluid collections can be loculated, and additional imaging such as an ultrasound or a CT of the chest may have to be obtained. As a general principle, the diagnosis is a combination of clinical, laboratory (microbiology), and radiological features and findings.

Prevention

Managing Blood Glucose Levels

Many risk factors in the development of DSWI are hard to modify, however several items were targeted for quality of care improvement in the perioperative period. Blood glucose control as a means of reducing DSWI has been studied extensively and proven to be effective in diabetic individuals (Zerr et al., 1997; Furnary, Zerr, Grunkemeier, & Starr, 1999). Glucose control has become mainstay of therapy in most ICU settings. At the same time, management of glucose following open-heart surgery has been implemented as a quality measure as part of the Surgical Care Improvement Project (SCIP). This has lead to the widespread adoption of active glucose control on cardiothoracic ICUs. It remains unclear what the exact upper limit of blood glucose should be in order to have a positive effect on the incidence of DSWI without causing harmful events such as hypoglycemia. It has been demonstrated in one randomized trial that intensive insulin therapy for perioperative glucose control in cardiac surgery patients does not have any benefit over conventional therapy targeting glucose levels under 200 mg/dL (Gandhi et al., 2007). In fact, an increase of adverse events was observed in the group receiving intensive insulin therapy with a target blood glucose between 80 and 100 mg/dL. It is now accepted that a glucose range of 140-200 mg/dL is considered optimal care for perioperative cardiac surgery patients (O'Connor, 2010). Similarly, new recommendations with revised blood glucose targets have been put forward by the American College of Physicians for all hospitalized patient populations (Qaseem, Humphrey, Chou, Snow, & Shekelle, 2011).

Decontaminating the Nasopharynx

As the primary causing organism is Staphylococcus aureus, decontamination of the nasopharynx using topical antibiotics (i.e. mupirocin) has been suggested as a preventive measure for wound infections. The application of mupirocin to the anterior nares is very effective in short-term eradication, and also effective against MRSA (Perl & Golub, 1998). While initial studies could show a benefit in reduction of DSWI, a more recent randomized trial could only demonstrate the eradicative effect, but no reduction in DSWI (Konvalinka, Errett, & Fong, 2006). Given the positive results of the initial trials, the lack of side effects, and the simplicity of this measure, it appears reasonable to incorporate topical mupirocin into a DSWI prevention bundle.

Decontaminating the Skin

Skin decontamination using chlorhexidine has been demonstrated to be effective in reducing Staphylococcus aureus microbial counts, but failed to reduce surgical site infections (Webster & Osborne, 2007). There has not been a convincing randomized trial to date, but again, given the simplicity of this measure and the theoretical advantage of eradicating bacteria (including MRSA) colonizing the patient's skin, it is advised to perform preoperative chlorhexidine washings. In addition to Staphylococcus aureus, chlorhexidine shows activity against coagulase-negative staphylococci and Gram-negative bacteria as well.

Giving Perioperative Antibiotics

Perioperative antibiotic prophylaxis is a key measure to prevent surgical site infections. Given the high incidence of staphylococci, using first generation cephalosporin with strong Gram-positive coverage is most important. This is further outlined in the guideline documents from the Society of Thoracic Surgeons (Edwards et al., 2006; Engelman et al., 2007). The timing of administration is also important, and the initial dose should be given within an hour before skin incision to ascertain adequate plasma levels. Intraoperative redoes regimens vary between antibiotics, i.e. cefazolin should be given every 3 hours and every 8 hours postoperatively. A meta-analysis looking specifically at drug choice could not demonstrate a benefit of prophylactic glycopeptide over beta-lactam antibiotics (Bolon et al., 2004). While a cephalosporin remains the primary agent for perioperative prophylaxis, it becomes more and more obvious that in the era of rising MRSA rates, the addition of a glycopeptide particularly in institutions with a high prevalence of MRSA is a feasible thing to do. In contrast to prophylaxis in other surgical specialties, cardiac surgery patients should receive antibiotics for a total of 48 hours postoperatively (Lador et al., 2012). In the thoracic surgery patient population, the frequent presence of an open airway must be taken into consideration. Here, the use of a second or third generation cephalosporin is advised for perioperative prophylaxis. Alternatively, a targeted antibiotic prophylaxis can be applied when intraoperative cultures are obtained (Schussler et al., 2008).

Other Measures to Prevent DSWI

The implantation of a gentamicin-impregnated sponge into the wound upon chest closure has been suggested to reduce wound infections, but this cannot be recommended at this time, as two larger studies independently showed no benefit (Bennett-Guerrero et al., 2010; Birgand et al., 2013). Using fixed plates instead of wires for sternal closure has been successfully used to prevent postoperative sternal complications and infections in high-risk patients (Song, Lohman, Renucci, Jeevanandam, & Raman, 2004; Snyder, Graham, Byers, & Holman, 2009). Similar to VAP, there is the notion to bundle preventive measures together to improve outcomes, as shown in a recent study (Miyahara et al., 2014). Whether to use bilateral mammary arteries for coronary bypass grafting is controversial. While studies have shown an increase in DSWI in diabetics (Savage et al., 2007), others could demonstrate a survival benefit likely due to the second arterial graft even in the diabetic subgroup (Puskas, Sadiq, Vassiliades, Kilgo, & Lattouf, 2012).

Treatment

Sternal Wound Infections

The traditional management of DSWI and mediastinitis involved surgical re-exploration followed by an open chest with subsequent dressing changes and washouts until deemed macroscopically cured. Then the sternum was reapproximated or a secondary closure using a muscle or omental flap was performed. This practice was in part responsible for the high morbidity and mortality of mediastinitis (Sarr, Gott, & Townsend, 1984). Open chest management results in an unstable thorax and invariably requires mechanical ventilation and prolonged immobilization. A major step forward was the introduction of closed suction-irrigation drainage, as this practice allowed sternal closure and continued therapy. While not a first-line therapy anymore, it is still successfully used in some institutions (Deschka et al., 2013). More recently, vacuum-assisted closure has been used to treat DSWI and mediastinitis, a treatment option, which evolved from chronic open wound therapy. Controlled suction is applied to the wound with the goal to enhance local perfusion and development of granulation tissue. The results in the post-sternotomy surgical population with DSWI or mediastinitis are very promising (Domkowski et al., 2003; Tocco et al., 2009). Despite the retrospective nature of most comparative studies regarding vacuum-assisted closure, it has become a first-line surgical therapy for DSWI, mediastinitis, and sternal osteomyelitis (Yu, Rippel, Smock, & Jarral, 2013). Ideally, surgical treatment should be based on clinical algorithms, and some institutions have suggested using biomarkers such as C-reactive protein levels to guide therapy (Sjögren, Malmsjö, Gustafsson, & Ingemansson, 2006).

If DSWI is suspected, a wound culture and mediastinal fluid is obtained and empiric antibiotic therapy is initiated, targeting the most common microorganisms in this setting, Gram-positive cocci, particularly Staphylococcus aureus. It is reasonable to empirically treat those patients with a first-generation cephalosporin such as cefazolin. In institutions with higher MRSA rates, vancomycin should be used or added. With the advent of MDR Gram-positive bacteria (Steinkraus, White, & Friedrich, 2007), newer antibiotics such as linezolid (Sacar et al., 2008) and daptomycin (Popov et al., 2011) may become more and more common in the antimicrobial therapy for DSWI.

Pleural Space Infections

Current treatment options for complicated effusions and empyema include iterative thoracentesis, chest tube placement for drainage, and surgical management via either open thoracotomy or video-assisted thoracoscopic surgery (VATS). In the early stages, antibiotic therapy alone or in combination with the intrapleural administration of fibrinolytic drugs may be sufficient. As a next step, thoracentesis may be considered, however this technique is mostly used for diagnostic purposes. Complicated effusions generally require continuous drainage via chest tubes, however, a recent study showed that thoracentesis alone could be a successful therapeutic alternative (Letheulle et al., 2013). Invasive surgical treatment involves either VATS visualization or open thoracotomy followed by lysis of adhesions and loculated fluid collections, drainage of effusion or pus, and excision of thickened visceral pleura, also known as decortication (Schweigert et al., 2014). There is beginning evidence showing improved patient outcomes with VATS versus the traditional open approach (Chambers, Routledge, Dunning, & Scarci, 2010).

Device-Related Infections

Driveline infections are the most common device-related infections and require antibiotic therapy for two to four weeks and optional surgical debridement depending on the clinical presentation. Antimicrobial therapy should primarily be based on culture results. If the device is deemed colonized with bacteria, a life-long suppressive antibiotic therapy is indicated (Nienaber et al., 2013). In case of more complicated courses of pump infection, i.e. inability to clear bacteria from the blood stream, pump explantation or exchange can be indicated, which carries significant morbidity. Consensus in diagnosis is important to initiate appropriate therapy, but despite adequate treatment, device-related infections are associated with reduced survival on assist device support (Koval, Thuita, Moazami, & Blackstone, 2014).

Infective Endocarditis

Background

Infective endocarditis is defined as an infection of the endothelium of the heart. It can also affect implanted prosthetic material such as pacemaker leads, valves, or cannulas. Its therapy has evolved substantially over the last century. While it was originally a fatal disease, the introduction of antibiotic therapy and more recently early surgical intervention changed the course of the disease dramatically (Thuny, Grisoli, Collart, Habib, & Raoult, 2012). Despite medical and surgical advances, in-hospital (15-20%) and 1-year (40%) mortality of endocarditis remain quite high. The most recent large cohort study revealed that endocarditis nowadays presents like a more acute disease than previously described. Patients are generally older with more comorbidities, also, staphylococcal infections are now much more common, so is prior exposure to healthcare (Murdoch et al., 2009). Valvular heart disease, either congenital or degenerative, and the presence of prosthetic valves are the major risk factors for developing endocarditis. Other patient factors include intravenous drug abuse, poor dentition causing recurrent transient bacteremia, immunosuppression, and the presence of indwelling catheters (i.e. dialysis lines) and other foreign intravascular material (i.e. pacemaker leads). Infected pacemaker leads frequently cause concomitant valvular infection necessitating early device removal (Athan et al., 2012).

Endocarditis usually develops as a result of bacteremia. The source of bacteremia is variable, but dental procedures and intravenous drug use seem to be among the common causing insults. Circulating bacteria then seed on damaged endothelium or prosthetic material, eventually causing an infected vegetation to develop in the heart. Damaged endothelium can occur in situations where there is either physical damage to the tissue or chronic inflammation such as in advanced degenerative or rheumatic valve disease.

After the initial bacteremia, there is often a delay of days to several weeks until clinical symptoms of endocarditis occur. The symptoms correlate with the degree of endocardial destruction. Acute valvular regurgitation is common and is poorly tolerated in the setting of a non-dilated ventricle. About a third of patients often present in advanced heart failure or cardiogenic shock and emergent surgical repair is usually required (Kiefer et al., 2011). Formation of a perivalvular abscess occurs in about 15% of cases (Murdoch et al., 2009), is typical for native aortic valve endocarditis, and often involves the entire aortic root. For prosthetic valve endocarditis, an abscess may be the only lesion, as the prosthetic material is often free of vegetations. Cardiac rhythm disorders, particularly heart block can be a sign of perivalvular abscess. Systemic embolization of endocarditic material can occur, most commonly to the brain. Clinically apparent cerebral embolic complications are seen in about 15-20% of patients and can preceded the actual diagnosis of endocarditis. Pulmonary emboli are observed in patients with right-sided endocarditis (Freedman, 1987; Petterson et al., 2014). In summary, the complications listed above are quite common and often times the reason patients with endocarditis require care in an ICU setting.

The majority of endocarditis cases is caused by Gram-positive microorganisms. The spectrum has changed significantly over the past decade (Slipczuk et al., 2013). Staphylococci are now considered the leading cause of endocarditis, whereas the incidence of streptococci is decreasing (Hoen et al, 2002; Selton-Suty et al., 2012). Healthcare-associated enterococcal endocarditis is also more common now, and vancomycin resistance is reported to be present in as much as 10% of isolated enterococcus strains (Chirouze et al., 2013). Coagulase-negative staphylococci remain a major factor in prosthetic valve endocarditis with a high incidence of methicillin resistance (Chu et al., 2009). In summary, these changes in causative organisms reflect an aging population with increasing and repeated healthcare contact, but also improved oral hygiene in industrialized countries.

Diagnosis

Early diagnosis is key, as delay of antibiotic therapy is linked to poor outcomes (Lodise, McKinnon, Swiderski, & Rybak, 2003). The diagnosis of endocarditis is dependent on clinical criteria, microbiological culture data, and echocardiographic findings. A summary of the diagnostic algorithm was first described as the Duke criteria and later modified by Li et al. (2000). The diagnostic sensitivity and specificity exceeds 80%. A fever and a new murmur are quite frequent, other signs are less common, however equally diagnostic (Table 10).

Aside from multiple sets of blood cultures, the microbiological diagnostic should include a serum sample to detect specific antibodies against Coxiella burnetii, Legionella pneumophila, and Mycoplasma pneumoniae. Blood culture results are highly variable and culture-negativity can entail therapeutic issues. Examples for causes of negative blood cultures in endocarditis are previous antibiotic therapy, intracellular bacteria, fungi, and other fastidious microorganisms. Modern molecular techniques such as polymerase chain reaction (PCR) are emerging and can help identify pathogens in culture-negative cases and also classify organisms in cases where contamination might be a concern (Millar & Moore, 2004). In some cases bacteria can only be cultured from excised valve tissue.

Imaging studies should begin with a transthoracic echocardiogram (TTE). This is a fast method to identify larger vegetations and valvular dysfunction (Habib et al., 2010). The classic echocardiographic

Table 10. Modified Duke Criteria for the diagnosis of infective endocarditis

Pathological Criteria (Need 1)	Clinical Criteria (Need 2 Major, 1 Major and 3 Minor, or 5 minor)
• Microorganism identified by culture or histology from vegetation, septic embolus, or abscess • Histological specimen from vegetation or abscess showing active endocarditis	*Major criteria* • 2 positive blood cultures with typical microorganism drawn at least 12 hours apart (or 1 positive blood culture for Coxiella burnetti or IgG titer > 1:800) • Evidence of endocardial involvement (new murmur, echocardiograpically detected intracardiac mass, abscess or valve dehiscence) *Minor criteria* • Fever > 38 °C • Vascular phenomena (septic emboli, Janeway lesions) • Immunological phenomena (Osler's nodes, Roth spots) • Predisposition to infective endocarditis (previous endocarditis, intravenous drug use) • Microbiological evidence not meeting major criteria

From: Li et al., Clinical Infectious Diseases, 2000

features include 1) and oscillating mass or vegetation on a valve or supporting structure, 2) abscess, 3) prosthetic valve dehiscence, and 4) new or worsening valvular regurgitation (Methangkool, Howard-Quijano, Ho, & Mahajan, 2014). In case of a negative TTE, a transesophageal echocardiogram (TEE) is indicated, as this modality is able to detect most vegetations, abscessed, and perforations. Especially in the setting of prosthetic valve endocarditis, TEE is the superior imaging modality. Newer techniques such as three-dimensional echocardiography, positron emission tomography (PET), and magnetic resonance imaging (MRI) can provide further information in difficult cases (Hansalia et al., 2009; Vind & Hess, 2010).

Given the frequency of cerebral emboli, a neurologic evaluation and potentially imaging studies may be necessary. This is particularly important in patients that are planned to have valve surgery and will undergo CPB. MRI is a highly sensitive diagnostic test for cerebral lesions and can potentially change clinical management (Duval et al., 2010; Novy et al., 2013; Goulenok et al., 2013).

Prevention

Traditionally, patients with preexisting cardiac conditions undergoing for example dental or gastrointestinal procedures, were to receive periprocedural prophylaxis with various antibiotics (Durack, 1995). These recommendations were based on expert opinion and data from animal studies. There is also the notion that for instance regular daily tooth brushing is more likely to cause bacteremia than a single dental procedure, and that antibiotic prophylaxis prevents few cases of endocarditis. Given the paucity of clinical evidence and the potential downsides of unnecessary administration of antibiotics, more recent guideline documents from the American Heart Association and the European Society of Cardiology restrict the use of periprocedural antibiotics. The only situation where antibiotic prophylaxis is still recommended is an invasive dental procedure in patients with a) a prosthetic valve, b) a history of infective endocarditis, c) unrepaired cyanotic congenital heart disease, d) certain repaired congenital heart defects using prosthetic material, or e) heart transplant recipients who develop valvular disease (Wilson et al., 2007; Habib et al., 2009; Nishimura et al., 2014). In Great Britain, antibiotic endocarditis prophylaxis is no longer recommended in any circumstance (Richey, Wray, & Stokes, 2008). Recent reports indicate that the incidence of infective endocarditis has not changed despite the dramatic change in guideline recommendations (Desimone et al., 2012). General skin and oral hygiene are thought to be important measures to reduce the risk of infection and endocarditis.

When choosing to administer prophylactic antibiotics, oral amoxicillin is still the recommended drug. This can be substituted by ampicillin or ceftriaxone if the intravenous route is preferred. Alternatives in the setting of penicillin allergy are cephalexin or clindamycin. In cases at increased risk for Staphylococcus aureus infection, i.e. frequent contact with healthcare, an appropriate staphylococcal antibiotic should be selected. Moreover, the increasing resistance of viridans streptococci may require a shift in antibiotic choice in the future (Thanavaro & Nixon, 2014).

Treatment

As mentioned above, despite advances in medical and surgical therapy, endocarditis carries a high mortality and early initiation of appropriate treatment is crucial. Delays in initiation of antibiotic therapy may result in complications such as sepsis and multiple organ dysfunction syndrome (MODS). Prompt antimicrobial therapy can also reduce the risk of septic emboli to the brain causing strokes by up to 65% (Dickerman et al., 2007). As a general principle, antibiotics should be started after the initial set of microbiological samples has been obtained. Therapy then has to be adjusted according to the culture results.

In terms of antibiotic drug choice, not very many things have changed over the past two decades, and the traditional agents still seem to play a major role in the treatment of endocarditis. Most guideline documents recommend a standard set of antibiotic drugs, and also specify potential combinations, and duration of therapy (Baddour et al., 2005; Wilson et al., 2007; Habib et al., 2009). Empirical treatment should be based on the severity of disease, whether a native or prosthetic valve is affected, and whether the patient has risk factors for MDR bacteria. In the light of increasing resistant Staphylococcus aureus infections, vancomycin should be part of the empiric therapy in all patients with suspected endocarditis presenting with severe sepsis in the cardiothoracic ICU (Table 11). It is however reasonable to initially treat clinically stable patients with amoxicillin or ceftriaxone only. Ceftriaxone likely provides better coverage of fastidious Gram-negative bacteria, such as bacilli out of the HACEK group (Haemophilus species, Aggregatibacter species, Cardiobacterium hominis, Eikenella corrodens, Kingella species) (Chambers et al., 2013). Vancomycin is also considered the first-line treatment in case of a severe penicillin allergy. Some Gram-negative bacteria are difficult to eradicate and early surgery is indicated. Similarly, fungal endocarditis generally requires dual antifungal coverage against yeast and mold as well as valve replacement. The mortality of fungal endocarditis is reported to be over 50% (Ellis, Al-Abdely, Sandridge, Greer, & Ventura, 2001).

Patients with suspected prosthetic valve endocarditis should receive rifampicin in addition to the standard regimen for synergistic purposes. If gentamicin is added, it should be dosed for actual body weight unless patients are severely obese, in which case the dose has to be reduced in order to avoid overdose. In contrast to other infections, in endocarditis gentamicin is often given twice daily for the treatment of endocarditis, however data to support one or the other strategy is lacking. The gentamicin serum levels should not exceed 1 mg/l before dosing and should be in the range of 3-5 mg/L after dosing of the drug. Vancomycin serum levels before dosing should be maintained between 15-20 mg/L.

Therapy duration is usually 4 weeks for uncomplicated native valve disease (streptococcal or HACEK infection) (6 weeks for prosthetic valve disease). Endocarditis due to Staphylococcus aureus and enterococcal infections should be treated for 6 weeks regardless of valve type involved. Newer antibiotics such as

Table 11. Example for empiric antibiotic therapy for infective endocarditis

Antibiotic Drug	Dose
Native valve endocarditis, stable clinical presentation	
Amoxicillin OR Ceftriaxone PLUS Gentamicin	2 gm q4 hours 2 gm q24 hours 1 mg/kg ABW q24 hours
Native valve endocarditis, severe sepsis, no risk factors for MDR bacteria	
Vancomycin PLUS Gentamicin	1.5-2 gm (loading dose), 15 mg/kg q12 hours (maintenance) 1 mg/kg IBW q12 hours
Native valve endocarditis, severe sepsis and risk factors for MDR bacteria	
Vancomycin PLUS Meropenem	1.5-2 gm (loading dose), 15 mg/kg q12 hours (maintenance) 2 gm q8 hours
Prosthetic valve endocarditis, pending or negative blood cultures	
Vancomycin PLUS Gentamicin PLUS Rifampicin	1.5-2 gm (loading dose), 15 mg/kg q12 hours (maintenance) 1 mg/kg IBW q12 hours 300-600 mg q12 hours
ABW = actual body weight, IBW = ideal body weight, MDR = multi-drug resistant	

From: Gould et al., Journal of Antimicrobial Chemotherapy, 2012

linezolid and daptomycin have also been studied in endocarditis. Linezolid seems to be at least as effective against MRSA as vancomycin and it could have a role as an alternative therapy for vancomycin-resistant enterococci (Patel, Rouse, Piper, & Steckelberg, 2001). Since linezolid is a bacteriostatic antibiotic, it should be administered in combination with a bactericidal agent. In one study, daptomycin has been described as non-inferior when compared with standard therapy (Fowler et al., 2006), but therapy failure and development of resistance have also been reported, particularly with daptomycin monotherapy (Arias et al., 2007; Twele et al., 2010). In rare cases of vancomycin and linezolid resistance, daptomycin has been successfully used in combination with tigecycline (Jenkins, 2007).

It is recommended that a surgical opinion should be obtained immediately after diagnosis of endocarditis independent of clinical presentation. The indication and timing of surgery is a much more complex issue and needs to be assessed in an individual case-by-case fashion. The most recent guidelines emphasize the importance of establishing a heart team to streamline the care of patients with valvular heart disease (Nishimura et al., 2014). This team is comprised of cardiac specialists from various clinical services, i.e. cardiac surgeons, cardiologists, critical care physicians, imaging specialists, and the purpose of this team is to integrate clinical data and expert information to provide optimal care for complex cardiac disease.

Indications for surgery have increased over the last years and early surgery is now performed in about 40-60% of patients with acute endocarditis (Table 12). The ultimate goal of surgical intervention is to treat acute and impending complications and to completely excise the infected tissue to eradicate infection. Mechanical and stented tissue valves both are acceptable options, and valve choice should be based on patient factors such as life expectancy and likelihood of compliance with chronic anticoagulation (Byrne et al., 2011). The use of bioprosthetic valves has increased over the last decade (Savage, Saha-Chaudhuri, Asher, Brennan, & Gammie, 2014). Some studies suggest different mortality for different types of valve prostheses, but this effect is likely due to patient factors prior to surgery (Nguyen et al., 2010; Savage et al., 2014). For aortic valve endocarditis complicated by aortic root abscess, cryopreserved homograft implantation has been successfully performed (Musci et al., 2010). For mitral valve endocarditis, leaflet repair and annuloplasty is always preferred over valve replacement, and excellent results have been reported for this approach (Zegdi et al., 2005). Right-sided endocarditis less often requires surgery, but if necessary, tricuspid repair should be attempted. Given the exponential increase in the use of cardiac implantable electronic devices (CIED), infectious complications related to those implants have become a growing issue. The American Heart Association therefore has issued a guideline document to guide therapy in patients with device infections (Baddour et al., 2010). In summary, patients with a CIED infection, or a CIED in the presence of infective endocarditis with a resistant microorganism, or endocarditis requiring surgical treatment should have complete removal of the device. Concomitant valve infection is common in the setting of an infected CIED and complete removal is associated with improved 1-year survival (Athan et al., 2012). If CIED re-implantation is clinically necessary, this should be delayed until after completion of antibiotic therapy for infective endocarditis. While driveline infection is the most common infectious complication after VAD implantation, bacteremia and subsequent endocarditis involving the device can occur. In this case, in addition to the initial six weeks of antibiotic therapy, chronic suppressive antimicrobial therapy is instituted. Device removal can be considered, but carries high perioperative morbidity (Nienaber et al., 2013).

Preoperative status seems to be a predictor of surgical outcome, especially lack of adequate antibiotic therapy, Staphylococcus aureus infection, comorbidities such as impaired renal function, and the presence of cerebral embolic complications (Chu et al., 2004; Grubitzsch et al., 2014; Pang et al., 2014).

Table 12. Indications for and timing of surgery in infective endocarditis

Indication	Timing
Heart failure	
• Aortic or mitral IE or PVE with severe acute regurgitation or valve obstruction or fistula causing refractory pulmonary edema or cardiogenic shock	Emergent
• Aortic or mitral IE with severe acute regurgitation or valve obstruction and persisting heart failure or echocardiographic signs of poor hemodynamic tolerance	Urgent
• Aortic or mitral IE or severe prosthetic dehiscence with severe regurgitation and no heart failure	Elective
• Right heart failure secondary to severe tricuspid regurgitation with poor response to diuretic therapy	Urgent versus elective
Uncontrolled infection	
• Locally uncontrolled infection (abscess, false aneurysm, fistula, enlarging vegetation)	Urgent
• Persistent fever and positive blood cultures > 7-10 days not related to an extracardiac cause	Urgent
• Infection caused by fungi or multiresistant organisms	Urgent versus elective
• PVE caused by staphylococci or Gram-negative bacteria (most cases od early PVE)	Urgent versus elective
Prevention of embolism	
• Aortic of mitral IE or PVE with large vegetations (> 10 mm) after 1 or more embolic episodes despite appropriate antibiotic therapy	Urgent
• Aortic or mitral IE or PVE with large vegetations (> 10 mm) and other predictors of complicated course (heart failure, persistent infection, abscess)	Urgent
• Aortic or mitral or PVE with isolated very large vegetations (> 15 mm)	Urgent
• Persistent tricuspid valve vegetations > 20 mm after recurrent pulmonary emboli	Urgent versus elective
Emergent surgery = within 24 hours, urgent surgery = within a few days, elective surgery = after 1-2 weeks of antibiotic therapy	
IE = infective endocarditis, PVE = prosthetic valve endocarditis	

From: Thuny et al., Lancet, 2012

Reported perioperative mortality is biased by patient characteristics and there are no randomized studies comparing outcomes of surgery versus medical therapy alone in endocarditis. Observational studies that attempt to correct for patient factors could demonstrate a survival benefit for patients undergoing surgery (Lalani et al., 2010).

Timing of surgery has always been a controversial topic. Even with a clear guideline-driven clinical indication for surgery, the ideal time point is difficult to determine. Some retrospective studies suggest a benefit when early surgery is performed (Funakoshi et al., 2011), others are equivocal when it comes to long-term results (Thuny et al., 2011). In a smaller randomized trial, patients assigned to having surgery within the first 48 hours after diagnosis had a significantly lower risk of death or embolic events than patients assigned to usual care. Despite the randomized nature of the study, the results should be looked at with caution, as this was a fairly healthy patient population with an unusually low mortality (Kang et al., 2012).

Neurological complications such as embolic strokes have traditionally been a driver for decision-making with regards to timing of surgery. While in the past early surgery was prohibitive in patients with embolic strokes due to the concern for hemorrhagic conversion on CPB, newer studies have shown comparable outcomes in patients with and without neurological complications at the time of surgery (Ruttmann et al., 2006; Thuny et al., 2007). Therefore, in the absence of severe neurologic damage, coma, or intracranial hemorrhage on imaging studies, early surgery is feasible and safe in patients with septic emboli or asymptomatic lesions visible on brain imaging (Wilson et al., 2007; Habib et al., 2009). Routine imaging is necessary to detect asymptomatic cerebral emboli and smaller hemorrhagic lesions, as they can pose significant risk even in the absence of clinical symptoms. Close perioperative neurological monitoring is necessary to detect hemorrhagic conversion, especially after starting anticoagulation (Misfeld et al., 2014).

Bloodstream Infections

Background

Catheter-related bloodstream infections can occur with any kind of indwelling line, but most commonly is related to central venous catheters. Every year, about 250,000 blood stream infections are detected in U.S. hospitals (Klevens et al., 2007). Most importantly, bloodstream infections are associated with a significant increase in hospital length-of-stay and cost of care (Stone, Braccia, & Larson, 2005). A rapid decline of Staphylococcus aureus central line-associated bloodstream infection (CLABSI) since about 2006 has been observed, while the incidence of CLABSI due to fungi, enterococci, and Gram-negative rods remained stable. This trend reflects the successful introduction of central line insertion bundles as a measure of infection prevention (Fagan, Edwards, Park, Fridkin, & Magill, 2013). Prevention bundles for CLABSI were introduced in 2008 after the Centers for Medicare & Medicaid Services (CMS) announced that they would no longer reimburse hospitals for expenses related to CLABSI.

CLABSI is defined by the CDC National Healthcare Safety Network (NHSN) as bacteremia with a recognized pathogen when the organism isolated from a blood culture is not related to infection at another site; or isolation of a common skin contaminant from two or more blood cultures associated with signs and symptoms of infection (fever, chills, or hypotension) that cannot be attributed to infection at another site (Horan, Andrus, & Dudeck, 2008). Infection develops after colonization of a catheter and biofilm formation, most commonly via an extraluminal route through bacteria originating from the skin at the insertion site (Safdar & Maki, 2004). Intraluminal infection through contaminated intravenous fluids or drugs or colonized infusion ports is also possible. Skin flora is a common cause for infection and can originate from the patient's own skin or from unwashed hands of staff. About 60% of CLABSI reported to the NHSN were caused by Gram-positive bacteria, 18% of isolates were Gram-negative, 12% were caused by fungi (Hidron et al., 2008). Fungal bloodstream infections are less frequent, but carry a significantly increased mortality (Kett, Azoulay, Echeverria, & Vincent, 2011).

Risk factors for CLABSI traditionally included prolonged hospitalization before catheter insertion, suboptimal sterility on insertion, prolonged duration of an indwelling catheter, preexisting microbial colonization at the insertion site, neutropenia, parenteral nutrition, femoral and jugular cannulation site, excessive manipulation of the catheter, and large-bore and multi-lumen catheters (Polderman & Girbes, 2002; Safdar, Kluger, & Maki, 2002). However, more recent studies were not able to reproduce those results likely due to the existing care bundles, maximum barrier precautions for modern central line placement, and advanced dressing techniques (Maki, Kluger, & Crnich, 2006).

Diagnosis

In new-onset fever on the ICU without any obvious non-infectious causes, blood cultures should be obtained to rule out bacteremia prior to initiation of antibiotic therapy. Alcoholic chlorhexidine skin preparation is essential before peripheral puncture. Alcohol or tincture of iodine are acceptable alternatives. About 25 mL of blood should be drawn from a single site, and 3 to 4 sets of blood cultures should be obtained within 24 hours after onset of fever. Per guideline recommendation from the Infectious Disease Society of America (IDSA), in patients with a central venous catheter, a separate blood culture should be drawn from a catheter port in addition to the peripheral puncture (Mermel et al., 2009). It is important to treat the catheter port from which the culture is obtained with the same sterile precautions as the skin.

Two distinct microbiological techniques have been described for the diagnosis of CLABSI, simultaneous blood culture and differential time to positivity. Simultaneous blood cultures are obtained from a catheter, ideally the distal port, and via a peripheral venipuncture. This method is considered both sensitive and specific for the diagnosis of CLABSI (Chatzinikolaou et al., 2004). The diagnostic cutoff is defined, so that the colony count from the catheter has to be at least 3-fold higher than from the peripheral culture. The second method also necessitates simultaneously drawn cultures from the catheter and from a peripheral site. Both cultures are incubated and nowadays continuously monitored using radiometric blood cultures systems (Blot et al., 1998). The differential time to positivity is then recorded, and the diagnosis is likely CLABSI when the culture from the catheter turns positive at least 120 minutes before the peripheral culture (Blot et al., 1999). Concomitant administration of antibiotics through the central venous catheter can lead to false negative results (Raad, Hanna, & Maki, 2007).

Another simple method is a single quantitative blood culture from a suspicious catheter, with a diagnostic cutoff of > 100 CFU/mL. This method has been questioned, as it was found to be non-specific when it comes to the differentiation between CLABSI and high-grade bacteremia. Withdrawal and culture of the suspicious catheter is a classic diagnostic method of CLABSI. Semi-quantitative culture of a 5 cm segment of the catheter tip showing > 15 CFU/mL reflects catheter colonization. Isolation of the same organism from a peripheral blood culture proves CLABSI. The downside of this method is the potential contamination upon catheter withdrawal through the skin, the necessity of catheter removal itself, and the fact that the roll-plate method only detects extraluminal colonization. Sonication of the catheter tip has been described as a quantitative method with the advantage of detecting both intra- and extraluminal colonization, with the diagnostic cutoff set at 100 CFU/mL (Raad, Sabbagh, Rand, & Sherertz, 1992). Obviously, these methods require the removal of the central venous catheter for diagnostic, not therapeutic reasons, which has become subject to controversial discussion. The IDSA still recommends catheter tip cultures, despite the evidence supporting this has been described as moderate at best. A more recent study including 975 patients showed that sonication is not superior to semi-quantitative analysis (Erb et al., 2014). Results like this combined with a modest positive predictive value further question the role of catheter tip cultures, and the test likely does not help the diagnosis (Peterson & Smith, 2014).

Prevention

Several guideline documents focus on the prevention of catheter-related bloodstream infections (O'Grady et al., 2011, Marschall et al., 2014). Basic strategies for CLABSI prevention include performance of proper hand hygiene before insertion, use of an all-in-one catheter kit, use of maximum barrier precautions during insertion (Hu, Lipsky, Veenstra, & Saint, 2004), antiseptic skin disinfection ideally with a 2% chlorhexidine solution (Vallés et al., 2008), and preferential cannulation of the subclavian vein. The choice of vein for access is obviously more complex in some clinical situations, and the subclavian vein may not always be the first choice due to pacemaker systems, deep vein thrombosis, or risk of pneumothorax in an unstable patient. In contrast to guideline recommendations, recent clinical trials have shown that, unless chronic access is planned, the three common insertion sites (subclavian, jugular, and femoral) carry a comparable risk of CLABSI (Deshpande et al., 2005; Marik, Flemmer, & Harrison, 2012). Therefore, the jugular vein remains the first choice given the ease of insertion and relatively low complication rate when ultrasound and pressure monitoring is used for insertion. Peripherally inserted central catheters (PICC) have been associated with a lower infection risk in the outpatient setting, but studies have shown that for inpatients and particularly in the ICU, the risk of developing CLABSI is comparable to traditionally inserted central venous catheters (Chopra, O'Horo, Rogers, Maki, & Safdar, 2013). The choice for PICC over a regularly inserted central line should not be considered a measure of infection control. Arterial lines are an underappreciated source of bloodstream infections and should be taken into consideration when an ICU patient develops new-onset fever suspicious for bacteremia. Sterile insertion technique similar to central line barrier precautions and choosing the radial over the femoral site seem to decrease the rate of infection (O'Horo, Maki, Krupp, & Safdar, 2014). Exchanging an existing catheter over a guidewire cannot be performed in a completely sterile fashion and therefore this technique should not be used when CLABSI is suspected.

After insertion of the catheter, measures to reduce CLABSI rate include disinfection of catheter hubs, daily evaluation and removal of catheters that are not necessary for the patient's care (Peredo et al., 2010; Weeks, Hsu, Yang, Sawyer, & Marsteller, 2014), and replacement of the administration tubing at intervals not longer than 96 hours, unless blood products or lipids were used via this set (Ullman et al., 2013). Topical or systemic antibiotic prophylaxis is not indicated for central line insertions and may potentially induce antimicrobial resistance. Routine or scheduled replacement of central venous catheters increases the risk of procedural complications, but does not decrease the incidence of CLABSI and is hence not recommended (Eyer, Brummitt, Crossley, Siegel, & Cerra, 1990).

Other preventive methods have been described that are currently only recommended in hospital settings that have an unacceptably high incidence of CLABSI. Several studies were performed evaluating the usefulness of impregnated catheters. Both antiseptic (chlorhexidine-silver sulfadiazine) and antibiotic (minocycline-rifampicin) coatings have been successfully studied (Lai et al., 2013). While both types of impregnated catheters appear to reduce CLABSI, recent meta-analyses concluded that most studies were small and difficult to compare given methodological limitations (Casey, Mermel, Nightingale, & Elliott, 2008; Hockenhull et al., 2009). Beneficial effects of anti-infective coating seem to be limited to ICU settings and are questionable in units where care bundles have been instituted as a measure of infection control. Therefore, central venous catheters treated with anti-infective agents are reserved for following situations: when units have a high CLABSI rate, in patients that have limited venous access and a history of CLABSI, and in patients that have a high risk of complications from CLABSI, i.e. recently implanted heart valve or vascular graft (Marschall et al., 2014). Many studies have investigated the effectiveness of chlorhexidine-impregnated sponges and other chlorhexidine-containing dressing materials. Chlorhexidine-gluconate impregnated sponges led to a reduction in CLABSI rates, even when those rates were already very low (Timsit et al., 2009; Timsit et al., 2012). For ICU care, it will likely become a general recommendation to use chlorhexidine-impregnated dressing materials. This is based on the fact that chlorhexidine washes have already been part of prior guidelines, and the incorporation of chlorhexidine in the dressing will eliminate frequent dressing changes that itself carry a risk of infection (Safdar et al., 2014).

Similar to the efforts around VAP prevention, the implementation of care bundles and the subsequent culture change was highly efficacious in reducing a detrimental clinical outcome, in this case CLABSI (Pronovost et al., 2006). The results reported in this landmark paper were replicated in other studies in various ICU settings (Peredo et al., 2010; Tang et al., 2014). As an example for the importance of culture change, some centers were able to show a sustained effect on CLABSI rates, even after the initial implantation and study phase was completed (Pronovost et al., 2010). Surveillance participation per the NHSN protocol is recommended in the consensus guidelines, particularly in the ICU setting. For the purpose of national comparison, rates should be expressed as CLABSI per 1,000 catheter days.

Treatment

Empiric antibiotic therapy is often initiated when CLABSI is suspected. The choice of antibiotic drug should be based on patient risk factors, underlying disease, severity of clinical presentation, and nature of the suspected intravascular device. Since Gram-positive bacteria are the most common cause of CLABSI, vancomycin is the first choice therapy, as this provides adequate coverage in case of methicillin resistance. There is some discussion in the literature about drifting vancomycin minimum inhibitory concentration (MIC) and increased risk of mortality. Although a higher MIC represents borderline resistance, the most recent meta-analysis addressing this problem could not demonstrate a link to increased mortality (Kalil, Van Schooneveld, Fey, & Rupp, 2014). In those cases, daptomycin is probably the most feasible alternative (Fowler Jr. et al., 2006). In contrast, for resistant enterococci, linezolid is likely the more effective choice than daptomycin (Patel & Gallagher, 2014). In order to initially provide broad Gram-negative coverage, a fourth generation cephalosporin or carbapenem should be added, and choice should be based on local microbial incidence and resistance patterns and patient factors, such as chronic lung disease (Gürntke et al., 2014). ICU patients with suspected femoral line infection should also receive empiric antifungal coverage. Invasive candidiasis carries a high mortality and immediate treatment is key (Kett et al., 2011). Local candida resistance patterns have to be taken into consideration when choosing the appropriate antifungal agent. More recently, Candida albicans resistant to fluconazole is an emerging issue, and in some institutions, empiric therapy with an echinocandine may be indicated, particularly when patients present critically ill (Dimopoulos, Antonopoulou, Armaganidis, & Vincent, 2013). Duration of antimicrobial therapy is described in detail in the most recent IDSA guidelines (Mermel et al., 2009). For short-term central venous catheters, therapy duration is around 7-14 days with the important exception of fungemia, where the therapy is 14 days after the first negative blood culture (Chahoud, Kanafani, & Kanj, 2013).

Aside from antibiotic therapy, catheter removal is the second important piece in the treatment of CLABSI. Short-term catheter, like those usually encountered on the ICU, should generally be removed if infected with the exception of uncomplicated infections caused by coagulase-negative staphylococci, where antibiotic lock therapy is thought to be a reasonable alternative. Finally, as part of the diagnostic workup, every patient with bacteremia should receive an echocardiogram to rule out endocarditis (Holland, Arnold, & Fowler Jr., 2014).

Urinary Tract Infections

Background

Most healthcare-associated urinary tract infections (UTI) are associated with the use of urinary catheters (CAUTI). On the ICU, as many as 95% of UTI cases are urinary catheter related (Weber et al., 2011). Virtually all patients on a CT surgical ICU will have a urinary catheter in place at some point during their perioperative course. CAUTI is associated with increased morbidity, mortality, and cost. Similar to VAP, CAUTI is subject to non-reimbursement by CMS since 2008 (Saint, Meddings, Calfee, Kowalski, & Krein, 2009), however the implementation of this policy has not led to reduced CAUTI rates thus far (Lee et al., 2012).

CAUTI are often caused by Gram-negative enterobacteria from endogenous perineal bacteria that cause ascending infection along the outside of the catheter (Tambyah, Halvorson, & Maki, 1999). Less commonly, bacteria are introduced intraluminal through for example a contaminated collection system. Contamination in these cases is usually due to inadequate hand hygiene of healthcare personnel. Among Gram-negative enterobacteria, Escherichia coli and Klebsiella species are the most common organisms. In the ICU setting, Enterococcus species, candida, and Pseudomonas aeruginosa are emerging pathogens. Escherichia coli isolates are increasingly resistant to fluoroquinolones and produce extended-spectrum beta-lactamases. In the same study, 12.5% of Klebsiella species isolates were carbapenem-resistant (Sievert et al., 2013). The clinical significance of enterococcus isolates from the urine is unclear, likewise, candida in the urine rarely represents infection. However, urinary catheter systems colonized with enterococci can function as a reservoir for the development of VRE. Staphylococcus is a rare cause of CAUTI and should prompt investigation for concomitant bloodstream infection or endocarditis. Biofilm formation on urinary catheter surfaces is possible. This presents a therapeutic challenge, as antibiotics poorly penetrate into the film (Saint & Chenoweth, 2003). Although bloodstream infections from CAUTI are rare, it is a clinically significant syndrome with a reported mortality as high as 33% (Chang et al., 2011). Several modifiable and non-modifiable risk factors for CAUTI exist, but the duration of catheterization is the main culprit (Table 13).

Diagnosis

Diagnosis of CAUTI can be a challenging process. Pyuria and bacteriuria are very common in the ICU setting, but this does not necessarily indicate a UTI (Tambyah & Maki, 2000). The diagnosis of UTI

Table 13. Risk factors for catheter-associated urinary tract infections

Modifiable	Non-Modifiable
• Duration of catheterization • Nonadherence to aseptic catheter care (i.e. opening a closed system) • Lower professional training of inserter • Catheter insertion outside of operating room	• Female sex • Severe underlying disease • Non-surgical disease • Age > 50 years • Diabetes mellitus • Serum creatinine > 2 mg/dL

From: Chenoweth et al., Infectious Disease Clinics of North America, 2014

requires clinical symptoms in conjunction with significant bacteriuria (Hooton et al., 2010). As many catheterized ICU patients are unable to express classic symptoms of UTI, fever may be the only clinical sign. A colony count of 10^3 CFU/mL is considered the threshold of significant bacteriuria in the diagnosis of CAUTI (Hooton et al., 2010). While catheter systems are considered a reservoir for often resistant microorganisms, mere bacteriuria rarely becomes symptomatic. Also, bacteriuria infrequently causes bloodstream infection or urosepsis (Tambyah & Maki, 2000), except for patient subgroups with certain comorbidities, such as neutropenia (Greene et al., 2012). Once nosocomial urinary tract-related bacteremia occurs, it carries a significant mortality and is often caused by MDR bacteria (Kang et al., 2011).

Prevention

Adherence to strict hand hygiene before and after patient contact is an overarching principle in the prevention of CAUTI, as it is in the prevention of other hospital-acquired infections (Pittet et al., 2009). As described above, the urinary tract and catheter systems of hospitalized patients and particularly ICU patients is a reservoir for MDR bacteria, especially enterobacteria and enterococci. Once a MDR microorganism is identified, contact precautions are indicated. The avoidance of broad-spectrum antibiotic therapy when not indicated is an important factor to address emerging MDR bacteria, and antibiotic stewardship programs can help to address this issue (Pollack & Srinivasan, 2014).

The most important strategy to prevent CAUTI is to limit the use of urinary catheters. Defining appropriate indications for urinary catheter placement is difficult in the acute care setting, and the inappropriateness of catheterization has been studied and described (Jain, Parada, David, & Smith, 1995; Apisarnthanarak et al., 2007). Urinary catheterization often is clinically necessary, i.e. in the perioperative management of anesthetized or sedated patients or to accurately measure urine output after cardiac surgery. In these cases, frequent assessment and early removal is critical. As physicians are often unaware of patients that have catheters in place for an extended period of time (Saint et al., 2000), nursing-driven protocols for early removal have become a common and successful practice (Crouzet et al., 2007; Fakih et al., 2008; Parry, Grant, & Sestovic, 2013). In addition to that, the advent of computerized order entry has brought forward electronic reminder systems that can effectively reduce the duration of catheterization (Cornia, Amory, Fraser, Saint, & Lipsky, 2003; Meddings, Rogers, Macy, & Saint, 2010).

For perioperative urinary catheter use, CMS has added catheter removal 24 hours after surgery to the list of SCIP quality measures. This is based on data that showed that after 2 days, patients were significantly more likely to develop CAUTI (Wald, Ma, Bratzler, & Kramer, 2008). Older patients have a higher likelihood of postoperative urinary retention, and are therefore at higher risk for catheterization and subsequent infection. Patients receiving regional analgesia via epidural catheters have a high risk for urinary retention (Baldini, Bagry, Aprikian, & Carli, 2009), however most of the evidence is derived from studies in patients with lumbar epidural catheters. Lumbar epidural analgesia has a significantly different neurophysiologic response than thoracic epidural analgesia. More recent studies have shown that early catheter removal can be performed safely in patient's receiving thoracic epidural analgesia, which led to a reduction in CAUTI (Zaouter, Kaneva, & Carli, 2009; Zaouter & Ouattara, 2014).

Strict aseptic technique while inserting and handling catheter systems is crucial for the prevention of CAUTI. Closed urine collection systems have been standard of care in U.S. hospitals for quite some time (Kunin & McCormack, 1966). For diagnostic urine samples, a designated sampling port should be accessed in an aseptic fashion instead of opening or disconnecting the system. Routine exchange of catheters is not recommended, except for mechanical reasons (Chenoweth & Saint, 2013). Antiseptic-impregnated urinary catheters as a means to reduce CAUTI have been studied (Johnson, Kuskowski, & Wilt, 2006). The most common coating materials contain nitrofurazone, minocycline, or rifampicin. While these catheters have been shown to reduce the rate of asymptomatic bacteriuria, a clear benefit in preventing CAUTI could not be demonstrated. The only indication for impregnated catheters are in settings or patient populations where CAUTI rate remains high despite adherence to aforementioned preventive measures. Similar to CLABSI prevention, preventive care bundles have been studied and successfully implemented for CAUTI (Saint et al., 2009; Saint et al., 2013).

Treatment

As a general principle, treatment for asymptomatic bacteriuria is not indicated, unless patients are pregnant or otherwise at high risk of developing complications, i.e. pyelonephritis or urosepsis. Similarly, asymptomatic candiduria also does not generally require treatment. If bacteriuria or funguria persists for more than 48 hours despite urinary catheter removal, development of UTI is likely and treatment should be initiated (Hooton et al., 2010). Initial empiric therapy depends on local microorganisms patterns and patient factors, i.e. long-term catheterization. A basic cephalosporin such as ceftriaxone is sufficient for community-acquired UTI or pyelonephritis. If the patient is unstable, a fluoroquinolone such as levofloxacine can be added. For CAUTI, initial empiric therapy should include broader Gram-negative coverage, i.e. ceftazidime. In case of previous catheterization or history of UTI, MDR bacteria are likely present and empiric therapy should be started using a carbapenem instead of a cephalosporin. Unfortunately, many patients are still inappropriately treated for asymptomatic bacteriuria, which has led to the development of MDR bacteria, with the bladder and long-term catheter systems as the reservoir (Cope et al., 2009). Focused educational efforts towards the appropriate use of urine cultures can effectively reduce the overuse of antibiotics (Pavese et al., 2009). The formation of biofilm on urinary catheters can make bacteria difficult to eradicate and promote the formation of MDR microorganisms. Therefore, urinary catheters should be removed or replaced if CAUTI is suspected if the catheter has been in place for more than 2 weeks. Duration of antibiotic therapy should be between 7 and 14 days depending on the response to therapy.

SYSTEMIC INFLAMMATORY RESPONSE FOLLOWING CARDIAC SURGERY

Background and Pathophysiology

Cardiac surgery is associated with a systemic inflammatory response syndrome (SIRS) that can potentially cause organ dysfunction (Paparella et al., 2002). This is often a consequence contact of blood with the surface of the CPB circuit and subsequent CPB-related effects such as translocation of endotoxin and ischemia-reperfusion. Certain underlying diseases and the surgical trauma itself are also important in the development and severity of SIRS. SIRS after cardiac surgery is generally the result of a non-infective insult, but has significant pathophysiologic overlap with sepsis (Cohen, 2002). SIRS as a consequence of CPB involves both the humoral and the cellular subsets of the innate immune system and can be divided into 2 distinct phases, the early and the late response. The early phase is triggered by blood contact with artificial surfaces, the late phase is driven primarily by endotoxemia and ischemia-reperfusion.

During the early phase, several protein systems and certain cells of the immune system are activated and interact in this very complex process leading to the distinct inflammatory response with the potential for coagulopathy, edema, inflammation, and end-organ damage. There are at least 5 different protein systems that are part of the initial response. The contact system is activated when blood comes into contact with negatively charged, non-endothelial surfaces. The activated factor XII eventually converts prekallikrein to kallikrein, which in turn activates intrinsic coagulation and neutrophils (Sainz, Pixley, & Colman, 2007). The activation of the intrinsic coagulation cascade upon contact leads to the formation of thrombin through activated factor X and several cofactors. The main endpoint is to form fibrin from fibrinogen and crosslink fibrin by activating factor XIII. Moreover, thrombin activates platelets and endothelial cells to help bind coagulation factors and promote hemostasis. On the other hand, the extrinsic coagulation pathway is initiated by an injured blood vessel where non-vascular cells are suddenly exposed to blood. Tissue-factor (TF) coming from these cells binds to factor VII and this complex ultimately leads to formation of activated factor X. The TF pathway in pro-inflammatory states, i.e. after cardiac surgery, is much more complex and includes cytokine-induced formation and expression of TF on circulating blood cells such as neutrophils (Engelmann, 2006). Another plasma protein group activated in the early phase of SIRS is the complement system, which comprises of at least 30 different circulating and membrane-bound proteins that support antibody-mediated immune response to infectious insults. 3 different pathways for the complement system have been described. The alternative pathway is the most important one when looking at CPB-induced complement activation. Contact of blood with the CPB circuit leads to hydrolytic conversion of C3 into C3a and C3b (Wan, Leclerc, & Vincent, 1997). The endpoint of the reaction is formation of the membrane attack complex and activation of neutrophils via C5. Complement activation is a feature of most surgical procedures, but it is a more pronounced after cardiac surgery with CPB and also correlates with the duration of CPB (Hirai, 2003). The magnitude of complement activation has clinical significance and correlates with subsequent organ dysfunction. The presumed underlying mechanisms include a complement-induced increase in vascular permeability and alterations in vasomotor tone. Furthermore, the membrane attack complex leads to cell lysis and may cause damage to endothelial cells, platelets, and even cardiomyocytes (Moat, Shore, & Evans, 1993). Finally, fibrinolysis is initiated in order to counterbalance the effects of thrombin generated via the coagulation cascades. Plasminogen is converted by tissue plasminogen activator (t-PA) into plasmin, a serine protease, which has the ability to disintegrate fibrin strands.

Several cell systems are activated as part of the initial phase of SIRS in cardiac surgery patients. First, the vascular endothelium plays a key role in the regulation of blood flow, vascular tone and integrity, and leukocyte adhesion and migration. Pro-inflammatory cytokines such as interleukin-1β (IL-1β) and tumor-necrosis factor-α (TNF-α) induce the expression of adhesion molecules to help leukocyte rolling and migration in this setting (Springer, 1994). Endothelial cells also produce hemostatic factors, i.e. anti-thrombin, thrombomodulin, and TF pathway inhibitor. Nitric oxide (NO) regulates endothelium-mediated vasodilation, which has been described as a protective mechanism in SIRS and sepsis. However, more deleterious effects of NO such as myocardial dysfunction have been linked to inducible NO synthase (iNOS), which is upregulated by CPB (Finkel et al., 1992). Inhibition of iNOS by for instance methylene blue can reverse refractory hypotension (Fischer & Levin, 2010). The complex and paradoxical effects of NO seem to be dependent on the timing, quantity, and source of production of the molecule. Small amounts of NO are produced by a constitutive endothelial NO synthase. The activity of this enzyme is suppressed in the early stages of inflammation to allow vasoconstriction and other processes like platelet adhesion to happen. After about 6 hours, iNOS upregulation occurs with the ultimate outcome of an increase in overall NO production, which goes along with an increase in the aforementioned pro-inflammatory cytokines (Bhagat, Hingorani, Palacios, Charles, & Vallance, 1999). Leukocyte activation is as key component of SIRS. During CPB, neutrophils are activated mostly by the contact and complement systems, but other factors such as cytokines, histamine, and direct contact with the endothelium play a role too. Direct endothelial contact leads to leukocyte rolling, expression of adhesion molecules, and ultimately a tight connection between the neutrophil and the endothelial cell (Zarbock & Ley, 2008). The pathological endpoint is microvascular occlusion with the potential for end-organ damage. A more complex mechanism facilitates the transmigration of neutrophils into the extracellular matrix, where they release additional cytotoxic material and can cause capillary leak, tissue edema, and cell death. These complex processes are likely responsible for end-organ dysfunction in the cardiac surgery patient (Clark, 2006). CPB has been shown to induce signaling changes in toll-like receptors (TLRs), a receptor group that regulates monocyte activation (Dybdahl et al., 2002). These changes lead to the release of a variety of pro-inflammatory cytokines with the potential to cause end-organ damage (Wan et al., 1997). Anti-inflammatory cytokines such as interleukin-10 (IL-10) play a role in attenuating the host response and can potentially limit the amount of injury (Giomarelli, Scolletta, Borrelli, & Biagioli, 2003). Monocytes also interact with the hemostatic system by forming complexes with platelets (Weerasinghe et al., 2006). Platelet activation secondary to CPB reduces the platelet count and causes dysfunction, which plays a critical role in post-CPB coagulopathy. This consumptive process occurs in addition to mechanical destruction by the CPB pumps and adhesion to the CPB circuit. Thrombin formed by the coagulation systems is another potent platelet activator (Despotis & Goodnough, 2000).

The late phase of SIRS is predominantly affected by ischemia-reperfusion and endotoxemia. Ischemia automatically occurs during CPB when an aortic cross-clamp is applied shutting down blood flow to the heart and the majority of the lungs. The reperfusion following cross-clamp release is associated with a marked inflammatory response within the previously ischemic tissues. Again, the common pathological features are increased capillary permeability, interstitial edema, coagulopathy, and end-organ dysfunction. The molecular mechanisms of ischemia-reperfusion injury were described above and are mostly related to the interaction between neutrophils and the endothelial layer. In addition to that, production of reactive oxygen species (ROS) and release of pro-inflammatory cytokines as well as prostacycline are part of the ischemia-reperfusion process. ROS are particularly injurious to the endothelium and other cell systems after reperfusion. A second mechanism described is the release of endotoxin (Kats,

Schönberger, Brands, Seinen, & van Oeveren, 2011). Endotoxins are lipopolysaccharides out of cell walls of Gram-negative bacteria. Translocation of bacteria from the gut is thought to be the primary source of circulating endotoxin, however measurement of this process in clinical studies has been very difficult (Riddington et al., 1996). Endotoxin itself activates complement, stimulates the release of pro-inflammatory cytokines, and increases NO levels.

Studies have linked an exaggerated inflammatory response after CPB with measurable adverse clinical outcomes. Patients tend to have more postoperative bleeding, need more pulmonary support, and gain more weight, likely secondary to capillary leak and tissue edema (Holmes 4th, 2002). Depending on the severity, SIRS can lead to MODS, as previously described for patients with sepsis (Marshall, 2001). The concept of SIRS is now well established after cardiac surgery, however studies showed variable results regarding the incidence of SIRS in this population when applying consensus SIRS/sepsis definitions. Modified criteria have been suggested to improve the diagnostic sensitivity (MacCallum, Finney, Gordon, Quinlan, & Evans, 2014). It is again important to understand that aside from CPB, there are other perioperative factors in cardiac surgery patients that can cause and enhance SIRS, i.e. surgical trauma, hemodilution, hypothermia, and other forms of reperfusion injury (Verma et al., 2002). Finally, fairly recent research has shown that the combined dysfunction of immune cells such as neutrophils and lymphocytes is an important predictor for the development of nosocomial infections, both in the setting of sepsis and after a non-infective insult (Conway Morris, 2013). Similarly, monocyte hyporesponsiveness and decreased TLR expression was associated with SIRS and an increased risk of developing pneumonia after cardiac surgery (Flier et al., 2014).

Management Strategies

Aside from the largely supportive treatment options, several pharmacologic and technical strategies have been described to approach perioperative SIRS in the cardiac surgical population. Among the pharmacologic interventions, the administration of corticosteroids is by far the best studied. Steroids have been shown to significantly reduce the magnitude of pro-inflammatory mediator release and also to augment the secretion of anti-inflammatory cytokines during CPB. Leukocyte and complement activation are also suppressed by supplemental corticosteroid administration (Chaney, 2002). The clinical relevance of this mechanism has been questioned, as we now know that factors other than CPB play a role in SIRS in cardiac surgery patients. In addition to that, the quality of clinical trials in this field has been negatively affected by sample size, poor study design, and clinical confounders. Therefore, meta-analyses of pooled data have been conducted that showed that steroids did significantly reduce the incidence of postop erative atrial fibrillation, perioperative bleeding, and ICU length of stay (Whitlock et al., 2008). Other meta-analyses could demonstrate similar beneficial effects on end-organ outcomes, but all together did lack a mortality difference (Ho & Tan, 2009; Dieleman et al., 2011). While these meta-analyses suggest a potential benefit with little harm, most authors concluded that well-designed randomized trials are necessary to answer the question whether corticosteroid administration truly provides a morbidity and mortality advantage for patients undergoing cardiac surgery with CPB. Two large randomized trials were recently initiated to address this problem, the Dexamethasone for Cardiac Surgery (DECS) and the Steroids In CaRdiac Surgery (SIRS) trials. The results of the DECS trial were recently published (Dieleman et al., 2012). This study in almost 4,500 patients receiving high-dose dexamethasone or placebo could not show a difference in the 30-day incidence of major adverse events. Similarly, smaller subtrials could not prove beneficial outcomes regarding the incidence of postoperative delirium (Sauër et al., 2014) and cognitive decline (Ottens et al., 2014). The SIRS trial results are anxiously awaited. Once completed, this will be one of the largest clinical trials in medicine enrolling 7,500 adult patients who will receive 2 doses of 250 mg intravenous methylprednisolone during cardiac surgery. The primary outcome measure will be 30-day mortality. Given the sample size and the careful design of this trial, it is thought that the results will have a significant impact on future indications for perioperative corticosteroids for cardiac surgery patients (Augoustides, 2012). Among the pharmacologic therapeutics, corticosteroids remain the only clinically relevant option. Other agents have been investigated, i.e. antioxidants and complement inhibitors, but most studies are either too small or have not shown any significant benefits (Verrier et al., 2004). Aprotinin, a protease inhibitor was ubiquitously used to prevent hyperfibrinolysis during cardiac operation. Secondarily, it was shown that it inhibited kallikrein, a key component of the contact system. Despite the theoretical advantages, aprotinin was removed from the market after 2 large and well-designed trials demonstrated an increased morbidity and mortality in patients receiving the drug (Mangano, Rieves, & Weiss, 2006; Fergusson et al., 2008).

Technical strategies to reduce the incidence of cardiac surgery-related SIRS include the use of heparin-bonded CPB circuits, ultrafiltration and other interventions around pump mechanics, blood conservation protocols and leukocyte filtration, and body temperature management. The use of heparin-bonded circuits is controversial. A meta-analysis including over 3,000 patients in 41 randomized trials could show a reduction of ventilation time and transfusion rates, however no other solid clinical outcomes were affected (Mangoush et al., 2007). Thus, the use of those circuits is highly variable. While ultrafiltration is common practice in pediatric cardiac surgery, it is used less frequently in adults. The most important scenario is the need for fluid removal in heart failure patients presenting for ventricular assist device implantation or transplantation. Its anti-inflammatory potential remains controversial (Bog'a et al., 2000). The question whether to use centrifugal or roller pump for CPB is still subject of debate. A meta-analysis including almost 2,000 patients could not find a difference in morbidity and mortality relative to the pump type (Saczkowski, Maklin, Mesana, Boodhwani, & Ruel, 2012). Blood transfusions certainly cause immunomodulation and are associated with an increased risk of infection (Rohde et al., 2014). Avoiding homologous blood products is an important quality measure after cardiac surgery. Hypothermia was found to delay the SIRS process in some studies, but eventually did not avoid it. While a significant reduction in pro-inflammatory mediators was demonstrated, the clinical outcome data is much less convincing. There is currently no evidence to support the routine use of hypothermia during CPB in order to attenuate the inflammatory response with the goal of improving patient outcomes. Moreover, normothermia is associated with a reduced risk of blood transfusion (Ho & Tan, 2011). Finally, avoiding CPB altogether, for example in the setting of off-pump coronary artery bypass (OPCAB) surgery, is a sensible approach to reduce SIRS caused by CPB. High-quality studies have shown that OPCAB surgery goes along with significantly reduced levels of pro-inflammatory cytokines, complement, and neutrophil and endothelial activation (Raja & Berg, 2007). A more recent trial showed that, ultimately, bypass surgery using CPB is associated with increased pro-inflammatory mediators, but the release of soluble endothelial adhesion molecules was the same as in OPCAB patients (Jongman et al., 2014). Unfortunately, most of the trials comparing bypass surgery with CPB with OPCAB surgery are not adequately designed or powered to address clinical outcomes. In summary, OPCAB is successfully used at experienced centers, but is not necessarily associated with improved patient outcomes. A randomized comparative trial would be ideal, but will be difficult to power to show a mortality difference.

FUTURE RESEARCH DIRECTIONS

As infections continue to have a big impact on perioperative morbidity and mortality in cardiac surgery patients and the introduction of new antibiotics are merely a reaction to an increase in resistant organisms, the focus of future research in this field will be on interventions and strategies that prevent or lower the risk for infections. The introduction and revision of preventive care bundles for VAP, CLABSI, and CAUTI is one example of the trend towards preventive medicine. Hand hygiene and other standard measures of infection control are now well established in the developed world, so the focus needs to be to make these a worldwide standard, but not to neglect ongoing staff education on these simple and effective interventions (De Bono, Heling, & Borg, 2014). Avoiding perioperative infections will also be of interest for healthcare economics, as non-reimbursement for hospital-acquired infections is adopted by more and more societies and governmental organizations.

More specific to the cardiac surgery population, several preventive strategies have been described and are very promising, but warrant further investigation in larger controlled trials. One example is screening tests to identify colonized patients before coming for surgery as a measure of improving individual patient outcome, but also as a measure of infection control (Segers et al., 2006). Another example, there is emerging evidence linking blood product administration with increased infection rates in general (Rohde et al., 2014) cardiac surgery patients (Horvath et al., 2013). Further studies are needed to specify the right target for perioperative blood glucose levels, particularly for non-diabetic patients, as the effect of tighter glucose control on DSWI rates is not well established in this population (O'Connor, 2010). There is promising work done in the field of SIRS after cardiac surgery with CPB. The preoperative administration of statins has been shown to attenuate the release of pro-inflammatory cytokines (Liakopoulos et al., 2006) and markers of myocardial damage (Martínez-Comendador et al., 2009) as well as reduce the incidence of postoperative new-onset atrial fibrillation (Jacob et al., 2014). At the same time, the anti-inflammatory potential has led to promising research in other clinical scenarios, i.e. atherosclerosis (Tousoulis et al., 2014) and sepsis (Dobesh & Olsen, 2014). A recent meta-analysis confirmed the beneficial effect of preoperative statin therapy and its impact on a wide variety of clinical outcomes (Kuhn et al., 2014). Finally, the results of an ongoing large randomized clinical trial on the use of corticosteroids in cardiac are potentially going to change practice to impact SIRS after cardiac surgery.

CONCLUSION

Postoperative infections remain a significant problem in patients undergoing cardiac and thoracic surgery admitted to the ICU. This population carries an increased risk for infection given the overall increased risk of infections in the ICU environment combined with the postoperative inflammatory response frequently seen after cardiac surgery. Effective measures of prevention, infection control, and quality improvement initiatives addressing specific infections such as pneumonia or catheter-associated bloodstream infection can help reduce the overall infection rate and potentially mortality. Early diagnosis and adequate antimicrobial treatment are crucial for therapy success. Strategies to attenuate the inflammatory response following cardiac surgery and bypass are currently limited, but new therapies could have an impact on clinical outcomes.

REFERENCES

Aarts, M. A., Hancock, J. N., Heyland, D., McLeod, R. S., & Marshall, J. C. (2008). Empiric antibiotic therapy for suspected ventilator-associated pneumonia: A systematic review and meta-analysis of randomized trials. *Critical Care Medicine*, *36*(1), 108–117. doi:10.1097/01.CCM.0000297956.27474.9D PMID:18007262

Abu-Salah, T., & Dhand, R. (2011). Inhaled antibiotic therapy for ventilator-associated tracheobronchitis and ventilator-associated pneumonia: An update. *Advances in Therapy*, *28*(9), 728–747. doi:10.1007/s12325-011-0051-z PMID:21833701

Alexiou, V. G., Ierodiakonou, V., Dimopoulos, G., & Falagas, M. E. (2009). Impact of patient position on the incidence of ventilator-associated pneumonia: A meta-analysis of randomized controlled trials. *Journal of Critical Care*, *24*(4), 515–522. doi:10.1016/j.jcrc.2008.09.003 PMID:19327314

Allou, N., Bronchard, R., Guglielminotti, J., Dilly, M. P., Provenchere, S., Lucet, J. C., & Montravers, P. et al. (2014). Risk factors for postoperative pneumonia after cardiac surgery and development of a preoperative risk score. *Critical Care Medicine*, *42*(5), 1150–1156. doi:10.1097/CCM.0000000000000143 PMID:24351376

American Thoracic Society. (2005). Guidelines for the management of adults with hospital-acquired, ventilator-associated, and healthcare-associated pneumonia. *American Journal of Respiratory and Critical Care Medicine*, *171*(4), 388–416. doi:10.1164/rccm.200405-644ST PMID:15699079

Apisarnthanarak, A., Rutjanawech, S., Wichansawakun, S., Ratanabunjerdkul, H., Patthranitima, P., Thongphubeth, K., & Fraser, V. J. et al. (2007). Initial inappropriate urinary catheters use in a tertiary-care center: Incidence, risk factors, and outcomes. *American Journal of Infection Control*, *35*(9), 594–599. doi:10.1016/j.ajic.2006.11.007 PMID:17980238

Arias, C. A., Torres, H. A., Singh, K. V., Panesso, D., Moore, J., Wanger, A., & Murray, B. (2007). Failure of daptomycin monotherapy for endocarditis caused by an Enterococcus faecium strain with vancomycin-resistant and vancomycin-susceptible subpopulations and evidence of in vivo loss of the vanA gene cluster. *Clinical Infectious Diseases*, *45*(10), 1343–1346. doi:10.1086/522656 PMID:17968832

Athan, E., Chu, V. H., Tattevin, P., Selton-Suty, C., Jones, P., & Naber, C. (2012). Clinical characteristics and outcome of infective endocarditis involving implantable cardiac devices. *Journal of the American Medical Association*, *307*(16), 1727–1735. doi:10.1001/jama.2012.497 PMID:22535857

Augoustides, J. G. T. (2012). The inflammatory response to cardiac surgery with cardiopulmonary bypass: Should steroid prophylaxis be routine? *Journal of Cardiothoracic and Vascular Anesthesia*, *26*(5), 952–958. doi:10.1053/j.jvca.2012.05.001 PMID:22765991

Backman, C., Zoutman, D. E., & Marck, P. B. (2008). An integrative review of the current evidence on the relationship between hand hygiene interventions and the incidence of healthcare-associated infections. *American Journal of Infection Control*, *36*(5), 33–48. doi:10.1016/j.ajic.2007.08.007 PMID:18241734

Baddour, L. M., Epstein, A. E., Erickson, C. C., Knight, B. P., Levison, M. E., Lockhart, P. B., & Taubert, K. A. et al. (2010). Update on cardiovascular implantable electronic device infections and their management: A scientific statement from the American Heart Association. *Circulation*, *121*(3), 458–477. doi:10.1161/CIRCULATIONAHA.109.192665 PMID:20048212

Baddour, L. M., Wilson, W. R., Bayer, A. S., Fowler, V. G. Jr, Bolger, A. F., Levison, M. E., & Taubert, K. A. et al. (2005). Infective endocarditis: Diagnosis, antimicrobial therapy, and management of complications: A statement for healthcare professionals from the Committee on Rheumatic Fever, Emdocarditis, and Kawasaki Disease, Council on Cardiovascular Disease in the Young, and the Councils on Clinical Cardiology, Stroke, and Cardiovascular Surgery and Anesthesia, American Heart Association: Endorsed by the Infectious Disease Society of America. *Circulation*, *111*(23), e394–e434. doi:10.1161/CIRCULATIONAHA.105.165564 PMID:15956145

Baldini, G., Bagry, H., Aprikian, A., & Carli, F. (2009). Postoperative urinary retention. Anesthetic and perioperative considerations. *Anesthesiology*, *110*(5), 1139–1157. doi:10.1097/ALN.0b013e31819f7aea PMID:19352147

Barr, J., Fraser, G. L., Puntillo, K., Ely, E. W., Gélinas, C., Dasta, J. F., & Jaeschke, R. et al. (2013). Clinical practice guidelines for the management of pain, agitation, and delirium in adult patients in the intensive care unit. *Critical Care Medicine*, *41*(1), 263–306. doi:10.1097/CCM.0b013e3182783b72 PMID:23269131

Bennett-Guerrero, E., Ferguson, T.B. Jr, Lin, M., Garg, J., Mark, D.B., & Scavo, V.A. Jr, … Corey, G.R., for the SWIPE-1 Trial Group. (2010). Effect of an implantable gentamicin-collagen sponge on sternal wound infections following cardiac surgery. A randomized trial. *Journal of the American Medical Association*, *304*, 755–762. doi:10.1001/jama.2010.1152 PMID:20716738

Bhagat, K., Hingorani, A. D., Palacios, M., Charles, I. G., & Vallance, P. (1999). Cytokine-induced venodilation in humans in vivo: eNOS masquerading as iNOS. *Cardiovascular Research*, *41*(3), 754–764. doi:10.1016/S0008-6363(98)00249-1 PMID:10435048

Birgand, G., Radu, C., Alkhoder, S., Al Attar, N., Raffoul, R., Dilly, M., & Lucet, J. et al. (2013). Does a gentamicin-impregnated collagen sponge reduce sternal wound infections in high-risk cardiac surgery patients? *Interactive Cardiovascular and Thoracic Surgery*, *16*(2), 134–142. doi:10.1093/icvts/ivs449 PMID:23115102

Blamoun, J., Alfakir, M., Rella, M. E., Wojcik, J. M., Solis, R. A., Anees Khan, M., & DeBari, V. A. (2009). Efficacy of an expanded ventilator bundle for the reduction of ventilator-associated pneumonia in the medical intensive care unit. *American Journal of Infection Control*, *37*(2), 172–175. doi:10.1016/j.ajic.2008.05.010 PMID:18945515

Blondet, J. J., & Beilman, G. J. (2007). Glycemic control and prevention of perioperative infection. *Current Opinion in Critical Care*, *13*(4), 421–427. doi:10.1097/MCC.0b013e32826388a1 PMID:17599013

Blot, F., Nitenberg, G., Chachaty, E., Raynard, B., Germann, N., Antoun, S., & Tancrède, C. et al. (1999). Diagnosis of catheter-related bacteraemia: A prospective comparison of the time to positivity of hub-blood versus peripheral-blood cultures. *Lancet*, *354*(9184), 1071–1077. doi:10.1016/S0140-6736(98)11134-0 PMID:10509498

Blot, F., Schmidt, E., Nitenberg, G., Tancrède, C., Leclercq, B., Laplanche, A., & Andremont, A. (1998). Earlier positivity of central-venous- versus peripheral-blood cultures is highly predictive of catheter-related sepsis. *Journal of Clinical Microbiology*, *36*, 105–109. PMID:9431930

Bog'a, M., Islamog'lu, F., Badak, I., Cikirikçiog'lu, M., Bakalim, T., Yag'di, T., & Hamulu, A. et al. (2000). The effects of modified hemofiltration on inflammatory mediators and cardiac performance in coronary artery bypass grafting. *Perfusion*, *15*(2), 143–150. doi:10.1177/026765910001500209 PMID:10789569

Bolon, M. K., Morlote, M., Weber, S. G., Koplan, B., Carmeli, Y., & Wright, S. B. (2004). Glycopeptides are no more effective than β-lactam agents for prevention of surgical site infection after cardiac surgery: A meta-analysis. *Clinical Infectious Diseases*, *38*(10), 1357–1363. doi:10.1086/383318 PMID:15156470

Boucher, H., Miller, L. G., & Razonable, R. R. (2010). Serious infections caused by methicillin-resistant Staphylococcus aureus. *Clinical Infectious Diseases*, *15*(S2), S183–S197. doi:10.1086/653519 PMID:20731576

Bouza, E., Alvarado, N., Alcalá, L., Pérez, M. J., Rincón, C., & Muñoz, P. (2007). A randomized and prospective study of 3 procedures for the diagnosis of catheter-related bloodstream infection without catheter withdrawal. *Clinical Infectious Diseases*, *44*(6), 820–826. doi:10.1086/511865 PMID:17304454

Bouza, E., Pérez, M. J., Muñoz, P., Rincón, C., Barrio, J. M., & Hortal, J. (2008). Continuous aspiration of subglottic secretions in the prevention of ventilator-associated pneumonia in the postoperative period of major heart surgery. *Chest*, *134*(5), 938–946. doi:10.1378/chest.08-0103 PMID:18641114

Boyce, J. M., Ligi, C., Kohan, C., Dumigan, D., & Havill, N. L. (2006). Lack of association between the increased incidence of Clostridium difficile-associated disease and the increasing use of alcohol-based hand scrubs. *Infection Control and Hospital Epidemiology*, *27*(5), 479–483. doi:10.1086/504362 PMID:16671029

Brims, F. J., Lansley, S. M., Waterer, G. W., & Lee, Y. C. (2010). Empyema thoracis. New insights into an old disease. *European Respiratory Review*, *19*(117), 220–228. doi:10.1183/09059180.00005610 PMID:20956197

Burke, J. P. (2003). Infection control – A problem for patient safety. *The New England Journal of Medicine*, *348*(7), 651–656. doi:10.1056/NEJMhpr020557 PMID:12584377

Byrne, J. G., Rezai, K., Sanchez, J. A., Bernstein, R. A., Okum, E., Leacche, M., & Higgins, R. S. D. et al. (2011). Surgical management of endocarditis: The Society of Thoracic Surgeons clinical practice guideline. *The Annals of Thoracic Surgery*, *91*(6), 2012–2019. doi:10.1016/j.athoracsur.2011.01.106 PMID:21620012

Cabrini, L., Plumari, V. P., Nobile, L., Olper, L., Pasin, S., Bocchino, S., & Zangrillo, A. et al. (2013). Non-invasive ventilation in cardiac surgery: A concise review. *Heart. Lung and Vessels*, *5*, 137–141. PMID:24364004

Carling, P. C., Parry, M. F., & Von Beheren, S. M.Healthcare Environmental Hygiene Study Group. (2008). Identifying opportunities to enhance environmental cleaning in 23 acute care hospitals. *Infection Control and Hospital Epidemiology*, *29*(1), 1–7. doi:10.1086/524329 PMID:18171180

Carrel, T. P., Eisinger, E., Vogt, M., & Turina, M. I. (2001). Pneumonia after cardiac surgery is predictable by tracheal aspirates but cannot be prevented by prolonged antibiotic prophylaxis. *The Annals of Thoracic Surgery*, *72*(1), 143–148. doi:10.1016/S0003-4975(01)02669-8 PMID:11465169

Casey, A. L., Mermel, L. A., Nightingale, P., & Elliott, T. S. (2008). Antimicrobial central venous catheters in adults: A systematic review and meta-analysis. *The Lancet Infectious Diseases*, *8*(12), 763–776. doi:10.1016/S1473-3099(08)70280-9 PMID:19022192

Chahoud, J., Kanafani, Z. A., & Kanj, S. S. (2013). Management of candidaemia and invasive candidiasis in critically ill patients. *International Journal of Antimicrobial Agents*, *42S*, S29–S35. doi:10.1016/j.ijantimicag.2013.04.008 PMID:23664579

Chalk, K., Meisel, C., Spies, C., Volk, T., Thuenemann, K., Linneweber, J., & Sander, M. et al. (2013). Dysfunction of alveolar macrophages after cardiac surgery: Predisposing factor for the development of postoperative pneumonia? – An observational study. *Critical Care (London, England)*, *17*, R285. doi:10.1186/cc13148 PMID:24321282

Chalmers, J. D., Rother, C., Salih, W., & Ewig, S. (2014). Healthcare-associated pneumonia does not accurately identify potentially resistant pathogens: A systematic review and meta-analysis. *Clinical Infectious Diseases*, *58*(3), 330–339. doi:10.1093/cid/cit734 PMID:24270053

Chambers, A., Routledge, T., Dunning, J., & Scarci, M. (2010). Is video-assisted thoracoscopic surgical decortication superior to open surgery in the management of adults with primary empyema? *Interactive Cardiovascular and Thoracic Surgery*, *11*(2), 171–177. doi:10.1510/icvts.2010.240408 PMID:20439299

Chambers, S. T., Murdoch, D., Morris, A., Holland, D., Pappas, P., Almela, M., & Chu, V. H. et al. (2013). HACEK infective endocarditis: Characteristics and outcomes from a large, mulit-national cohort. *PLoS ONE*, *8*(5), e63181. doi:10.1371/journal.pone.0063181 PMID:23690995

Chaney, M. A. (2002). Corticosteroids and cardiopulmonary bypass: A review of clinical investigations. *Chest*, *121*(3), 921–931. doi:10.1378/chest.121.3.921 PMID:11888978

Chang, R., Greene, M. T., Chenoweth, C. E., Kuhn, L., Shuman, E., Rogers, M. A. M., & Saint, S. (2011). Epidemiology of hospital-acquired urinary tract-related bloodstream infection at a university hospital. *Infection Control and Hospital Epidemiology*, *32*(11), 1127–1129. doi:10.1086/662378 PMID:22011543

Chatzinikolaou, I., Hanna, H., Hachem, R., Alakech, B., Tarrand, J., & Raad, I. (2004). Differental quantitative blood cultures for the diagnosis of catheter-related bloodstream infections associated with short- and long-term catheters: A prospective study. *Diagnostic Microbiology and Infectious Disease*, *50*(3), 167–172. doi:10.1016/j.diagmicrobio.2004.07.007 PMID:15541601

Chenoweth, C., & Saint, S. (2013). Preventing catheter-associated urinary tract infections in the intensive care unit. *Critical Care Clinics*, *29*(1), 19–32. doi:10.1016/j.ccc.2012.10.005 PMID:23182525

Chirouze, C., Athan, E., Alla, F., Chu, V. H., Corey, G. R., & Selton-Suty, C. (2013). Enterococcal endocarditis in the beginning of the 21st century: An analysis from the International Collaboration on Endocarditis – Prospective cohort study. *Clinical Microbiology and Infection*, *19*(12), 1140–1147. doi:10.1111/1469-0691.12166 PMID:23517406

Chlebicki, M. P., & Safdar, N. (2007). Topical chlorhexidine for the prevention of ventilator-associated pneumonia: A meta-analysis. *Critical Care Medicine*, *35*(2), 595–602. doi:10.1097/01.CCM.0000253395.70708.AC PMID:17205028

Chopra, V., O'Horo, J. C., Rogers, M. A. M., Maki, D. G., & Safdar, N. (2013). The risk of bloodstream infection associated with peripherally inserted central catheters compared with central venous catheters in adults: A systematic review and meta-analysis. *Infection Control and Hospital Epidemiology*, *34*(9), 908–918. doi:10.1086/671737 PMID:23917904

Chu, V. H., Cabell, C. H., Benjamin, D. K. Jr, Kuniholm, E. F., Fowler, V. G. Jr, Engemann, J., & Wang, A. et al. (2004). Early predictors of in-hospital death in infective endocarditis. *Circulation*, *109*(14), 1745–1749. doi:10.1161/01.CIR.0000124719.61827.7F PMID:15037538

Chu, V. H., Miro, J. M., Hoen, B., Cabell, C. H., Pappas, P. A., Jones, P., & Fowler, V. G. et al. (2009). Coagulase-negative staphylococcal prosthetic valve endocarditis – A contemporary update based on the International Collaboration on Endocarditis: Prospective cohort study. *Heart (British Cardiac Society)*, *95*(7), 570–576. doi:10.1136/hrt.2008.152975 PMID:18952633

Clark, S. C. (2006). Lung injury after cardiopulmonary bypass. *Perfusion*, *21*(4), 225–228. doi:10.1191/0267659106pf872oa PMID:16939116

Cohen, J. (2002). The immunopathogenesis of sepsis. *Nature*, *420*(6917), 885–891. doi:10.1038/nature01326 PMID:12490963

Conway Morris, A., Anderson, N., Brittan, M., Wilkinson, T. S., McAuley, D. F., Antonelli, J., & Simpson, A. J. et al. (2013). Combined dysfunctions of immune cells predict nosocomial infection in critically ill patients. *British Journal of Anaesthesia*, *111*(5), 778–787. doi:10.1093/bja/aet205 PMID:23756248

Cope, M., Cevallos, M. E., Cadle, R. M., Darouiche, R. O., Musher, D. M., & Trautner, B. W. (2009). Inappropriate treatment of catheter-associated asymptomatic bacteriuria in a tertiary care hospital. *Clinical Infectious Diseases*, *48*(9), 1182–1188. doi:10.1086/597403 PMID:19292664

Cornia, P. B., Amory, J. K., Fraser, S., Saint, S., & Lipsky, B. A. (2003). Computer-based order entry decreased duration of indwelling urinary catheterization in hospitalized patients. *The American Journal of Medicine*, *114*(5), 404–407. doi:10.1016/S0002-9343(02)01568-1 PMID:12714131

Craven, D. E., Lei, Y., Ruthazer, R., Sarwar, A., & Hudcova, J. (2013). Incidence and outcomes of ventilator-associated tracheobronchitis and pneumonia. *The American Journal of Medicine*, *126*(6), 542–549. doi:10.1016/j.amjmed.2012.12.012 PMID:23561632

Croce, M. A., Swanson, J. M., Magnotti, L. J., Claridge, J. A., Weinberg, J. A., Wood, G. C., & Fabian, T. C. et al. (2006). The futility of the clinical pulmonary infections score in trauma patients. *The Journal of Trauma*, *60*(3), 523–527. doi:10.1097/01.ta.0000204033.78125.1b PMID:16531849

Crouzet, J., Bertrand, X., Venier, A. G., Badoz, M., Husson, C., & Talon, D. (2007). Control of the duration of urinary catheterization: Impact on catheter-associated urinary tract infection. *The Journal of Hospital Infection*, *67*(3), 253–257. doi:10.1016/j.jhin.2007.08.014 PMID:17949851

Davies, C. W., Kearney, S. E., Gleeson, F. V., & Davies, R. J. (1999). Predictors of outcome and long-term survival in patients with pleural infections. *American Journal of Respiratory and Critical Care Medicine*, *160*(5), 1682–1687. doi:10.1164/ajrccm.160.5.9903002 PMID:10556140

De Bono, S., Heling, G., & Borg, M. A. (2014). Organizational culture and its implications for infection prevention and control in healthcare institutions. *The Journal of Hospital Infection*, *86*(1), 1–6. doi:10.1016/j.jhin.2013.10.007 PMID:24309419

De Smet, A. M. G. A., Kluytmans, J. A. J. W., Cooper, B. S., Mascini, E. M., Benus, R. F. J., van der Werf, T. S., & Bonten, M. J. M. et al. (2009). Decontamination of the digestive tract and oropharynx in ICU patients. *The New England Journal of Medicine*, *360*(1), 20–31. doi:10.1056/NEJMoa0800394 PMID:19118302

Deschka, H., Erler, S., El-Ayoubi, L., Vogel, C., Vöhringer, L., & Wimmer-Greinecker, G. (2013). Suction-irrigation drainage: An underestimated therapeutic option for surgical treatment of deep sternal wound infections. *Interactive Cardiovascular and Thoracic Surgery*, *17*(1), 85–89. doi:10.1093/icvts/ivt078 PMID:23529753

Deshpande, K. S., Hatem, C., Ulrich, H. L., Currie, B. P., Aldrich, T. K., Bryan-Brown, C. W., & Kvetan, V. (2005). The incidence of infectious complications of central venous catheters at the subclavian, internal jugular, and femoral sites in an intensive care unit population. *Critical Care Medicine*, *33*(1), 13–20. doi:10.1097/01.CCM.0000149838.47048.60 PMID:15644643

Desimone, D. C., Tleyjeh, I. M., Correa de Sa, D. D., Anavekar, N. S., Lahr, B. D., Sohail, M. R., & Baddour, L. M. et al. (2012). Incidence of infective endocarditis caused by viridans group streptococci before and after publication of the 2007 American Heart Association's endocarditis prevention guidelines. *Circulation*, *126*(1), 60–64. doi:10.1161/CIRCULATIONAHA.112.095281 PMID:22689929

Despotis, G. J., & Goodnough, L. T. (2000). Management approaches to platelet-related microvascular bleeding in cardiothoracic surgery. *The Annals of Thoracic Surgery*, *70*(2), S20–S32. doi:10.1016/S0003-4975(00)01604-0 PMID:10966007

Dickerman, S.A., Abrutyn, E., Barsic, B., Bouza, E., Cecchi, E., & Moreno, A., … Cabell, C.H., for the ICE Investigators. (2007). The relationship between the initiation of antimicrobial therapy and the incidence of stroke in infective endocarditis: An analysis from the ICE Prospective Cohort Study Group (ICE-PCS). *American Heart Journal*, *154*, 1086–1094. PMID:18035080

Dieleman, J. M., Nierich, A. P., Rosseel, P. M., van der Maaten, J. M., Hofland, J., & Diephuis, J. C. (2012). Intraoperative high-dose dexamethasone for cardiac surgery. A randomized controlled trial. *Journal of the American Medical Association*, *308*(17), 1761–1767. doi:10.1001/jama.2012.14144 PMID:23117776

Dieleman, J. M., van Paassen, J., van Dijk, D., Arbous, M., Kalkman, C. J., Vandenbroucke, J. P., & Dekkers, O. M. et al. (2011). Prophylactic corticosteroids for cardiopulmonary bypass in adults. *Cochrane Database of Systematic Reviews*, CD005566. PMID:21563145

Diez, C., Koch, D., Kuss, O., Silber, R., Friedrich, I., & Boergermann, J. (2007). Risk factors for mediastinitis after cardiac surgery – A retrospective analysis of 1700 patients. *Journal of Cardiothoracic Surgery*, *2*(1), 23. doi:10.1186/1749-8090-2-23 PMID:17511885

Dimopoulos, G., Poulakou, G., Pneumatikos, I. A., Armaganidis, A., Kollef, M. H., & Matthaiou, D. K. (2013). Short- vs long-duration antibiotic regimens for ventilator-associated pneumonia. A systematic review and meta-analysis. *Chest*, *144*(6), 1759–1767. doi:10.1378/chest.13-0076 PMID:23788274

Dobesh, P. P., & Olsen, K. M. (2014). Statins role in the prevention and treatment of sepsis. *Pharmacological Research*, *88*, 31–40. doi:10.1016/j.phrs.2014.04.010 PMID:24794878

Dobler, C. C., & Waterer, G. (2013). Healthcare-associated pneumonia: A US disease or relevant to the Asia Pacific, too? *Respirology (Carlton, Vic.)*, *18*(6), 923–932. doi:10.1111/resp.12132 PMID:23714303

Domkowski, P. W., Smith, M. L., Gonyon, D. L. Jr, Drye, C., Wooten, M. K., Levin, L. S., & Wolfe, W. G. (2003). Evaluation of vacuum-assisted closure in the treatment of poststernotomy mediastinitis. *The Journal of Thoracic and Cardiovascular Surgery*, *126*(2), 386–390. doi:10.1016/S0022-5223(03)00352-0 PMID:12928634

Duckro, A. N., Blom, D. W., Lyle, E. A., Weinstein, R. A., & Hayden, M. K. (2005). Transfer of vancomycin-resistant enterococci via health care worker hands. *Archives of Internal Medicine*, *165*(3), 302–307. doi:10.1001/archinte.165.3.302 PMID:15710793

Durack, D. T. (1995). Prevention of infective endocarditis. *The New England Journal of Medicine*, *332*(1), 38–44. doi:10.1056/NEJM199501053320107 PMID:7990863

Duval, X., Iung, B., Klein, I., Brochet, E., Thabut, G., & Arnoult, F., … Leport, C., for the IMAGE (Resonance Magnetic Imaging at the Acute Phase of Endocarditis) Study Group. (2010). Efficacy of cerebral magnetic resonance imaging on clinical decisions in infective endocarditis: A prospective study. *Annals of Internal Medicine*, *152*, 497–504. doi:10.7326/0003-4819-152-8-201004200-00006 PMID:20404380

Dybdahl, B., Wahba, A., Lien, E., Flo, T. H., Waage, A., Qureshi, N., & Sundan, A. et al. (2002). Inflammatory response after open heart surgery: Release of heat-shock protein 70 and signaling through toll-like receptor-4. *Circulation*, *105*(6), 685–690. doi:10.1161/hc0602.103617 PMID:11839622

Edwards, F. H., Engelman, R. M., Houck, P., Shahian, D. M., & Bridges, C. R. (2006). The Society of Thoracic Surgeons practice guideline series: Antibiotic prophylaxis in cardiac surgery, part I: Duration. *The Annals of Thoracic Surgery*, *81*(1), 397–404. doi:10.1016/j.athoracsur.2005.06.034 PMID:16368422

Eggimann, P., & Revelly, J. (2006). Should antibiotic combinations be used to treat ventilator-associated pneumonia? *Seminars in Respiratory and Critical Care Medicine*, *27*(01), 68–81. doi:10.1055/s-2006-933675 PMID:16508883

El Solh, A. A., Bhora, M., Pineda, L., & Dhillon, R. (2006). Nosocomial pneumonia in elderly patients following cardiac surgery. *Respiratory Medicine*, *100*(4), 729–736. doi:10.1016/j.rmed.2005.07.011 PMID:16126381

Ellis, M. E., Al-Abdely, H., Sandridge, A., Greer, W., & Ventura, W. (2001). Fungal endocarditis: Evidence in the world literature, 1965-1995. *Clinical Infectious Diseases*, *32*(1), 50–62. doi:10.1086/317550 PMID:11118386

Engelman, R., Shahian, D., Shemin, R., Guy, T. S., Bratzler, D., Edwards, F., & Bridges, C. et al. (2007). The Society of Thoracic Surgeons practice guideline series: Antibiotic prophylaxis in cardiac surgery, part II: Antibiotic choice. *The Annals of Thoracic Surgery*, *83*(4), 1569–1576. doi:10.1016/j.athoracsur.2006.09.046 PMID:17383396

Engelmann, B. (2006). Initiation of coagulation by tissue factor carriers in blood. *Blood Cells, Molecules & Diseases*, *36*(2), 188–190. doi:10.1016/j.bcmd.2005.12.020 PMID:16473535

Eom, J. S., Lee, M., Chun, H., Choi, H. J., Jung, S., Kim, Y., & Lee, J. S. et al. (2014). The impact of a ventilator bundle on preventing ventilator-associated pneumonia: A multicenter study. *American Journal of Infection Control*, *42*(1), 34–37. doi:10.1016/j.ajic.2013.06.023 PMID:24189326

Erb, S., Frei, R., Schregenberger, K., Dangel, M., Nogarth, D., & Widmer, A. F. (2014). Sonication for diagnosis of catheter-related infection is not better than traditional roll-plate culture: A prospective cohort study with 975 central venous catheters. *Clinical Infectious Diseases*, *59*(4), 541–544. doi:10.1093/cid/ciu352 PMID:24825872

Ewig, S., Welte, T., & Torres, A. (2012). Is healthcare-associated pneumonia a distinct entity needing specific therapy? *Current Opinion in Infectious Diseases*, *25*(2), 166–175. doi:10.1097/QCO.0b013e32835023fb PMID:22248977

Eyer, S., Brummitt, C., Crossley, K., Siegel, R., & Cerra, F. (1990). Catheter-related sepsis: Prospective, randomized study of three methods of long-term catheter maintenance. *Critical Care Medicine*, *18*(10), 1073–1079. doi:10.1097/00003246-199010000-00005 PMID:2209033

Fagan, R. P., Edwards, J. R., Park, B. J., Fridkin, S. K., & Magill, S. S. (2013). Incidence trends in pathogen-specific central line-associated bloodstream infections in US intensive care units, 1990-2010. *Infection Control and Hospital Epidemiology*, *34*(9), 893–899. doi:10.1086/671724 PMID:23917902

Fakih, M. G., Dueweke, C., Meisner, S., Berriel-Cass, D., Savoy-Moore, R., Brach, N., & Saravolatz, L. D. et al. (2008). Effect of nurse-led multidisciplinary roundson reducing the unnecessary use of urinary catheterization in hospitalized patients. *Infection Control and Hospital Epidemiology*, *29*(9), 815–819. doi:10.1086/589584 PMID:18700831

Fergusson, D. A., Hébert, P. C., Mazer, C. D., Fremes, S., MacAdams, C., Murkin, J. M., & Pretorius, R. et al. (2010). A comparison of aprotinin and lysine analogues in high-risk cardiac surgery. *The New England Journal of Medicine*, *358*(22), 2319–2331. doi:10.1056/NEJMoa0802395 PMID:18480196

Filsoufi, F., Castillo, J. G., Rahmanian, P. B., Broumand, S. R., Silvay, G., Carpentier, A., & Adams, D. H. (2009). Epidemiology of deep sternal wound infection in cardiac surgery. *Journal of Cardiothoracic and Vascular Anesthesia*, *23*(4), 488–494. doi:10.1053/j.jvca.2009.02.007 PMID:19376733

Finkel, M. S., Oddis, C. V., Jacob, T. D., Watkins, S. C., Hattler, B. G., & Simmons, R. L. (1992). Negative inotropic effects of cytokines on the heart mediated by nitric oxide. *Science*, *257*(5068), 387–389. doi:10.1126/science.1631560 PMID:1631560

Fischer, G. W., & Levin, M. A. (2010). Vasoplegia during cardiac surgery: Current concepts and management. *Seminars in Thoracic and Cardiovascular Surgery*, *22*(2), 140–144. doi:10.1053/j.semtcvs.2010.09.007 PMID:21092891

Fitch, Z. W., & Whitman, G. J. R. (2014). Incidence, risk, and prevention of ventilator-associated pneumonia in adult cardiac surgery patients: A systematic review. *Journal of Cardiac Surgery*, *29*(2), 196–203. doi:10.1111/jocs.12260 PMID:24304223

Flier, S., Concepcion, A. N., Versteeg, D., Kappen, T. H., Hoefer, I. E., de Lange, D. W., & Buhre, W. F. et al. (2014). Monocyte hyporesponsiveness and toll-like receptor expression profiles in coronary artery bypass grafting and its clinical implications for postoperative inflammatory response and pneumonia. *European Journal of Anaesthesiology*, *31*, 1–12. PMID:24225728

Floros, P., Sawhney, R., Vrtik, M., Hinton-Bayre, A., Weimers, P., Senewiratne, S., & Shah, P. et al. (2011). Risk factors and management approach for deep sternal wound infection after cardiac surgery at a tertiary medical centre. *Heart Lung and Circulation*, *20*(11), 712–717. doi:10.1016/j.hlc.2011.08.001 PMID:21906999

Fournier, P. E., Drancourt, M., Colson, P., Rolain, J. M., La Scola, B., & Raoult, D. (2013). Modern clinical microbiology: New challenges and solutions. *Nature Reviews. Microbiology*, *11*(8), 574–585. doi:10.1038/nrmicro3068 PMID:24020074

Fowler, V. G. Jr, Boucher, H. W., Corey, R. G., Abrutyn, E., Karchmer, A. W., Rupp, M. E., & Cosgrove, S. E. et al. (2006). Daptomycin versus standard therapy for bacteremia and endocarditis caused by Staphylococcus aureus. *The New England Journal of Medicine*, *355*(7), 653–665. doi:10.1056/NEJMoa053783 PMID:16914701

Fowler, V. G. Jr, O'Brien, S. M., Muhlbaier, L. H., Corey, G. R., Ferguson, T. B., & Peterson, E. D. (2005). Clinical predictors of major infections after cardiac surgery. *Circulation*, *112*, I-358–I-365. PMID:16159846

Freedman, L. R. (1987). The pathogenesis of infective endocarditis. *The Journal of Antimicrobial Chemotherapy*, *20*(Suppl A), 1–6. doi:10.1093/jac/20.suppl_A.1 PMID:3316154

Funakoshi, S., Kaji, S., Yamamuro, A., Tani, T., Kinoshita, M., Okada, Y., & Furukawa, Y. (2011). Impact of early surgery in the active phase on long-term outcomes in left-sided native valve infective endocarditis. *The Journal of Thoracic and Cardiovascular Surgery*, *142*(4), 836–842. doi:10.1016/j.jtcvs.2011.01.040 PMID:21397271

Furnary, A. P., Zerr, K. J., Grunkemeier, G. L., & Starr, A. (1999). Continuous intravenous insulin infusion reduces the incidence of deep sternal wound infection in diabetic patients after cardiac surgical procedures. *The Annals of Thoracic Surgery*, *67*(2), 352–362. doi:10.1016/S0003-4975(99)00014-4 PMID:10197653

Gastmeier, P., Geffers, C., Brandt, C., Zuschneid, I., Sohr, D., Schwab, F., & Rüden, H. et al. (2006). Effectiveness of a nationwide nosocomial infection surveillance system for reducing nosocomial infections. *The Journal of Hospital Infection*, *64*(1), 16–22. doi:10.1016/j.jhin.2006.04.017 PMID:16820247

Gelijns, A. C., Moskowitz, A. J., Acker, M. A., Argenziano, M., Geller, N. L., Puskas, J. D., & Blackstone, E. H. et al. (2014). Management practices and major infections after cardiac surgery. *Journal of the American College of Cardiology*, *64*(4), 372–381. doi:10.1016/j.jacc.2014.04.052 PMID:25060372

Giomarelli, P., Scolletta, S., Borrelli, E., & Biagioli, B. (2003). Myocardial and lung injury after cardiopulmonary bypass: Role of interleukin (IL)-10. *The Annals of Thoracic Surgery*, *76*(1), 117–123. doi:10.1016/S0003-4975(03)00194-2 PMID:12842524

Girard, T. D., Kress, J. P., Fuchs, B. D., Thomason, J. W. W., Schweickert, W. D., Pun, B. T., & Ely, W. E. et al. (2008). Efficacy and safety of a paired sedation and ventilator weaning protocol for mechanically ventilated patients in intensive care (Awakening and Breathing Controlled trial): A randomised controlled trial. *Lancet*, *371*(9607), 126–134. doi:10.1016/S0140-6736(08)60105-1 PMID:18191684

Girou, E., Loyeau, S., Legrand, P., Oppein, F., & Brun-Buisson, C. (2002). Efficacy of handrubbing with alcohol based solution versus standard handwashing with antiseptic soap: Randomised clinical trial. *British Medical Journal*, *325*(7360), 362. doi:10.1136/bmj.325.7360.362 PMID:12183307

Goldstein, D. J., Naftel, D., Holman, W., Bellumkonda, L., Pamboukian, S. V., Pagani, F. D., & Kirklin, J. (2012). Continuous-flow devices and percutaneous site infections: Clinical outcomes. *The Journal of Heart and Lung Transplantation*, *31*(11), 1151–1157. doi:10.1016/j.healun.2012.05.004 PMID:22766022

Goulenok, T., Klein, I., Mazighi, M., Messika-Zeitoun, D., Alexandra, J. F., Mourvillier, B., & Duval, X. et al. (2013). Infective endocarditis with symptomatic cerebral complications; Contribution of cerebral magnetic resonance imaging. *Cerebrovascular Diseases (Basel, Switzerland)*, *35*(4), 327–336. doi:10.1159/000348317 PMID:23615478

Greene, M. T., Chang, R., Kuhn, L., Rogers, M. A. M., Chenoweth, C. E., Shuman, E., & Saint, S. (2012). Predictors of hospital-acquired urinary tract-related bloodstream infection. *Infection Control and Hospital Epidemiology*, *33*(10), 1001–1007. doi:10.1086/667731 PMID:22961019

Grgurich, P. E., Hudcova, J., Lei, Y., Sarwar, A., & Craven, D. E. (2013). Diagnosis of ventilator-associated pneumonia: Controversies and working toward a gold standard. *Current Opinion in Infectious Diseases*, *26*(2), 140–150. doi:10.1097/QCO.0b013e32835ebbd0 PMID:23411419

Grubitzsch, H., Schaefer, A., Melzer, C., Wernecke, K. D., Gabbieri, D., & Konertz, W. (2014). Outcome after surgery for prosthetic valve endocarditis and the impact of preoperative treatment. *The Journal of Thoracic and Cardiovascular Surgery*, *148*(5), 2052–2059. doi:10.1016/j.jtcvs.2014.05.025 PMID:24951022

Gürntke, S., Kohler, C., Steinmetz, I., Pfeifer, Y., Eller, C., Gastmeier, P., & Leistner, R. et al. (2014). Molecular epidemiology of extended-spectrum beta-lactamase (ESBL)-positive Klebsiella pneumonia from bloodstream infections and risk factors for mortality. *Journal of Infection and Chemotherapy*, *20*(12), 817–819. doi:10.1016/j.jiac.2014.08.012 PMID:25224765

Habib, G., Badano, L., Tribouilloy, C., Vilacosta, I., Zamorano, J. L., Galderisi, M., & Aakhus, S. et al. (2010). Recommendations for the practice of echocardiography in infective endocarditis. *European Journal of Echocardiography*, *11*(2), 202–219. doi:10.1093/ejechocard/jeq004 PMID:20223755

Habib, G., Hoen, B., Tornos, P., Thuny, F., Prendergast, B., Vilacosta, I., & van Camp, G. et al. (2009). Guidelines on the prevention, diagnosis, and treatment of infective endocarditis (new version 2009): The Task Force on the Prevention, Diagnosis, and Treatment of Infective Endocarditis of the European Society of Cardiology (ESC). *European Heart Journal, 30*(19), 2369–2413. doi:10.1093/eurheartj/ehp285 PMID:19713420

Hannan, M. M., Husain, S., Matner, F., Danziger-Isakov, L., Drew, R. J., Corey, G. R., & Mooney, M. L. et al. (2011). Working formulation for the standardization of definitions of infections in patients using ventricular assist devices. *The Journal of Heart and Lung Transplantation, 30*(4), 375–384. doi:10.1016/j.healun.2011.01.717 PMID:21419995

Hansalia, S., Biswas, M., Dutta, R., Hage, F. G., Hsiung, M. C., Nanda, N. C., & Yin, W. H. et al. (2009). The value of live/real time three-dimensional transesophageal echocardiography in the assessment of valvular regurgitation. *Echocardiography (Mount Kisco, N.Y.), 26*(10), 1264–1273. doi:10.1111/j.1540-8175.2009.01042.x PMID:19929872

Harbarth, S., Fankhauser, C., Schrenzel, J., Christenson, J., Gervaz, P., Bandiera-Clerc, C., & Pittet, D. et al. (2008). Universal screening for methicillin-resistant Staphylococcus aureus at hospital admission and nosocomial infection in surgical patients. *Journal of the American Medical Association, 299*, 1149–1157. doi:10.1001/jama.299.10.1149 PMID:18334690

He, S., Chen, B., Li, W., Yan, J., Chen, L., Wang, X., & Xiao, Y. (2014). Ventilator-associated pneumonia after cardiac surgery: A meta-analysis and systematic review. *The Journal of Thoracic and Cardiovascular Surgery, 148*(6), 3148–3155.e5. doi:10.1016/j.jtcvs.2014.07.107 PMID:25240522

Heilmann, C., Stahl, R., Schneider, C., Sukhodolya, T., Siepe, M., Olschewski, M., & Beyersdorf, F. (2013). Wound complications after median sternotomy: A single-center study. *Interactive Cardiovascular and Thoracic Surgery, 16*(5), 643–648. doi:10.1093/icvts/ivs554 PMID:23355648

Hess, D. R. (2005). Noninvasive positive-pressure ventilation and ventilator-associated pneumonia. *Respiratory Care, 50*, 924–929. PMID:15972113

Heyland, D. K., Dodek, P., Muscedere, J., Day, A., & Cook, D.Canadian Critical Care Trials Group. (2008). Randomized trial of combination versus monotherapy for the empiric treatment for suspected ventilator-associated pneumonia. *Critical Care Medicine, 36*(3), 737–744. doi:10.1097/01.CCM.0B013E31816203D6 PMID:18091545

Hidron, A. I., Edwards, J. R., Patel, J., Horan, T. C., Sievert, D. M., Pollock, D. A., & Fridkin, S. K. (2008). NHSN annual update: Antimicrobial-resistant pathogens associated with healthcare-associated infections: Annual summary of data reported to the National Healthcare Safety Network at the Centers for Disease Control and Prevention, 2006-2007. *Infection Control and Hospital Epidemiology, 29*(11), 996–1011. doi:10.1086/591861 PMID:18947320

Hirai, S. (2003). Systemic inflammatory response syndrome after cardiac surgery under cardiopulmonary bypass. *Annals of Thoracic and Cardiovascular Surgery, 9*, 365–370. PMID:15003097

Ho, K. M., & Tan, J. A. (2009). Benefits and risks of corticosteroid prophylaxis in adult cardiac surgery: A dose-response meta-analysis. *Circulation*, *119*(14), 1853–1866. doi:10.1161/CIRCULATIONAHA.108.848218 PMID:19332460

Ho, K. M., & Tan, J. A. (2011). Benefits and risks of maintaining normothermia during cardiopulmonary bypass in adult cardiac surgery: A systematic review. *Cardiovascular Therapeutics*, *29*(4), 260–279. doi:10.1111/j.1755-5922.2009.00114.x PMID:20041882

Hockenhull, J. C., Dwan, K. M., Smith, G. W., Gamble, C. L., Boland, A., Walley, T. J., & Dickson, R. C. (2009). The clinical effectiveness of central venous catheters treated with anti-infective agents in preventing catheter-related bloodstream infections: A systematic review. *Critical Care Medicine*, *37*(2), 702–712. doi:10.1097/CCM.0b013e3181958915 PMID:19114884

Hoen, B., Alla, F., Selton-Suty, C., Béguinot, I., Bouvet, A., & Briançon, S., … Vandenesch, F., for the Association pour l'Etude et la Prévention de l'Endocardite Infectieuse (AEPEI) Study Group. (. (2002). Changing profile of infective endocarditis. Results of a 1-year survey in France. *Journal of the American Medical Association*, *288*, 75–81. doi:10.1001/jama.288.1.75 PMID:12090865

Holland, T. L., Arnold, C., & Fowler, V. G. Jr. (2014). Clinical management of Staphylococcus aureus bacteremia. A review. *Journal of the American Medical Association*, *312*(13), 1330–1341. doi:10.1001/jama.2014.9743 PMID:25268440

Holmes, J. H. IV, Connolly, N. C., Paull, D. L., Hill, M. E., Guyton, S. W., Ziegler, S. F., & Hall, R. A. (2002). Magnitude of the inflammatory response to cardiopulmonary bypass and its relation to adverse clinical outcomes. *Inflammation Research*, *51*(12), 579–586. doi:10.1007/PL00012432 PMID:12558191

Hooton, T. M., Bradley, S. F., Cardenas, D. D., Colgan, R., Geerlings, S. E., Rice, J. C., & Nicolle, L. E. et al. (2010). Diagnosis, prevention, and treatment of catheter-associated urinary tract infection in adults: 2009 international clinical practice guidelines from the Infectious Diseases Society of America. *Clinical Infectious Diseases*, *50*(5), 625–663. doi:10.1086/650482 PMID:20175247

Horan, T. C., Andrus, M., & Dudeck, M. A. (2008). CDC/NHSN surveillance definition of healthcare-associated infection and criteria for specific types of infections in the acute care setting. *American Journal of Infection Control*, *36*(5), 309–332. doi:10.1016/j.ajic.2008.03.002 PMID:18538699

Hortal, J., Gianella, M., Pérez, M. J., Barrio, J. M., Desco, M., Bouza, E., & Muñoz, P. (2009). Incidence and risk factors for ventilator-associated pneumonia after major heart surgery. *Intensive Care Medicine*, *35*(9), 1518–1525. doi:10.1007/s00134-009-1523-3 PMID:19557389

Hu, K. K., Lipsky, B. A., Veenstra, D. L., & Saint, S. (2004). Using maximal sterile barriers to prevent central venous catheter-related infection: A systematic evidence-based review. *American Journal of Infection Control*, *32*(3), 142–146. doi:10.1016/j.ajic.2003.10.006 PMID:15153925

Huang, S., Datta, R., & Platt, R. (2006). Risk of acquiring antibiotic-resistant bacteria from previous room occupants. *Archives of Internal Medicine*, *166*(18), 1945–1951. doi:10.1001/archinte.166.18.1945 PMID:17030826

Huang, S. S., Yokoe, D. S., Hinrichsen, V. L., Spurchise, L. S., Datta, R., Miroshnik, I., & Platt, R. (2006). Impact of routine intensive care unit surveillance cultures and resultant barrier precautions on hospital-wide methicillin-resistant Staphylococcus aureus bacteremia. *Clinical Infectious Diseases*, *43*(8), 971–978. doi:10.1086/507636 PMID:16983607

Hugonnet, S., Chevrolet, J., & Pittet, D. (2007). The effect of workload on infection risk in critically ill patients. *Critical Care Medicine*, *35*(1), 76–81. doi:10.1097/01.CCM.0000251125.08629.3F PMID:17095946

Hulzebos, E. H., Helders, P. J., Favié, N. J., De Bie, R. A., Brutel de la Riviere, A., & Van Meeteren, N. L. (2006). Preoperative intensive inspiratory muscle training to prevent postoperative pulmonary complications in high-risk patients undergoing CABG surgery: A randomized clinical trial. *Journal of the American Medical Association*, *296*(15), 1851–1857. doi:10.1001/jama.296.15.1851 PMID:17047215

Ibañez, J., Riera, M., Anezaga, R., Herrero, J., Colomar, A., & Campillo-Artero, C. … Bonnin, O. (2014). Long-term mortality after pneumonia in cardiac surgery patients.: A propensity-matched analysis. *Journal of Intensive Care Medicine*; Advance online publication. doi:10.1177/0885066614523918

Iregui, M., Ward, S., Sherman, G., Fraser, V., & Kollef, M. (2002). Clinical importance of delays in the initiation of appropriate antibiotic treatment for ventilator-associated pneumonia. *Chest*, *122*(1), 262–268. doi:10.1378/chest.122.1.262 PMID:12114368

Jabbar, U., Leischner, J., Kasper, D., Gerber, R., Sambol, S. P., Parada, J. P., & Gerding, D. N. et al. (2010). Effectiveness of alcohol-based hand rubs for removal of Clostridium difficile spores from hands. *Infection Control and Hospital Epidemiology*, *31*(6), 565–570. doi:10.1086/652772 PMID:20429659

Jacob, K. A., Nathoe, H. M., Dieleman, J. M., van Osch, D., Kluin, J., & van Dijk, D. (2014). Inflammation in new-onset atrial fibrillation after cardiac surgery. *European Journal of Clinical Investigation*, *44*(4), 402–408. doi:10.1111/eci.12237 PMID:24387767

Jarvis, W. R. (2003). Benchmarking for prevention: The Centers for Disease Control and Prevention's National Nosocomial Infections Surveillance (NNIS) system experience. *Infection*, *31*(Suppl 2), 44–48. PMID:15018472

Jenkins, I. (2007). Linezolid- and vancomycin-resistant Enterococcus faecium endocarditis: Successful treatment with tigecycline and daptomycin. *Journal of Hospital Medicine*, *5*(5), 343–344. doi:10.1002/jhm.236 PMID:17935250

Jernigan, J. A., Titus, M. G., Gröschel, D. H., Getchell-White, S., & Farr, B. M. (1996). Effectiveness of contact isolation during a hospital outbreak of methicillin-resistant Staphylococcus aureus. *American Journal of Epidemiology*, *143*(5), 496–504. doi:10.1093/oxfordjournals.aje.a008770 PMID:8610665

Johnson, J. R., Kuskowski, M. A., & Wilt, T. J. (2006). Systematic review: Antimicrobial urinary catheters to prevent catheter-associated urinary tract infection in hospitalized patients. *Annals of Internal Medicine*, *144*(2), 116–126. doi:10.7326/0003-4819-144-2-200601170-00009 PMID:16418411

Jongman, R. M., Zijlstra, J. G., Kok, W. F., van Harten, A. E., Mariani, M. A., Moser, J., & van Meurs, M. et al. (2014). Off-pump CABG surgery reduces systemic inflammation compared wth on-pump surgery but does not change systemic endothelial responses: A prospective randomized study. *Shock (Augusta, Ga.)*, *42*, 121–128. doi:10.1097/SHK.0000000000000190 PMID:24727871

Kaki, R., Elligsen, M., Walker, S., Simor, A., Palmay, L., & Daneman, N. (2011). Impact of antibiotic stewardship in critical care: A systematic review. *The Journal of Antimicrobial Chemotherapy*, *66*(6), 1223–1230. doi:10.1093/jac/dkr137 PMID:21460369

Kalanuria, A. A., Zai, W., & Mirski, M. (2014). Ventilator-associated pneumonia in the ICU. *Critical Care (London, England)*, *18*(2), 208. doi:10.1186/cc13775 PMID:25029020

Kalil, A. C., Van Schooneveld, T. C., Fey, P. D., & Rupp, M. E. (2014). Association between vancomycin minimum inhibitory concentration and mortality among patients with Staphylococcus aureus bloodstream infections. A systematic review and meta-analysis. *Journal of the American Medical Association*, *312*(15), 1552–1564. doi:10.1001/jama.2014.6364 PMID:25321910

Kang, C., Chung, D. R., Son, J. S., Ko, K. S., Peck, K. R., & Song, J.Korean Network for Study of Infectious Diseases (KONSID). (2011). Clinical significance of nosocomial acquisition in urinary tract-related bacteremia caused by gram-negative bacilli. *American Journal of Infection Control*, *39*(2), 135–140. doi:10.1016/j.ajic.2010.03.022 PMID:21176996

Kang, D., Kim, Y., Kim, S., Sun, B. J., Kim, D., Yun, S., & Sohn, D. et al. (2012). Early surgery versus conventional treatment for infective endocarditis. *The New England Journal of Medicine*, *366*(26), 2466–2473. doi:10.1056/NEJMoa1112843 PMID:22738096

Kats, S., Schönberger, J. P., Brands, R., Seinen, W., & van Oeveren, W. (2011). Endotoxin release in cardiac surgery with cardiopulmonary bypass: Pathophysiology and possible therapeutic strategies. An update. *European Journal of Cardio-Thoracic Surgery*, *39*(4), 451–458. doi:10.1016/j.ejcts.2010.06.011 PMID:20663682

Kendall, A., Landers, T., Kirk, J., & Young, E. (2012). Point-of-care hand hygiene: Preventing infection behind the curtain. *American Journal of Infection Control*, *40*(4), S3–S10. doi:10.1016/j.ajic.2012.02.009 PMID:22546271

Kett, D. H., Azoulay, E., Echeverria, P. M., & Vincent, J.Extended Prevalence of Infection in the ICU Study. (2011). Candida bloodstream infections in intensive care units: Analysis of the extended prevalence of infection in intensive care unit study. *Critical Care Medicine*, *39*(4), 665–670. doi:10.1097/CCM.0b013e318206c1ca PMID:21169817

Kett, D. H., Cano, E., Quartin, A. A., Mangino, J. E., Zervos, M. J., Peyrani, P., & Ramirez, J. A. et al. (2011). Implementation of guidelines for management of possible multidrug-resistant pneumonia in intensive care: An observational, multicentre cohort study. *The Lancet Infectious Diseases*, *11*(3), 181–189. doi:10.1016/S1473-3099(10)70314-5 PMID:21256086

Keusch, G. T. (2003). The history of nutrition: Malnutrition, infection and immunity. *The Journal of Nutrition*, *133*, 336S–340S. PMID:12514322

Kiefer, T., Park, L., Tribouilloy, C., Cortes, C., Casillo, R., Chu, V., & ICE-PCS Investigators, et al.. (2011). Association between valvular surgery and mortality among patients with infective endocarditis complicated by heart failure. *Journal of the American Medical Association*, *306*(20), 2239–2247. doi:10.1001/jama.2011.1701 PMID:22110106

Klevens, R. M., Edwards, J. R., Richards, C. L. Jr, Horan, T. C., Gaynes, R. P., Pollock, D. A., & Cardo, D. M. (2007). Estimating health care-associated infections and deaths in U.S. hospitals, 2002. *Public Health Reports*, *122*, 160–166. PMID:17357358

Klompas, M. (2007). Does this patient have ventilator-associated pneumonia? *Journal of the American Medical Association*, *297*(14), 1583–1593. doi:10.1001/jama.297.14.1583 PMID:17426278

Klompas, M. (2010). Prevention of ventilator-associated pneumonia. *Expert Review of Anti-Infective Therapy*, *8*(7), 791–800. doi:10.1586/eri.10.59 PMID:20586564

Klompas, M. (2013). Complications of mechanical ventilation – The CDC's new surveillance paradigm. *The New England Journal of Medicine*, *368*(16), 1472–1475. doi:10.1056/NEJMp1300633 PMID:23594002

Klompas, M., Branson, R., Eichenwald, E. C., Greene, L. R., Howell, M. D., Lee, G., & Berenholtz, S. M. et al. (2014). Strategies to prevent ventilator-associated pneumonia in acute care hospitals: 2014 update. *Infection Control and Hospital Epidemiology*, *35*(8), 915–936. doi:10.1086/677144 PMID:25026607

Klompas, M., Speck, K., Howell, M. D., Greene, L. R., & Berenholtz, S. M. (2014). Reappraisal of routine oral care with chlorhexidine gluconate for patients receiving mechanical ventilation: Systematic review and meta-analysis. *JAMA Internal Medicine*, *174*(5), 751–761. doi:10.1001/jamainternmed.2014.359 PMID:24663255

Kollef, M. H., Afessa, B., Anzueto, A., Veremakis, C., Kerr, K. M., & Margolis, B. D. (2008). Silver-coated endotracheal tubes and incidence of ventilator-associated pneumonia. The NASCENT randomized trial. *Journal of the American Medical Association*, *300*(7), 805–813. doi:10.1001/jama.300.7.805 PMID:18714060

Kollef, M. H., Sharpless, L., Vlasnik, J., Pasque, C., Murphy, D., & Fraser, V. J. (1997). The impact of nosocomial infections on patient outcomes following cardiac surgery. *Chest*, *112*(3), 666–675. doi:10.1378/chest.112.3.666 PMID:9315799

Konvalinka, A., Errett, L., & Fong, I. W. (2006). Impact of treating Staphylococcus aureus nasal carriers on wound infections in cardiac surgery. *The Journal of Hospital Infection*, *64*(2), 162–168. doi:10.1016/j.jhin.2006.06.010 PMID:16930768

Koval, C. E., Thuita, L., Moazami, N., & Blackstone, E. (2014). Evolution and impact of drive-line infection in a large cohort of continuous-flow ventricular assist device recipients. *The Journal of Heart and Lung Transplantation*, *33*(11), 1164–1172. doi:10.1016/j.healun.2014.05.011 PMID:25034793

Kress, J. P., Pohlman, A. S., O'Connor, M. F., & Hall, J. B. (2000). Daily interruption of sedative infusions in critically ill patients undergoing mechanical ventilation. *The New England Journal of Medicine*, *342*(20), 1471–1477. doi:10.1056/NEJM200005183422002 PMID:10816184

Kubota, H., Miyata, H., Motomura, N., Ono, M., Takamoto, S., Harii, K., & Kyo, S. et al. (2013). Deep sternal wound infections after cardiac surgery. *Journal of Cardiothoracic Surgery*, *8*, 132. PMID:23688324

Kuhn, E. W., Liakopoulos, O. J., Stange, S., Deppe, A., Slottosch, I., Choi, Y., & Wahlers, T. (2014). Preoperative statin therapy in cardiac surgery: A meta-analysis of 90000 patients. *European Journal of Cardio-Thoracic Surgery*, *45*(1), 17–26. doi:10.1093/ejcts/ezt181 PMID:23562936

Kumar, A. (2009). Optimizing antimicrobial therapy in sepsis and septic shock. *Critical Care Clinics*, *25*(4), 733–751. doi:10.1016/j.ccc.2009.08.004 PMID:19892250

Kumar, A., Roberts, D., Wood, K. E., Light, B., Parillo, J. E., Sharma, S., & Cheang, M. et al. (2006). Duration of hypotension before initiation of effective antimicrobial therapy is the critical determinant of survival in human septic shock. *Critical Care Medicine*, *34*(6), 1589–1596. doi:10.1097/01.CCM.0000217961.75225.E9 PMID:16625125

Kunin, C. M., & McCormack, R. C. (1966). Prevention of catheter-induced urinary-tract infections by sterile closed drainage. *The New England Journal of Medicine*, *274*(21), 1155–1161. doi:10.1056/NEJM196605262742101 PMID:5934951

Lacherade, J. C., De Jonghe, B., Guezennec, P., Debbat, K., Hayon, J., Monsel, A., & Bastuji-Garin, S. et al. (2010). Intermittent subglottic secretion drainage and ventilator-associated pneumonia: A multicenter trial. *American Journal of Respiratory and Critical Care Medicine*, *182*(7), 910–917. doi:10.1164/rccm.200906-0838OC PMID:20522796

Lador, A., Nasir, H., Mansur, N., Sharoni, E., Biderman, P., Leibovici, L., & Paul, M. (2012). Antibiotic prophylaxis in cardiac surgery: Systematic review and meta-analysis. *The Journal of Antimicrobial Chemotherapy*, *67*(3), 541–550. doi:10.1093/jac/dkr470 PMID:22083832

Lai, N. M., Chaiyakunapruk, N., Lai, N. A., O'Riordan, E., Pau, W. S. C., & Saint, S. (2013). Catheter impregnation, coating or bonding for reducing central venous catheter-related infections in adults. *Cochrane Database of Systematic Reviews*, CD007878. PMID:23740696

Larmann, J., & Theilmeier, G. (2004). Inflammatory response to cardiac surgery: Cardiopulmonary bypass versus non-cardiopulmonary bypass surgery. *Best Practice & Research. Clinical Anaesthesiology*, *18*(3), 425–438. doi:10.1016/j.bpa.2003.12.004 PMID:15212337

Latham, R., Lancaster, A. D., Covington, J. F., Pirolo, J. S., & Thomas, C. S. Jr. (2001). The association of diabetes and glucose control with surgical-site infections among cardiothoracic surgery patients. *Infection Control and Hospital Epidemiology*, *22*(10), 607–612. doi:10.1086/501830 PMID:11776345

Lee, G. M., Kleinman, K., Soumerai, S. B., Tse, A., Cole, D., Fridkin, S. K., & Jha, A. K. et al. (2012). Effect of nonpayment for preventable infections in U.S. hospitals. *The New England Journal of Medicine*, *367*(15), 1428–1437. doi:10.1056/NEJMsa1202419 PMID:23050526

Letheulle, J., Tattevin, P., Saunders, L., Kerjouan, M., Léna, H., Descrues, B., & Jouneau, S. et al. (2013). Iterative thoracentesis as first-line treatment of complicated parapneumonic effusion. *PLoS ONE*, *9*(1), e84788. doi:10.1371/journal.pone.0084788 PMID:24400113

Li, J. S., Sexton, D. J., Mick, N., Nettles, R., Fowler, V. G. Jr, Ryan, T., & Corey, G. R. et al. (2000). Proposed modifications to the Duke criteria for the diagnosis of infective endocarditis. *Clinical Infectious Diseases*, *30*(4), 633–638. doi:10.1086/313753 PMID:10770721

Liakopoulos, O. J., Dörge, H., Schmitto, J. D., Nagorsnik, U., Grabedünkel, J., & Schoendube, F. A. (2006). Effects of preoperative statin therapy on cytokines after cardiac surgery. *The Thoracic and Cardiovascular Surgeon*, *54*(4), 250–254. doi:10.1055/s-2006-923836 PMID:16755446

Livermore, D. M. (2005). Minimising antibiotic resistance. *The Lancet Infectious Diseases*, *5*(7), 450–459. doi:10.1016/S1473-3099(05)70166-3 PMID:15978531

Lodise, T. P., McKinnon, P. S., Swiderski, L., & Rybak, M. J. (2003). Outcomes analysis of delayed antibiotic treatment for hospital-acquired Staphylococcus aureus bacteremia. *Clinical Infectious Diseases*, *36*(11), 1418–1423. doi:10.1086/375057 PMID:12766837

Lola, I., Levidiotou, S., Petrou, A., Arnaoutoglou, H., Apostolakis, E., & Papadopoulos, G. S. (2011). Are there independent predisposing factors for postoperative infections following open heart surgery? *Journal of Cardiothoracic Surgery*, *6*(1), 151. doi:10.1186/1749-8090-6-151 PMID:22082355

Lorente, L., Lecuona, M., Jimenez, A., Mora, M. L., & Sierra, A. (2007). Influence of an endotracheal tube with polyurethane cuff and subglottic secretion drainage on pneumonia. *American Journal of Respiratory and Critical Care Medicine*, *176*(11), 1079–1083. doi:10.1164/rccm.200705-761OC PMID:17872488

Luna, C. M., Aruj, P., Niederman, M. S., Garzón, J., Violi, D., & Prignoni, A. (2006). Appropriateness and delay to initiate therapy in ventilator-associated pneumonia. *The European Respiratory Journal*, *27*(1), 158–164. doi:10.1183/09031936.06.00049105 PMID:16387949

MacCallum, N. S., Finney, S. J., Gordon, S. E., Quinlan, G. J., & Evans, T. W. (2014). Modified criteria for the systemic inflammatory response syndrome improves their utility following cardiac surgery. *Chest*, *145*(6), 1197–1203. doi:10.1378/chest.13-1023 PMID:24576975

Magill, S. S., Klompas, M., Balk, R., Burns, S. M., Deutschman, C. S., Diekema, D., & Lipsett, P. et al. (2013). Developing a new, national approach to surveillance for ventilator-associated events. *Critical Care Medicine*, *41*(11), 2467–2475. doi:10.1097/CCM.0b013e3182a262db PMID:24162674

Maki, D. G., Kluger, D. M., & Crnich, C. J. (2006). The risk of bloodstream infection in adults with different intravascular devices: A systematic review of 200 published prospective studies. *Mayo Clinic Proceedings*, *81*(9), 1159–1171. doi:10.4065/81.9.1159 PMID:16970212

Mangano, D. T., Rieves, R. D., & Weiss, K. D. (2006). Judging the safety of aprotinin. *The New England Journal of Medicine*, *355*(21), 2261–2262. doi:10.1056/NEJMc066520 PMID:17124031

Mangoush, O., Purkayastha, S., Haj-Yahia, S., Kinross, J., Hayward, M., Bartolozzi, F., & Athanasiou, T. et al. (2007). Heparin-bonded circuits versus nonheparin-bonded circuits: An evaluation of their effect on clinical outcomes. *European Journal of Cardio-Thoracic Surgery*, *31*(6), 1058–1069. doi:10.1016/j.ejcts.2007.01.029 PMID:17306555

Marik, P. E., Flemmer, M., & Harrison, W. (2012). The risk of catheter-related bloodstream infection with femoral venous catheters as compared to subclavian and internal jugular venous catheters: A systematic review of the literature and meta-analysis. *Critical Care Medicine*, *40*(8), 2479–2485. doi:10.1097/CCM.0b013e318255d9bc PMID:22809915

Mariya Joseph, N., Sistla, S., Kumar Dutta, T., Shankar Badhe, A., Rasitha, D., & Chandra Parija, S. (2012). Outcome of ventilator-associated pneumonia: Impact of antibiotic therapy and other factors. *Australasian Medical Journal*, *5*, 135–140. PMID:22905055

Marschall, J., Mermel, L. A., Fakih, M., Hadaway, L., Kallen, A., O'Grady, N. P., & Yokoe, D. S. et al. (2014). Strategies to prevent central line-associated infections in acute care hospitals: 2014 update. *Infection Control and Hospital Epidemiology*, *35*(7), 753–771. doi:10.1086/676533 PMID:24915204

Marshall, J. C. (2001). Inflammation, coagulopathy, and the pathogenesis of multiple organ dysfunction syndrome. *Critical Care Medicine*, *29*, S99–S106. doi:10.1097/00003246-200107001-00032 PMID:11445742

Martinez, J. A., Nicolas, J. M., Marco, F., Horcajada, J. P., Garcia-Seggara, G., & Trilla, A. (2006). Comparison of antimicrobial cycling and mixing strategies in two medical intensive care units. *Critical Care Medicine*, *34*, 275–279. PMID:16424711

Martínez-Comendador, J. M., Alvarez, J. R., Mosquera, I., Sierra, S., Adrio, B., Carro, J. G., & Bengochea, J. et al. (2009). Preoperative statin treatment reduces systemic inflammatory response and myocardial damage in cardiac surgery. *European Journal of Cardio-Thoracic Surgery*, *36*(6), 998–1005. doi:10.1016/j.ejcts.2009.05.022 PMID:19581104

Mauermann, W. J., Sampathkumar, P., & Thompson, R. L. (2008). Sternal wound infections. *Best Practice & Research. Clinical Anaesthesiology*, *22*(3), 423–436. doi:10.1016/j.bpa.2008.04.003 PMID:18831296

McFarlane, H. J., MacDonald, J., Collins, T. C., Molyneaux, P. J., & Carman, W. F. (2009). Severe pneumonia after cardiac surgery as a result of infection with parainfluenza virus type 4. *Journal of Cardiothoracic and Vascular Anesthesia*, *23*(1), 84–86. doi:10.1053/j.jvca.2008.02.008 PMID:18834791

McWilliams, D., Weblin, J., Atkins, G., Bion, J., Williams, J., & Elliott, C. … Snelson, C. (2014). Enhancing rehabilitation of mechanically ventilated patients in the intensive care unit: A quality improvement project. *Journal of Critical Care*; Advance online publication. doi:10.1016/j.jcrc.2014.09.018

Meddings, J., Rogers, M. A., Macy, M., & Saint, S. (2010). Systematic review and meta-analysis: Reminder systems to reduce catheter-associated urinary tract infections and urinary catheter use in hospitalized patients. *Clinical Infectious Diseases*, *51*(5), 550–560. doi:10.1086/655133 PMID:20673003

Mehta, S., Burry, L., Cook, D., Fergusson, D., Steinberg, M., & Granton, J. (2012). Daily sedation interruption in mechanically ventilated critically ill patients cared for with a sedation protocol. A randomized controlled trial. *Journal of the American Medical Association*, *308*(19), 1985–1992. doi:10.1001/jama.2012.13872 PMID:23180503

Mermel, L. A., Allon, M., Bouza, E., Craven, D. E., Flynn, P., O'Grady, N. P., & Warren, D. K. et al. (2009). Clinical practice guidelines for the diagnosis and management of intravascular catheter-related infection: 2009 update by the Infectious Disease Society of America. *Clinical Infectious Diseases*, *49*(1), 1–45. doi:10.1086/599376 PMID:19489710

Methangkool, E., Howard-Quijano, K., Ho, J. K., & Mahajan, A. (2014). Infective endocarditis: The importance of intraoperative echocardiography. *Anesthesia and Analgesia*, *119*(1), 35–40. doi:10.1213/ANE.0000000000000195 PMID:24945122

Michalopoulos, A., Geroulanos, S., Rosmarakis, E. S., & Falagas, M. E. (2006). Frequency, characteristics, and predictors of microbiologically documented nosocomial infections after cardiac surgery. *European Journal of Cardio-Thoracic Surgery*, *29*(4), 456–460. doi:10.1016/j.ejcts.2005.12.035 PMID:16481186

Mietto, C., Pinciroli, R., Patel, N., & Berra, L. (2013). Ventilator-associated pneumonia: Evolving definitions and preventive strategies. *Respiratory Care*, *58*(6), 990–1003. doi:10.4187/respcare.02380 PMID:23709196

Millar, B. C., & Moore, J. E. (2004). Current trends in the molecular diagnosis of infective endocarditis. *European Journal of Clinical Microbiology & Infectious Diseases*, *23*(5), 353–365. doi:10.1007/s10096-004-1132-6 PMID:15112074

Misfeld, M., Girrbach, F., Etz, C. D., Binner, C., Aspern, K. V., Dohmen, P. M., & Mohr, F. et al. (2014). Surgery for infective endocarditis complicated by cerebral embolism; A consecutive series of 375 patients. *The Journal of Thoracic and Cardiovascular Surgery*, *147*(6), 1837–1846. doi:10.1016/j.jtcvs.2013.10.076 PMID:24837722

Miyahara, K., Matsuura, A., Takemura, H., Mizutani, S., Saito, S., & Toyama, M. (2014). Implementation of bundled interventions greatly decreases deep sternal wound infection following cardiovascular surgery. *The Journal of Thoracic and Cardiovascular Surgery*, *148*(5), 2381–2388. doi:10.1016/j.jtcvs.2014.04.005 PMID:24820192

Moat, N. E., Shore, D. F., & Evans, T. W. (1993). Organ dysfunction and cardiopulmonary bypass: The role of complement and complement regulatory proteins. *European Journal of Cardio-Thoracic Surgery*, *7*(11), 563–573. doi:10.1016/1010-7940(93)90241-3 PMID:8297608

Murdoch, D. R., Corey, G. R., Hoen, B., Miró, J. M., Fowler, V. G. Jr, & Bayer, A. S. (2009). Clinical presentation, etiology, and outcome of infective endocarditis in the 21st century. The International Collaboration on Endocarditis – Prospective cohort study. *Archives of Internal Medicine*, *169*(5), 463–473. doi:10.1001/archinternmed.2008.603 PMID:19273776

Muscedere, J., Dodek, P., Keenan, S., Fowler, R., Cook, D., & Heyland, D. (2008). Comprehensive evidence-based clinical practice guidelines for ventilator-associated pneumonia: Prevention. *Journal of Critical Care*, *23*(1), 126–137. doi:10.1016/j.jcrc.2007.11.014 PMID:18359430

Muscedere, J., Rewa, O., Mckechnie, K., Jiang, X., Laporta, D., & Heyland, D. K. (2011). Subglottic secretion drainage for the prevention of ventilator-associated pneumonia: A systematic review and meta-analysis. *Critical Care Medicine*, *39*(8), 1985–1991. doi:10.1097/CCM.0b013e318218a4d9 PMID:21478738

Musci, M., Weng, Y., Hübler, M., Amiri, A., Pasic, M., Kosky, S., & Hetzer, R. et al. (2010). Homograft aortic root replacement in native or prosthetic active infective endocarditis: Twenty-year single-center experience. *The Journal of Thoracic and Cardiovascular Surgery*, *139*(3), 665–673. doi:10.1016/j.jtcvs.2009.07.026 PMID:19767017

Nguyen, D. T., Delahaye, F., Obadia, J., Duval, X., Selton-Suty, C., Carteaux, J., & Alla, F. et al. (2010). Aortic valve replacement for active infective endocarditis: 5-year survival comparison of bioprostheses, homografts and mechanical prostheses. *European Journal of Cardio-Thoracic Surgery*, *37*(5), 1025–1032. doi:10.1016/j.ejcts.2009.11.035 PMID:20036573

Nienaber, J. J. C., Kusne, S., Riaz, T., Walker, R. C., Baddour, L. M., Wright, A. J., & Sohail, M. R. et al. (2013). Clinical manifestations and management of left ventricular assist device-associated infections. *Clinical Infectious Diseases*, *57*(10), 1438–1448. doi:10.1093/cid/cit536 PMID:23943820

Nishimura, R. A., Otto, C. M., Bonow, R. O., Carabello, B. A., Erwin, J. P. III, Guyton, R. A., & Thomas, J. D. et al. (2014). 2014 AHA/ACC guideline for the management of patients with valvular heart disease. *Journal of the American College of Cardiology*, *63*(22), e57–e185. doi:10.1016/j.jacc.2014.02.536 PMID:24603191

Novy, E., Sonneville, R., Mazighi, M., Klein, I. F., Mariotte, E., Mourvillier, B., & Wolff, M. et al. (2013). Neurological complications of infective endocarditis: New breakthroughs in diagnosis and management. *Medecine et Maladies Infectieuses*, *43*(11-12), 443–450. doi:10.1016/j.medmal.2013.09.010 PMID:24215865

O'Connor, C. J. (2010). Glycemic control during cardiac surgery: A moving target? *Current Opinion in Anaesthesiology*, *23*, 47–48. doi:10.1097/ACO.0b013e328333c115 PMID:19858716

O'Grady, N. P., Alexander, M., Burns, L. A., Dellinger, E. P., Garland, J., Heard, S. O., & Saint, S. et al. (2011). Guidelines for the prevention of intravascular catheter-related infections. *Clinical Infectious Diseases*, *52*(9), e162–e193. doi:10.1093/cid/cir257 PMID:21460264

O'Horo, J. C., Maki, D. G., Krupp, A. E., & Safdar, N. (2014). Arterial catheters as a source of bloodstream infection: A systematic review and meta-analysis. *Critical Care Medicine*, *42*(6), 1334–1339. doi:10.1097/CCM.0000000000000166 PMID:24413576

Oostdijk, E. A. N., Kesecioglu, J., Schultz, M. J., Visser, C. E., de Jonge, E., van Essen, E. H. R., & Bonten, M. J. M. et al. (2014). Effects of decontamination of the oropharynx and digestive tract on antibiotic resistance in ICUs. A randomized clinical trial. *Journal of the American Medical Association*, *312*, 1429–1437. doi:10.1001/jama.2014.7247 PMID:25271544

Ottens, T. H., Dieleman, J. M., Sauër, A. C., Peelen, L. M., Nierich, A. P., de Groot, W. J., & van Dijk, D. et al. (2014). Effects of dexamethasone on cognitive decline after cardiac surgery. *Anesthesiology*, *121*(3), 492–500. doi:10.1097/ALN.0000000000000336 PMID:25225745

Palmer, L. B., & Smaldone, G. C. (2014). Reduction of bacterial resistance with inhaled antibiotics in the intensive care unit. *American Journal of Respiratory and Critical Care Medicine*, *189*(10), 1225–1233. doi:10.1164/rccm.201312-2161OC PMID:24646034

Pang, P. Y., Sin, Y. K., Lim, C. H., Tan, T. E., Lim, S. L., Chao, V. T., & Chua, Y. L. (2014). Surgical management of infective endocarditis: An analysis of early and late outcomes. *European Journal of Cardio-Thoracic Surgery*; Advance online publication. doi:10.1093/ejcts/ezu281 PMID:25027271

Paparella, D., Yau, T. M., & Young, E. (2002). Cardiopulmonary bypass induced inflammation: Pathophysiology and treatment. An update. *European Journal of Cardio-Thoracic Surgery*, *21*(2), 232–244. doi:10.1016/S1010-7940(01)01099-5 PMID:11825729

Parks, N. A., Magnotti, L. J., Weinberg, J. A., Zarzaur, B. L., Schroeppel, T. J., Swanson, J. M., & Croce, M. A. et al. (2012). Use of the clinical pulmonary infection score to guide therapy for ventilator-associated pneumonia risks antibiotic overexposure in patients with trauma. *Journal of Trauma and Acute Care Surgery*, *73*(1), 52–58. doi:10.1097/TA.0b013e31825ac37b PMID:22743372

Parry, M. F., Grant, B., & Sestovic, M. (2013). Successful reduction in catheter-associated urinary tract infections: Focus on nurse-directed catheter removal. *American Journal of Infection Control*, *41*(12), 1178–1181. doi:10.1016/j.ajic.2013.03.296 PMID:23768439

Pasquina, P., Tramèr, M. R., & Walder, B. (2003). Prophylactic respiratory physiotherapy after cardiac surgery: Systematic review. *British Medical Journal*, *327*(7428), 1379. doi:10.1136/bmj.327.7428.1379 PMID:14670881

Patel, R., & Gallagher, J. C. (2014). Vancomycin-resistant enterococcal bacteremia pharmacotherapy. *The Annals of Pharmacotherapy*; Advance online publication. doi:10.1177/1060028014556879 PMID:25352037

Patel, R., Rouse, M. S., Piper, K. E., & Steckelberg, J. M. (2001). Linezolid therapy of vancomycin-resistant Enterococcus faecium experimental endocarditis. *Antimicrobial Agents and Chemotherapy*, *45*(2), 621–623. doi:10.1128/AAC.45.2.621-623.2001 PMID:11158767

Pavese, P., Saurel, N., Labarère, J., Decouchon, C., Vittoz, J., Foroni, L., & François, P. et al. (2009). Does an educational session with an infectious diseases physician reduce the use of inappropriate antibiotic therapy for inpatients with positive urine culture results? A controlled before-and-after study. *Infection Control and Hospital Epidemiology*, *30*(6), 596–599. doi:10.1086/597514 PMID:19419329

Peredo, R., Sabatier, C., Villagrá, A., González, J., Hernández, C., Pérez, F., & Vallés, J. et al. (2010). Reduction in catheter-related bloodstream infections in critically ill patients through a multiple system intervention. *European Journal of Clinical Microbiology & Infectious Diseases*, *29*(9), 1173–1177. doi:10.1007/s10096-010-0971-6 PMID:20533071

Perencevich, E. N., Fisman, D. N., Lipsitch, M., Harris, A. D., Morris, J. G. Jr, & Smith, D. L. (2004). Projected benefits of active surveillance for vancomycin-resistant enterococci in intensive care units. *Clinical Infectious Diseases*, *38*(8), 1108–1115. doi:10.1086/382886 PMID:15095215

Perl, T. M., & Golub, J. E. (1998). New approaches to reduce Staphylococcus aureus nosocomial infection rates: Treating S. aureus nasal carriage. *The Annals of Pharmacotherapy*, *32*(1), S7–S16. doi:10.1177/106002809803200104 PMID:9475834

Peterson, L. R., & Smith, B. A. (2014). Non-utility of catheter tip cultures for the diagnosis of central line-associated blood stream infection (CLABSI). *Clinical Infectious Diseases*; Advance online publication. doi:10.1093/cid/ciu845 PMID:25355902

Petterson, G. B., Hussain, S. T., Shrestha, S. K., Gordon, S., Fraser, T. G., Ibrahim, K. S., & Blackstone, E. H. (2014). Infective endocarditis: An atlas of disease progression for describing, staging, coding, and understanding the pathology. *The Journal of Thoracic and Cardiovascular Surgery*, *147*(4), 1142–1149. doi:10.1016/j.jtcvs.2013.11.031 PMID:24507402

Pincock, T., Bernstein, P., Warthman, S., & Holst, E. (2012). Bundling hand hygiene interventions and measurement to decrease health care-associated infections. *American Journal of Infection Control*, *40*(4), S18–S27. doi:10.1016/j.ajic.2012.02.008 PMID:22546269

Pittet, D., Allegranzi, B., & Boyce, J.World Health Organization World Alliance for Patient Safety Challenge Core Group of Experts. (2009). The World Health Organization guidelines on hand hygiene in health care and their consensus recommendations. *Infection Control and Hospital Epidemiology*, *30*(7), 611–622. doi:10.1086/600379 PMID:19508124

Poch, D. S., & Ost, D. E. (2009). What are the important risk factors for healthcare-associated pneumonia? *Seminars in Respiratory and Critical Care Medicine*, *30*(01), 26–35. doi:10.1055/s-0028-1119806 PMID:19199184

Poelaert, J., Depuydt, P., De Wolf, A., Van de Velde, S., Herck, I., & Blot, S. (2008). Polyurethane cuffed endotracheal tubes to prevent early postoperative pneumonia after cardiac surgery: A pilot study. *The Journal of Thoracic and Cardiovascular Surgery*, *135*(4), 771–776. doi:10.1016/j.jtcvs.2007.08.052 PMID:18374755

Poelaert, J., Haentjens, P., & Blot, S. (2014). Association among duration of mechanical ventilation, cuff material of endotracheal tube, and postoperative nosocomial pneumonia in cardiac surgical patients: A prospective study. *The Journal of Thoracic and Cardiovascular Surgery*, *148*(4), 1622–1627. doi:10.1016/j.jtcvs.2014.05.085 PMID:25127550

Polderman, K. H., & Girbes, A. R. (2002). Central venous catheter use. Part 2: Infectious complications. *Intensive Care Medicine*, *28*(1), 18–28. doi:10.1007/s00134-001-1156-7 PMID:11818995

Pollack, L. A., & Srinivasan, A. (2014). Core elements of hospital antibiotic stewardship programs from the Centers for Disease Control and Prevention. *Clinical Infectious Diseases*, *59*(Suppl 3), S97–S100. doi:10.1093/cid/ciu542 PMID:25261548

Popov, A. F., Schmitto, J. D., Jebran, A. F., Bireta, C., Friedrich, M., Rajaruthnam, D., & Schoendube, F. A. et al. (2011). Treatment of gram-positive deep sternal wound infections in cardiac surgery – Experiences with daptomycin. *Journal of Cardiothoracic Surgery*, *6*(1), 112. doi:10.1186/1749-8090-6-112 PMID:21929771

Pronovost, P., Needham, D., Berenholtz, S., Sinopoli, D., Chu, H., Cosgrove, S., & Goeschel, C. et al. (2006). An intervention to decrease catheter-related bloodstream infections in the ICU. *The New England Journal of Medicine*, *355*(26), 2725–2732. doi:10.1056/NEJMoa061115 PMID:17192537

Pronovost, P. J., Goeschel, C. A., Colantuoni, E., Watson, S., Lubomski, L. H., Berenholtz, S. M., & Needham, D. et al. (2010). Sustaining reductions in catheter related bloodstream infections in Michigan intensive care units; Observational study. *British Medical Journal*, *340*(feb04 1), c309. doi:10.1136/bmj.c309 PMID:20133365

Pugin, J., Auckenthaler, R., Mili, N., Janssens, J. P., Lew, P. D., & Suter, P. M. (1991). Diagnosis of ventilator-associated pneumonia by bacteriologic analysis of bronchoscopic and nonbronchoscopic "blind" bronchoalveolar lavage fluid. *The American Review of Respiratory Disease*, *143*(5_pt_1), 1121–1129. doi:10.1164/ajrccm/143.5_Pt_1.1121 PMID:2024824

Puskas, J. D., Sadiq, A., Vassiliades, T. A., Kilgo, P. D., & Lattouf, O. M. (2012). Bilateral internal thoracic artery grafting is associated with significantly improved long-term survival, even among diabetic patients. *The Annals of Thoracic Surgery*, *94*(3), 710–716. doi:10.1016/j.athoracsur.2012.03.082 PMID:22677228

Qaseem, A., Humphrey, L. L., Chou, R., Snow, V., & Shekelle, P.Clinical Guidelines Committee of the American College of Physicians. (2011). Use of intensive insulin therapy for the management of glycemic control in hospitalized patients: A clinical practice guideline from the American College of Physicians. *Annals of Internal Medicine*, *154*(4), 260–267. doi:10.7326/0003-4819-154-4-201102150-00007 PMID:21320941

Raad, I., Hanna, H., & Maki, D. (2007). Intravascular catheter-related infections: Advances, in diagnosis, prevention, and management. *The Lancet Infectious Diseases*, *7*(10), 645–657. doi:10.1016/S1473-3099(07)70235-9 PMID:17897607

Radrizzani, D., Bertolini, G., Facchini, R., Simini, B., Bruzzone, P., Zanforlin, G., & Iapichino, G. et al. (2006). Early enteral immunonutrition vs. parenteral nutrition in critically ill patients without severe sepsis: A randomized clinical trial. *Intensive Care Medicine*, *32*(8), 1191–1198. doi:10.1007/s00134-006-0238-y PMID:16788808

Raja, S. G., & Berg, G. A. (2007). Impact of off-pump coronary artery bypass surgery on systemic inflammation: Current best available evidence. *Journal of Cardiac Surgery*, *22*(5), 445–455. doi:10.1111/j.1540-8191.2007.00447.x PMID:17803591

Rapp-Kesek, D., Ståhle, E., & Karlsson, T. (2004). Body mass index and albumin in the preoperative evaluation of cardiac surgery patients. *Clinical Nutrition (Edinburgh, Lothian)*, *23*(6), 1398–1404. doi:10.1016/j.clnu.2004.06.006 PMID:15556262

Rea-Neto, A., Youssef, N. C. M., Tuche, F., Brunkhorst, F., Ranieri, V. M., Reinhart, K., & Sakr, Y. (2008). Diagnosis of ventilator-associated pneumonia; A systematic review of the literature. *Critical Care (London, England)*, *12*(2), R56. doi:10.1186/cc6877 PMID:18426596

Resar, R., Pronovost, P., Haraden, C., Simmonds, T., Rainey, T., & Nolan, T. (2005). Using a bundle approach to improve ventilator care processes and reduce ventilator-associated pneumonia. *Joint Commission Journal on Quality and Patient Safety*, *31*, 243–248. PMID:15960014

Richey, R., Wray, D., & Stokes, T.Guideline Development Group. (2008). Prophylaxis against infective endocarditis: Summary of NICE guidance. *British Medical Journal*, *336*(7647), 770–771. doi:10.1136/bmj.39510.423148.AD PMID:18390528

Riddington, D. W., Venkatesh, B., Bolvin, C. M., Bonser, R. S., Elliott, T. S., Marshall, T., & Bion, J. F. et al. (1996). Intestinal permeability, gastric intramucosal pH, and systemic endotoxemia in patients undergoing cardiopulmonary bypass. *Journal of the American Medical Association*, *275*(13), 1007–1012. doi:10.1001/jama.1996.03530370045029 PMID:8596232

Risnes, I., Abdelnoor, M., Almdahl, S. M., & Svennevig, J. L. (2010). Mediastinitis after coronary artery bypass grafting risk factors and long-term survival. *The Annals of Thoracic Surgery*, *89*(5), 1502–1510. doi:10.1016/j.athoracsur.2010.02.038 PMID:20417768

Robiscek, A., Beaumont, J. L., Paule, S. M., Hacek, D. M., Thomson, R. B. Jr, Kaul, K. L., & Peterson, L. R. et al. (2008). Universal surveillance for methicillin-resistant Staphylococcus aureus in 3 affiliated hospitals. *Annals of Internal Medicine*, *148*(6), 409–418. doi:10.7326/0003-4819-148-6-200803180-00003 PMID:18347349

Rohde, J. M., Dimcheff, D. E., Blumberg, N., Saint, S., Langa, K. M., Kuhn, L., & Rogers, M. A. M. et al. (2014). Health care-associated infection after red blood cell transfusion. A systematic review and meta-analysis. *Journal of the American Medical Association*, *311*(13), 1317–1326. doi:10.1001/jama.2014.2726 PMID:24691607

Ruttmann, E., Willeit, J., Ulmer, H., Chevtchik, O., Höfer, D., Poewe, W., & Müller, L. C. et al. (2006). Neurological outcome of septic cardioembolic stroke after infective endocarditis. *Stroke*, *37*(8), 2094–2099. doi:10.1161/01.STR.0000229894.28591.3f PMID:16794213

Sacar, M., Sacar, S., Kaleli, I., Cevahir, N., Teke, Z., Kavas, S. T., & Turgut, H. et al. (2008). Efficacy of linezolid in the treatment of mediastinitis due to methicillin-resistant Staphylococcus aureus: An experimental study. *International Journal of Infectious Diseases*, *12*, 396–401. PMID:18162429

Saczkowski, R., Maklin, M., Mesana, T., Boodhwani, M., & Ruel, M. (2012). Centrifugal pump and roller pump in adult cardiac surgery: A meta-analysis of randomized controlled trials. *Artificial Organs*, *36*(8), 668–676. doi:10.1111/j.1525-1594.2012.01497.x PMID:22804106

Safdar, N., Dezfoulian, C., Collard, H. R., & Saint, S. (2005). Clinical and economic consequences of ventilator-associated pneumonia: A systematic review. *Critical Care Medicine*, *33*(10), 2184–2193. doi:10.1097/01.CCM.0000181731.53912.D9 PMID:16215368

Safdar, N., Kluger, D. M., & Maki, D. G. (2002). A review of risk factors for catheter-related bloodstream infection caused by percutaneously inserted, noncuffed central venous catheters: Implications for preventive strategies. *Medicine; Analytical Reviews of General Medicine, Neurology, Psychiatry, Dermatology, and Pediatries*, *81*(6), 466–479. doi:10.1097/00005792-200211000-00007 PMID:12441903

Safdar, N., & Maki, D. G. (2004). The pathogenesis of catheter-related bloodstream infection with noncuffed short-term central venous catheters. *Intensive Care Medicine*, *30*(1), 62–67. doi:10.1007/s00134-003-2045-z PMID:14647886

Safdar, N., O'Horo, J. C., Ghufran, A., Bearden, A., Didier, M. E., Chateau, D., & Maki, D. G. (2014). Chlorhexidine-impregnated dressing for prevention of catheter-related bloodstream infection: A meta-analysis. *Critical Care Medicine*, *42*(7), 1703–1713. doi:10.1097/CCM.0000000000000319 PMID:24674924

Saint, S., & Chenoweth, C. E. (2003). Biofilms in catheter-associated urinary tract infections. *Infectious Disease Clinics of North America*, *17*(2), 411–432. doi:10.1016/S0891-5520(03)00011-4 PMID:12848477

Saint, S., Greene, M. T., Kowalski, C. P., Watson, S. R., Hofer, T. P., & Krein, S. L. (2013). Preventing catheter-associated urinary tract infection in the United States. A national comparative study. *JAMA Internal Medicine*, *173*(10), 874–879. doi:10.1001/jamainternmed.2013.101 PMID:23529579

Saint, S., Meddings, J. A., Calfee, D., Kowalski, C. P., & Krein, S. L. (2009). Catheter-associated urinary tract infection and the Medicare rule changes. *Annals of Internal Medicine*, *150*(12), 877–884. doi:10.7326/0003-4819-150-12-200906160-00013 PMID:19528567

Saint, S., Olmsted, R. N., Fakih, M. G., Kowalski, C. P., Watson, S. R., Sales, A. E., & Krein, S. L. (2009). Translating health care-associated urinary tract infection prevention research into practice via the bladder bundle. *Joint Commission Journal on Quality and Patient Safety*, *35*, 449–455. PMID:19769204

Saint, S., Wiese, J., Amory, J. K., Bernstein, M. L., Patel, U. D., Zemencuk, J. K., & Hofer, T. P. et al. (2000). Are physicians aware of which of their patients have indwelling urinary catheters? *The American Journal of Medicine*, *109*(6), 476–480. doi:10.1016/S0002-9343(00)00531-3 PMID:11042237

Sainz, I. M., Pixley, R. A., & Colman, R. W. (2007). Fifty years of research on the plasma kallikrein-kinin system: From protein structure and function to cell biology and in-vivo pathophysiology. *Thrombosis and Haemostasis*, *98*, 77–83. PMID:17597995

Sandiumenge, A., Diaz, E., Bodi, M., & Rello, J. (2003). Therapy of ventilator-associated pneumonia. A patient-based approach based on the ten rules of "The Tarragona Strategy". *Intensive Care Medicine*, *29*, 876–883. PMID:12677369

Sarr, M. G., Gott, V. L., & Townsend, T. R. (1984). Mediastinal infection after cardiac surgery. *The Annals of Thoracic Surgery*, *38*(4), 415–423. doi:10.1016/S0003-4975(10)62300-4 PMID:6385892

Sauër, A. C., Slooter, A. J. C., Veldhuijzen, D. S., van Eijk, M. M. J., Devlin, J. W., & van Dijk, D. (2014). Intraoperative dexamethasone and delirium after cardiac surgery: A randomized clinical trial. *Anesthesia and Analgesia*, *119*(5), 1046–1052. doi:10.1213/ANE.0000000000000248 PMID:24810262

Savage, E. B., Grab, J. D., O'Brien, S. M., Ali, A., Okum, E. J., Perez-Tamayo, A., & Higgins, R. S. D. et al. (2007). Use of both internal thoracic arteries in diabetic patients increases deep sternal wound infections. *The Annals of Thoracic Surgery*, *83*(3), 1002–1007. doi:10.1016/j.athoracsur.2006.09.094 PMID:17307448

Savage, E. B., Saha-Chaudhuri, P., Asher, C. R., Brennan, J. M., & Gammie, J. S. (2014). Outcomes and prosthesis choice for active aortic valve infective endocarditis: Analysis of the Society of Thoracic Surgeons Adult Cardiac Surgery Database. *The Annals of Thoracic Surgery*, *98*(3), 806–814. doi:10.1016/j.athoracsur.2014.05.010 PMID:25085561

Schurink, C. A., Van Nieuwenhoven, C. A., Jacobs, J. A., Rozenberg-Arska, M., Joore, H. C., Buskens, E., & Bonten, M. J. et al. (2004). Clinical pulmonary infection score for ventilator-associated pneumonia: Accuracy and inter-observer variability. *Intensive Care Medicine*, *30*(2), 217–224. doi:10.1007/s00134-003-2018-2 PMID:14566455

Schussler, O., Dermine, H., Alifano, M., Casetta, A., Coignard, S., Roche, N., & Regnard, J. F. et al. (2008). Should we change antibiotic prophylaxis for lung surgery? Postoperative pneumonia is the critical issue. *The Annals of Thoracic Surgery*, *86*(6), 1727–1734. doi:10.1016/j.athoracsur.2008.08.005 PMID:19021965

Schweigert, M., Solymosi, N., Dubecz, A., Fernández, M. J., Stadlhuber, R., Ofner, D., & Stein, H. J. (2014). Surgery for parapneumonic pleural empyema – What influence does the rising prevalence of multimorbidity and advanced age has on the current outcome? *The Surgeon*. doi:10.1016/j.surge.2014.05.002 PMID:24930000

Segers, P., Speekenbrink, R. G. H., Ubbink, D. T., van Ogtrop, M. L., & de Mol, B. A. (2006). Prevention of nosocomial infection in cardiac surgery by decontamination of the nasopharynx and oropharynx with chlorhexidine gluconate. *Journal of the American Medical Association*, *296*(20), 2460–2466. doi:10.1001/jama.296.20.2460 PMID:17119142

Selton-Suty, C., Célard, M., Le Moing, V., Doco-Lecompte, T., Chirouze, C., Iung, B., & Hoen, B. et al. (2012). Preeminence of Staphylococcus aureus in infective endocarditis: A 1-year population-based survey. *Clinical Infectious Diseases*, *54*(9), 1230–1239. doi:10.1093/cid/cis199 PMID:22492317

Sharma, V., Deo, S. V., Stulak, J. M., Durham, L. A. III, Daly, R. C., Park, S. J., & Joyce, L. D. et al. (2012). Driveline infections in left ventricular assist devices: Implications for destination therapy. *The Annals of Thoracic Surgery*, *94*(5), 1381–1386. doi:10.1016/j.athoracsur.2012.05.074 PMID:22818961

Sheng, W., Xing, Q., Hou, W., Sun, L., Niu, Z., Lin, M., & Chi, Y. (2014). Independent risk factors for ventilator-associated pneumonia after cardiac surgery. *Journal of Investigative Surgery*, *27*(5), 256–261. doi:10.3109/08941939.2014.892652 PMID:24660655

Shi, Z., Xie, H., Wang, P., Zhang, Q., Wu, Y., Chen, E., & Furness, S. et al. (2013). Oral hygiene for critically ill patients to prevent ventilator-associated pneumonia. *Cochrane Database of Systematic Reviews*, CD008367. PMID:23939759

Sievert, D. M., Ricks, P., Edwards, J. R., Schneider, A., Patel, J., Srinivasan, A., & Fridkin, S. et al. (2013). Antimicrobial-resistant pathogens associated with healthcare-associated infections: Summary of data reported to the National Healthcare Safety Network at the Centers for Disease Control and Prevention, 2009-2010. *Infection Control and Hospital Epidemiology*, *34*(1), 1–14. doi:10.1086/668770 PMID:23221186

Silvestri, L., van Saene, H. K., Casarin, A., Berlot, G., & Gullo, A. (2008). Impact of selective decontamination of the digestive tract on carriage and infection due to Gram-negative and Gram-positive bacteria: A systematic review of randomised controlled trials. *Anaesthesia and Intensive Care*, *36*, 324–338. PMID:18564793

Sjögren, J., Malmsjö, M., Gustafsson, R., & Ingemansson, R. (2006). Poststernotomy mediastinitis: A review of conventional surgical treatments, vacuum-associated closure therapy and presentation of the Lund University Hospital mediastinitis algorithm. *European Journal of Cardio-Thoracic Surgery*, *30*(6), 898–905. doi:10.1016/j.ejcts.2006.09.020 PMID:17056269

Snyder, C. W., Graham, L. A., Byers, R. E., & Holman, W. L. (2009). Primary sternal plating to prevent sternal wound complications after cardiac surgery: Early experience and patterns of failure. *Interactive Cardiovascular and Thoracic Surgery*, *9*(5), 763–766. doi:10.1510/icvts.2009.214023 PMID:19710069

Song, D. H., Lohman, R. F., Renucci, J. D., Jeevanandam, V., & Raman, J. (2004). Primary sternal plating in high-risk patients prevents mediastinitis. *European Journal of Cardio-Thoracic Surgery*, *26*(2), 367–372. doi:10.1016/j.ejcts.2004.04.038 PMID:15296898

Springer, T. A. (1994). Traffic signals for lymphocyte recirculation leukocyte emigration: The multistep paradigm. *Cell*, *76*(2), 301–314. doi:10.1016/0092-8674(94)90337-9 PMID:7507411

Srinivasan, A., Song, X., Ross, T., Merz, W., Brower, R., & Perl, T. M. (2002). A prospective study to determine whether cover gowns in addition to gloves decrease nosocomial transmission of vancomycin-resistant enterococci in an intensive care unit. *Infection Control and Hospital Epidemiology*, *23*(8), 424–428. doi:10.1086/502079 PMID:12186206

Steinkraus, G., White, R., & Friedrich, L. (2007). Vancomycin MIC creep in non-vancomycin-intermediate Staphylococcus aureus (VISA), vancomycin-susceptible clinical methicillin-resistant S. aureus (MRSA) blood isolates from 2001-05. *The Journal of Antimicrobial Chemotherapy*, *60*(4), 788–794. doi:10.1093/jac/dkm258 PMID:17623693

Stone, P. W., Braccia, D., & Larson, E. (2005). Systematic review of economic analyses of health care-associated infections. *American Journal of Infection Control*, *33*(9), 501–509. doi:10.1016/j.ajic.2005.04.246 PMID:16260325

Stone, P. W., Pogorzelska-Maziarz, M., Herzig, C. T. A., Weiner, L. M., Furuya, E. Y., Dick, A., & Larson, E. (2014). State of infection prevention in US hospitals enrolled in the National Health and Safety Network. *American Journal of Infection Control*, *42*(2), 94–99. doi:10.1016/j.ajic.2013.10.003 PMID:24485365

Surawicz, C. M., Brandt, L. J., Binion, D. G., Ananthakrishnan, A. N., Curry, S. R., Gilligan, P. H., & Zuckerbraun, B. S. et al. (2013). Guidelines for diagnosis, treatment, and prevention of Clostridum difficile infections. *The American Journal of Gastroenterology*, *108*(4), 478–498. doi:10.1038/ajg.2013.4 PMID:23439232

Tambyah, P. A., Halvorson, K. T., & Maki, D. G. (1999). A prospective study of pathogenesis of catheter-associated urinary tract infections. *Mayo Clinic Proceedings*, *74*(2), 131–136. doi:10.4065/74.2.131 PMID:10069349

Tambyah, P. A., & Maki, D. G. (2000). Catheter-associated urinary tract infection is rarely symptomatic. A prospective study of 1497 catheterized patients. *Archives of Internal Medicine*, *160*(5), 678–682. doi:10.1001/archinte.160.5.678 PMID:10724054

Tang, H., Lin, H., Lin, Y., Leung, P., Chuang, Y., & Lai, C. (2014). The impact of central line insertion bundle on central line-associated bloodstream infection. *BMC Infectious Diseases*, *14*(1), 356. doi:10.1186/1471-2334-14-356 PMID:24985729

Thanavaro, K. L., & Nixon, J. V. (2014). Endocarditis 2014: An update. *Heart & Lung*, *43*(4), 334–337. doi:10.1016/j.hrtlng.2014.03.009 PMID:24780242

Thuny, F., Avierinos, J., Tribouilloy, C., Giorgi, R., Casalta, J., Milandre, L., & Habib, G. et al. (2007). Impact of cerebrovascular complications on mortality and neurologic outcome during infective endocarditis: A prospective multicentre study. *European Heart Journal*, *28*(9), 1155–1161. doi:10.1093/eurheartj/ehm005 PMID:17363448

Thuny, F., Beurtheret, S., Mancini, J., Gariboldi, V., Casalta, J., Riberi, A., & Habib, G. et al. (2011). The timing of surgery influences mortality and morbidity in adults with severe complicated infective endocarditis: A propensity analysis. *European Heart Journal*, *32*(16), 2027–2033. doi:10.1093/eurheartj/ehp089 PMID:19329497

Thuny, F., Grisoli, D., Collart, F., Habib, G., & Raoult, D. (2012). Management of infective endocarditis: Challenges and perspectives. *Lancet*, *379*(9819), 965–975. doi:10.1016/S0140-6736(11)60755-1 PMID:22317840

Timsit, J., Mimoz, O., Mourvillier, B., Souweine, B., Garrouste-Orgeas, M., Alfandari, S., & Lucet, J. et al. (2012). Randomized controlled trial of chlorhexidine dressing and highly adhesive dressing for preventing catheter-related infections in critically ill adults. *American Journal of Respiratory and Critical Care Medicine*, *186*(12), 1272–1278. doi:10.1164/rccm.201206-1038OC PMID:23043083

Timsit, J., Schwebel, C., Bouadma, L., Geffroy, A., Garrouste-Orgeas, M., Pease, S., & Dressing Study Group, et al.. (2009). Chlorhexidine-impregnated sponges and less frequent dressing changes for prevention of catheter-related infections in critically ill adults: A randomized controlled trial. *Journal of the American Medical Association*, *301*(12), 1231–1241. doi:10.1001/jama.2009.376 PMID:19318651

Tocco, M. P., Constantino, A., Ballardini, M., D'Andrea, C., Masala, M., Merico, E., & Sordini, P. et al. (2009). Improved results of the vacuum-assisted closure and Nitinol clips sternal closure after postoperative deep sternal wound infection. *European Journal of Cardio-Thoracic Surgery*, *35*(5), 833–838. doi:10.1016/j.ejcts.2008.12.036 PMID:19216084

Toumpoulis, I. K., Anagnostopoulos, C. E., DeRose, J. J., & Swistel, D. G. (2005). The impact of deep sternal wound infection on long-term survival after coronary artery bypass grafting. *Chest*, *127*(2), 464–471. doi:10.1378/chest.127.2.464 PMID:15705983

Tousoulis, D., Psarros, C., Demosthenous, M., Patel, R., Antoniades, C., & Stefanadis, C. (2014). Innate and adaptive inflammation as a therapeutic target in vascular disease. *Journal of the American College of Cardiology*, *63*(23), 2491–2502. doi:10.1016/j.jacc.2014.01.054 PMID:24613322

Twele, L., Moyen, E., Zhang, K., Dalton, B., Church, D., & Conly, J. (2010). Methicillin-resistant Staphylococcus aureus endocarditis and de novo development of daptomycin resistance during therapy. *The Canadian Journal of Infectious Diseases & Medical Microbiology = Journal Canadien des Maladies Infectieuses et de la Microbiologie Medicale / AMMI Canada*, *21*, 89–93. PMID:21629617

Udy, A. A., Roberts, J. A., & Lipman, J. (2013). Clinical implications of antibiotic pharmacokinetic principles in the critically ill. *Intensive Care Medicine*, *39*(12), 2070–2082. doi:10.1007/s00134-013-3088-4 PMID:24045886

Ullman, A. J., Cooke, M. L., Gillies, D., Marsh, N. M., Daud, A., McGrail, M. R., & Rickard, C. M. et al. (2013). Optimal timing for intravascular administration set replacement. *Cochrane Database of Systematic Reviews*, CD003588. PMID:24037784

Vallés, J., Fernández, I., Alcaraz, D., Chacón, E., Cazorla, A., Canals, M., & Morón, A. et al. (2008). Prospective randomized trial of 3 antiseptic solutions for prevention of catheter colonization in an intensive care unit for adult patients. *Infection Control and Hospital Epidemiology*, *29*(9), 847–853. doi:10.1086/590259 PMID:18665819

Verma, S., Fedak, P. W., Weisel, R. D., Butany, J., Rao, V., Maitland, A., & Yau, T. M. et al. (2002). Fundamentals of reperfusion injury for the clinical cardiologist. *Circulation*, *105*(20), 2332–2336. doi:10.1161/01.CIR.0000016602.96363.36 PMID:12021216

Verrier, E. D., Shernan, S. K., Taylor, K. M., Van de Werf, F., Newman, M. F., Chen, J. C., & Levy, J. H. et al.for the PRIMO-CABG Investigators. (2004). Terminal complement blockade with pexelizumab during coronary artery bypass graft surgery requiring cardiopulmonary bypass: A randomized trial. *Journal of the American Medical Association*, *291*(19), 2319–2327. doi:10.1001/jama.291.19.2319 PMID:15150203

Vind, S. H., & Hess, S. (2010). Possible role of PET/CT in infective endocarditis. *Journal of Nuclear Cardiology*, *17*(3), 516–519. doi:10.1007/s12350-009-9174-x PMID:19953353

Wald, H. L., Ma, A., Bratzler, D. W., & Kramer, A. M. (2008). Indwelling urinary catheter use in the postoperative period: Analysis of the National Surgical Infection Prevention Project data. *Archives of Surgery*, *143*(6), 551–557. doi:10.1001/archsurg.143.6.551 PMID:18559747

Walkey, A. J., O'Donnell, M. R., & Wiener, R. S. (2011). Linezolid vs glycopeptide antibiotics for the treatment of suspected methicillin-resistant Staphylococcus aureus nosocomial pneumonia: A meta-analysis of randomized controlled trials. *Chest*, *139*(5), 1148–1155. doi:10.1378/chest.10-1556 PMID:20864609

Wan, S., Leclerc, J. L., & Vincent, J. L. (1997). Inflammatory response to cardiopulmonary bypass: Mechanisms involved and possible therapeutic strategies. *Chest*, *112*(3), 676–692. doi:10.1378/chest.112.3.676 PMID:9315800

Warren, D. K., Zack, J. E., Mayfield, J. L., Chen, A., Prentice, D., Fraser, V. J., & Kollef, M. H. (2004). The effect of an education program on the incidence of central venous catheter-associated bloodstream infection in a medical ICU. *Chest*, *126*(5), 1612–1618. doi:10.1378/chest.126.5.1612 PMID:15539735

Weber, D. J., Sickbert-Bennett, E. E., Gould, C. V., Brown, V. M., Huslage, K., & Rutala, W. A. (2011). Incidence of catheter-associated and non-catheter-associated urinary tract infections in a healthcare system. *Infection Control and Hospital Epidemiology*, *32*(8), 822–823. doi:10.1086/661107 PMID:21768769

Webster, J., & Osborne, S. (2007). Preoperative bathing or showering with skin antiseptics to prevent surgical site infections. *Cochrane Database of Systematic Reviews*, CD004985. PMID:17443562

Weeks, K. R., Hsu, Y. J., Yang, T., Sawyer, M., & Marsteller, J. A. (2014). Influence of a multifaceted intervention on central line days in intensive care units: Results of a national multisite study. *American Journal of Infection Control*, *42*(10Suppl), S197–S202. doi:10.1016/j.ajic.2014.06.003 PMID:25239710

Weerasinghe, A., Athanasiou, T., Philippidis, P., Day, J., Mandal, K., Warren, O., & Taylor, K. et al. (2006). Platelet-monocyte pro-coagulant interactions in on-pump coronary surgery. *European Journal of Cardio-Thoracic Surgery*, *29*(3), 312–318. doi:10.1016/j.ejcts.2005.11.036 PMID:16423536

Whitlock, R. P., Chan, S., Devereaux, J. P., Sun, J., Rubens, F. D., Thorlund, K., & Teoh, K. H. T. (2008). Clinical benefit of steroid use in patients undergoing cardiopulmonary bypass: A meta-analysis of randomized trials. *European Heart Journal*, *29*(21), 2592–2600. doi:10.1093/eurheartj/ehn333 PMID:18664462

Widmer, A. F. (2000). Replace hand washing with use of a waterless alcohol hand rub? *Clinical Infectious Diseases*, *31*(1), 136–143. doi:10.1086/313888 PMID:10913411

Wilson, W., Taubert, K. A., Gewitz, M., Lockhart, P. B., Baddour, L. M., Levison, M., & Durack, D. T. et al. (2007). Prevention of infective endocarditis: Guidelines from the American Heart Association: A guideline from the American Heart Association Rheumatic Fever, Endocarditis, and Kawasaki Disease Committee, Council on Cardiovascular Disease in the Young, and the Council on Clinical Cardiology, Council on Cardiovascular Surgery and Anesthesia, and the Quality of Care and Outcomes Research Interdisciplinary Working Group. *Circulation*, *116*(15), 1736–1754. doi:10.1161/CIRCULATIONAHA.106.183095 PMID:17446442

Wip, C., & Napolitano, L. (2009). Bundles to prevent ventilator-associated pneumonia: How valuable are they? *Current Opinion in Infectious Diseases*, *22*(2), 159–166. doi:10.1097/QCO.0b013e3283295e7b PMID:19276975

Wunderink, R. G., Niederman, M. S., Kollef, M. H., Shorr, A. F., Kunkel, M. J., Baruch, A., & Chastre, J. et al. (2012). Linezolid in methicillin-resistant Staphylococcus aureus nosocomial pneumonia: A randomized, controlled study. *Clinical Infectious Diseases*, *54*(5), 621–629. doi:10.1093/cid/cir895 PMID:22247123

Yu, A. W., Rippel, R. A., Smock, E., & Jarral, O. A. (2013). In patients with post-sternotomy mediastinitis is vacuum-assisted closure superior to conventional therapy? *Interactive Cardiovascular and Thoracic Surgery*, *17*(5), 861–866. doi:10.1093/icvts/ivt326 PMID:23912622

Zack, J. E., Garrison, T., Trovillion, E., Clinkscale, D., Coopersmith, C. M., Fraser, V. J., & Kollef, M. H. (2002). Effect of an education program aimed at reducing the occurrence of ventilator-associated pneumonia. *Critical Care Medicine*, *30*(11), 2407–2412. doi:10.1097/00003246-200211000-00001 PMID:12441746

Zaouter, C., Kaneva, P., & Carli, F. (2009). Less urinary tract infection by earlier removal of bladder catheter in surgical patients receiving thoracic epidural analgesia. *Regional Anesthesia and Pain Medicine*, *34*(6), 542–548. doi:10.1097/AAP.0b013e3181ae9fac PMID:19916208

Zaouter, C., & Ouattara, A. (2014). How long is a transurethral catheter necessary in patients undergoing thoracotomy and receiving thoracic epidural analgesia? Literature review. *Journal of Cardiothoracic and Vascular Anesthesia*; Advance online publication. doi:10.1053/j.jcva.2014.05.022 PMID:25287748

Zarbock, A., & Ley, K. (2008). Mechanisms and consequences of neutrophil interaction with the endothelium. *American Journal of Pathology*, *172*(1), 1–7. doi:10.2353/ajpath.2008.070502 PMID:18079440

Zarbock, A., Mueller, E., Netzer, S., Gabriel, A., Feindt, P., & Kindgen-Milles, D. (2009). Prophylactic nasal continuous positive airway pressure following cardiac surgery protects from postoperative pulmonary complications. *Chest*, *135*(5), 1252–1259. doi:10.1378/chest.08-1602 PMID:19017864

Zegdi, R., Debièche, M., Latrémouille, C., Lebied, D., Chardigny, C., Grinda, J., & Fabiani, J. et al. (2005). Long-term results of mitral valve repair in active endocarditis. *Circulation*, *111*(19), 2532–2536. doi:10.1161/01.CIR.0000165122.08660.1A PMID:15867185

Zerr, K. J., Furnary, A. P., Grunkemeier, G. L., Bookin, S., Kanhere, V., & Starr, A. (1997). Glucose control lowers the risk of wound infection in diabetics after open heart operations. *The Annals of Thoracic Surgery*, *63*, 356–361. doi:10.1016/S0003-4975(96)01044-2 PMID:9033300

Zilberberg, M. D., Shorr, A. F., & Kollef, M. H. (2009). Implementing quality improvements in the intensive care unit: Ventilator bundle as an example. *Critical Care Medicine*, *37*(1), 305–309. doi:10.1097/CCM.0b013e3181926623 PMID:19050626

ADDITIONAL READING

Barsanti, M. C., & Woeltje, K. F. (2009). Infection prevention in the intensive care unit. *Infectious Disease Clinics of North America*, *23*(3), 703–725. doi:10.1016/j.idc.2009.04.012 PMID:19665091

Bedeir, K., Reardon, M., & Ramlawi, B. (2014). Infective endocarditis: Perioperative management and surgical principles. *The Journal of Thoracic and Cardiovascular Surgery*, *147*(4), 133–141. doi:10.1016/j.jtcvs.2013.11.022 PMID:24412256

Chenoweth, C. E., Gould, C. V., & Saint, S. (2014). Diagnosis, management, and prevention of catheter-associated urinary tract infections. *Infectious Disease Clinics of North America*, *28*(1), 105–119. doi:10.1016/j.idc.2013.09.002 PMID:24484578

Craven, D. E., Lei, Y., Ruthazer, R., Sarwar, A., & Hudcova, J. (2013). Incidence and outcomes of ventilator-associated tracheobronchitis and pneumonia. *The American Journal of Medicine*, *126*(6), 542–549. doi:10.1016/j.amjmed.2012.12.012 PMID:23561632

De Pascale, G., Bello, G., Tumbarello, M., & Antonelli, M. (2012). Severe pneumonia in intensive care: Cause, diagnosis, treatment and management: A review of the literature. *Current Opinion in Pulmonary Medicine*, *18*(3), 213–221. doi:10.1097/MCP.0b013e328351f9bd PMID:22388582

Erwin, J. P., & Otto, C. M. (2014). Infective endocarditis: Old problem, new guidelines and still much to learn. *Heart (British Cardiac Society)*, *100*(13), 996–998. doi:10.1136/heartjnl-2014-305836 PMID:24794421

Fitch, Z. W., & Whitman, G. J. R. (2014). Indidence, risk, and prevention of ventilator-associated pneumonia in adult cardiac surgery patients: A systematic review. *Journal of Cardiac Surgery*, *29*(2), 196–203. doi:10.1111/jocs.12260 PMID:24304223

Fournier, P. E., Drancourt, M., Colson, P., Rolain, J. M., La Scola, B., & Raoult, D. (2013). Modern clinical microbiology: New challenges and solutions. *Nature Reviews. Microbiology*, *11*(8), 574–585. doi:10.1038/nrmicro3068 PMID:24020074

Klompas, M., Branson, R., Eichenwald, E. C., Greene, L. R., Howell, M. D., Lee, G., & Berenholtz, S. M. et al. (2014). Strategies to prevent ventilator-associated pneumonia in acute care hospitals: 2014 update. *Infection Control and Hospital Epidemiology*, *35*(8), 915–936. doi:10.1086/677144 PMID:25026607

Lador, A., Nasir, H., Mansur, N., Sharoni, E., Biderman, P., Leibovici, L., & Paul, M. (2012). Antibiotic prophylaxis in cardiac surgery: Systematic review and meta-analysis. *The Journal of Antimicrobial Chemotherapy*, *67*(3), 541–550. doi:10.1093/jac/dkr470 PMID:22083832

Laffey, J. G., Boylan, J. F., & Cheng, D. C. H. (2002). The systemic inflammatory response to cardiac surgery. *Anesthesiology*, *97*(1), 215–252. doi:10.1097/00000542-200207000-00030 PMID:12131125

Lepelletier, D., Bourigault, C., Roussel, J. C., Lasserre, C., Leclère, B., Corvec, S., & Despins, P. et al. (2013). Epidemiology and prevention of surgical site infections after cardiac surgery. *Medecine et Maladies Infectieuses*, *43*(10), 403–409. doi:10.1016/j.medmal.2013.07.003 PMID:23988675

Lorente, L., Blot, S., & Rello, J. (2010). New issues and controversies in the prevention of ventilator-associated pneumonia. *American Journal of Respiratory and Critical Care Medicine*, *182*(7), 870–876. doi:10.1164/rccm.201001-0081CI PMID:20448095

Magill, S. S., Klompas, M., Balk, R., Burns, S. M., Deutschman, C. S., Diekema, D., & Lipsett, P. et al. (2013). Developing a new, national approach to surveillance for ventilator-associated events. *Critical Care Medicine*, *41*(11), 2467–2475. doi:10.1097/CCM.0b013e3182a262db PMID:24162674

Martin, G. S. (2012). Sepsis, severe sepsis and septic shock: Changes in incidence, pathogens and outcomes. *Expert Review of Anti-Infective Therapy*, *10*(6), 701–706. doi:10.1586/eri.12.50 PMID:22734959

Mauermann, W. J., Sampathkumar, P., & Thompson, R. L. (2008). Sternal wound infections. *Best Practice & Research. Clinical Anaesthesiology*, *22*(3), 423–436. doi:10.1016/j.bpa.2008.04.003 PMID:18831296

Mietto, C., Pinciroli, R., Patel, N., & Berra, L. (2013). Ventilator-associated pneumonia: Evolving definitions and preventive strategies. *Respiratory Care*, *58*(6), 990–1003. doi:10.4187/respcare.02380 PMID:23709196

Nienaber, J., Wilhelm, M. P., & Sohail, M. R. (2013). Current concepts in the diagnosis and managements of left ventricular assist device infections. *Expert Review of Anti-Infective Therapy*, *11*(2), 201–210. doi:10.1586/eri.12.163 PMID:23409825

Petterson, G. B., Hussain, S. T., Shrestha, S. K., Gordon, S., Fraser, T. G., Ibrahim, K. S., & Blackstone, E. H. (2014). Infective endocarditis: An atlas of disease progression for describing, staging, coding, and understanding the pathology. *The Journal of Thoracic and Cardiovascular Surgery*, *147*(4), 1142–1149. doi:10.1016/j.jtcvs.2013.11.031 PMID:24507402

Pittet, D., Allegranzi, B., Sax, H., Dharan, S., Pessoa-Silva, C. L., Donaldson, L., & Boyce, J. M.WHO Global Patient Safety Challenge, World Alliance for Patient Safety. (2006). Evidence-based model for hand transmission during patient care and the role of improved practices. *The Lancet Infectious Diseases*, *6*(10), 641–652. doi:10.1016/S1473-3099(06)70600-4 PMID:17008173

Prendergast, B. D., & Tornos, P. (2010). Surgery for infective endocarditis: Who and when? *Circulation*, *121*(9), 1141–1152. doi:10.1161/CIRCULATIONAHA.108.773598 PMID:20212293

Thuny, F., Gaubert, J., Jacquier, A., Tessonnier, L., Cammilleri, S., Raoult, D., & Habib, G. (2013). Imaging investigations in infective endocarditis: Current approach and perspectives. *Archives of Cardiovascular Disease*, *106*(1), 52–62. doi:10.1016/j.acvd.2012.09.004 PMID:23374972

Thuny, F., Grisoli, D., Collart, F., Habib, G., & Raoult, D. (2012). Management of infective endocarditis: Challenges and perspectives. *Lancet*, *379*(9819), 965–975. doi:10.1016/S0140-6736(11)60755-1 PMID:22317840

Weber, D. J., & Rutala, W. A. (2011). Central line-associated blood stream infections: Prevention and management. *Infectious Disease Clinics of North America*, *25*(1), 77–102. doi:10.1016/j.idc.2010.11.012 PMID:21315995

KEY TERMS AND DEFINITIONS

Antibiotic Resistance: Capability of a microorganism to reduce or neutralize the efficacy of an antibiotic substance.

Care Bundle: Combining evidence-based interventions to prevent infection and improve outcomes.

Colony Forming Unit (CFU): A method to quantify the growth of an isolated microorganism.

Infection Control: Prevention (hygiene), monitoring (surveillance), and management (isolation) in the healthcare environment.

Ischemia-Reperfusion Injury: The fact that reperfusion of an ischemic organ or region causes additional tissue damage.

Minimum Inhibitory Concentration (MIC): The lowest concentration of an antibiotic drug that will inhibit the visible growth of an isolated microorganism.

Systemic Inflammatory Response Syndrome (SIRS): Host response to an infectious or non-infectious insult featuring systemic symptoms such as cardiovascular instability.

Chapter 20
Hematology and Transfusion

Zarah Antongiorgi
UCLA, USA

Vadim Gudzenko
UCLA, USA

ABSTRACT

The cardiac perioperative period presents a unique clinical scenario where the risk of life-threatening hemorrhage is balanced against the risk of thrombosis. Management practices are in a continual flux as practitioners respond to evidence showing the serious harms independently associated with anemia, bleeding and transfusion of blood (Ranucci, Aronson, et al., 2011a). Despite comprehensive transfusion guideline recommendations rates of blood transfusion range from 7.8% to 92.8% across US hospitals (Bennett-Guerrero et al., 2010). In this chapter we navigate the complex hemostasis and transfusion issues in cardiac surgery to provide clinicians a comprehensive understanding of the coagulation system in this specialized population. We emphasize a multidisciplinary team approach focused on risk stratification with preoperative optimization to minimize coagulopathy and bleeding followed by a tailored and conservative use of blood products for maximum patient benefit.

INTRODUCTION

Cardiac surgery is associated with a high potential for life-threatening bleeding. The propensity to bleed is multifactorial and dependent on the combined effects of the surgical intervention, the application of antithrombotic and antiplatelet therapies as part of the medical management for cardiovascular disease plus the resultant hemodilution and associated coagulopathy predictably following CPB. While most cardiac patients tolerate the coagulation alteration secondary to implementation of CPB, up to half will receive a blood transfusion totaling up to 2.5 million blood transfusions a year (Speiss, 2002). When life-threatening bleeding occurs, timely blood product administration supports the hemodynamics, reverses coagulopathy and treats anemia to restore hemoglobin and ensure adequate delivery of oxygen

DOI: 10.4018/978-1-4666-8603-8.ch020

to tissues. Multiple studies have demonstrated the negative consequences of anemia in cardiac surgery patients including increased renal failure, strokes and mortality (Carson et al., 2011; Loor et al., 2012; van Straten et al., 2009).

In the non-bleeding cardiac surgery patient with anemia no data supports a universally applicable hemoglobin level at which to transfuse and our ability to measure oxygen levels at organs is scarce. The transfusion of blood in anemic patients should help in oxygen delivery to tissues but there is evidence that transfused blood fails to increase tissue oxygen utilization (Suttner et al., 2004). In addition, the potential infectious, inflammatory and immunomodulatory effects of blood transfusion cannot be underestimated. The evidence for worsened outcomes after transfusion of even a single unit of blood in cardiac surgical patients continues to grow and includes increased risk of infection, sepsis, renal failure, prolonged mechanical ventilation and mortality (Koch et al., 2006; Murphy et al., 2007; van Straten et al., 2009). With a greater concern for the risks of transfusion, tolerance of anemia emerged and several randomized control trials were performed comparing liberal and restrictive transfusion strategies in a variety of clinical settings showing no mortality benefit with a higher hemoglobin (Carson et al., 2011; Hajjar et al., 2010; Hébert et al., 1999; Villanueva et al., 2013)

The true relative risk of allogenic blood transfusion versus anemia is unknown and there is marked variation in transfusion practices across hospitals. Evaluating the cardiac patients receiving transfusions has identified that 80% of blood products are being used in only 10-20% of all patients (V. A. Ferraris & Ferraris, 1995). Risk factors for blood transfusion after cardiac surgery include emergency surgery, low preoperative hematocrit, older age, female sex, length of cardiopulmonary bypass time, complexity of surgery, poor left ventricular function, insulin dependent diabetes and renal insufficiency (Despotis et al., 1996; V. A. Ferraris et al., 2011). Identifying modifiable risk factors while developing tools and techniques to optimize patients pre-operatively combined with coagulopathy prevention to minimize bleeding and reliance on transfusion as treatment for anemia forms the basis of effective Patient Blood Management (PBM) protocols. Curtailing bleeding and transfusion involves timely cessation of pre-operative anticoagulation medications, special considerations with hemodilution on CPB, employing pharmacologic therapies directed at minimizing fibrinolysis, implementing goal directed hemostatic therapy practices using alternatives to traditional blood components for coagulopathy reversal and prioritizing leukoreduced and newer blood products to diminish inflammatory or immunomodulatory effects. A multidisciplinary team should be responsible for the execution of the Patient Blood Management protocols as teams, not individuals, care for cardiac patients in the Operating Room (OR) and the Intensive Care Unit (ICU).

Chapter Objectives:

- Define and review the coagulation abnormalities present in the post-cardiac surgery patient
- Review the pharmacologic management of coagulopathy in the cardiac surgery patient
- Review the consequences of anemia, bleeding and blood transfusion in cardiac surgery patients
- Review strategies for the management of the bleeding cardiac surgery patient
- Define the rationale and indications for currently available blood and blood component therapy
- Review strategies for blood conservation in cardiac surgery
- Review future research and emerging trends in the hematologic issues affecting cardiac surgery patients

BLEEDING, COAGULOPATHY, AND ANEMIA

Several hematologic insults occur that increase the risk of bleeding in cardiac surgery with 3-10% of patients experiencing excessive postoperative bleeding (Whitlock, Crowther, & Ng, 2005). One series looking at 16,000 patients' chest tube output in the first 12 hours showed risk of operative mortality was 3 times higher in major bleeders and with every incremental increase of 100 mL the mortality risk increased by 12% (Ranucci, Baryshnikova, Castelvecchio, Pelissero, 2013). While the definition of hemorrhage is ill defined, it increases the need for re-exploration and this is often the corollary used to track significant hemorrhage. Re-operation occurs in 2-8% of cardiac patients and is associated with prolonged mechanical ventilation and hospital stay, higher rates of renal failure and decreased survival (Vivacqua et al., 2011). A retrospective analysis of 1188 patients following cardiac surgery with CPB found 6.4% experienced post-operative hemorrhage defined by chest tube drainage exceeding 200 ml/hr for one hour or > 2 ml/kg/hr for two consecutive hours within the first 6 hours after operation (Christensen, Dziewior, Kempel, & Heymann, 2012). Patients with excessive bleeding were significantly more likely to experience stroke, require re-exploration and not survive to 30 days. Further analysis defined 495 ml of chest tube output within the first 24 hours post-operatively as the threshold level of bleeding most predictive of reduced 30-day mortality. In this series, 84% of patients experiencing post-operative hemorrhage received red blood cell transfusion compared to 25% of patients without hemorrhage, reinforcing the fact that bleeding is not the only indication guiding blood transfusion. Up to 25% of transfusions in cardiac surgery are considered inappropriate (Goodnough, Soegiarso, Birkmeyer, & Welch, 1993).

Bleeding in cardiac surgery occurs due to surgical and medical reasons. Surgical sites at risk for bleeding include suture lines at anastomotic sites, side branches of conduits, substernal soft tissues and periostium and cannulation sites (Bojar, 2011). Re-exploration is associated with significant morbidity and increased mortality, but delaying re-exploration more than 12 hours exposes patients to more vasopressors, more blood products and the risk of low cardiac output syndrome with subsequent organ failure (Choong, Gerrard, Goldsmith, Dunningham, & Vuylsteke, 2007; Karthik, Grayson, McCarron, Pullan, & Desmond, 2004). Approximately 60-70% of post-operative bleeding requiring return to the OR is surgical in nature however non-surgical bleeding from coagulopathy heralds much higher risk of worsened outcomes including death (Hall et al., 2001).

The management of medical bleeding is much more challenging given the complexity of the coagulation system, especially after cardiac surgery. The basic components of successful hemostasis include primary measures of platelet aggregation at a site of injury and secondary measures of fibrin cross-linking to create clot. The classic coagulation model originated in the 1960s with the description of the parallel extrinsic and intrinsic pathways, each with a cascade of zymogen activation leading to a common pathway creating the critical prothrombinase complex composed of Factors Xa, Va plus calcium on a phospholipid membrane (Davie & Ratnoff, 1964). Prothrombinase complex is responsible for converting prothrombin (factor II) to thrombin that catalyzes conversion of fibrinogen (Factor I) into fibrin. Thrombin is also critical for activation of platelets and other factors, importantly Factor XIII, which is necessary for taking cross-linked fibrin monomers and polymerizing the links to form a stable clot resistant to lysis. The extrinsic pathway is initiated when trauma exposes vascular subendothelium to reveal tissue factor (TF), also called thromboplastin, which binds and forms complexes with Factor VII to allow activation of Factor X and initiation of prothrombinase complex formation. The intrinsic pathway starts with Factor XII, high molecular weight kininogen and prekallekrein activation following blood interaction with artificial surfaces or launching of the complement system. This leads to Factor XI activation which then utilizes and activates Factors VIII and IX to activate Factors X and V to create the prothrombinase complex. (Figure 1)

Since the description of the profactor model of hemostasis, an in vivo cell-based model has been proposed which describes hemostasis as a function of cell membranes occurring in three overlapping phases: initiation, amplification and propagation (Hoffman & Monroe, 2007) (Figure 2).

The ***initiation phase*** involves an injured cell bearing tissue factor that combines with Factor VII to activate Factors IX plus X and V to form prothrombinase complex that produces small amounts of thrombin. The ***amplification phase*** uses collagen at the site of tissue injury to bind free von Willebrand Factor (vWF), which then acts to capture platelets via attachment to glycoprotein receptors. Once adhered, platelets are stimulated by the localized thrombin leading to expression of several additional glycoprotein receptors including GIb and GIIb/IIIa that attract Factors VIII, vWF, and XI and promotes platelet aggregation (Rinder, Bohnert, & Rinder 1991). The activated platelet membrane serves as a stage for concentrated thrombin mediated factor activation and subsequent creation of prothrombinase complex necessary for even more thrombin production. Activated platelets also undergo conformational change causing release of potent platelet agonists – thromboxane A2 (TXA2) and adenosine diphosphate (ADP). ADP specifically works on platelets at P2Y1 and P2Y12 receptors and causes release of granules containing procoagulant substances like vWF and FVa to further sustain and intensify coagulant actions and thrombin production on the membrane surface. The ***propagation phase*** results when accelerated prothrombinase complex production on the activated platelet surface produces a massive localized thrombin burst sufficient for fibrin production and clot formation. A single thrombin activated platelet can expose more than 12,000 copies of GIIb/IIIa receptors for platelet aggregation and fibrinogen binding for rapid fibrin clot formation (Tanaka, Key & Levy, 2009).

As soon as the coagulation cascade is initiated, simultaneous activation of the fibrinolysis system is occurring to limit the extent of clot formation in the body. In response to TF generation, endothelial cells release tissue factor pathway inhibitor (TFPI) which neutralizes Factor Xa when combined with VIIa:TF complexes. Antithrombin III (ATIII) is a serine protease inhibitor released in response to TF that works to deactivate thrombin (Factor IIa) and Factors XIIa, XIa and Xa. Additionally, the procoagulant effects of thrombin are balanced by the triggered release of tissue plasminogen activator (tPA) to catalyze the cleavage of plasminogen to plasmin, the enzyme responsible for the degradation of fibrin clot into inactive fragments known as D-dimers. Plasmin also neutralizes Factors Va and VIIIa and alters platelet glycoprotein receptors to impair platelet aggregation. Free thrombin may also travel away from the vascular injury site and bind to thrombomodulin on endothelial surfaces where it can activate Protein C, a serine protease that disables the critical coagulation Factors Va and VIIa. Even in the absence of active coagulation, endothelial cells are constantly producing anti-coagulant substances like nitric oxide, prostacyclin and ecto-ADPase to attenuate platelet activity, heparan cofactors for antithrombin mediated factor inhibition and even tPA release.(Achneck et al., 2010)

Laboratory measurements used to evaluate coagulation include the prothrombin time (PT) and the activated partial thromboplastin time (aPTT). By adding tissue factor to plasma the PT detects reductions in extrinsic pathway Factors VII, X, V and prothrombin. The aPTT has a low TF assay plus the addition of a contact system activator to mimic the intrinsic pathway and detect deficiencies in Factors XII, XI, IX, VIII and V. Factor levels must fall below 50% for PT prolongation while most intrinsic factor levels must fall below 35% for aPTT prolongation to occur.(Tanaka et al., 2009) Clinically the extent of bleed-

Figure 1. Coagulation cascade with pharmacologic agent application. PCC: Prothrombin complex concentrates. TF: Tissue Factor, rFVIIa: Recombinant Factor VII, vWF: von Willebrand Factor, DDAVP: Desmopressin, HMWK: High molecular weight kininogen.

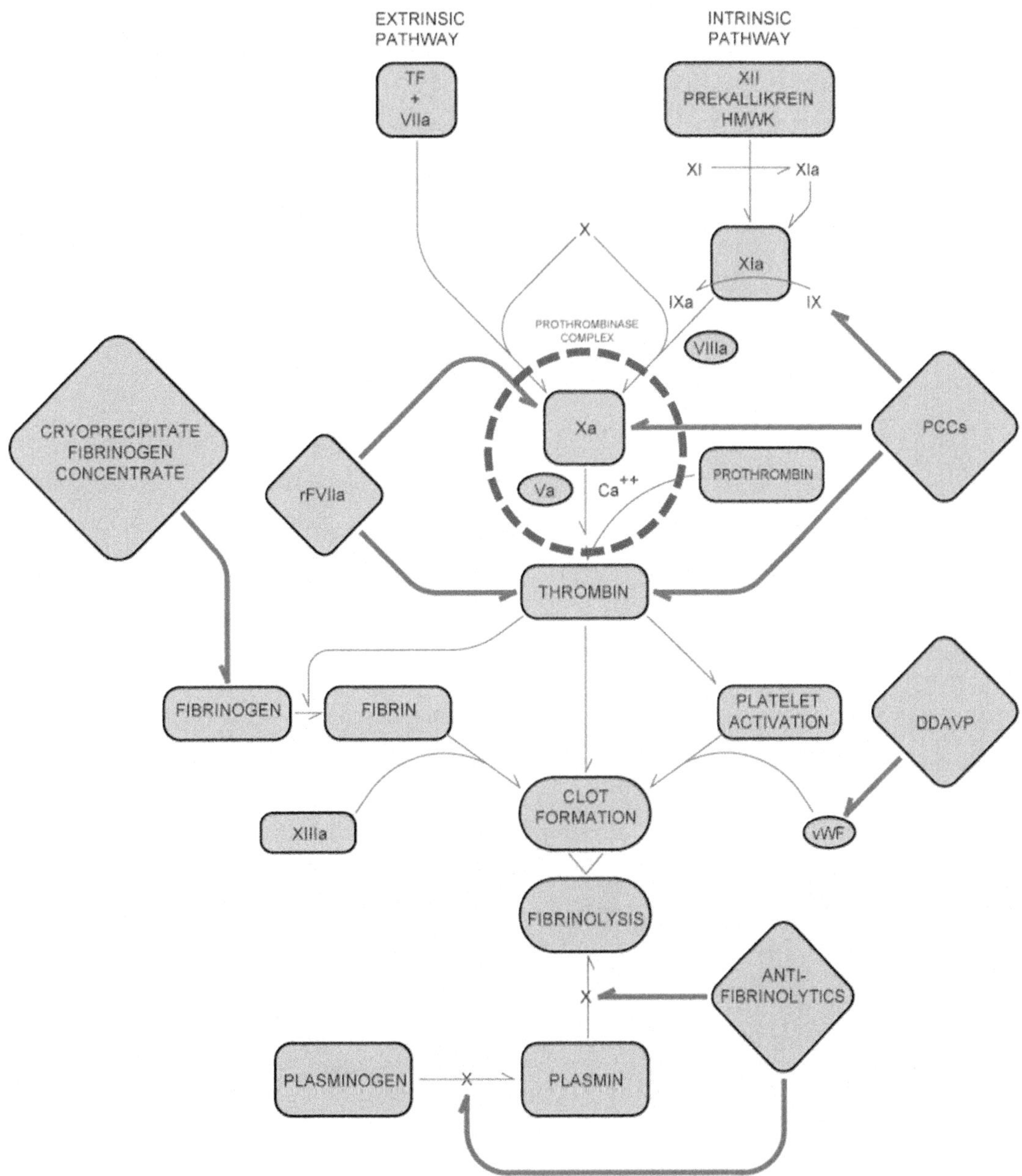

Figure 2. Cell based model of coagulation.TF: tissue factor, GIb and GIIb/IIIa: glycoprotein receptor, ADP: adenosine dephosphate, TXA2: Thromoxane A2.

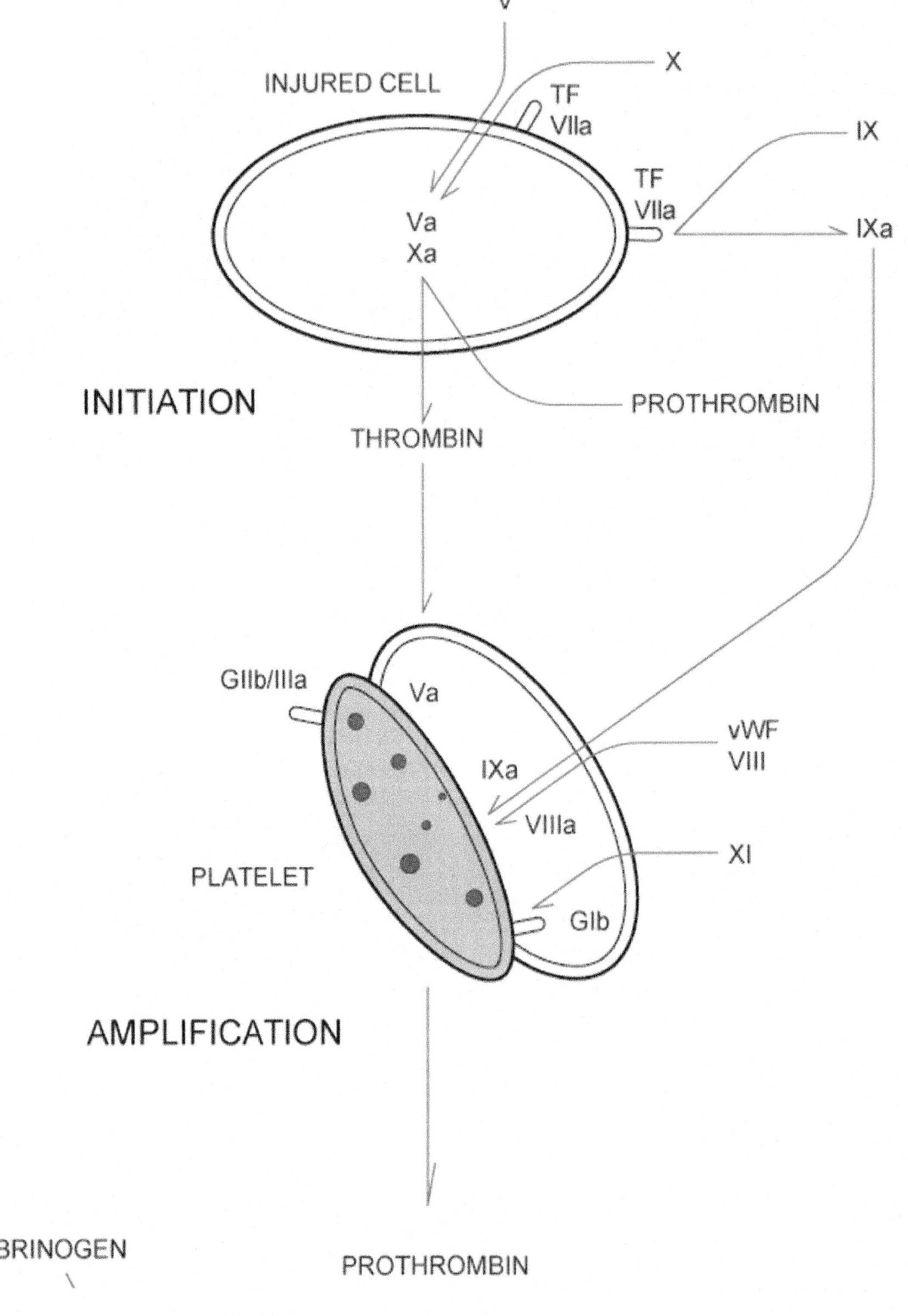

ing may be counterintuitive based on the measured PT and aPTT values. This divergence is because the PT and aPTT do not reflect the in vivo interaction of coagulation factors with platelets or fibrinogen and reveal no information about clot stability since the tests are stopped before the action of Factor XIIIa.

Activated Clotting Time (ACT) is another point-of-care (POC) test that is easy to perform in the OR or ICU to measure overall time to clot but provides very little insight on the exact mechanisms causing prolongation. Thromboelastography (TEG) or thromboelastrometry (ROTEM) are qualitative measurements of clotting that reflect the relationship of platelets, fibrinogen and coagulation factors to each other in clot stability. Specific antiplatelet drug effects from ASA, ADP or GIIb/IIIa receptor inhibitors are not detected by TEG but platelet function assays using whole blood impedence aggregrometry can distinguish such platelet defects when assessing perioperative platelet dysfunction.(Görlinger et al., 2013) Details regarding techniques for coagulation monitoring are covered in Chapter 32.

Cardiopulmonary Bypass Coagulopathy

The necessity for cardiopulmonary bypass (CPB) in cardiac surgery wreaks havoc on the hematologic balance in the body with insult severity increasing proportionally to the length of time spent on CPB. First, blood exposure to the extracorporeal circuit instigates massive activation of the intrinsic coagulation pathway with resultant thrombin formation. Anticoagulation with heparin prior to CPB is requisite to prevent instantaneous clotting. Heparin works by enhancing the inhibitory effects of antithrombin III to block new thrombin formation. Despite heparin, thrombin generation occurs within minutes of CPB initiation and is so profound that levels stay elevated for weeks to months.(Brister, Ofosu, & Buchanan, 1993) During CPB, fibrinogen and fibrin are deposited onto the extracorporeal membrane and are capable of binding thrombin, which renders it resistant to ATIII/heparin inhibition. Thrombin remains operational in this adhered state and continues to activate platelets enabling factor assemblage of prothrombinase complex and thus more thrombin creation.(Paparella, Brister, & Buchanan, 2004) Following surgical incision the wound and pericardium in particular release large amounts of tissue factor causing activation of the extrinsic cascade and additional thrombin formation.(Chung et al., 1996) In addition to coagulation pathway activation, a strong inflammatory response occurs to CPB with leukocyte activation and release of similar acute phase reactants produced in sepsis including interleukin-1, tumor necrosis factor and endotoxin. Tissue factor expression on cells and production by monocytes is enhanced in this proinflammatory state. (Paparella, Yau, & Young, 2002)

Heparin is essential to prevent thrombogenesis, but other measures to ensure adequate oxygenation and perfusion include the use of hemodilution to decrease blood viscosity and improve microcirculatory flow. Despite decreasing oxygen carrying capacity, adequate oxygen delivery can be maintained on CPB with hematocrit of 22-24%.(Makar, Taylor, Zhao, Farrohi, & Trimming, 2010) Along with anemia, the consequence of hemodilution is a reduction in platelets and coagulation factors. A dilutional coagulopathy becomes problematic after reversal of heparin and cessation of CPB when the potential for bleeding becomes paramount. Accurate dosing of protamine for reversal of heparin is a critical step since underdosing or overdosing can exacerbate bleeding tendency. Protamine neutralizes the effects of heparin but it also affects platelet aggregation by altering vWF and GIb interactions.(Lindblad, Wakefield, Whitehouse, & Stanley, 1988) A profound fibrinolytic response is also seen with CPB initiation due to a thrombin triggered surge in t-PA production and fibrin mediated stimulation of synthesis in macrophages, monocytes, fibroblasts and endothelial cells.(Rozental & Shore-Lesserson, 2012) Plasmin activity is hyperactive with extensive fibrin degradation such that D-dimer levels can remain elevated for months following surgery.

Thrombocytopathy and thrombocytopenia reflects the most highlighted coagulation disturbance after CPB. Platelet numbers are reduced by 30-50% due to hemodilution, organ sequestration, consumption and destruction by shear forces. Extensive platelet activation by thrombin, the extracorporeal membrane and high plasmin concentrations causes platelets to empty of all their procoagulant granule stores leaving them essentially ineffective. Platelets are stripped of critical receptor activity through circuit-bound fibrinogen tethering platelets at GIIb/IIIa receptors, heparin blocked binding of vWF at GIb receptors, and alpha-adrenergic receptor unresponsiveness to catecholamine stimulation. (Rozental & Shore-Lesserson, 2012)

Pharmacologic Management of Coagulopathy (Figure 1)

Antifibrinolytics

Antifibrinolytics have been proven to thwart bleeding from CPB associated coagulopathy by decreasing consumption of coagulation factors and platelets. Synthetic lysine analogues epsilon-aminocaproic acid (EACA) and tranexamic acid (TA) act by binding to plasminogen and preventing production of plasmin. Aprotinin is a bovine derived serine protease inhibitor with broad activity including inhibition of plasmin, thrombin, kallikerin, activated protein C and FXIa creating an excellent profile that promotes hemostasis with preservation of existing clots plus added anti-inflammatory actions. In a Cochrane meta-analysis all three drugs were shown to decrease bleeding, blood transfusions and re-operation rates compared to placebo without significant risks of thrombotic complications. (Henry, 2011) In 2008 aprotinin was withdrawn from the market following studies documenting increased renal failure and mortality with use in high-risk surgical patients.(Fergusson et al., 2008; Mangano, Tudor, Dietzel, Multicenter Study of Perioperative Ischemia Research Group, Ischemia Research and Education Foundation, 2006) Much controversy followed but in 2011 the Canadian government performed an extensive investigation and reapproved its use with strict guidelines for use in only low-risk patients. A recent propensity-matched cohort study comparing surgeries before and after the aprotinin withdrawal demonstrated increased bleeding, acute kidney injury and 30 day mortality in the non-aprotinin group. (Walkden, Verheyden, Goudie, & Murphy, 2013) Whether or not aprotinin will regain broad use, newer serine proteases are being developed including CU2010 and DX-88, both potent inhibitors of kallikrein with potential for expanded anti-inflammatory effects.(Rozental & Shore-Lesserson, 2012) In the mean time, despite proven efficacy of EACA and TA, investigations are ongoing into ideal dosing patterns in cardiac surgery especially since seizures have been documented with TA at higher doses.(Koster & Schirmer, 2011; Ngaage & Bland, 2010)

Desmopressin

The arginine vasopressin analog desmopressin acetate acts on the V2-receptor to release vWF, FVIII precursors and tPA from endothelial cells with definite benefit for patients with von Willebrand disease and potential benefits for patients with acquired defects in platelet function. Evidence for reducing post-operative bleeding has been sparse and most guidelines do not recommend the prophylactic use of

DDAVP. (V. A. Ferraris et al., 2011) A recent review assessing the utility of DDVAP in cardiac surgery in curbing post-operative blood loss and transfusions showed potential benefit for patients who received ASA preoperatively, had CPB times exceeding 140 minutes or evidence of abnormalities on platelet function assays.(Wademan & Galvin, 2014) Some benefit from preoperative use of DDAVP has been demonstrated in patients undergoing aortic valve replacement.(Steinlechner et al., 2011)

Hemostatic Factors

The search for procoagulant agents targeting specific hemostatic deficiencies in perioperative coagulopathy is ongoing.

The most discussed and widely used in cardiac surgery is recombinant activated ***factor VII (rFVIIa)***, a drug only FDA approved for treatment in hemophiliacs with inhibitors to Factors VIII and IX. The mechanism of action includes enhancement of TF:VIIa complex formation, direct binding and activation of Factor X on activated platelet surface membranes without TF presence and profound thrombin propagation.(G. A. Allen, Hoffman, Roberts, & Monroe, 2002) Use in cardiac surgery is technically "off label" and often reserved for severe coagulopathic bleeding unresponsive to other measures. A small randomized control trial looking at safety and efficacy of different doses of rFVIIa versus placebo for massive bleeding after cardiac surgery demonstrated decreased transfusion and re-operation rates in the treatment arms, but also a trend not reaching statistical significance for increased critical adverse events including stroke, thromboembolism and death.(Gill et al., 2009) Following this, a safety review of 35 randomized placebo controlled studies of off-label use of rFVIIa demonstrated equal rates of venoembolism but increased rates of arterial embolic events, especially in patients older than 65 years and those being treated for spontaneous central nervous system bleeding.(Levi, Levy, Andersen, & Truloff, 2010) Given the lack of definitive data demonstrating the safety and efficacy of rFVIIa in cardiac surgery, and the cost of $1000/mg, administration should be limited to life threatening bleeding not receptive to normal therapy following a thorough risk/benefit analysis. Recommendations to decrease risk and maximize benefit would be using doses of 30 – 60 mcg/kg, a fraction of that used for hemophiliacs, giving it early in resuscitation with redosing after 2 hours and avoiding use in patients with thrombophilia or presence of vascular foreign bodies.(Rozental & Shore-Lesserson, 2012)

Factor XIII is the final enzyme in the coagulation cascade responsible for cross-linking of fibrin monomers to form a solid fibrin polymer. Additional purported effects include anti-inflammatory properties with ability to reduce tissue permeability and edema.(Wozniak, Noll, Akintürk, Thul, & Müller, 2001) Several studies have shown CPB induced reduction of FXIII levels correlating with increased bleeding but two small studies demonstrated improvement in bleeding and transfusion requirement when FXIII was added to antifibrinolytic therapy at the conclusion of CPB.(Gödje, Gallmeier, Schelian, Grünewald, & Mair, 2006; Gödje, Haushofer, Lamm, & Reichart, 1998) Karkouti et al. (2013) performed a phase II, randomized double-blinded, placebo-controlled trial evaluating two different doses of FXIII given at the conclusion of CPB to patients with moderate risk for post-operative bleeding. Factor XIII levels tested at CPB conclusion showed a 40% drop in all groups with subsequent increase in levels only in treatment groups 30 minutes after administration. Antifibrinolytic therapy was also employed with tranexamic acid. Despite this, there were no differences in transfusion requirements or re-operation rates between groups.(Karkouti et al., 2013) Further studies are needed to assess the utility of FXIII in bleeding after cardiac surgery.

Prothrombin Complex Concentrates (PCC) represent a group of coagulation factor formulations containing variable concentrations of the Vitamin K dependent factors II, VII, IX, X with more contemporary products containing anticoagulants protein C, protein S, heparin and antithrombin III to balance the risk of thrombosis.(Sørensen, Spahn, Innerhofer, Spannagl, & Rossaint, 2011) Initially used for hemophiliacs with factor inhibitors, PCCs are now approved for warfarin reversal in the setting of bleeding. There are 3- and 4-factor PCCs available with the main difference being additional presence of FVII. FEIBA, Bebulin and Profilnine are 3-factor formulations available in the US and the only 4-factor PCC, Kcentra, was FDA approved in May 2013. The use of PCC for warfarin reversal is well established and the most current guidelines support using PCC formulations containing FVIIa over FFP for acute reversal.(V. A. Ferraris et al., 2011) In terms of PCC application in the management of post-cardiac surgery hemorrhage, one case report documents successful use of 4-factor Beriplex as a rescue agent for severe post-op bleeding in patients with Child-Pugh Class B cirrhosis.(Stuklis, O'Shaughnessy, & Ohri, 2001) Another retrospective review that included 7 cardiac patients with life-threatening post-op bleeding failing conventional therapy, documented decreased transfusion needs after Beriplex administration.(Bruce & Nokes, 2008) More recently Song et al (2014) published a review of 25 cardiac patients with severe post-operative hemorrhage refractory to conventional interventions who received a 4-factor derivation of FEIBA, which included rFVIIa. FEIBA was administered before chest closure based on the surgeons' clinical evaluation of hemostasis following traditional measures with blood products. The results showed a statistically significant decline in blood product administration following FEIBA administration with 100% successful primary chest closure, 0% re-operation rate and only 1 documented thrombotic complication noted.(Song et al., 2014) While these studies are promising in terms of efficacy they do not fully evaluate safety and additional research is needed to accurately characterize the thromboembolic risks of these drugs in cardiac surgery patients.

Fibrinogen is a critical and rate limiting component of clot formation. It is the first factor that diminishes in cases of significant bleeding and low levels have been shown to strongly predict bleeding and transfusion requirements following cardiac surgery.(Karlsson et al., 2008) Although commercial preparations of fibrinogen are available their use is only approved for treatment of severe hypofibrinogenemia. Safety and efficacy trials have been performed and demonstrate that compared to alternative forms of fibrinogen replacement, fresh frozen plasma (FFP) or cryoprecipitate, purified fibrinogen concentrates provide a quicker, lower volume, non-infectious and targeted intervention for bleeding. (Rahe-Meyer & Sørensen, 2011) A single-center placebo-controlled randomized control trial explored intraoperative fibrinogen use in high-risk aortic surgery and demonstrated significantly lower rates of blood transfusions in the treatment arm.(Rahe-Meyer et al., 2013) Use for treatment of excessive surgical bleeding is occurring but robust studies supporting this activity are not completed yet as reported in a recent Cochrane review.(Wikkelsø, 2013)

Antiplatelet and Anticoagulants in the Perioperative Period

The influence of antithrombotic and antiplatelet therapy on perioperative cardiac bleeding can be significant. Decisions regarding the timing of cessation and reinitiation for these medications should be guided by balancing the relative risk of bleeding against the risk of thrombosis and ischemia. Recent guidelines regarding antiplatelet medications, including ASA and P2Y12 inhibitors, were published for patients undergoing CABG procedures.(Sousa-Uva et al., 2014) Aspirin therapy has been associated with increased bleeding, but benefits for graft patency after CABG appear to outweigh the risks supporting continuation of low-dose ASA up until surgery and restarting within 6-24 hours afterward.(Jacob, Smedira, Blackstone, Williams, & Cho, 2011) For patients at high risk of bleeding, ASA may be stopped 3-5 days preoperatively. (Sun et al., 2008) The more complicated situations arise for patients on dual antiplatelet therapy (DAPT) with ASA plus a P2Y12 inhibitor like clopidogrel, ticagrelor or prasurgrel a mainstay following Acute Coronary Syndrome (ACS) and Percutaneous Coronary Intervention (PCI). DAPT cessation perioperatively places patients at risk for thrombotic and ischemic events but continuation is associated with increased bleeding and blood transfusion.(Ascione et al., 2005) Most guidelines agree that for non-urgent surgery, there should be 5-7 days of cessation of P2Y12 inhibitors prior to operating. (V. A. Ferraris et al., 2011; Hillis et al., 2011; Sousa-Uva et al., 2014) For patients presenting with acute coronary syndrome with ongoing ischemia, hemodynamic instability, complex coronary artery disease or recent stenting, bridging antiplatelet therapy with intravenous P2Y12 inhibitor cangrelor or GIIb/IIIa inhibitors tirofiban or eptifibatide is an option as these medications can be stopped within hours of OR time.(Savonitto et al., 2010) Additionally, the use of preoperative platelet function assays allows timing of surgery to be more informed with studies showing evidence for reduction in surgical delay.(Mahla et al., 2012)

Vitamin K antagonists like warfarin are usually stopped within 4 days of planned surgery. Given the multiple options for reversal, Vitamin K, FFP, PCC and the ease of transition up until surgical time with unfractionated heparin infusion, it is rarely a factor in increasing perioperative bleeding. The newer generation of oral anticoagulants being developed to replace warfarin, such as direct thrombin inhibitors like dabigatran and FXa inhibitors like rivaroxaban or apixiban, represent new challenges since there is no validated way to measure drug activity and there are no targeted reversal agents available. There is evidence that these drugs can be monitored via thromboelastrography and there has been some success with using PCC for reversal.(Artang, Galloway, & Nielsen, 2014; Mazer, 2014)

Anemia: Pre-Op, Intraop, Post-Op

The World Health Organization defines severe anemia as a hemoglobin level below 8 g/dL. The physiologic and clinical significance of anemia is best studied in patients who are unable to utilize blood transfusion. Wesikopf and Silverman evaluated correlating hemoglobin level and mortality in Jehovah's Witness patients refusing transfusion and found in patients with cardiovascular disease Hgb 6 – 7 g/dL marked the threshold for mortality increase and patients anemic to 3 - 4 g/dL only survived half the time.(Weiskopf & Silverman, 2013) A study of over 10,000 CABG patients found significantly higher mortality in patients with preoperative anemia per WHO guidelines.(van Straten et al., 2009) Etiologies of anemia in preoperative cardiac patients include hospital acquired, iron deficiency and anemia of chronic disease with prevalence ranging 22 to 30%.(Karkouti et al., 2008b) Preoperative anemia is the biggest predictor of nadir hematocrit levels during CPB with lower levels portending increased risk of stroke, renal insufficiency, longer mechanical ventilation and mortality.(Karkouti et al., 2005; Loor et al., 2012) Interestingly at least one retrospective analysis of 10,000 non-emergent, non-anemic patients found that the absolute hematocrit number was not associated with worsened outcomes, but instead a relative drop from the patients baseline hemoglobin of 50% or more intraoperatively was associated with an increased composite risk of hospital death, stroke and renal failure.(Karkouti, Wijeysundera, Beattie, Reducing Bleeding in Cardiac Surgery (RBC) Investigators, 2008a) Interventions to treat preoperative anemia include iron supplementation and recombinant human erythropoetin (EPO) therapy. Short course of EPO therapy prior to cardiac surgery, at least 4 – 6 days to allow time for effect, is associated with avoidance of blood transfusion in cardiac surgery patients.(Alghamdi, Albanna, Guru, & Brister, 2006a) Even a single preoperative IV administration of recombinant erythropoietin together with supplemental iron can significantly decrease the rate of PRBC transfusion in anemic patients undergoing valvular heart surgery.(Yoo et al., 2011) The use of long-term epogen therapy carries a risk of thrombotic complications and use in cardiovascular revascularization patients should be thoughtfully considered. Targeting a preoperative hematocrit of 30% is reasonable and recommended, especially in the setting of autologous blood donation.(Nalla, Freedman, Hare, & Mazer, 2012)

Even in the absence of massive bleeding or extreme hemodilution cardiac surgical patients experience a hemoglobin drift with the maximum drop occurring by postoperative day 3 – 4 with 79% of patients recovering almost half of the loss one week after surgery.(George et al., 2012) Evaluating anemia in patients from the IMAGINE study, which looked at ACE inhibitor use after CABG, postoperative anemia was common with 94% of patients within the first 6 days of surgery and 19% having levels below 9 g/dL.(Westenbrink et al., 2011) When the same patients were evaluated 50 days after surgery, 44% were still anemic and every 1 g/dL drop in hemoglobin was associated with a 13% increased risk of major adverse cardiac event. An observational study of cardiac surgery patients who did not receive blood transfusion admitted for rehabilitation found patients with initial hemoglobin levels below 10 g/dL performed worse on initial 6 minute walk tests compared to patients with higher hemoglobin levels but this deficit was overcome by the end of their stay, supporting a policy to restrict blood transfusions to lower hemoglobin levels.(Ranucci, La Rovere, et al., 2011b)

Transfusions

From the 1940s to the 1980s, despite the paucity of evidence endorsing the benefit of blood, transfusion was considered such a life saving therapy that the known 10% risk of hepatitis transmission did not dissuade transfusions to reach the arbitrary goal of 10 g/dL.(D. J. Allen & Chae-Kim, 2002; Speiss, 2002) There are numerous retrospective studies demonstrating a breadth of grave consequences associated with blood transfusion in cardiac surgery including increased early and short term mortality.(Murphy & Angelini, 2006) At least one prospective study following almost 12,000 isolated CABG patients confirmed retrospective study findings of increased renal failure, prolonged ventilatory support, serious infections, cardiac complications and neurologic events with RBC transfusion.(Koch et al., 2006) A more recent retrospective analysis of more than 8500 cardiac surgery patients in the United Kingdom compared infection rates, ischemic complications, hospital costs and survival in patients who had received red blood cell transfusions to those who had not.(Murphy et al., 2007) After adjusting for co-morbidities patients who had received blood suffered an over 3-fold increase in infectious and ischemic complications and a 6-fold mortality increase, regardless of nadir hematocrit levels. The most compelling evidence for abandoning liberal transfusion strategies comes from the Transfusion Requirement After Cardiac Surgery (TRACS) trial, the first prospective randomized control trial comparing a restrictive strategy with transfusion threshold of hematocrit 24%, compared to a liberal strategy with transfusion threshold of 30%.(Hajjar et al., 2010) 502 patients were analyzed after randomization with the restrictive strategy patients averaging Hct of 28.4% while the liberal strategy averaged 31.8%. There was no difference between the groups in a composite end point encompassing 30-day mortality, cardiogenic shock, renal failure requiring dialysis and acute respiratory distress syndrome. Regardless of assigned transfusion strategy, when evaluating patients who received blood there was significant harm with blood transfusion with every unit of blood associated with a 1.2 fold increase in 30-day mortality. Additionally, patients who ultimately needed red blood cells received more FFP intraoperatively presumably from more severe coagulopathy and raises the question of how transfusion of other blood products affect outcomes.

A retrospective study of 4500 on-pump CABG patients looking at hospital mortality found a 12-fold increased mortality after FFP transfusion, a 13-fold increase after platelets and a 5-fold increase after RBC transfusion.(Ranucci, Pazzaglia, Bianchini, Bozzetti, & Isgrò, 2008) Another retrospective study of over 5000 CABG patients attempted to create a more robust model of transfusion risk on long-term mortality by incorporating several established risk factors, including renal insufficiency and preoperative hemoglobin, and different blood components.(Bjursten, Dardashti, Ederoth, Brondén, & Algotsson, 2013) Follow up at 7.5 years revealed that transfusion of FFP was associated with decreased survival, transfusion of red blood cells had no effect on survival while platelets improved survival. In another evaluation of over 5000 CABG and valve surgery patients, a lasting negative effect on mortality was demonstrated where transfusion of any blood, platelets or FFP product resulted in a median time to death of 0.83 years compared to 4.68 years in non-transfused patients.(Bhaskar, Dulhunty, Mullany, & Fraser, 2012)

When investigating the cause of worsened outcomes after transfusion in cardiac surgery, the rare transmission of HIV (1:2-8 million) or hepatitis C (1:2 million) or hemolytic transfusion reactions (1:100,000) are not implicated even though this is what we often highlight when consenting patients for transfusion.(Nalla et al., 2012) The increased infectious complications are actually attributed to the immunosuppressive and proinflammatory features of transfusion. Donor leukocytes present in stored RBCs contain significant levels of immunoregulatory molecules that impair actions of T-helper cells and natural killer cells. These contaminant donor white blood cells produce inflammatory markers that add to the already pronounced cytokine release after CPB and cause an additional injury to the already vulnerable endothelium. Transfusion of a single unit of blood after CPB can propagate cytokine levels fifteen-fold.(Fransen, Maessen, Dentener, Senden, & Buurman, 1999) In this state, patients are particularly susceptible to transfusion related respiratory sequelae as the CPB induced endothelial injury attracts and adheres neutrophils that release lytic enzymes and platelet aggregators within lung parenchyma to cause capillary damage and leakage. Transfusion associated circulatory overload (TACO) is a rare but possible consequence of massive transfusion in patients with limited cardiovascular reserve leading to pulmonary edema. Despotis et al collected data from studies and FDA reports to estimate transfusion related mortality in cardiac patients and found TRALI (transfusion related acute lung injury), the number one reported cause of transfusion related death in all comers, to be responsible for up to 50 deaths per million units transfused in cardiac surgery patients. Bacterial infections accounted for up to 100 deaths while as many as 15,000 deaths per million transfused units were attributed to WBC mediated mechanisms (Despotis, Eby, & Lublin, 2008). Leukoreduction of RBCs has been advocated to reduce some of these immune-mediated consequences based on studies demonstrating reduction of infection and even mortality but a true causal relationship is difficult to determine (Bilgin et al., 2007). While current guidelines endorse the practice of pre-storage leukoreduction, Canada and most European countries perform universal leukoreduction but the United States has yet to implement standardization (V. A. Ferraris et al., 2011). Another mechanism at play is the effect of storage duration on transfusion outcomes. The clinical consequences of the "storage lesion" which encompasses the metabolic and biochemical changes that occur in stored blood was evaluated by comparing cardiac surgery patients who received fresher versus older blood and found a significant increase in respiratory failure, renal failure, sepsis and both short term and long term mortality in patients receiving blood stored greater than two weeks (Koch et al., 2008). The physiologic explanation of this phenomenon is related to impaired offloading of oxygen from depletion of 2,3 disphosphoglycerate (DPG) in stored blood combined with the altered rheology of transfused erythrocytes which prevents smooth flow in capillaries within the microcirculation of critical organs (Murphy & Angelini, 2006). The recently published Red Cell Storage Duration Study (RECESS) randomized 1098 patients undergoing complex cardiac surgery to receive blood less than 10 days old or blood stored greater than 21 days. Results from the study showed no significant difference in organ dysfunction or mortality between the groups. (Steiner et. al., 2015).

Patient Blood Management

Patient Blood Management (PBM) encompasses employing a variety of evidence-based medical and surgical strategies aimed at preserving hemoglobin levels, minimizing blood loss, and carefully targeting transfusions to avoid unnecessary exposure to blood products. The World Health Organization and the Joint Commission have individually promoted utilization of PBM as a means to boost patient safety and clinical outcomes (Goodnough & Shander, 2012). Despite the availability of comprehensive, evidence-based blood conservation guidelines from the Society of Thoracic Surgeons and Society of Cardiovascular Anesthesiologists, when surveying over 1000 institutions only 26% reported adopting at least one practice change from the guidelines (Likosky et al., 2010). Guidelines raise awareness and instigate conversations but the actual drive for change requires agreement and cooperation among the multiple disciplines and professions involved in caring for these patients including cardiac surgeons, anesthesiologists, critical care physicians, perfusionists, nurses, transfusion medicine practitioners, pharmacists and laboratory personnel (Hessel & Levy, 2010). Reluctance to adopt clinical practice changes comes from the multitude of unanswered questions and perceived lack of evidence in regards to PBM application in cardiac surgery (Ranucci, Aronson, et al., 2011a). What we do know is a solitary practitioner dictating transfusion practices based on personal clinical judgment exposes more patients to unnecessary transfusions compared with algorithm driven protocols (Avidan et al., 2004). When blood conservation strategies have been applied and studied across multiple cardiac centers in the US, transfusion rates go down, morbidity and mortality decrease and thousands of dollars are saved (LaPar et al., 2013; Moskowitz et al., 2010).

The details and exact components of PBM protocols will vary based on an institution's resources and specific patient population but three main pillars are cited that span the entire surgical experience 1) erythropoiesis promotion, 2) minimizing bleeding, 3) optimizing tolerance of anemia (Goodnough & Shander, 2012; Shander et al., 2012). Identifying and treating anemia might mean initiation of iron, B12 or folate supplementation, cessation of medications that may cause anemia, consideration of erythropoieses stimulating therapies or postponement of surgery until anemia is better managed. Identifying those at risk for blood transfusion can be facilitated by using such validated scoring systems as the Transfusion Risk Understanding Scoring Tool (TRUST) which calculates a percent likelihood of transfusion based on risk factors including female gender, preoperative anemia, age > 65 years, renal insufficiency, and repeat or complex cardiac surgery (Alghamdi, Davis, Brister, Corey, & Logan, 2006b). Intraoperative considerations include adjustments to CPB practices including using intraoperative autologous donation

(IAD), applying retrograde autologous priming (RAP) with smaller priming volumes to avoid excessive hemodilution and the use of cell salvage techniques all of which formed the foundation for a successful conservation program at Cornell University with recently published results demonstrating reductions in blood transfusions, post-operative bleeding, reoperation and respiratory failure rates (Avgerinos, Debois, & Salemi, 2014). Minimizing bleeding requires quick and reliable diagnosis of coagulation abnormalities followed by targeted hemotherapy. Utilization of viscoelastic and aggregometric point-of-care (POC) testing, specifically ROTEM and Multiplate, with restrictive hemoglobin thresholds was shown to reduce bleeding, reduce blood product utilization and improve 6-month mortality compared to conventional laboratory testing in 100 coagulopathic cardiac surgery patients.(Weber et al., 2012) A follow-up review by Görlinger et al (2013) evaluating 16 studies, covering 8507 cardiac patients using viscoelastic and aggregometric POC testing in combination with algorithms prioritizing specific coagulation factor concentrates over blood therapy confirmed these positive benefits and introduced a pyramid approach to hemostatic therapy practices hemostatic therapeutic interventions starts from the bottom of the pyramid and continues to the top until hemostasis is achieved. Given the infrastructure required to implement the technology for POC testing, the pharmacy and blood bank approval needed for factor concentrates, many institutions are still relying on traditional laboratory testing and blood component therapy, including the University of California. Adopted intraoperative and postoperative transfusion algorithms (Figure 3) include targeted therapies based on specific laboratory values in the clinical context of bleeding and anemia. The negotiated hemoglobin transfusion thresholds fall in line with STS/SCA guidelines but also consider clinical scenarios of hypovolemia or inadequate oxygenation delivery via measured mixed venous oxygen saturations in the decision process.

Figure 3. Stepwise algorithm for intraoperative and postoperative transfusion of PRBC and blood components developed and adapted by University of California blood conservation initiative. Algorithm emphasized multidisciplinary approach towards patient blood management (PBM).

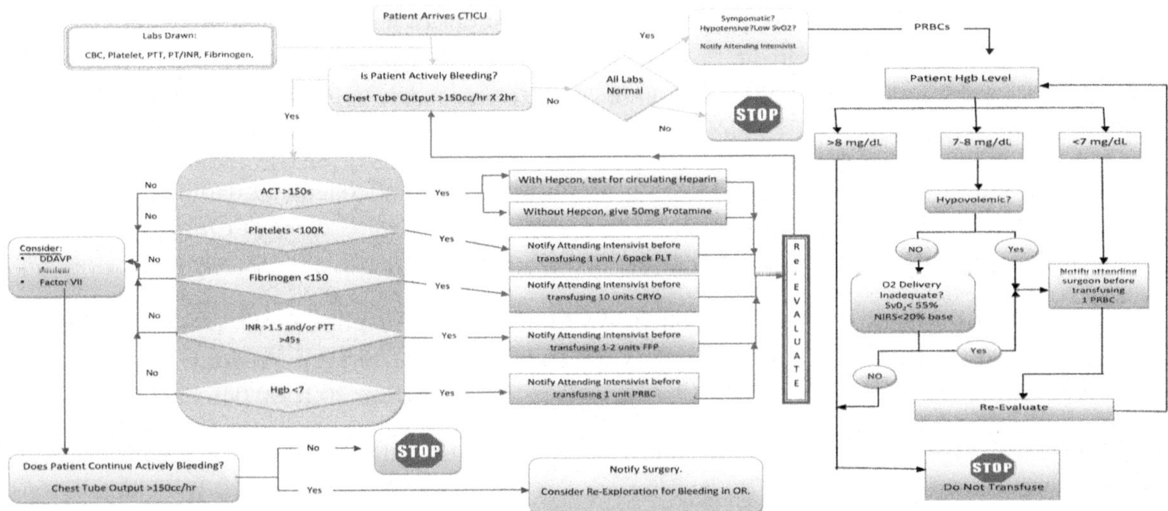

CONCLUSION

Cardiac surgical patients are exposed to a variety of hematologic alterations due to preoperative administration of anticoagulant and antiplatelet medications, institution of CPB with intraoperative use of anticoagulants, coagulation factors and blood components. Despite decades of cardiac surgical practice and significant accumulated evidence, there is still considerable controversy regarding optimal use of blood components and transfusion practice. The future direction of transfusion practice will be based on multidisciplinary protocols that prioritize judicious use of blood component therapy based on reliable and easily accessible POC systems.

REFERENCES

Achneck, H. E., Sileshi, B., Parikh, A., Milano, C. A., Welsby, I. J., & Lawson, J. H. (2010). Pathophysiology of bleeding and clotting in the cardiac surgery patient: From vascular endothelium to circulatory assist device surface. *Circulation*, *122*(20), 2068–2077. doi:10.1161/CIRCULATIONAHA.110.936773 PMID:21098468

Alghamdi, A. A., Albanna, M. J., Guru, V., & Brister, S. J. (2006a). Does the use of erythropoietin reduce the risk of exposure to allogeneic blood transfusion in cardiac surgery? A systematic review and meta-analysis. *Journal of Cardiac Surgery*, *21*(3), 320–326. doi:10.1111/j.1540-8191.2006.00241.x PMID:16684074

Alghamdi, A. A., Davis, A., Brister, S., Corey, P., & Logan, A. (2006b). Development and validation of Transfusion Risk Understanding Scoring Tool (TRUST) to stratify cardiac surgery patients according to their blood transfusion needs. *Transfusion*, *46*(7), 1120–1129. doi:10.1111/j.1537-2995.2006.00860.x PMID:16836558

Allen, D. J., & Chae-Kim, S. H. (2002). Risks and complications of neuraxial anesthesia and the use of anticoagulation in the surgical patient. ... *(Baylor University Medical* .... Allen, G. A., Hoffman, M., Roberts, H. R., & Monroe, D. M. (2002). Recombinant activated factor VII: Its mechanism of action and role in the control of hemorrhage. *Canadian Journal of Anaesthesia*, *49*(10), S7–S14. PMID:12546000

Artang, R., Galloway, G., & Nielsen, J. D. (2014). Monitoring novel anticoagulants dabigatran, rivaroxaban and apixabain using thrombelastography. *Journal of the American College of Cardiology*, *63*(12), A439. doi:10.1016/S0735-1097(14)60439-3

Ascione, R., Ghosh, A., Rogers, C. A., Cohen, A., Monk, C., & Angelini, G. D. (2005). In-hospital patients exposed to clopidogrel before coronary artery bypass graft surgery: A word of caution. *The Annals of Thoracic Surgery*, *79*(4), 1210–1216. doi:10.1016/j.athoracsur.2004.09.046 PMID:15797051

Avgerinos, D. V., Debois, W., & Salemi, A. (2014). Blood conservation strategies in cardiac surgery: More is better. *European Journal of Cardio-Thoracic Surgery*, *46*(5), 865–870. doi:10.1093/ejcts/ezt661 PMID:24482391

Avidan, M. S., Alcock, E. L., Da Fonseca, J., Ponte, J., Desai, J. B., Despotis, G. J., & Hunt, B. J. (2004). Comparison of structured use of routine laboratory tests or near-patient assessment with clinical judgement in the management of bleeding after cardiac surgery. *British Journal of Anaesthesia*, *92*(2), 178–186. doi:10.1093/bja/aeh037 PMID:14722166

Bennett-Guerrero, E., Zhao, Y., O'Brien, S. M., Ferguson, T. B., Peterson, E. D., Gammie, J. S., & Song, H. K. (2010). Variation in use of blood transfusion in coronary artery bypass graft surgery. *Journal of the American Medical Association*, *304*(14), 1568–1575. doi:10.1001/jama.2010.1406 PMID:20940382

Bhaskar, B., Dulhunty, J., Mullany, D. V., & Fraser, J. F. (2012). Impact of blood product transfusion on short and long-term survival after cardiac surgery: More evidence. *The Annals of Thoracic Surgery*, *94*(2), 460–467. doi:10.1016/j.athoracsur.2012.04.005 PMID:22626751

Bilgin, Y. M., van de Watering, L. M. G., Eijsman, L., Versteegh, M. I. M., van Oers, M. H. J., & Brand, A. (2007). Is increased mortality associated with post-operative infections after leukocytes containing red blood cell transfusions in cardiac surgery? An extended analysis. *Transfusion Medicine (Oxford, England)*, *17*(4), 304–311. doi:10.1111/j.1365-3148.2007.00746.x PMID:17680957

Bjursten, H., Dardashti, A., Ederoth, P., Brondén, B., & Algotsson, L. (2013). Increased long-term mortality with plasma transfusion after coronary artery bypass surgery. *Intensive Care Medicine*, *39*(3), 437–444. doi:10.1007/s00134-012-2723-9 PMID:23052960

Bojar, R. M. (2011). *Manual of Perioperative Care in Adult Cardiac Surgery*. John Wiley & Sons.

Brister, S. J., Ofosu, F. A., & Buchanan, M. R. (1993). Thrombin generation during cardiac surgery: Is heparin the ideal anticoagulant? *Thrombosis and Haemostasis*, *70*(2), 259–262. PMID:8236131

Bruce, D., & Nokes, T. J. C. (2008). Prothrombin complex concentrate (Beriplex P/N) in severe bleeding: Experience in a large tertiary hospital. *Critical Care (London, England)*, *12*(4), R105. doi:10.1186/cc6987 PMID:18706082

Carson, J. L., Terrin, M. L., Noveck, H., Sanders, D. W., Chaitman, B. R., & Rhoads, G. G. et al.. (2011). Liberal or Restrictive Transfusion in High-Risk Patients after Hip Surgery. *The New England Journal of Medicine*, 111214140020001. PMID:22168590

Choong, C. K., Gerrard, C., Goldsmith, K. A., Dunningham, H., & Vuylsteke, A. (2007). Delayed re-exploration for bleeding after coronary artery bypass surgery results in adverse outcomes. *European Journal of Cardio-Thoracic Surgery*, *31*(5), 834–838. doi:10.1016/j.ejcts.2007.02.001 PMID:17360191

Christensen, M. C., Dziewior, F., Kempel, A., & von Heymann, C. (2012). Increased chest tube drainage is independently associated with adverse outcome after cardiac surgery. *Journal of Cardiothoracic and Vascular Anesthesia*, *26*(1), 46–51. doi:10.1053/j.jvca.2011.09.021 PMID:22100857

Chung, J. H., Gikakis, N., Rao, A. K., Drake, T. A., Colman, R. W., & Edmunds, L. H. (1996). Pericardial blood activates the extrinsic coagulation pathway during clinical cardiopulmonary bypass. *Circulation*, *93*(11), 2014–2018. doi:10.1161/01.CIR.93.11.2014 PMID:8640976

Davie, E. W., & Ratnoff, O. D. (1964). Waterfall sequence for intrinsic blood clotting. *Science*, *145*(3638), 1310–1312. doi:10.1126/science.145.3638.1310 PMID:14173416

Despotis, G., Eby, C., & Lublin, D. M. (2008). A review of transfusion risks and optimal management of perioperative bleeding with cardiac surgery. *Transfusion*, *48*(1Suppl), 2S–30S. doi:10.1111/j.1537-2995.2007.01573.x PMID:18302579

Despotis, G. J., Filos, K. S., Zoys, T. N., Hogue, C. W., Spitznagel, E., & Lappas, D. G. (1996). Factors associated with excessive postoperative blood loss and hemostatic transfusion requirements: A multivariate analysis in cardiac surgical patients. *Anesthesia and Analgesia*, *82*(1), 13–21. PMID:8712388

Fergusson, D. A., Hébert, P. C., Mazer, C. D., Fremes, S., MacAdams, C., Murkin, J. M., & Pretorius, R. et al. (2008). A comparison of aprotinin and lysine analogues in high-risk cardiac surgery. *The New England Journal of Medicine*, *358*(22), 2319–2331. doi:10.1056/NEJMoa0802395 PMID:18480196

Ferraris, V. A., Brown, J. R., Despotis, G. J., Hammon, J. W., Reece, T. B., & Saha, S. P. et al.. (2011). 2011 update to the Society of Thoracic Surgeons and the Society of Cardiovascular Anesthesiologists blood conservation clinical practice guidelines. *The Annals of Thoracic Surgery*, *91*(3), 944–982. PMID:21353044

Ferraris, V. A., & Ferraris, S. P. (1995). Limiting excessive postoperative blood transfusion after cardiac procedures. A review. *Texas Heart Institute Journal*, *22*(3), 216–230. PMID:7580359

Fransen, E., Maessen, J., Dentener, M., Senden, N., & Buurman, W. (1999). Impact of blood transfusions on inflammatory mediator release in patients undergoing cardiac surgery. *Chest*, *116*(5), 1233–1239. doi:10.1378/chest.116.5.1233 PMID:10559080

George, T. J., Beaty, C. A., Kilic, A., Haggerty, K. A., Frank, S. M., Savage, W. J., & Whitman, G. J. (2012). Hemoglobin drift after cardiac surgery. *The Annals of Thoracic Surgery*, *94*(3), 703–709. doi:10.1016/j.athoracsur.2012.03.038 PMID:22609121

Gill, R., Herbertson, M., Vuylsteke, A., Olsen, P. S., von Heymann, C., Mythen, M., & Schmidt, T. A. et al. (2009). Safety and Efficacy of Recombinant Activated Factor VII: A Randomized Placebo-Controlled Trial in the Setting of Bleeding After Cardiac Surgery. *Circulation*, *120*(1), 21–27. doi:10.1161/CIRCULATIONAHA.108.834275 PMID:19546387

Gödje, O., Gallmeier, U., Schelian, M., Grünewald, M., & Mair, H. (2006). Coagulation factor XIII reduces postoperative bleeding after coronary surgery with extracorporeal circulation. *The Thoracic and Cardiovascular Surgeon*, *54*(1), 26–33. doi:10.1055/s-2005-872853 PMID:16485185

Gödje, O., Haushofer, M., Lamm, P., & Reichart, B. (1998). The effect of factor XIII on bleeding in coronary surgery. *The Thoracic and Cardiovascular Surgeon*, *46*(5), 263–267. doi:10.1055/s-2007-1010236 PMID:9885116

Goodnough, L. T., & Shander, A. (2012). Patient blood management. *Anesthesiology*, *116*(6), 1367–1376. doi:10.1097/ALN.0b013e318254d1a3 PMID:22487863

Goodnough, L. T., Soegiarso, R. W., Birkmeyer, J. D., & Welch, H. G. (1993). Economic impact of inappropriate blood transfusions in coronary artery bypass graft surgery. *The American Journal of Medicine*, *94*(5), 509–514. doi:10.1016/0002-9343(93)90086-5 PMID:8498396

Görlinger, K., Shore-Lesserson, L., Dirkmann, D., Hanke, A. A., Rahe-Meyer, N., & Tanaka, K. A. (2013). Management of hemorrhage in cardiothoracic surgery. *Journal of Cardiothoracic and Vascular Anesthesia*, *27*(4Suppl), S20–S34. doi:10.1053/j.jvca.2013.05.014 PMID:23910533

Hajjar, L. A., Vincent, J.-L., Galas, F. R. B. G., Nakamura, R. E., Silva, C. M. P., Santos, M. H., & Auler, J. O. C. et al. (2010). Transfusion requirements after cardiac surgery: The TRACS randomized controlled trial. *Journal of the American Medical Association*, *304*(14), 1559–1567. doi:10.1001/jama.2010.1446 PMID:20940381

Hall, T. S., Brevetti, G. R., Skoultchi, A. J., Sines, J. C., Gregory, P., & Spotnitz, A. J. (2001). Re-exploration for hemorrhage following open heart surgery differentiation on the causes of bleeding and the impact on patient outcomes. *Annals of Thoracic and Cardiovascular Surgery*, *7*(6), 352–357. PMID:11888475

Hébert, P. C., Wells, G., Blajchman, M. A., Marshall, J., Martin, C., Pagliarello, G., & Yetisir, E. et al. (1999). A multicenter, randomized, controlled clinical trial of transfusion requirements in critical care. Transfusion Requirements in Critical Care Investigators, Canadian Critical Care Trials Group. *The New England Journal of Medicine*, *340*(6), 409–417. doi:10.1056/NEJM199902113400601 PMID:9971864

Henry, D. A. (Ed.). (2011). Anti-fibrinolytic use for minimising perioperative allogeneic blood transfusion. *Cochrane Database of Systematic Reviews*, (1): CD001886. PMID:21249650

Hessel, E. A. II, & Levy, J. H. (2010). Guidelines for perioperative blood transfusion and conservation in cardiac surgery: Lessons and challenges. *Anesthesia and Analgesia*, *111*(6), 1555–1559. doi:10.1213/ANE.0b013e3181fbb386 PMID:21106971

Hillis, L. D., Smith, P. K., Anderson, J. L., Bittl, J. A., Bridges, C. R., Byrne, J. G., et al. (2011). *2011 ACCF/AHA Guideline for Coronary Artery Bypass Graft Surgery: a report of the American College of Cardiology Foundation/American Heart Association Task Force on Practice Guidelines* (Vol. 124, pp. e652–735). ACCF/AHA.

Hoffman, M., & Monroe, D. M. (2007). Coagulation 2006: A modern view of hemostasis. *Hematology/Oncology Clinics of North America*, *21*(1), 1–11. doi:10.1016/j.hoc.2006.11.004 PMID:17258114

Jacob, M., Smedira, N., Blackstone, E., Williams, S., & Cho, L. (2011). Effect of timing of chronic preoperative aspirin discontinuation on morbidity and mortality in coronary artery bypass surgery. *Circulation*, *123*(6), 577–583. doi:10.1161/CIRCULATIONAHA.110.957373 PMID:21282503

Karkouti, K., Djaiani, G., Borger, M. A., Beattie, W. S., Fedorko, L., Wijeysundera, D., & Karski, J. et al. (2005). Low hematocrit during cardiopulmonary bypass is associated with increased risk of perioperative stroke in cardiac surgery. *The Annals of Thoracic Surgery*, *80*(4), 1381–1387. doi:10.1016/j.athoracsur.2005.03.137 PMID:16181875

Karkouti, K., von Heymann, C., Jespersen, C. M., Korte, W., Levy, J. H., Ranucci, M., & Song, H. K. et al. (2013). Efficacy and safety of recombinant factor XIII on reducing blood transfusions in cardiac surgery: A randomized, placebo-controlled, multicenter clinical trial. *The Journal of Thoracic and Cardiovascular Surgery, 146*(4), 927–939. doi:10.1016/j.jtcvs.2013.04.044 PMID:23820174

Karkouti, K., Wijeysundera, D. N., & Beattie, W. S.Reducing Bleeding in Cardiac Surgery (RBC) Investigators. (2008a). Risk associated with preoperative anemia in cardiac surgery: A multicenter cohort study. *Circulation, 117*(4), 478–484. doi:10.1161/CIRCULATIONAHA.107.718353 PMID:18172032

Karkouti, K., Wijeysundera, D. N., Yau, T. M., McCluskey, S. A., van Rensburg, A., & Beattie, W. S. (2008b). The influence of baseline hemoglobin concentration on tolerance of anemia in cardiac surgery. *Transfusion, 48*(4), 666–672. doi:10.1111/j.1537-2995.2007.01590.x PMID:18194382

Karlsson, M., Ternström, L., Hyllner, M., Baghaei, F., Nilsson, S., & Jeppsson, A. (2008). Plasma fibrinogen level, bleeding, and transfusion after on-pump coronary artery bypass grafting surgery: A prospective observational study. *Transfusion, 48*(10), 2152–2158. doi:10.1111/j.1537-2995.2008.01827.x PMID:18657083

Karthik, S., Grayson, A. D., McCarron, E. E., Pullan, D. M., & Desmond, M. J. (2004). Reexploration for bleeding after coronary artery bypass surgery: risk factors, outcomes, and the effect of time delay. *The Annals of Thoracic Surgery, 78*(2), 527–34– discussion 534.

Koch, C. G., Li, L., Duncan, A. I., Mihaljevic, T., Cosgrove, D. M., Loop, F. D., & Blackstone, E. H. et al. (2006). Morbidity and mortality risk associated with red blood cell and blood-component transfusion in isolated coronary artery bypass grafting. *Critical Care Medicine, 34*(6), 1608–1616. doi:10.1097/01.CCM.0000217920.48559.D8 PMID:16607235

Koch, C. G., Li, L., Sessler, D. I., Figueroa, P., Hoeltge, G. A., Mihaljevic, T., & Blackstone, E. H. (2008). Duration of red-cell storage and complications after cardiac surgery. *The New England Journal of Medicine, 358*(12), 1229–1239. doi:10.1056/NEJMoa070403 PMID:18354101

Koster, A., & Schirmer, U. (2011). Re-evaluation of the role of antifibrinolytic therapy with lysine analogs during cardiac surgery in the post aprotinin era. *Current Opinion in Anaesthesiology, 24*(1), 92–97. doi:10.1097/ACO.0b013e32833ff3eb PMID:20881484

LaPar, D. J., Crosby, I. K., Ailawadi, G., Ad, N., Choi, E., Spiess, B. D., et al. (2013). Blood product conservation is associated with improved outcomes and reduced costs after cardiac surgery. *The Journal of Thoracic and Cardiovascular Surgery, 145*(3), 796–803– discussion 803–4.

Levi, M., Levy, J. H., Andersen, H. F., & Truloff, D. (2010). Safety of recombinant activated factor VII in randomized clinical trials. *The New England Journal of Medicine, 363*(19), 1791–1800. doi:10.1056/NEJMoa1006221 PMID:21047223

Likosky, D. S., FitzGerald, D. C., Groom, R. C., Jones, D. K., Baker, R. A., Shann, K. G., & Body, S. C. et al. (2010). Effect of the perioperative blood transfusion and blood conservation in cardiac surgery clinical practice guidelines of the Society of Thoracic Surgeons and the Society of Cardiovascular Anesthesiologists upon clinical practices. *Anesthesia and Analgesia, 111*(2), 316–323. doi:10.1213/ANE.0b013e3181e329f1 PMID:20488928

Lindblad, B., Wakefield, T. W., Whitehouse, W. M., & Stanley, J. C. (1988). The effect of protamine sulfate on platelet function. *Scandinavian Journal of Thoracic and Cardiovascular Surgery*, *22*(1), 55–59. doi:10.3109/14017438809106052 PMID:3387950

Loor, G., Li, L., Sabik, J. F. III, Rajeswaran, J., Blackstone, E. H., & Koch, C. G. (2012). Nadir hematocrit during cardiopulmonary bypass: End-organ dysfunction and mortality. *The Journal of Thoracic and Cardiovascular Surgery*, *144*(3), 654–662.e4. doi:10.1016/j.jtcvs.2012.03.058 PMID:22507841

Mahla, E., Suarez, T. A., Bliden, K. P., Rehak, P., Metzler, H., Sequeira, A. J., & Gurbel, P. A. et al. (2012). Platelet function measurement-based strategy to reduce bleeding and waiting time in clopidogrel-treated patients undergoing coronary artery bypass graft surgery: The timing based on platelet function strategy to reduce clopidogrel-associated bleeding related to CABG (TARGET-CABG) study. *Circulation: Cardiovascular Interventions*, *5*(2), 261–269. doi:10.1161/CIRCINTERVENTIONS.111.967208 PMID:22396581

Makar, M., Taylor, J., Zhao, M., Farrohi, A., & Trimming, M. (2010). *Perioperative Coagulopathy, Bleeding, and Hemostasis During Cardiac Surgery A Comprehensive Review*. ICU Director.

Mangano, D. T., Tudor, I. C., & Dietzel, C.Multicenter Study of Perioperative Ischemia Research Group, Ischemia Research and Education Foundation. (2006). The risk associated with aprotinin in cardiac surgery. *The New England Journal of Medicine*, *354*(4), 353–365. doi:10.1056/NEJMoa051379 PMID:16436767

Mazer, C. D. (2014). Blood conservation in cardiac surgery: Guidelines and controversies. *Transfusion and Apheresis Science*, *50*(1), 20–25. doi:10.1016/j.transci.2013.12.008 PMID:24529682

Moskowitz, D. M., McCullough, J. N., Shander, A., Klein, J. J., Bodian, C. A., Goldweit, R. S., & Ergin, M. A. (2010). The impact of blood conservation on outcomes in cardiac surgery: Is it safe and effective? *The Annals of Thoracic Surgery*, *90*(2), 451–458. doi:10.1016/j.athoracsur.2010.04.089 PMID:20667328

Murphy, G. J., & Angelini, G. D. (2006). Indications for blood transfusion in cardiac surgery. *The Annals of Thoracic Surgery*, *82*(6), 2323–2334. doi:10.1016/j.athoracsur.2006.06.020 PMID:17126171

Murphy, G. J., Reeves, B. C., Rogers, C. A., Rizvi, S. I. A., Culliford, L., & Angelini, G. D. (2007). Increased mortality, postoperative morbidity, and cost after red blood cell transfusion in patients having cardiac surgery. *Circulation*, *116*(22), 2544–2552. doi:10.1161/CIRCULATIONAHA.107.698977 PMID:17998460

Nalla, B. P., Freedman, J., Hare, G. M. T., & Mazer, C. D. (2012). Update on blood conservation for cardiac surgery. *Journal of Cardiothoracic and Vascular Anesthesia*, *26*(1), 117–133. doi:10.1053/j.jvca.2011.07.024 PMID:22000983

Ngaage, D. L., & Bland, J. M. (2010). Lessons from aprotinin: Is the routine use and inconsistent dosing of tranexamic acid prudent? Meta-analysis of randomised and large matched observational studies. *European Journal of Cardio-Thoracic Surgery*, *37*(6), 1375–1383. doi:10.1016/j.ejcts.2009.11.055 PMID:20117944

Paparella, D., Brister, S. J., & Buchanan, M. R. (2004). Coagulation disorders of cardiopulmonary bypass: A review. *Intensive Care Medicine*, *30*(10), 1873–1881. doi:10.1007/s00134-004-2388-0 PMID:15278267

Paparella, D., Yau, T. M., & Young, E. (2002). Cardiopulmonary bypass induced inflammation: Pathophysiology and treatment. An update. *European Journal of Cardio-Thoracic Surgery*, *21*(2), 232–244. doi:10.1016/S1010-7940(01)01099-5 PMID:11825729

Rahe-Meyer, N., Solomon, C., Hanke, A., Schmidt, D. S., Knoerzer, D., Hochleitner, G., & Pichlmaier, M. et al. (2013). Effects of fibrinogen concentrate as first-line therapy during major aortic replacement surgery: A randomized, placebo-controlled trial. *Anesthesiology*, *118*(1), 40–50. doi:10.1097/ALN.0b013e3182715d4d PMID:23249928

Rahe-Meyer, N., & Sørensen, B. (2011). For: Fibrinogen concentrate for management of bleeding. *Journal of Thrombosis and Haemostasis*, *9*(1), 1–5. doi:10.1111/j.1538-7836.2010.04099.x PMID:20946151

Ranucci, M., Aronson, S., Dietrich, W., Dyke, C. M., Hofmann, A., Karkouti, K., & von Heymann, C. et al. (2011a). Patient blood management during cardiac surgery: Do we have enough evidence for clinical practice? *The Journal of Thoracic and Cardiovascular Surgery*, *142*(2), 249.e1–249.e32. doi:10.1016/j.jtcvs.2011.04.007 PMID:21605874

Ranucci, M., Baryshnikova, E., Castelvecchio, S., & Pelissero, G.Surgical and Clinical Outcome Research (SCORE) Group. (2013). Major bleeding, transfusions, and anemia: The deadly triad of cardiac surgery. *The Annals of Thoracic Surgery*, *96*(2), 478–485. doi:10.1016/j.athoracsur.2013.03.015 PMID:23673069

Ranucci, M., La Rovere, M. T., Castelvecchio, S., Maestri, R., Menicanti, L., Frigiola, A., & Febo, O. et al. (2011b). Postoperative anemia and exercise tolerance after cardiac operations in patients without transfusion: What hemoglobin level is acceptable? *The Annals of Thoracic Surgery*, *92*(1), 25–31. doi:10.1016/j.athoracsur.2011.02.058 PMID:21592458

Ranucci, M., Pazzaglia, A., Bianchini, C., Bozzetti, G., & Isgrò, G. (2008). Body size, gender, and transfusions as determinants of outcome after coronary operations. *The Annals of Thoracic Surgery*, *85*(2), 481–486. doi:10.1016/j.athoracsur.2007.10.014 PMID:18222248

Rozental, T., & Shore-Lesserson, L. (2012). Pharmacologic management of coagulopathy in cardiac surgery: An update. *Journal of Cardiothoracic and Vascular Anesthesia*, *26*(4), 669–679. doi:10.1053/j.jvca.2012.03.030 PMID:22608465

Savonitto, S., D'Urbano, M., Caracciolo, M., Barlocco, F., Mariani, G., Nichelatti, M., & De Servi, S. et al. (2010). Urgent surgery in patients with a recently implanted coronary drug-eluting stent: A phase II study of "bridging" antiplatelet therapy with tirofiban during temporary withdrawal of clopidogrel. *British Journal of Anaesthesia*, *104*(3), 285–291. doi:10.1093/bja/aep373 PMID:20047898

Shander, A., Van Aken, H., Colomina, M. J., Gombotz, H., Hofmann, A., Krauspe, R., & Spahn, D. R. et al. (2012). Patient blood management in Europe. *British Journal of Anaesthesia*, *109*(1), 55–68. doi:10.1093/bja/aes139 PMID:22628393

Song, H. K., Tibayan, F. A., Kahl, E. A., Sera, V. A., Slater, M. S., Deloughery, T. G., & Scanlan, M. M. (2014). Safety and efficacy of prothrombin complex concentrates for the treatment of coagulopathy after cardiac surgery. *The Journal of Thoracic and Cardiovascular Surgery*, *147*(3), 1036–1040. doi:10.1016/j.jtcvs.2013.11.020 PMID:24365268

Sørensen, B., Spahn, D. R., Innerhofer, P., Spannagl, M., & Rossaint, R. (2011). Clinical review: Prothrombin complex concentrates -evaluation of safety and thrombogenicity. *Critical Care (London, England), 15*(1), 201. doi:10.1186/cc9311 PMID:21345266

Sousa-Uva, M., Storey, R., Huber, K., Falk, V., Leite-Moreira, A. F., Amour, J., & Collet, J.-P. et al. (2014). Expert position paper on the management of antiplatelet therapy in patients undergoing coronary artery bypass graft surgery. *European Heart Journal, 35*(23), 1510–1514. doi:10.1093/eurheartj/ehu158 PMID:24748565

Speiss, B. D. (2002). Transfusion and outcome in heart surgery. *The Annals of Thoracic Surgery, 74*(4), 986–987. doi:10.1016/S0003-4975(02)03906-1 PMID:12400732

Steiner, M. E., Ness, P. M., Assman, S. F., Triulzi, D. J., Sloan, S. R., & Delaney, M. et al.. (2015). Effects of red-cell storage duration on patients undergoing cardiac surgery. *The New England Journal of Medicine, 372*(15), 1419–1429. doi:10.1056/NEJMoa1414219 PMID:25853746

Steinlechner, B., Zeidler, P., Base, E., Birkenberg, B., Ankersmit, H. J., Spannagl, M., & Jilma, B. et al. (2011). Patients with severe aortic valve stenosis and impaired platelet function benefit from preoperative desmopressin infusion. *The Annals of Thoracic Surgery, 91*(5), 1420–1426. doi:10.1016/j.athoracsur.2011.01.052 PMID:21439546

Stuklis, R. G., O'Shaughnessy, D. F., & Ohri, S. K. (2001). Novel approach to bleeding in patients undergoing cardiac surgery with liver dysfunction. *European Journal of Cardio-Thoracic Surgery: Official Journal of the European Association for Cardio-Thoracic Surgery, 19*(2), 219–220. doi:10.1016/S1010-7940(00)00641-2 PMID:11167117

Sun, J. C. J., Whitlock, R., Cheng, J., Eikelboom, J. W., Thabane, L., Crowther, M. A., & Teoh, K. H. T. (2008). The effect of pre-operative aspirin on bleeding, transfusion, myocardial infarction, and mortality in coronary artery bypass surgery: A systematic review of randomized and observational studies. *European Heart Journal, 29*(8), 1057–1071. doi:10.1093/eurheartj/ehn104 PMID:18346962

Suttner, S., Piper, S. N., Kumle, B., Lang, K., Röhm, K. D., Isgro, F., & Boldt, J. (2004). The influence of allogeneic red blood cell transfusion compared with 100% oxygen ventilation on systemic oxygen transport and skeletal muscle oxygen tension after cardiac surgery. *Anesthesia and Analgesia, 99*(1), 2–11. doi:10.1213/01.ANE.0000120163.44315.47 PMID:15281492

Tanaka, K. A., Key, N. S., & Levy, J. H. (2009). Blood coagulation: Hemostasis and thrombin regulation. *Anesthesia and Analgesia, 108*(5), 1433–1446. doi:10.1213/ane.0b013e31819bcc9c PMID:19372317

van Straten, A. H. M., Hamad, M. A. S., van Zundert, A. J., Martens, E. J., Schönberger, J. P. A. M., & de Wolf, A. M. (2009). Preoperative hemoglobin level as a predictor of survival after coronary artery bypass grafting: A comparison with the matched general population. *Circulation, 120*(2), 118–125. doi:10.1161/CIRCULATIONAHA.109.854216 PMID:19564556

Villanueva, C., Colomo, A., Bosch, A., Concepción, M., Hernandez-Gea, V., Aracil, C., & Guarner, C. et al. (2013). Transfusion strategies for acute upper gastrointestinal bleeding. *The New England Journal of Medicine, 368*(1), 11–21. doi:10.1056/NEJMoa1211801 PMID:23281973

Vivacqua, A., Koch, C. G., Yousuf, A. M., Nowicki, E. R., Houghtaling, P. L., Blackstone, E. H., & Sabik, J. F. III. (2011). Morbidity of bleeding after cardiac surgery: Is it blood transfusion, reoperation for bleeding, or both? *The Annals of Thoracic Surgery*, *91*(6), 1780–1790. doi:10.1016/j.athoracsur.2011.03.105 PMID:21619974

Wademan, B. H., & Galvin, S. D. (2014). Desmopressin for reducing postoperative blood loss and transfusion requirements following cardiac surgery in adults. *Interactive Cardiovascular and Thoracic Surgery*, *18*(3), 360–370. doi:10.1093/icvts/ivt491 PMID:24263581

Walkden, G. J., Verheyden, V., Goudie, R., & Murphy, G. J. (2013). Increased perioperative mortality following aprotinin withdrawal: A real-world analysis of blood management strategies in adult cardiac surgery. *Intensive Care Medicine*, *39*(10), 1808–1817. doi:10.1007/s00134-013-3020-y PMID:23863975

Weiskopf, R. B., & Silverman, T. A. (2013). Balancing potential risks and benefits of hemoglobin-based oxygen carriers. *Transfusion*, *53*(10), 2327–2333. PMID:23869543

Westenbrink, B. D., Kleijn, L., de Boer, R. A., Tijssen, J. G., Warnica, W. J., Baillot, R., & van Gilst, W. H. et al. (2011). Sustained postoperative anaemia is associated with an impaired outcome after coronary artery bypass graft surgery: Insights from the IMAGINE trial. *Heart (British Cardiac Society)*, *97*(19), 1590–1596. doi:10.1136/heartjnl-2011-300118 PMID:21757458

Whitlock, R., Crowther, M. A., & Ng, H. J. (2005). Bleeding in cardiac surgery: Its prevention and treatment--an evidence-based review. *Critical Care Clinics*, *21*(3), 589–610. doi:10.1016/j.ccc.2005.04.003 PMID:15992674

Wikkelsø, A. (Ed.). (2013). Fibrinogen concentrate in bleeding patients. *Cochrane Database of Systematic Reviews*, *8*, CD008864. PMID:23986527

Wozniak, G., Noll, T., Akintürk, H., Thul, J., & Müller, M. (2001). Factor XIII prevents development of myocardial edema in children undergoing surgery for congenital heart disease. *Annals of the New York Academy of Sciences*, *936*(1), 617–620. doi:10.1111/j.1749-6632.2001.tb03549.x PMID:11460520

Yoo, Y.-C., Shim, J.-K., Kim, J.-C., Jo, Y.-Y., Lee, J.-H., & Kwak, Y.-L. (2011). Effect of single recombinant human erythropoietin injection on transfusion requirements in preoperatively anemic patients undergoing valvular heart surgery. *Anesthesiology*, *115*(5), 929–937. doi:10.1097/ALN.0b013e318232004b PMID:22027622

KEY TERMS AND DEFINITIONS

Anemia: According to WHO anemia is a condition in which the number of red blood cells is insufficient to meet the body's oxygenation needs. For an adult female, anemia is defined as an Hgb level below 12 g/dl while adult males are considered anemic when levels fall below 13 g/dl. An Hgb level below 8 g/dl is considered severe anemia.

Coagulopathy: Condition in which the blood's ability to clot is impaired. Due to fine balance of coagulation system, a higher propensity for clot formation is also considered a coagulopathy.

Patient Blood Management (PBM): Patient centered evidence based multidisciplinary approach to blood transfusion focused on erythropoiesis promotion, minimizing bleeding, and optimizing tolerance of anemia.

Prothrombin Complex Concentrate (PCC): Combination of several coagulation factors derived from human plasma. Primarily used for reversal of Coumadin and in cases of severe coagulopathy. Multiple products are commercially available, primarily divided in three-factors (II, IX and X) and four-factors (II, VII, IX and X) preparations.

Thromboelastography and Thromboelastrometry: Point of care test using viscoelastic technique for qualitative assessment of the entire coagulation system encompassing the interaction of platelets and coagulation factors in clot formation and fibrinolysis.

Transfusion Associated Circulatory Overload (TACO): Volume overload from excessive administration of blood products. TACO is clinically characterized by hypertension, pulmonary edema and increased filling pressures.

Transfusion Related Acute Lung Injury (TRALI): Immune mediated syndrome characterized by acute respiratory distress following blood transfusion.

Chapter 21
Endocrine and Metabolic Management in the Cardiothoracic ICU

Rifka C. Schulman
Long Island Jewish Medical Center, USA

Jeffrey I. Mechanick
Icahn School of Medicine at Mount Sinai, USA

ABSTRACT

In this chapter, we review several important endocrine disorders frequently encountered in patients undergoing cardiothoracic surgery. Hyperglycemia, common in patients with and without diabetes mellitus (DM) in the perioperative period, has been linked to poor outcomes. Use of an intravenous insulin infusion early in the postoperative course, followed by transition to subcutaneous insulin, with maintenance of moderate glycemic targets (100-180 mg/dL) is currently the standard of care. Oral intake should be encouraged in the postoperative period, but if not possible, nutrition support with enteral nutrition should be considered. Critical illness related corticosteroid insufficiency (CIRCI) should be suspected in critically ill patients with refractory hypotension requiring vasopressors, especially in the setting of septic shock. Although diagnositic criteria are controversial, if suspected, empiric treatment with corticosteroids should be initiated. Nonthyroidal illness syndrome (NTIS) is common in critically ill patients and thyroid function tests should be interpreted with caution in this population.

INTRODUCTION

Endocrine and metabolic problems are among the many complex medical issues that face the cardiothoracic surgical patient. While at first glance these issues may appear minor, compared to obvious imperatives such as cardiac and pulmonary function, a deeper understanding of endocrine/metabolic pathophysiology will enhance overall care and clinical outcomes. The first objective of this chapter is to review the metabolic effects of stress endured by the CTICU patient, with an understanding of the various stages

DOI: 10.4018/978-1-4666-8603-8.ch021

of critical illness that may be traversed depending on the severity of illness. Subsequently, the chapter will explore four key topics: 1) tight glycemic control, 2) nutrition support, 3) adrenal insufficiency, and 4) abnormal thyroid function. For each of these important areas, the relevant literature will be reviewed and optimal management strategies presented.

BACKGROUND

While significant and recent advances in cardiothoracic surgical care have optimized patient outcomes, these patients sustain varying degrees of critical illness in the post-operative period. From a metabolic perspective, patients can be understood in terms of four sequential stages of critical illness, each with a unique hormonal and metabolic milieu: acute critical illness (ACI), prolonged acute critical illness (PACI), chronic critical illness (CCI), and recovery from critical illness (RCI) (Hollander & Mechanick, 2006; Schulman & Mechanick, 2012).

ACI follows a stressor (e.g., surgery, infection, or trauma) that triggers the "stress response," characterized by enhanced secretion of "stress hormones" (e.g., cortisol, glucagon, and growth hormone), catecholamines, and cytokines (tumor necrosis factor-α [TNF-α], interleukin-1 [IL-1], and interleukin-6 [IL-6]) (Singer, De Santis, & Vitale, 2004). Increased levels of cytokines shift reverse-phase reactants (e.g., albumin, transferrin, and cortisol-binding globulin) to acute-phase reactants (e.g., C-reactive protein and immunoglobulins). This hormonal milieu diverts substrates from anabolic to catabolic pathways, stimulating gluconeogenesis, lipolysis, and proteolysis of skeletal muscle, while inhibiting peripheral glucose uptake, to ensure an adequate supply of substrates (Chang & Bistrian, 1998; Marques, & Langouche, 2012). These metabolic changes create a state of insulin resistance, frequently leading to hyperglycemia in critically ill patients (Mechanick, 2006).

PACI, beginning at around day 3 of critical illness, is characterized by a persistent stress response, with maintenance of inflammation, catabolism, and insulin resistance. While ACI is considered an adaptive response, conferred by evolutionary mechanisms, the persistence of critically ill patients in the intensive care unit (ICU), repeatedly avoiding death by artificial means, is largely due to technological innovations, which have no evolutionary precedent. Persistent immune-neuroendocrine (INA) output results in excessive tissue breakdown, hyperglycemia, and hypoalbuminemia.

CCI, beginning with tracheotomy at around day 10-14 of critical illness, represents a unique maladaptive physiological state characterized by prolonged mechanical ventilation, kwashiorkor-like malnutrition, stress hyperglycemia, neuroendocrine dysfunction, impaired wound healing, immune deficiency, metabolic bone disease, critical illness myopathy and polyneuropathy, neurocognitive dysfunction, and excessive symptom burden for patients (Hollander & Mechanick, 2006; Nelson, Meier, & Litke, 2004).

RCI is defined by successful liberation from mechanical ventilation and promotes amelioration of inflammation and a return from catabolism to anabolism. Survivors frequently suffer from persistent organ dysfunction and impaired quality of life. Patients in the cardiothoracic ICU ideally recover from critical illness within a few days postoperatively, directly following ACI. However, some patients follow a more complicated course with prolonged mechanical ventilation.

GLYCEMIC CONTROL

Pathophysiology

Hyperglycemia and insulin resistance are common features of critical illness, resulting as part of the stress response in an effort to maintain adequate availability of glucose. Blood glucose (BG) levels > 110 mg/dL were identified in 98.7% of a cohort of cardiovascular surgery patients (Van den Berghe, Wouters, & Weekers, 2001). In patients who are young, lean, and fasting, as would have been the case from an evolutionary perspective, the stress response can maintain serum glucose in the normal range. However, as is more often the case in the modern day cardiothoracic ICU, patients are older and obese, have multiple comorbidities, and receive many interacting medications and possibly nutrition support, the last frequently leading to hyperglycemia even in patients without a history of diabetes mellitus (DM) (Boonen & Van den Berghe, 2014). Stress hyperglycemia – the appearance of hyperglycemia under periods of stress in the absence of DM -- is typically reversible and of short duration in the postoperative period (Dungan, Braithwaite, & Preiser, 2009). Insulin requirements generally decrease proportional to improvements in clinical status and time after surgery. Stress hyperglycemia is an entity with increasing relevance in conjunction with clinical outcomes. Patients with pre-existing type-1 or -2 DM usually require increased amounts of insulin in the perioperative period, with gradual return to baseline insulin dosing with resolution of the metabolic stress.

In the post-operative or critically ill patient, hyperglycemia is related to cytokine- and hormone-mediated insulin resistance, combined with impaired glucose uptake (GLUT transporters) (Langouche, & Van den Berghe, 2006). Hyperglycemia has been found to induce harm by multiple mechanisms, including pro-inflammatory effects, oxidative tissue injury, endothelial dysfunction, and pancreatic ß-cell apoptosis (Mechanick, 2006). In the cardiothoracic patient, hyperglycemia inhibits myocardial glycolysis and enhances free fatty acid metabolism, resulting in a deficit of glycolysis-derived ATP and the potential for membrane destabilization and arrhythmias (Furnary, Gao, & Grunkemeier, 2003). Furthermore, increased levels of cytokines induced by hyperglycemia can stimulate a postoperative capillary leak syndrome, leading to pulmonary edema and prolonged requirements for mechanical ventilation (Lazar, Chipkin, & Fitzgerald, 2004). Insulin corrects hyperglycemia but has additional salutary effects including anabolism, suppression of reactive oxygen species, and vasodilation via generation of nitric oxide (Le Roith, 2004).

While the adverse effects of hyperglycemia in the cardiothoracic ICU patient are evident, hypoglycemia has become increasingly recognized as a critical factor surrounding glycemic control. Acute hypoglycemia activates the sympathetic nervous system and stimulates secretion of counter-regulatory hormones (i.e., glucagon and epinephrine) resulting in hemodynamic shifts and altering regional blood flow as a protective response to defend the brain from neuroglycopenia (Wright, & Frier, 2008). While in otherwise healthy, young adults, these effects may be transient, patients with pre-existing endothelial dysfunction may suffer from enhanced vascular damage (i.e., myocardial and/or cerebral ischemia). Furthermore, severe hypoglycemia may result in seizures, loss of consciousness or coma. Hypoglycemia is associated with characteristic effects on the myocardium. During acute hypoglycemia, an increased heart rate, systolic blood pressure, cardiac output, and contractility, compromise the cardiovascular system. Hypoglycemia is associated with arrhythmias, which may predispose to sudden cardiac death (Snell-Bergeon, & Wadwa, 2012).

Historical Perspective

General ICU

The evidence base on glycemic control in the ICU has shifted clinical practice patterns several times in recent years, with important relevance for the cardiothoracic ICU. While traditional thinking considered stress hyperglycemia a physiologic response to critical illness, the landmark Leuven study by Van den Berghe et al. (2001), the first randomized controlled trial on blood glucose (BG) control in critical illness, showed improved morbidity and mortality in a surgical ICU with intensive insulin therapy (IIT) using an intravenous (IV) insulin infusion, targeting BG of 80-110 mg/dL, compared to the traditional approach (BG < 215 mg/dL). Of note 62% of patients in this study had undergone cardiac surgery. A subsequent study in the Leuven medical ICU by Van den Berghe showed improved morbidity but not mortality in the tight glycemic control group (Van den Berghe, Wilmer, & Hermans, 2006). Following the results of these studies, worldwide clinical practice adopted the concept of tight glycemic control in the ICU.

In subsequent years, the findings of Van den Berghe et al. could not be consistently replicated. Notably, the large multicenter Normoglycemia in Intensive Care Evaluation-Survival Using Glucose Algorithm Regulation (NICE-SUGAR) study showed an increased mortality and 13-fold increased rate of severe hypoglycemia in the tight control group (80-108 mg/dL) compared to the moderate control group (140-180 mg/dL) (NICE-SUGAR Study Investigators, 2009). A *post hoc* analysis of the NICE-SUGAR study database showed a strong association between moderate and severe hypoglycemia and the risk of death (NICE-SUGAR Study Investigators, 2012). Subsequent to NICE-SUGAR, clinical practice shifted again, with moderate glucose control (140-180 mg/dL) representing the new recommended glucose target for critically ill patients (Moghissi, Korytkowski, & DiNardo, 2009).

A number of important differences in the Leuven and NICE-SUGAR study designs help with interpretation of the disparate results. The Leuven studies were highly standardized, with well-trained nurses, frequent BG measurements using whole arterial blood and a blood gas analyzer, a dedicated central venous line lumen, and accurate syringe pump for IV insulin (Boonen & Van den Berghe, 2014). NICE-SUGAR, reflecting more typical clinical practice, was not standardized, with different levels of staff training and utilizing many types of glucose measurements. The discrepant results of these studies show that optimal and safe glucose targets may vary by institution or hospital unit, based on resources, training and infrastructure, especially in regards to monitoring for and treatment of hypoglycemia (Weiss & Mechanick, 2011). Additionally, the delivery of nutrition support was optimized in the Leuven studies but not in NICE-SUGAR: 19 kcal/kg/d versus 11 kcal/kg/d, respectively (Berger & mechanick, 2010). The ability to safely attain tight glycemic control without excessive risk of hypoglycemia may depend on the delivery of adequate nutrition (Scurlock, Raikhelkar, & Mechanick 2010).

In addition to the correlations between uncontrolled hyperglycemia and hypoglycemia with outcomes in the critically ill, a third significant glycemic variable has been identified. Increased glycemic variability, using standard deviation, range, or other metrics, has been recognized as a strong independent predictor of mortality in ICU patients (Krinsley, 2008; Hermanides, Vriesendorp, & Bosman, 2010). Therefore, consideration should be made not just to optimize the mean BG, or avoid hypoglycemia, in the ICU patient, but also to maintain stability and avoid large swings in glucose values.

Recently a number of studies have reported a differential mortality effect related to diabetes status. Van den Berghe G, Wilmer A, & Milants (2006), using a pooled database of the 2 seminal Leuven studies, found that IIT reduced mortality in all patients except for those with pre-existing DM. In A large retrospective multicenter cohort study of medical and surgical ICU patients, DM status and glucose targets were critically assessed (Krinsley, Egi, & Kiss, 2013). Among patients without DM, a mean BG of 80-140 mg/dL was associated with a decreased mortality compared to higher glucose levels. However, among patients with DM, a mean BG of 80-110 mg/dL correlated with an increased risk of mortality compared to 110-180 mg/dL. In a cohort of patients with CCI, tighter glycemic control was correlated with improved outcomes in patients with stress hyperglycemia but not with DM (Schulman, Moshier, & Rho, 2014). Furthermore, the utilization of Hemoglobin A1c (A1c) to determine optimal glucose targets in the ICU has been suggested, but will require additional study (Egi, Bellomo, & Stachowski, 2011).

Patients with pre-existing DM may adapt to the harmful effects of hyperglycemia over time via downregulation of GLUT transporters (Klip, Tsakiridis, Marrette, 1994). Conversely, patients without DM prior to hospitalization, but with new and transient stress hyperglycemia due to critical illness, may experience a higher level of glycemia-related toxicity. Therefore, a lower glucose target may be appropriate for patients with stress hyperglycemia, while a higher target may be appropriate for patients with pre-existing DM.

Cardiothoracic ICU

Diabetes and pre-diabetes are highly prevalent in the cardiothoracic surgical population. This is consistent with the increased prevalence of DM in the general population and the known relationship between uncontrolled DM and coronary artery disease. The relationships among DM, glycemic status, and coronary artery bypass graft (CABG) outcomes account for increased perioperative morbidity, mortality, and recurrent angina in patients with DM (Szabo, Hakanson, & Svedjeholm, 2002; Carson, Scholz, & Chen, 2002). Previously, these associations were thought to be irreversible and a function of preoperative comorbidities with DM (e.g., obesity, hypertension, peripheral vascular disease, and chronic kidney disease). Subsequently, evidence showed that uncontrolled hyperglycemia in the preoperative (Anderson, Brismar, & Barr, 2005), intraoperative (Doenst, Wijeysundera, & Karkouti, 2005), and postoperative (McAlister, Man, & Bistritz, 2003) periods was linked to higher morbidity and mortality in patients both with and without DM.

A landmark study by Furnary et al. (2003) examined the effect of perioperative glycemic control in patients with DM undergoing CABG (n=3554). Patients were treated with subcutaneous insulin for BG < 200 mg/dL (1987-1991), IV insulin for BG 150-200 mg/dL (1991-1998), and IV insulin for BG 100-150 mg/dL (1998-2001). Both glucose control and mortality were found to be significantly lower with IV insulin, with a multivariable analysis identifying IIT as independently protective against death. Overall mortality in this DM population was 2.5% in the IIT group, and 5.3% in the subcutaneous insulin group, demonstrating a 57% reduction (p<0.0001). In fact, Furnary et al. showed that IIT eliminated the increased hospital mortality associated with DM status after CABG. Of note, individual daily average glucose level from the operative day and from post-operative day (POD) 1 and 2, were each independent predictors of death, but not the glucose on POD 3; this supports application of the 4-stage model of critical illness in this cardiac surgery population.

Lazar et al. (2004) prospectively randomized DM patients undergoing CABG to receive IIT with a modified glucose-insulin-potassium solution (BG target 125-200 mg/dL) compared to standard therapy with subcutaneous insulin (BG target < 250 mg/dL) in the perioperative period. Tighter control with IIT resulted in many short-term benefits, including reduced length of stay, incidence of atrial fibrillation, and need for vasopressor support. Importantly, long-term benefits of IIT included significantly reduced

2-year mortality and decreased episodes of recurrent ischemia and wound infections. Optimized perioperative glycemic control has also been correlated with significantly decreased rates of sternal wound infections (Zerr, Furnary, & Grunkemeier, 1997; Hruska, Smith, & Hendy, 2005).

The use of more aggressive glycemic control (90-120 mg/dL) was prospectively compared to moderate glycemic control (120-180 mg/dL) in a cohort of patients with DM undergoing CABG and receiving IV insulin in the perioperative period (Lazar, McDonnell, & Chipkin, 2011). There was no significant difference in clinical outcomes, but a higher incidence of hypoglycemia was noted in the tighter control group. Therefore this aggressive level of control provided no added benefit but increased harm.

Interestingly, a cohort of cardiothoracic surgery patients demonstrated that absence of an adequate early postoperative stress response (BG $\geq$ 120 mg/dL) was associated with increased ICU mortality (Via, Scurlock, & Adams, 2010). In this same cohort, patients who recovered from ACI or PACI had lower average BG levels early in the ICU course than patients who recovered from CCI, indicating an association between poorer glucose control and prolonged ICU course.

Management Strategies

Prior to cardiothoracic surgery, an A1c level should be drawn regardless of DM status to identify normal preoperative glycemic control (< 5.7%), pre-diabetes (5.7-6.4%) or pre-existing or occult DM ($\geq$ 6.5%). Patients with a history of DM that is tightly controlled may have lower A1c levels. The type of DM (1 vs. 2) should be identified, as patients with type 1 DM always require basal insulin to prevent the risk of diabetic ketoacidosis. It is important to check the A1c prior to surgery to obtain the most accurate result. The A1c value is extremely useful to predict patterns of hyperglycemia in the perioperative period and for planning DM management at discharge.

Patients with a history of DM should be instructed on how to manage their oral hypoglycemic agents and/or insulin prior to surgery. Oral DM medications and non-insulin injectables should be held approximately 24 hours prior to surgery (Lazar, McDonnell, & Chipkin, 2009). Recent use of a sulfonylurea agent may increase the risk of hypoglycemia when fasting (McDonnell, Alexanian, & White, 2012). Patients previously on an insulin regimen should be instructed to hold their pre-meal rapid-acting insulin (lispro, aspart, or glulisine) dose on the morning of surgery when they are fasting. Basal insulin (glargine, detemir, or NPH) should still be given the night before or the morning of surgery. Some practitioners maintain the usual doses of basal insulin, while others recommend a partial dose reduction to avoid hypoglycemia (e.g. 80% of the usual dose). Patients using a continuous subcutaneous insulin pump should discontinue the pump and transition to an intravenous insulin infusion just prior to surgery. Patients with grossly uncontrolled and/or newly diagnosed DM, or with BG > 180 mg/dL, can also be started on IV insulin prior to surgery, which should lower BG to the target range within 4-8 hours. Attention should be paid to renal function as the risk of hypoglycemia is increased in the setting of chronic kidney disease and acute kidney injury.

In the perioperative period, IV insulin allows for rapid titrating of insulin as requirements can fluctuate in response to stress and various medications, some of which are routinely given in dextrose. A nurse-driven insulin infusion protocol should be utilized for titration of the insulin infusion. Many insulin protocols exist, but the important elements include hourly BG monitoring and higher order algorithms, such as using of the rate of change of BG values and the current insulin infusion rate to determine changes in insulinization (McDonnell et al., 2012). A number of effective IIT protocols have been described in the literature (Van den Berghe et al., 2001; Furnary et al., 2003; Goldberg, Siegel, & Sherwin, 2004;

Via et al., 2010). The accuracy of point-of-care glucose meters in an ICU setting is sub-optimal and if used, should be confirmed with serum glucose values regularly. The Society for Thoracic Surgeons (STS) guidelines recommend that all patients with DM, or any patient with BG > 180 mg/dL regardless of DM status, should be initiated on IV insulin in the operating room and for at least 24 hours post-operatively to maintain a BG ≤ 180 mg/dL (Lazar et al., 2009). BG < 100 mg/dL should typically be avoided to prevent hypoglycemia. More frequent glucose monitoring (every 30-60 minutes) should be performed intra-operatively, and may need to be monitored every 15 minutes during the administration of cardioplegia and systemic cooling and rewarming. Patients who require 3 or more days of ICU care due to need for mechanical ventilation, inotropes, anti-arrhythmic drugs, renal replacement therapy, intra-aortic balloon pump or left ventricular assist device support, should be considered for tighter glucose targets if this can be achieved safely.

The Surgical Care Improvement Project (SCIP) is a national quality benchmark, requiring BG ≤ 180 mg/dL during the time period 18-24 hours following cardiothoracic surgery (Fry, 2008; QualityNet.org). A multidisciplinary approach including involvement of cardiothoracic surgery, endocrinology, anesthesiology, nursing and pharmacy is recommended to achieve optimal glycemic control in the perioperative period (McDonnell et al., 2012). Furthermore, a panel of insulin protocols to address different challenges in glycemic control for the CTICU patient is beneficial and utilized at the Mount Sinai Hospital (Table 1).

Consultation by an inpatient diabetes service is helpful to coordinate the transition off of intravenous to subcutaneous insulin and to optimize medication management for discharge. Alternatively a protocol can be devised for the routine transition process, tailored to individual hospital settings. Ideally IV insulin should be continued until POD 2 when the stress response has partially dissipated, insulin requirements have decreased, and SCIP benchmarks have been completed. Patients should also be extubated, off vasopressors, and ready to receive nutrition prior to discontinuation of IV insulin.

At the time of transition from IV to subcutaneous insulin, a basal insulin should be administered subcutaneously followed by discontinuation of the insulin drip 2 hours later, to allow time for the basal

Table 1. Cardiometabolic support protocols utilized at the Mount Sinai Hospital cardiothoracic ICU and stepdown units

Cardiometabolic Support Protocols
Screening with Hemoglobin A1C
Intraoperative insulin drip protocol
Postoperative insulin drip protocol • For patients in the immediate postoperative period (ACI, PACI)
"Patch protocol" to correct hyperglycemia if SCIP benchmark is in danger of violation
Transition protocol from intravenous to subcutaneous insulin with oral nutrition • e.g. Lispro pre-meal 3 times daily and once daily glargine
Transition protocol from intravenous to subcutaneous insulin with enteral nutrition • e.g. NPH every 6 hours plus lispro correction scale every 6 hours
CCI subcutaneous insulin protocol • For ongoing management of glycemic control with enteral and/or parenteral nutrition
Protocol for transition off insulin or to discharge oral medications on the wards
Hypoglycemia protocol

ACI = acute critical illness; PACI = prolonged acute critical illness; CCI = chronic critical illness.

insulin to take effect. This step is important to prevent hyperglycemia given the short half life (7 minutes) of intravenous regular insulin. The basal insulin dose can be determined according to a transition protocol, if available, or calculated based on insulin drip requirements. In addition to basal insulin, pre-meal (nutritional or bolus) insulin and a correction scale should be ordered, both utilizing rapid-acting insulin. Most hospitals have a number of correctional scales to select from based on the patient's insulin requirements. This method of using basal, pre-meal, and correction insulin is referred to as basal-bolus or multiple dose insulin (MDI) therapy, and is the mainstay of inpatient DM management. Patients who are not eating should not receive nutritional insulin, but can still receive correction insulin for hyperglycemia. Patients who are receiving continuous enteral nutrition (EN) can be managed with basal insulin, including NPH every 6 hours as an option, in conjunction with a correction scale administered every 3-6 hours. Patients receiving parenteral nutrition (PN) can have regular insulin placed into the PN bag, generally starting with 0.1 unit of insulin per gram of dextrose. Various approaches to this transition process have been described in the literature (McDonnell et al., 2012, Dungan, Hall, & Schuster, 2011). Caution should be made to avoid hypoglycemia, and the utilization of a hypoglycemia protocol (i.e. nurse education, IV dextrose at the bedside) can be effective to quickly normalize any downward trend in blood glucose. Other strategies for insulin management are summarized in Table 2.

Once patients leave the cardiothoracic ICU and are transferred to a step-down or regular hospital unit, standard inpatient glycemic goals should be targeted: A fasting and pre-meal BG 100-140 mg/dL and a random BG < 180 mg/dL, with avoidance of hypoglycemia (BG < 70 mg/L) (Moghissi et al. 2009; Umpierrez, Hellman, & Korytkowski, 2012). Point-of-care glucose should be monitored before meals and at bedtime. Daily titration of insulin doses may be required to maintain BG in the target range.

Glycemic status and elevated A1c are predictors of increased postoperative hyperglycemia and glucose variability after CABG (Masla, Gottschalk, & Durieux, 2011). Patients with a history of uncontrolled DM, and/or requiring large doses or insulin at home would be expected to have significant insulin requirements postoperatively. However, what may be surprising is that patients without DM may require large doses of insulin in the first few postoperative days due to stress hyperglycemia. The A1c value is important for these patients as insulin requirements will drop significantly each postoperative day, and proactive lowering of the basal-bolus insulin regimen is required when BG are in the target range to avoid hypoglycemia. Patients with stress hyperglycemia usually can be discharged home off of DM medication. Patients noted to have pre-diabetes should be counseled on lifestyle modification and diabetes prevention and to follow up with their primary care physician. An A1c will also guide the clinician regarding discharge planning for patients with DM: if the A1c is > 7.0% consideration for optimization of the prior home regimen should be made. Patients with A1c > 9% should usually be sent home on an insulin regimen and follow up closely with endocrinology as an outpatient. If resuming oral agents at

Table 2. Additional strategies for insulin titration

Strategy	Definition
Cross-titration	Initiate or increase subcutaneous insulin regimen while decreasing IV insulin infusion
Co-titration	Increase nutrition support prescription while simultaneously increasing insulin regimen
Counter-titration	Increase nutrition support prescription while lowering insulin doses (utilized for hypoglycemia) or Decrease nutrition support prescription while increasing insulin doses (utilized for hyperglycemia)

discharge, caution should be made to check for any new contraindications for the use of these agents (Table 3). Patients with type 1 DM should always be sent home on an insulin regimen including basal and nutritional insulin or resume use of an insulin pump. DM education should be started early on in the hospital stay once a high A1c has been identified.

NUTRITION SUPPORT

Challenges in the ICU

The provision of adequate macro- and micronutrients is of great importance during critical illness but is often suboptimally executed. Determination of nutritional requirements in the ICU population is challenging. The use of indirect calorimetry to determine energy requirements is the gold standard, but requires technical expertise and is unavailable at many institutions. Alternatively, predictive equations

Table 3. Oral and non-insulin injectable diabetes medications and contraindications

Class	Name	Mechanism of Action (Route)	Side Effects	Contraindications
Biguanides	Metformin	Decrease insulin resistance (oral)	Gastrointestinal Lactic acidosis (rare)	Creatinine >1.4 (females) Creatinine > 1.5 (males) Severe congestive heart failure Cirrhosis
Sulfonylureas	Glipizide Glyburide Glimepiride	Increase release of insulin from beta cells (oral)	Hypoglycemia Weight gain	Elderly Alcohol abuse Renal insufficency
Meglitinides	Repaglinide Nateglinide	Increase release of insulin from beta cells (oral)	Hypoglycemia Weight gain	Caution in decreased renal function[a]
DPP4 inhibitors	Sitagliptin, Saxagliptin, Linagliptin	Decrease glucagon Increase insulin (oral)	Pancreatitis	Pancreatitis Dose adjust for renal impairment
GLP 1 agonists	Exenatide, Liraglutide	Decrease glucagon Increase insulin slow gastric empyting (subcutaneous)	Gastrointestinal Pancreatitis	Pancreatitis Avoid with GFR < 30 mL/min
Alpha glucosidase inhibitor	Acarbose	Prevent intestinal absorption of glucose (oral)	Gastrointestinal	Cirrhosis Gastrointestinal disorders
Thiazolidine-diones	Pioglitazone	Decrease insulin resistance (oral)	Edema Weight gain Exacerbated heart failure Bladder cancer fractures	Congestive heart failure
SGLT2 inhibitor	Canagliflozin	Inhibit glucose reabsorption in the kidney (oral)	Urinary tract and genital infections Polyuria	Avoid in the elderly and with renal impairment

[a]Meglitinides are short acting and preferred over sulfonylureas in patients with renal impairment and in the elderly to avoid hypoglycemia.

may be used, or simple formulas, such as 20–25 kcal/kg/day and 1.2–1.5 g/kg/d protein. However, such weight-based formulas may be inaccurate due to edema, sarcopenia, and obesity. Losses of nitrogen through diarrhea, vomiting, wound or ostomy drainage, and hemodialysis confound the calculation of protein requirements. Monitoring of nutritional status is also difficult given inaccuracy of weight due to fluid retention. Furthermore, hypoalbuminemia correlates with the severity of inflammation and may be more a marker of metabolic stress than nutritional status.

Underfeeding is common in the ICU setting due to hesitation to initiate nutrition support, under-prescribing by practitioners, and logistical reasons. For instance, the amount of enteral feeds actually received by the patient is often lower than that prescribed due to holding of nutrition for procedures or gastrointestinal intolerance. Underfeeding has been associated with an increased mortality, infectious rate, duration of mechanical ventilation, and ICU length of stay (Stapleton, Jones, & Heyland, 2007). Of note, underfeeding of energy and protein are distinct entities, with prescription of adequate amounts of each necessary for optimal outcome (Weijs, Stapel, & de Groot, 2012). Additionally, sufficient lipid intake (> 1 g/kg/week) is necessary to prevent essential fatty acid deficiency (Mascioli, Lopes, & Champagne, 1996)

Conversely, overfeeding has been implicated with multiple harmful effects (Schulman & Mechanick, 2013). Overfeeding of dextrose exacerbates stress hyperglycemia and may potentiate fluid retention, hypertriglyceridemia, hepatic steatosis, and hypercapnia. Overfeeding of protein may predispose to azotemia and hypertonic dehydration. Lipid excess can induce cholestasis. Parenteral lipid may exert an immunosuppressive effect, potentially predisposing to bacterial and fungal growth in the setting of poor aseptic precautions (Mirtallo, Dasta, & Kleinschmidt, 2010).

Another potential complication of nutrition support is refeeding hypophosphatemia or a more fulminant refeeding syndrome, owing to elevations in insulin with carbohydrate delivery. Both of these conditions are more often observed in chronic and/or severe malnutrition and can manifest severe hypophosphatemia. Refeeding syndrome can also manifest hypokalemia, hypomagnesemia, thiamine deficiency, redistribution of other micronutrients, fluid overload, and multi-organ dysfunction (Skipper, 2012). Patients at risk for the development of refeeding syndrome should be managed with initially low and then gradually increasing levels of nutrition support, combined with close monitoring of volume status and aggressive repletion of electrolytes, especially phosphate.

Management Strategies

Patients who are recovering from ACI and who are able to take oral nutrition should be optimized using this route. Nutritional assessment by a registered dietitian should be requested for all high-risk patients, especially the elderly, those with comorbidities, pre-existing malnutrion, and/or impairment of the GI tract. If necessary, nutritional shakes can supplement inadequate oral intake, and specialized formulas used as needed (e.g. diabetes or renal preparations).

Patients who progress through later stages of critical illness (PACI and CCI), who remain mechanically ventilated for a prolonged period, typically require nutrition support. The gastrointestinal tract should be used to provide EN If accessible and functional. Tolerance of gastric residuals up to 500 mL appears to be safe and is recommended (Montejo, Minambres, & Bordeje, 2010). If needed a post-pyloric feeding tube can be placed when standard enteral feeds via nasogastric tube are not tolerated. If all efforts to utilize the gastrointestinal tract fail, then PN support should be prescribed according to the patient's clinical and biochemical status.

Significant controversy in the literature has surrounded the optimal timing to consider adding PN when EN is insufficient to provide nutritional requirements. Over the years disagreement in the clinical practice guidelines between The American Society for Parenteral and Enteral Nutrition (ASPEN) and The European Society for Clinical Nutrition and Metabolism (ESPEN) existed regarding late (after 7 days) vs. early (after 2 days) initiation of PN, respectively (Martindale, McClave, & Vanek, 2009; Singer, Berger, & Van den Berghe, 2009). However, recently, the EPaNIC trial, a large multicenter randomized controlled trial, showed that late initiation of PN resulted in a shorter ICU length of stay, a reduced rate of infections, and no difference in mortality compared to early use of PN (Casaer, Mesotten, & Hermans, 2011). This trial along with others, have produced more of a consensus among the experts: hypocaloric nutrition may be acceptable during the first week in the ICU (ACI and early PACI) but nutrition should certainly be optimized during the later stages of critical illness (Casaer & Van den Berghe, 2014).

Of note, a prospective randomized controlled trial from Geneva (Heidegger, Graf, & Thibault, 2011) demonstrated improved clinical outcomes with supplemental PN, added after ICU day 3 only if EN is < 60% of target, and in patients estimated to stay >5 days in the ICU. This study utilized indirect calorimetry to determine calorie targets and individualized PN formulas. This is in contrast to the above study by Casaer et al. (2011) which did not utilize indirect calorimetry for energy determinations, used standardized PN formulas and concentrated dextrose (D20W) infusions, and included lower risk ICU patients. Further studies are needed to better elucidate the potential benefits of supplemental PN in the sickest of ICU patients unable to meet nutritional requirements through the enteral route.

ADRENAL INSUFFICIENCY

Pathophysiology

Regardless of the etiology, critical illness is a severe form of physiological stress. One essential component of the acute stress response involves activation of the hypothalamic-pituitary-adrenal (HPA) axis culminating in the accelerated production of cortisol from the adrenal cortex. This response is mediated by secretion of corticotropin-releasing hormone (CRH) and arginine vasopressin (AVP) from the hypothalamus, stimulating secretion of adrenocorticotropic hormone (ACTH) from the anterior pituitary. Acute stress-induced hypercortisolism, with a loss of the diurnal pattern of secretion, is considered a beneficial and protective response. Hypercortisolism shifts metabolism from anabolic to catabolic pathways to provide needed energy; gluconeogenesis and lipolysis are stimulated and peripheral glucose uptake is suppressed, leading to increased serum blood glucose and free fatty acid levels. Cortisol promotes hemodynamic stability via intravascular fluid retention and by improving sensitivity of vascular smooth muscle to vasopressor agents. Additionally cortisol's anti-inflammatory effect may prevent overstimulation of the inflammatory cascade via downregulation of cytokines (Van den Berghe, 2002; Marik, Pastores, & Annane, 2008; Boonen & Van den Berghe, 2014).

While the traditional understanding of hypercortisolism in critical illness was presumed to be ACTH-driven, the related factors are now considered to be more complex. While patients with ACI demonstrate both elevated ACTH and cortisol levels, hypothalamic-pituitary suppression is identified beginning around day 3-5 of critical illness (PACI), notably with low levels of ACTH. One explanation for the paradoxical maintenance of hypercortisolism despite low levels of ACTH in the later stages of critical illness, relates to direct humoral stimulation of the adrenal gland via pro-inflammatory cytokines or endothelin-1 (Bornstein, Engeland, & Ehrhart-Bornstein, 2008; Vermes, Beishuizen, & Hampsink, 1995). Importantly, recent studies have demonstrated reduced cortisol clearance (Boonen, Vervenne, & Meersseman, 2013) in critical illness via suppression of principal cortisol-metabolizing enzymes: ring A reductases (5β-reductase and 5α-reductase) in the liver and 11β-hydroxysteroid dehydrogenase type 2 (11β-HSD2). These enzymes convert cortisol to cortisone in the kidney and are suppressed by increased levels of serum bile acids, characteristic of critical illness (Vanwijngaerden, Wayters, & Langouche, 2011).

The definition and diagnostic approach to adrenal insufficiency in the ICU has been a controversial topic. The overall incidence of adrenal insufficiency in a surgical ICU population was reported at 0.66%, but increased to 6% in the subset of patients with an ICU stay ≥ 14 days, and 11% in the subset with age > 55 years and ICU stay ≥ 14 days (Barquist & Kirton, 1997). In ICU patients with severe sepsis and septic shock, the prevalence of adrenal insufficiency was as high as 60% (Annane, Maxime, & Ibrahim, 2006). Such discrepancies in reported prevalence likely stem from discordant criteria used to make the diagnosis of adrenal insufficiency in different patient populations. While impaired adrenal function in the ICU may occasionally be attributable to structural damage of the adrenal or pituitary glands due to hemorrhage or infarction, the majority of cases are thought to result from reversible dysfunction of the HPA axis.

The term, "relative adrenal insufficiency," or more recently, "critical illness related corticosteroid insufficiency" (CIRCI) has been used to describe an insufficient corticosteroid activity for the severity of illness of a particular patient (Marik, 2009). While the involved mechanisms are complex and not fully understood, an array of factors may be involved, including suppression of the HPA axis and acquired glucocorticoid resistance. Increased levels of TNF-α and IL-1 seen in critical illness may be linked to the reversible HPA axis dysfunction of CIRCI (Gaillard, 1990). Septic shock has been associated with nitric oxide synthase induced neuronal apoptosis of the hypothalamus (Sharshar, Gray, & Lorin de la Grandmaison, 2003). The use of etomidate for tracheal intubation has been linked to higher frequency of temporary adrenal suppression but is not consistently linked to worse outcomes (Freund, Jabre, & Mourad, 2014). Corticosteroid tissue resistance refers to the inability of activated glucocorticoid receptors to downregulate the transcription of inflammatory mediators, despite the presence of hypercortisolism (Meduri & Yates, 2004).

Greater than 90% of circulating cortisol is bound to proteins: primarily corticosteroid-binding globulin (CBG), and to a lesser degree, albumin (Hamrahian, Oseni, & Arafah, 2004). One of the characteristic metabolic shifts of acute illness is the shift from reverse phase reactant to acute phase reactant production in the liver, commonly resulting in hypoalbuminemia and significant reductions in CBG in critically ill patients. Reduced levels of binding proteins would be expected to reduce serum total cortisol levels (the standard assay measured) while not necessarily affecting free cortisol values. Therefore, free cortisol levels may be more predictive of beneficial response to steroid therapy in patients suspected of having CIRCI (Hamrahian et al., 2004).

Diagnosis

Absolute adrenal insufficiency classically presents with symptoms of fatigue, weakness, listlessness, orthostatic dizziness, weight loss, nausea, vomiting and anorexia, with salt-craving and hyperpigmentation specific for primary adrenal insufficiency. Common laboratory abnormalities include hyponatremia, hyperkalemia, hypoglycemia, and mild eosinophilia (Oelkers, 1996). This clinical presentation is in contrast with that of CIRCI, in which the most common manifestation is hypotension refractory to intravenous fluids, requiring use of vasopressor agents (Marik, 2009). CIRCI should be suspected in any critically ill patient requiring vasopressor support. There is no consistent pattern of hemodynamic parameters in CIRCI, possibly reflecting variability in the underlying disease state.

The precise level of serum cortisol required for sufficient adrenal function in the critically ill patient is unclear. A random cortisol of less than 15 or 25 mcg/dL in a highly stressed patient has been suggested as a diagnostic threshold for relative adrenal insufficiency (Cooper & Stewart, 2003; Marik & Zaloga, 2003). Although stressed patients are thought to lose the normal diurnal pattern of cortisol secretion, serum cortisol tests are limited by the timing of measurement, as large hourly fluctuations have been reported (Marik, 2009).

The use of a cosyntropin stimulation test for the diagnosis of adrenal insufficiency in critically ill patients has been well studied. This dynamic test consists of the administration of cosyntropin, a synthetic ACTH, at 250 mcg intravenously with serum cortisol assessed at times zero, 30 minutes and 60 minutes. In the unstressed subject, adrenal insufficiency is indicated by a maximally stimulated cortisol less than 18-20 mcg/dL (Oelkers, 1996). In a cohort of patients with septic shock, a Δ max cortisol (highest cortisol value minus time zero value) ≤ 9 mcg/dL was associated with worse 28-day mortality (Annane, Sebille, & Troche 2000).

One criticism of the 250 mcg cosyntropin test relates to the supraphysiologic dose used and whether subtle levels of adrenal dysfunction could be missed. A "low dose" 1 mcg cosyntropin test has been suggested and has been shown to diagnose CIRCI in patients who would be considered to have adequate adrenal function according to the "high dose" test (Siraux, De Backer, & Yalavatti, 2005; Burry, Little, & Hallett, 2013). Nevertheless, the 1 mcg test is not as well studied in association with clinical outcomes as the 250 mcg test, and is therefore not recommended for the diagnosis of CIRCI in clinical practice (Marik et al. 2008).

The use of free cortisol in place of total cortisol has been suggested for the diagnosis of adrenal insufficiency in the critically ill patient. Hamrahian et al.(2004) showed that in an ICU cohort subnormal baseline and cosyntropin-stimulated serum total cortisol levels were common in patients with hypoproteinemia, but free cortisol levels were found to be high-normal or elevated. A baseline serum free cortisol threshold of 2.0 mcg/dL, or 3.1 mcg/dL after cosyntropin stimulation, was suggested to identify patients at risk for CIRCI. Critiques of this study include the absence of patients with severe septic shock, the population with the strongest correlation between adrenal dysfunction and outcome (Polderman, van Zanten, & Girbes, 2004). Additionally, the free cortisol assay is technically difficult and not widely available. Studies of interstitial cortisol obtained via micro-dialysis catheter placed into subcutaneous adipose tissue, in a cohort of mechanically ventilated patients with sepsis, showed moderate correlation between total and free cortisol with interstitial levels (Vassiliadi, Ilias, & Tzanela, 2013). In this study, a total cortisol < 10 mcg/dL and a free cortisol < 0.8 mcg/dL correlated with interstitial cortisol values in the lowest quartile. The routine use of free cortisol to guide clinical decision-making is still being studied.

Annane et al. (2006) utilized metyrapone, known to block the final step of cortisol synthesis (conversion of 11β-deoxycortisol to cortisol) to critically assess diagnostic methods for CIRCI in a population of patients with sepsis. This study found that optimal predictors of adrenal insufficiency were a random total cortisol < 10 mcg/dL or a Δ max cortisol after cosyntropin 250 mcg of ≤ 9 mcg/dL. These diagnostic criteria are recommended for assessment of CIRCI by a consensus statement from the American College of Critical Care Medicine (Marik et al. 2008).

Management Strategies

In addition to the controversies surrounding diagnosis of CIRCI, a lack of consensus on when and how to treat with corticosteroids has persisted. Several decades ago, short courses of high-dose corticosteroid treatment (10,000 – 40,000 mg of hydrocortisone per day) in patients with ARDS and severe sepsis were studied, but found to be linked to higher mortality and rates of complications such as super-infection (Cronin, Cook, & Carlet, 1995). More recently, longer courses of lower and more physiological doses of hydrocortisone (200 – 300 mg per day), termed "stress dose," were studied in a number of randomized controlled trials and found to be efficacious with a consistent benefit on survival and reversal of shock (Minneci, Deans, & Banks, 2004). Additionally, use of stress dose hydrocortisone in septic shock has been shown to improve quality of life in survivors and reduce the incidence of post-traumatic stress disorder (Schelling, Stoll, & Kapfhammer, 1999).

One important placebo-controlled, randomized, double-blinded, parallel trial in France, studied the use of hydrocortisone 50mg intravenously every 6 hours and fludrocortisone 50 mcg orally once daily for a 7 day course in a cohort of patient with septic shock (Annane, Sebille, & Charpentier, 2002). Among non-responders to the cosyntropin stimulation test (Δ max cortisol ≤ 9 mcg/dL), presumably indicative of CIRCI, treatment with hydrocortisone and fludrocortisone significantly reduced the risk of death and the use of vasopressor support, without an increase in adverse events.

Subsequently, the corticosteroid therapy of septic shock (CORTICUS) study was a multicenter, randomized, double-blinded, placebo-controlled trial, studying the use of hydrocortisone 50mg intravenously every 6 hours vs. placebo over 5 days, followed by tapering doses over 6 days in a cohort of patients with septic shock (Sprung, Annane, & Keh, 2008). At 28 days, there was no significant difference in mortality in the 2 groups, regardless of responsiveness to cosyntropin testing, contrary to the prior findings of Annane et al. (2002). Patients receiving hydrocortisone did benefit from faster resolution of shock compared to placebo, but suffered increased rates of super-infection.

The CORTICUS study differed from the earlier French study in several ways:

- Patients in the French study were sicker, with an entry requirement to the study of a blood pressure less than 90 mm Hg for greater than 1 hour despite intravenous fluids and vasopressor support.
- Enrollment in the French study was allowed only within 8 hours after fulfilling criteria for septic shock, while in CORTICUS, a 72-hour window was used.
- Fludrocortisone was not included in the CORTICUS study since 200mg of hydrocortisone per day is thought to provide sufficient mineralocorticoid activity itself.
- In the French study treatment was stopped abruptly after 7 days, while in CORTCIUS therapy was tapered from days 5 to 11.

In summary, the combined findings of these studies indicate that benefit from hydrocortisone is most pronounced among patients treated early after the onset of septic shock and who remain hypotensive despite vasopressor therapy (Sprung et al., 2008). Interestingly, a recent consensus statement on this issue recommends avoiding the use of a cosyntropin stimulation test or other biochemical measurements due to poor test performance. Rather, treatment decisions should be based on clinical features, namely patients in septic shock unresponsive to vasopressor therapy (Marik et al., 2008). Dexamethasone is not recommended for treatment of CIRCI because of associated prolonged suppression of the HPA axis.

Recent data suggest that even lower doses of corticosteroids may be optimal for the treatment of CIRCI. Results from stable isotope studies show a 24-hour cortisol production of about 60 mg per day in critically ill patients with SIRS, compared to about 30 mg per day in controls (Boonen et al. 2013; Boonen et al., 2014). The use of the lowest possible effective dose of corticosteroid is important because of the many potential adverse effects of prolonged corticosteroid use in the critically ill patient, including hyperglycemia, myopathy, loss of lean body mass, and bone loss. Whether treatment with these lower doses correlates with outcomes is of interest and will require further study.

ABNORMAL THYROID FUNCTION

The nonthyroidal illness syndrome (NTIS) has been well described and refers to a constellation of thyroid lab abnormalities frequently seen in patients without true thyroid disease. This syndrome is frequently encountered in the ICU (Adler & Wartofsky, 2007). Varying degrees of NTIS may be seen in as many as 75% of hospitalized patients. The severity of NTIS appears to be proportional to the severity of illness and has been associated with increased mortality in ICU patients (Wang, Pan, & Wang, 2012).

During ACI, there is a decrease in serum levels of the active hormone, triiodothyronine (T_3) and an increase in reverse T_3, which appears to be mediated by suppressed action of the type-1 deiodinase that peripherally converts thyroxine (T_4) to T_3. The low T_3 is typically accompanied by a normal level of T_4 and thyroid stimulating hormone (TSH). Factors that may stimulate this low-T_3 state include an absence of nutrition and elevated levels of inflammatory cytokines. This response to starvation may be beneficial during ACI by reducing the energy expenditure (Boonen & Van den Berghe, 2014). This effect may be related to worsened outcomes with early parenteral nutrition in the ICU (Langouche, Vander Perre, & Marques, 2013).

During PACI and CCI, hypothalamic-pituitary suppression produces a biochemical picture that could be confused with central hypothyroidism: low or low-normal T_4 and TSH in addition to continued low T_3. These effects may be mimicked or exacerbated by the presence of medications known to suppress hypothalamic function, such as corticosteroids and dopamine. In comparison to the potentially adaptive nature of NTIS acutely, it is suspected that NTIS in the later stages of critical illness without evolutionary precedent may represent a maladaptive response. NTIS rarely produces a completely suppressed TSH as seen in hyperthyroidism or in actual central hypothyroidism (Bao, Oiknine, & Fisher, 2012). If recovery from critical illness occurs, a bolstered hypothalamic-pituitary response may produce a temporary and mild TSH elevation.

Given the common occurrence of NTIS, thyroid function studies should ideally only be assessed in ICU patients with a clinical picture consistent with hypo- or hyperthyroidism. Hypothyroidism should be suspected in patients with hypothermia, bradycardia, hypotension, prior neck surgery, or difficulty weaning off of the ventilator. True hypothyroidism is suspected by the presence of an elevated TSH. When the TSH elevation is only mild (< 10 U/mL), true hypothyroidism should be differentiated from a resolving NTIS, which can also have a mild TSH elevation in the recovery phase (Mechanick & Brett, 2002). A positive anti-thyroid peroxidase (TPO) antibody titer, consistent with Hashimoto's thyroiditis, in conjunction with a repeat TSH that is continuing to rise, helps substantiate the need for treatment with levothyroxine (synthetic T_4). Extreme caution should be taken when replacing thyroid hormone in a patient with active ischemia; very low doses (12.5-25 mcg daily) of levothyroxine should be initiated and titrated up as tolerated with close monitoring. The use of liothyronine (synthetic T_3) for routine thyroid replacement is not recommended as this is the active hormone and may predispose cardiac patients to increased arrhythmias. Treatment of NTIS with levothyroxine or liothyronine is controversial and is not currently recommended (Adler et al., 2007; De Groot, 2006). The use of hypothalamic releasing factors (e.g. thyrotropin releasing hormone [TRH]) to correct hypothalamic suppression has been investigated but requires validation in clinical trials (Van den Berghe, Baxter, & Weekers, 2002).

New onset hyperthyroidism is extremely rare in the ICU, but should be considered in the differential for unexplained tachycardia, atrial fibrillation, weight loss, hyperthermia, and heat intolerance. Patients receiving amiodarone should have baseline thyroid function testing, given the associated occurrence of hypo- and hyperthyroidism.

When indicated, levothyroxine should be administered "on an empty stomach" to enhance absorption. For patients who can take medication orally, the drug should be in the morning at least 30 minutes prior to food or other medications. Patients receiving enteral nutrition who require treatment with levothyroxine, should have tube feeds cycled over 20–23 hours, to permit delivery of levothyroxine in the absence of nutrition. If the gastrointestinal tract is nonfunctional or malabsorption is suspected, intravenous levothyroxine can be administered at 50–80% of the usual oral dose (Mechanick et al., 2002). Patients suspected to have myxedema coma, or profound hypothyroidism with altered mental status and hemodynamic instability, should always be treated with intravenous levothyroxine. Doses should be determined based on cardiac status, age, and severity of hypothyroidism (clinical and biochemical) with the assistance of an endocrinologist.

FUTURE RESEARCH DIRECTIONS

While much progress has been made in recent years toward understanding key endocrine and metabolic issues facing the cardiothoracic patient, further research is still required to clarify a number of management issues. As reviewed above, the notion of differing glycemic targets for patients with DM vs. stress hyperglycemia (higher vs. lower, respectively), is of interest and will require further validation in prospective studies, especially in the cardiothoracic ICU population. The increasing consensus surrounding delayed use of PN in the first week of critical illness is a result of recent and ongoing studies designed to clarify an issue that has long been controversial. Autophagy, a protective pathway involving removal of cellular debris and damaged organelles, may be negatively affected by parenteral nutrients during ACI, and will require further investigation (Vanhorebeek, Gunst, & Derde, 2011). Finally, whether even lower and more physiologic doses of "stress dose" hydrocortisone are efficacious for treatment of CIRCI requires further investigation.

CONCLUSION

As described above, abnormal endocrine and metabolic parameters are extremely common in the cardiothoracic ICU population. These abnormalities are present in varying degrees during the 4 metabolic stages of critical illness. The significance of optimized glycemic control following cardiac surgery to promote the best possible patient outcomes is now appreciated. Use of IIT with an IV insulin infusion followed by careful transition to subcutaneous basal-bolus insulin is the standard of care in the CTICU. Oral nutrition should be encouraged, but if not possible, nutrition support should be provided to meet energy and protein targets. Diagnosis and treatment of adrenal and thyroid disorders in the CTICU can be challenging; differentiating "typical" values of critical illness from a true endocrine disorder is difficult but important to prevent morbidity and mortality. The involvement of an endocrinologist or an endocrinology team in the management of these issues is beneficial and should be considered.

REFERENCES

Adler, S. M., & Wartofsky, L. (2007). The nonthyroidal illness syndrome. *Endocrinology and Metabolism Clinics of North America*, *36*(3), 657–672. doi:10.1016/j.ecl.2007.04.007 PMID:17673123

Anderson, R. E., Brismar, K., Barr, G., & Ivert, T. (2005). Effects of cardiopulmonary bypass on glucose homestasis after coronary artery bypass surgery. *European Journal of Cardio-Thoracic Surgery*, *28*(3), 425–430. doi:10.1016/j.ejcts.2005.05.025 PMID:16054822

Annane, D., Maxime, V., Ibrahim, F., Alvarez, J. C., Abe, E., & Boudou, P. (2006). Diagnosis of adrenal insufficiency in severe sepsis and septic shock. *American Journal of Respiratory and Critical Care Medicine*, *174*(12), 1319–1326. doi:10.1164/rccm.200509-1369OC PMID:16973979

Annane, D., Sebille, V., Charpentier, C., Bollaert, P. E., Francois, B., Korach, J. M., & Bellissant, E. et al. (2002). Effect of treatment with low doses of hydrocortisone and fludrocortisone on mortality in patients with septic shock. *Journal of the American Medical Association*, *288*(7), 862–871. doi:10.1001/jama.288.7.862 PMID:12186604

Annane, D., Sebille, V., Troche, G., Raphael, J. C., Gajdos, P., & Bellissant, E. (2000). A 3-level prognostic classification in septic shock based on cortisol levels and cortisol response to corticotropin. *Journal of the American Medical Association*, *283*(8), 1038–1045. doi:10.1001/jama.283.8.1038 PMID:10697064

Bao, S., Oiknine, R., & Fisher, S. J. (2012). Differentiating nonthyroidal illness syndrome from central hypothyroidism in the acutely ill hospitalized patient. *Endocrine*, *42*(3), 758–760. doi:10.1007/s12020-012-9685-0 PMID:22562722

Barquist, E., & Kirton, O. (1997). Adrenal insufficiency in the surgical intensive care unit patient. *Journal of Trauma and Acute Care Surgery*, *42*(1), 27–31. doi:10.1097/00005373-199701000-00006 PMID:9003254

Berger, M. M., & Mechanick, J. I. (2010). Continuing controversy in the intensive care unit: Why tight glycemic control, nutrition support, and nutritional pharmacology are each necessary therapeutic considerations. *Current Opinion in Clinical Nutrition and Metabolic Care*, *13*(2), 167–169. doi:10.1097/MCO.0b013e328335f2e0 PMID:20075721

Boonen, E., & Van den Berghe, G. (2014). Endocrine responses to critical illness: Novel insights and therapeutic implications. [Epub ahead of print]. *The Journal of Clinical Endocrinology and Metabolism*, jc20134115. PMID:24517153

Boonen, E., Vervenne, H., Meersseman, P., Andrew, R., Mortier, L., Declercq, P. E., & Van den Berghe, G. et al. (2013). Reduced cortisol metabolism during critical illness. *The New England Journal of Medicine*, *368*(16), 1477–1488. doi:10.1056/NEJMoa1214969 PMID:23506003

Bornstein, S. R., Engeland, W. C., Ehrhart-Bornstein, M., & Herman, J. P. (2008). Dissociation of ACTH and glucocorticoids. *Trends in Endocrinology and Metabolism*, *19*(5), 175–180. doi:10.1016/j.tem.2008.01.009 PMID:18394919

Burry, L., Little, A., Hallett, D., & Mehta, S. (2013). Detection of critical illness-related corticosteroid insufficiency using a 1 μg adrenocorticotropic hormone test. *Shock (Augusta, Ga.)*, *39*(2), 144–148. PMID:23324883

Carson, J., Scholz, P., Chen, A., Peterson, E., Gold, J., & Schneider, S. (2002). Diabetes mellitus increases short-term mortality and morbidity in patients undergoing coronary artery bypass graft surgery. *Journal of the American College of Cardiology*, *40*(3), 418–423. doi:10.1016/S0735-1097(02)01969-1 PMID:12142105

Casaer, M. P., Mesotten, D., Hermans, G., Wouters, P. J., Schetz, M., Meyfroidt, G., & Van den Berghe, G. et al. (2011). Early versus late parenteral nutrition in critically ill adults. *The New England Journal of Medicine*, *365*(6), 506–517. doi:10.1056/NEJMoa1102662 PMID:21714640

Casaer, M. P., & Van den Berghe, G. (2014). Nutrition in the acute phase of critical illness. *The New England Journal of Medicine*, *370*(13), 1227–1236. doi:10.1056/NEJMra1304623 PMID:24670169

Chang, H. R., & Bistrian, B. (1998). The role of cytokines in the catabolic consequences of infection and injury. *Journal of Parenteral and Enteral Nutrition*, *22*(3), 156–166. doi:10.1177/0148607198022003156 PMID:9586794

Cooper, M. S., & Stewart, P. M. (2003). Corticosteroid insufficiency in acutely ill patients. *The New England Journal of Medicine*, *348*(8), 727–734. doi:10.1056/NEJMra020529 PMID:12594318

Cronin, L., Cook, D. J., Carlet, J., Heyland, D. K., King, D., Lansang, M. A., & Fisher, C. J. Jr. (1995). Corticosteroid treatment for sepsis: A critical appraisal and meta-analysis of the literature. *Critical Care Medicine*, *23*(8), 1430–1439. doi:10.1097/00003246-199508000-00019 PMID:7634816

De Groot, L. (2006). Non-thyroidal illness syndrome is a manifestation of hypothalamic-pituitary dysfunction, and in view of current evidence, should be treated with appropriate replacement therapies. *Critical Care Clinics*, *22*(1), 57–86. doi:10.1016/j.ccc.2005.10.001 PMID:16399020

Doenst, T., Wijeysundera, D., Karkouti, K., Zechner, C., Maganti, M., Rao, V., & Borger, M. A. (2005). Hyperglycemia during cardiopulmonary bypass is an independent risk factor for mortality in patients undergoing cardiac surgery. *The Journal of Thoracic and Cardiovascular Surgery*, *130*(4), 1144–1149. doi:10.1016/j.jtcvs.2005.05.049 PMID:16214532

Dungan, K., Hall, C., Schuster, D., & Osei, K. (2011). Comparison of 3 algorithms for basal insulin in transitioning from intravenous to subcutaneous insulin in stable patients after cardiothoracic surgery. *Endocrine Practice*, *17*(5), 753–758. doi:10.4158/EP11027.OR PMID:21550950

Dungan, K. M., Braithwaite, S. S., & Preiser, J. C. (2009). Stress hyperglycemia. *Lancet*, *373*(9677), 1798–1807. doi:10.1016/S0140-6736(09)60553-5 PMID:19465235

Egi, M., Bellomo, R., Stachowski, E., French, C. J., Hart, G. K., Taori, G., & Bailey, M. et al. (2011). The interaction of chronic and acute glycemia with mortality in critically ill patients with diabetes. *Critical Care Medicine*, *39*(1), 105–111. doi:10.1097/CCM.0b013e3181feb5ea PMID:20975552

Freund, Y., Jabre, P., Mourad, J., Lapostolle, F., Reuter, P. G., Woimant, M., & Adnet, F. et al. (2014). Relative adrenal insufficiency in critically ill patient after rapid sequence intubation: KETASED ancillary study. *Journal of Critical Care*; epub ahead of print. PMID:24508204

Fry, D. E. (2008). Surgical site infections and the surgical care improvement project (SCIP): Evolution of national quality measures. *Surgical Infections*, *9*(6), 579–584. doi:10.1089/sur.2008.9951 PMID:19216670

Furnary, A. P., Gao, G., Grunkemeier, G. L., Wu, Y., Zerr, K. J., Bookin, S. O., & Starr, A. et al. (2003). Continuous insulin infusion reduces mortality in patients with diabetes undergoing coronary artery bypass grafting. *The Journal of Thoracic and Cardiovascular Surgery*, *125*(5), 1007–1021. doi:10.1067/mtc.2003.181 PMID:12771873

Gaillard, R. C., Turnill, D., Sappino, P., & Muller, A. F. (1990). Tumor necrosis factor alpha inhibits the hormonal response of the pituitary gland to hypothalamic releasing factors. *Endocrinology*, *127*(1), 101–106. doi:10.1210/endo-127-1-101 PMID:2163305

Goldberg, P. A., Siegel, M. D., Sherwin, R. S., Halickman, J. I., Lee, M., Bailey, V. A., & Inzucchi, S. E. et al. (2004). Implementation of a safe and effective insulin infusion protocol in a medical intensive care unit. *Diabetes Care*, *27*(2), 461–467. doi:10.2337/diacare.27.2.461 PMID:14747229

Hamrahian, A. H., Oseni, T. S., & Arafah, B. M. (2004). Measurements of serum free cortisol in critically ill patients. *The New England Journal of Medicine*, *350*(16), 1629–1638. doi:10.1056/NEJMoa020266 PMID:15084695

Heidegger, C. P., Graf, S., Thibault, R., Darmon, P., Berger, M., & Pichard, C. (2011). Supplemental parenteral nutrition (SPN) in intensive care unit (ICU) patients for optimal energy coverage: Improved clinical outcome. *Clinical Nutrition Supplements*, *1*(1), 2–3. doi:10.1016/S1744-1161(11)70006-0

Hermanides, J., Vriesendorp, T. M., Bosman, R. J., Zandstra, D. F., Hoekstra, J. B., & DeVries, J. H. (2010). Glucose variability is associated with intensive care unit mortality. *Critical Care Medicine*, *38*(3), 838–842. doi:10.1097/CCM.0b013e3181cc4be9 PMID:20035218

Hollander, J. M., & Mechanick, J. I. (2006). Nutrition support and the chronic critical illness syndrome. *Nutrition in Clinical Practice*, *21*(6), 587–604. doi:10.1177/0115426506021006587 PMID:17119165

Hruska, L. A., Smith, J. M., Hendy, M. P., Fritz, V. L., & McAdams, S. (2005). Continuous insulin infusion reduces infectious complications in diabetics following coronary surgery. *Journal of Cardiac Surgery*, *20*(5), 403–407. doi:10.1111/j.1540-8191.2005.200472.x PMID:16153268

Klip, A., Tsakiridis, T., Marrette, A., & Ortiz, P. A. (1994). Regulation of expression of glucose transporters by glucose: A review of studies in vivo and in cell cultures. *The FASEB Journal*, *8*, 43–53. PMID:8299889

Krinsley, J. S. (2009). Glycemic variability and mortality in critically ill patients: The impact of diabetes. *Journal of Diabetes Science and Technology*, *3*(6), 1292–1301. doi:10.1177/193229680900300609 PMID:20144383

Krinsley, J. S., Egi, M., Kiss, A., Devendra, A. N., Schuetz, P., Maurer, P. M., & Bellomo, R. et al. (2013). Diabetic status and the relation of the three domains of glycemic control to mortality in critically ill patients: An international multicenter cohort study. *Critical Care (London, England)*, *17*(2), R37. doi:10.1186/cc12547 PMID:23452622

Langouche, L., & Van den Berghe, G. (2006). Glucose metabolism and insulin therapy. *Critical Care Clinics*, *22*(1), 119–129. doi:10.1016/j.ccc.2005.09.005 PMID:16399023

Langouche, L., Vander Perre, S., Marques, M., Boelen, A., Wouters, P. J., Casaer, M. P., & Van den Berghe, G. (2013). Impact of early nutrient restriction during critical illness on the nonthyroidal illness syndrome and its relation with outcome: A randomized, controlled clinical study. *The Journal of Clinical Endocrinology and Metabolism*, *98*(3), 1006–1013. doi:10.1210/jc.2012-2809 PMID:23348400

Lazar, H. L., Chipkin, S. R., Fitzgerald, C. A., Bao, Y., Cabral, H., & Apstein, C. S. (2004). Tight glycemic control in diabetic coronary artery bypass graft patients improves perioperative outcomes and decreases recurrent ischemic events. *Circulation*, *109*(12), 1497–1502. doi:10.1161/01.CIR.0000121747.71054.79 PMID:15006999

Lazar, H. L., McDonnell, M. M., Chipkin, S., Fitzgerald, C., Bliss, C., & Cabral, H. (2011). Effects of aggressive versus moderate glycemic control on clinical outcomes in diabetic coronary artery bypass graft patients. *Annals of Surgery*, *254*(3), 458–464. doi:10.1097/SLA.0b013e31822c5d78 PMID:21865944

Lazar, H. L., McDonnell, M. M., Chipkin, S., Furnary, A. P., Engelman, R. M., Sadhu, A. R., & Shemin, R. J. et al. (2009). The Society for Thoracic Surgeons practice guideline series: Blood glucose management during adult cardiac surgery. *The Annals of Thoracic Surgery*, *87*(2), 663–669. doi:10.1016/j.athoracsur.2008.11.011 PMID:19161815

Le Roith, D. (2004). Molecular mechanisms by which metabolic control may improve outcomes. *Endocrine Practice*, *10*(2Supple), 57–62. doi:10.4158/EP.10.S2.57 PMID:15251642

Marik, P. E. (2009). Critical illness-related corticosteroid insufficiency. *Chest*, *135*(1), 181–193. doi:10.1378/chest.08-1149 PMID:19136406

Marik, P. E., Pastores, S. M., Annane, D., Meduri, G. U., Sprung, C. L., Arlt, W., & Vogeser, M. et al. American College of Critical Care Medicine. (2008). Recommendations for the diagnosis and management of corticosteroid insufficiency in critically ill adult patients: Consensus statements from an international task force by the American College of Critical Care Medicine. *Critical Care Medicine*, *36*(6), 1937–1949. doi:10.1097/CCM.0b013e31817603ba PMID:18496365

Marik, P. E., & Zaloga, G. P. (2003). Adrenal insufficiency during septic shock. *Critical Care Medicine*, *31*(1), 141–145. doi:10.1097/00003246-200301000-00022 PMID:12545007

Marques, M. B., & Langouche, L. (2012). Endocrine, Metabolic, and Morphologic Alterations of Adipose Tissue During Critical Illness. *Critical Care Medicine*. PMID:23135416

Martindale, R. G., McClave, S. A., Vanek, V. W., McCarthy, M., Roberts, P., Taylor, B., & Cresci, G. et al. (2009). Guidelines for the provision and assessment of nutrition support therapy in the adult critically ill patient: Society of Critical Care Medicine and American Society for Parenteral and Enteral Nutrition: executive summary. *Critical Care Medicine*, *37*(5), 1757–1761. doi:10.1097/CCM.0b013e3181a40116 PMID:19373044

Mascioli, E. A., Lopes, S. M., Champagne, C., & Driscoll, D. F. (1996). Essential fatty acid deficiency and home total parenteral nutrition patients. *Nutrition (Burbank, Los Angeles County, Calif.)*, *12*(4), 245–249. doi:10.1016/S0899-9007(96)90850-3 PMID:8862529

Masla, M., Gottschalk, A., Durieux, M. E., & Groves, D. S. (2011). HbA1c and diabetes predict perioperative hyperglycemia and glycemic variability in on-pump coronary artery bypass graft patients. *Journal of Cardiothoracic and Vascular Anesthesia*, *25*(5), 799–803. doi:10.1053/j.jvca.2010.09.028 PMID:21111636

McAlister, F. A., Man, J., Bistritz, L., Amad, H., & Tandon, P. (2003). Diabetes and coronary artery bypass surgery: An examination of perioperative glycemic control and outcomes. *Diabetes Care*, *26*(5), 1518–1524. doi:10.2337/diacare.26.5.1518 PMID:12716815

McDonnel, M. E., Alexanian, S. M., White, L., & Lazar, H. L. (2012). A primer for achieving glycemic control in the cardiac surgical patient. *Journal of Cardiac Surgery*, *27*(4), 470–477. doi:10.1111/j.1540-8191.2012.01471.x PMID:22640228

Mechanick, J. I. (2006). Metabolic Mechanisms of stress hyperglycemia. *Journal of Parenteral and Enteral Nutrition*, *30*(2), 157–163. doi:10.1177/0148607106030002157 PMID:16517960

Mechanick, J. I., & Brett, E. M. (2002). Nutrition support of the chronically critically ill patient. *Critical Care Clinics*, *18*(3), 597–618. doi:10.1016/S0749-0704(02)00006-4 PMID:12140915

Mechanick, J. I., & Brett, E. M. (2002). Endocrine and metabolic issues in the management of the chronically critically ill patient. *Critical Care Clinics*, *18*(3), 619–641. doi:10.1016/S0749-0704(02)00005-2 PMID:12140916

Meduri, G. U., & Yates, C. R. (2004). Systemic inflammation-associated glucocorticoid resistance and outcome of ARDS. *Annals of the New York Academy of Sciences*, *1024*(1), 24–53. doi:10.1196/annals.1321.004 PMID:15265772

Minneci, P. C., Deans, K. J., Banks, S. M., Eichacker, P. Q., & Natanson, C. (2004). Meta-analysis: The effect of steroids on survival and shock during sepsis depends on the dose. *Annals of Internal Medicine*, *141*(1), 47–56. doi:10.7326/0003-4819-141-1-200407060-00014 PMID:15238370

Mirtallo, J. M., Dasta, J. F., Kleinschmidt, K. C., & Varon, J. (2010). State of the art review: intravenous fat emulsions: current applications, safety profile, and clinical implications. *The Annals of Pharmacotherapy*, *44*, 688–700. PMID:20332339

Moghissi, E. S., Korytkowski, M. T., DiNardo, M., Einhorn, D., Hellman, R., Hirsch, I. B., & Umpierrez, G. E. et al. (2009). American Association of Clinical Endocrinologists and American Diabetes Association consensus statement on inpatient glycemic control. *Diabetes Care*, *32*(6), 1119–1131. doi:10.2337/dc09-9029 PMID:19429873

Montejo, J. C., Minambres, E., Bordeje, L., Mesejo, A., Acosta, J., Heras, A., & Manzanedo, R. et al. (2010). Gastric residual volume during enteral nutrition in ICU patients: The REGANE study. *Intensive Care Medicine*, *36*(8), 1386–1393. doi:10.1007/s00134-010-1856-y PMID:20232036

Nelson, J. E., Meier, D. E., Litke, A., Natale, D. A., Siegel, R. E., & Morrison, R. S. (2004). The symptoms burden of chronic critical illness. *Critical Care Medicine*, *32*(7), 1527–1534. doi:10.1097/01.CCM.0000129485.08835.5A PMID:15241097

NICE-SUGAR Study Investigators. (2009). Intensive versus conventional glucose control in critically ill patients. *The New England Journal of Medicine*, *360*(13), 1283–1297. doi:10.1056/NEJMoa0810625 PMID:19318384

NICE-SUGAR Study Investigators. (2012). Hypoglycemia and risk of death in critically ill patients. *The New England Journal of Medicine*, *367*(12), 1108–1118. doi:10.1056/NEJMoa1204942 PMID:22992074

Oelkers, W. (1996). Adrenal insufficiency. *The New England Journal of Medicine*, *335*(16), 1206–1212. doi:10.1056/NEJM199610173351607 PMID:8815944

Polderman, K. H., van Zanten, A., & Girbes, A. R. J. (2004). Free cortisol and critically ill patients. *The New England Journal of Medicine*, *351*(4), 395–397. doi:10.1056/NEJM200407223510419 PMID:15278953

Schelling, G., Stoll, C., Kapfhammer, H. P., Rothenhäusler, H. B., Krauseneck, T., Durst, K., & Briegel, J. et al. (1999). The effect of stress doses of hydrocortisone during septic shock on posttraumatic stress disorder and health-related quality of life in survivors. *Critical Care Medicine*, *27*(12), 2678–2683. doi:10.1097/00003246-199912000-00012 PMID:10628609

Schulman, R. C., & Mechanick, J. I. (2012). Metabolic and nutrition support in the chronic critical illness syndrome. *Respiratory Care*, *57*(6), 958–977. doi:10.4187/respcare.01620 PMID:22663970

Schulman, R. C., & Mechanick, J. I. (2013). Can Nutrition Support Interfere with Recovery from Acute Critical Illness? *World Review of Nutrition and Dietetics*, *105*, 69–81. doi:10.1159/000341272 PMID:23075588

Schulman, R. C., Moshier, E. L., Rho, L., Casey, M. F., Godbold, J. H., & Mechanick, J. I. (2014). Association of Glycemic Control Parameters with Clinical Outcomes in Chronic Critical Illness. [Epub ahead of print]. *Endocrine Practice*, *20*(9), 884–893. doi:10.4158/EP13324.OR PMID:24641919

Scurlock, C. S., Raikhelkar, J., & Mechanick, J. (2010). Parenteral nutrition in the critically ill patient [letter]. *The New England Journal of Medicine*, *362*(1), 81–84, author reply 83–84. doi:10.1056/NEJMc0909589 PMID:20054053

Sharshar, T., Gray, F., Lorin de la Grandmaison, G., Hopkinson, N. S., Ross, E., Dorandeu, A., & Annane, D. et al. (2003). Apoptosis of neurons in cardiovascular autonomic centres triggered by inducible nitric oxide synthase after death from septic shock. *Lancet*, *362*(9398), 1799–1805. doi:10.1016/S0140-6736(03)14899-4 PMID:14654318

Singer, M., De Santis, V., Vitale, D., & Jeffcoate, W. (2004). Multiorgan failure is an adaptive, endocrine-mediated, metabolic response to overwhelming systemic inflammation. *Lancet*, *364*(9433), 545–548. doi:10.1016/S0140-6736(04)16815-3 PMID:15302200

Singer, P., Berger, M. M., Van den Berghe, G., Biolo, G., Calder, P., Forbes, A., & Pichard, C. et al. (2009). ESPEN guidelines on parenteral nutrition: Intensive care. *Clinical Nutrition (Edinburgh, Lothian)*, *28*(4), 387–400. doi:10.1016/j.clnu.2009.04.024 PMID:19505748

Siraux, V., De Backer, D., Yalavatti, G., Melot, C., Gervy, C., Mockel, J., & Vincent, J. L. (2005). Relative adrenal insufficiency in patients with septic shock: Comparison of low-dose and conventional corticotropin tests. *Critical Care Medicine*, *33*, 2479–2486. doi:10.1097/01.CCM.0000185641.87051.7C PMID:16276169

Skipper, A. (2012). Refeeding syndrome or refeeding hypophosphatemia: A systematic review of cases. *Nutrition in Clinical Practice*, *27*(1), 34–40. doi:10.1177/0884533611427916 PMID:22307490

Snell-Bergeon, J. K., & Wadwa, R. P. (2012). Hypoglycemia, diabetes, and cardiovascular disease. *Diabetes Technology & Therapeutics*, *14*(S1Supple 1), S51–S58. doi:10.1089/dia.2012.0031 PMID:22650225

Sprung, C. L., Annane, D., Keh, D., Moreno, R., Singer, M., Freivogel, K., & Briegel, J. et al. (2008). Hydrocortisone therapy for patients with septic shock. *The New England Journal of Medicine*, *358*(2), 111–124. doi:10.1056/NEJMoa071366 PMID:18184957

Stapleton, R. D., Jones, N., & Heyland, D. K. (2007). Feeding critically ill patients: What is the optimal amount of energy? *Critical Care Medicine*, *5*(9Suppl), 535–540. doi:10.1097/01.CCM.0000279204.24648.44 PMID:17713405

Surgical Care Improvement Project, version 4.3 (2014). *Specifications Manual for National Hospital Inpatient Quality Measures*. QualityNet.org.

Szabo, Z., Hakanson, E., & Svedjeholm, R. (2002). Early postoperative outcome and medium-term survival in 540 diabetic and 2239 nondiabetic patients undergoing coronary artery bypass grafting. *The Annals of Thoracic Surgery*, *74*(3), 712–719. doi:10.1016/S0003-4975(02)03778-5 PMID:12238829

Umpierrez, G. E., Hellman, R., Korytkowski, M. T., Kosiborod, M., Maynard, G. A., Montori, V. M., & Van den Berghe, G. et al. (2012). Management of hyperglycemia in hospitalized patients in non-critical care setting: An Endocrine Society clinical practice guideline. *The Journal of Clinical Endocrinology and Metabolism*, *97*(1), 16–38. doi:10.1210/jc.2011-2098 PMID:22223765

Van den Berghe, G. (2002). Neuroendocrine pathobiology of chronic critical illness. *Critical Care Clinics*, *18*(3), 509–528. doi:10.1016/S0749-0704(02)00007-6 PMID:12140911

Van den Berghe, G., Baxter, R. C., Weekers, F., Wouters, P., Bowers, C. Y., Iranmanesh, A., & Bouillon, R. et al. (2002). The combined administration of GH-releasing peptide-2 (GHRP-2), TRH and GnRH to men with prolonged critical illness evokes superior endocrine and metabolic effects compared to treatment with GHRP-2 alone. *Horumon To Rinsho*, *56*, 655–669. PMID:12030918

Van den Berghe, G., Wilmer, A., Hermans, G., Meersseman, W., Wouters, P. J., Milants, I., & Bouillon, R. et al. (2006). Intensive insulin therapy in the medical ICU. *The New England Journal of Medicine*, *354*(5), 449–461. doi:10.1056/NEJMoa052521 PMID:16452557

Van den Berghe, G., Wilmer, A., Milants, I., Wouters, P. J., Bouckaert, B., Bruyninckx, F., & Schetz, M. et al. (2006). Intensive insulin therapy in mixed medical/surgical intensive care units. *Diabetes*, *55*(11), 3151–3159. doi:10.2337/db06-0855 PMID:17065355

Van den Berghe, G., Wouters, P., Weekers, F., Verwaest, C., Bruyninckx, F., Schetz, M., & Bouillon, R. et al. (2001). Intensive insulin therapy in the critically ill patients. *The New England Journal of Medicine*, *345*(19), 1359–1367. doi:10.1056/NEJMoa011300 PMID:11794168

Vanhorebeek, I., Gunst, J., Derde, S., Derese, I., Boussemaere, M., Guiza, F., & Van den Berghe, G. et al. (2011). Insufficient activation of autophagy allows cellular damage to accumulate in critically ill patients. *The Journal of Clinical Endocrinology and Metabolism*, *96*(4), E633–E645. doi:10.1210/jc.2010-2563 PMID:21270330

Vanwijngaerden, Y. M., Wauters, J., Langouche, L., Vander Perre, S., Liddle, C., Coulter, S., & Mesotten, D. et al. (2011). Critical illness evokes elevated circulating bile acids related to altered hepatic transporter and nuclear receptor expression. *Hepatology (Baltimore, Md.)*, *54*(5), 1741–1752. doi:10.1002/hep.24582 PMID:21800341

Vassiliadi, D. A., Ilias, I., Tzanela, M., Nikitas, N., Theodorakopoulou, M., Kopteridea, P., & Dimopoulou, I. et al. (2013). Interstitial cortisol obtained by microdialysis in mechanically ventilated septic patients: Correlations with total and free serum cortisol. *Journal of Critical Care*, *28*, 158–165. PMID:22981531

Vermes, I., Beishuizen, A., Hampsink, R. M., & Haanen, C. (1995). Dissociation of plasma adrenocorticotropin and cortisol levels in critically ill patients: Possible role of endothelin and atrial natriuretic hormone. *The Journal of Clinical Endocrinology and Metabolism*, *80*(4), 1238–1242. PMID:7714094

Via, M. A., Scurlock, C., Adams, D. H., Weiss, A. J., & Mechanick, J. I. (2010). Impaired postoperative hyperglycemic stress response associated with increased mortality in patients in the cardiothoracic surgery intensive care unit. *Endocrine Practice*, *16*(5), 798–804. doi:10.4158/EP10017.OR PMID:20350912

Wang, F., Pan, W., Wang, H., Wang, S., Pan, S., & Ge, J. (2012). Relationship between thyroid function and ICU mortality: A prospective observation study. *Critical Care (London, England)*, *16*(1), R11. doi:10.1186/cc11151 PMID:22257427

Weijs, P. J., Stapel, S. N., de Groot, S. D., Driessen, R. H., de Jong, E., Girbes, A. R., & Beishuizen, A. et al. (2012). Optimal protein and energy nutrition decreases mortality in mechanically ventilated, critically ill patients: A prospective observational cohort study. *Journal of Parenteral and Enteral Nutrition*, *36*(1), 60–68. doi:10.1177/0148607111415109 PMID:22167076

Weiss, A. J., & Mechanick, J. M. (2011). Glycemic control: How tight in the intensive care unit? *Seminars in Thoracic and Cardiovascular Surgery*, *23*(1), 1–4. doi:10.1053/j.semtcvs.2011.04.006 PMID:21807288

Wright, R. J., & Frier, B. M. (2008). Vascular disease and diabetes: Is hypoglycaemia an aggravating factor? *Diabetes/Metabolism Research and Reviews*, *24*(5), 353–363. doi:10.1002/dmrr.865 PMID:18461635

Zerr, K. J., Furnary, A. P., Grunkemeier, G. L., Bookin, S., Kanhere, V., & Starr, A. (1997). Glucose control lowers the risk of wound infection in diabetics after open heart operations. *The Annals of Thoracic Surgery*, *63*, 356–361. doi:10.1016/S0003-4975(96)01044-2 PMID:9033300

ADDITIONAL READING

Adler, S. M., & Wartofsky, L. (2007). The nonthyroidal illness syndrome. *Endocrinology and Metabolism Clinics of North America*, *36*(3), 657–672. doi:10.1016/j.ecl.2007.04.007 PMID:17673123

Annane, D., Sebille, V., Charpentier, C., Bollaert, P. E., Francois, B., Korach, J. M., & Bellissant, E. et al. (2002). Effect of treatment with low doses of hydrocortisone and fludrocortisone on mortality in patients with septic shock. *Journal of the American Medical Association*, *288*(7), 862–871. doi:10.1001/jama.288.7.862 PMID:12186604

Boonen, E., & Van den Berghe, G. (2014). Endocrine responses to critical illness: Novel insights and therapeutic implications. [Epub ahead of print]. *The Journal of Clinical Endocrinology and Metabolism*, jc20134115. PMID:24517153

Boonen, E., Vervenne, H., Meersseman, P., Andrew, R., Mortier, L., Declercq, P. E., & Van den Berghe, G. et al. (2013). Reduced cortisol metabolism during critical illness. *The New England Journal of Medicine*, *368*(16), 1477–1488. doi:10.1056/NEJMoa1214969 PMID:23506003

Casaer, M. P., Mesotten, D., Hermans, G., Wouters, P. J., Schetz, M., Meyfroidt, G., & Van den Berghe, G. et al. (2011). Early versus late parenteral nutrition in critically ill adults. *The New England Journal of Medicine*, *365*(6), 506–517. doi:10.1056/NEJMoa1102662 PMID:21714640

Casaer, M. P., & Van den Berghe, G. (2014). Nutrition in the acute phase of critical illness. *The New England Journal of Medicine*, *370*(13), 1227–1236. doi:10.1056/NEJMra1304623 PMID:24670169

Egi, M., Bellomo, R., Stachowski, E., French, C. J., Hart, G. K., Taori, G., & Bailey, M. et al. (2011). The interaction of chronic and acute glycemia with mortality in critically ill patients with diabetes. *Critical Care Medicine*, *39*(1), 105–111. doi:10.1097/CCM.0b013e3181feb5ea PMID:20975552

Furnary, A. P., Gao, G., Grunkemeier, G. L., Wu, Y., Zerr, K. J., Bookin, S. O., & Starr, A. et al. (2003). Continuous insulin infusion reduces mortality in patients with diabetes undergoing coronary artery bypass grafting. *The Journal of Thoracic and Cardiovascular Surgery*, *125*(5), 1007–1021. doi:10.1067/mtc.2003.181 PMID:12771873

Hamrahian, A. H., Oseni, T. S., & Arafah, B. M. (2004). Measurements of serum free cortisol in critically ill patients. *The New England Journal of Medicine*, *350*(16), 1629–1638. doi:10.1056/NEJMoa020266 PMID:15084695

Hollander, J. M., & Mechanick, J. I. (2006). Nutrition support and the chronic critical illness syndrome. *Nutrition in Clinical Practice*, *21*(6), 587–604. doi:10.1177/0115426506021006587 PMID:17119165

Krinsley, J. S. (2009). Glycemic variability and mortality in critically ill patients: The impact of diabetes. *Journal of Diabetes Science and Technology*, *3*(6), 1292–1301. doi:10.1177/193229680900300609 PMID:20144383

Krinsley, J. S., Egi, M., Kiss, A., Devendra, A. N., Schuetz, P., Maurer, P. M., & Bellomo, R. et al. (2013). Diabetic status and the relation of the three domains of glycemic control to mortality in critically ill patients: An international multicenter cohort study. *Critical Care (London, England)*, *17*(2), R37. doi:10.1186/cc12547 PMID:23452622

Lazar, H. L., Chipkin, S. R., Fitzgerald, C. A., Bao, Y., Cabral, H., & Apstein, C. S. (2004). Tight glycemic control in diabetic coronary artery bypass graft patients improves perioperative outcomes and decreases recurrent ischemic events. *Circulation*, *109*(12), 1497–1502. doi:10.1161/01.CIR.0000121747.71054.79 PMID:15006999

Lazar, H. L., McDonnell, M. M., Chipkin, S., Furnary, A. P., Engelman, R. M., Sadhu, A. R., & Shemin, R. J. et al. (2009). The Society for Thoracic Surgeons practice guideline series: Blood glucose management during adult cardiac surgery. *The Annals of Thoracic Surgery*, *87*(2), 663–669. doi:10.1016/j.athoracsur.2008.11.011 PMID:19161815

Le Roith, D. (2004). Molecular mechanisms by which metabolic control may improve outcomes. *Endocrine Practice*, *10*(2Supple), 57–62. doi:10.4158/EP.10.S2.57 PMID:15251642

Marik, P. E., Pastores, S. M., Annane, D., Meduri, G. U., Sprung, C. L., Arlt, W., & Vogeser, M. et al. American College of Critical Care Medicine. (2008). Recommendations for the diagnosis and management of corticosteroid insufficiency in critically ill adult patients: Consensus statements from an international task force by the American College of Critical Care Medicine. *Critical Care Medicine*, *36*(6), 1937–1949. doi:10.1097/CCM.0b013e31817603ba PMID:18496365

Martindale, R. G., McClave, S. A., Vanek, V. W., McCarthy, M., Roberts, P., Taylor, B., & Cresci, G. et al. (2009). Guidelines for the provision and assessment of nutrition support therapy in the adult critically ill patient: Society of Critical Care Medicine and American Society for Parenteral and Enteral Nutrition: executive summary. *Critical Care Medicine*, *37*(5), 1757–1761. doi:10.1097/CCM.0b013e3181a40116 PMID:19373044

McDonnel, M. E., Alexanian, S. M., White, L., & Lazar, H. L. (2012). A primer for achieving glycemic control in the cardiac surgical patient. *Journal of Cardiac Surgery*, *27*(4), 470–477. doi:10.1111/j.1540-8191.2012.01471.x PMID:22640228

Mechanick, J. I. (2006). Metabolic Mechanisms of stress hyperglycemia. *Journal of Parenteral and Enteral Nutrition*, *30*(2), 157–163. doi:10.1177/0148607106030002157 PMID:16517960

Moghissi, E. S., Korytkowski, M. T., DiNardo, M., Einhorn, D., Hellman, R., Hirsch, I. B., & Umpierrez, G. E. et al. (2009). American Association of Clinical Endocrinologists and American Diabetes Association consensus statement on inpatient glycemic control. *Diabetes Care*, *32*(6), 1119–1131. doi:10.2337/dc09-9029 PMID:19429873

NICE-SUGAR Study Investigators. (2009). Intensive versus conventional glucose control in critically ill patients. *The New England Journal of Medicine*, *360*(13), 1283–1297. doi:10.1056/NEJMoa0810625 PMID:19318384

Schulman, R. C., & Mechanick, J. I. (2012). Metabolic and nutrition support in the chronic critical illness syndrome. *Respiratory Care*, *57*(6), 958–977. doi:10.4187/respcare.01620 PMID:22663970

Schulman, R. C., & Mechanick, J. I. (2013). Can Nutrition Support Interfere with Recovery from Acute Critical Illness? *World Review of Nutrition and Dietetics*, *105*, 69–81. doi:10.1159/000341272 PMID:23075588

Singer, P., Berger, M. M., Van den Berghe, G., Biolo, G., Calder, P., Forbes, A., & Pichard, C. et al. (2009). ESPEN guidelines on parenteral nutrition: Intensive care. *Clinical Nutrition (Edinburgh, Lothian)*, *28*(4), 387–400. doi:10.1016/j.clnu.2009.04.024 PMID:19505748

Snell-Bergeon, J. K., & Wadwa, R. P. (2012). Hypoglycemia, diabetes, and cardiovascular disease. *Diabetes Technology & Therapeutics*, *14*(S1Supple 1), S51–S58. doi:10.1089/dia.2012.0031 PMID:22650225

Umpierrez, G. E., Hellman, R., Korytkowski, M. T., Kosiborod, M., Maynard, G. A., Montori, V. M., & Van den Berghe, G. et al. (2012). Management of hyperglycemia in hospitalized patients in non-critical care setting: An Endocrine Society clinical practice guideline. *The Journal of Clinical Endocrinology and Metabolism*, *97*(1), 16–38. doi:10.1210/jc.2011-2098 PMID:22223765

Van den Berghe, G., Wilmer, A., Hermans, G., Meersseman, W., Wouters, P. J., Milants, I., & Bouillon, R. et al. (2006). Intensive insulin therapy in the medical ICU. *The New England Journal of Medicine*, *354*(5), 449–461. doi:10.1056/NEJMoa052521 PMID:16452557

Van den Berghe, G., Wouters, P., Weekers, F., Verwaest, C., Bruyninckx, F., Schetz, M., & Bouillon, R. et al. (2001). Intensive insulin therapy in the critically ill patients. *The New England Journal of Medicine*, *345*(19), 1359–1367. doi:10.1056/NEJMoa011300 PMID:11794168

Vanhorebeek, I., Gunst, J., Derde, S., Derese, I., Boussemaere, M., Guiza, F., & Van den Berghe, G. et al. (2011). Insufficient activation of autophagy allows cellular damage to accumulate in critically ill patients. *The Journal of Clinical Endocrinology and Metabolism*, *96*(4), E633–E645. doi:10.1210/jc.2010-2563 PMID:21270330

KEY TERMS AND DEFINITIONS

Acute Critical Illness (ACI): The initial metabolic phase of critical illness (about day 0-3), characterized by the acute stress response.

Chronic Critical Illness (CCI): The third metabolic phase of critical illness, designated to begin at the time of tracheostomy and reflecting a highly inflammatory state, associated with persistent multi-organ dysfunction.

Critical Illness-Related Corticosteroid Insufficiency (CIRCI): The relative deficiency of corticosteroid activity in the setting of increased requirements due to critical illness.

Diabetes Mellitus (DM): A disease of insufficient or ineffective insulin production leading to high glucose levels and predisposing to multiple complications and mortality.

Intensive Insulin Therapy: Utilization of an intravenous insulin infusion protocol to main blood glucose in a narrow range.

Nonthyroidal Illness Syndrome (NTIS): A constellation of thyroid function abnormalities commonly seen in the critically ill, resulting from systemic illness, and in the absence of true thyroid disease.

Nutrition Support: The provision of macro- and micronutrients via enteral and/or parenteral nutrition when oral intake is insufficient.

Prolonged Acute Critical Illness (PACI): The second phase of critical illness, occurring when the patient remains critically ill for a prolonged period with persistent stress response (about day 3-14).

Recovery from Critical Illness (RCI): The final phase of critical illness, beginning at the time of liberation from mechanical ventilation and culminating with hospital discharge.

Stress Hyperglycemia: The temporary occurrence of hyperglycemia, commonly seen in critical illness, in the absence of meeting criteria for diabetes mellitus.

Section 5

Surgical Techniques and Postoperative Concerns

Chapter 22
Coronary Artery Disease

Rakesh C. Arora
University of Manitoba, Canada

Rohit Singal
University of Manitoba, Canada

ABSTRACT

Coronary artery bypass grafting (CABG), first introduced in 1968, is now one of the most common surgical procedures and the most common cardiac procedures worldwide. It is estimated that over 800,000 CABG surgeries are performed worldwide each year. The goals of CABG are to reduce mortality, prevent the progress of heart failure and reduce symptoms associated with coronary artery disease. This chapter deals with cardiac critical care issues that pertain to the patient undergoing CABG and potential post-operative complications.

INTRODUCTION

Coronary artery bypass grafting (CABG), first introduced in 1968 (Favaloro), is now one of the most common surgical procedures and the most common cardiac procedures worldwide. It is estimated that over 800,000 CABG surgeries are performed worldwide each year. CABG is a procedure in which one or more stenosed (or occluded) coronary arteries are bypassed with an alternate blood vessel conduit to re-establish normal blood flow to the myocardium. Bypass grafts are typically done using an artery, such as internal mammary artery (IMA), radial artery (RA) or gastroepiploic artery (GEA); or vein (most commonly the greater saphenous vein from the leg). CABG is typically performed with the use of cardiopulmonary bypass (CPB) and cardioplegic arrest (most commonly using a mixture of blood and crystalloid with a high concentration of potassium) to permit the creation of the anastomosis on an arrested heart. In the past two to three decades, other techniques such as the performance of bypass grafts on a beating heart using off-pump coronary artery bypass (OPCAB) or through minimally invasive direct coronary bypass grafting (MIDCAB) have been developed. The goals of CABG are to reduce mortality, prevent the progress of heart failure and reduce symptoms associated with coronary artery disease. This chapter deals with cardiac critical care issues that pertain to the patient undergoing CABG and potential post-operative complications.

DOI: 10.4018/978-1-4666-8603-8.ch022

TYPES OF CONDUITS USED FOR CABG

Patients currently being referred for surgical revascularization are increasingly complex and have a greater burden of co-morbidity and coronary artery disease than in the previous eras of cardiac surgery (Farkouh et al., 2008; Kapur et al., 2010; Mohr et al., 2013; Serruys et al., 2009). Due to the characteristics and long-term patency, the choice of conduits used for coronary artery bypass grafting impacts long-term outcomes, especially with the increasingly complex patient population (Cheng & Slaughter, 2013). Generally, conduits for bypass grafts are taken from one of four areas of the body: saphenous vein grafts (SVG) from the lower limbs, internal mammary arteries (IMA) from the chest wall, radial arteries (RA) from the forearm and infrequently gastroepiploic arteries (GEA) from the abdomen.

Arterial grafts have demonstrated longer patency than veins which translates to better long-term survival, fewer reoperations, a lower rate of myocardial infarction and less recurrent angina compared to vein grafts (Buxton et al., 2009; Cheng & Slaughter, 2013; Desai et al., 2007; Desai, Cohen, Naylor, & Fremes, 2004; Hayward & Buxton, 2007; Loop et al., 1986; Takagi et al., 2014; Weiss, Zhao, Tian, Taggart, & Yan, 2013).

Internal Mammary Artery (IMA): The internal mammary arteries course on the left and right side of the sternum. Unlike vein or radial artery grafts, IMAs are usually not removed from their original position. They often remain connected to their natural site of origin and only one end is separated from the chest wall (*in-situ*). The distal end is then anastomosed to one of the coronary arteries. The IMAs appear to be inherently "biologically privileged" as a conduit for CABG. They demonstrate resistance to the development of atherosclerosis, a thinner medial layer with less smooth muscle making it less prone to spasm, a more resistant endothelium protecting it against injury during conduit harvest and reduced proliferative response to known mitogens and pulsatile mechanical stretch (Buxton et al., 2009; Cheng & Slaughter, 2013; Tatoulis, Buxton, & Fuller, 2004).

Most commonly the IMA is used for bypassing the left anterior descending (LAD) coronary artery due to superior early and late survival after CABG (Buxton et al., 2009; Desai et al., 2007; Hayward & Buxton, 2007; Loop et al., 1986). Furthermore, use of the right IMA (RIMA) in addition to the left IMA (LIMA) otherwise known as bilateral internal mammary artery (BIMA) grafting confers additional survival advantage over the use of just the LIMA for CABG (Lytle et al., 2004; D P Taggart, D'Amico, & Altman, 2001; Takagi et al., 2014; Weiss et al., 2013). A landmark trial in 2001 by Lytle and colleagues found that the use of BIMA over LIMA conferred a survival benefit ($p < 0.0001$) of 89% versus 87% at 7 years, 81% versus 78% at 10 years, 67% versus 58% at 15 years, and 50% versus 37% at 20 years. Patency of both the LIMA and RIMA are exceptional with 10-year patency rates ranging from 88-95% depending on the territory grafted (where the higher patency value corresponds to the LIMA to LAD configuration)(Lytle et al., 2004; Tatoulis et al., 2004; Tatoulis, Buxton, & Fuller, 2011; Weiss et al., 2013; Zacharias et al., 2009).

While using the RIMA there are concerns regarding length, the ability to use it to the circumflex system and the potential risk for increased sternal complication, however recent improvements in surgical techniques have addressed many of these issues. Skeletonization of the IMA has been shown to improve length, reduce compromise of sternal blood flow, decreasing sternal infections and complications, even in diabetic patients (Tatoulis et al., 2004; Tranbaugh et al., 2014). Furthermore, excellent patency rates have been demonstrated when utilized as a "free" graft and anastomosed in a "Y" fashion to the LIMA (Nasso et al., 2009; Tranbaugh et al., 2014).

Radial Artery (RA): Multiple studies have shown that maximizing the use of arterial conduits may yield improved clinical outcomes (Deb et al., 2012; Desai et al., 2004; Nasso et al., 2009; Tatoulis et al., 2004; Zacharias et al., 2009). Therefore, in addition to the use of LIMA to the LAD and the RIMA to a separate coronary territory, other arterial conduits have been investigated for their utility in CABG. The RA, taken from the inner forearm, is an arterial conduit initially described by Carpentier in 1973 (Carpentier, Guermonprez, Deloche, Frechette, & DuBost, 1973). Early enthusiasm for this conduit was tempered by concerns that radial-artery grafts were prone to spasm and functional occlusion and their use was abandoned for many years (Geha, Krone, McCormick, & Baue, 1975). Interestingly, in 1992, Acar and colleagues provided an update to this initial series of patients demonstrating that previously reported occluded or narrowed RA grafts were patent at 18 years' follow-up (Acar et al., 1992). Furthermore, they also reported a series of patients receiving RA grafts using a refined harvesting technique and pharmacologic measures to minimize spasm that revitalized interest in the RA as an additional arterial conduit.

In 2004, the RAPS investigators undertook a multicenter RCT to determine the relative patency rate of radial-artery and saphenous-vein grafts (Desai et al., 2004). Angiographic data was available for 440 of the randomized patients at one-year demonstrating superior patency of the RA over the SVG (91.8% vs. 86.4%; p=0.009), with a larger effect seen in women and in patients with diabetes in subsequent analyses (Desai et al., 2007), but a diffuse narrowing of the RA graft (the angiographic "string sign") was present in 7.0% of studied RA grafts (vs. only 0.9% SVG; p=0.001). In further sub-analyses it was determined that RA patency depends on the severity of native-vessel stenosis due to the effect on competitive flow from the patient's native coronary arteries, female gender, diabetes, peripheral vascular disease (PVD), lack of statin use and the use of a single anti-platelet (Deb et al., 2012; Desai et al., 2007; Hata et al., 2011). As such, RA grafts should preferentially be used for target vessels with high-grade lesions (80% stenosis, preferably 90%) to maintain short and long-term patency (Achouh & Acar, 2013; Deb et al., 2012; Desai et al., 2007) .

Subsequent data from large RCTs and meta-analyses suggest that RA patency is comparable to SVG patency in the short term but is likely superior over the medium term and long term (Achouh & Acar, 2013; Collins, Webb, Chong, & Moat, 2008; Desai et al., 2007, 2004; Nasso et al., 2009; Rehman, Yi, & Taggart, 2013; Tranbaugh et al., 2014). This conclusion is still a subject of ongoing debate (see RAPCO trial (Hayward & Buxton, 2007; Hayward et al., 2010) and other (Dreifaldt et al., 2013)). The use of a RA before the use of a RIMA is more controversial as there is conflicting data on long-term benefit of one over another (Achouh et al., 2012; Nasso et al., 2009; Navia et al., 2014; Tatoulis et al., 2004; Tranbaugh et al., 2014), and as such, choice of the second arterial conduit is often dictated by the patient's coronary disease severity and patient and surgeon preferences (Tranbaugh et al., 2014).

Radial Artery Spasm: While from a technical standpoint the RA is an attractive conduit to use as it is both easy to dissect and to handle for bypass grafting, its susceptibility to vasospasm remains as an impediment to wide-spread use for CABG. Postoperative RA vasospasm, reported to be as high as 5-10%, is believed to be secondary to its thick muscular medial layer and innervated adventitial layer that makes it more susceptible to vasoconstrictor influence (Attaran, John, & El-Gamel, 2008; He, 2013). Therefore the avoidance of high-dose intravenous vasopressor therapy in the OR and ICU, though not substantiated in clinical study, makes intuitive sense. For graft spasm prophylaxis, the use of both intraoperative and postoperative strategies has been described. The intraoperative use of an organ-bath solution of verapamil, nitroglycerin, heparin and sodium bicarbonate (He, 2013) and a postoperative nitroglycerin infusion (Chanda, Brichkov, & Canver, 2000) and/or an oral or intravenous calcium channel blocker (such as diltiazem or nicardipine) are commonly used (Attaran et al., 2008; He, 2013). Postoperative anti-spasm prophylaxis is typically continued for up to 6-12 months. This may include: nifedipine 20 mg twice a day; or verapamil 120-240 mg per day; or diltiazem at an appropriate low dose (Attaran et al., 2008; Deb et al., 2012; He, 2013), however there is currently no clear agreement as to the optimal agent nor links to clinical outcome data. Nonetheless, previous surveys have demonstrated that prophylaxis against spasm of RA grafts is practiced in over 95% of responding sites with the duration of anti-spasm therapy varied from several weeks up to six months (Myers & Fremes, 2003).

Other Arterial Conduits: The gastroepiploic artery (GEA) to the stomach or the inferior epigastric artery (IEA) from the abdominal wall are other arterial conduit options for grafting, though rarely used unless the above described conduits are unavailable or inadequate. Similar to the RA, the GEA has a thick smooth muscle media that is prone to spasm. Furthermore, harvest of the either the GEA or IEA arteries requires intra-abdominal entry or an extra abdominal incision, which may increase operative time and may be associated with additional complications. With regards to patency, the GEA has undergone more extensive study than the IEA. Patency rate are analogous to RA graft with 92-98% and 80—90% at one and five years respectively, though lower when grafted to the LAD territory (Malvindi, Jacob, Kallikourdis, & Vitale, 2007; Suma et al., 2007).

Saphenous Vein Grafts (SVG): Despite support for the use of multiple arterial conduits for coronary revascularization, recent large randomized trials suggest that the use of a total arterial conduit strategy (i.e. an arterial conduit to every graft coronary territory) is infrequently employed (15-20%) (Farkouh et al., 2012; Kapur et al., 2010; Serruys et al., 2009). The saphenous vein remains a commonly used conduit for bypass grafts due the relative abundance of conduit, reasonable caliber, and technical ease of use when creating an anastomosis to the coronary artery. However, short and long-term patency is typically inferior to the IMA graft, in particular to the LAD and this has a direct impact on patient survival (Loop et al., 1986). Acute thrombosis, neo-intimal hyperplasia and accelerated atherosclerosis have been proposed as the three principle mechanisms leading to SVG failure (Harskamp, Lopes, Baisden, de Winter, & Alexander, 2013). Approximately 15-20% of vein grafts occlude in the first year, half of which acutely occlude in the first two weeks following surgery. Subsequent annual occlusion rate appears to be time and mechanism dependent with annual occlusion rate of 1% to 2% in years one and six, and 4% to 5% in years six to ten following CABG. At 10 years, approximately 60% of vein grafts are patent (Campeau et al., 1984; Fitzgibbon et al., 1996; Shah et al., 2003). However, our understanding of SVG failure has improved over time. In a review of 3715 graft angiograms in 1607 patients with symptomatic angina, Shah and colleagues (2003) identified improved long-term SVG patency in older patients with good left ventricular function, anastomosed to large-caliber arteries on the left system and when grafted with a small-diameter vein (i.e. veins are harvested from the calf because they are a better size match to the coronary arteries) were associated with the best outcome. A further study by Hayward et al, found 5-year patency of over 80% when an SVG is anastomosed to the largest non-LAD artery and statin therapy is given (Hayward & Buxton, 2007). Furthermore, in a recent randomized trial, Dreifaldt et al. (2013) demonstrated that use of a "no-touch" technique for SVG harvest had a superior patency rate to RA grafts (95% vs. 84%) at a mean follow-up of 36 months.

WHO SHOULD BE UNDERGOING CABG?

In 2011, the American College of Cardiology Foundation and the American Heart Association Task Force (ACCF/AHA) on Practice Guidelines provided an update to their joint statement on guidelines for coronary artery bypass graft surgery (Hillis et al., 2011). The current CABG guidelines state CABG is the preferred treatment (Class I recommendation) for:

- Patients with significant (>50% diameter stenosis), unprotected left main (LM) coronary artery stenosis.
- In patients with significant (>70% diameter) stenoses in 3 major coronary arteries (with or without involvement of the proximal left anterior descending (LAD) artery) or in the proximal LAD plus 1 other major coronary artery.
- In patients undergoing non-coronary cardiac surgery with greater than or equal to 50% luminal diameter narrowing of the left main coronary artery or greater than or equal to 70% luminal diameter narrowing of other major coronary arteries.
- Emergency CABG is recommended in patients with acute myocardial infarction (MI) in whom:
    - Primary percutaneous coronary intervention (PCI) has failed or cannot be performed and with coronary anatomy suitable for CABG
    - Persistent ischemia of a significant area of myocardium at rest and/or hemodynamic instability refractory to nonsurgical therapy is present
    - Undergoing surgical repair of a post-infarction mechanical complication of MI, such as ventricular septal rupture, mitral valve insufficiency because of papillary muscle infarction and/or rupture, or free wall rupture
    - In patients with cardiogenic shock and who are suitable for CABG
    - Survivors of sudden death with presumed ischemic-mediated ventricular tachycardia
    - CABG (or PCI) with one or more significant (>70% diameter) coronary artery stenoses amenable in patients who have unacceptable angina despite guideline-directed medical therapy

PERCUTANEOUS CORONARY INTERVENTION (PCI) OR CABG?

Since the introduction of percutaneous transluminal coronary angioplasty (PTCA) in the 1970's (Grüntzig, Senning, & Siegenthaler, 1979), there has been intense debate of using a less invasive percutaneous coronary intervention (PCI) versus coronary artery bypass grafting (CABG) for single , multi and left main coronary artery disease (Bansilal et al., 2012; Brener et al., 2004; Buszman et al., 2008; (BARI) Investigators, 1996; Ferreira, Peter, Salerno, Bolooki, & de Marchena, 2003; Hannan et al., 2008; Kapur et al., 2010; Morice et al., 2002; Morrison et al., 2001; Rodriguez et al., 2001; Serruys et al., 2005, 2009; David P Taggart, 2006). A consistent message in the majority of randomized clinical trials has been similar outcomes with regards to short-term mortality and cerebrovascular events, CABG appears to be associated with improved long-term survival and decreased need for repeat revascularization (Mohr et al., 2013; Serruys et al., 2005; The BARI Investigators, 2007).

Trials You Should Know

The Arterial Revascularization Therapy Study (ARTS): In 2005, Serruys and colleagues published five-year outcomes of their study in which 1205 patients were randomized to CABG (n = 605) or PCI with stent implantation (n = 600) (Serruys et al., 2005). The primary clinical end point was freedom from major adverse cardiac and cerebrovascular events (MACCE) at one year with MACCE at five-year follow-up constituting the final secondary end point. The authors reported that there was no difference in one-year or five-year survival (mortality in both groups was 2.6% at one year and 8% at five years). A limitation of this study, however, was that approximately 70% of the patients had single or double-vessel coronary artery disease and normal left ventricular function and therefore were unlikely to see any mortality benefit from surgery (Taggart, 2006). However there was a reduction in the need for re-intervention (30% versus 9%) in favor of CABG.

The Surgery or Stent (SoS) trial: The SoS trial sought to examine the impact of acute coronary syndromes (ACS) on the relative benefits of coronary artery bypass grafting (CABG) versus stent-assisted percutaneous coronary intervention (PCI) with bare metal stents.(Zhang et al., 2005) Patients with multi-vessel disease were randomly assigned to CABG (n = 500) or stent-assisted PCI (n = 488). The impact of treatment on one-year outcomes was compared in ACS and non-ACS subgroups. The authors reported a higher cost associated with CABG, however the one-year health status (as measured by the Seattle Angina Questionnaire (Spertus et al., 1995; Spertus, Winder, Dewhurst, Deyo, & Fihn, 1994)) was better with CABG and rates of repeat revascularization were higher in the PCI group (ACS, 15.5% vs 7.1%, P =.04; non-ACS, 18.0% vs 3.2%, p = 0.001), particularly in patients with concurrent diabetes.

The Synergy between PCI with Taxus and Cardiac Surgery (SYNTAX) trial: With the advent of drug-eluting stents (DES)(Ferreira et al., 2003; Kastrati et al., 2007; Serruys, Kutryk, & Ong, 2006; Spaulding, Daemen, Boersma, Cutlip, & Serruys, 2007) newer studies have sought to determine the superiority of CABG versus PCI revascularization for multi-vessel coronary artery disease. The Percutaneous Coronary Intervention versus Coronary-Artery Bypass Grafting for Severe Coronary Artery Disease (a.k.a. Synergy between PCI with Taxus and Cardiac Surgery (SYNTAX) trial), was a randomized controlled trial of 1,800 patients with multivessel coronary disease that compared CABG versus PCI using contemporary generation drug-eluting stents (Serruys et al., 2009). Interestingly, this study was designed as a non-inferiority comparison for the primary end point of any a major adverse cardiac or cerebrovascular event (i.e. MACCE: death from any cause, stroke, myocardial infarction, or repeat revascularization) at 12-month periods after randomization. The study found no difference in repeat infarctions or survival, however higher rates of strokes were seen in the CABG group. Still, with regards to the study's primary endpoint, major adverse cardiac or cerebrovascular events at 12 months were significantly higher in the DES group (17.8% versus 12.4% for CABG; P=0.002). This was primarily driven by a higher repeat revascularization in the PCI group (13.5% vs. 5.9%, P<0.001) and as a result, the criterion for non-inferiority was not met.

In 2013, the SYNTAX investigators reported their five-year composite rate of major adverse cardiac and cerebrovascular events (MACCE) using Kaplan-Meier analysis on an intention-to-treat basis. The authors reported estimates of MACCE of 26.9% in the CABG group versus 37.3% in the PCI group (p<0·0001). Furthermore, estimates of myocardial infarction (3.8% in the CABG group vs 9.7% in the PCI group; p<0·0001) and repeat revascularisation (13.7% vs. 25.9%; p<0·0001) were significantly increased with PCI versus CABG. The difference in cerebrovascular events seen at 12 months was no longer present in the 5-year analysis (3.5% in the CABG group vs. 3.0% in the PCI group; p = 0.66). An important output of this study was the categorization of coronary artery disease burden into three groups: low (SYNYAX Score of 0-22), intermediate (SYNTAX Score of 23-32) and high (SYNTAX Score of ≥ 33) (see www.syntaxscore.com). The authors have concluded that CABG should remain the standard of care for patients with complex lesions (high or intermediate SYNTAX scores). For patients with less complex disease (low SYNTAX scores) or left main coronary disease (low or intermediate SYNTAX scores), PCI is an acceptable alternative (although associated with higher need for revascularization). There is still ongoing debate over these conclusions.

The FREEDOM (Future Revascularization Evaluation in Patients With Diabetes Mellitus—Optimal Management of Multi-vessel Disease): With the evolution of drug-eluting stents, reports have demonstrated a potential need for repeat revascularization in patients with concurrent diabetes and multi-vessel CAD (Kapur et al., 2010; Serruys et al., 2009). To this end, Farkouh and the FREEDOM Trial Investigators (2012)reported the results in which they sought to determine whether aggressive medical therapy with DES-PCI was superior to CABG in patients with diabetes and multi-vessel CAD. A total of 1900 patients were randomized to PCI with drug-eluting stents or CABG. Also, there was an attempt following guideline-driven targets for lipid, blood pressure and glycemic control in all enrolled patients. The primary outcome measure was a composite of death from any cause, non-fatal myocardial infarction or non-fatal stroke with a minimum follow-up for two years. Importantly, the mean SYNTAX score was 26.2±8.6, indicating at least intermediate coronary disease complexity. The authors observed the rate of myocardial infarction and death from any cause was significantly higher in the PCI group than in the CABG group (respectively 13.9% vs. 6%; p < 0.001 for MI and 14.9% vs 10.6%; p < 0.049 for death), whereas the rate of stroke was significantly higher in the CABG group (5.2% CABG vs. 2.4% PCI; p < 0.03). The higher relative risk of stroke among patients undergoing CABG was primarily evident only in the early post-procedural period. With reference to their primary outcome, CABG was found to be superior to PCI with DES in patients with diabetes and advanced (predominantly three- vessel) coronary artery disease. The study results affirm the utility of multi-vessel CABG over PCI in diabetic patients (Taggart, 2013).

The Heart Team: An important output from the most recent CAD interventional (Farkouh et al., 2012; Mohr et al., 2013; Serruys et al., 2009) and other cardiac clinical trials (Leon et al., 2010; Makkar et al., 2012; Miller et al., 2012; Svensson et al., 2013) has been the development of the "heart team" concept. This has been described as a process of shared decision making between an interventional cardiologist and a cardiac surgeon during the evaluation of a patient's suitability for intervention. Indeed, the most recent version of the ACCF/AHA Practice Guidelines for CAD has endorsed the Heart Team approach to revascularization in patients with unprotected left main or complex CAD as a Class I recommendation. We at the St. Boniface Hospital in Winnipeg, Canada have further evolved this concept to involve a larger number of key-stakeholders in the decision making process. Patients that are deemed "complex" are referred to a panel consisting of a cardiologist, an interventional cardiologist, a cardiac surgeon, a cardiac anesthesiologist and a cardiac critical care specialist (see Figures 1-3). Prior to presentation of a patient to the panel, a formal referral document which includes a standardized assessment of frailty (Rockwood et al., 2005), cardiac risk prediction score (Nashef et al., 2012) and other pertinent history and investigations is completed. Lastly, panel discussions are held as educational rounds in which all house-staff are permitted to attend.

Figure 1. Example WHRA Cardiac Sciences Complex Case Rounds Referral Form, Page 1

Guidelines for referral are **complex patients when the best treatment option is uncertain**. May include left main coronary disease; 3 vessel coronary disease; adult congenital disease, complex valve cases, redo cardiac surgery cases, high surgical risk; adverse patient factors including frailty, cognitive impairment, significant comorbid disease number; and therapeutic uncertainty

Question to be addressed:
I. CABG Vs. PCI Vs. Medical II. Valve Surgery Vs. TEVI Vs. Medical III. Transplantation
IV. VAD V. Pericardectomy VI. Adverse Event ____________
VII. Other

Therapeutic Problem:
a. Angina b. Congestive Heart Failure c. Asymptomatic LV Dysfunction d. Asymptomatic CAD e. Other

Diagnostic Category:
a. CAD b. Valvular Disease c. Mixed CAD Valvular Disease d. Congenital
e. Pericardial f. Cardiomyopathy g. Other

Referring MD Name (print): ____________ Presenting MD Name (print): ____________

Date of Cardiac Cath [D D M M M Y Y Y Y] Date of CT [D D M M M Y Y Y Y]

Date of ECHO [D D M M M Y Y Y Y] Date of MRI [D D M M M Y Y Y Y]

Dementia *(see back of form)* ☐ None ☐ Mild ☐ Moderate ☐ Severe

Euroscore II Parameters

Age ______ Gender ______ Weight ______ Serum Creatinine ______ umol/L

Extra Cardiac Arteriopathy .... ☐ Yes ☐ No
(claudication, carotid occlusion or >50% stenosis, amputation for peripheral vascular disease previous/planned intervention)

Clinical Frailty Score *(see back of form)* .... ______

Previous Cardiac Surgery .... ☐ Yes ☐ No

Chronic Lung Disease .... ☐ Yes ☐ No
(long term use bronchodilators or steroids)

Active Endocarditis .... ☐ Yes ☐ No
(antibiotic or endocarditis at time of surgery)

Critical Preoperative State .... ☐ Yes ☐ No
(pre-op ventricular tachycardia or ventricular fibrillation or aborted sudden death, cardiac massage, inotropes or IABP, anuria or oliguria <10ml/hr)

Diabetic requiring Insulin .... ☐ Yes ☐ No

NYHA Class *(see back of form)* .... ☐ I ☐ II ☐ III ☐ IV

CCS Class *(see back of form)* .... ☐ I ☐ II ☐ III ☐ IV

LV Function *(see back of form)* .... ☐ Good ☐ Moderate ☐ Poor ☐ Very Poor

MI < 90 days .... ☐ Yes ☐ No

Pulmonary hypertension ☐ No ☐ Moderate (PA systolic 31-55 mmHg) ☐ Severe (PA systolic >55 mmHg)

Urgency: .... ☐ Elective ☐ Urgent ☐ Emergency ☐ Salvage

Elective, Urgent (stable, cannot be sent home), **Emergency** (Must be done today), **Salvage** (CPR/ECMO preop)

Weight of Intervention: .... ☐ CABG ☐ Non-CABG ☐ 2 Procedures ☐ > two 2 Procedures

Surgery on Thoracic Aorta .... ☐ Yes ☐ No

July 14, 2014 7102-4174-4 Page 1 of 3

OFF-PUMP CORONARY ARTERY BYPASS GRAFTING (OPCAB)

Adverse clinical events associated with coronary artery bypass surgery (CABG) have been attributed to deleterious effects of cardiopulmonary bypass (CPB) including inflammation, macroemboli (aortic cannulation), microemboli and non-physiologic flow. While the use of CPB to perform CABG remains the "gold standard", the performance of OPCAB garnered intensive enthusiasm following its introduction in an to attempt to avoid these adverse events. This enthusiasm, though marked at the turn of the century, has waned over the last decade in the absence of definitive supportive studies, the concern regarding incomplete revascularization and the increasing technical demands related to OPCAB. The procedure

Figure 2. Example WHRA Cardiac Sciences Complex Case Rounds Referral Form, Page 2

For patients with liver disease:

	Measure	1 point	2 points	3 points
Child-Pugh score	Total bilirubin μmol/l	<34	34-50	>50
	Plasma albumin, g/l	>35	28-35	<28
	PT INR	<1.7	1.71-2.30	> 2.30
	Ascites *(see back of form)*	None	Mild	Moderate to Severe
	Encephalopathy *(see back of form)*	None	Grade I-II (or suppressed with Rx)	Grade III-IV (or refractory)

Other significant comorbity or concerns not listed above ______________________

Clinical Frailty Scale:

1 Very Fit	Robust, active, energetic, motivated, exercise regularly
2 Well	No active disease, less fit than category 1, exercise occasionally, e.g. seasonally
3 Managing Well	Medical problems well controlled, not regularly active beyond routine walking
4 Vulnerable	Not dependent for daily help, symptoms limit activities
5 Mildly Frail	Evident slowing, transportation, heavy housework, medications, shopping, walking, meal preparation
6 Moderately Frail	Help with all outside activities, keeping house, stairs, bathing, minimal assistance dressing
7 Severely Frail	Completely dependent for personal care (physical or cognitive; stable not high risk of dying < 6 mon
8 Very Severely Frail	Completely dependent, approaching end of life, could not recover even from a minor illness
9 Terminally ill	Life expectancy <6 months

CMAJ 2005; 173(5):489-95

Dementia Scoring:

Mild	forgetting details of recent event though remembers event, repeating same question/story, social withdrawal
Moderate	recent memory very impaired, can remember past life events well, personal care with prompting
Severe	cannot do personal care without help

LV Function: Good (LVEF > 50%) Moderate (LVEF 31-50%) Poor (LVEF 21-30%) Very Poor (< 21%)

NYHA Class: I (no dyspnea in ordinary activity) II (slight limitation during ordinary activity) III (marked limitation during ordinary activity) IV (symptoms at rest)

CCS Class: 0 (no angina) I (angina during strenuous activity) II (angina during moderate physical activity) III (angina with everyday living activities) IV (angina at rest)

Ascites grades:
1: mild, only visible on ultrasound and CT
2: moderate symmetrical distension of abdomen detectable with flank bulging and shifting dullness
3: directly visible, large or gross ascites with marked abdominal distension

Hepatic encephalopathy:
1: Trivial lack awareness; euphoria or anxiety; shortened attention span; impaired simple math
2: Lethargy/apathy; minimal disorientation time/place; min personality change; inappropriate behavior
3: Somnolence-semi stupor but responsive to verbal stimuli; confusion; gross disorientation

Child-Pugh Points	Life Expectancy years	Perioperative Mortality
A = 5-6	15-20	10%
B = 7-9	4-14	30%
C = 10-15	4-14	80%

Journal of Hepatology 2005; 42: S100–S107; Lancet 2008; 371: 838–51

CABG	Coronary Artery Bypass Surgery
CCS	Canadian Cardiovascular Society
ECHO	Echocardiogram
eGRF	estimated glomerular filtration rate
IABP	Intra Aortic Balloon pump
LV	Left ventricle
MI	Myocardial Infarction
NYHA	New York Heart Association
PA	Pulmonary Artery
PCI	Percutaneous Coronary Intervention
RV	Right ventricle
TAVI	Transthetei Aortic Valve Implantation
VAD	Ventricular Assisted Device

Page 2 of 3

now occurs approximately 10-20% of the time in North American centres (Polomsky & Puskas, 2012). The purported benefit of OPCAB in many non-randomized clinical studies included reduced use of resources, reduced blood loss and transfusion, reduced postoperative atrial fibrillation, reduced release of biochemical markers of myocardial damage, reduced early neurocognitive dysfunction, reduced renal insufficiency and shorter length of hospitalization (Angelini, Taylor, Reeves, & Ascione, 2002; Puskas et al., 2004). Earlier clinical trials, including several large retrospective analyses and meta-analyses, have demonstrated surgical outcomes in patients undergoing OPCAB to be comparable to results achieved

Figure 3. Example WHRA Cardiac Sciences Complex Case Rounds Referral Form, Page 3

Date of Rounds [ ][ ][ ][ ][ ][ ][ ][ ][ ]
D D M M M Y Y Y Y

Completed by the Chairperson

Referring MD: ____________________

Syntax Score ____________ EuroSCORE II ____________

Dementia: ____________ Clinical Frailty Score: ____________

1. **Outcome of Discussion**
   a. CABG recommended
   b. Valve surgery recommended
   c. TAVR recommended
   d. PCI recommended
   e. Further investigation recommended
      i. Cardiac MR
      ii. Cardiac CT
      iii. DSE
      iv. MIBI
      v. GXT
      vi. Other: ____________________
   f. Medical therapy recommended
   g. Palliative care / Pain Control only
   h. Other: ____________________

2. **Discussion Vote**
   a. Unanimous decision
   b. Majority vote
   c. No conclusion could be reached

Page 3 of 3

with "traditional" CABG with the use of CPB. On the other hand, some studies have shown that patients receiving OPCAB have a higher risk of incomplete revascularization and graft failure than patients receiving a standard CABG (Khan et al., 2004; Nathoe et al., 2003).

Trials You Should Know

Two large retrospective trials have examined the outcome of OPCAB in large datasets. A retrospective study in New York state examined outcomes in 68,000 CABG patients where 9000 procedures were performed with the OPCAB technique from 1997 to 2000 (Racz et al., 2004). Within the limitations of the somewhat heterogeneous nature of the two groups (i.e. patients in the OPCAB group were typically older, female and had higher rates of low left ventricular ejection fraction, greater co-morbidity, peripheral vascular disease, calcific aortic disease, CHF and renal dysfunction whereas the conventional CABG group had more extensive coronary disease and a higher incidence of shock), risk-adjusted mortality, perioperative MI, wound infection, renal failure requiring dialysis and respiratory failure were not different. There were, however, higher rates of: stroke (2.0% versus 1.6%, p=0.003), bleeding requiring reoperation (2.2% versus 1.6%, $p<0.001$) and longer hospital length of stay (one median day) in the standard CABG group. Conversely, higher risk of gastrointestinal complications (1.2% versus 0.9%, p=0.003) was observed in the OPCAB group. Importantly, patients in the standard CABG group had a higher survival rate (89.6% versus 88.8%, $p=0.022$) and freedom from repeat revascularization (percutaneous coronary intervention or CABG, 84.7% versus 82.1%, $p<0.0001$). The issue of a surgeon "learning curve" may have influenced early inter-group differences as data from the last two years of the study (i.e. excluding the first year) did not show any survival benefit of the on-pump versus the OPCAB group.

A second large retrospective study of 17401 patients (of which 7283 underwent an OPCAB procedure) undergoing CABG between 1999-2001 undertook propensity matching in all patients with multivessel disease to minimize selection bias (Mack et al., 2004). In the propensity-matched groups, the mortality rate was 2.2% in the OPCAB group, versus 3.7% in the CPB group ($p<0.001$). In addition, the rates of complications (such as blood products, wound infection, stroke, gastrointestinal and respiratory complications, renal failure, MI, and multi-organ failure) were significantly lower in the OPCAB group. These authors concluded that OPCAB is associated with less morbidity and mortality and patients at high risk derived the most benefit (i.e. women, older adults, and patients undergoing reoperation).

Reston et al., have previously presented a meta-analysis of short-term and mid-term outcomes following OPCAB (Reston, Tregear, & Turkelson, 2003). At the time of their review, the authors identified 53 studies of OPCAB patients that included ten randomized controlled trials, five prospective controlled studies and 38 retrospective controlled studies. They observed that rates of perioperative myocardial infarction, stroke, reoperation for bleeding, renal failure and mortality were lower after OPCAB than after conventional CABG. Midterm (3 to 25 months) angina recurrence did not appear to differ between treatments. A trend of lower re-intervention rates with conventional CABG, and lower overall mortality with OPCAB in more experienced centers was also seen. The authors concluded that more studies are required before firm conclusions can be drawn concerning the effect of OPCAB on midterm mortality, angina recurrence and repeat intervention.

Since 2009, four major randomized controlled trials have been published, increasing the level of evidence significantly (see Table1).

The largest trial of these is the 'Effects of Off-Pump and On-Pump Coronary-Artery Bypass Grafting at 1 Year' study (a.k.a. The CORONARY Trial) (Lamy et al., 2013). In this trial, the authors sought to understand the impact of OPCAB in a wide range of patients. Patients were enrolled if they were: age of 70 years or more, had peripheral arterial disease, cerebrovascular disease or carotid stenosis of 70% or more of the luminal diameter or renal insufficiency. Patients 60 to 69 years of age were also eligible if they had at least one of the following risk factors: diabetes requiring treatment with an oral hypoglycemic agent or insulin, the need for urgent revascularization after an acute coronary syndrome, left ventricular ejection fraction of 35% or less or a recent history of smoking (<1 year before randomization); patients 55 to 59 years of age were eligible if they had at least two of those risk factors. The

Table 1. Recent randomized controlled trials examining OPCAB and conventional CABG

Study	Patient Sample Size	Outcome
Off-Pump Coronary Artery Bypass Surgery Is Associated With Worse Arterial and Saphenous Vein Graft Patency and Less Effective Revascularization Results From the Veterans Affairs Randomized On/Off Bypass (ROOBY) Trial - Shroyer et al., 2009)	Multicenter, randomized trial, 2203 patients to urgent of elective CABG patients to either off-pump or on-pump procedures. Primary Outcome: *Short-term: Composite of death or complications (reoperation, new mechanical support, cardiac arrest, coma, stroke, or renal failure) before discharge or within 30 days after surgery. Long-term (Oneyear): Composite of death from any cause, a repeat revascularization procedure, or a nonfatal myocardial infarction*	There was no significant difference between off-pump and on-pump CABG in the rate of the 30-day composite outcome. The off-pump group had worse composite outcomes and poorer graft patency than did patients in the on-pump group at 1 year.
On-Pump Versus Off-Pump Coronary Artery Bypass Surgery in Elderly Patients Results From the Danish On-Pump Versus Off-Pump Randomization Study (The DOORS Study - Houlind et al., 2012)	Multicenter, randomized trial, 900 patients >70 years of age were assigned to conventional CABG or OPCAB surgery. Primary Outcomes: *Combined end point of mortality, myocardial infarction, or stroke within 30 days.*	Note: No major differences in intermediate-term (6-month) mortality or HRQoL were found (secondary end-points)
Off-Pump versus On-Pump Coronary-Artery Bypass Grafting in Elderly Patients (GOPCABE Study - Diegeler et al., 2013)	2539 patients, aged 75 years and older undergoing elective, first-time CABG were randomized to conventional CABG (1268 patients) or OPCAB (1271 patients). Primary Outcomes: *A composite of death, stroke, myocardial infarction, repeat revascularization, or new renal-replacement therapy at 30 days and at 12 months after surgery.*	There was no significant difference between on-pump CABG and OPCAB in the composite outcome of death, stroke, myocardial infarction, repeat revascularization, or new renal-replacement therapy at either 30 days or 12 months after surgery.
Effects of Off-Pump and On-Pump Coronary-Artery Bypass Grafting at 1 Year (CORONARY Trial -Lamy et al., 2013)	4752 patients were enrolled at 79 hospitals in 19 countries and were randomly assigned to undergo either off-pump CABG (2375 patients) or on-pump CABG (2377 patients). Primary Outcomes: *Life and cognitive function at discharge, at 30 days, and at 1 year and clinical outcomes at 1 year. The second co-primary outcome consisted of the first co-primary outcome plus the rate of repeat coronary revascularization at a mean of 5 years (data still pending).*	No significant difference between off-pump and on-pump CABG with respect to the primary composite outcome, the rate of repeat coronary revascularization, quality of life, or neurocognitive function at 1- year.

CABG = coronary artery bypass grafting; HRQoL = health related quality of life; OPCAB = off-pump coronary artery bypass grafting procedure.

investigators observed no significant differences between off-pump and on-pump CABG with respect to the primary composite outcome, the rate of repeat coronary revascularization, quality of life, or neurocognitive function at one–year.

Summary: It remains uncertain whether OPCAB is associated with a distinct advantage or whether the outcome with OPCAB is similar or identical to that achieved by CABG with CPB. Large, well designed randomized trials have failed to demonstrate a significant difference between techniques, leaving the decision as to whether or not to pursue OPCAB to institutions and surgeons based on their own experience and beliefs. Despite this, a practical utility for OPCAB remains in cases where patients have severely calcified or diseased aortas in which manipulation or clamping of the aorta can be associated with dire neurological consequences. In these populations the use of OPCAB may be advantageous.

MINIMALLY INVASIVE DIRECT CORONARY ARTERY BYPASS (MIDCAB)

Minimally invasive direct coronary artery bypass (MIDCAB) surgery is an option for patients who specifically require a left internal mammary artery (LIMA) bypass graft to the left anterior descending (LAD) coronary artery (Calafiore et al., 1996; Subramanian, Mccabe, Geller, Hospital, & York, 1997). The MIDCAB is usually performed through a small left anterior thoracotomy using an off-pump technique. This technique can also be performed as part of a staged hybrid procedure where other coronary vessels are revascularized using a catheter-based percutaneous coronary intervention technique either at the same time or in a delayed fashion. The purported benefits of minimally invasive bypass surgery include a smaller incision, a smaller scar, reduced risk of infection, decreased recovery time and a shorter hospital stay (Ruel et al., 2014). However, it does not provide any benefit over OPCAB performed via a conventional median sternotomy (Rogers et al., 2013).

COMPLICATIONS FOLLOWING CORONARY ARTERY BYPASS SURGERY

Since the early days of CABG, the tracking and the identification of risk factors for mortality has been the focus of many studies. However, the prospective tracking of other complications such as major vascular events, cardiac surgery associated kidney injury and delirium, has been less robust with variable and unclear event definitions. A study from nearly two decades ago demonstrated that when events are examined in a formal and prospective manner, the rates of perioperative complications are higher than previously believed.(Roach et al., 1996) Indeed, review of the literature will show a wide range of adverse outcomes over the past 20 years (see Table 2).

PERIOPERATIVE MYOCARDIAL INJURY

Myocardial infarction after cardiac surgery differs from that observed in the classic non-operative acute coronary syndrome (ACS) setting. In the cardiac surgery setting there may be an element of plaque instability. Activation of complement, coagulation and cytokine cascades facilitate activation of leukocytes, platelets and endothelial cells resulting in thrombosis, myocardial injury and cell death (Levy & Tanaka, 2003). Perioperative myocardial infarction may result, however, from intraoperative ischemia and reperfusion injury, coronary embolization, spasm and small vessel thrombosis (Thygesen et al., 2012).

The detection of perioperative myocardial infarction after cardiac surgery is difficult. The development of a new Q wave on the electrocardiogram (ECG) is strongly suggestive of a worse outcome. In a report from the Coronary Artery Surgery Study (CASS), the 62 patients who had a Q wave myocardial infarction had a higher mortality in-hospital (9.7 versus 1.0% in the 1278 patients without a Q wave myocardial infarction) (Chaitman et al., 1983). Myocardial infarction defined by new Q waves occurs in 4-5% of patients (Chaitman et al., 1983; Yokoyama et al., 2000). In contrast, a real-time diagnosis of perioperative myocardial infarction in cardiac surgery is challenging, since cardiac enzyme/biomarker elevation occurs universally as a result of the procedure and since ST-segment ECG changes may reflect post-operative pericardial inflammation. This is demonstrated by the wide range of event rates that have been reported (ranging from 0.1% to 7.7%; see Table 2).

Table 2. Perioperative vascular event rate in cardiac surgery patients

Author	Study Type	Patient population	Enrolment years	N	Mortality	MI	Cardiac arrest	Stroke
Roach et al., 1996	Prospective observational	Elective CABG	Sep 1991 to Sep 1993	2108	NR	NR	NR	63/2108 (3.0%)
el-Banayosy et al., 1998	Retrospective chart review	3476 CABG 734 Valve procedure 422 CABG + Valve procedure 336 Other procedures	Jan 1993-Dec 1994	4968	NR	NR	113 (2.3%) [CABG: 74 (2.1%); Valve: 17 (2.3%); CABG+Valve: 10 (2.4%); Other: 12 (3.6%)]	NR
Wahr et al., 1999	Prospective observational	Elective CABG	Sep 1991-Sep 1993	2402	86 (3.6%)	NR	84 (3.5%)	NR
Stamou et al., 2001	Retrospective analysis	CABG only with < 4 grafts	Sep 1989-Jun 1999	16,528	NR	NR	NR	333 (2.0%)
Mackay, Powell, Osgathorp, & Rozario, 2002	Prospective audit	Patients from a specialist cardiothoracic hospital	1995-2001	11,100	NR	NR	818 (7.4%)	NR
D. T. Mangano, 2002	Prospective cohort	CABG	Nov 1996-June 2000	5065	164 (3.2%)	185 (3.7%)	NR	92 (1.8%)
McKhann et al., 2004	Prospective cohort	CABG with or without concurrent procedure	Jan 1997-Dec 2000	2711	65 (2.4%)	NR	NR	73 (2.7%)
DeFoe et al., 2003	Prospective observational	Elective, urgent and emergency CABG	1997-2000	7134	128 (1.8%)	NR	NR	86 (1.2%)
Nalysnyk, Fahrbach, Reynolds, Zhao, & Ross, 2003	Systematic review	Isolated CABG	1990-2003	205,717	3497 (1.7%)	4937 (2.4%)	NR	2674 (1.3%)
Anyanwu, Filsoufi, Salzberg, Bronster, & Adams, 2007	Retrospective analysis of prospectively-collected data	All cardiac surgeries listed in New York State database	1998-2004	5085	286 (5.6%)	NR	NR	134 (2.6%) [CABG: (1.7%); Valve: (1.8%); CABG+Valve: (4.4%); Ascending aorta: (4.6%)]
L. M. Martin et al., 2008	Prospective cohort	Elective cardiac surgery	2001-2006	836	NR	1 (0.1%)	NR	6 (0.7%)
Singh et al., 2008	STS Database analysis	CABG only From STS Database	2004-2006	370,793	7045 (1.9%)	NR	NR	NR
Liakopoulos et al., 2008	Systematic review and meta-analysis	All cardiac surgeries	1999-2007	31,725	920 (2.9%)	1301 (4.17%)	NR	761 (2.4%)

continued on following page

Table 2. Continued

Author	Study Type	Patient population	Enrolment years	N	Mortality	MI	Cardiac arrest	Stroke
Li, Zheng, & Hu, 2009	Prospective cohort	CABG with or without concurrent procedure	Jan 2004-Dec 2005	9248 [8120 CABG only]	302 (3.27%) [180 (2.22%) in CABG only group]	NR	NR	NR
Mohammed et al., 2009	Prospective cohort	CABG only	2006-2007	847	9 (1.1%)	17 (2.0%)	NR	NR
Guney et al., 2008	Prospective cohort	CABG only	Feb 1998-Oct 2004	10,993	NR	NR	179 (1.6%)	NR
Garvin et al., 2010	Prospective cohort	Primary on-pump CABG	Aug 2001-May 2006	1403	12 (0.86%)	108 (7.7%)	16 (1.1%)	17 (1.2%)
Duncan et al., 2010	Retrospective analysis of prospectively collected data	On-pump CABG or valve procedures	Oct 2005-May 2007	4302	73 (1.7%)	43 (1.0%)	NR	NR

Still, the most common and prognostically relevant major complication after cardiac surgery is myocardial injury (defined by an elevated creatinine kinase myocardial band fraction or troponin measurement)(Domanski et al., 2011), which can impact both short and long-term mortality (Domanski et al., 2011; Lurati Buse et al., 2010; Petäjä, Salmenperä, Pulkki, & Pettilä, 2009). Although some elevation of cardiac enzymes (e.g. CK-MB and troponin) occurs commonly in patients undergoing cardiac surgery, studies suggest moderate and higher rises in cardiac enzymes and biomarkers have important prognostic implications (Moussa et al., 2013; Petäjä et al., 2009; Preeshagul et al., 2013; Søraas et al., 2012; Thygesen et al., 2012). In a meta-analysis by Petaja and colleagues that included 29,483 patients from 23 articles, a CK-MB greater than 5 times the upper limit of normal resulted in an increased mortality over the next 40 months (Petäjä et al., 2009). From this meta-analysis, high rises in CK-MB occur in approximately 20% of patients.

A meta-analysis by Domanski and colleagues (2011) examined the impact of elevated postoperative troponin I. This included an analysis of data from two RCTs that included approximately 250 international centres. However this also posed a problem in that many different troponin I assays would have been used across the 250 centers. Likewise in the Lurati Buse meta-analysis twelve different troponin assays were evaluated and strikingly different proportion of patients had elevations (i.e., 2.2% to 40.6%) across the studies (Lurati Buse et al., 2010). Recently, the Vascular Events In Non-cardiac Surgery Patients Cohort Evaluation (VISION) Study Group published results on the relationship of 4th generation troponin T (TnT) assays and 30-day mortality in 15133 patients undergoing non-cardiac surgery (Devereaux et al., 2012). They identified a relationship with peak TnT in the first 3 days following non-cardiac surgery and 30-day mortality. This study, therefore, highlights the need to determine the relationship of the current generation troponin assay measurement and post-operative mortality following cardiac surgery. Studies to determine this relationship are currently underway at the time of writing of this chapter (Vascular Events In Surgery patIents cOhort evaluatioN – Cardiac Surgery. ClinicalTrials.gov Identifier: NCT01842568)

POSTOPERATIVE CARDIAC ARREST

The incidence of cardiac arrest after cardiac surgery is around 0.7—2.9% (Anthi et al., 1998; Birdi, Chaudhuri, Lenthall, Reddy, & Nashef, 2000; el-Banayosy et al., 1998; Lottes et al., 2007; Mackay et al., 2002) and has reduced in recent years. Importantly, successful resuscitation to hospital discharge in this group of patients has been reported between 17—79%, a far higher proportion than described in other settings (Dunning et al., 2009). The purported rationale for superior survival in the cardiac surgery patient is the high incidence of potentially reversible causes for the arrest. Ventricular fibrillation (VF) accounts for the rhythm in 25—50% of cases and in the cardiothoracic intensive care unit setting this is immediately identified and treated. In addition, tamponade and major bleeding account for many arrests and both conditions may be quickly relieved by prompt resuscitation and emergency resternotomy where appropriate (Dunning et al., 2006, 2009; Mackay et al., 2002). Furthermore, the early institution of extra-corporeal membrane oxygenation (ECMO) during resuscitative efforts has been described (Gologorsky et al., 2010), however further study is required to determine survival benefit.

New Guidelines for Cardiac Advanced Life Support in the Cardiac Surgery Patient

In 2007, the Clinical Guideline Committee of the European Association for Cardio-Thoracic Surgery (EACTS) initiated a process to create a set of clear clinical guidelines to apply specifically to resuscitation after cardiac surgery. A formal guideline statement was published in 2009 (Dunning et al., 2009). The provided protocol (Figure 4) is a modification of the 2005 European Resuscitation Council advanced life support cardiac arrest algorithm (Soar et al., 2005) and is recommended to be used in the ICU. An important element of this new guideline is the identification of the 6 key-roles of the ICU cardiac arrest team to promote successful resuscitation in the cardiac surgery patient (Figure 5). There are several notable deviations from the "standard" ACLS resuscitation guidelines (Field et al., 2010; Hazinski et al., 2010), notably with regards to the timing of initiating closed chest cardiopulmonary resuscitation (CPR), epinephrine and atropine administration, epicardial pacing, chest re-opening. At the time of writing of this chapter, the American Heart Association Guidelines for Cardiopulmonary Resuscitation and Emergency Cardiovascular Care Science have stated that "there is insufficient evidence on epinephrine dose, anti-arrhythmic use, and other routine pharmacological interventions to recommend deviating from standard resuscitation guidelines when cardiac arrest occurs after cardiac surgery," however it may be "...reasonable to perform resternotomy in an appropriately staffed and equipped intensive care unit"(Vanden Hoek et al., 2010).

NEUROLOGIC COMPLICATIONS

Neurologic complications have been a recognized concern since the inception of cardiac surgery (Gilma, 1965; for recent review see McDonagh et al., 2014)).

Ischemic or Embolic Cerebral Event: In 1996, Roach and colleagues described rates of adverse cerebral outcomes after CABG in 2108 patients across 24 centers. They observed the rate of adverse cerebral outcomes was 6.1% with resultant substantial increases in mortality, length of stay and resource utilization (Roach et al., 1996). In more recent clinical trials, rates of perioperative stroke has been reported to

Figure 4. Proposed algorithm for approach to hypotension emergencies and cardiac arrest following cardiac surgery. Reproduced with permission from Oxford University Press.

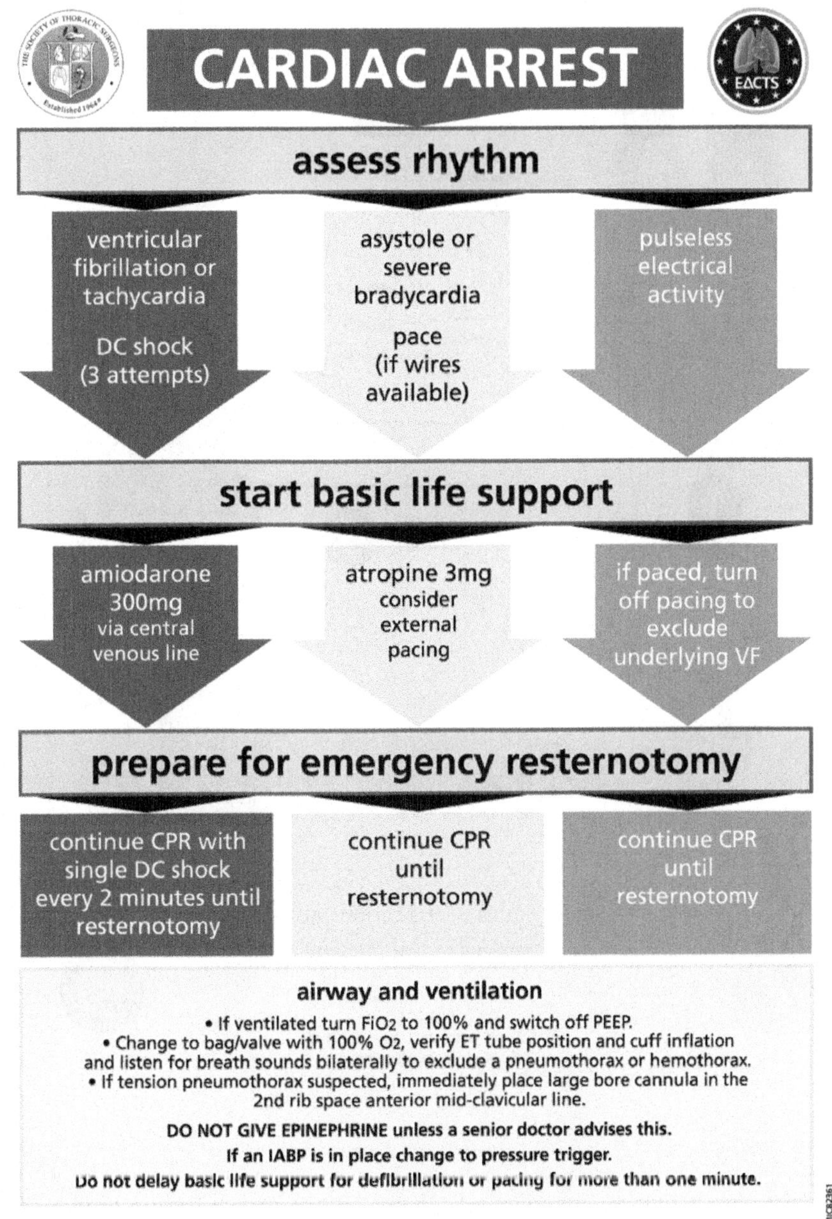

range from 2.2-5.2% (Farkouh et al., 2012; Serruys et al., 2009). Intraoperatively, several strategies are employed with the hopes of minimizing the risk of ischemic and embolic events: maintenance of a higher mean arterial blood pressure (Gold et al., 1995), using cerebral oximetry monitoring and intervening with different techniques for low cerebral saturation (Denault, Deschamps, & Murkin, 2007; Murkin & Arango, 2009; Palmbergen, van Sonderen, Keyhan-Falsafi, Keunen, & Wolterbeek, 2012; Slater et al., 2009), the use of transesophageal echocardiography and epiaortic ultrasound scanning to identify and avoid manipulation of aortic atheromatous disease (Hillis et al., 2011), the use of neuraxial anesthetic

Figure 5. Diagram of proposed six key roles for managing cardiac arrest following cardiac surgery. Reproduced with permission from Oxford University Press.

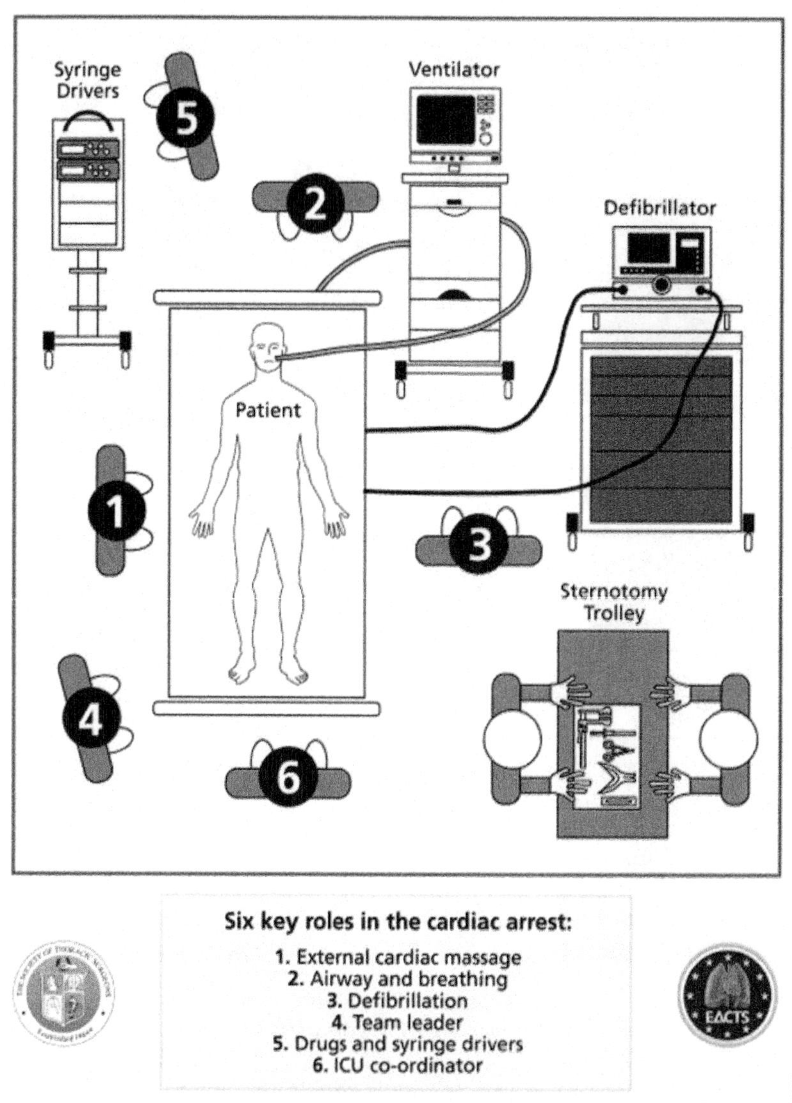

adjuncts (Svircevic et al., 2011), maintenance of a hemoglobin concentration higher than 60 g/L (or 6 g/dL) on cardiopulmonary bypass and at least 70 g/L (or 7 g/dL) postoperatively (Ferraris et al., 2007) and rationalized control of blood glucose (less than 9.99 mmol/L)(Hillis et al., 2011).

The "Porcelain Aorta": During coronary artery bypass grafting, manipulation of the ascending aorta can cause atheromatous embolism from a severely diseased ascending aorta. A patient with an "egg-shell" or significantly calcified aorta is at particularly high-risk with a rate of stroke reported to be as high as nearly 30% (Wareing, Davila-Roman, Barzilai, Murphy, & Kouchoukos, 1992). The time points where embolism can occur are: (1) during arterial cannulation of the aorta, (2) cross-clamping of the aorta, and (3) partial (or side-biting) clamping of the proximal ascending aorta for construction of the proximal anastomosis (Leyh, Bartels, Nötzold, & Sievers, 1999). Several techniques, either in isolation or more commonly in some combination, have been proposed to reduce the risk of athero-embolism through the avoidance of manipulation of a heavily calcified ascending aorta and aortic arch. These include: single-clamp technique, placement of proximal saphenous vein grafts (SVG) to the internal mammary artery (IMA) or the innominate artery, complete arterial revascularization with pedicled arterial grafts, hypothermic fibrillatory arrest avoiding clamping of the ascending aorta, replacement of the ascending aorta, aortic endarterectomy, patch aortoplasty, and arterial cannulation of the axillary artery (Akins, 1984; Bittner & Savitt, 2001; Cirillo et al., 2009; Culliford, Colvin, Rohrer, Baumann, & Spencer, 1986; Leyh et al., 1999; Sabik, Lytle, McCarthy, & Cosgrove, 1995; Wareing et al., 1992). As discussed above, the use of an OPCAB or hybrid MIDCAB technique are alternate approaches to perform aortic "no-touch"procedures, however high quality evidence as to whether this reduces perioperative strokes is unclear.

Delirium: Delirium is an acute confusional state characterized by fluctuating mental status, inattention, and either disorganized thinking or altered level of consciousness (Bergeron, Dubois, Dumont, Dial, & Skrobik, 2001; Ely et al., 2001, 2004; Innouye, Dyck, Alessi, & Balkin, 1990; Inouye et al., 1999). It has long been recognized as a complication of cardiac surgery, and is more common among elderly patients and those with greater co-morbid disease burden (Gokgoz et al., 1997; Kornfeld, Heller, Frank, & Moskowitz, 1974; van der Mast & Roest, 1996). The occurrence of postoperative delirium is often dismissed by the heath-care team as it has been traditionally been believed to be a transient and benign entity. In recent years, however, increasing attention has been paid to the negative effect of delirium on post-operative outcomes, including long-term survival, freedom from hospital readmission and reduced cognitive and functional recovery (Gottesman et al., 2010; Koster, Hensens, Schuurmans, & van der Palen, 2012; Koster, Hensens, & van der Palen, 2009; Loponen et al., 2008; B.-J. Martin, Buth, Arora, & Baskett, 2012; Rudolph et al., 2006, 2010; Saczynski et al., 2012; van Dijk et al., 2000). Despite its strong association with adverse post-operative events, delirium is an often under-recognized source of end-organ dysfunction. In the absence of an active screening program, delirium goes undiagnosed in greater than 70% of cases (Katznelson et al., 2010; Pisani, 2003). When utilizing a systematic methodology of delirium screening in the cardiothoracic ICU with either the confusion assessment method for the intensive care unit (CAM-ICU)(Ely et al., 2001, 2004) or the intensive care delirium screening checklist (ICDSC)(Bergeron et al., 2001). Current estimates of rate of postoperative delirium is approximately 20 to 25% patients (Arenson, MacDonald, Grocott, Hiebert, & Arora, 2013; Koster, Hensens, Schuurmans, & van der Palen, 2013; McPherson et al., 2013; Rudolph et al., 2009). Increasingly, cardiac surgical procedures are being performed on older patients with recent coronary syndromes, higher New York Heart Association classifications, lower left ventricular ejection fractions and cardiogenic shock; all of which are associated with increased rates of postoperative delirium. Therefore, it is likely that the incidence of post-operative delirium will continue to increase secondary to the aging demographic of the "typical" cardiac surgery patient.

Despite the numerous adverse consequences associated with its occurrence, to date postoperative delirium is neither preventable nor effectively treated with existing management strategies (Riker et al., 2009; Shehabi et al., 2010). One approach, therefore, is to attempt to develop predictive models that seek to identify potentially modifiable risk factors associated with the occurrence of post-operative delirium. Rudolph and colleagues (2009) identified 4 risk factors associated with an increased risk of postoperative delirium following cardiac surgery: prior stroke or transient ischemic attack, low Mini Mental State Examination score, abnormal serum albumin, and depression (via use of the Geriatric Depression Scale (Rinaldi et al., 2003)). Others have further identified elevated preoperative surgical risk scores, older age (≥70 years), number of comorbidities, history of delirium, alcohol use, type of surgery, blood transfusion, mechanical ventilation and infection as additional risk factors (Arenson et al., 2013; Koster et al., 2013; B.-J. Martin, Buth, Arora, & Baskett, 2010). Lastly, McPherson (2013) identified that the use of chemical restraints via use of benzodiazepines or the use of physical restraints/restraining devices predisposed patients to a greater risk of delirium, pointing to potential areas of quality improvement in the cardiac surgical ICU.

CARDIAC SURGERY ASSOCIATED ACUTE KIDNEY INJURY

Acute kidney injury (AKI) is a serious and potentially life-threatening complication in critically ill adults. After cardiac surgery with cardiopulmonary bypass (CPB), severe renal injury (i.e. requirement for dialysis) occurs in ~2% of patients and is associated with a 60% mortality risk (Chertow et al., 1997; Thakar, Arrigain, Worley, Yared, & Paganini, 2005). Milder degrees of kidney failure, occurring in up to 17% of patients, are associated independently with a 19-fold increase in short-term mortality (C. M. Mangano et al., 1998). The two currently used definitions of cardiac surgery associated acute kidney injury (CSA-AKI) are the RIFLE (Risk, Injury, Failure, Loss, and End-stage kidney disease) criteria (Bellomo, Kellum, & Ronco, 2007; Bellomo, Ronco, Kellum, Mehta, & Palevsky, 2004) and the Acute Kidney Injury Network (AKIN) criteria (Mehta et al., 2007). The RIFLE classification defines three grades of severity of AKI (Risk, Injury and Failure) based on changes to serum creatinine and urine output and two clinical out- comes (Loss, End-stage). The AKIN group has sought to increase the sensitivity of the RIFLE criteria by recommending that a smaller change in serum creatinine (≥26.2 µmol/L) be used as the threshold to define the presence of AKI (see Table 3).

In 2012, the KDIGO (Kidney Disease: Improving Global Outcomes) AKI working group published further criteria for the definition and classification of AKI that is meant to serve as combination of AKIN and RIFLE definitions.(Kidney Disease: Improving Global Outcomes (KDIGO) CKD Work Group, 2012) Specific to the cardiac surgery patient:

Table 3. A comparison of the different definition and classification schemes for CSA-AKI

Scoring System	Serum Creatinine Criteria	Urine Output Criteria
RIFLE		
Stage 1	Increase in serum creatinine ≥1.5X baseline or >25% decrease in eGFR	<0.5 mL/kg/h for ≥6h
Stage 2	Increase in serum creatinine ≥2.0X baseline or >50% decrease in eGFR	<0.5 mL/kg/h for ≥12 h
Stage 3	Increase in serum creatinine ≥3.0X baseline or >75% decrease in eGFR or an absolute serum creatinine ≥354 µmol/L with an acute rise of at least 44 µmol/L	<0.3 mL/kg/h ≥24h or anuria ≥12 h
AKIN		
Stage 1	Increase in serum creatinine ≥26.2 µmol/L or increase to ≥150–199% (1.5- to 1.9-fold) from baseline	<0.5 mL/kg/h for ≥6h
Stage 2	Increase in serum creatinine to 200–299% (>2–2.9 fold) from baseline	<0.5 mL/kg/h for ≥12 h
Stage 3	Increase in serum creatinine to ≥300% (≥3-fold) from baseline or serum creatinine ≥354 µmol/L with an acute rise of at least 44 µmol/L or initiation of RRT	<0.3 mL/kg/h ≥24h or anuria ≥12 h

eGFR= estimated glomerular filtration rate; RRT = renal replacement therapy

- Increase in serum creatinine by ≥ 26.5 µM (0.3 mg/dl) within 48 hours; or
- Increase in serum creatinine to ≥1.5 times baseline within 7 days

Kidney injury can occur before, during, or after the operation. Multiple factors can insult the kidney including hemodynamic instability, inflammation, hemolysis and nephrotoxic agents. In the setting of cardiac surgery the majority of renal injury arises intraoperatively during cardiopulmonary bypass (Thakar et al., 2005). Indeed, a renal tubular injury signal is measurable shortly after the initiation of CPB (Ho et al., 2012; Loef et al., 2005). CSA-AKI results from the interplay between patient susceptibility to renal injury and intra-operative renal insults. The evolution of ischemic AKI is conceptually divided into initiation, extension, maintenance and repair phases. The initiation phase is the period immediately following an ischemic insult in which reversible tubular injury begins and glomerular filtration (GFR) drops abruptly. At the tissue level ATP depletion, generation of reactive oxygen species and induction of inflammatory mechanisms contribute to sub-lethal epithelial and endothelial damage. If the ischemic insult is brief and mild, the injury remains sub-lethal and rapid recovery of organ function ensues. Prolonged/severe ischemia followed by reperfusion, however, leads to an extension phase characterized by microvascular damage, tubule cell death, desquamation and luminal obstruction. This leads to further decline in GFR. The injured endothelial and epithelial cells amplify inflammatory cascades. The maintenance phase is characterized by a dynamic equilibrium between waning injury and evolving repair mechanisms. The balance between cell survival and death determines the severity and duration of this phase. GFR reaches its nadir in the maintenance phase. The recovery phase is characterized by improvement in GFR and reestablishment of tubular epithelium (Sutton, Fisher, & Molitoris, 2002). While several serum and urine biomarkers have been sought (Bagshaw & Gibney, 2008) (such as neutrophil gelatinase–associated lipocalin (NGAL), kidney injury molecule-1 (KIM-1), and interleukin-18) none of these have been proved to provide reliable or timely prediction of impending AKI to assist with the development of strategies to mitigate AKI progression.

Karkouti and colleagues (2009) reported a multicenter cohort of 3500 adult patients who underwent cardiac surgery at seven hospitals to identify potentially modifiable risk factors associated with cardiac surgery associate acute kidney injury (CSA-AKI). Using multivariate logistic regression analysis they identified three potentially modifiable variables that were independently and strongly associated with AKI. These variables were preoperative anemia, perioperative red blood cell transfusions and surgical re-exploration. Karkouti et al. (2009) reason that while the kidney has a capacity to tolerate isolated insults such as hypoperfusion, a combination of several insults or risk factors (multiple hits) is necessary for CSA-AKI to occur. Therefore, strategies that seek to mitigate preoperative anemia, perioperative red blood cell transfusions and surgical re exploration may offer protection against this complication, however further study is required to substantiate this approach.

BLEEDING AND TRANSFUSION

It is well established that severe postoperative bleeding leads to increased morbidity and mortality in cardiac surgery patients and is a relatively common complication of cardiac surgery. It is associated with renal failure, sepsis, neurological impairment, acute respiratory distress syndrome and death. Risk scores to predict patients at high risk of bleeding have been generated (The Papworth Bleeding Risk Score (Vuylsteke et al., 2011)); where risk factors associated with bleeding include urgent or emergent surgery, non CABG cardiac surgery, lower body mass index and older age.

The relationship between peri-operative blood transfusions and post-operative morbidity is increasingly recognized though the exact nature of it is still under examination. Kock and colleagues examined outcomes of blood transfusions in 11,963 patients who underwent isolated CABG at a single centre from 1995 to 2002 (Koch et al., 2006). In this population 49% of patients received at least one blood transfusion of which roughly half were given in the operating room and half in the postoperative ICU. The analysis of this large sample of data revealed that there was a dose dependent relationship between blood transfusions and all morbidities including in-hospital mortality, infection, renal complications, neurologic complications and prolonged ventilator support. The authors concluded, however, that the retrospective nature of the analysis limits the ability to attribute these morbidities entirely to the transfusion themselves despite the fact that transfusion showed up significantly in all the statistical models utilized. This is substantiated by the fact that risk factors for receiving transfusion in their population were older age, smaller size, low pre-operative hematocrit and patients undergoing re-operative surgery, clearly a higher risk group.

It is no surprise, with this level of evidence that recommendations and practices regarding postoperative transfusion triggers are variable and broad. For example, the 2011 STS update on blood conservation and practice guidelines states that there is no indication for transfusion at a hemoglobin concentration greater than 10 g/dL, and that transfusion is likely indicated at a value less than 6 g/dL and even 7 g/dL, although this recommendation is not supported by quality evidence (Ferraris et al., 2011). As such, there is a need for a proper RCT to shed light on the impact of blood tranfusions on complications post CABG. The 'Transfusion Requirements in Cardiac Surgery III (TRICS-III, ClinicalTrials.gov identifier NCT02042898) is an international, multi-centre randomized controlled trial in cardiac surgery patients comparing a restrictive transfusion strategy with a liberal strategy to assess differences in an appropriate composite outcome; it is underway with the intention of enrolling over 3500 patients and will hopefully provide this very important information.

CONCLUSION

Ischemic heart disease is a major cause of morbidity and mortality throughout the world. With an aging population, older patients are increasingly being considered for surgical revascularization. Therefore it is important for those involved in cardiothoracic perioperative care to be well versed in conduct of the CABG procedure and the potential complications that can occur in the early postoperative period.

ACKNOWLEDGMENT

Rakesh C. Arora has received an unrestricted educational grant from Pfizer Canada Inc. He has also received research salary support from the Manitoba Health Research Council, Manitoba Medical Service Foundation and the Department of Surgery at the University of Manitoba. Dr. Arora the current chair of the CANadian CARdiovascular critical carE (CANCARE) Society and the President of the American Delirium Society at the time of writing of this chapter.

We would like to thank Drs. Claudio Rigatto, Julie Ho, Paul Komenda and Navdeep Tangri from the Manitoba Renal Program for their assistance with material related to CSA-AKI.

We would like to thank Drs. Andre Lamy, Richard Whitlock (McMaster University – Hamilton, Canada), Jean-Francois Legare (Dalhousie University – Halifax, Canada) and Ansar Hassan (Saint John, New Brunswick, Canada) for assistance with material related to Complications Following Cardiac Surgery.

We would like to thank Mr. Bryce Alexander and Mr. Andrew Stammers for their assistance in proof-reading and formatting.

REFERENCES

Acar, C., Jebara, V. A., Portoghese, M., Beyssen, B., Pagny, J. Y., & Grare, P. … Guermonprez, J. L. (1992). Revival of the radial artery for coronary artery bypass grafting. *The Annals of Thoracic Surgery, 54*(4), 652–9; discussion 659–60. Retrieved from http://www.ncbi.nlm.nih.gov/pubmed/1358040

Achouh, P., & Acar, C. (2013). Twenty-year fate of the radial artery graft. *Annals of Cardiothoracic Surgery*, *2*(4), 481–484. doi:10.3978/j.issn.2225-319X.2013.07.13 PMID:23977626

Achouh, P., Isselmou, K. O., Boutekadjirt, R., D'Alessandro, C., Pagny, J.-Y., Fouquet, R., & Acar, C. et al. (2012). Reappraisal of a 20-year experience with the radial artery as a conduit for coronary bypass grafting. *European Journal of Cardio-Thoracic Surgery : Official Journal of the European Association for Cardio-Thoracic Surgery*, *41*(1), 87–92. doi:10.1016/j.ejcts.2011.05.027 PMID:21900019

Akins, C. W. (1984). Noncardioplegic myocardial preservation for coronary revascularization. *The Journal of Thoracic and Cardiovascular Surgery*, *88*(2), 174–181. Retrieved from http://www.ncbi.nlm.nih.gov/pubmed/6611456 PMID:6611456

Angelini, G. D., Taylor, F. C., Reeves, B. C., & Ascione, R. (2002). Early and midterm outcome after off-pump and on-pump surgery in Beating Heart Against Cardioplegic Arrest Studies (BHACAS 1 and 2): A pooled analysis of two randomised controlled trials. *Lancet*, *359*(9313), 1194–1199. doi:10.1016/S0140-6736(02)08216-8 PMID:11955537

Anthi, A., Tzelepis, G. E., Alivizatos, P., Michalis, A., Palatianos, G. M., & Geroulanos, S. (1998). Unexpected cardiac arrest after cardiac surgery: Incidence, predisposing causes, and outcome of open chest cardiopulmonary resuscitation. *Chest*, *113*(1), 15–19. http://www.ncbi.nlm.nih.gov/pubmed/9440561 doi:10.1378/chest.113.1.15 PMID:9440561

Anyanwu, A. C., Filsoufi, F., Salzberg, S. P., Bronster, D. J., & Adams, D. H. (2007). Epidemiology of stroke after cardiac surgery in the current era. *The Journal of Thoracic and Cardiovascular Surgery*, *134*(5), 1121–1127. doi:10.1016/j.jtcvs.2007.06.031 PMID:17976438

Arenson, B. G., MacDonald, L. A., Grocott, H. P., Hiebert, B. M., & Arora, R. C. (2013). Effect of intensive care unit environment on in-hospital delirium after cardiac surgery. *The Journal of Thoracic and Cardiovascular Surgery*, *146*(1), 172–178. doi:10.1016/j.jtcvs.2012.12.042 PMID:23317943

Attaran, S., John, L., & El-Gamel, A. (2008). Clinical and potential use of pharmacological agents to reduce radial artery spasm in coronary artery surgery. *The Annals of Thoracic Surgery*, *85*(4), 1483–1489. doi:10.1016/j.athoracsur.2007.10.042 PMID:18355566

Bagshaw, S. M., & Gibney, R. T. N. (2008). Conventional markers of kidney function. *Critical Care Medicine*, *36*(4Suppl), S152–S158. doi:10.1097/CCM.0b013e318168c613 PMID:18382187

Bansilal, S., Farkouh, M. E., Hueb, W., Ogdie, M., Dangas, G., Lansky, A. J., & Fuster, V. et al. (2012). The Future REvascularization Evaluation in patients with Diabetes mellitus: optimal management of Multivessel disease (FREEDOM) trial: clinical and angiographic profile at study entry. *American Heart Journal*, *164*(4), 591–599. doi:10.1016/j.ahj.2012.06.012 PMID:23067919

Bellomo, R., Kellum, J., & Ronco, C. (2007). Defining and classifying acute renal failure: From advocacy to consensus and validation of the RIFLE criteria. *Intensive Care Medicine*, *33*(3), 409–413. doi:10.1007/s00134-006-0478-x PMID:17165018

Bellomo, R., Ronco, C., Kellum, J. A., Mehta, R. L., & Palevsky, P. (2004). Acute renal failure - definition, outcome measures, animal models, fluid therapy and information technology needs: the Second International Consensus Conference of the Acute Dialysis Quality Initiative (ADQI) Group. *Critical Care (London, England)*, *8*(4), R204–12. doi:10.1186/cc2872

Bergeron, N., Dubois, M. J., Dumont, M., Dial, S., & Skrobik, Y. (2001). Intensive Care Delirium Screening Checklist: Evaluation of a new screening tool. *Intensive Care Medicine*, *27*(5), 859–864. doi:10.1007/s001340100909 PMID:11430542

Birdi, I., Chaudhuri, N., Lenthall, K., Reddy, S., & Nashef, S. A. (2000). Emergency reinstitution of cardiopulmonary bypass following cardiac surgery: Outcome justifies the cost. *European Journal of Cardio-Thoracic Surgery : Official Journal of the European Association for Cardio-Thoracic Surgery*, *17*(6), 743–746. http://www.ncbi.nlm.nih.gov/pubmed/10856870 doi:10.1016/S1010-7940(00)00453-X PMID:10856870

Bittner, H. B., & Savitt, M. A. (2001). Management of porcelain aorta and calcified great vessels in coronary artery bypass grafting with off-pump and no-touch technology. *The Annals of Thoracic Surgery*, *72*(4), 1378–1380. http://www.ncbi.nlm.nih.gov/pubmed/11603471 doi:10.1016/S0003-4975(01)02568-1 PMID:11603471

Brener, S. J., Lytle, B. W., Casserly, I. P., Schneider, J. P., Topol, E. J., & Lauer, M. S. (2004). Propensity analysis of long-term survival after surgical or percutaneous revascularization in patients with multivessel coronary artery disease and high-risk features. *Circulation*, *109*(19), 2290–2295. doi:10.1161/01.CIR.0000126826.58526.14 PMID:15117846

Buszman, P. E., Kiesz, S. R., Bochenek, A., Peszek-Przybyla, E., Szkrobka, I., Debinski, M., & Tendera, M. et al. (2008). Acute and late outcomes of unprotected left main stenting in comparison with surgical revascularization. *Journal of the American College of Cardiology*, *51*(5), 538–545. doi:10.1016/j.jacc.2007.09.054 PMID:18237682

Buxton, B. F., Hayward, P., Newcomb, A. E., Moten, S., Seevanayagam, S., & Gordon, I. (2009). Choice of conduits for coronary artery bypass grafting: Craft or science? *European Journal of Cardio-Thoracic Surgery : Official Journal of the European Association for Cardio-Thoracic Surgery*, *35*(4), 658–670. doi:10.1016/j.ejcts.2008.10.058 PMID:19231230

Calafiore, a M., Giammarco, G. D., Teodori, G., Bosco, G., D'Annunzio, E., Barsotti, a, ... Contini, M. (1996). Left anterior descending coronary artery grafting via left anterior small thoracotomy without cardiopulmonary bypass. *The Annals of Thoracic Surgery, 61*(6), 1658–63; discussion 1664–5. Retrieved from http://www.ncbi.nlm.nih.gov/pubmed/8651765

Campeau, L., Enjalbert, M., Lespérance, J., Bourassa, M. G., Kwiterovich, P. Jr, Wacholder, S., & Sniderman, A. (1984). The relation of risk factors to the development of atherosclerosis in saphenous-vein bypass grafts and the progression of disease in the native circulation. A study 10 years after aortocoronary bypass surgery. *The New England Journal of Medicine, 311*(21), 1329–1332. doi:10.1056/NEJM198411223112101 PMID:6333635

Carpentier, A., Guermonprez, J. L., Deloche, A., Frechette, C., & DuBost, C. (1973). The aorta-to-coronary radial artery bypass graft. A technique avoiding pathological changes in grafts. *The Annals of Thoracic Surgery, 16*(2), 111–121. http://www.ncbi.nlm.nih.gov/pubmed/4582222 doi:10.1016/S0003-4975(10)65825-0 PMID:4582222

Chaitman, B. R., Alderman, E. L., Sheffield, L. T., Tong, T., Fisher, L., & Mock, M. B. ... Killip, T. (1983). Use of survival analysis to determine the clinical significance of new Q waves after coronary bypass surgery. *Circulation, 67*(2), 302–9. Retrieved from http://www.ncbi.nlm.nih.gov/pubmed/6600217

Chanda, J., Brichkov, I., & Canver, C. C. (2000). Prevention of radial artery graft vasospasm after coronary bypass. *The Annals of Thoracic Surgery, 70*(6), 2070–2074. http://www.ncbi.nlm.nih.gov/pubmed/11156122 doi:10.1016/S0003-4975(00)02001-4 PMID:11156122

Cheng, A., & Slaughter, M. S. (2013). How I choose conduits and configure grafts for my patients-rationales and practices. *Annals of Cardiothoracic Surgery, 2*(4), 527–532. doi:10.3978/j.issn.2225-319X.2013.07.17 PMID:23977632

Chertow, G. M., Lazarus, J. M., Christiansen, C. L., Cook, E. F., Hammermeister, K. E., Grover, F., & Daley, J. (1997). Preoperative renal risk stratification. *Circulation, 95*(4), 878–884. http://www.ncbi.nlm.nih.gov/pubmed/9054745 doi:10.1161/01.CIR.95.4.878 PMID:9054745

Cirillo, M., Messina, A., Dalla Tomba, M., Brunelli, F., Mhagna, Z., Villa, E., & Troise, G. et al. (2009). A new no-touch aorta technique for arterial-source, off-pump coronary surgery. *The Annals of Thoracic Surgery, 88*(4), e46–e47. doi:10.1016/j.athoracsur.2009.07.045 PMID:19766780

Collins, P., Webb, C. M., Chong, C. F., & Moat, N. E. (2008). Radial artery versus saphenous vein patency randomized trial: Five-year angiographic follow-up. *Circulation, 117*(22), 2859–2864. doi:10.1161/CIRCULATIONAHA.107.736215 PMID:18506009

Comparison of coronary bypass surgery with angioplasty in patients with multivessel disease. The Bypass Angioplasty Revascularization Investigation (BARI) Investigators. (1996). *The New England Journal of Medicine, 335*(4), 217–25. doi:10.1056/NEJM199607253350401

Culliford, A. T., Colvin, S. B., Rohrer, K., Baumann, F. G., & Spencer, F. C. (1986). The atherosclerotic ascending aorta and transverse arch: a new technique to prevent cerebral injury during bypass: experience with 13 patients. *The Annals of Thoracic Surgery, 41*(1), 27–35. http://www.ncbi.nlm.nih.gov/pubmed/3942429 doi:10.1016/S0003-4975(10)64492-X PMID:3942429

Deb, S., Cohen, E., Singh, S. K., Une, D., Laupacis, A., & Fremes, S. E. (2012). Radial artery and saphenous vein patency more than 5 years after coronary artery bypass surgery: Results from RAPS (Radial Artery Patency Study). *Journal of the American College of Cardiology*, *60*(1), 28–35. doi:10.1016/j.jacc.2012.03.037 PMID:22742399

DeFoe, G. R., Krumholz, C. F., DioDato, C. P., Ross, C. S., Olmstead, E. M., Groom, R. C., & O'Connor, G. T. et al. (2003). Lowest core body temperature and adverse outcomes associated with coronary artery bypass surgery. *Perfusion*, *18*(2), 127–133. doi:10.1191/0267659103pf660oa PMID:12868791

Denault, A., Deschamps, A., & Murkin, J. M. (2007). A proposed algorithm for the intraoperative use of cerebral near-infrared spectroscopy. *Seminars in Cardiothoracic and Vascular Anesthesia*, *11*(4), 274–281. doi:10.1177/1089253207311685 PMID:18270192

Desai, N. D., Cohen, E. A., Naylor, C. D., & Fremes, S. E. (2004). A randomized comparison of radial-artery and saphenous-vein coronary bypass grafts. *The New England Journal of Medicine*, *351*(22), 2302–2309. doi:10.1056/NEJMoa040982 PMID:15564545

Desai, N. D., Naylor, C. D., Kiss, A., Cohen, E., Feder-Elituv, R., Miwa, S., & Fremes, S. E. et al. (2007). Impact of patient and target-vessel characteristics on arterial and venous bypass graft patency: Insight from a randomized trial. *Circulation*, *115*(6), 684–691. doi:10.1161/CIRCULATIONAHA.105.567495 PMID:17283268

Devereaux, P. J., Chan, M. T. V., Alonso-Coello, P., Walsh, M., Berwanger, O., Villar, J. C., & Yusuf, S. et al. (2012). Association between postoperative troponin levels and 30-day mortality among patients undergoing noncardiac surgery. *Journal of the American Medical Association*, *307*(21), 2295–2304. doi:10.1001/jama.2012.5502 PMID:22706835

Diegeler, A., Börgermann, J., Kappert, U., Breuer, M., Böning, A., Ursulescu, A., & Hilker, M. et al. (2013). Off-pump versus on-pump coronary-artery bypass grafting in elderly patients. *The New England Journal of Medicine*, *368*(13), 1189–1198. doi:10.1056/NEJMoa1211666 PMID:23477657

Domanski, M. J., Mahaffey, K., Hasselblad, V., Brener, S. J., Smith, P. K., Hillis, G., & Farkouh, M. E. et al. (2011). Association of myocardial enzyme elevation and survival following coronary artery bypass graft surgery. *Journal of the American Medical Association*, *305*(6), 585–591. doi:10.1001/jama.2011.99 PMID:21304084

Dreifaldt, M., Mannion, J. D., Bodin, L., Olsson, H., Zagozdzon, L., & Souza, D. (2013). The no-touch saphenous vein as the preferred second conduit for coronary artery bypass grafting. *The Annals of Thoracic Surgery*, *96*(1), 105–111. doi:10.1016/j.athoracsur.2013.01.102 PMID:23684156

Duncan, A. E., Abd-Elsayed, A., Maheshwari, A., Xu, M., Soltesz, E., & Koch, C. G. (2010). Role of intraoperative and postoperative blood glucose concentrations in predicting outcomes after cardiac surgery. *Anesthesiology*, *112*(4), 860–871. doi:10.1097/ALN.0b013e3181d3d4b4 PMID:20216389

Dunning, J., Fabbri, A., Kolh, P. H., Levine, A., Lockowandt, U., Mackay, J., & Nashef, S. A. M. et al. (2009). Guideline for resuscitation in cardiac arrest after cardiac surgery. *European Journal of Cardio-Thoracic Surgery : Official Journal of the European Association for Cardio-Thoracic Surgery*, *36*(1), 3–28. doi:10.1016/j.ejcts.2009.01.033 PMID:19297185

Dunning, J., Nandi, J., Ariffin, S., Jerstice, J., Danitsch, D., & Levine, A. (2006). The Cardiac Surgery Advanced Life Support Course (CALS): Delivering significant improvements in emergency cardiothoracic care. *The Annals of Thoracic Surgery*, *81*(5), 1767–1772. doi:10.1016/j.athoracsur.2005.12.012 PMID:16631670

el-Banayosy, A., Brehm, C., Kizner, L., Hartmann, D., Körtke, H., Körner, M. M., … Körfer, R. (1998). Cardiopulmonary resuscitation after cardiac surgery: a two-year study. *Journal of Cardiothoracic and Vascular Anesthesia, 12*(4), 390–2. Retrieved from http://www.ncbi.nlm.nih.gov/pubmed/9713724

Ely, E. W., Margolin, R., Francis, J., May, L., Truman, B., Dittus, R., … Inouye, S. K. (2001). Evaluation of delirium in critically ill patients: Validation of the Confusion Assessment Method for the Intensive Care Unit (CAM-ICU), *29*(7).

Ely, E. W., Shintani, A., Truman, B., Speroff, T., Gordon, S. M., Harrell, F. E., & Dittus, R. S. et al. (2004). Delirium as a predictor of mortality in mechanically ventilated patients in the intensive care unit. *Journal of the American Medical Association*, *291*(14), 1753–1762. doi:10.1001/jama.291.14.1753 PMID:15082703

Farkouh, M. E., Dangas, G., Leon, M. B., Smith, C., Nesto, R., Buse, J. B., & Fuster, V. et al. (2008). Design of the Future REvascularization Evaluation in patients with Diabetes mellitus: Optimal management of Multivessel disease (FREEDOM) Trial. *American Heart Journal*, *155*(2), 215–223. doi:10.1016/j.ahj.2007.10.012 PMID:18215589

Farkouh, M. E., Domanski, M., Sleeper, L., Siami, F. S., Dangas, G., Mack, M., & Fuster, V. et al. (2012). Strategies for multivessel revascularization in patients with diabetes. *The New England Journal of Medicine*, *367*(25), 2375–2384. doi:10.1056/NEJMoa1211585 PMID:23121323

Favaloro, R. G. (1968). Saphenous vein autograft replacement of severe segmental coronary artery occlusion: Operative technique. *The Annals of Thoracic Surgery*, *5*(4), 334–339. http://www.ncbi.nlm.nih.gov/pubmed/5647919 doi:10.1016/S0003-4975(10)66351-5 PMID:5647919

Ferraris, V., Ferraris, S. P., Saha, S. P., Hessel, E. a, Haan, C. K., Royston, B. D., … Body, S. (2007). Perioperative blood transfusion and blood conservation in cardiac surgery: The Society of Thoracic Surgeons and The Society of Cardiovascular Anesthesiologists clinical practice guideline. *The Annals of Thoracic Surgery*, *83*(5Suppl), S27–S86. doi:10.1016/j.athoracsur.2007.02.099 PMID:17462454

Ferraris, V., Brown, J. R., Despotis, G. J., Hammon, J. W., Reece, T. B., Saha, S. P., … Shann, K. G. (2011). 2011 update to the Society of Thoracic Surgeons and the Society of Cardiovascular Anesthesiologists blood conservation clinical practice guidelines. *The Annals of Thoracic Surgery, 91*(3), 944–82. doi:10.1016/j.athoracsur.2010.11.078

Ferreira, A. C., Peter, A., Salerno, T., Bolooki, H., & de Marchena, E. (2003). Clinical impact of drug-eluting stents in changing referral practices for coronary surgical revascularization in a tertiary care center. *The Annals of Thoracic Surgery, 75*(2), 485–9. Retrieved from http://www.ncbi.nlm.nih.gov/pubmed/12607658

Field, J. M., Hazinski, M. F., Sayre, M. R., Chameides, L., Schexnayder, S. M., Hemphill, R., & Vanden Hoek, T. L. et al. (2010). Part 1: executive summary: 2010 American Heart Association Guidelines for Cardiopulmonary Resuscitation and Emergency Cardiovascular Care. *Circulation*, *122*(18Suppl 3), S640–S656. doi:10.1161/CIRCULATIONAHA.110.970889 PMID:20956217

Fitzgibbon, G. M., Kafka, H. P., Leach, A. J., Keon, W. J., Hooper, G. D., & Burton, J. R. (1996). Coronary bypass graft fate and patient outcome: Angiographic follow-up of 5,065 grafts related to survival and reoperation in 1,388 patients during 25 years. *Journal of the American College of Cardiology*, *28*(3), 616–626. http://www.ncbi.nlm.nih.gov/pubmed/8772748 doi:10.1016/0735-1097(96)00206-9 PMID:8772748

Garvin, S., Muehlschlegel, J. D., Perry, T. E., Chen, J., Liu, K., Fox, A. A., & Body, S. C. et al. (2010). Postoperative activity, but not preoperative activity, of antithrombin is associated with major adverse cardiac events after coronary artery bypass graft surgery. *Anesthesia and Analgesia*, *111*(4), 862–869. doi:10.1213/ANE.0b013e3181b7908c PMID:19820236

Geha, A. S., Krone, R. J., McCormick, J. R., & Baue, A. E. (1975). Selection of coronary bypass. Anatomic, physiological, and angiographic considerations of vein and mammary artery grafts. *The Journal of Thoracic and Cardiovascular Surgery*, *70*(3), 414–431. Retrieved from http://www.ncbi.nlm.nih.gov/pubmed/240984 PMID:240984

Gilman, S.GILMAN. (1965). Cerebral Disorders after open-heart operations. *The New England Journal of Medicine*, *272*(10), 489–498. doi:10.1056/NEJM196503112721001 PMID:14250198

Gokgoz, L., Gunaydin, S., Sinci, V., Unlu, M., & Boratav, C. Babacan, a, … Ersoz, a. (1997). Psychiatric complications of cardiac surgery postoperative delirium syndrome. *Scandinavian Cardiovascular Journal : SCJ, 31*(4), 217–22. Retrieved from http://www.ncbi.nlm.nih.gov/pubmed/9291540

Gold, J. P., Charlson, M. E., Williams-Russo, P., Szatrowski, T. P., Peterson, J. C., & Pirraglia, P. A. … Barbut, D. (1995). Improvement of outcomes after coronary artery bypass. A randomized trial comparing intraoperative high versus low mean arterial pressure. *The Journal of Thoracic and Cardiovascular Surgery, 110*(5), 1302–11; discussion 1311–4. Retrieved from http://www.ncbi.nlm.nih.gov/pubmed/7475182

Gologorsky, E., Macedo, F. I. B., Carvalho, E. M., Gologorsky, A., Ricci, M., & Salerno, T. a. (2010). Postoperative cardiac arrest after heart surgery: Does extracorporeal perfusion support a paradigm change in management? *Anesthesiology Research and Practice*, *2010*. doi:10.1155/2010/937215 PMID:20798770

Gottesman, R. F., & Grega, M. a, Bailey, M. M., Pham, L. D., Zeger, S. L., Baumgartner, W. a, … McKhann, G. M. (2010). Delirium after coronary artery bypass graft surgery and late mortality. *Annals of Neurology*, *67*(3), 338–344. doi:10.1002/ana.21899 PMID:20373345

Grüntzig, A. R., Senning, A., & Siegenthaler, W. E. (1979). Nonoperative dilatation of coronary-artery stenosis: Percutaneous transluminal coronary angioplasty. *The New England Journal of Medicine*, *301*(2), 61–68. doi:10.1056/NEJM197907123010201 PMID:449946

Guney, M. R., Ketenci, B., Yapici, F., Sokullu, O., Firat, M. F., Uyarel, H., & Demirtas, M. et al. (2008). Results of treatment methods in cardiac arrest following coronary artery bypass grafting. *Journal of Cardiac Surgery*, *24*(3), 227–233. doi:10.1111/j.1540-8191.2008.00760.x PMID:19040406

Hannan, E. L., Wu, C., Walford, G., Culliford, A. T., Gold, J. P., Smith, C. R., & Jones, R. H. et al. (2008). Drug-eluting stents vs. coronary-artery bypass grafting in multivessel coronary disease. *The New England Journal of Medicine*, *358*(4), 331–341. doi:10.1056/NEJMoa071804 PMID:18216353

Harskamp, R. E., Lopes, R. D., Baisden, C. E., de Winter, R. J., & Alexander, J. H. (2013). Saphenous vein graft failure after coronary artery bypass surgery: Pathophysiology, management, and future directions. *Annals of Surgery*, *257*(5), 824–833. doi:10.1097/SLA.0b013e318288c38d PMID:23574989

Hata, M., Yoshitake, I., Wakui, S., Unosawa, S., Kimura, H., Hata, H., & Shiono, M. (2011). Long-term patency rate for radial artery vs. saphenous vein grafts using same-patient materials. *Circulation Journal : Official Journal of the Japanese Circulation Society, 75*(6), 1373–7. Retrieved from http://www.ncbi.nlm.nih.gov/pubmed/21467657

Hayward, P., & Buxton, B. F. (2007). Contemporary coronary graft patency: 5-year observational data from a randomized trial of conduits. *The Annals of Thoracic Surgery*, *84*(3), 795–799. doi:10.1016/j.athoracsur.2007.04.028 PMID:17720377

Hayward, P., Gordon, I. R., Hare, D. L., Matalanis, G., Horrigan, M. L., Rosalion, A., & Buxton, B. F. (2010). Comparable patencies of the radial artery and right internal thoracic artery or saphenous vein beyond 5 years: Results from the Radial Artery Patency and Clinical Outcomes trial. *The Journal of Thoracic and Cardiovascular Surgery*, *139*(1), 60–65, discussion 65–67. doi:10.1016/j.jtcvs.2009.09.043 PMID:20106358

Hazinski, M. F., Nolan, J. P., Billi, J. E., Böttiger, B. W., Bossaert, L., de Caen, A. R., & Zideman, D. et al. (2010). Part 1: Executive summary: 2010 International Consensus on Cardiopulmonary Resuscitation and Emergency Cardiovascular Care Science With Treatment Recommendations. *Circulation*, *122*(16Suppl 2), S250–S275. doi:10.1161/CIRCULATIONAHA.110.970897 PMID:20956249

He, G.-W. (2013). Arterial grafts: Clinical classification and pharmacological management. *Annals of Cardiothoracic Surgery*, *2*(4), 507–518. doi:10.3978/j.issn.2225-319X.2013.07.12 PMID:23977630

Hillis, L. D., Smith, P. K., Anderson, J. L., Bittl, J., Bridges, C. R., Byrne, J. G., & Winniford, M. D. et al. (2011). ACCF/AHA Guideline for Coronary Artery Bypass Graft Surgery: executive summary: a report of the American College of Cardiology Foundation/American Heart Association Task Force on Practice Guidelines. *Circulation*, *124*(23), 2610–2642. doi:10.1161/CIR.0b013e31823b5fee PMID:22064600

Ho, J., Reslerova, M., Gali, B., Nickerson, P. W., Rush, D. N., Sood, M. M., & Rigatto, C. et al. (2012). Serum creatinine measurement immediately after cardiac surgery and prediction of acute kidney injury. *American Journal of Kidney Diseases : The Official Journal of the National Kidney Foundation*, *59*(2), 196–201. doi:10.1053/j.ajkd.2011.08.023 PMID:21967775

Houlind, K., Kjeldsen, B. J., Madsen, S. N., Rasmussen, B. S., Holme, S. J., Nielsen, P. H., & Mortensen, P. E. (2012). On-pump versus off-pump coronary artery bypass surgery in elderly patients: Results from the Danish on-pump versus off-pump randomization study. *Circulation*, *125*(20), 2431–2439. doi:10.1161/CIRCULATIONAHA.111.052571 PMID:22523305

Innouye, S., Dyck, C., Alessi, C., & Balkin, S. (1990). Clarifying confusion: the confusion assessment. *Ann Intern Med*. Retrieved from http://scholar.google.com/scholar?hl=en&btnG=Search&q=intitle:Clarifying+confusion:+the+confusion+assessment#1

Inouye, S. K., Bogardus, S. T. Jr, Charpentier, P. A., Leo-Summers, L., Acampora, D., Holford, T. R., & Cooney, L. M. Jr. (1999). A multicomponent intervention to prevent delirium in hospitalized older patients. *The New England Journal of Medicine*, *340*(9), 669–676. doi:10.1056/NEJM199903043400901 PMID:10053175

Kapur, A., Hall, R. J., Malik, I. S., Qureshi, A. C., Butts, J., de Belder, M., & Beatt, K. J. et al. (2010). Randomized comparison of percutaneous coronary intervention with coronary artery bypass grafting in diabetic patients. 1-year results of the CARDia (Coronary Artery Revascularization in Diabetes) trial. *Journal of the American College of Cardiology*, *55*(5), 432–440. doi:10.1016/j.jacc.2009.10.014 PMID:20117456

Karkouti, K., Wijeysundera, D. N., Yau, T. M., Callum, J. L., Cheng, D. C., Crowther, M., & Beattie, W. S. et al. (2009). Acute kidney injury after cardiac surgery: Focus on modifiable risk factors. *Circulation*, *119*(4), 495–502. doi:10.1161/CIRCULATIONAHA.108.786913 PMID:19153273

Kastrati, A., Mehilli, J., Pache, J., Kaiser, C., Valgimigli, M., Kelbaek, H., & Schömig, A. et al. (2007). Analysis of 14 trials comparing sirolimus-eluting stents with bare-metal stents. *The New England Journal of Medicine*, *356*(10), 1030–1039. doi:10.1056/NEJMoa067484 PMID:17296823

Katznelson, R., Djaiani, G., Tait, G., Wasowicz, M., Sutherland, A. M., Styra, R., … Beattie, W. S. (2010). Hospital administrative database underestimates delirium rate after cardiac surgery. *Canadian Journal of Anaesthesia = Journal Canadien D'anesthésie*, *57*(10), 898–902. doi:10.1007/s12630-010-9355-8

Khan, N. E., De Souza, A., Mister, R., Flather, M., Clague, J., Davies, S., & Pepper, J. et al. (2004). A randomized comparison of off-pump and on-pump multivessel coronary-artery bypass surgery. *The New England Journal of Medicine*, *350*(1), 21–28. doi:10.1056/NEJMoa031282 PMID:14702424

Kidney DiseaseImproving Global Outcomes (KDIGO) CKD Work Group. (2012). Notice. *Kidney International. Supplement*, *2*(1), 1–138. doi:10.1038/kisup.2012.1 PMID:25028630

Koch, C. G., Li, L., Duncan, A. I., Mihaljevic, T., Cosgrove, D. M., Loop, F. D., & Blackstone, E. H. et al. (2006). Morbidity and mortality risk associated with red blood cell and blood-component transfusion in isolated coronary artery bypass grafting. *Critical Care Medicine*, *34*(6), 1608–1616. doi:10.1097/01.CCM.0000217920.48559.D8 PMID:16607235

Kornfeld, D. S., Heller, S. S., & Frank, K. a, & Moskowitz, R. (1974). Personality and psychological factors in postcardiotomy delirium. *Archives of General Psychiatry*, *31*(2), 249–53. Retrieved from http://www.ncbi.nlm.nih.gov/pubmed/4853590

Koster, S., Hensens, A. G., Schuurmans, M. J., & van der Palen, J. (2012). Consequences of delirium after cardiac operations. *The Annals of Thoracic Surgery*, *93*(3), 705–711. doi:10.1016/j.athoracsur.2011.07.006 PMID:21992939

Koster, S., Hensens, A. G., Schuurmans, M. J., & van der Palen, J. (2013). Prediction of delirium after cardiac surgery and the use of a risk checklist. *European Journal of Cardiovascular Nursing : Journal of the Working Group on Cardiovascular Nursing of the European Society of Cardiology*, *12*(3), 284–292. doi:10.1177/1474515112450244 PMID:22694810

Koster, S., Hensens, A. G., & van der Palen, J. (2009). The long-term cognitive and functional outcomes of postoperative delirium after cardiac surgery. *The Annals of Thoracic Surgery*, *87*(5), 1469–1474. doi:10.1016/j.athoracsur.2009.02.080 PMID:19379886

Lamy, A., Devereaux, P. J., Prabhakaran, D., Taggart, D. P., Hu, S., Paolasso, E., & Yusuf, S. et al. (2013). Effects of off-pump and on-pump coronary-artery bypass grafting at 1 year. *The New England Journal of Medicine*, *368*(13), 1179–1188. doi:10.1056/NEJMoa1301228 PMID:23477676

Leon, M. B., Smith, C. R., Mack, M., Miller, D. C., Moses, J. W., Svensson, L. G., & Pocock, S. et al. (2010). Transcatheter aortic-valve implantation for aortic stenosis in patients who cannot undergo surgery. *The New England Journal of Medicine*, *363*(17), 1597–1607. doi:10.1056/NEJMoa1008232 PMID:20961243

Levy, J. H., & Tanaka, K. A. (2003). Inflammatory response to cardiopulmonary bypass. *The Annals of Thoracic Surgery*, *75*(2), S715–S720. http://www.sciencedirect.com/science/article/pii/000349759391048R doi:10.1016/S0003-4975(02)04701-X PMID:12607717

Leyh, R. G., & Bartels, C. Nötzold, a, & Sievers, H. H. (1999). Management of porcelain aorta during coronary artery bypass grafting. *The Annals of Thoracic Surgery, 67*(4), 986–8. Retrieved from http://www.ncbi.nlm.nih.gov/pubmed/11603471

Li, Y., Zheng, Z., & Hu, S. (2009). The Chinese coronary artery bypass grafting registry study: Analysis of the national multicentre database of 9248 patients. *Heart (British Cardiac Society)*, *95*(14), 1140–1144. doi:10.1136/hrt.2008.146563 PMID:18632834

Liakopoulos, O. J., Choi, Y.-H., Haldenwang, P. L., Strauch, J., Wittwer, T., Dörge, H., & Wahlers, T. et al. (2008). Impact of preoperative statin therapy on adverse postoperative outcomes in patients undergoing cardiac surgery: A meta-analysis of over 30,000 patients. *European Heart Journal*, *29*(12), 1548–1559. doi:10.1093/eurheartj/ehn198 PMID:18506053

Loef, B. G., Epema, A. H., Smilde, T. D., Henning, R. H., Ebels, T., Navis, G., & Stegeman, C. (2005). Immediate postoperative renal function deterioration in cardiac surgical patients predicts in-hospital mortality and long-term survival. *Journal of the American Society of Nephrology : JASN*, *16*(1), 195–200. doi:10.1681/ASN.2003100875 PMID:15563558

Loop, F. D., Lytle, B. W., Cosgrove, D. M., Stewart, R. W., Goormastic, M., Williams, G. W., & Sheldon, W. C. et al. (1986). Influence of the internal-mammary-artery graft on 10-year survival and other cardiac events. *The New England Journal of Medicine*, *314*(1), 1–6. doi:10.1056/NEJM198601023140101 PMID:3484393

Loponen, P., Luther, M., Wistbacka, J.-O., Nissinen, J., Sintonen, H., Huhtala, H., & Tarkka, M. R. (2008). Postoperative delirium and health related quality of life after coronary artery bypass grafting. *Scandinavian Cardiovascular Journal : SCJ*, *42*(5), 337–344. doi:10.1080/14017430801939217 PMID:18609064

Lottes, A. E., Rundell, A. E., Geddes, L., Kemeny, A. E., Otlewski, M. P., & Babbs, C. F. (2007). Sustained abdominal compression during CPR raises coronary perfusion pressures as much as vasopressor drugs. *Resuscitation, 75*(3), 515–524. doi:10.1016/j.resuscitation.2007.05.012 PMID:17630090

Lurati Buse, G. a, Koller, M. T., Grapow, M., Bolliger, D., Seeberger, M., & Filipovic, M. (2010). The prognostic value of troponin release after adult cardiac surgery - a meta-analysis. *European Journal of Cardio-Thoracic Surgery : Official Journal of the European Association for Cardio-Thoracic Surgery, 37*(2), 399–406. doi:10.1016/j.ejcts.2009.05.054 PMID:19699102

Lytle, B. W., Blackstone, E. H., Sabik, J. F., Houghtaling, P., Loop, F. D., & Cosgrove, D. M. (2004). The effect of bilateral internal thoracic artery grafting on survival during 20 postoperative years. *The Annals of Thoracic Surgery, 78*(6), 2005–12; discussion 2012–4. doi:10.1016/j.athoracsur.2004.05.070

Mack, M. J., Pfister, A., Bachand, D., Emery, R., Magee, M. J., Connolly, M., & Subramanian, V. (2004). Comparison of coronary bypass surgery with and without cardiopulmonary bypass in patients with multivessel disease. *The Journal of Thoracic and Cardiovascular Surgery, 127*(1), 167–173. doi:10.1016/j.jtcvs.2003.08.032 PMID:14752427

Mackay, J. H., Powell, S. J., Osgathorp, J., & Rozario, C. J. (2002). Six-year prospective audit of chest reopening after cardiac arrest. *European Journal of Cardio-Thoracic Surgery : Official Journal of the European Association for Cardio-Thoracic Surgery, 22*(3), 421–425. http://www.ncbi.nlm.nih.gov/pubmed/12204734 doi:10.1016/S1010-7940(02)00294-4 PMID:12204734

Makkar, R. R., Fontana, G. P., Jilaihawi, H., Kapadia, S., Pichard, A. D., Douglas, P. S., & Leon, M. B. et al. (2012). Transcatheter aortic-valve replacement for inoperable severe aortic stenosis. *The New England Journal of Medicine, 366*(18), 1696–1704. doi:10.1056/NEJMoa1202277 PMID:22443478

Malvindi, P. G., Jacob, S., Kallikourdis, A., & Vitale, N. (2007). What is the patency of the gastroepiploic artery when used for coronary artery bypass grafting? *Interactive Cardiovascular and Thoracic Surgery, 6*(3), 397–402. doi:10.1510/icvts.2007.155259 PMID:17669877

Mangano, C. M., Diamondstone, L. S., Ramsay, J. G., Aggarwal, A., Herskowitz, A., & Mangano, D. T. (1998). Renal dysfunction after myocardial revascularization: Risk factors, adverse outcomes, and hospital resource utilization. The Multicenter Study of Perioperative Ischemia Research Group. *Annals of Internal Medicine, 128*(3), 194–203. http://www.ncbi.nlm.nih.gov/pubmed/9454527 doi:10.7326/0003-4819-128-3-199802010-00005 PMID:9454527

Mangano, D. T. (2002). Aspirin and mortality from coronary bypass surgery. *The New England Journal of Medicine, 347*(17), 1309–1317. doi:10.1056/NEJMoa020798 PMID:12397188

Martin, B.-J., Buth, K. J., Arora, R. C., & Baskett, R. J. F. (2010). Delirium as a predictor of sepsis in post-coronary artery bypass grafting patients: A retrospective cohort study. *Critical Care (London, England), 14*(5), R171. doi:10.1186/cc9273 PMID:20875113

Martin, B.-J., Buth, K. J., Arora, R. C., & Baskett, R. J. F. (2012). Delirium: A cause for concern beyond the immediate postoperative period. *The Annals of Thoracic Surgery, 93*(4), 1114–1120. doi:10.1016/j.athoracsur.2011.09.011 PMID:22200370

Martin, L. M., Halpin, L. S., Barnett, S. D., Speir, A. M., Hunt, S. L., Mukherjee, N., & Ad, N. (2008). The association between early outcome, health-related quality of life, and survival following elective open-heart surgery. *The Journal of Cardiovascular Nursing*, *23*(5), 432–442. doi:10.1097/01.JCN.0000317453.10521.5b PMID:18728516

McDonagh, D. L., Berger, M., Mathew, J. P., Graffagnino, C., Milano, C., & Newman, M. F. (2014). Neurological complications of cardiac surgery. *Lancet Neurology*, *13*(May), 490–502. doi:10.1016/S1474-4422(14)70004-3 PMID:24703207

McKhann, G. M., Grega, M., Borowicz, L. M. Jr, Selnes, O., Baumgartner, W., & Royall, R. M. (2004). Encephalopathy and Stroke After Coronary Artery Bypass Grafting. *Current Treatment Options in Cardiovascular Medicine*, *6*(3), 171–178. http://www.ncbi.nlm.nih.gov/pubmed/15096308 doi:10.1007/s11936-996-0011-0 PMID:15096308

McPherson, J., Wagner, C. E., Boehm, L. M., Hall, J. D., Johnson, D. C., Miller, L. R., & Pandhvaripande, P. P. et al. (2013). Delirium in the cardiovascular ICU: Exploring modifiable risk factors. *Critical Care Medicine*, *41*(2), 405–413. doi:10.1097/CCM.0b013e31826ab49b PMID:23263581

Mehta, R. L., Kellum, J., Shah, S. V., Molitoris, B. A., Ronco, C., Warnock, D. G., & Levin, A. (2007). Acute Kidney Injury Network: Report of an initiative to improve outcomes in acute kidney injury. *Critical Care (London, England)*, *11*(2), R31. doi:10.1186/cc5713 PMID:17331245

Miller, D. C., Blackstone, E. H., Mack, M. J., Svensson, L. G., Kodali, S. K., Kapadia, S., & Smith, C. R. et al. (2012). Transcatheter (TAVR) versus surgical (AVR) aortic valve replacement: Occurrence, hazard, risk factors, and consequences of neurologic events in the PARTNER trial. *The Journal of Thoracic and Cardiovascular Surgery*, *143*(4), 832–843.e13. doi:10.1016/j.jtcvs.2012.01.055 PMID:22424519

Mohammed, A., Agnihotri, A. K., van Kimmenade, R. R. J., Martinez-Rumayor, A., Green, S. M., Quiroz, R., & Januzzi, J. L. (2009). Prospective, comprehensive assessment of cardiac troponin T testing after coronary artery bypass graft surgery. *Circulation*, *120*(10), 843–850. doi:10.1161/CIRCULATIONAHA.108.837278 PMID:19704098

Mohr, F. W., Morice, M.-C., Kappetein, A. P., Feldman, T. E., Ståhle, E., Colombo, A., & Serruys, P. W. et al. (2013). Coronary artery bypass graft surgery versus percutaneous coronary intervention in patients with three-vessel disease and left main coronary disease: 5-year follow-up of the randomised, clinical SYNTAX trial. *Lancet*, *381*(9867), 629–638. doi:10.1016/S0140-6736(13)60141-5 PMID:23439102

Morice, M.-C., Serruys, P. W., Sousa, J. E., Fajadet, J., Ban Hayashi, E., Perin, M., & Falotico, R. et al. (2002). A randomized comparison of a sirolimus-eluting stent with a standard stent for coronary revascularization. *The New England Journal of Medicine*, *346*(23), 1773–1780. doi:10.1056/NEJMoa012843 PMID:12050336

Morrison, D., Sethi, G., Sacks, J., Henderson, W., Grover, F., Sedlis, S., & Lewis, D. et al. (2001). Percutaneous coronary intervention versus coronary artery bypass graft surgery for patients with medically refractory myocardial ischemia and risk factors for adverse outcomes with bypass: A multicenter, randomized trial. *Journal of the American College of Cardiology*, *38*(1), 143–149. doi:10.1016/S0735-1097(01)01366-3 PMID:11451264

Moussa, I. D., Klein, L. W., Shah, B., Mehran, R., Mack, M. J., Brilakis, E. S., & Stone, G. W. et al. (2013). Consideration of a new definition of clinically relevant myocardial infarction after coronary revascularization: An expert consensus document from the Society for Cardiovascular Angiography and Interventions (SCAI). *Journal of the American College of Cardiology*, *62*(17), 1563–1570. doi:10.1016/j.jacc.2013.08.720 PMID:24135581

Murkin, J. M., & Arango, M. (2009). Near-infrared spectroscopy as an index of brain and tissue oxygenation. *British Journal of Anaesthesia*, *103*(Suppl), i3–i13. doi:10.1093/bja/aep299 PMID:20007987

Myers, M. G., & Fremes, S. E. (2003). Prevention of radial artery graft spasm: A survey of Canadian surgical centres. *The Canadian Journal of Cardiology*, *19*(6), 677–681. Retrieved from http://www.ncbi.nlm.nih.gov/pubmed/12772018 PMID:12772018

Nalysnyk, L., Fahrbach, K., Reynolds, M. W., Zhao, S. Z., & Ross, S. (2003). Adverse events in coronary artery bypass graft (CABG) trials: A systematic review and analysis. *Heart (British Cardiac Society)*, *89*(7), 767–772. http://www.pubmedcentral.nih.gov/articlerender.fcgi?artid=1767742&tool=pmcentrez&rendertype=abstract doi:10.1136/heart.89.7.767 PMID:12807853

Nashef, S. M., Roques, F., Sharples, L. D., Nilsson, J., Smith, C., Goldstone, A. R., & Lockowandt, U. (2012). EuroSCORE II. *European Journal of Cardio-Thoracic Surgery : Official Journal of the European Association for Cardio-Thoracic Surgery*, *41*(4), 734–44; discussion 744–5. doi:10.1093/ejcts/ezs043

Nasso, G., Coppola, R., Bonifazi, R., Piancone, F., Bozzetti, G., & Speziale, G. (2009). Arterial revascularization in primary coronary artery bypass grafting: Direct comparison of 4 strategies--results of the Stand-in-Y Mammary Study. *The Journal of Thoracic and Cardiovascular Surgery*, *137*(5), 1093–1100. doi:10.1016/j.jtcvs.2008.10.029 PMID:19379973

Nathoe, H. M., van Dijk, D., Jansen, E. W. L., Suyker, W. J. L., Diephuis, J. C., van Boven, W.-J., & de Jaegere, P. P. T. et al. (2003). A comparison of on-pump and off-pump coronary bypass surgery in low-risk patients. *The New England Journal of Medicine*, *348*(5), 394–402. doi:10.1056/NEJMoa021775 PMID:12556542

Navia, D., Vrancic, M., Piccinini, F., Camporrotondo, M., Thierer, J., Gil, C., & Benzadon, M. (2014). Is the second internal thoracic artery better than the radial artery in total arterial off-pump coronary artery bypass grafting? A propensity score-matched follow-up study. *The Journal of Thoracic and Cardiovascular Surgery*, *147*(2), 632–638. doi:10.1016/j.jtcvs.2013.02.012 PMID:23566513

Palmbergen, W., van Sonderen, A., Keyhan-Falsafi, A. M., Keunen, R. W. M., & Wolterbeek, R. (2012). Improved perioperative neurological monitoring of coronary artery bypass graft patients reduces the incidence of postoperative delirium: The Haga Brain Care Strategy. *Interactive Cardiovascular and Thoracic Surgery*, *15*(4), 671–677. doi:10.1093/icvts/ivs317 PMID:22778141

Petäjä, L., Salmenperä, M., Pulkki, K., & Pettilä, V. (2009). Biochemical injury markers and mortality after coronary artery bypass grafting: A systematic review. *The Annals of Thoracic Surgery*, *87*(6), 1981–1992. doi:10.1016/j.athoracsur.2008.12.063 PMID:19463650

Pisani, M. (2003). Underrecognition of Preexisting Cognitive Impairment by Physicians in Older ICU Patients<xref rid="AFF1">*</xref>. *CHEST Journal*, *124*(6), 2267. doi:10.1378/chest.124.6.2267

Polomsky, M., & Puskas, J. D. (2012). Off-pump coronary artery bypass grafting--the current state. *Circulation Journal : Official Journal of the Japanese Circulation Society, 76*(4), 784–90. Retrieved from http://www.ncbi.nlm.nih.gov/pubmed/22451446

Preeshagul, I., Gharbaran, R., Jeong, K. H., Abdel-Razek, A., Lee, L. Y., Elman, E., & Suh, K. S. (2013). Potential biomarkers for predicting outcomes in CABG cardiothoracic surgeries. *Journal of Cardiothoracic Surgery, 8*(1), 176. doi:10.1186/1749-8090-8-176 PMID:23866777

Puskas, J. D., Williams, W. H., Mahoney, E. M., Huber, P. R., Block, P. C., Duke, P. G., & Guyton, R. A. et al. (2004). Off-pump vs conventional coronary artery bypass grafting: early and 1-year graft patency, cost, and quality-of-life outcomes: a randomized trial. *Journal of the American Medical Association, 291*(15), 1841–1849. doi:10.1001/jama.291.15.1841 PMID:15100202

Racz, M. J., Hannan, E. L., Isom, O. W., Subramanian, V., Jones, R. H., Gold, J. P., & Rose, E. A. et al. (2004). A comparison of short- and long-term outcomes after off-pump and on-pump coronary artery bypass graft surgery with sternotomy. *Journal of the American College of Cardiology, 43*(4), 557–564. doi:10.1016/j.jacc.2003.09.045 PMID:14975463

Rehman, S. M., Yi, G., & Taggart, D. P. (2013). The radial artery: Current concepts on its use in coronary artery revascularization. *The Annals of Thoracic Surgery, 96*(5), 1900–1909. doi:10.1016/j.athoracsur.2013.06.083 PMID:24090580

Reston, J. T., Tregear, S. J., & Turkelson, C. M. (2003). Meta-analysis of short-term and mid-term outcomes following off-pump coronary artery bypass grafting. *The Annals of Thoracic Surgery, 76*(5), 1510–1515. doi:10.1016/S0003-4975(03)01195-0 PMID:14602277

Riker, R. R., Shehabi, Y., Bokesch, P. M., Ceraso, D., Wisemandle, W., Koura, F., & Rocha, M. G. et al. (2009). Dexmedetomidine vs midazolam for sedation of critically ill patients: A randomized trial. *Journal of the American Medical Association, 301*(5), 489–499. doi:10.1001/jama.2009.56 PMID:19188334

Rinaldi, P., Mecocci, P., Benedetti, C., Ercolani, S., Bregnocchi, M., Menculini, G., & Cherubini, A. et al. (2003). Validation of the Five-Item Geriatric Depression Scale in Elderly Subjects in Three Different Settings. *Journal of the American Geriatrics Society, 51*(5), 694–698. doi:10.1034/j.1600-0579.2003.00216.x PMID:12752847

Roach, G. W., Kanchuger, M., Mangano, C. M., Newman, M., Nussmeier, N., Wolman, R., & Ley, C. et al. (1996). Adverse cerebral outcomes after coronary bypass surgery. Multicenter Study of Perioperative Ischemia Research Group and the Ischemia Research and Education Foundation Investigators. *The New England Journal of Medicine, 335*(25), 1857–1863. doi:10.1056/NEJM199612193352501 PMID:8948560

Rockwood, K., Song, X., MacKnight, C., Bergman, H., Hogan, D. B., McDowell, I., & Mitnitski, A. (2005). A global clinical measure of fitness and frailty in elderly people. *CMAJ : Canadian Medical Association Journal, 173*(5), 489–95. doi:10.1503/cmaj.050051

Rodriguez, A., Bernardi, V., Navia, J., Baldi, J., Grinfeld, L., Martinez, J., … O'Neill, W. (2001). Argentine Randomized Study: Coronary Angioplasty with Stenting versus Coronary Bypass Surgery in patients with Multiple-Vessel Disease (ERACI II): 30-day and one-year follow-up results. ERACI II Investigators. *Journal of the American College of Cardiology, 37*(1), 51–8. Retrieved from http://www.ncbi.nlm.nih.gov/pubmed/11153772

Rogers, C. A., Pike, K., Angelini, G. D., Reeves, B. C., Glauber, M., Ferrarini, M., & Murphy, G. J. (2013). An open randomized controlled trial of median sternotomy versus anterolateral left thoracotomy on morbidity and health care resource use in patients having off-pump coronary artery bypass surgery : The Sternotomy Versus Thoracotomy (STET) trial. *The Journal of Thoracic and Cardiovascular Surgery, 146*(2), 306–316.e9. doi:10.1016/j.jtcvs.2012.04.020 PMID:22944093

Rudolph, J. L., Inouye, S. K., Jones, R. N., Yang, F. M., Fong, T. G., Levkoff, S. E., & Marcantonio, E. R. (2010). Delirium: An independent predictor of functional decline after cardiac surgery. *Journal of the American Geriatrics Society, 58*(4), 643–649. doi:10.1111/j.1532-5415.2010.02762.x PMID:20345866

Rudolph, J. L., Jones, R. N., Grande, L. J., Milberg, W. P., King, E. G., Lipsitz, L. A., & Marcantonio, E. R. et al. (2006). Impaired executive function is associated with delirium after coronary artery bypass graft surgery. *Journal of the American Geriatrics Society, 54*(6), 937–941. doi:10.1111/j.1532-5415.2006.00735.x PMID:16776789

Rudolph, J. L., Jones, R. N., Levkoff, S. E., Rockett, C., Inouye, S. K., Sellke, F. W., & Marcantonio, E. R. et al. (2009). Derivation and validation of a preoperative prediction rule for delirium after cardiac surgery. *Circulation, 119*(2), 229–236. doi:10.1161/CIRCULATIONAHA.108.795260 PMID:19118253

Ruel, M., Shariff, M., Lapierre, H., Goyal, N., Dennie, C., Sadel, S. M., & McGinn, J. T. Jr et al.. (2014). Results of the Minimally Invasive Coronary Artery Bypass Grafting Angiographic Patency Study. *The Journal of Thoracic and Cardiovascular Surgery, 147*(1), 203–208. doi:10.1016/j.jtcvs.2013.09.016 PMID:24183338

Sabik, J. F., Lytle, B. W., McCarthy, P. M., & Cosgrove, D. M. (1995). Axillary artery: An alternative site of arterial cannulation for patients with extensive aortic and peripheral vascular disease. *The Journal of Thoracic and Cardiovascular Surgery, 109*(5), 885–890, discussion 890–891. http://www.ncbi.nlm.nih.gov/pubmed/7739248 doi:10.1016/S0022-5223(95)70312-8 PMID:7739248

Saczynski, J. S., Marcantonio, E. R., Quach, L., Fong, T. G., Gross, A., Inouye, S. K., & Jones, R. N. (2012). Cognitive trajectories after postoperative delirium. *The New England Journal of Medicine, 367*(1), 30–39. doi:10.1056/NEJMoa1112923 PMID:22762316

Serruys, P. W., Kutryk, M. J. B., & Ong, A. T. L. (2006). Coronary-artery stents. *The New England Journal of Medicine, 354*(5), 483–495. doi:10.1056/NEJMra051091 PMID:16452560

Serruys, P. W., Morice, M.-C., Kappetein, A. P., Colombo, A., Holmes, D. R., Mack, M. J., & Mohr, F. W. et al. (2009). Percutaneous coronary intervention versus coronary-artery bypass grafting for severe coronary artery disease. *The New England Journal of Medicine, 360*(10), 961–972. doi:10.1056/NEJMoa0804626 PMID:19228612

Serruys, P. W., Ong, A. T. L., & van Herwerden, L. a, Sousa, J. E., Jatene, A., Bonnier, J. J. R. M., … Unger, F. (2005). Five-year outcomes after coronary stenting versus bypass surgery for the treatment of multivessel disease: The final analysis of the Arterial Revascularization Therapies Study (ARTS) randomized trial. *Journal of the American College of Cardiology*, *46*(4), 575–581. doi:10.1016/j.jacc.2004.12.082 PMID:16098418

Shah, P. J., Gordon, I., Fuller, J., Seevanayagam, S., Rosalion, A., Tatoulis, J., & Buxton, B. F. et al. (2003). Factors affecting saphenous vein graft patency: Clinical and angiographic study in 1402 symptomatic patients operated on between 1977 and 1999. *The Journal of Thoracic and Cardiovascular Surgery*, *126*(6), 1972–1977. doi:10.1016/S0022-5223(03)01276-5 PMID:14688715

Shehabi, Y., Botha, J. A., Ernest, D., Freebairn, R. C., Reade, M., Roberts, B. L., & Seppelt, I. (2010). Clinical application, the use of dexmedetomidine in intensive care sedation, *13*(2), 40–50.

Shroyer, A. L., Grover, F. L., Hattler, B., Collins, J. F., McDonald, G. O., Kozora, E., & Novitzky, D. et al. (2009). On-pump versus off-pump coronary-artery bypass surgery. *The New England Journal of Medicine*, *361*(19), 1827–1837. doi:10.1056/NEJMoa0902905 PMID:19890125

Singh, M., Gersh, B. J., Li, S., Rumsfeld, J. S., Spertus, J., O'Brien, S. M., & Peterson, E. D. et al. (2008). Mayo Clinic Risk Score for percutaneous coronary intervention predicts in-hospital mortality in patients undergoing coronary artery bypass graft surgery. *Circulation*, *117*(3), 356–362. doi:10.1161/CIRCULATIONAHA.107.711523 PMID:18172033

Slater, J. P., Guarino, T., Stack, J., Vinod, K., Bustami, R. T., Brown, J. M. III, & Parr, G. V. S. et al. (2009). Cerebral oxygen desaturation predicts cognitive decline and longer hospital stay after cardiac surgery. *The Annals of Thoracic Surgery*, *87*(1), 36–44, discussion 44–45. doi:10.1016/j.athoracsur.2008.08.070 PMID:19101265

Soar, J., Deakin, C. D., Nolan, J. P., Abbas, G., Alfonzo, A., Handley, A. J., & Thies, K. et al. (2005). European Resuscitation Council guidelines for resuscitation 2005. Section 7. Cardiac arrest in special circumstances. *Resuscitation*, *67*(Suppl 1), S135–S170. doi:10.1016/j.resuscitation.2005.10.004 PMID:16321711

Søraas, C. L., Friis, C., Engebretsen, K. V. T., Sandvik, L., Kjeldsen, S. E., & Tønnessen, T. (2012). Troponin T is a better predictor than creatine kinase-MB of long-term mortality after coronary artery bypass graft surgery. *American Heart Journal*, *164*(5), 779–785. doi:10.1016/j.ahj.2012.05.027 PMID:23137510

Spaulding, C., Daemen, J., Boersma, E., Cutlip, D. E., & Serruys, P. W. (2007). A pooled analysis of data comparing sirolimus-eluting stents with bare-metal stents. *The New England Journal of Medicine*, *356*(10), 989–997. doi:10.1056/NEJMoa066633 PMID:17296825

Spertus, J. a, Winder, J. a, Dewhurst, T. a, Deyo, R. a, & Fihn, S. D. (1994). Monitoring the quality of life in patients with coronary artery disease. *The American Journal of Cardiology*, *74*(12), 1240–4. Retrieved from http://www.ncbi.nlm.nih.gov/pubmed/7977097

Spertus, J. a, Winder, J. a, Dewhurst, T. a, Deyo, R. a, Prodzinski, J., McDonell, M., & Fihn, S. D. (1995). Development and evaluation of the Seattle Angina Questionnaire: a new functional status measure for coronary artery disease. *Journal of the American College of Cardiology, 25*(2), 333–41. Retrieved from http://www.ncbi.nlm.nih.gov/pubmed/7829785

Stamou, S. C., Hill, P. C., Dangas, G., Pfister, J., Boyce, S. W., Dullum, M. K. C., & Silver, B. et al. (2001). Stroke after coronary artery bypass: Incidence, predictors, and clinical outcome. *Stroke, 32*(7), 1508–1513. doi:10.1161/01.STR.32.7.1508 PMID:11441193

Subramanian, V. A., Mccabe, J. C., Geller, C. M., Hospital, L. H., & York, N. (1997). Grafting : Two-Year Clinical Experience, *4975*(97).

Suma, H., Tanabe, H., Takahashi, A., Horii, T., Isomura, T., Hirose, H., & Amano, A. (2007). Twenty years experience with the gastroepiploic artery graft for CABG. *Circulation, 116*(11Suppl), I188–I191. doi:10.1161/CIRCULATIONAHA.106.678813 PMID:17846302

Sutton, T. A., Fisher, C. J., & Molitoris, B. A. (2002). Microvascular endothelial injury and dysfunction during ischemic acute renal failure. *Kidney International, 62*(5), 1539–1549. doi:10.1046/j.1523-1755.2002.00631.x PMID:12371954

Svensson, L. G., Tuzcu, M., Kapadia, S., Blackstone, E. H., Roselli, E. E., Gillinov, A. M., & Lytle, B. W. et al. (2013). A comprehensive review of the PARTNER trial. *The Journal of Thoracic and Cardiovascular Surgery, 145*(3Suppl), S11–S16. doi:10.1016/j.jtcvs.2012.11.051 PMID:23410766

Svircevic, V., Nierich, A. P., Moons, K. G. M., Diephuis, J. C., Ennema, J. J., Brandon Bravo Bruinsma, G. J., & van Dijk, D. et al. (2011). Thoracic epidural anesthesia for cardiac surgery: A randomized trial. *Anesthesiology, 114*(2), 262–270. doi:10.1097/ALN.0b013e318201d2de PMID:21239976

Taggart, D. P. (2006). Thomas B. Ferguson Lecture. Coronary artery bypass grafting is still the best treatment for multivessel and left main disease, but patients need to know. *The Annals of Thoracic Surgery, 82*(6), 1966–1975. doi:10.1016/j.athoracsur.2006.06.035 PMID:17126093

Taggart, D. P. (2013). The FREEDOM trial: A definitive answer to coronary artery bypass grafting or stents in patients with diabetes and multivessel coronary artery disease. *European Journal of Cardio-Thoracic Surgery : Official Journal of the European Association for Cardio-Thoracic Surgery, 44*(6), 978–979. doi:10.1093/ejcts/ezt450 PMID:24047712

Taggart, D. P., D'Amico, R., & Altman, D. G. (2001). Effect of arterial revascularisation on survival: A systematic review of studies comparing bilateral and single internal mammary arteries. *Lancet, 358*(9285), 870–875. doi:10.1016/S0140-6736(01)06069-X PMID:11567701

Takagi, H., Goto, S.-N., Watanabe, T., Mizuno, Y., Kawai, N., & Umemoto, T. (2014). A meta-analysis of adjusted hazard ratios from 20 observational studies of bilateral versus single internal thoracic artery coronary artery bypass grafting. *The Journal of Thoracic and Cardiovascular Surgery*, 1–10. doi:10.1016/j.jtcvs.2014.01.010 PMID:24521973

Tatoulis, J., Buxton, B. F., & Fuller, J. (2004). Patencies of 2127 arterial to coronary conduits over 15 years. *The Annals of Thoracic Surgery, 77*(1), 93–101. doi:10.1016/S0003-4975(03)01331-6 PMID:14726042

Tatoulis, J., Buxton, B. F., & Fuller, J. (2011). The right internal thoracic artery: The forgotten conduit--5,766 patients and 991 angiograms. *The Annals of Thoracic Surgery*, *92*(1), 9–15, discussion 15–17. doi:10.1016/j.athoracsur.2011.03.099 PMID:21718825

Thakar, C. V., Arrigain, S., Worley, S., Yared, J.-P., & Paganini, E. P. (2005). A clinical score to predict acute renal failure after cardiac surgery. *Journal of the American Society of Nephrology : JASN*, *16*(1), 162–168. doi:10.1681/ASN.2004040331 PMID:15563569

The BARI Investigators. (2007). The final 10-year follow-up results from the BARI randomized trial. *Journal of the American College of Cardiology*, *49*(15), 1600–1606. doi:10.1016/j.jacc.2006.11.048 PMID:17433949

The Syntax Score. (n.d.).

Thygesen, K., Alpert, J. S., Jaffe, A. S., Simoons, M. L., Chaitman, B. R., White, H. D., & Mendis, S. et al. (2012). Third universal definition of myocardial infarction. *European Heart Journal*, *33*(20), 2551–2567. doi:10.1093/eurheartj/ehs184 PMID:22922414

Tranbaugh, R. F., Dimitrova, K. R., Lucido, D. J., Hoffman, D. M., Dincheva, G. R., Geller, C. M., & Swistel, D. G. et al. (2014). The second best arterial graft: A propensity analysis of the radial artery versus the free right internal thoracic artery to bypass the circumflex coronary artery. *The Journal of Thoracic and Cardiovascular Surgery*, *147*(1), 133–140. doi:10.1016/j.jtcvs.2013.08.040 PMID:24100104

Van der Mast, R. C., & Roest, F. H. (1996). Delirium after cardiac surgery: A critical review. *Journal of Psychosomatic Research*, *41*(1), 13–30. http://www.ncbi.nlm.nih.gov/pubmed/8887815 doi:10.1016/0022-3999(96)00005-0 PMID:8887815

Van Dijk, D., Keizer, A. M. A., Diephuis, J. C., Durand, C., Vos, L. J., & Hijman, R. (2000). Neurocognitive dysfunction after coronary artery bypass surgery: A systematic review. *The Journal of Thoracic and Cardiovascular Surgery*, *120*(4), 632–639. doi:10.1067/mtc.2000.108901 PMID:11003741

Vanden Hoek, T. L., Morrison, L. J., Shuster, M., Donnino, M., Sinz, E., Lavonas, E. J., & Gabrielli, A. et al. (2010). Part 12: cardiac arrest in special situations: 2010 American Heart Association Guidelines for Cardiopulmonary Resuscitation and Emergency Cardiovascular Care. *Circulation*, *122*(18Suppl 3), S829–S861. doi:10.1161/CIRCULATIONAHA.110.971069 PMID:20956228

Vuylsteke, A., Pagel, C., Gerrard, C., Reddy, B., Nashef, S., Aldam, P., & Utley, M. (2011). The Papworth Bleeding Risk Score: A stratification scheme for identifying cardiac surgery patients at risk of excessive early postoperative bleeding. *European Journal of Cardio-Thoracic Surgery : Official Journal of the European Association for Cardio-Thoracic Surgery*, *39*(6), 924–930. doi:10.1016/j.ejcts.2010.10.003 PMID:21094051

Wahr, J. A., Parks, R., Boisvert, D., Comunale, M., Fabian, J., Ramsay, J., & Mangano, D. T. (1999). Preoperative serum potassium levels and perioperative outcomes in cardiac surgery patients. Multicenter Study of Perioperative Ischemia Research Group. *Journal of the American Medical Association*, *281*(23), 2203–2210. doi:10.1001/jama.281.23.2203 PMID:10376573

Wareing, T. H., Davila-Roman, V. G., Barzilai, B., Murphy, S. F., & Kouchoukos, N. T. (1992). Management of the severely atherosclerotic ascending aorta during cardiac operations. A strategy for detection and treatment. *The Journal of Thoracic and Cardiovascular Surgery*, *103*(3), 453–462. Retrieved from http://www.ncbi.nlm.nih.gov/pubmed/1545544 PMID:1545544

Weiss, A. J., Zhao, S., Tian, D. H., Taggart, D. P., & Yan, T. D. (2013). A meta-analysis comparing bilateral internal mammary artery with left internal mammary artery for coronary artery bypass grafting. *Annals of Cardiothoracic Surgery*, *2*(4), 390–400. doi:10.3978/j.issn.2225-319X.2013.07.16 PMID:23977614

Yokoyama, Y., Chaitman, B. R., Hardison, R. M., Guo, P., Krone, R., & Stocke, K. … Detre, K. M. (2000). Association between new electrocardiographic abnormalities after coronary revascularization and five-year cardiac mortality in BARI randomized and registry patients. *The American Journal of Cardiology, 86*(8), 819–24. Retrieved from http://www.ncbi.nlm.nih.gov/pubmed/11024394

Zacharias, A., Schwann, T., Riordan, C. J., Durham, S. J., Shah, A. S., & Habib, R. H. (2009). Late results of conventional versus all-arterial revascularization based on internal thoracic and radial artery grafting. *The Annals of Thoracic Surgery*, *87*(1), 19–26.e2. doi:10.1016/j.athoracsur.2008.09.050 PMID:19101262

Zhang, Z., Spertus, J., Mahoney, E. M., Booth, J., Nugara, F., Stables, R. H., & Weintraub, W. S. (2005). The impact of acute coronary syndrome on clinical, economic, and cardiac-specific health status after coronary artery bypass surgery versus stent-assisted percutaneous coronary intervention: 1-year results from the stent or surgery (SoS) trial. *American Heart Journal*, *150*(1), 175–181. doi:10.1016/j.ahj.2005.01.019 PMID:16084166

Chapter 23
Aortic Valvular Disease

Eric Leo Sarin
Emory University, USA

Vinod H. Thourani
Emory University, USA

ABSTRACT

Broadly speaking, pathology is categorized as being primarily related to valvular stenosis (AS) or regurgitation (AR), but a diseased valve may often exhibit both. The predilection of degenerative disease of the aortic valve, particularly stenosis, for the elderly has resulted in a steadily increasing prevalence as the population ages. As general life expectancy increases in the United States and other western countries, surgery to correct aortic valve disease will increase. As more elderly patients with more comorbidities present for surgery their intraoperative and perioperative care will become more complex. This chapter discusses ways for the practicing intensivist to facilitate identification and treatment in the immediate peri-operative period.

INTRODUCTION

Surgery to repair a dysfunctional aortic valve remains the most common indication for valvular heart surgery. Broadly speaking, pathology is categorized as being primarily related to valvular stenosis (AS) or regurgitation (AR), but a diseased valve may often exhibit both. The predilection of degenerative disease of the aortic valve, particularly stenosis, for the elderly has resulted in a steadily increasing prevalence as the population ages. As general life expectancy increases in the United States and other western countries, surgery to correct aortic valve disease will increase. As more elderly patients with more comorbidities present for surgery their intraoperative and perioperative care will become more complex.

In general, symptomatic patients should be offered surgical correction. However, many elderly patients with severe AS have significant medical comorbidities. In the past, this has resulted in a significant minority of patients not being referred for surgery. The advent of transcatheter aortic valve replacement (TAVR) has offered promise as a durable therapeutic option for those patients previously considered to be at increased risk for traditional surgery.

DOI: 10.4018/978-1-4666-8603-8.ch023

The goal of this chapter to is to provide an overview of the epidemiology and pathophysiology of adult aortic valve disease followed by a discussion of the operative procedures performed to correct this pathology. Emphasis will be placed on potential complications and their manifestations in the immediate peri-operative period to facilitate identification and treatment for the practicing intensivist.

Aortic Stenosis (AS)

AS is the result of gradual thickening and calcification of the aortic leaflets over time. As the leaflets subsequently become less pliable and resist normal movement, a transvalvular gradient develops. This process is multifactorial and influenced by clinical factors (age, gender, hypertension) patient habits (smoking), and genetic factors (Boon, Cheriex, Lodder, & Kessels, 1997; Stewart et al., 1997; Thanassoulis et al., 2013). A congenitally bicuspid aortic valve, which is found in approximately 1.4% of the population, is the most common cause of symptomatic AS in patients less than 70 years of age(Go et al., 2013; Roberts & Ko, 2005). The mechanical stress on the bicuspid valve predisposes these patients to earlier calcific degeneration. In a population based study, bicuspid aortic valve patients were far more likely to progress to valve replacement (24.4% in 20 years) then the general population (Michelena et al., 2008).

Progression of stenosis is reflected by a reduction of aortic valve area (AVA) and an increase in transvalvular gradients and flow velocities. This process is typically slow with an average annual decrease in AVA of 0.1cm/yr and an increase mean gradient of 5-8 mmHg (Brener, Duffy, Thomas, & Stewart, 1995; Nassimiha, Aronow, Ahn, & Goldman, 2001; Otto et al., 1997). Over time, the increase in left ventricular systolic pressure needed to overcome the stenotic valve increases left ventricular wall stress with resultant left ventricular hypertrophy. When left untreated the left ventricle eventually decompensates with resultant heart failure symptoms. Guidelines for operative intervention in the setting of aortic stenosis are listed in the accompanying table.

The natural history of aortic stenosis was classically described by Ross and Braunwald in 1968 (Ross & Braunwald, 1968). The authors defined the symptom triad of angina, syncope, and heart failure as harbingers of advanced disease with well-defined associated morbidity and mortality. Expected survival after the development of these symptoms is dismal and has been subsequently corroborated by multiple authors (Cheitlin et al., 1979; Davies, Gershlick, & Balcon, 1991; Otto, Pearlman, & Gardner, 1989; Turina, Hess, Sepulcri, & Krayenbuehl, 1987). Despite pathophysiologic similarities to atherosclerosis, attempts to curb AS progression with statin therapy have been unsuccessful in randomized trials (Cowell et al., 2005; Rossebo et al., 2008) and at present, no effective medical therapies exist. The only definitive therapy remains relief of the mechanical obstruction with valve replacement.

The prevalence of AS mirrors the aging population. An often cited study by Nkomo and colleagues pooled results of four large population based studies in the United States. The authors found AS in less than 0.2% of patients under age 65, in 1.3% of those between age 65 and 74, and in 2.8% of those 75 and older(Nkomo et al., 2006). This correlation with age is consistent across industrialized nations and has been confirmed by other authors (Eveborn, Schirmer, Heggelund, Lunde, & Rasmussen, 2013; Lindroos, Kupari, Heikkila, & Tilvis, 1993; Nkomo et al., 2006; Stewart et al., 1997).

This fact coupled with increasing life expectancies across the Western world has led to some startling projections. In the United State alone, there will be an estimated 72 million people over age 65 by 2030 (Iung & Vahanian, 2014). Similar population-based increases are being projected in France and the United Kingdom as well.

Figure 1. Decision algorithm for patients with aortic stenosis. Reprinted with permission from 2014 AHA/ACC Guidelines for Management of Patients with Valvular Heart Disease.

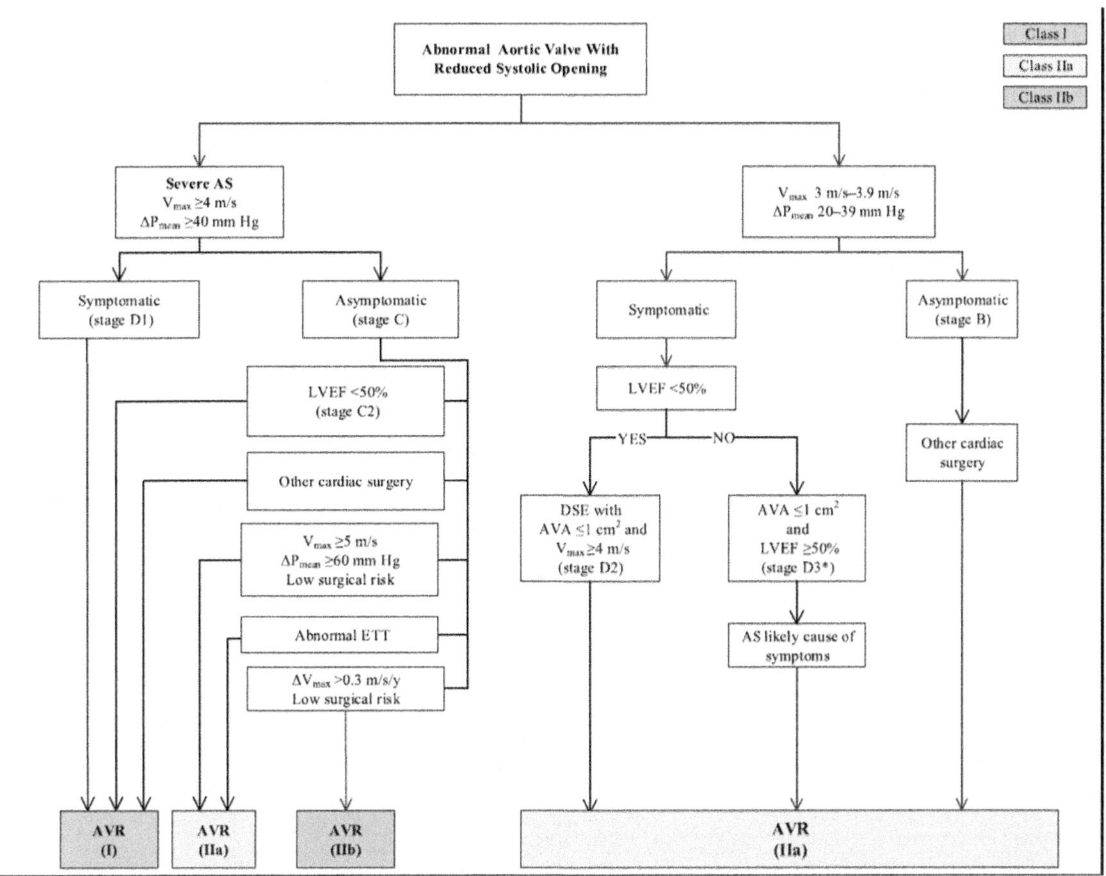

Unsurprisingly, increasing patient age is often accompanied by significant comorbid conditions. This association has already begun to manifest itself in patients undergoing open surgery. A review of 108,687 aortic valve replacements from the Society of Thoracic Surgeons Database noted that from 1997-2006 the mean age of patients increased (65.9 vs. 67.9, p <.001) as did the predicted risk of mortality (2.75% vs. 3.25%, p<.001). Despite the changes, the actual observed mortality decreased by 24% over the same time period (Brown et al., 2009). Despite the surgical success with progressively more difficult patients there is a still a large group that remains untreated (Dua, Dang, Shaker, Varadarajan, & Pai, 2011; Freed et al., 2010).

Aortic Regurgitation (AR)

Valvular dysfunction related to insufficient leaflet coaptation and regurgitation is another indication for aortic valve replacement. AR is less common than AS. In the aforementioned population study it had prevalence of 0.5%(Nkomo et al., 2006) which is comparable to similar studies(Reid, Anton-Culver, Yunis, & Gardin, 2007; Singh et al., 1999).

Figure 2. Increasing prevalence of AS according to age in population based studies. Reprinted with permission from Canadian Journal of Cardiology, 2014.

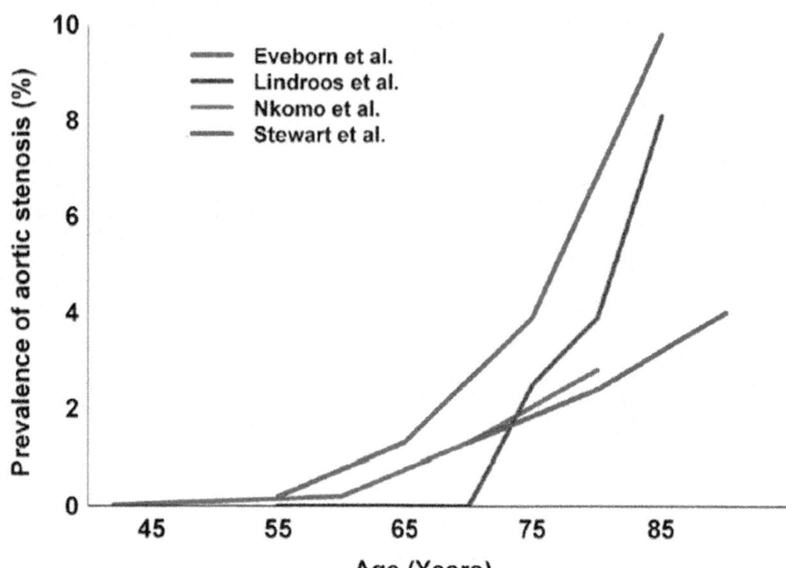

The pathophysiology of these patients is different from their stenotic counterparts. The underlying etiology is related to dilatation of the aortic root structures with relatively normal leaflets or in the presence of a congenitally bicuspid valve. These patients develop volume overload of the left ventricle which subsequently progresses to left ventricular dilatation.

The acuity of onset and degree of regurgitation has an enormous impact on the patient's preoperative clinical status. Typically the normal progression for patients is very gradual with long asymptomatic periods for patients with mild and even moderate AR. Once the AR is severe, patients begin presenting with signs and symptoms of heart failure. Patient's often present with fatigue, orthopnea, and other progressive signs of a failing heart. Although patients with aortic insufficiency may have a longer asymptomatic period than their stenotic counterparts, there is often a rapid, progressive decline in clinical status following the onset of symptoms.

Acute onset of severe regurgitation in the setting of endocarditis can result in a rapid hemodynamic collapse of the left ventricle that is simply unable to accommodate the rapid increase in volume overload. The criteria for operative intervention in the setting of aortic regurgitation are listed in the accompanying figure

SURGICAL AORTIC VALVE REPLACEMENT (SAVR)

Once the decision has been made to proceed with open surgery the most common approach is aortic valve replacement using either a mechanical or bioprosthetic valve prosthesis on an arrested heart using cardiopulmonary bypass. While full median sternotomy remains the most common approach, recent attempts to minimize the surgical trauma to the patient have resulted in minimally invasive techniques.

Figure 3. Decision algorithm for patients with aortic regurgitation. Reprinted with permission from 2014 AHA/ACC Guidelines for Management of Patients with Valvular Heart Disease).

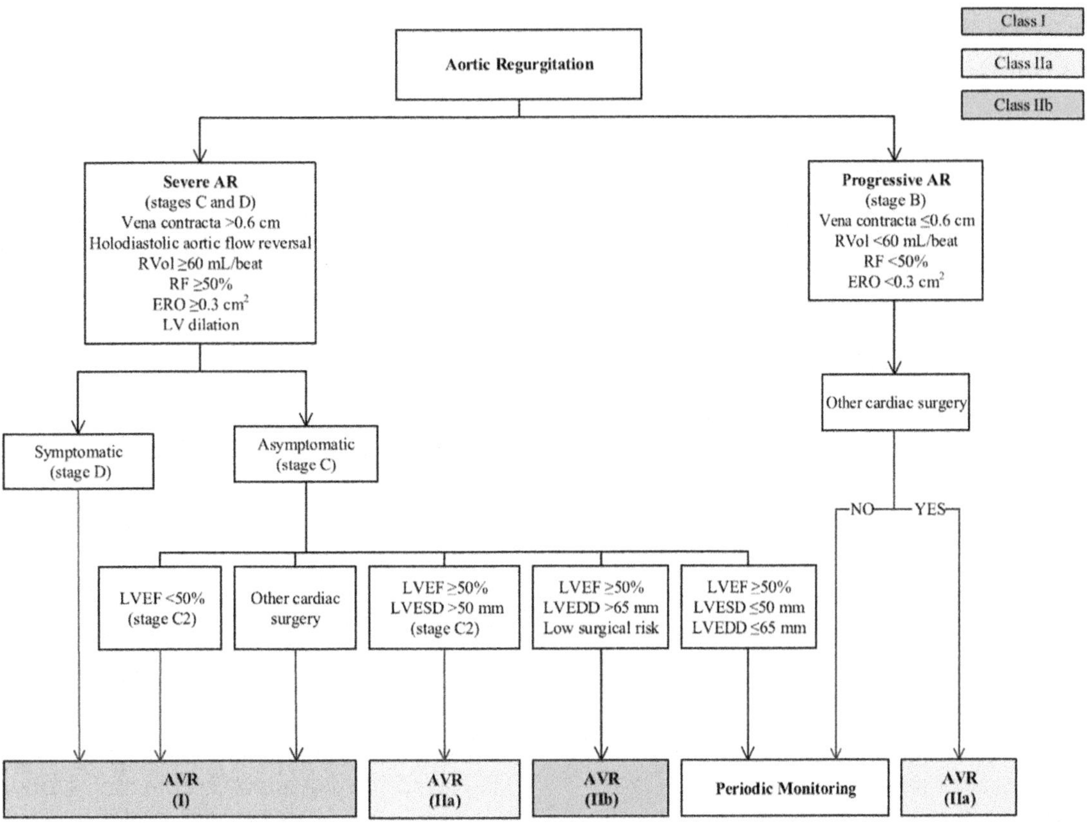

Approaching the valve via either an upper partial sternotomy or right anterior minithoracotomy have proven safe and effective with comparable results compared with traditional open replacement (Furukawa et al., 2014; Phan, Xie, Di Eusanio, & Yan, 2014).

Isolated Aortic Valve Replacement

Whether performed via full median sternotomy or minimally invasive approach the conduct of aortic valve replacement itself remains the same. After the institution of cardiopulmonary bypass, the ascending aorta is clamped and the heart is arrested using a combination of antegrade and retrograde cardioplegia. The aorta is opened transversely to expose the native valve. Diseased leaflets are completely excised to expose the native annulus with careful attention paid to remove any and all particulate debris that may result from valve debridement. Sutures are full-thickness, brought through the annulus from the ventricular side, and then through the sewing ring of the prosthetic valve. The valve is then carefully seated so that it sits snugly in a supra-annular position. The aortotomy is then closed with a running prolene suture.

As with all cardiac surgery, meticulous myocardial protection is of the utmost importance. Strategies for myocardial protection are as varied as the options for valve replacement. There are multiple effective techniques, but the ultimate success of the operation rests not so much on the protection strategy chosen, but rather its effective implementation. Particularly in these patients, that may present with either a severely hypertrophied ventricle or one with depressed myocardial function at baseline. Failure to adequately protect the myocardium throughout the procedure can have catastrophic results.

Outcomes

Recent data from the STS database describes the mortality for isolated SAVR in all patients as less than 3%. In patients with minimal risk, the mortality approaches 1% or less (Holmes et al., 2012). The incidence of stroke decreased from 1.7% to 1.2% in the STS database from 1997 to 2006 (Brown et al., 2009) which is consistent with other reviews of the STS dataset (O'Brien et al., 2009). In general the other risks following AVR are relatively low, heart block requiring PPM (<1%), renal failure requiring dialysis (0.7%), perioperative MI (2%) and their incidence has remained consistently acceptable for the last 30 years (Lytle et al., 1989).

Long-term survival following excellent aortic valve replacement is generally quite good. Likosky and colleagues reported on 7584 patients that underwent AVR or AVR/CABG. Median survival following isolated AVR in patients less than 80 years old at the time of surgery was 11.5 years(Likosky et al., 2009). For older patients aged 80-84 or ≥ 85 years of age, median survival approximated that for the general population, 6.8 years for 80-84 year olds, and 6.2 years for those 85 and older. Typically, the vast majority return to an acceptable quality of life. Multiple surveys of octogenarians post-AVR have reported that the vast majority are able to live at home (95%) with a normal quality of life (93%) (Huber, Goeber, Berdat, Carrel, & Eckstein, 2007), and feel that surgery was a good choice (92%)(Kolh, Lahaye, Gerard, & Limet, 1999).

The addition of comorbid conditions and their associated severity will obviously have a negative impact on peri-operative outcomes. This was illustrated by a recent study reporting outcomes following SAVR in high-risk (STS PROM >10%) patients. Patients had a mean STS PROM of 16.3% which was almost identical to the actual post-operative mortality of 16.4% (Thourani et al., 2011). Furthermore, the incidence of stroke (4.1%), renal failure requiring dialysis (8.2%) and multi-system organ failure (6.9%) were all increased.

Mechanical vs. Tissue Valves

The decision regarding which type of prosthetic valve to use has been a subject of great debate for many years (Badhwar, Ofenloch, Rovin, van Gelder, & Jacobs, 2012; Vicchio et al., 2008; Weber et al., 2012). In general the operating surgeon has to weigh the risks and benefits on a patient by patient basis. Younger patients without a contraindication for lifelong anticoagulation should be considered for a mechanical valve. Similarly, older patients may be more suitable for a bioprosthetic valve. The surgeon needs to consider the risks and benefits of the annual risk of bleeding complications versus structural degeneration of a bioprosthetic valve requiring reoperation later in life.

The rapid development of TAVR has also presented us with the ability to perform a valve in valve replacement for a failing bioprosthetic valve. Although early results appear promising it would be premature for surgeons to widely adopt this paradigm without the benefit of long-term durability data from TAVR valves.

Whether the chosen prosthetic is mechanical or biologic, conduct of the operation is identical. Mechanical valves can be somewhat more difficult to seat. Additionally, since some models will have leaflets that will that will extend below the annular plane in the open position, appropriate orientation within the aortic annulus is important. At the time of placement, the surgeon atraumatically tests the mechanical valve leaflets to make sure they are able to fully open and close without difficulty. The commissural posts on a bioprosthetic valve must be oriented anatomically within the patient's native annulus to avoid obscuring or obstructing the patient's native coronary arteries. Additionally, an improperly placed aortotomy i.e. too low will make closure over the valve at the end of the procedure very difficult.

Ascending Aortic Replacement

Concomitant replacement of the ascending aorta can often be done in combination with aortic valve replacement, the 'Wheat procedure', or in combination with a full root replacement. Indications for common aortic replacement are described by the society guidelines (Svensson et al., 2013). In general, an aorta measuring 5-5.5 cm in maximum diameter should be replaced. Special consideration can be given to patients with aortas of smaller diameter with suspected connective tissue disorder. There is a growing body of evidence to suggest the patient's with a bicuspid aortic valve should have aggressive treatment of the proximal ascending aorta at the time of surgical replacement. In the setting of concomitant aortic replacement, the ICU team should inquire about target MAPs in the post-operative period as some surgeons may want to keep them on the lower side to minimize suture line oozing and to protect fragile aortic tissue.

Small Aortic Root

Prosthetic valves have been continually refined over the years to continue to improve the effective orifice area of the valve. However in the setting of a small native aortic root and annulus, the surgeon may be confronted with the possibility of not being able to put a large enough valve in place. The potential for patient prosthetic mismatch (PPM) and its subsequent clinical significance has been widely studied (Blackstone et al., 2003; Blais et al., 2003; Jamieson et al., 2010; Moon et al., 2006; Pibarot & Dumesnil, 2000; Tasca et al., 2006). When the surgeon is confronted with a small annulus, there are a few options for increasing valve area.

A stentless valve improves its effective orifice area by removing the supporting frame used to support most bioprosthetic valves. It is a slightly more technically demanding operation, but does have the benefit of lower transvalvular gradients compared to stented bioprostheses. Post-operative care for these patients is identical to those undergoing stented valve replacements.

In situations where the annulus is simply too small, there are techniques to enlarge the aortic annulus. Posterior annular enlargements are typically done by incising the aorta in the non-coronary sinus down to the level of the aortic annulus and onto the subaortic curtain. A more aggressive enlargement can continue down onto the anterior leaflet of the mitral valve but this is rarely necessary. A patch reconstruction is then performed to account for the defect and the enlarged orifice is used to implant an appropriately sized valve. Annular enlargement solely in the non-coronary sinus is known as a Nick's procedure, while enlargement in the commisure between the left and non-coronary cusps is referred to as a Manougian

Since both enlargement techniques involve the non-coronary cusp they are often confused and described using either surgeon's name. Posterior annular enlargement is a relatively simple method for minimizing the risks associated with patient prosthetic mismatch. Recent reviews of outcomes following

Figure 4. Manougian-type annular enlargement of aortic root

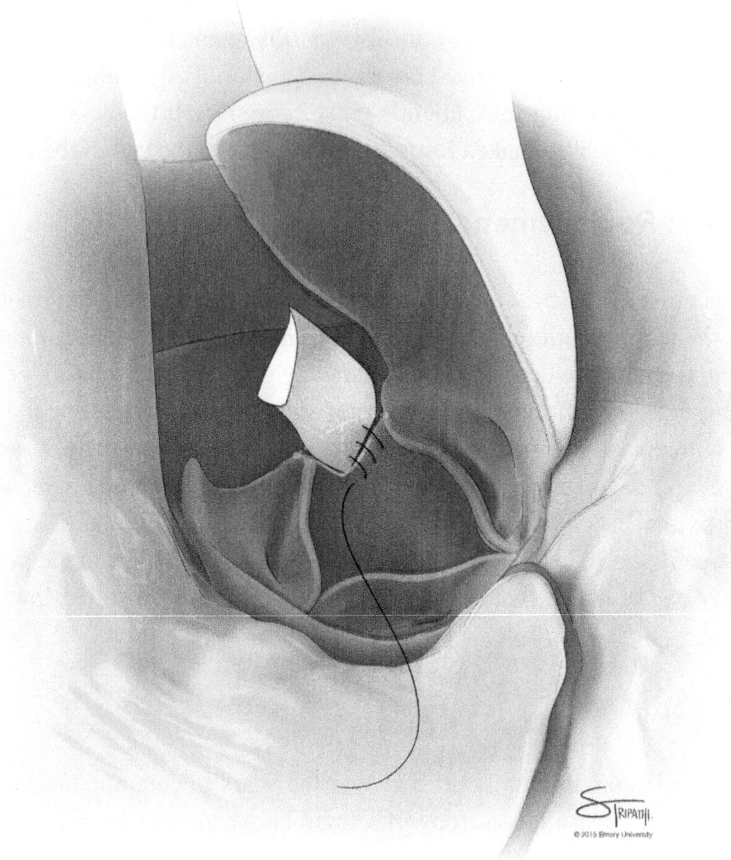

annular enlargement are favorable with no added operative risk and improved transvalvular gradients (Coutinho, Correia, Pauperio, de Oliveira, & Antunes, 2011; Dhareshwar et al., 2007).

The method of anterior annular enlargement is referred to as the Konno-Rastan procedure. This technique is primarily used in pediatric patients where a more dramatic enlargement may be required. This is done in the right coronary cusp on the pulmonary artery side of the right coronary artery. The incision extends through the annulus and into the ventricular septum with a second incision required to open the right ventricle. This location is inherently more challenging as it places the native right coronary and the conduction system at risk. Following the seating of the upsized valve, two patches are used to close the ventricular septal defect, the right ventriculotomy, and the aortotomy.

Root Replacement

Patients who have concomitant disease of aortic root should also undergo aortic root replacement. This can be done with either a biologic or mechanical valved conduit. Dissection is more involved requiring excision of the aortic sinuses in addition to the valve leaflets. Great care is taken to preserve a button of aortic tissue around the ostium of both the left and right main coronary arteries. The dissection for root replacement puts multiple cardiac structures at risk. The left atrium, right atrium, left ventricle, right ventricle, right ventricular outflow tract, main pulmonary artery, and right pulmonary artery may all be injured. Visualization must be maintained by the surgeon for any inadvertent injury during the dissection. These injured areas can often be very difficult to identify and repair once the cross-clamp has been released. Additionally, reimplantation of the coronary arteries is potentially subject to complication. Care must be taken to adequately mobilize an appropriate length of the coronary artery to prevent malpositioning or kinking once the aortic root has been pressurized. Again, repair of bleeding, particularly from the left coronary button can be very difficult to repair once the cross-clamp is removed. As the dissection is more involved and the surgeries have a longer associated ischemic time, patients will generally require more inotropic and vasoactive support following the cessation of bypass.

INTRAOPERATIVE COMPLICATIONS

Most significant intraoperative complications relating to technique will be recognized before the patient leaves the room. Clinically significant bleeding is typically readily apparent following removal of the cross-clamp and during weaning from cardiopulmonary bypass. Issues related to valve placement i.e. paravalvular leak will be demonstrated by transesophageal echocardiography as well as immediate ventricular distention following removal of the clamp. Issues related to myocardial preservation or improperly implanted coronary arteries will manifest as cardiogenic shock with or without associated arrhythmias. The experienced aortic valve surgeon should recognize the signs of potential trouble early and began a systematic investigation to identify and treat the cause. Efforts to remedy these problems may require return to cardiopulmonary bypass or even re-arresting the heart and re-doing the valve and/or root replacements. Either one of the scenarios will result in a patient whose postoperative care will be significantly more complex because of the extended nature of the procedure.

Coronary Malperfusion

Obstruction of the native coronary ostia via the sewing ring or the struts of the bioprosthetic valve can cause significant myocardial dysfunction. Low-lying coronaries may be suggested by the cardiac catheterization but it is incumbent upon the surgeon to carefully identify the origins of both right and left main coronary ostia at the time of surgery. Positioning of the valve must take the location of the origins of the ostia into consideration. Commonly these obstructions can be somewhat dynamic in nature, with symptoms only becoming apparent during periods of relative hypotension as part of the physiologic ebb and flow of the post-bypass period. The surgeon must be 100% confident in coronary perfusion before making the decision to close the chest.

Maintaining a higher mean arterial blood pressure may be necessary and an IABP may help to augment perfusion, but if coronary malperfusion remains a significant issue, a single vein bypass to the affected distribution is required. This can be done off-pump if the heart will tolerate positioning, otherwise a return to cardiopulmonary bypass with or without cardiac arrest is warranted. Reopening of the aorta with removal and repositioning of the valve should only be attempted if the surgeon is confident that the malperfusion is related to a technical error. Often times these replacements were difficult procedures technically and the chances of affecting the outcome by re-replacing the valve are limited.

Following aortic root replacement, malpositioning of the coronary buttons can result in significant limitations in coronary perfusion. Steps to avoid these complications should be taken to insure adequate mobilization of the coronary buttons and appropriate placement with regard to the final root geometry when the cross-clamp is removed. As with mechanical obstruction by a prosthetic valve, the simplest solution is often a single vein bypass to the affected distribution done off-pump. Repeat aortic cross-clamping with repeat cardioplegic arrest of the heart to reposition the button in question is a large undertaking that places the patient at significantly increased risk. Typically, following vein bypass, resolution of the malperfusion is immediately noticeable with improved hemodynamics allowing safe weaning from cardiopulmonary bypass.

Paravalvular Leak

Paravalvular leak detected by TEE following cross-clamp removal represent a small minority of cases. The location and severity of a jet must be thoroughly evaluated by the echocardiographer. The decision about whether or not to root to return to bypass and repair the valve is based on several factors. A straightforward valve replacement with a leak in a readily accessible location i.e. the non-coronary sinus should be managed aggressively. However if the procedure was technically challenging secondary to excessive annular calcification and the leak is small and in a difficult to access location on either the left or right coronary cusp these patients can be treated expectantly. Postoperatively, they'll need to be followed for signs of hemolysis related to turbulent flow. Sometimes during follow-up these patients will present for reoperation based on either heart failure symptoms or substantial hemolysis if the jet worsens over time. Since this leak is outside the valve frame, a valve in valve TAVR procedure is not an option. In this instance, the surgeon will have to consider the risks of repeat sternotomy and redo valve replacement in the context of the patient's clinical condition. Experience with catheter-based interventions and leak closure using specialized devices is promising (Nietlispach et al., 2010; Taramasso et al., 2014), but should be reserved for those patients who represent a prohibitive operative risk.

Heart Block

The native conduction system lies in close proximity to the aortic annulus in the region of the right and non-commissural post. Surgeons must practice great care when placing their annular sutures at this level as too deep of a bite will affect the conduction system.

Heart block related to suture placement is typically readily apparent once the heart has been reperfused. Surgeons must provide reliable epicardial pacing for the immediate perioperative period. In some instances, once local tissue edema and swelling subsides post surgery, one may see a restoration of normal conduction. However a small percentage of patients will progress to require permanent pacemaker implantation. The intensivist's immediate interrogation of the adequacy of the epicardial pacing wires should be confirmed. Facility and ready access for a pacing wire via the pulmonary artery catheter should also be arranged. In lieu of this, transcutaneous pacing can be performed in the sedated patient.

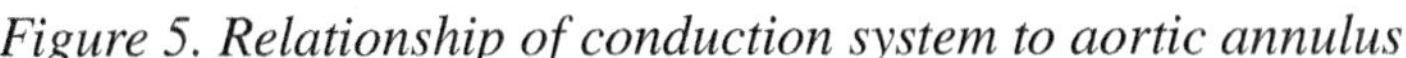

Figure 5. Relationship of conduction system to aortic annulus

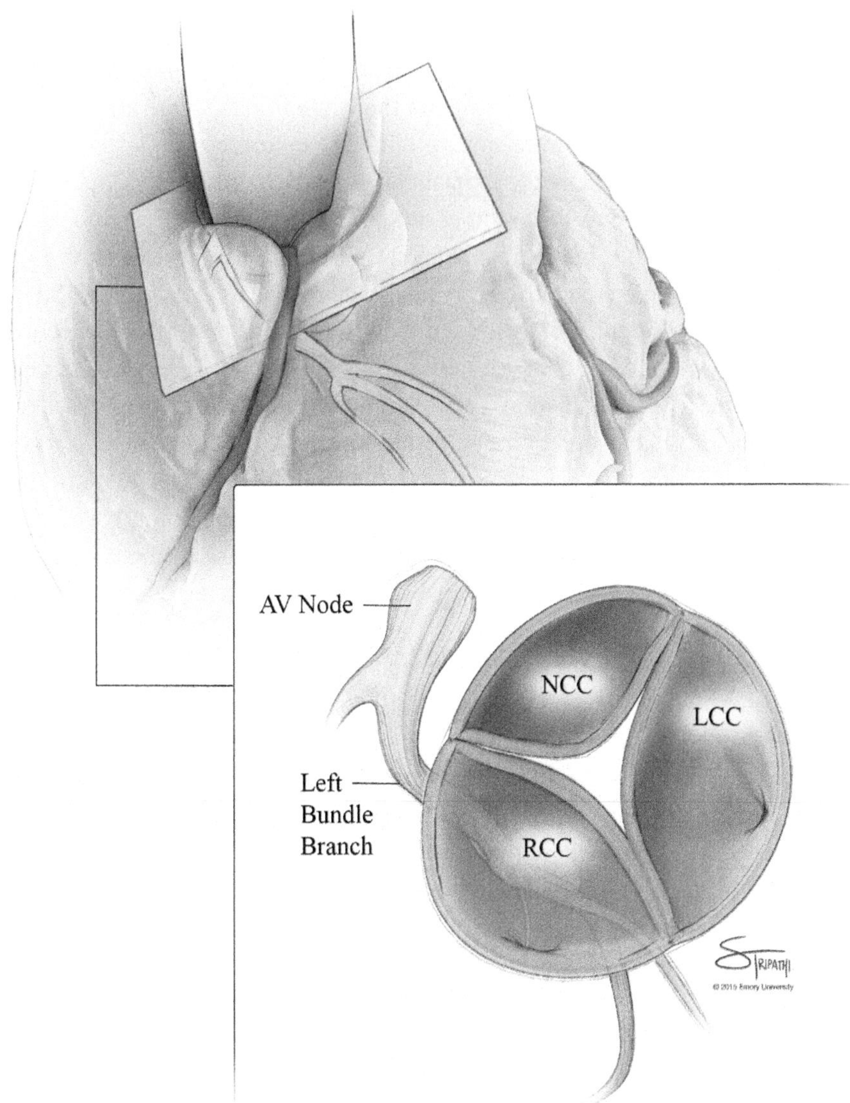

TRANSCATHETER AORTIC VALVE REPLACEMENT (TAVR)

The introduction of transcatheter aortic valve replacement in 2002 has initiated a remarkable era of innovation and rapid proliferation of technologies related to this novel approach. The prospect of an effective aortic valve replacement that does not require the physiologic trauma of cardiopulmonary bypass represents a tremendous advance for patients with this disease. Initial studies in Europe and the United States focused on the application of this technology in more elderly, frail patients who were deemed to not be candidates for surgery, or for whom surgery was associated with a much higher than normal risk. Multiple clinical studies to date, including two large well-controlled prospective randomized studies have confirmed the effectiveness of the technique with apparent benefits when compared to open surgical aortic valve replacement.

The Placement of Aortic Transcatheter Valves or PARTNER trial established the significance and potential 'game-changing' effects of TAVR therapy in the United States. One arm of the study randomized 358 patients with severe AS who were not candidates for surgery (Cohort B) to TAVR with an Edwards SAPIEN valve versus optimal medical management with balloon valvuloplasty. A significantly decreased mortality for TAVR patients was seen at one year (30.7% vs. 50.7%) and at 2 year follow-up (43.4% vs. 68%)(Leon et al., 2010). This finding shaped future trials as it was no longer considered ethical to randomize these patients to medical therapy alone. The results of Cohort A of the PARTNER trial demonstrated that in high risk patients (STS risk score of 10%) TAVR could achieve comparable short- and mid-term results to SAVR, albeit with a higher risk of bleeding complications (Smith et al., 2011).

The CoreValve Extreme Risk US Pivotal Trial examined the Medtronic CoreValve device in extreme risk/ inoperable patients as a single arm study. At one year, the incidence of all-cause mortality and major stroke was 26%. Major vascular complications were lower (8.2%) and permanent pacemaker placement was higher (21.6%) when compared to the PARTNER trial (Popma et al., 2014). The high risk arm of the study was the first to demonstrate a survival advantage at one year for TAVR (14.2%) vs. SAVR (19.1%)(Adams et al., 2014). This finding bolstered the growing body of evidence supporting this approach in high risk patients.

There are several variations in both the available technologies as well as the routes of delivery with which the intensivist must be familiar with in order to effectively manage these patients postoperatively. The valves themselves can be broadly classified as either being balloon-expandable or self-expandable in nature. The Edwards SAPIEN is the most common example of a balloon-expandable valve while Medtronic's CoreValve is the first of what will likely be many self-expanding valves. The engineering differences of these two valves affect where they sit in the aortic root as well as the associated complications with their use. All of these valves are made from pericardial tissue and do not require Coumadin anticoagulation postoperatively.

OPERATIVE TECHNIQUES

A variety of access sites for deployment have been described. The default route is the retrograde transfemoral approach. When anatomic factors preclude this approach, well-described alternative access sites include the transapical, transaortic, or subclavian routes. As each access site is associated with its own particular risks and benefits, it is incumbent on the modern intensivist to have a thorough understanding of the methods for each of the access sites and the associated complications

Transfemoral TAVR (TF)

Transfemoral delivery is the least invasive approach and has become the procedure of choice in patients with appropriate vasculature. Vascular access is obtained in the bilateral groins. Utilizing pre-operative imaging, the delivery sheath is placed on the side where the artery is at least the minimum required diameter, has the least amount of calcification, and is without excessive tortuousity. The non-delivery side provides arterial access to provide angiography during valve placement and deployment, as well as venous access to place a temporary pacing catheter in the right ventricle. The ability to provide consistent pacing capture is critical for a safe TAVR deployment.

The femoral artery on the implant-side can be accessed by direct surgical cutdown or percutaneously depending on surgeon preference. Once appropriate intra-arterial wire access is confirmed, serial dilators are passed and the delivery sheath is advanced into the descending aorta. The patient is systemically heparinized to an ACT of > 250 seconds and the aortic valve is crossed with a wire to provide access to the left ventricle. The wire placed in the left ventricular cavity has circular curve to minimize the risk of perforation during the procedure. Pre-dilatation of the aortic valve with balloon valvuloplasty is performed under rapid ventricular pacing (generally 180-220 beats/minute) in anticipation of valve placement.

The valve delivery system is inserted and advanced to the appropriate trans-annular position. A combination of fluoroscopy and echocardiography is used to confirm appropriate positioning. The SAPIEN valve is ideally positioned to span the tips of the aortic leaflets to the aortic annulus or below. The longer CoreValve is positioned so that the inflow portion is approximately 4-6 mm below the annulus, while its distal extent rests in the ascending aorta. Once appropriate positioning is confirmed, a Sapien valve is deployed using a long cine-fluoroscopic run under rapid ventricular pacing and controlled inflation/deflation of the delivery balloon. The CoreValve system does not commonly require rapid ventricular pacing during deployment, although increasing the heart rate to 100-120 bpm can facilitate placement.

After deployment, proper valve position is assessed with echocardiography and angiography. Valve placement that is either too high or too low in the annulus may require placement of a second valve. A trace or mild amount of paravalvular leak is expected after TAVR with the first generation devices. Paravalvular leak in an appropriately positioned valve can be treated with balloon post-dilatation to expand the valve frame and improve apposition to the native valve.

Transapical TAVR (TA)

The TA approach has served as the primary alternative access route for the Sapien valve. In patients with significant peripheral vascular disease, the TA TAVR represents a very effective option. Relative contraindications for this approach are severe COPD with a FEV1% predicted < 30% or a left ventricular ejection fraction < 20%.

The patient is placed supine on the operating room table and femoral artery and vein access is achieved as described for the TF approach. A 4-5 cm left anterolateral thoracotomy is made in the 5th or 6th intercostal space to expose the apex of the left ventricle. Intravenous lidocaine is administered and two pledgeted 3-0 prolene pursestring sutures are placed in the ventricle just cephalad to the apex and lateral to the LAD. The pursestring sutures into the myocardium should be deep stitches, but not transmural in order to avoid ventricular tearing.

Needle access to the left ventricle is obtained and a guidewire is passed antegradely across the aortic valve, and into the descending aorta. The delivery system is carefully advanced into the left ventricle. Balloon aortic valvuloplasty can be performed with or without rapid ventricular pacing. Subsequent positioning, deployment, and post-assessment of the valve is similar to that described for TF-TAVR. After confirming adequate valve position and function, the apical sutures are tied down using rapid ventricular pacing. Once access site hemostasis is confirmed, a small flexible chest tube is placed in the left pleural space and the thoracotomy is closed in a routine fashion.

Transaortic TAVR (TAo)

The transaortic approach is gaining increasing popularity as an alternative access site for both balloon expanded and self-expanding valves. The TAo approach is advantageous because it avoids a thoracotomy in patients with poor respiratory function and thus is generally less painful than the TA approach. The TAo approach is contraindicated in patients with a heavily calcified, 'porcelain' aorta or in an otherwise hostile mediastinum (i.e. patients with a history of cobalt radiation). It can also be technically challenging in the setting of a prior sternotomy, especially if the patient has patent grafts from a previous CABG.

The patient is placed supine on the operating room table. Femoral access for pacing access and aortography is obtained. The pre-op CT scan provides valuable information regarding the anatomy of the ascending aorta. Ideally a 7 cm distance from the proposed cannulation site to the annulus is present to ensure adequate space for valve deployment. A standard mini-sternotomy incision is made. The distal ascending aorta is exposed and two aortic purse strings are placed at the base of the innominate artery. A counter-incision at the base of the neck will help obtain a more comfortable angle of approach for the delivery catheter The valve is crossed with a wire and subsequent positioning, deployment, and post-assessment of the valve is similar to a TF approach. The pericardium is left open, a small flexible chest tube is left in place, and the sternotomy is closed in a standard fashion.

Subclavian/Trans-Axillary TAVR

The trans-subclavian approach was popularized as an alternative access route for the CoreValve device. An axillary arterial approach provides a few distinct advantages compared to other alternative access routes. It remains less invasive as it does not require entering the thoracic space and presents an appealing alternative for a frail, older patient in whom a TF approach is limited by anatomy. Additionally, it is suitable in cases of aortic calcification, or severe ventricular and pulmonary dysfunction which would limit other alternative approaches.

Standard femoral arterial and venous access is obtained. Surgical cutdown for axillary artery exposure should be familiar to most cardiac surgeons as it is routinely employed as an arterial inflow cannulation site in the setting of aortic surgery. An oblique incision is made below the clavicle and the axillary artery is exposed. The artery can be cannulated directly or via a synthetic graft sewn on in an end to side fashion. The delivery sheath is carefully advanced into the aortic arch and TAVR deployment proceeds following the usual protocol. At the conclusion of the procedure following removal of the delivery sheath, vascular control of the access site is obtained and selective angiography can be used to confirm vessel integrity at the access site.

Less Common Routes

In those patients who are not suitable for any of the more common access routes described there are alternatives for TAVR deployment that have been used in much smaller numbers. A transcarotid approach can be used if a patient has a right common carotid artery diameter of at least 8mm without evidence of stenosis (Guyton, Block, Thourani, Lerakis, & Babaliaros, 2013). The right common carotid artery is exposed with a longitudinal neck incision similar to that used for carotid endarterectomy. All patients have distal cerebral perfusion maintained with a passive shunt from the femoral artery with patch closure of the carotid at the completion of the procedure.

Recently, a trans-caval approach has been described (Greenbaum et al., 2014). Access is obtained in the common femoral vein and then an aorto-caval fistula is created via the inferior vena cava. Once arterial access is obtained in the infra-renal abdominal aorta, deployment proceeds similar to a TF TAVR. In a series of 19 patients, the approach achieved successful valve deployment in 17 patients but with a high rate of blood transfusion (79%) and vascular complications (33%).

TAVR COMPLICATIONS

Despite its minimally invasive approach, procedural complications associated with TAVR can be substantial and are associated with considerable morbidity and mortality. The Valve Academic Research Consortium-2 (VARC-2) criteria provide standardized definitions for evaluating studies of TAVR use (Kappetein et al., 2012). As with any surgical procedure, thorough pre-procedural planning is of the utmost importance when trying to minimize complications.

Neurologic

TAVR is unique in that it requires the manipulation of large bore catheters in the ascending aorta and aortic arch as well as across a heavily calcified aortic valve. This coupled with balloon expansion and fracture of the calcified aortic leaflets likely represents the etiology for the bulk of acute neurologic events. The incidence of cerebrovascular events during the 30-day period after TAVR ranges from 3% to 7%.(Thomas et al., 2010). The majority of these (50–70%) are peri-procedural and occur within 24 hours of the procedure. The original PARTNER study demonstrated an increased incidence of peri-procedural stroke following TAVR when compared to SAVR.(Miller et al., 2012; Smith et al., 2011) and a recent meta-analysis compiled an overall 30-day stroke rate 3.3±1.8 (Eggebrecht et al., 2012). The type of device used does not seem to impact stroke incidence, but increased operator experience does correlate with lower event rates (Athappan et al., 2014).

As interest in stroke following in TAVR has grown, a surprising discovery has been the incidence of new cerebral ischemic lesions following TAVR. Recent studies which obtained diffusion-weighted MRIs on patients before and after TAVR demonstrated new lesions in up to 75% of patients post-TAVR(Fairbairn et al., 2012; Rodes-Cabau et al., 2011). The vast majority of these lesions are not associated with clinical evidence of a neurologic event and there was no difference in the number and size of lesions when comparing the TF and the TA approach (Rodes-Cabau et al., 2011).

Given the temporal relationship of neurologic events to the procedure itself, a baseline neurologic exam should be performed as quickly as possible upon arrival to the ICU. Weaning of sedation should be performed as quickly as the clinical condition allows to facilitate serial examination. Evidence of a new neurologic deficit should be managed in the standard fashion. Procedural aspects associated with neurologic events include balloon post-dilatation and valve embolization(Nombela-Franco et al., 2012) and the intensivist should employ heightened scrutiny in these settings. Oral ant-platelet therapy (ASA/Clopidogrel) should be initiated as soon as considered safe with regards to post-operative bleeding.

Since much of the embolic phenomena are peri-procedural, there have been multiple new technologies developed to minimize neurologic sequelae. These devices can be categorized in two broad categories:

Deflectors which prevent passage of emboli to the cerebrovascular system by redirecting them to the lower half of the body and filtration/retrieval devices which capture and collect emboli for removal from the systemic circulation.

The two main deflector devices, the Embrella (Edwards Lifesciences) and the Triguard (Keystone Heart, Ltd.) along with the Montage Dual Filter (Claret Medical, Inc.) represent the current leaders in the field of neuroprotection technology. All 3 devices have been used in small patient series with acceptable results and excellent success with deployment and retrieval. However, larger randomized trials are needed to determine their clinical utility for the TAVR population.

Vascular

Complications related to the arterial access site have been a frequent problem since the early days of this technology. Direct vascular injury is primarily related to the large diameter sheaths needed to deliver the valve. Data from the original PARTNER trial spotlighted the significance of this problem. For the high risk cohort A patients, major vascular complications occurred in 11% of TAVR patients compared to 3.2% in SAVR patients (Smith et al., 2011). In the non-operative cohort B patients, 16.2% of TF TAVR patients had a major vascular event within 30 days compared to 1.1% of patients randomized to standard medical therapy (Leon et al., 2010). The implications of these complications are significant with a four-fold increase in 30 day mortality (14.1% vs. 3.1%) demonstrated in the PARTNER patients (Genereux et al., 2012).

One difficulty when comparing results of earlier studies is the different definitions of bleeding and vascular access complications. The VARC-2 criteria represent consensus opinion for these definitions and should be the standard used for reporting TAVR complications.

Over time, better patient screening and selection coupled with increased operator experience has resulted in improved outcomes. This has also been paralleled by improvements in the associated technology

Table 1. Bleeding definitions for TAVR procedures. Reprinted with permission from VARC-2 Guidelines, European Heart Journal, 2012

Bleeding
Life-threatening or disabling bleeding
Fatal bleeding *(BARC type 5)* OR
Bleeding in a critical organ, such as intracranial, intraspinal, intraocular, or pericardial necessitating pericardiocentesis, or intramuscular with compartment syndrome *(BARC type 3b and 3c)* OR
Bleeding causing hypovolemic shock or severe hypotension requiring vasopressors or surgery *(BARC type 3b)* OR
Overt source of bleeding with drop in hemoglobin >5 g/dL or whole blood or packed red blood cells (RBCs) transfusion >4 units *(BARC type 3b)*
Major bleeding (BARC type 3a)
Overt bleeding either associated with a drop in the hemoglobin level of at least 3.0 g/dl or requiring transfusion of two or three units of whole blood/RBC, or causing hospitalization or permanent injury, or requiring surgery AND
Does not meet criteria of life-threatening or disabling bleeding
Minor bleeding (BARC type 2 or 3a, depending on the severity)
Any bleeding worthy of clinical mention (e.g. access site hematoma) that does not qualify as life-threatening, disabling, or major

BARC = Bleeding Academic Research Consortium (29); RBC = red blood cell

Table 2. Definitions of vascular access complications. Reprinted with permission from VARC-2 Guidelines, European Heart Journal, 2012

Vascular Access Site and Access-Related Complications
Major vascular complications
Any aortic dissection, aortic rupture, annulus rupture, left ventricle perforation, or new apical aneurysm/pseudo-aneurysm OR
Access site or access-related vascular injury (dissection, stenosis, perforation, rupture, arterio-venous fistula, pseudoaneurysm, hematoma, irreversible nerve injury, compartment syndrome, percutaneous closure device failure)*leading to* death, life-threatening or major bleeding [a], visceral ischemia, or neurological impairment OR
Distal embolization (non-cerebral) from a vascular source requiring surgery or resulting in amputation or irreversible end-organ damage OR
The use of unplanned endovascular or surgical intervention *associated* with death, major bleeding, visceral ischemia or neurological impairment OR
Any new ipsilateral lower extremity ischemia documented by patient symptoms, physical exam, and/or decreased or absent blood flow on lower extremity angiogram OR
Surgery for access site-related nerve injury OR
Permanent access site-related nerve injury
Minor vascular complications
Access site or access-related vascular injury (dissection, stenosis, perforation, rupture, arterio-venous fistula, pseudoaneuysms, hematomas, percutaneous closure device failure) *not leading to* death, life-threatening or major bleeding, visceral ischemia, or neurological impairment OR
Distal embolization treated with embolectomy and/or thrombectomy and not resulting in amputation or irreversible end-organ damage OR
Any unplanned endovascular stenting or unplanned surgical intervention not meeting the criteria for a major vascular complication OR
Vascular repair or the need for vascular repair (via surgery, ultrasound-guided compression, transcatheter embolization, or stent-graft)
Percutaneous closure device failure
Failure of a closure device to achieve hemostasis at the arteriotomy site leading to alternative treatment (other than manual compression or adjunctive endovascular ballooning)

with smaller diameter delivery devices now available. However, ongoing blood loss should always be a consideration in the unstable postoperative patient. Because of the varied sites of access, investigation for bleeding may require different modalities.

Transfemoral access with poor hemostatic control may develop a retroperitoneal hematoma that could go undiagnosed at the bedside. If this is suspected, it must be diagnosed and treated expeditiously. A CT scan will readily demonstrate the bleeding. In some institutions, organized protocols dictate a return to the hybrid operating room or cardiac catheterization lab with angiography to evaluate for the bleeding source. This offers the potential benefit of therapeutic intervention at the same time if a bleeding source is identified.

Bleeding related to transapical access can be significant and may initially manifest as excessive chest tube drainage. However, in the setting of a clotted chest tube the first indication may be opacification or "white out" of the left lung field on chest x-ray. Patients with dense pleural adhesions may even present with tamponade physiology. This should be treated with a return to the operating room and exploration as passive maneuvers (PEEP, increased tidal volume) are unlikely to control an arterial bleeding source.

Postoperative bleeding after TAo access will present much like bleeding after a standard sternotomy. Chest tube output as well as an enlarged mediastinal silhouette should alert the intensivist to a possible problem. While bleeding may be related to sternal closure or mediastinal soft tissue, one must remember that there is an aortic cannulation site which, if it is the culprit, will require a return to the operating room and definitive surgical closure.

Subclavian access is unlikely to represent a significant source of occult bleeding since there is no potential space for blood to accumulate. A significant bleed at this site will present with a large associated hematoma and possibly even neurologic changes of the affected extremity if enough pressure is exerted on the cords of the brachial plexus.

Vascular complications are not limited solely to access site bleeding. Perforation of either ventricle related to mechanical trauma has been reported with TAVR. Presentation in the immediate peri-operative period will be consistent with tamponade physiology and readily diagnosed by bedside echocardiography. Expedient drainage should be performed and persistent bleeding that does not respond to conservative management should prompt a return to the operating room for definitive repair.

Dissection related to an access site or mechanical trauma anywhere along the arterial tree is also a consideration. Significant dissection involving the femoral or subclavian artery will present with signs of arterial insufficiency in the affected limb. Diminished peripheral pulses, delayed capillary refill, and an asymmetric neurovascular exam should prompt further investigation. Central aortic dissection site related to TAo access is usually recognized in the operating room but could be confirmed with either CT scanning or echocardiography in the post-operative period.

Conduction Abnormalities

As previously depicted, the close proximity of the native conduction system to the aortic annulus puts it at risk following aortic valve replacement. Due to the engineering design of TAVR valves, which require the use of radial force to achieve placement, new conduction abnormalities are seen more frequently than with SAVR. In addition, the particular design features of the balloon-expandable and self-expanding valves lead to consistent differences in the need for permanent pacemakers between the two technologies.

A recent meta-analysis of 41 studies involving over 11,000 TAVR patients illustrates this difference between devices. Among the series of CoreValve implants reviewed, the median incidence of PPM placement was 28% compared with 6% for SAPIEN implants. The authors presented unadjusted estimates which ascribed a 2.5- fold higher risk of PPM need for a CoreValve compared to SAPIEN. In addition, pre-operative first degree A-V block, left anterior hemi-block, and right bundle branch block were all predictive of an increased need for PPM (Siontis et al., 2014). The conduction abnormalities are usually apparent early in the recovery period and, as illustrated in another meta-analysis, more than 90% of the PPM implantations occur within the first week following surgery (Erkapic et al., 2012).

In the immediate post-procedure period, knowledge of the device implanted and its associated effects on conduction are mandatory. Part of the exchange in the ICU should include any information regarding acute changes in conduction during the procedure. Additionally, the intensivist should compare the EKG obtained on arrival in the ICU to one obtained pre-op. A change in conduction should prompt heightened awareness of possible bradyarrythmias requiring pacing.

Typically, an experienced TAVR team will leave temporary venous access in place in patients who are at increased risk. However, the ICU staff needs to have a contingency plan in place for rapid heart rate support should it become necessary.

Paravalvular Regurgitation

Paravalvular regurgitation (PVR) of some degree has been very common in the early TAVR experience. A significant difference between TAVR and high risk SAVR patients in Cohort A of the PARTNER study persisted at 2 year follow-up with more than 50% of TAVR patients having at least mild PVR(Kodali et al., 2012). This is significant because even mild residual PVR was associated with a 10-15% higher 2 year mortality. This association between residual PVR and mortality has been confirmed by other authors(Moat et al., 2011; Sinning et al., 2012; Tamburino et al., 2011) with a recent literature review identifying AR >2+ as a significant independent predictor of short- and long-term mortality(Genereux, Head, et al., 2013).

Acute transvalvular regurgitation may occur due to incomplete valve closure when the valve is deployed in the setting of systemic arterial hypotension and this improves when the blood pressure is increased. The valve also may simply require a brief period of time (minutes) to "warm up" and achieve full leaflet mobility. A third scenario for transvalvular AR may be due to an over-hanging native aortic leaflet which can prevent closure of the TAVR valve leaflets. This scenario particularly affected the first generation SAPIEN valve, whose default leaflet position was in an open configuration. The valve relied on back pressure during diastole to close the leaflets and if native tissue impaired the back flow, significant central AR was present. In this event, the operator would attempt to close the TAVR valve leaflets by placing a pigtail catheter in each aortic cusp. If this is unsuccessful, another TAVR valve should be deployed just aortic to the initial TAVR valve in order to adequately displace the native aortic leaflets. Subsequent generations of the SAPIEN valve (SAPIEN XT, SAPIEN 3) altered the leaflet design to a 'semi-closed' position and this has become less of a problem. The length of the CoreValve's stent frame prevents overhanging tissue from altering valve function.

The pathophysiology linking PVR and mortality is an area of ongoing investigation. Most, if not all, of the newer generation valves have design features to minimize PVR. Additionally, the importance of minimizing PVR is a well-accepted doctrine among TAVR practitioners. Patients with significant (³2+ AR) in a valve deployed at the appropriate height, can be treated with balloon post-dilatation to further expand the valve into the native valve tissue. If a valve is deployed either too high or too low, a second valve deployed inside the first can extend the 'seal zone' thereby reducing PVR. The risk/ benefit of further intervention to increase the radial force of the valve must be weighed against the possibility of stroke and annular disruption by the heart team. Knowledge of the presence and severity of residual PVR is an important part of the transition to care in the ICU. Trace or mild PVR will not have much impact on the immediate post-procedure management. However, PVR of severity of 2+ or greater will need attention with regard to afterload reduction and possible chronotropic therapy to optimize the volume status of the left ventricle.

Acute Kidney Injury

The origin of AKI following TAVR is multi-factorial and related to predisposing conditions such as diabetes mellitus, pre-existing chronic kidney disease, and peripheral vascular disease. There are also operative events including iatrogenic atheroemboli and hypoperfusion during valve deployment which can contribute to the development of AKI. In the PARTNER study, in addition to their other comorbidities, 11.1% of TAVR-treated patients in Cohort A and 5.6% of TAVR-treated patients in Cohort B presented with baseline creatinine greater than 2 mg/dL(Leon et al., 2010; Smith et al., 2011).

The VARC-2 grading criteria stratify AKI into three stages based on degree of increase in serum creatinine and severity of oliguria/anuria.

The increase in creatinine must occur within 48 h.

Utilizing this criteria, the incidence of significant AKI, defined as Stage 2 or 3, after TAVR has been reported to be 8.3%(Genereux, Kodali, et al., 2013). In this same study, 50% of patients with significant AKI required dialysis. Patients in the significant AKI group also had a substantial increase in all-cause mortality at 30 days (44.4% vs. 3%). This dramatic increase in mortality has been echoed by multiple other studies (Takagi et al., 2013).

The TA approach for TAVR has been associated with an increased risk for AKI in some series (Barbash et al., 2012). A recent meta-analysis highlighted a significantly higher incidence of renal replacement therapy following TA-TAVR (8.2%) vs. TF-TAVR (2.8%)(Khatri et al., 2013). When interpreting these results it is important to remember that TA patients, by definition, have a higher burden of atherosclerotic vascular disease. The increased incidence of AKI is more likely related to the underlying severity of their vascular disease and not the route of TAVR deployment.

Prevention of AKI in the TAVR population begins during the procedure. Manual hand injections instead of power injections for aortography will decrease the overall contrast load during the procedure. Additionally, optimizing hydration status should start during the procedure. While great care should be taken with volume administration for patients with AS and heart failure symptoms, most patients presenting for an elective TAVR are on the 'less-hydrated' side at the beginning of the procedure. Ventricular filling status on echocardiography and LVEDP measurements from left heart catheterization provide excellent information regarding volume status that can be used to guide treatment.

After arrival in the ICU, care should be taken to minimize nephrotoxic agents in patients at risk. Maintaining adequate arterial pressure to optimize renal perfusion should be an understood goal of the immediate post-operative period. Any deviation in urine output or significant rise from baseline creatinine level should prompt an aggressive investigation.

Table 3. Definitions for acute kidney injury. Reprinted with permission from VARC-2 Guidelines, European Heart Journal, 2012.

Acute Kidney Injury (AKIN Classification)
Stage 1
Increase in serum creatinine to 150–199% (1.5–1.99 x increase compared with baseline) OR increase of >0.3 mg/dl (>26.4 mmol/l) OR
Urine output <0.5 ml/kg/h for >6 but <12 h
Stage 2
Increase in serum creatinine to 200–299% (2.0–2.99 × increase compared with baseline) OR
Urine output <0.5 ml/kg/h for >12 but <24 h
Stage 3
Increase in serum creatinine to >300% (>3 × increase compared with baseline) OR serum creatinine of >4.0 mg/dl (>354 mmol/l) with an acute increase of at least 0.5 mg/dl (44 mmol/l) OR
Urine output <0.3 ml/kg/h for >24 h OR
Anuria for > 12 h

LESS COMMON COMPLICATIONS

Many of the intra-procedural complications related to TAVR have decreased as experience with the technique has grown. While certain technologic improvements have facilitated this, much of it is simply attributable to growing experience with what is essentially a very new technique. The following intra-procedural complications may still occur, but they have become less frequent as operators have become savvier with the potential pitfalls of the TAVR procedure.

Valve Embolization

Valve embolization most commonly affects balloon-expanded valves and is typically due to the loss of pacing capture during deployment. However, it can affect both types of valve if they are badly mal-positioned or grossly undersized. Avoiding valve embolization begins with meticulous multi-modality imaging (multi-slice CT and TEE) coupled with thorough understanding of the sizing requirements of the valve to be implanted. Confirmation of reliable pacing capture prior to valve deployment is mandatory. Careful valve positioning using a slow, controlled deployment will help the operator make subtle adjustments to ensure the best possible location for the valve.

In the event of gross malpositioning, maintaining wire access is of paramount importance. This will allow the valve to be recaptured with a balloon and repositioned distally. Typically, a safe location is anywhere distal to the left subclavian artery in the descending thoracic aorta or immediately proximal to the common iliac bifurcation in the abdominal aorta. After the embolized valve is secured, a 2nd valve may be implanted in the annulus to complete the TAVR. Valve embolization into the left ventricle is less common and almost always requires surgical intervention for removal.

Coronary Occlusion

Myocardial infarction is a rare, yet catastrophic complication during TAVR and occurs in less than 1% of patients (Ribeiro et al., 2013) (Leon et al., 2010). Acute, aorto-ostial coronary occlusion may be treated effectively with immediate percutaneous coronary intervention (PCI) or emergent peripheral cardiopulmonary bypass followed by PCI. Left main coronary artery occlusion is most likely, although right coronary artery obstruction has also been described. Percutaneous intervention can be facilitated in high-risk cases by placing a 0.014-inch coronary interventional wire and/or balloon into the coronary artery at risk prior to deployment of the new valve. Prevention remains the mainstay of treatment for this dreadful complication. Coronary artery orifice < 12mm as determined by a high-definition CT scan should prompt concern. In such scenarios, performing a BAV with a concomitant root angiogram may discern the potential for coronary artery occlusion.

Cardiac Tamponade

Tamponade can result from cardiac perforation of either the right or left ventricle during placement of the pacemaker, wire manipulation, or by the nosecone of the TAVR delivery system. Large inspiratory drops in systemic arterial pressure (pulsus paradoxus) suggest a hemodynamically significant effusion and echocardiography will be confirmatory. Treatment with pericardiocentesis is often all that is needed since bleeding is often self-limited. However, if it is related to a larger diameter device surgical exploration may be required.

FUTURE DIRECTIONS

Surgical treatment of aortic valve disease represents a mainstay of modern cardiothoracic surgery. Our understanding of the epidemiology of aortic valve pathology, coupled with projections for worldwide population growth suggests that the need for therapy will grow substantially in the coming decades. In the light of the exciting new technology advances, it is important to remember that SAVR represents the gold standard for all low and intermediate operative risk patients at this time.

The rapid evolution of TAVR is an incredibly exciting development in the field of structural heart disease. The ability to deliver effective treatment to older patients with more comorbidities represents a true sea-change in the way we view this disease. Over the next two years in the United States alone we can expect to see half dozen new valves beginning clinical trials. Furthermore, technological advances will allow us to progressively mitigate the associated risks of the procedure thereby making it more appealing for the broader population.

There are currently two ongoing trials in the United States, one utilizing SAPIEN and one CoreValve, which are investigating the efficacy of TAVR treatment in patient's at intermediate risk for complications (i.e. STS risk of 3-8%). The results of these trials will have a huge impact and how we manage aortic stenosis in the years to come. Additionally, new valve types have been developed for the treatment of primary aortic insufficiency. This requires a different type of engineering since the calcified, rigid annulus of AS is not present to provide fixation. As this technology evolves the ability to treat all pathologies related to the aortic valve will become available.

Treatment of aortic valve disease represents a rapidly moving target and with each new technologic advance, associated risks and complications will become apparent. The modern intensivist will be challenged to keep abreast of each new device and the potentially new challenges they may present in the post-operative period. When one stops to consider that this technology is just a decade old, we can reasonably anticipate a continuous and rapid evolution that will mandate continued attention.

REFERENCES

Adams, D. H., Popma, J. J., Reardon, M. J., Yakubov, S. J., Coselli, J. S., Deeb, G. M., & Oh, J. K. et al. (2014). Transcatheter aortic-valve replacement with a self-expanding prosthesis. *The New England Journal of Medicine*, *370*(19), 1790–1798. doi:10.1056/NEJMoa1400590 PMID:24678937

Athappan, G., Gajulapalli, R. D., Sengodan, P., Bhardwaj, A., Ellis, S. G., Svensson, L., & Kapadia, S. R. et al. (2014). Influence of transcatheter aortic valve replacement strategy and valve design on stroke after transcatheter aortic valve replacement: A meta-analysis and systematic review of literature. *Journal of the American College of Cardiology*, *63*(20), 2101–2110. doi:10.1016/j.jacc.2014.02.540 PMID:24632286

Badhwar, V., Ofenloch, J. C., Rovin, J. D., van Gelder, H. M., & Jacobs, J. P. (2012). Noninferiority of closely monitored mechanical valves to bioprostheses overshadowed by early mortality benefit in younger patients. *The Annals of Thoracic Surgery*, *93*(3), 748–753. doi:10.1016/j.athoracsur.2011.12.032 PMID:22364968

Barbash, I. M., Ben-Dor, I., Dvir, D., Maluenda, G., Xue, Z., Torguson, R., & Waksman, R. et al. (2012). Incidence and predictors of acute kidney injury after transcatheter aortic valve replacement. *American Heart Journal*, *163*(6), 1031–1036. doi:10.1016/j.ahj.2012.01.009 PMID:22709757

Blackstone, E. H., Cosgrove, D. M., Jamieson, W. R., Birkmeyer, N. J., Lemmer, J. H. Jr, Miller, D. C., & Chai, A. et al. (2003). Prosthesis size and long-term survival after aortic valve replacement. *The Journal of Thoracic and Cardiovascular Surgery*, *126*(3), 783–796. doi:10.1016/S0022-5223(03)00591-9 PMID:14502155

Blais, C., Dumesnil, J. G., Baillot, R., Simard, S., Doyle, D., & Pibarot, P. (2003). Impact of valve prosthesis-patient mismatch on short-term mortality after aortic valve replacement. *Circulation*, *108*(8), 983–988. doi:10.1161/01.CIR.0000085167.67105.32 PMID:12912812

Boon, A., Cheriex, E., Lodder, J., & Kessels, F. (1997). Cardiac valve calcification: Characteristics of patients with calcification of the mitral annulus or aortic valve. *Heart (British Cardiac Society)*, *78*(5), 472–474. doi:10.1136/hrt.78.5.472 PMID:9415006

Brener, S. J., Duffy, C. I., Thomas, J. D., & Stewart, W. J. (1995). Progression of aortic stenosis in 394 patients: Relation to changes in myocardial and mitral valve dysfunction. *Journal of the American College of Cardiology*, *25*(2), 305–310. doi:10.1016/0735-1097(94)00406-G PMID:7829781

Brown, J. M., O'Brien, S. M., Wu, C., Sikora, J. A., Griffith, B. P., & Gammie, J. S. (2009). Isolated aortic valve replacement in North America comprising 108,687 patients in 10 years: changes in risks, valve types, and outcomes in the Society of Thoracic Surgeons National Database. *Journal of Thoracic and Cardiovascular Surgery, 137*(1), 82-90. doi: S0022-5223(08)01409-8 [pii] 10.1016/j.jtcvs.2008.08.015

Cheitlin, M. D., Gertz, E. W., Brundage, B. H., Carlson, C. J., Quash, J. A., & Bode, R. S. Jr. (1979). Rate of progression of severity of valvular aortic stenosis in the adult. *American Heart Journal*, *98*(6), 689–700. doi:10.1016/0002-8703(79)90465-4 PMID:495418

Coutinho, G. F., Correia, P. M., Pauperio, G., de Oliveira, F., & Antunes, M. J. (2011). Aortic root enlargement does not increase the surgical risk and short-term patient outcome? *European Journal of Cardio-Thoracic Surgery*, *40*(2), 441–447. doi:10.1016/j.ejcts.2010.11.064 PMID:21236693

Cowell, S. J., Newby, D. E., Prescott, R. J., Bloomfield, P., Reid, J., Northridge, D. B., & Boon, N. A.Lipid Lowering Trial, Impact on Regression Investigators. (2005). A randomized trial of intensive lipid-lowering therapy in calcific aortic stenosis. *The New England Journal of Medicine*, *352*(23), 2389–2397. doi:10.1056/NEJMoa043876 PMID:15944423

Davies, S. W., Gershlick, A. H., & Balcon, R. (1991). Progression of valvar aortic stenosis: A long-term retrospective study. *European Heart Journal*, *12*(1), 10–14. PMID:2009886

Dhareshwar, J., Sundt, T. M. III, Dearani, J. A., Schaff, H. V., Cook, D. J., & Orszulak, T. A. (2007). Aortic root enlargement: What are the operative risks? *The Journal of Thoracic and Cardiovascular Surgery*, *134*(4), 916–924. doi:10.1016/j.jtcvs.2007.01.097 PMID:17903507

Dua, A., Dang, P., Shaker, R., Varadarajan, P., & Pai, R. G. (2011). Barriers to surgery in severe aortic stenosis patients with Class I indications for aortic valve replacement. *The Journal of Heart Valve Disease*, *20*(4), 396–400. PMID:21863651

Eggebrecht, H., Schmermund, A., Voigtlander, T., Kahlert, P., Erbel, R., & Mehta, R. H. (2012). Risk of stroke after transcatheter aortic valve implantation (TAVI): A meta-analysis of 10,037 published patients. *EuroIntervention*, *8*(1), 129–138. doi:10.4244/EIJV8I1A20 PMID:22391581

Erkapic, D., De Rosa, S., Kelava, A., Lehmann, R., Fichtlscherer, S., & Hohnloser, S. H. (2012). Risk for permanent pacemaker after transcatheter aortic valve implantation: A comprehensive analysis of the literature. *Journal of Cardiovascular Electrophysiology*, *23*(4), 391–397. doi:10.1111/j.1540-8167.2011.02211.x PMID:22050112

Eveborn, G. W., Schirmer, H., Heggelund, G., Lunde, P., & Rasmussen, K. (2013). The evolving epidemiology of valvular aortic stenosis. the Tromso study. *Heart (British Cardiac Society)*, *99*(6), 396–400. doi:10.1136/heartjnl-2012-302265 PMID:22942293

Fairbairn, T. A., Mather, A. N., Bijsterveld, P., Worthy, G., Currie, S., Goddard, A. J., & Greenwood, J. P. et al. (2012). Diffusion-weighted MRI determined cerebral embolic infarction following transcatheter aortic valve implantation: Assessment of predictive risk factors and the relationship to subsequent health status. *Heart (British Cardiac Society)*, *98*(1), 18–23. doi:10.1136/heartjnl-2011-300065 PMID:21737581

Freed, B. H., Sugeng, L., Furlong, K., Mor-Avi, V., Raman, J., Jeevanandam, V., & Lang, R. M. (2010). Reasons for nonadherence to guidelines for aortic valve replacement in patients with severe aortic stenosis and potential solutions. *The American Journal of Cardiology*, *105*(9), 1339–1342. doi:10.1016/j.amjcard.2009.12.056 PMID:20403489

Furukawa, N., Kuss, O., Aboud, A., Schonbrodt, M., Renner, A., Hakim Meibodi, K., & Borgermann, J. et al. (2014). Ministernotomy versus conventional sternotomy for aortic valve replacement: Matched propensity score analysis of 808 patients. *European Journal of Cardio-Thoracic Surgery*, *46*(2), 221–226, discussion 226–227. doi:10.1093/ejcts/ezt616 PMID:24446478

Genereux, P., Head, S. J., Hahn, R., Daneault, B., Kodali, S., Williams, M. R., & Leon, M. B. et al. (2013). Paravalvular leak after transcatheter aortic valve replacement: The new Achilles' heel? A comprehensive review of the literature. *Journal of the American College of Cardiology*, *61*(11), 1125–1136. doi:10.1016/j.jacc.2012.08.1039 PMID:23375925

Genereux, P., Head, S. J., Van Mieghem, N. M., Kodali, S., Kirtane, A. J., Xu, K., & Leon, M. B. et al. (2012). Clinical outcomes after transcatheter aortic valve replacement using valve academic research consortium definitions: A weighted meta-analysis of 3,519 patients from 16 studies. *Journal of the American College of Cardiology*, *59*(25), 2317–2326. doi:10.1016/j.jacc.2012.02.022 PMID:22503058

Genereux, P., Kodali, S. K., Green, P., Paradis, J. M., Daneault, B., Rene, G., & Williams, M. R. et al. (2013). Incidence and effect of acute kidney injury after transcatheter aortic valve replacement using the new valve academic research consortium criteria. *The American Journal of Cardiology*, *111*(1), 100–105. doi:10.1016/j.amjcard.2012.08.057 PMID:23040657

Go, A. S., Mozaffarian, D., Roger, V. L., Benjamin, E. J., Berry, J. D., Borden, W. B., & Turner, M. B. et al.Stroke Statistics, Subcommittee. (2013). Heart disease and stroke statistics--2013 update: A report from the American Heart Association. *Circulation*, *127*(1), e6–e245. doi:10.1161/CIR.0b013e31828124ad PMID:23239837

Greenbaum, A. B., O'Neill, W. W., Paone, G., Guerrero, M. E., Wyman, J. F., Cooper, R. L., & Lederman, R. J. (2014). Caval-aortic access to allow transcatheter aortic valve replacement in otherwise ineligible patients: Initial human experience. *Journal of the American College of Cardiology*, *63*(2525 Pt A), 2795–2804. doi:10.1016/j.jacc.2014.04.015 PMID:24814495

Guyton, R. A., Block, P. C., Thourani, V. H., Lerakis, S., & Babaliaros, V. (2013). Carotid artery access for transcatheter aortic valve replacement. *Catheterization and Cardiovascular Interventions*, *82*(4), E583–E586. doi:10.1002/ccd.24596 PMID:22887932

Holmes, D. R. Jr, Mack, M. J., Kaul, S., Agnihotri, A., Alexander, K. P., Bailey, S. R., & Thomas, J. D. et al. (2012). 2012 ACCF/AATS/SCAI/STS expert consensus document on transcatheter aortic valve replacement. *Journal of the American College of Cardiology*, *59*(13), 1200–1254. doi:10.1016/j.jacc.2012.01.001 PMID:22300974

Huber, C. H., Goeber, V., Berdat, P., Carrel, T., & Eckstein, F. (2007). Benefits of cardiac surgery in octogenarians--a postoperative quality of life assessment. *European Journal of Cardio-Thoracic Surgery*, *31*(6), 1099–1105. doi:10.1016/j.ejcts.2007.01.055 PMID:17369044

Iung, B., & Vahanian, A. (2014). Epidemiology of Acquired Valvular Heart Disease. *The Canadian Journal of Cardiology*, *30*(9), 962–970. doi:10.1016/j.cjca.2014.03.022 PMID:24986049

Jamieson, W. R., Ye, J., Higgins, J., Cheung, A., Fradet, G. J., Skarsgard, P., & Lichtenstein, S. V. et al. (2010). Effect of prosthesis-patient mismatch on long-term survival with aortic valve replacement: Assessment to 15 years. *The Annals of Thoracic Surgery*, *89*(1), 51–58, discussion 59. doi:10.1016/j.athoracsur.2009.08.070 PMID:20103205

Kappetein, A. P., Head, S. J., Genereux, P., Piazza, N., van Mieghem, N. M., Blackstone, E. H., & Leon, M. B. et al. (2012). Updated standardized endpoint definitions for transcatheter aortic valve implantation: The Valve Academic Research Consortium-2 consensus document. *Journal of the American College of Cardiology*, *60*(15), 1438–1454. doi:10.1016/j.jacc.2012.09.001 PMID:23036636

Khatri, P. J., Webb, J. G., Rodes-Cabau, J., Fremes, S. E., Ruel, M., Lau, K., & Ko, D. T. et al. (2013). Adverse effects associated with transcatheter aortic valve implantation: A meta-analysis of contemporary studies. *Annals of Internal Medicine*, *158*(1), 35–46. doi:10.7326/0003-4819-158-1-201301010-00007 PMID:23277899

Kodali, S. K., Williams, M. R., Smith, C. R., Svensson, L. G., Webb, J. G., & Makkar, R. R. et al. Investigators, Partner Trial. (2012). Two-year outcomes after transcatheter or surgical aortic-valve replacement. *The New England Journal of Medicine*, *366*(18), 1686–1695. doi:10.1056/NEJMoa1200384 PMID:22443479

Kolh, P., Lahaye, L., Gerard, P., & Limet, R. (1999). Aortic valve replacement in the octogenarians: Perioperative outcome and clinical follow-up. *European Journal of Cardio-Thoracic Surgery*, *16*(1), 68–73. doi:10.1016/S1010-7940(99)00146-3 PMID:10456406

Leon, M. B., Smith, C. R., Mack, M., Miller, D. C., Moses, J. W., Svensson, L. G., & Pocock, S. et al. (2010). Transcatheter aortic-valve implantation for aortic stenosis in patients who cannot undergo surgery. *The New England Journal of Medicine*, *363*(17), 1597–1607. doi:10.1056/NEJMoa1008232 PMID:20961243

Likosky, D. S., Sorensen, M. J., Dacey, L. J., Baribeau, Y. R., Leavitt, B. J., DiScipio, A. W., & O'Connor, G. T. et al.Northern New England Cardiovascular Disease Study, Group. (2009). Long-term survival of the very elderly undergoing aortic valve surgery. *Circulation*, *120*(11Suppl), S127–S133. doi:10.1161/CIRCULATIONAHA.108.842641 PMID:19752357

Lindroos, M., Kupari, M., Heikkila, J., & Tilvis, R. (1993). Prevalence of aortic valve abnormalities in the elderly: an echocardiographic study of a random population sample. *Journal of the American College of Cardiology, 21*(5), 1220-1225. doi: 0735-1097(93)90249-Z [pii]

Lytle, B. W., Cosgrove, D. M., Taylor, P. C., Goormastic, M., Stewart, R. W., Golding, L. A., & Loop, F. D. et al. (1989). Primary isolated aortic valve replacement. Early and late results. *The Journal of Thoracic and Cardiovascular Surgery*, *97*(5), 675–694. PMID:2709860

Michelena, H. I., Desjardins, V. A., Avierinos, J. F., Russo, A., Nkomo, V. T., Sundt, T. M., & Enriquez-Sarano, M. et al. (2008). Natural history of asymptomatic patients with normally functioning or minimally dysfunctional bicuspid aortic valve in the community. *Circulation*, *117*(21), 2776–2784. doi:10.1161/CIRCULATIONAHA.107.740878 PMID:18506017

Miller, D. C., Blackstone, E. H., Mack, M. J., Svensson, L. G., Kodali, S. K., Kapadia, S., . . . Executive, Committee. (2012). Transcatheter (TAVR) versus surgical (AVR) aortic valve replacement: occurrence, hazard, risk factors, and consequences of neurologic events in the PARTNER trial. *Journal of Thoracic and Cardiovascular Surgery, 143*(4), 832-843 e813. doi: 10.1016/j.jtcvs.2012.01.055

Moat, N. E., Ludman, P., de Belder, M. A., Bridgewater, B., Cunningham, A. D., Young, C. P., & Mullen, M. J. et al. (2011). Long-term outcomes after transcatheter aortic valve implantation in high-risk patients with severe aortic stenosis: The U.K. TAVI (United Kingdom Transcatheter Aortic Valve Implantation) Registry. *Journal of the American College of Cardiology*, *58*(20), 2130–2138. doi:10.1016/j.jacc.2011.08.050 PMID:22019110

Moon, M. R., Pasque, M. K., Munfakh, N. A., Melby, S. J., Lawton, J. S., Moazami, N., & Damiano, R. J. Jr et al.. (2006). Prosthesis-patient mismatch after aortic valve replacement: Impact of age and body size on late survival. *The Annals of Thoracic Surgery*, *81*(2), 481–488, discussion 489. doi:10.1016/j.athoracsur.2005.07.084 PMID:16427836

Nassimiha, D., Aronow, W. S., Ahn, C., & Goldman, M. E. (2001). Rate of progression of valvular aortic stenosis in patients > or = 60 years of age. *American Journal of Cardiology, 87*(6), 807-809, A809.

Nietlispach, F., Johnson, M., Moss, R. R., Wijesinghe, N., Gurvitch, R., Tay, E. L., & Webb, J. G. et al. (2010). Transcatheter closure of paravalvular defects using a purpose-specific occluder. *JACC: Cardiovascular Interventions, 3*(7), 759–765. doi:10.1016/j.jcin.2010.04.013 PMID:20650438

Nishimura, R. A., Otto, C. M., Bonow, R. O., Carabello, B. A., Erwin, J. P. III, Guyton, R. A., & Thomas, J. D. et al. (2014). 2014 AHA/ACC guideline for the management of patients with valvular heart disease: executive summary: a report of the American College of Cardiology/American Heart Association Task Force on Practice Guidelines. *Journal of the American College of Cardiology, 63*(22), 2438–2488. doi:10.1016/j.jacc.2014.02.537 PMID:24603192

Nkomo, V. T., Gardin, J. M., Skelton, T. N., Gottdiener, J. S., Scott, C. G., & Enriquez-Sarano, M. (2006). Burden of valvular heart diseases: A population-based study. *Lancet, 368*(9540), 1005–1011. doi:10.1016/S0140-6736(06)69208-8 PMID:16980116

Nombela-Franco, L., Webb, J. G., de Jaegere, P. P., Toggweiler, S., Nuis, R. J., Dager, A. E., & Rodes-Cabau, J. et al. (2012). Timing, predictive factors, and prognostic value of cerebrovascular events in a large cohort of patients undergoing transcatheter aortic valve implantation. *Circulation, 126*(25), 3041–3053. doi:10.1161/CIRCULATIONAHA.112.110981 PMID:23149669

O'Brien, S. M., Shahian, D. M., Filardo, G., Ferraris, V. A., Haan, C. K., Rich, J. B., . . . Anderson, R. P. (2009). The Society of Thoracic Surgeons 2008 cardiac surgery risk models: part 2--isolated valve surgery. *Annals of Thoracic Surgery, 88*(1 Suppl), S23-42. doi: S0003-4975(09)01059-5 [pii] 10.1016/j.athoracsur.2009.05.056

Otto, C. M., Burwash, I. G., Legget, M. E., Munt, B. I., Fujioka, M., Healy, N. L., & Schwaegler, R. G. et al. (1997). Prospective study of asymptomatic valvular aortic stenosis. Clinical, echocardiographic, and exercise predictors of outcome. *Circulation, 95*(9), 2262–2270. doi:10.1161/01.CIR.95.9.2262 PMID:9142003

Otto, C. M., Pearlman, A. S., & Gardner, C. L. (1989). Hemodynamic progression of aortic stenosis in adults assessed by Doppler echocardiography. *Journal of the American College of Cardiology, 13*(3), 545–550. doi:10.1016/0735-1097(89)90590-1 PMID:2918158

Phan, K., Xie, A., Di Eusanio, M., & Yan, T. D. (2014). A Meta-Analysis of Minimally Invasive Versus Conventional Sternotomy for Aortic Valve Replacement. *The Annals of Thoracic Surgery, 98*(4), 1499–1511. doi:10.1016/j.athoracsur.2014.05.060 PMID:25064516

Pibarot, P., & Dumesnil, J. G. (2000). Hemodynamic and clinical impact of prosthesis-patient mismatch in the aortic valve position and its prevention. *Journal of the American College of Cardiology, 36*(4), 1131–1141. doi:10.1016/S0735-1097(00)00859-7 PMID:11028462

Popma, J. J., Adams, D. H., Reardon, M. J., Yakubov, S. J., Kleiman, N. S., & Heimansohn, D. et al.. CoreValve United States Clinical, Investigators. (2014). Transcatheter Aortic Valve Replacement Using A Self-Expanding Bioprosthesis in Patients With Severe Aortic Stenosis at Extreme Risk for Surgery. *Journal of the American College of Cardiology*. doi:10.1016/j.jacc.2014.02.556

Reid, C. L., Anton-Culver, H., Yunis, C., & Gardin, J. M. (2007). Prevalence and clinical correlates of isolated mitral, isolated aortic regurgitation, and both in adults aged 21 to 35 years (from the CARDIA study). *The American Journal of Cardiology*, *99*(6), 830–834. doi:10.1016/j.amjcard.2006.10.048 PMID:17350376

Ribeiro, H. B., Webb, J. G., Makkar, R. R., Cohen, M. G., Kapadia, S. R., Kodali, S., & Rodes-Cabau, J. et al. (2013). Predictive factors, management, and clinical outcomes of coronary obstruction following transcatheter aortic valve implantation: Insights from a large multicenter registry. *Journal of the American College of Cardiology*, *62*(17), 1552–1562. doi:10.1016/j.jacc.2013.07.040 PMID:23954337

Roberts, W. C., & Ko, J. M. (2005). Frequency by decades of unicuspid, bicuspid, and tricuspid aortic valves in adults having isolated aortic valve replacement for aortic stenosis, with or without associated aortic regurgitation. *Circulation*, *111*(7), 920–925. doi:10.1161/01.CIR.0000155623.48408.C5 PMID:15710758

Rodes-Cabau, J., Dumont, E., Boone, R. H., Larose, E., Bagur, R., Gurvitch, R., & Webb, J. G. et al. (2011). Cerebral embolism following transcatheter aortic valve implantation: Comparison of transfemoral and transapical approaches. *Journal of the American College of Cardiology*, *57*(1), 18–28. doi:10.1016/j.jacc.2010.07.036 PMID:21185496

Ross, J. Jr, & Braunwald, E. (1968). Aortic stenosis. *Circulation*, *38*(1Suppl), 61–67. PMID:4894151

Rossebo, A. B., Pedersen, T. R., Boman, K., Brudi, P., Chambers, J. B., Egstrup, K., & Willenheimer, R. et al. (2008). Intensive lipid lowering with simvastatin and ezetimibe in aortic stenosis. *The New England Journal of Medicine*, *359*(13), 1343–1356. doi:10.1056/NEJMoa0804602 PMID:18765433

Singh, J. P., Evans, J. C., Levy, D., Larson, M. G., Freed, L. A., Fuller, D. L., & Benjamin, E. J. et al. (1999). Prevalence and clinical determinants of mitral, tricuspid, and aortic regurgitation (the Framingham Heart Study). *The American Journal of Cardiology*, *83*(6), 897–902. doi:10.1016/S0002-9149(98)01064-9 PMID:10190406

Sinning, J. M., Hammerstingl, C., Vasa-Nicotera, M., Adenauer, V., Lema Cachiguango, S. J., Scheer, A. C., & Werner, N. et al. (2012). Aortic regurgitation index defines severity of peri-prosthetic regurgitation and predicts outcome in patients after transcatheter aortic valve implantation. *Journal of the American College of Cardiology*, *59*(13), 1134–1141. doi:10.1016/j.jacc.2011.11.048 PMID:22440213

Siontis, G. C., Juni, P., Pilgrim, T., Stortecky, S., Bullesfeld, L., Meier, B., & Windecker, S. et al. (2014). Predictors of permanent pacemaker implantation in patients with severe aortic stenosis undergoing TAVR: A meta-analysis. *Journal of the American College of Cardiology*, *64*(2), 129–140. doi:10.1016/j.jacc.2014.04.033 PMID:25011716

Smith, C. R., Leon, M. B., Mack, M. J., Miller, D. C., Moses, J. W., Svensson, L. G., & Pocock, S. J. et al. (2011). Transcatheter versus surgical aortic-valve replacement in high-risk patients. *The New England Journal of Medicine*, *364*(23), 2187–2198. doi:10.1056/NEJMoa1103510 PMID:21639811

Stewart, B. F., Siscovick, D., Lind, B. K., Gardin, J. M., Gottdiener, J. S., Smith, V. E., & Otto, C. M. et al. (1997). Clinical factors associated with calcific aortic valve disease. Cardiovascular Health Study. *Journal of the American College of Cardiology*, *29*(3), 630–634. doi:10.1016/S0735-1097(96)00563-3 PMID:9060903

Svensson, L. G., Adams, D. H., Bonow, R. O., Kouchoukos, N. T., Miller, D. C., O'Gara, P. T., & Williams, M. R. et al. (2013). Aortic valve and ascending aorta guidelines for management and quality measures. *The Annals of Thoracic Surgery*, *95*(6Suppl), S1–S66. doi:10.1016/j.athoracsur.2013.01.083 PMID:23688839

Takagi, H., Niwa, M., Mizuno, Y., Goto, S. N., & Umemoto, T. (2013). Incidence, predictors, and prognosis of acute kidney injury after transcatheter aortic valve implantation: A summary of contemporary studies using Valve Academic Research Consortium definitions. *International Journal of Cardiology*, *168*(2), 1631–1635. doi:10.1016/j.ijcard.2013.01.273 PMID:23453450

Tamburino, C., Capodanno, D., Ramondo, A., Petronio, A. S., Ettori, F., Santoro, G., & Ussia, G. P. et al. (2011). Incidence and predictors of early and late mortality after transcatheter aortic valve implantation in 663 patients with severe aortic stenosis. *Circulation*, *123*(3), 299–308. doi:10.1161/CIRCULATIONAHA.110.946533 PMID:21220731

Taramasso, M., Maisano, F., Latib, A., Denti, P., Guidotti, A., Sticchi, A., & Alfieri, O. (2014). *Conventional surgery and transcatheter closure via surgical transapical approach for paravalvular leak repair in high-risk patients: results from a single-centre experience*. European Heart Journal Cardiovascular Imaging; doi:10.1093/ehjci/jeu105

Tasca, G., Mhagna, Z., Perotti, S., Centurini, P. B., Sabatini, T., Amaducci, A., & Pibarot, P. et al. (2006). Impact of prosthesis-patient mismatch on cardiac events and midterm mortality after aortic valve replacement in patients with pure aortic stenosis. *Circulation*, *113*(4), 570–576. doi:10.1161/CIRCULATIONAHA.105.587022 PMID:16401767

Thanassoulis, G., Campbell, C. Y., Owens, D. S., Smith, J. G., Smith, A. V., Peloso, G. M., & Post, W. S. et al. (2013). Genetic associations with valvular calcification and aortic stenosis. *The New England Journal of Medicine*, *368*(6), 503–512. doi:10.1056/NEJMoa1109034 PMID:23388002

Thomas, M., Schymik, G., Walther, T., Himbert, D., Lefevre, T., Treede, H., & Wendler, O. et al. (2010). Thirty-day results of the SAPIEN aortic Bioprosthesis European Outcome (SOURCE) Registry: A European registry of transcatheter aortic valve implantation using the Edwards SAPIEN valve. *Circulation*, *122*(1), 62–69. doi:10.1161/CIRCULATIONAHA.109.907402 PMID:20566953

Thourani, V. H., Ailawadi, G., Szeto, W. Y., Dewey, T. M., Guyton, R. A., Mack, M. J., . . . Bavaria, J. E. (2011). Outcomes of surgical aortic valve replacement in high-risk patients: a multiinstitutional study. *Annals of Thoracic Surgery, 91*(1), 49-55; discussion 55-46. doi: 10.1016/j.athoracsur.2010.09.040

Turina, J., Hess, O., Sepulcri, F., & Krayenbuehl, H. P. (1987). Spontaneous course of aortic valve disease. *European Heart Journal*, *8*(5), 471–483. PMID:3609042

Vicchio, M., Della Corte, A., De Santo, L. S., De Feo, M., Caianiello, G., Scardone, M., & Cotrufo, M. (2008). Tissue versus mechanical prostheses: Quality of life in octogenarians. *The Annals of Thoracic Surgery*, *85*(4), 1290–1295. doi:10.1016/j.athoracsur.2007.12.039 PMID:18355512

Weber, A., Noureddine, H., Englberger, L., Dick, F., Gahl, B., Aymard, T., & Carrel, T. P. et al. (2012). Ten-year comparison of pericardial tissue valves versus mechanical prostheses for aortic valve replacement in patients younger than 60 years of age. *The Journal of Thoracic and Cardiovascular Surgery*, *144*(5), 1075–1083. doi:10.1016/j.jtcvs.2012.01.024 PMID:22341653

Chapter 24
Surgical Management of Mitral Valve Disease

Robin Varghese
Icahn School of Medicine at Mount Sinai, USA

ABSTRACT

Surgery for the mitral valve has increased over the last decade, with a focus on an increasing number of valve repairs for degenerative mitral valve disease. This chapter discusses the surgical management of mitral valve disease with a focus on the pathology of mitral valve stenosis and regurgitation. With an examination into the pathophysiology of the lesions. Subsequently a discussion regarding the various surgical techniques for mitral valve surgery followed by the major and minor complications of surgery are reviewed to provide the Intensivist with an overview of possible complications. Finally a look at the future direction of the field is briefly examined.

INTRODUCTION

With the advent of reliable valve repair, and better bioprosthetic valve replacement technology the incidence of mitral valve surgery has increased over the last decade.

Mitral valve lesions can broadly be divided into two main categories – those being regurgitation and stenosis. Trends in mitral valve surgery have shown an increase in the number of regurgitant lesions being repaired and for those valves requiring replacement a movement to the increasing use of bioprosthetic valves over mechanical valves (Gammie, Sheng et al., 2009). Indeed the management of patients after surgery on the mitral valve can be challenging especially in cases of left ventricular dysfunction and dilatation. In this chapter we will review a basic understanding of mitral valve anatomy and etiologies of mitral valve lesions and their importance in managing the postoperative patient. In addition an understanding of surgical indications and techniques will be discussed including valve replacement, and repair in a variety of conditions and their effect on postoperative care. A major focus will be placed on intraoperative and postoperative considerations and potential complications that the Intensivist must be cognizant of when managing patients after mitral valve surgery. Finally a focus on future research and novel strategies for addressing mitral valve disease will be reviewed.

DOI: 10.4018/978-1-4666-8603-8.ch024

EPIDEMIOLOGY

The incidence of the spectrum of mitral valve disease etiologies has changed over the last two decades with a fall in the number of cases of mitral stenosis secondary to rheumatic disease (Olson, Subramanian et al 1987). The incidence of mitral stenosis in the United States is the least common of all cardiac valve lesions and is estimated to be 0.1% with the frequency being evenly distributed among decades of life after the age of 50 (Nkomo, Gardin et al., 2006) The incidence of mitral regurgitation on the contrary is the most common cardiac valve lesion with an estimated incidence of 1.7% in the United States and having an increasing incidence with age. Surgical treatment for mitral stenosis has predominantly been mechanical valve replacement in the younger to middle-aged population, however this trend has changed towards an increasing use of bioprosthetic valve replacement Gammie, Sheng et al., 2009). In addition there has been a trend toward increasing mitral valve repair for mitral regurgitation secondary to degenerative (organic) mitral valve disease.

VALVE ANATOMY

The mitral valve is composed of a number of structures that function together allowing the valve to open in diastole and close in systole. There are five main components to allowing the mitral valve to function correctly: The valve leaflets, annulus, chordae tendineae, papillary muscles and the left ventricular wall. As the heart progresses through the cardiac cycle these components move together allowing for a competent valve. Anatomic or physiological changes to one or more of these components may lead to valve dysfunction.

There are two leaflets that comprise the mitral valve - anterior and posterior (Ranganathan, Lam et al., 1970). The region where the leaflets meet in continuity is referred to as the commissures. Although the leaflets are shaped differently they comprise the same surface area. The leaflets coapt along the rough zone which is thicker compared to the thinner atrial zone. Where the leaflets insert into the atrium is known as the annulus of the valve. The anterior aspect of the annulus is supported by the fibrous skeleton of the heart and as one moves towards the posterior annulus in a counterclockwise direction the fibrous support diminishes and eventually is absent leading to a more fragile region along the posterior annulus which is prone to dilatation (Wilcox & Anderson, 2004).

The chordae tendineae of the valve attach the leaflets to the papillary muscles. The chordae are divided into three main types depending on where they attach onto the leaflets (Lam, Ranganathan et al., 1970).

The primary chordae insert very close to the free margin of the leaflet edge. Secondary chordae attach to the leaflets usually in their mid portion in the ventricular side. Finally basal chordae extend from the ventricular wall or papillary muscle and insert at the base of the posterior leaflet.

Two large groups of papillary muscles are usually present – the anterolateral papillary muscle and posteromedial papillary muscle. Both muscle heads insert into the ventricular wall. These papillary muscles provide anchoring of the chordae that are also attached to the valve leaflets. The papillary muscles allow the left ventricle to play an important role in the function of the mitral valve. As the left ventricle contracts the papillary muscles also contract to avoid excess slack in the chordae and hence preventing the leaflets from prolapsing into the atrium resulting in mitral regurgitation.

In adults the mitral valve orfice is 4-6cm^2 when measured in cross-section (Iung, Gohlke-Barwolf et al., 2002).

ETIOLOGY OF MITRAL VALVE DISEASE

Mitral Stenosis

The most common cause of mitral stenosis (MS) in the world remains rheumatic disease, although it's incidence in the United States has fallen dramatically over the last two decades (Olson, Subramanian et al., 1987). Signs and symptoms of stenosis usually present decades after the initial pharyngitis from Group A streptococci. The characteristic pathophysiological changes in the valve involve calcification of the leaflets commencing at the commissures and chordae. As the commissures fuse the valve orifice contracts leaving a small central orifice. Chordae tendinae calcify and shorten leading to restriction of valve motion (Mann, Zipes et al., 2014). Other less common causes of MS include congenital MS, obstructive tumors, annular calcification, and large vegetations.

Mitral Regurgitation

Unlike stenosis, mitral regurgitation (MR) has a wide variety of etiologies, the most common being degenerative disease which composes of fibroelastic deficiency and Barlow's syndrome. Other causes include endocarditis, connective tissue disorders, rheumatic disease, ischemic heart disease, and annular dilatation. Given the varied causes of MR the Carpentier functional classification allows for a uniform method by which the valve pathology may be understood (Carpentier, Adams & Filsoufi, 2010). The valve dysfunction is divided into three categories: Type I dysfunction describes a valve with normal leaflet motion through the cardiac cycle. In this case the usual cause of valve dysfunction is annular dilatation. Type II dysfunction describes a valve with excess leaflet motion where either one or both leaflets prolapse above the plane of the annulus. This is often the most common finding in degenerative valve pathologies and may be secondary to chordal rupture/elongation. Finally type III dysfunction corresponds to a valve that has restricted leaflet motion and is divided into two categories depending on whether the restriction occurs in systole or diastole. Type IIIa dysfunction consists of a valve that has restricted motion in diastole and usually is a result of rheumatic valve disease. Type IIIb dysfunction describes a valve with restricted motion in systole and is often a result of ischemic heart disease leading to tethering of the chordae due to ventricular dilation or a wall motion abnormality.

PREOPERATIVE PRESENTATION AND HEMODYNAMICS

Mitral Stenosis

Mitral stenosis is classified into three categories – mild, moderate and severe. The degree of stenosis is based on measurements of valve orifice area, and transvalvular gradients **(Table 1).** The most common presentation in MS is dyspnea on exertion and palpitations. Symptoms initially occur with exercise when heart rate is increased. This leads to an increased circulating blood volume in the presence of a shorter diastolic filling time. In MS, ventricular filling is delayed and so it is dependent on the diastolic filling time to maximize preload. Hence as patient's exercise or increase their activity levels the relative tachycardia shortens diastole therefore decreasing ventricular filling leading to a diminished cardiac output. The residual "excess" volume left behind in the atrium leads to an increased left atrial pressure

Table 1. Classification of severity in mitral valve disease

	Mild	Moderate	Severe
Mitral Stenosis	MG < 5 mmHg MVA >1.5cm^2 DPHT: <150ms	MG 5-10mmHg MVA 1.0-1.5cm^2 DPHT: 150-220ms	MG >10mmHg MVA <1.0cm^2 DPHT: >220ms
Mitral Regurgitation	Vena contraca <0.3cm ERV <30ml EROA: <0.20cm^2	Vena contracta 0.3-0.7cm ERV: <60ml EROA: < 0.40cm^2	Vena contracta ≥0.7 ERV: ≥60ml EROA: ≥ 0.40cm^2

MG: mean gradient, MVA: mitral valve area, DPHT: diastolic pressure-half time, ERV: effective regurgitant volume, EROA: effective regurgitant orifice area

(LAP) which inturn leads to a fall in the transpulmonary gradient. This may result in capillary leak and symptoms of pulmonary congestion. In cases of severe mitral stenosis acute tachycardia can lead to pulmonary edema. Although in the presence of a normal heart the atrial kick provides about 25% of to the ventricular preload, in cases if severe mitral stenosis the atrial kick can contribute up to 40% or more of ventricular preload. Hence in atrial tachy-arrhythmmias such as atrial flutter or atrial fibrillation acute symptoms of dyspnea and orthopnea can occur secondary to acute pulmonary congestion. Hence it is of vital importance to maintain atrial-ventricular synchrony with a slower heart rate to maximize ventricular preload in the setting of a fixed obstruction. Patients are often recommended to be maintained on antiarrhythmics such as beta blockers or calcium channel blockers to maintain sinus rhythm with a slower rate to maximize diastolic filling time prior to surgical correction.

Patients with MS exhibit altered left atrial pressures and over time subsequent increases in right atrial pressures. The left atrial pressure waveform shows a prominent atrial contraction (a wave) with a gradual pressure decline during diastole during ventricular filling (gradual y descent) (Choi, Bacharach et al., 1995). In patients with increased pulmonary vascular resistance (PVR), pulmonary arterial pressures will be elevated a volume overload ensues. This increased PAP can lead to inadequate emptying of the right ventricle (RV) and hence an elevated JVP is often found at central venous pressures rise. The left ventricular diastolic pressure is normal in the majority of patients with isolated MS and reduced in the remaining patients. Measurements of Left ventricular (LV) systolic performance revealed a slight reduction in these parameters likely due to reduced preload and increased afterload (Choi, Bacharach et al., 1995). Despite this, measurements in ventricular contractility is normal in the majority of patients. Compared with the LV, the changes in the left atrium are marked.

Increased volume and pressure load on the left atrium leads to atrial dilatation and fibrosis of the atrial wall. This results in disorganization of the atrial muscle bundles which result in rhythm disturbances secondary to differing atrial conduction velocities and refractory periods. These conduction disturbances can result in atrial fibrillation which is an independent predictor of severity of MS (Moreyra, Wilson et al., 1998).

Mitral Regurgitation

MR is classified into three degrees of severity – mild, moderate and severe. The degree of severity is based on objective parameters such as effective regurgitation volume, effective regurgitation orifice area, proximal isovelocity surface area, and vena contracta (**Table 1**) (Zoghbi, Enriquez-Sarano et al., 2003). Qualitative methods include, reversal of flow in the pulmonary veins, left atrial enlargement, presence of multiple large regurgitant jets by color Doppler. As with MS symptoms with mitral regurgitation are most often dyspnea on exertion and palpitations. The degree of regurgitation is dynamic as a number of factors can worsen or improve the degree of regurgitation. As left atrial pressure is markedly lower than systemic pressure a large portion (up to 50%) of the total regurgitation volume is ejected in the left atrium prior to the aortic valve opening. As afterload increases the amount of regurgitant volume increases. The size of the regurgitant orifice area in the most important predictor in the amount of regurgitation. Increasing contractility decreased the ventricular chamber size bringing the mitral leaflets closer to together and hence decreasing this regurgitant orifice. On the other hand factors that lead the dilatation of the LV such as volume overload or ischemia may worsen the degree of MR. In the early phase of the disease process the LV compensates for the MR but emptying more completely as a portion of blood is ejected back against the low left atrial pressure. Over time as the left ventricle dilates it continues to compensate until the dilatation occurs out of proportion with an increase in LV mass. This leads to an increased end diastolic volume (EDV), and although the forward stroke volume may remain mostly unchanged, given the increased EDV the effective ejection fraction begins to fall. At this course of the disease, patients continue to increase the circulating blood volume to maintain forward stroke volume, which eventually results in rising LAP and a lowering of the transpulmonary gradient with volume overload leading to pulmonary congestion and the symptoms of heart failure. Compensation can be maintained for years however on average most patient will develop symptoms with 7 years (Rosenhek, Rader et al., 2006).

Clear data exists illustrating that as left ventricular ejection fraction (LVEF) falls below 40% it is difficult to improve LV function back to normal and in the majority of cases EF falls postoperatively. Furthermore preoperative ejection fraction above 60% is a predictor of long-term survival (Enriquez-Sarano, Tajik et al., 1994).

INDICATIONS FOR SURGICAL INTERVENTION

Mitral Stenosis

By enlarge surgical intervention for mitral stenosis is based on guidelines provided by the American Heart Association/American College of Cardiology (ACC/AHA) (Nishimura, Otto et al., 2014). The basic premise of the guidelines is that intervention is not required until symptoms develop and in a large number of cases percutaneous mitral balloon commisurotomy (PMBC) is the initial therapy of choice when intervention is required. Not all valves are amenable to PMBC and Wilkin's scoring system can be used to assist in predicting which valves are most likely to achieve success from PMBC (Wilkins, Weyman et al., 1988) (Padial, Abascal et al., 1999). Particularly valves with moderate MR at the outset, severely calcified leaflets are not recommended for PMBC. In addition the presence of left atrial clot is a contraindication to PMBC. These patients should be referred for surgical repair/replacement of the valve in addition to atrial thrombectomy if needed.

Mitral Regurgitation

Similar to MS surgical intervention for MR is based on guidelines provided by the American Heart Association/American College of Cardiology (Nishimura, Otto et al., 2014). Unlike MS, surgical intervention for severe MR is advocated based on changes in LV size and function in addition to valve reparability and symptoms. It is currently recommended to perform MV Repair for asymptomatic patients with severe MR if valve the likelihood of valve repairability is >95% and operative mortality is <1%. If this is not the case then patients should either be referred to specialized centers than can offer these results or patients may undergo careful monitoring until symptoms develop or changes in EF or LV size occur. The survival advantage of repair over replacement diminishes as patients age and hence some argue for replacement in the elderly with complex regurgitant valves as the replacement will last the patient's lifetime, despite the increased risk of stroke and endocarditis compared with repair, arguing that if a repair fails early a reoperation in the elderly comes is significant morbidity. Although not present in the American guidelines, the European Society of Cardiology/European Association for Cardio-Thoracic Surgery (ESC/EACTS) guidelines consider atrial fibrillation and left atrial size in the decision-making for surgical intervention (Vahanian, Alfieri et al., 2012).

SURGICAL TECHNIQUES AND CONTROVERSIES

Incision and Cannulation Options

The two main approaches for mitral valve exposure is the standard full or partial median sternotomy or a left anterior thoracotomy. A right anterior thoracotomy approach has been mostly abandoned in favor of the previously stated options.

The full median sternotomy approach can be done with a full skin incision (18-25 centimeters) or small skin incision 8-11cm for cosmesis. With the smaller incision small cannulae for cardiopulmonary bypass are required which likely necessitate the use of vaccum assisted drainage. With a thoracotomy approach a 5-10cm incision is made in the 4 or 5th intercostal space and cardiopulmonary bypass often established peripherally via the femoral artery/vein and often times the superior vena cava is cannulated via the right internal jugular vein. Relative contrandications to a thoracotomy approach to valve repair include previous surgical entry into the right thoracic cavity, poor pulmonary function with inability to tolerate single-lung ventilation, and concominant cardiac surgical procedures where greater exposure to the heart is required. Depending on the size of the aortic cannulae a formal incision will be required in the groin. In general cannulae which are 19 French or larger require a femoral cut-down and primary repair of the arterial cannulation site. Larger arterial cannulae provide less resistance and hence less shearing forces on the component blood cells. Furthermore larger cannulae decrease the maximum velocity at which the blood is ejected out of the aortic cannulae thereby minimizing the possibility of arterial injury. In the same way smaller and longer venous cannulae increase resistance and hence decrease venous drainage into the cardiopulmonary bypass reservoir. Often times to compensate vacuum-assisted drainage is required to improve the venous drainage. Once the heart is exposed the mitral valve can be accessed by two common techniques. One is via dissection of the interatrial (Sondergaard's) groove followed by an incision directly in the the left atrium. The second common option is to enter the right atrium followed by an incision in the interatrial septum which arrives one into the left atrium. A less common approach is via the left atrial room behind the ascending aorta. This option is sometimes employed when the aorta is transected for aortic root work that is concomitantly required.

With the exception of the rarely employed left atrial roof technique bicaval cannulation is required to establish adequate drainage from both the superior vena cava (SVC) and inferior vena cava (IVC) and exposure of the mitral valve often leads to torsion on the great veins which may lead to obstruction of drainage from these vessels if a single cannulae is placed in the right atrium. Once the heart is arrested and the valve is exposed the surgeon should inspect the CVP to ensure it is low suggesting that drainage of the SVC is adequate. They should also communicate with the perfusionist to ensure that there hasn't been a change in drainage due to malpositioned cannulae after the valve has been exposed with retractors.

The incision type can also vary the cardioplegia strategy for arresting and protecting the heart during the operation. The two modes of cardioplegia delivery are the antegrade cardioplegia delivery method where the cardioplegia solution is directed in the ascending aorta below the cross clamp and into the coronary arteries. This is obviously dependent on a competent aortic valve and no proximal stenosis in the main coronary arteries. The retrograde cardioplegia delivery method requires the insertion of a catheter into the coronary sinus which cardioplegia is delivery in "backwards" fashion to through the veins to the capillaries and then drains back to the arteries and through the left and right main coronary ostia. This method is beneficial when the aortic valve in incompetent which is often the case when the left atrium is retracted to expose the mitral valve. Concerns with this method arise if the catheter is placed beyond the middle cardiac vein which drains the right ventricle. Theoretically there can be very little cardioplegia delivery to the middle cardiac vein. Fortunately a number of the commonly used cannaulae allow for blood drainage to pass backwards from the cannuale tip and ensure delivery to the middle cardiac vein. Cardioplegia can also be administered warm or cold with the majority of centers using cold cardioplegia in the range of 4°C. Most standard cardioplegia solutions should be administered every 20-30 minutes. Some cardioplegia solution have been shown to require longer time intervals between redosing. At each dose it is of utmost importance for the surgeon to ensure that the cardioplegia is being delivered. In mitral valve surgery this is usually via the retrograde catheter. Confirmation of delivery can be achieved by seeing return of cardioplegia into the left ventricle which has leaked down from the coronary ostia through the aortic valve, distention of the middle cardiac vein in the inferior wall of the right ventricle. If using a myocardial temperature probe a fall in myocardial temperature should ensue shortly after delivery when cold cardioplegia is administered. Finally a lack of cardiac activity throughout the operation is suggesting of adequate delivery.

The incision type is also important to consider when managing the postoperative valve patient in that it pain issues will be different. There may be multiple incisions with a thoracotomy approach but only one with a sternotomy approach. If major bleeding occurred postoperatively via a sternotomy approach opening the chest at the bedside is easier for the surgical team to control bleeding with manual pressure and also carryout intracardiac massage if needed. On the other hand if major hemorrhage occurred via a mini-thoracotomy the incision may require being extended and despite this, adequate lighting may not be available to locate bleeding in the deep thorax. Alternatively an emergency sternotomy could be performed and the intensive care unit should have adequate equipment and protocols in place to address this scenario.

Valve Replacement and Repair

Mitral valve replacement is an established and safe way to address mitral stenosis or mitral regurgitation when repair durability is of concern. Mitral valve repair with various mechanical prosthesis began in the 1960's and bioprosthetic valves followed in the 1970's. Mechanical valves have been shown to possess longer freedom from structural failure, but require life-long anticoagulation with warfarin and make an audible click each time the valve closes. Bioprosthetic valve can be used without long-term warfarin therapy, but have a durability between 8-20 years depending on patient age. These factors come into play when deciding on valve choice with the patient. The most commonly used bioprosthetic valves include a porcine valve and a valve constructed from bovine pericardium. Both valves show excellent durability which increases with patient age.

Valve replacement for mechanical valves requires careful assessment to ensure that any chordal/leaflet preservation will not impede with mechanical leaflet function. This is less of a concern with bioproshtetic valve replacement. In both cases once the valve is sutured in place it should be tested to ensure adequate opening and closing prior to closing the atrium.

Most degenerative valves can be repaired in valve centers with appropriate expertise. Unlike valve replacement the annuloplasty sutures are non-plegetted and serve to decrease the annular size as well as secure the annuloplasty ring in place. The sutures in both valve replacement and repair are placed near important cardiac structures which can result in complications if injured during this process (see figure 1). The selection of ring sizing in mitral valve repair is done based on the intercommissural distance as well as the length of the anterior leaflet from the mid point at the annulus to it's free edge. Valve repair techniques can involve resection of unsupported or damaged leaflet tissue, use of sliding plasty, placement of neochordae, closure of gaps between leaflet segments, and commissuroplasty (Varghese & Adams, 2011).

Concomitant tricuspid valve surgery for moderate TR or tricuspid annular dilatation is performed at varying incidences based on surgeon preference. The current retrospective observational data suggests a tricuspid annuloplasty may decrease the incidence of future tricuspid regurgitation but a clinical trial has not been performed to date (Anyanwu, Chikwe et al., 2008), (Dreyfus, Corbi et al., 2005).

Once the valve repair/replacement is completed and atria are closed the heart is appropriately de-aired and the cross clamp removed under low flow conditions.

Ventricular pacing wires are recommended in all cases in the event of heart block or bradycardia postoperatively. An atrial pacing wires is beneficial in cases of LV or RV dysfunction to improve preload and provide AV synchrony optimal ventricular contraction. Occasionally a very friable atrium may dissuade the surgical team from placing an atrial wire.

Figure 1.

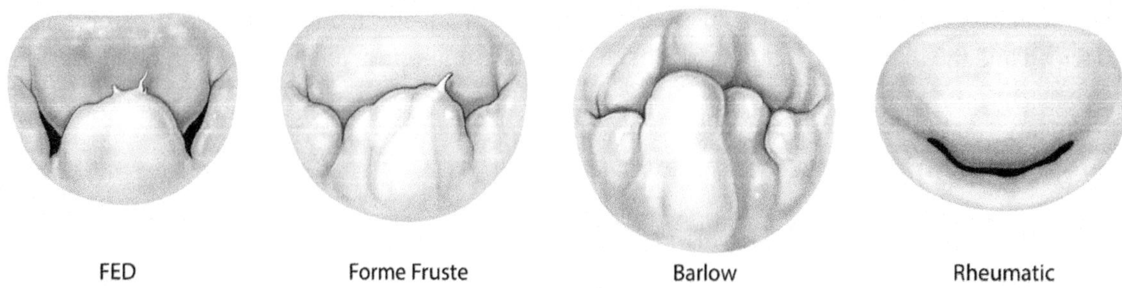

Figure 2.

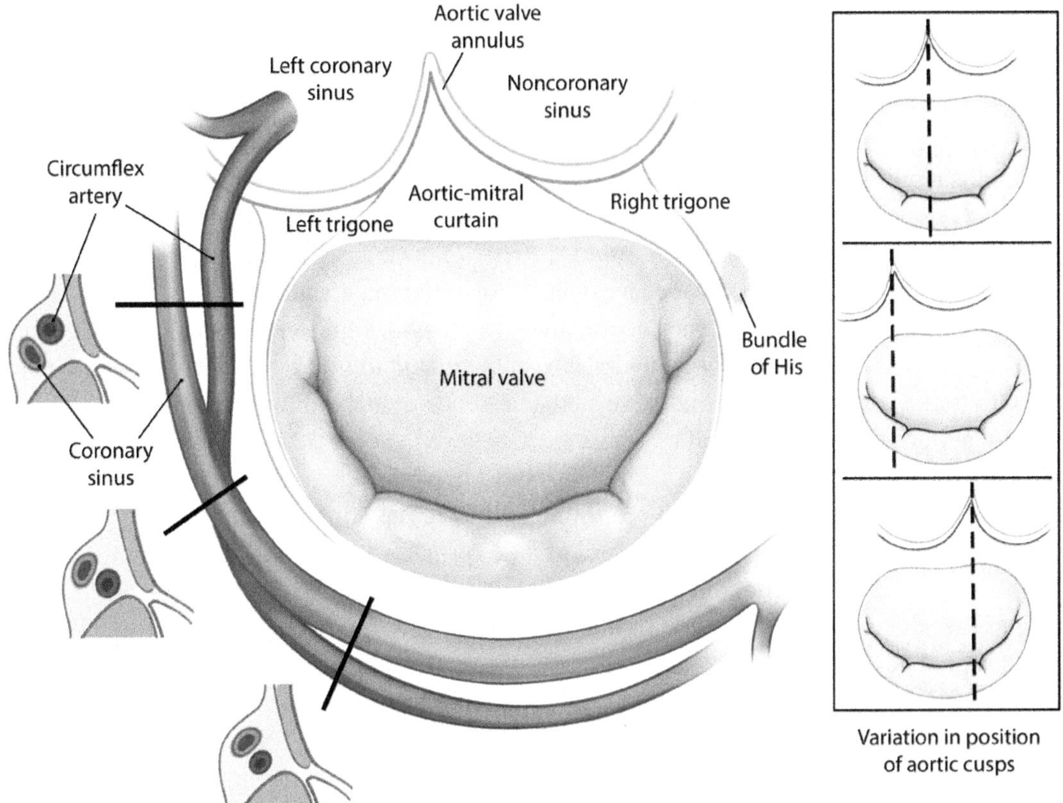

COMPLICATIONS

Heart Block: Permanent complete heart block with mitral valve surgery is uncommon ranging between 2-4%, while temporary second-degree or third-degree block occurs more frequently in the perioperative period. Hence all patients should receive temporary pacing wires. Ensuring appropriate sensing of the ventricular wire is important to avoid inappropriate discharge of the pacemaker during ventricular repolarization which may lead to Torsades de Pointes.

Residual MR: Residual mitral regurgitation after valve repair predicts valve durability. In the majority of cases elective valve repairs with residual MR will lead to the surgeon arresting the heart again to readdress the residual regurgitation. In cases where the valve repair is palliative such as that in an elderly patient with severe mitral annular calcification (MAC), or in a young patient where the only other option would be replacement, residual MR may be accepted as replacement is not a good option or not safely possible.

Low Cardiac Output Syndrome (LCOS): This may occur for a variety of reasons including preoperative poor LV function, ventricular stunning from prolonged cross-clamp time, poor myocardial protection, coronary injury or a combination of these (Varghese, Itagaki et al., 2014). A new regional lateral wall motion abnormality raises concern for circumflex coronary artery injury. In some cases flow can be seen on Transesophageal Echocardiography (TEE). As discussed previously injury to the circumflex coronary artery can occur from valve annuloplasty or replacement sutures leading to a "kink" or outright suture compression of the circumflex artery. If this occurs the wall motion abnormality occurs within minutes of removing the cross clamp and when weaning from cardiopulmonary bypass. The options to the surgeon include opening the left atrium to remove the sutures in this area and reinsert new sutures or bypass the circumflex coronary artery. If there is localized inferior wall hypokinesis and a tricuspid valve repair was performed the surgeon must always consider injury to the right coronary artery prior to its main bifurcation (Varghese, Akujuo & Adams, 2010). In these cases the anterior RV wall may possess normal function as the compression occurs further down the main right coronary artery. These cases are often more difficult to detect as they do not always arise with significant hemodynamic compromise and a small amount of inferior wall hypokinesis can be related to micro air emboli down the coronary artery. Often times the distinguishing factor is the presence of arrhythmias when there is injury to the right coronary artery. The options in this case are to relieve the obstruction by removing the offending suture and replacing it or performing a coronary artery bypass of the right coronary artery. Global LV dysfunction suggests stunning of the myocardium. In these cases support with inotropes is required and occasionally an intra aortic balloon pump is placed do further assist the heart.

Right Ventricular Dysfunction: RV dysfunction can be difficult problem to manage. Furthermore when it ensues or worsens after arrival in the intensive care unit, it can be a difficult problem to diagnose and should be on the forefront of the Intensivist's mind. Temporary intraoperative RV dysfunction can occur early due to micro air emboli into the right coronary artery which sits anterior in the aortic call and hence by gravity is more likely to collect micro air from the LV during de-airing of the heart. This usually resolves quick with reperfusion of the heart and once the air has been passed through the coronary tree. Persistent RV dysfunction can be seen both by direct examination of the right ventricle in the surgical field and on TEE. After appropriate reperfusion a distended minimally contracting RV raises concern for a more persistent RV that will require medical support. If this fails, mechanical support with IABP can be considered, or rarely temporary assist devices.

Aortic Valve Injury: The presence of new aortic insufficiency after mitral valve repair or replacement is concerning for a leaflet injury secondary to a suture in the anterior annulus grabbing the non-coronary or left coronary leaflets of the aortic valve. The management here usually involves arresting the heart and replacing the inciting suture and also inspecting the aortic valve to ensure that it does not need additional repair. Occasionally valve replacement may be required.

Bleeding from Atrioventricular (AV) Groove Disruption: The AV groove along the posterior annulus of the mitral valve is devoid of much fibrous tissue. Hence it is less robust and more prone to injury and disruption of the AV groove. This most commonly occurs in elderly females with fragile atrial tissue. This complication first arises usually after the cross-clamp has been removed and the patient is weaned from cardiopulmonary bypass. A large amount of red blood collects in the pericardial well. The exact location is often difficult to determine as the bleeding is arising from the AV groove at the base of the heart. Given the gravity and treatment for AV disruptions the surgeon should ensure that bleeding is not arising from the atrial suture line, or the left atrial appendage if it was manipulated (ligated, excised) during the operation. If an AV groove disruption is the most likely concern the treatment is re-arrest the heart, remove the prothetic mitral valve/ring, repair the tear with a patch, place one size smaller valve or If previously repaired, replace the valve with an undersized prosthesis. This may still not repair the tear and the patient may continue to bleed requiring surgical packing, massive transfusions and an open-chest to the ICU. Avoiding hypertension is imperative in this situation as the systemic afterload increases ventricular systolic pressures that in turn apply pressure on the fragile repair site.

Systolic Anterior Motion (SAM): SAM refers to displacement of the free-edge of the anterior leaflet into the left ventricular outflow tract (LVOT) during systole (Carpentier, Adams & Filsoufi, 2010). This can result in LVOT obstruction that ranges from mild to severe and can also lead to MR as the coaptation line is disrupted. SAM can occur primarily prior to valve repair as a result of hypertrophic cardiomyopathy or it may occur secondarily to valve repair. Factors that narrow the distance between the coaptation line and the LVOT increase the risk for SAM. Therefore predictors for SAM after mitral valve repair include a hyperdynamic LV, small ventricular size, thickened basal septum, long posterior leaflet and a narrow aorto-mitral angle (<120^{0}) (Varghese, Itagaki et al., 2014). Management of SAM always starts with medical therapy which aims to maximize ventricular filling thereby increasing the distance from the anterior leaflet and the LVOT. Specifically these measures including: increasing preload, decreasing heart rate, increasing afterload and decreasing contractility (which is usually hyperdynamic). A detailed algorithm for the management of SAM is shown in Figure 3 & 4. With medical therapy the majority of SAM will resolve. Occasionally re-repair of the valve is required for severe cases of SAM. Upon arrival

Figure 3.

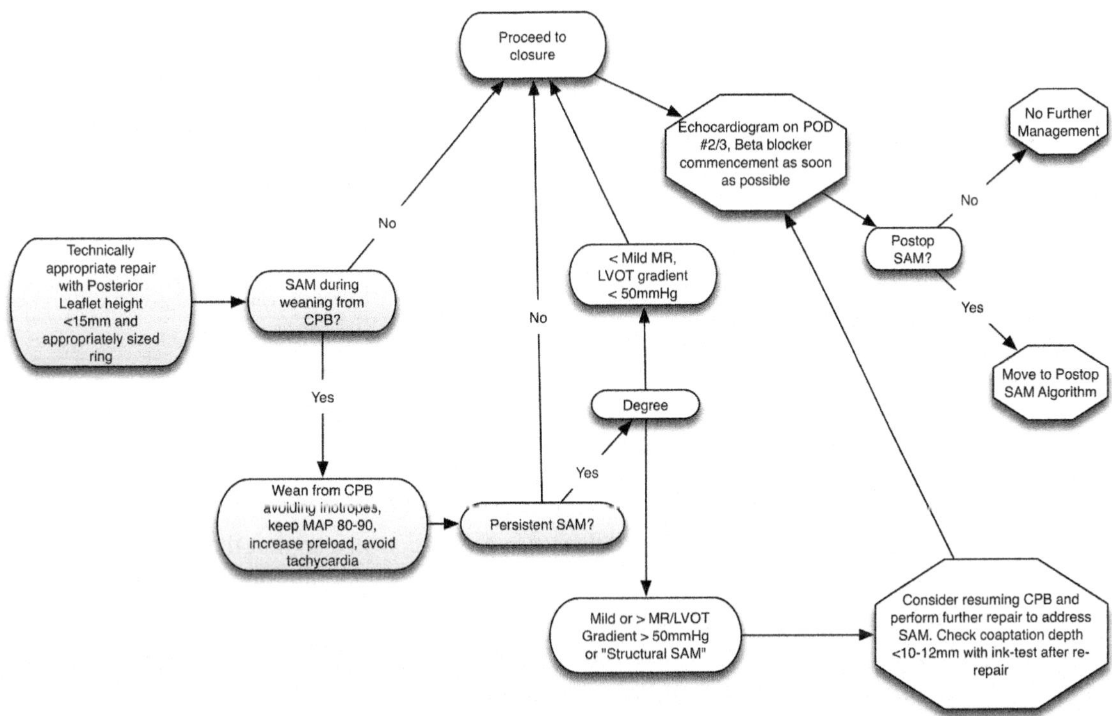

Figure 4.

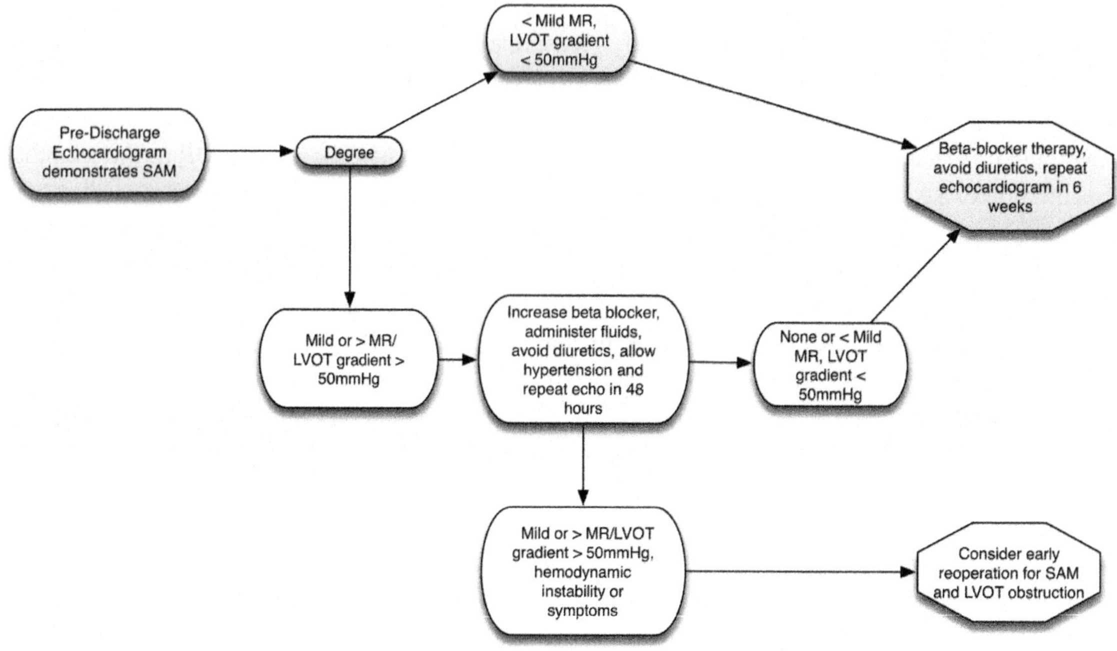

Table 2. Comparison of Sternotomy and thoracotomy incisions

	Sternotomy	Right Thoracotomy
Usual incision length	8-20 cm	5-10cm
Additional Incisions	None	Peripheral cannulation, stab incision for cross clamp
Cannulation strategies	Ascending aorta and direct SVC and IVC (via right atrium)	Axillary/femoral artery femoral vein, internal jugular
Concomitant procedures	All cardiac procedures	Tricuspid valve and ablation procedures
Relative contraindications	None	Previous right thorax surgery, inability to tolerate single lung ventilation

SVC: superior vena cava, IVC inferior vena cava

to the ICU the intensive care team should be made aware of this concern so that these medical interventions can be maintained during the postoperative period. Cases where volume status has fallen, afterload is decreased and inotropes are started for concern of LCOS can lead to acute pulmonary edema, hypoxia and acute respiratory failure. Occasionally re-repair of the valve is required during the same operation or in the future for unresolving SAM (Varghese, Anyanwu et al., 2012).

REFERENCES

Anyanwu, A. C., Chikwe, J., & Adams, D. H. (2008). Tricuspid valve repair for treatment and prevention of secondary tricuspid regurgitation in patients undergoing mitral valve surgery. *Current Cardiology Reports*, *10*(2), 110–117. doi:10.1007/s11886-008-0020-6 PMID:18417011

Carpentier, A., Adams, D. H., & Filsoufi, F. (2010). *Carpentier's Reconstructive Valve Surgery*. Saunders Elsevier.

Choi, B. W., Bacharach, S. L., Barbour, D. J., Leon, M. B., McCarthy, K. E., & Bonow, R. O. (1995). Left ventricular systolic dysfunction diastolic filling characteristics and exercise cardiac reserve in mitral stenosis. *The American Journal of Cardiology*, *75*(7), 526–529. doi:10.1016/S0002-9149(99)80599-2 PMID:7864006

Dreyfus, G. D., Corbi, P. J., Chan, K. M., & Bahrami, T. (2005). Secondary tricuspid regurgitation or dilatation: Which should be the criteria for surgical repair? *The Annals of Thoracic Surgery*, *79*(1), 127–132. doi:10.1016/j.athoracsur.2004.06.057 PMID:15620928

Enriquez-Sarano, M., Tajik, A. J., Schaff, H. V., Orszulak, T. A., Bailey, K. R., & Frye, R. L. (1994). Echocardiographic prediction of survival after surgical correction of organic mitral regurgitation. *Circulation*, *90*(2), 830–837. doi:10.1161/01.CIR.90.2.830 PMID:8044955

Gammie, J. S., Sheng, S., Griffith, B. P., Peterson, E. D., Rankin, J. S., O'Brien, S. M., & Brown, J. M. (2009). Trends in mitral valve surgery in the United States: Results from the Society of Thoracic Surgeons Adult Cardiac Surgery Database. *The Annals of Thoracic Surgery*, *87*(5), 1431–1437, discussion 1437–1439. doi:10.1016/j.athoracsur.2009.01.064 PMID:19379881

Iung, B., Gohlke-Barwolf, C., Tornos, P., Tribouilloy, C., Hall, R., Butchart, E., & Vahanian, A. (2002). Recommendations on the management of the asymptomatic patient with valvular heart disease. *European Heart Journal*, *23*(16), 1253–1266. doi:10.1053/euhj.2002.3320 PMID:12698958

Lam, J. H., Ranganathan, N., Wigle, E. D., & Silver, M. D. (1970). Morphology of the human mitral valve. I. Chordae tendineae: A new classification. *Circulation*, *41*(3), 449–458. doi:10.1161/01.CIR.41.3.449 PMID:5415982

Mann D. L., Zipes, D. P., Libby, P., Bonow, R. O., & Braunwald, E. (2014). *Braunwald's Heart Disease*. Elsevier.

Moreyra, A. E., Wilson, A. C., Deac, R., Suciu, C., Kostis, J. B., Ortan, F., & Mahalingham, B. et al. (1998). Factors associated with atrial fibrillation in patients with mitral stenosis: A cardiac catheterization study. *American Heart Journal*, *135*(1), 138–145. doi:10.1016/S0002-8703(98)70354-0 PMID:9453533

Nishimura, R. A., Otto, C. M., Bonow, R. O., Carabello, B. A., Erwin, J. P. III, Guyton, R. A., & Thomas, J. D. et al. (2014). Erwin JPr, Guyton RA, O'Gara PT, Ruiz CE, Skubas NJ, Sorajja P, Sundt TMr, Thomas JD. 2014 AHA/ACC guideline for the management of patients with valvular heart disease: executive summary: a report of the American College of Cardiology/American Heart Association Task Force on Practice Guidelines. *Journal of the American College of Cardiology*, *63*(22), 2438–2488. doi:10.1016/j.jacc.2014.02.537 PMID:24603192

Nkomo, V. T., Gardin, J. M., Skelton, T. N., Gottdiener, J. S., Scott, C. G., & Enriquez-Sarano, M. (2006). Burden of valvular heart diseases: A population-based study. *Lancet*, *368*(9540), 1005–1011. doi:10.1016/S0140-6736(06)69208-8 PMID:16980116

Olson, L. J., Subramanian, R., Ackermann, D. M., Orszulak, T. A., & Edwards, W. D. (1987). Surgical pathology of the mitral valve: A study of 712 cases spanning 21 years. *Mayo Clinic Proceedings*, *62*(1), 22–34. doi:10.1016/S0025-6196(12)61522-5 PMID:3796056

Padial, L. R., Abascal, V. M., Moreno, P. R., Weyman, A. E., Levine, R. A., & Palacios, I. F. (1999). Echocardiography can predict the development of severe mitral regurgitation after percutaneous mitral valvuloplasty by the Inoue technique. *The American Journal of Cardiology*, *83*(8), 1210–1213. doi:10.1016/S0002-9149(99)00061-2 PMID:10215286

Ranganathan, N., Lam, J. H., Wigle, E. D., & Silver, M. D. (1970). Morphology of the human mitral valve. II. The value leaflets. *Circulation*, *41*(3), 459–467. doi:10.1161/01.CIR.41.3.459 PMID:5415983

Rosenhek, R., Rader, F., Klaar, U., Gabriel, H., Krejc, M., Kalbeck, D., & Baumgartner, H. et al. (2006). Outcome of watchful waiting in asymptomatic severe mitral regurgitation. *Circulation*, *113*(18), 2238–2244. doi:10.1161/CIRCULATIONAHA.105.599175 PMID:16651470

Tribouilloy, C. M., Enriquez-Sarano, M., Schaff, H. V., Orszulak, T. A., Bailey, K. R., Tajik, A. J., & Frye, R. L. (1999). Impact of preoperative symptoms on survival after surgical correction of organic mitral regurgitation: Rationale for optimizing surgical indications. *Circulation*, *99*(3), 400–405. doi:10.1161/01.CIR.99.3.400 PMID:9918527

Vahanian, A., Alfieri, O., Andreotti, F., Antunes, M. J., Baron-Esquivias, G., Baumgartner, H., & Zembala, M. et al. (2012). Guidelines on the management of valvular heart disease (version 2012). *European Heart Journal*, *33*(19), 2451–2496. doi:10.1093/eurheartj/ehs109 PMID:22922415

Varghese, R., & Adams, D.H. (2014). Techniques in repairing posterior leaflet prolapse. *Operative Techniques in Thoracic and Cardiovascular Surgery* (pp. 293-308). Academic Press.

Varghese, R., Akujuo, A., & Adams, D. H. (2010). Right coronary artery injury after tricuspid valve repair. *Seminars in Thoracic and Cardiovascular Surgery*, *22*(2), 189–190. doi:10.1053/j.semtcvs.2010.09.004 PMID:21092900

Varghese, R., Anyanwu, A. C., Itagaki, S., Milla, F., Castillo, J., & Adams, D. H. (2012). Management of systolic anterior motion after mitral valve repair: An algorithm. *The Journal of Thoracic and Cardiovascular Surgery*, *143*(4Suppl), S2–S7. doi:10.1016/j.jtcvs.2012.01.063 PMID:22423603

Varghese, R., Itagaki, S., Anyanwu, A. C., Milla, F., & Adams, D. H. (2014). Predicting early left ventricular dysfunction after mitral valve reconstruction: The effect of atrial fibrillation and pulmonary hypertension. *The Journal of Thoracic and Cardiovascular Surgery*, *148*(2), 422–427. doi:10.1016/j.jtcvs.2013.08.073 PMID:24176266

Varghese, R., Itagaki, S., Anyanwu, A. C., Trigo, P., Fischer, G., & Adams, D. H. (2014). Predicting systolic anterior motion after mitral valve reconstruction: Using intraoperative transoesophageal echocardiography to identify those at greatest risk. *European Journal of Cardio-Thoracic Surgery*, *45*(1), 132–137, discussion 137–138. doi:10.1093/ejcts/ezt234 PMID:23657548

Wilcox, B. R. (2004). *Surgical Anatomy of the Heart*. Cambridge, UK: Cambridge University Press.

Wilkins, G. T., Weyman, A. E., Abascal, V. M., Block, P. C., & Palacios, I. F. (1988). Percutaneous balloon dilatation of the mitral valve: An analysis of echocardiographic variables related to outcome and the mechanism of dilatation. *British Heart Journal*, *60*(4), 299–308. doi:10.1136/hrt.60.4.299 PMID:3190958

Zoghbi, W. A., Enriquez-Sarano, M., Foster, E., Grayburn, P. A., Kraft, C. D., Levine, R. A., & Weissman, N. J. et al. (2003). Recommendations for evaluation of the severity of native valvular regurgitation with two-dimensional and Doppler echocardiography. *Journal of the American Society of Echocardiography*, *16*(7), 777–802. doi:10.1016/S0894-7317(03)00335-3 PMID:12835667

ADDITIONAL READING

Carpentier, A., Adams, D. H., & Filsoufi, F. (2010). *Carpentier's Reconstructive Valve Surgery*. Saunders Elsevier.

Nishimura, R. A., Otto, C. M., Bonow, R. O., Carabello, B. A., Erwin, J. P. III, Guyton, R. A., & Thomas, J. D. et al. (2014). AHA/ACC guideline for the management of patients with valvular heart disease: executive summary: a report of the American College of Cardiology/American Heart Association Task Force on Practice Guidelines. *Journal of the American College of Cardiology*, *63*(22), 2438–2488. doi:10.1016/j.jacc.2014.02.537 PMID:24603192

Vahanian, A., Alfieri, O., Andreotti, F., Antunes, M. J., Baron-Esquivias, G., Baumgartner, H., & Zembala, M. et al. (2012). Guidelines on the management of valvular heart disease (version 2012). *European Heart Journal*, 33. PMID:22922415

Varghese, R., Anyanwu, A. C., Itagaki, S., Milla, F., Castillo, J., & Adams, D. H. (2012). Management of systolic anterior motion after mitral valve repair: An algorithm. *The Journal of Thoracic and Cardiovascular Surgery*, *143*(4Suppl), S2–S7. doi:10.1016/j.jtcvs.2012.01.063 PMID:22423603

Chapter 25
Thoracic Aortic Disease

Berhane Worku
New York Methodist Hospital, USA & New York Presbyterian Hospital, USA & Weil Cornell Medical College, USA

Leonard Girardi
New York Presbyterian Hospital, USA & Weil Cornell Medical College, USA

ABSTRACT

Thoracic aortic disease most commonly presents in the form of aneurysmal dilation or dissection of the ascending or descending thoracic aorta, most commonly secondary to degenerative disease and hypertension. Several genetic connective tissue disorders are commonly associated as well. Treatment is focused on blood pressure control and surgical repair. Surgical repair of thoracic aortic disease presents unique risks, including neurologic injury involving the brain or spinal cord, and several adjuncts are available to mitigate against this risk. This chapter discusses commonly associated risk factors, preoperative testing, surgical repair, and postoperative management of thoracic aortic disease along with strategies for minimizing neurologic injury.

INTRODUCTION

With current cardiopulmonary bypass techniques, surgery for thoracic aortic disease has become much more common, with low morbidity and mortality rates. Ascending aortic aneurysm repair can be performed with ~2% operative mortality rate (Cohn et. al. 1996). Increasingly complex procedures on the aortic root, including replacement with a valved conduit with coronary reimplantation and valve sparing root replacement are performed with similar outcomes. Aortic arch aneurysms requiring a period of circulatory arrest for repair pose additional neurologic risks, and several adjuncts to standard cardiopulmonary bypass techniques including deep hypothermia, antegrade, and retrograde cerebral perfusion, have been utilized to reduce stroke risks. Similarly, descending thoracic aortic aneurysm repair is associated with increased paraplegia risk due to spinal cord ischemia and again a variety of techniques to reduce this risk

DOI: 10.4018/978-1-4666-8603-8.ch025

are similarly available. The decision to undertake repair requires an assessment of the risks of surgery versus those of rupture or dissection if observation is chosen. As operative risks decrease, this balance is shifted in favor of earlier operation.

BACKGROUND

Aortic aneurysms are most commonly degenerative in nature, secondary to cystic medial necrosis in which there is a loss of elastic tissue in the aortic wall. Vascular myocytes in the media undergo necrosis, and are replaced by cystic accumulations. Risk factors are similar to those of atherosclerosis, including smoking, hypertension, hypercholesterolemia, and diabetes. Connective tissue diseases such as Marfan, Loewy-Dietz, and Ehlers-Danlos syndromes, bicuspid aortic valve disease, and certain infections also predispose to aneurysm formation.

Marfan syndrome is an autosomal dominant disease caused by mutation of the gene encoding fibrillin-1, a glycoprotein component of the extracellular matrix. Clinical features most commonly include aortic root dilation along with dilation and dissection of the remaining aorta, mitral valve prolapse, ocular and orthopedic manifestations, and spontaneous pneumothorax. These patients are prone to more rapid growth, rupture, and dissection of their aneurysms. A positive family history and pregnancy may increase this risk, and beta blocker therapy significantly reduces it. Most patients eventually die from complications of aortic aneurysm disease (Pomianowski & Elefteriades 2013).

Loeys-Dietz syndrome is an autosomal disease caused by mutation of the gene encoding the transforming growth factor beta receptor, and may present in a fashion similar to Marfan syndrome, although with heightened severity. Patients commonly demonstrate the triad of hypertelorism, bifid uvula, and widespread arterial aneurysm formation. Aneurysm formation may occur at an earlier age than in Marfan syndrome (Pomianowski & Elefteriades 2013).

Ehlers-Danlos syndrome is an autosomal dominant disease caused by mutation of the gene encoding type III collagen. Clinical manifestations include skin hyperelasticity and fragility leading to easy bleeding, joint hypermobility, aneurysms of medium and large sized vessels prone to rupture, and visceral perforation. Again, most patients eventually die of from arterial aneurysm rupture (Pomianowski & Elefteriades 2013).

Bicuspid aortic valve is the most common congenital cardiac malformation, occurring in 1-2% of the population. This entity appears to have a familial association, although no inheritable mutation has been identified. The bicuspid aortic valve may function normally, but is prone to stenosis or regurgitation. In addition, these patients have a poorly understood propensity to ascending and aortic root aneurysm and dissection formation (Verma & Siu 2014).

Mycotic aneurysms, most commonly from syphilis infection, is now uncommon with current antimicrobial therapy. The ascending aorta is most commonly involved, with destruction of the media and saccular aneurysm formation (Lopes, Almeida, Dias, Pinho, & Maciel 2008). Inflammatory aortitis is most commonly secondary to giant cell or temporal arteritis. Granulomatous inflammation of the media involving medium and large sized arteries can lead to aneurysm formation. Takayasu's arteritis most commonly leads to stenosis of the aortic arch and its branches, but may lead to aneurysm formation. Several other autoimmune inflammatory conditions may also lead to aortic aneurysm formation (Pagni, Ganzel, Williams, Slater, & Trivedi 2012).

ASCENDING AORTIC ANEURYSMS

Classification

The aortic annulus is a fibrous structure connecting the left ventricle to the aorta. There are three aortic valve leaflets or cusps, the left, right, and noncoronary leaflets. The sinotubular junction is just above the commisures and marks the beginning of the ascending aorta. The aortic root is between the aortic annulus and the sinotubular junction and contains the three sinuses of Valsalva, also named after their corresponding leaflet as the left, right, and noncoronary sinuses. The left main coronary artery arises from the left sinus and the right coronary artery from the right sinus. The ascending aorta extends to the origin of the innominate artery, after which the aortic arch begins.

Aneurysms may involve the aortic root, the ascending aorta, or the arch in isolation or in combination. Aneurysms that involve the sinotubular junction and thus splay the commisures of the aortic valve apart may cause aortic regurgitation, as may dilation of the aortic annulus. Different techniques are required to repair each kind of aneurysm, with or without valve repair or replacement, and will be discussed below.

Etiology

Ascending aortic aneurysms are most commonly degenerative in nature, secondary to cystic medial necrosis. Patients with connective tissue disorders and those with bicuspid aortic valve disease are prone to their development. Specifically, Marfan syndrome is associated with aortic root aneurysms (figure 1). Mycotic aneurysms and aneurysms related to autoimmune disease also tend to localize to the ascending aorta.

Presentation

Most ascending aortic aneurysms are asymptomatic, with the aneurysm discovered incidentally on radiographic imaging. Patients may complain of chest pain and those with significant aortic regurgitation may present with signs of heart failure. Patients with aortic arch aneurysms may present with hoarseness secondary to stretching of the left recurrent laryngeal nerve as it wraps around the distal arch at the ligamentum arteriosum. Dysphagia may be caused by compression of the esophagus posteriorly, known as dysphagia lusoria. Physical exam is usually unremarkable, but occasionally a pulsatile mass may be palpated in the lower neck.

Preoperative Evaluation

Angiography has historically been the gold standard for evaluation of the thoracic aorta. In recent years axial imaging with computed tomographic angiography (CTA) or magnetic resonance imaging (MRI) has supplanted angiography, and provides excellent detail with regards to aneurysm extent, presence of dissection or rupture, and associated abnormalities. Aortic aneurysms are predisposed to rupture or dissection, and size is the best predictor of this, with the cumulative risk of rupture, dissection, or death increasing from 5.8% at 4-4.9cm to 8.1% at 5-5.9cm to 15.6% at >6cm (Davies et. al. 2002). Thus, repair is usually recommended at 5.5cm, at which point the risk of surgery is less than the risk of aneurysm related complications. In the setting of significant aortic regurgitation due to aneurysmal dilation of the

Figure 1.

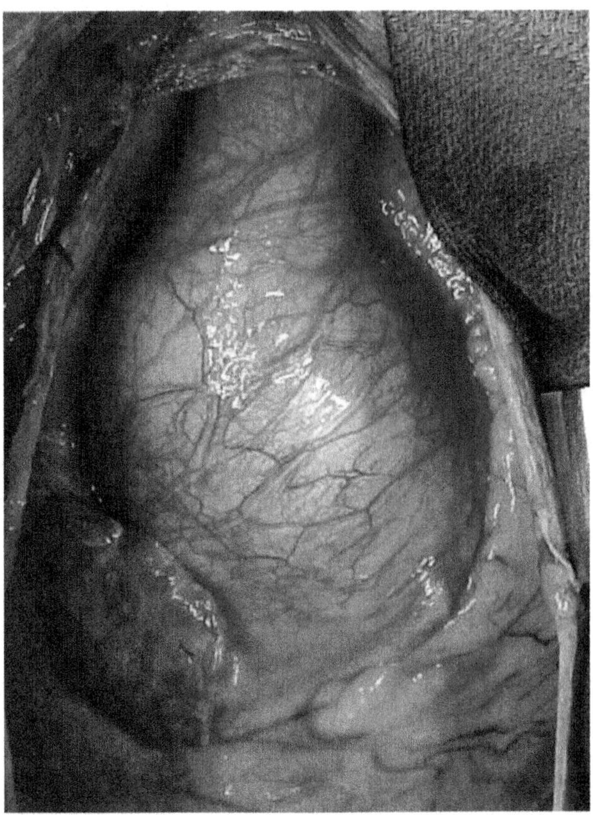

sinotubular junction, repair may be undertaken at a size of 5cm. Patients undergoing other concomitant cardiac surgery should undergo aneurysm repair at a size of 5cm. In patients with Marfan syndrome or other defined connective tissue disorders, repair may also be undertaken at 5cm. In the setting of aortic valve replacement for bicuspid valve disease, concomitant aortic aneurysm repair is performed at 4.5cm.

Echocardiography can assess the size of the aortic annulus, aortic root, sinotubular junction, and proximal ascending aorta. The degree of aortic regurgitation and its mechanism can be determined, with assessment of leaflet prolapse or fenestrations, as well as annular or sinotubular junction dilation. Left ventricular function and size can be assessed, as can other valvular pathology. Cardiac catheterization may identify significant coronary artery disease requiring concomitant revascularization. An aortogram performed during catheterization can be helpful in determining proximal arch involvement, which will affect surgical management as discussed below. Preoperative workup is otherwise as for other cardiac procedures.

Operative Technique

Ascending aortic aneurysm repair is performed with standard cardiopulmonary bypass techniques as for coronary or valvular procedures, with circulatory arrest utilized in the setting of an arch aneurysm as discussed below. Operative technique is therefore focused on an expeditious and hemostatic repair that minimizes cardiac ischemic time while avoiding postoperative bleeding. In addition, aneurysmal dilation of the sinotubular junction can predispose to significant aortic regurgitation by splaying apart the commisures. Therefore, a critical decision must be made as to whether to replace the aortic valve or whether restoration of the sinotubular junction to normal dimensions with aneurysm repair alone is sufficient to correct aortic regurgitation.

General endotracheal anesthesia and standard monitoring devices including foley catheter, swan-ganz catheter, and arterial line are utilized. Median sternotomy and standard aortic and venous cannulation are carried out. The aorta is crossclamped and the heart arrested in standard fashion. If the aneurysm is isolated to the ascending aorta, it is resected to the sinotubular junction and replaced with a Dacron graft. If the sinotubular junction is dilated with resulting aortic regurgitation, and the aortic valve leaflets are otherwise normal, reducing the sinotubular junction to a normal diameter by anastomosis to an appropriately sized graft will frequently correct the regurgitation. If there is significant aortic stenosis or regurgitation not amenable to repair as described, aortic valve replacement is performed, and the aorta replaced as described.

Aortic root aneurysms are commonly associated with Marfan syndrome and require graft replacement with reimplantation of the coronaries, with or without aortic valve replacement. In the setting of normal aortic cusps, valve sparing aortic root replacement may be considered. The ascending aorta and aortic root are excised and the aortic leaflets preserved. The coronary arteries are similarly preserved with a button of aortic wall. A Dacron graft of appropriate diameter is attached to the aortic annulus with interrupted pledgeted sutures. The aortic valve is resuspended within the graft. The coronaries are reimplanted into the graft and the distal anastomosis performed to the aorta (figure 2a-h). If the aortic valve leaflets are abnormal, complete aortic root replacement is performed with a composite valved conduit. The aortic root and leaflets are excised, and the coronaries preserved with a button of aortic wall. A Dacron graft with valve attached is secured to the aortic annulus with interrupted pledgeted sutures. The coronaries are reattached to the graft and the distal anastomosis performed to the native aorta (figure 3).

In the pediatric or young adult population, the Ross procedure is another option for aortic root replacement. The aortic root is replaced with patient's pulmonic valve and pulmonary artery, and the pulmonic valve replaced with a pulmonary homograft. The benefit is very high durability and lack of need for anticoagulation. In children, the pulmonic autograft will grow with the patient. It is also suitable for active infective endocarditis when foreign material is undesirable. However, the procedure is more technically demanding and not performed by many. In addition, it should not be used in patients with Marfan syndrome due to the possibility of aneurysmal dilation of the autograft. Finally, aortic homograft is another option for aortic root replacement, especially in the setting of active infection. Drawbacks include poor durability with early calcification and failure requiring reoperation.

In order to replace the aortic arch, circulation must be arrested and the brain protected. Strategies for circulatory arrest include deep hypothermia with antegrade or retrograde cerebral protection. If antegrade cerebral perfusion is chosen, arterial cannulation is via the axillary artery, approached via a subclavicular incision. An 8mm graft is sewn end to side and the graft is cannulated (figure 4a). A dual stage venous cannula in the right atrium is used for venous drainage unless additional procedures requiring alternative cannulation approaches are to be performed. The patient is placed on cardiopulmonary bypass and systemically cooled to 18 degrees Celsius. During this period of cooling, the heart will normally fibrillate. If significant aortic regurgitation is present, the left ventricle will distend during this time. A left ventricular vent is thus mandatory prior to cooling, and if inadequate to prevent left ventricular distention, the aorta must be clamped, and any cardiac or proximal aortic repairs may be undertaken while systemic cooling commences. When systemic temperatures reach 18 degrees Celsius as measured by bladder,

Figure 2.

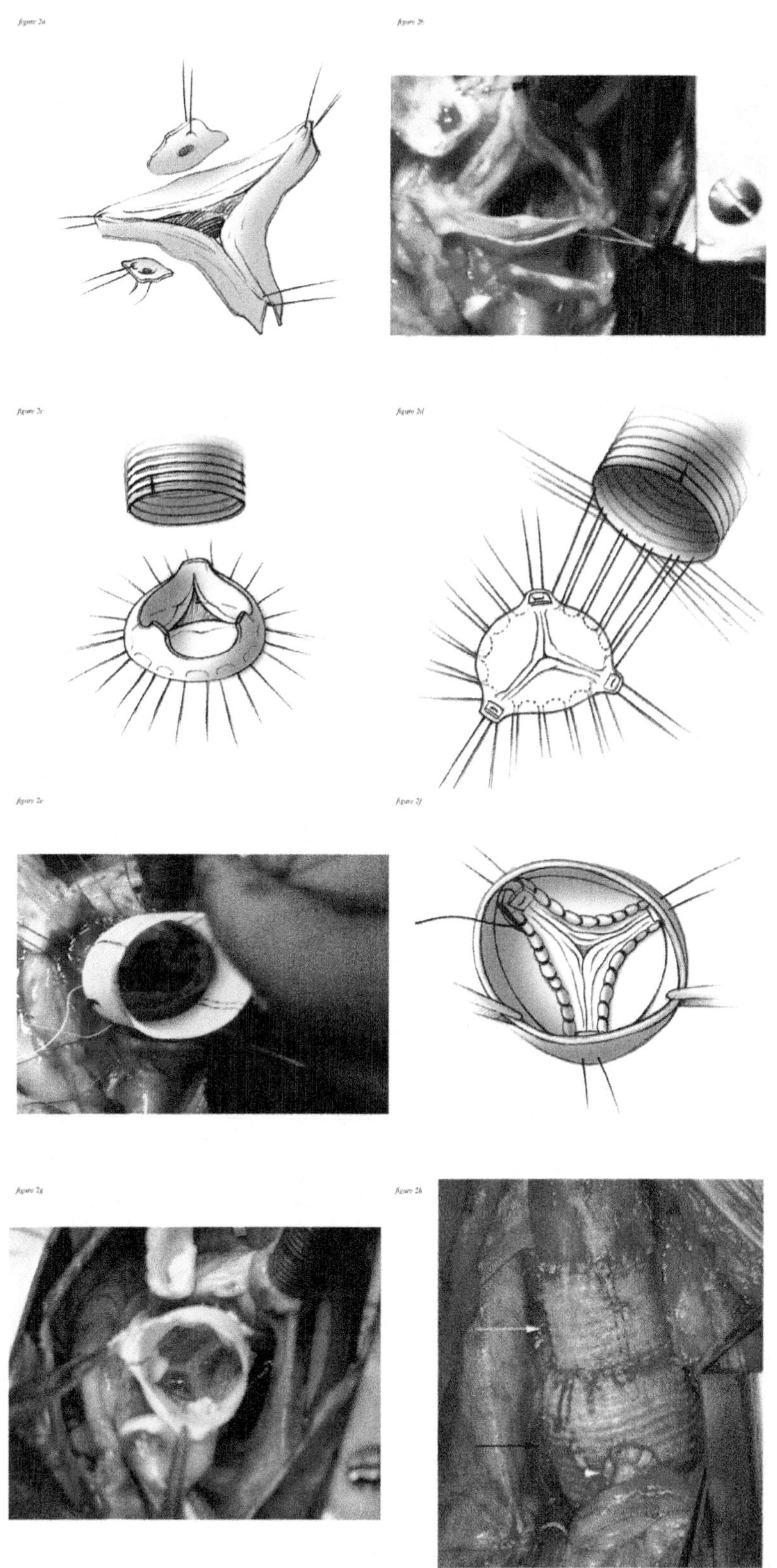

Figure 3.

figure 3a

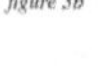

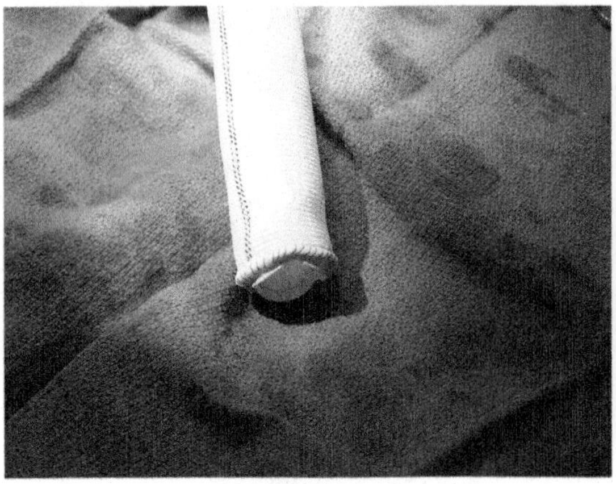

figure 3b

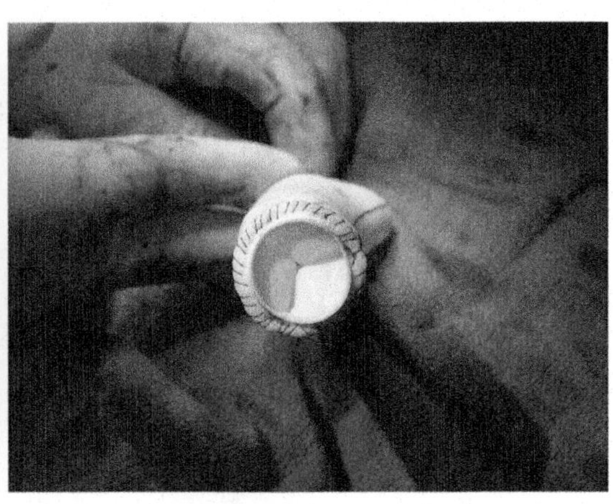

figure 3c

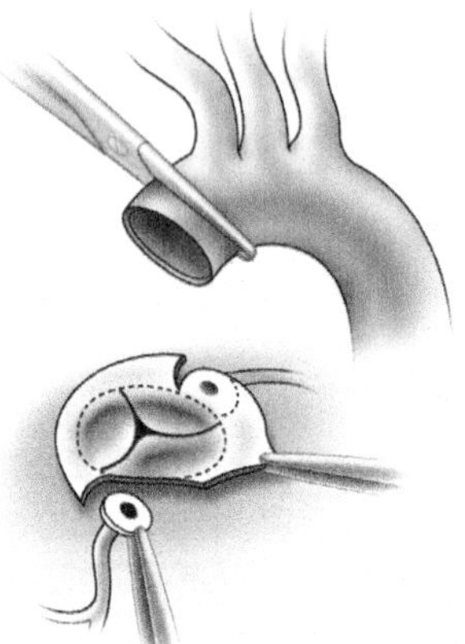

figure 3d

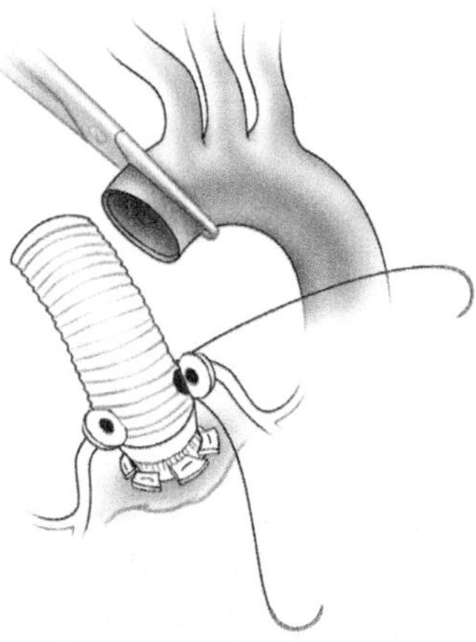

figure 3e

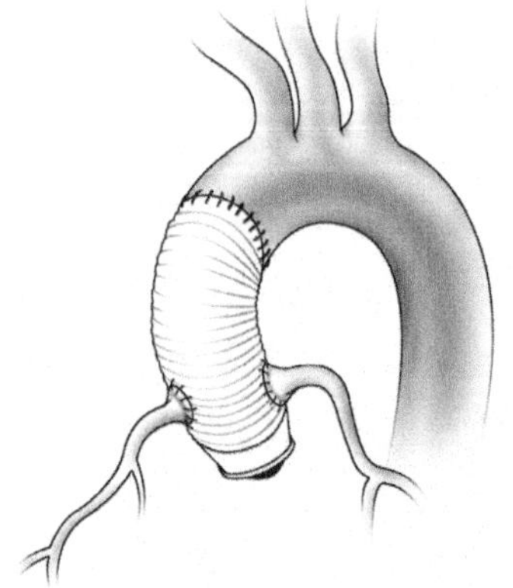

Figure 4.

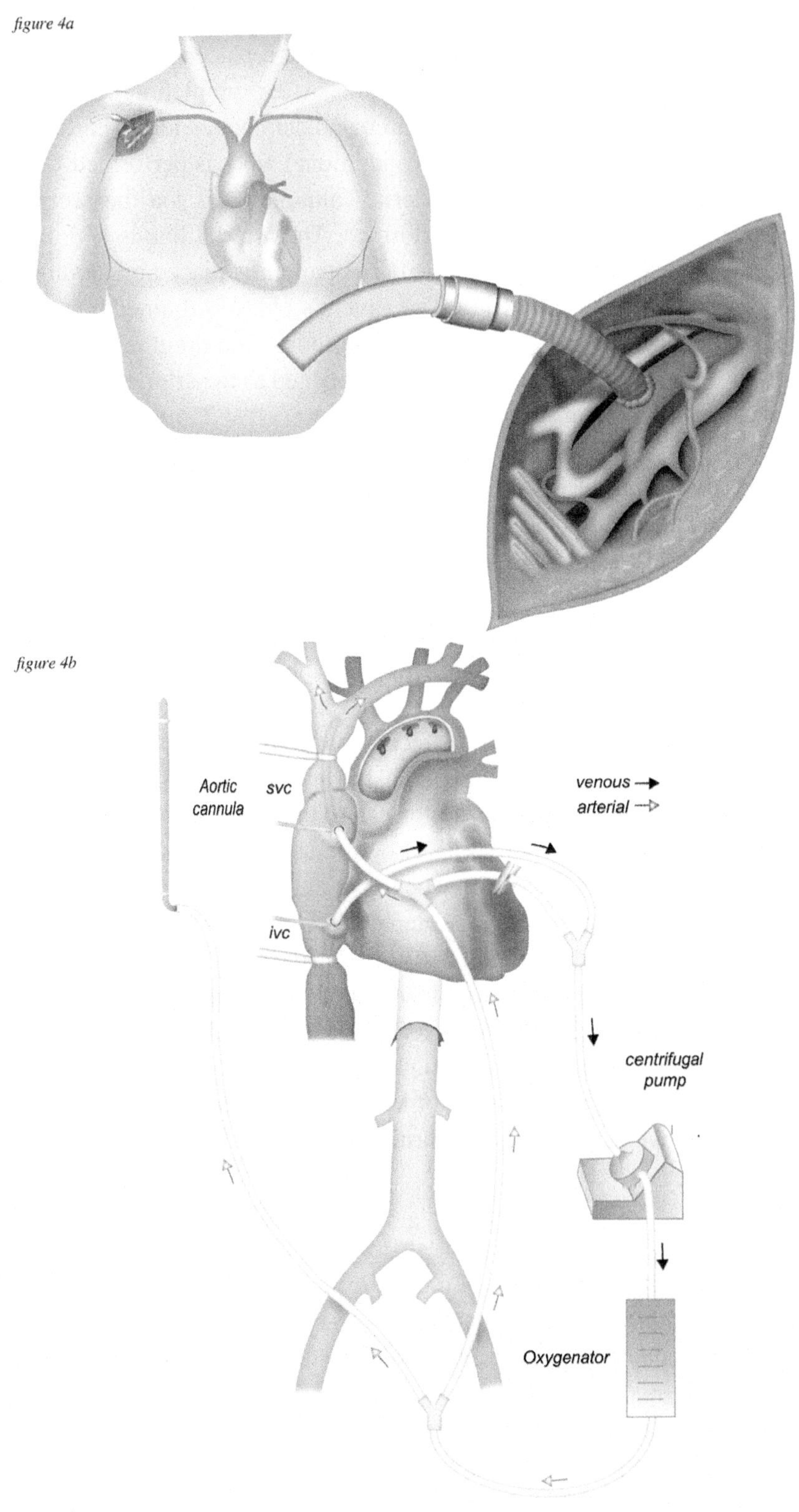
figure 4a
figure 4b
Aortic
cannula
svc
ivc
venous
arterial
centrifugal
pump
Oxygenator

rectal, or tympanic temperatures, usually after 30-40 minutes of cooling, methohexital is administered to achieve electroencephalographic (EEG) silence. The patient' blood is drained into the pump. The innominate artery is clamped and the arch aneurysm resected and replaced. During the distal anastomosis, the brain is perfused via the right axillary artery cannula. After completion of the distal anastomosis, the innominate artery is unclamped, the graft is deaired and clamped, and full cardiopulmonary bypass is resumed while the proximal anastomosis and any additional work is performed.

If retrograde cerebral perfusion is chosen, arterial cannulation is via the ascending aorta or the femoral artery. Bicaval venous cannulation is performed. The arterial line is Y'd to the superior vena cava cannula, with the connection initially clamped. The patient is placed on cardiopulmonary bypass and systemically cooled to 18 degrees Celsius. The patient's blood is drained into the pump. The arch aneurysm resected and replaced. During the distal anastomosis, the brain is perfused via the superior vena cava. The superior vena cava cannula is snared and opened to the arterial line. Retrograde cerebral perfusion is commenced with central venous pressure maintained at 25mmHg. After completion of the distal anastomosis, the arterial cannula is placed in the side arm of the graft, and the graft is deaired and clamped. Retrograde cerebral perfusion is discontinued and the superior vena cava cannula opened to the venous line, and full cardiopulmonary bypass is resumed while the proximal anastomosis and any additional work is performed (figure 4b). If the femoral artery cannulation was selected initially, the artery is repaired at this time.

The operative technique for aortic arch replacement depends on the extent of the arch aneurysm. For aneurysms involving the proximal arch, a hemiarch replacement may be performed in which the aortic arch is divided from the level of the innominate artery to roughly the midpoint of the lesser curve of the aortic arch. The graft thus constitutes half of the reconstructed arch, and the arch vessels are left intact (figure 5a-b). For aneurysms involving the entire arch, the arch is transected distal to the left subclavian artery and resected. The distal anastomosis is performed to the descending aorta. The arch vessels may be left together on an "island" if not splayed apart by the aneurysm and the island sewn to the graft (figure 5c-e). Alternatively, the arch vessels may be reimplanted separately into the graft (figure 5f). In the setting of a known descending aneurysm, the elephant trunk technique may be employed, in which a length of graft is initially invaginated onto itself and placed in the descending aorta. The folded edge used for the distal anastomosis. The graft is then unfolded out of the descending aorta and the proximal and arch anastomoses performed. A length of graft is left in the descending aorta for use during subsequent thoracotomy and descending aortic replacement (figure 5g-k). In either setting, the proximal anastomosis may be to the sinotubular junction in the setting of a normal aortic root. If aortic root replacement was undertaken as described above, a graft to graft anastomosis is performed.

Brain Protection

During any procedure requiring replacement of the aortic arch, a period of circulatory arrest is required. The risk of stroke after such procedures is increased but several adjuncts have reduced this risk to acceptable levels, including antegrade/retrograde cerebral perfusion, deep hypothermia, and induction of EEG silence.

The risk of stroke from a period of circulatory arrest is influenced by the length of brain ischemia time, by embolization of air or particulate material from aortic atheroma, and from residual brain metabolism. The risk of stroke rises significantly after 30-45 minutes of circulatory arrest. By perfusing the right axillary artery and clamping the innominate artery, the brain receives oxygenated blood at systemic

Figure 5.

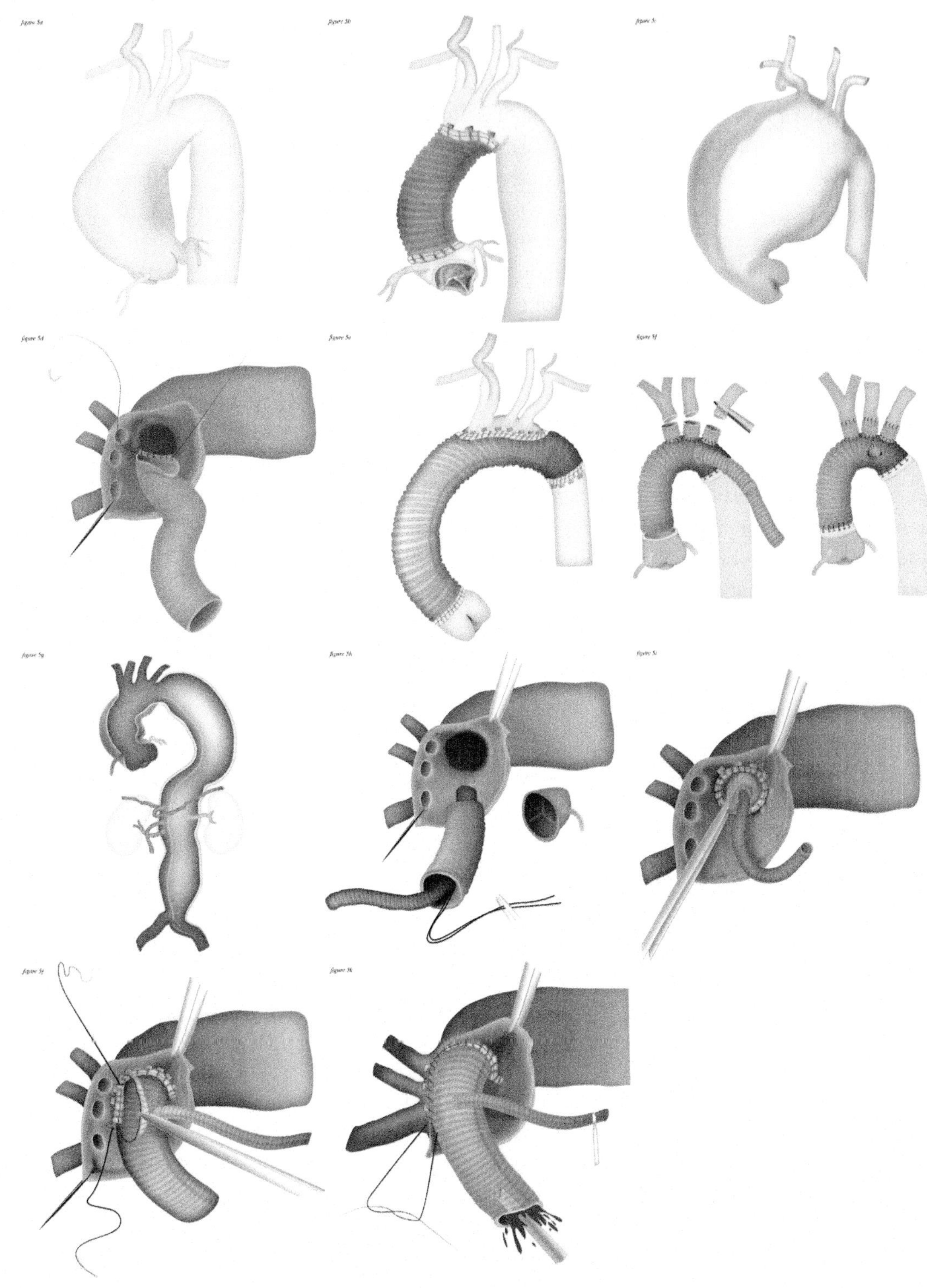

perfusion pressures while maintaining a nearly bloodless aortic arch. The only caveat is that a patent circle of Willis must be present to perfuse the left brain. The downside is the time required to dissect the axillary artery and sew a graft to it. With retrograde cerebral perfusion, the superior vena cava cannula is perfused with arterial blood during the period of circulatory arrest. Because of the risk of brain edema with venous hypertension, perfusion pressures of 25mmHg are used, and it is thus likely that benefit is derived from maintenance of cerebral hypothermia and flushing air and particulate material retrograde, reducing the risk of embolic stroke. Antegrade cerebral perfusion is theoretically protective especially with longer circulatory arrest times. However, in a recent study 879 patients undergoing aortic arch surgery utilizing retrograde cerebral perfusion were retrospectively analyzed. Hemiarch repair was performed in 671 patients and total arch repair n 208. Although total arch patients had longer circulatory arrest times (39 vs 21 minutes, $p < .001$), the incidence of transient (3.0 vs 2.4%, $p < .813$) and permanent (1.3% vs 1.9%, $p< .519$) neurologic dysfunction was similar in both groups and mortality was actually higher in the hemiarch group (4.8% vs 0.5%, $p < .003$). Long term survival was similar in both groups (Girardi, Shavladze, Sedrakyan, & Neragi 2014). Thus, extensive aneurysms can safely be repaired utilizing retrograde cerebral perfusion when circulatory arrest times are kept under 40-45 minutes.

If circulatory arrest alone or with retrograde cerebral perfusion is to be used and the axillary artery not cannulated, direct aortic cannulation is preferable to femoral cannulation to prevent retrograde embolization of aortic atheroma (figure 6). Deep hypothermia to 18 degrees Celsius is utilized to reduce brain metabolism. During cooling and rewarming, a 10 degrees Celsius maximum gradient is allowed between systemic blood temperature and core body temperature as measured by bladder, rectal, or tympanic temperatures. Packing the head in ice reduces brain rewarming by ambient temperatures. Methohexital 500mg is administered prior to induction of circulatory arrest to achieve EEG silence.

Postoperative Management

Postoperative management after ascending aortic aneurysm repair is similar to that for routine cardiac surgery with a few exceptions. A history of significant hypertension and subsequent left ventricular hypertrophy and diastolic dysfunction is commonplace. Fluctuating hemodynamics in such patients is best treated with volume resuscitation. Ischemic electrocardiographic changes and hemodynamic instability after an aortic root replacement must raise concern for kinking of a coronary artery due to reimplantation at an inappropriate height on the aortic graft. This requires return to the operating room for revision. Renal failure is a well described complication after circulatory arrest due to renal ischemia. Preexisting renal insufficiency and older age are risk factors. Postoperatively, a dopamine infusion may be used. Renal failure postoperatively may require temporary or permanent hemodialysis. Finally, stroke is the most significant concern after circulatory arrest. Postoperatively, sedation is held immediately and neurologic status assessed hourly or more as needed. Seizures are treated with dilantin and correction of metabolic disturbances. Repeated seizures or neurologic deficits warrant head imaging when the patient is hemodynamically stable enough to be transported. Treatment consists of induced hypertension to improve cerebral perfusion, but is otherwise expectant unless hemorrhagic complications or severe edema warrant neurosurgical intervention.

In a study of 115 patients undergoing ascending aortic aneurysm repair, 20 (17%) of whom required circulatory arrest, overall operative mortality was 1.7%, and was similar amongst patients undergoing concomitant root repair (1.8%), separate valve replacement and supracoronary ascending aortic replacement

Figure 6.

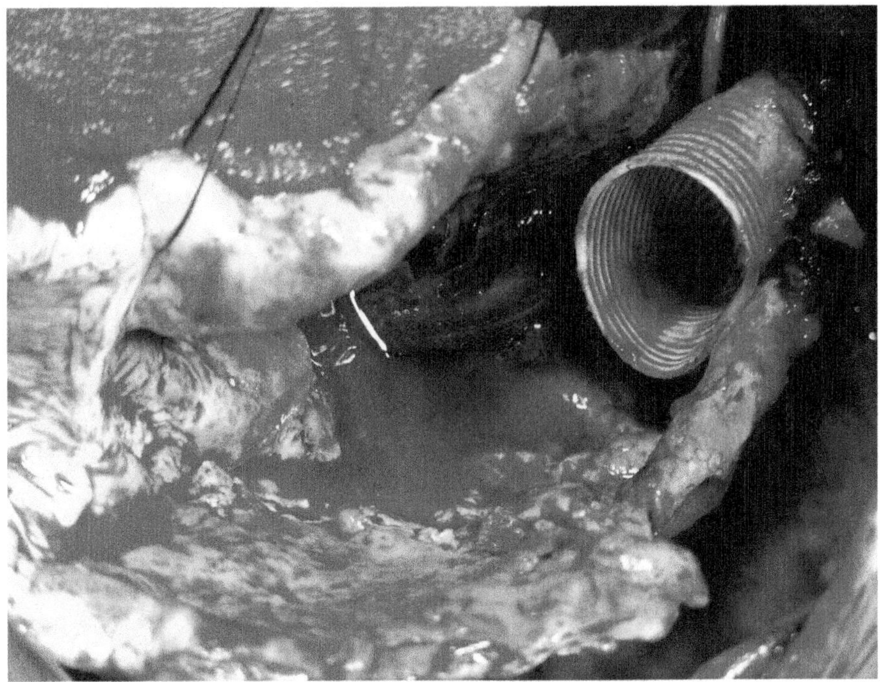

(2%), and isolated supracoronary ascending aortic replacement (0%). The overall bleeding complication rate was 3%, the stroke rate was 2%, and myocardial infarction rate was 1% (Cohn et. al., 1996). Thus, with current myocardial protection and circulatory arrest techniques and postoperative care, ascending aortic and aortic arch surgery can be performed with low complication rates and excellent survival.

ASCENDING AORTIC DISSECTION

Introduction

Type A dissections involve the ascending aorta with or without involvement of the descending aorta. They usually present with chest pain radiating to the back and abdomen; hypertension is usually an accompanying feature. Untreated, mortality is high, estimated at 25% at 24 hours, 50% at 48 hours, 80% at one week, and 95% at one month. Management is urgent surgical repair in almost all cases.

Classification

Aortic dissections are commonly characterized by the Stanford classification scheme into type A dissections, involving the ascending with or without the descending aorta, and type B, involving only the descending aorta. The DeBakey classification scheme categorizes dissections into type I, involving the ascending and descending aorta, type II, involving only the ascending aorta, and type III involving only the descending aorta. Intramural hematoma (IMH) is a variant of classic aortic dissection caused by rupture of the vaso vasorum in the aortic media. Penetrating aortic ulcer (PAU) is similarly another variant caused by rupture of an atherosclerotic plaque into the media. Both may evolve into a classic dissection or rupture.

Etiology

Type A dissection starts as an initial tear, usually located just distal to the sinotubular junction and usually associated with hypertension, which allows blood to track within the media creating a false lumen. Propagation of the dissection usually occurs distally, but may extend retrograde to involve the coronary arteries and aortic annulus. The false lumen usually remains patent as a result of secondary tears or fenestrations in the distal flap that allow for blood reentry into the true lumen. If no reentry sites exist, the false lumen may thrombose. Branch vessels may become obstructed by progression of the dissection flap. Connective tissue disorders, bicuspid aortic valve disease and aortic coarctation are associated conditions. Iatrogenic dissection may be precipitated by cardiac catheterization or transcatheter aortic valve implantation. Illicit drug use and pregnancy may also precipitate aortic dissection due associated to hemodynamic changes.

Presentation

The most common presenting symptom in type A dissection is severe, tearing chest pain which may radiate to the back or abdomen, associated with hypertension. Hypotension is rare and should raise concern for rupture. Acute complications most commonly result from rupture with tamponade. Tamponade may also be secondary to transudation of fluid through the aortic wall into the pericardial space. Acute severe aortic regurgitation due to retrograde involvement of the aortic annulus is the next most common acute complication. Acute myocardial infarction from retrograde involvement of the coronary arteries may also occur, involving the right coronary artery most commonly.

Malperfusion syndromes may result from compression of the true lumen by the false lumen, or by occlusion of branch vessels by the dissection flap or extension of the dissection into a branch vessel. Stroke may occur, and altered mental status may be even more common. If the dissection progresses to the descending aorta paraplegia may occur secondary to spinal cord ischemia from interruption of intercostal arteries. Lower extremity ischemia with a peripheral pulse deficit, renal ischemia presenting with oliguria or flank pain, and visceral ischemia presenting as pain out of proportion to physical exam may result. In the chronic phase, type A dissections may progress to aneurysm formation, the management of which is as described above.

Preoperative Evaluation

The key to diagnosis of type A dissection is a high level of suspicion, as presenting characteristics may vary and delays in diagnosis can be rapidly fatal. Angiography has historically been the gold standard test although in recent years CTA or MRI have supplanted this, both because of the level of detail offered and their noninvasiveness. MRI is less commonly used due to longer image acquisition time, limited patient access during the study, and limited availability. Gadolinium is not mandatory for visualizing a dissection. CTA requires intravenous contrast but may delineate the extent of a dissection, branch vessel involvement, patency of the false lumen, presence of an IMH or PAU, and pericardial or pleural effusion or mediastinal hematoma suggesting leak. When CTA is performed for suspected aortic dissection, the study should always include the chest, abdomen, and pelvis to include the proximal femoral arteries. Transesophageal echocardiography is also excellent for demonstrating type A dissections. Limitations include the need for sedation, potential hemodynamic alterations, user dependence, and inability to visualize branch vessel involvement below the diaphragm. Coronary catheterization is not indicated as it rarely changes management and incurs a significant delay.

Management

Operative intervention is indicated in almost all cases of type A dissection to prevent the known sequelae of rupture, myocardial infarction, acute severe aortic regurgitation, stroke, or other malperfusion syndromes. Patients presenting with major stroke or coma or those with significant comorbidities with limited life expectancy may be considered for nonoperative management, although this is controversial. The goal of the operation is to replace the dissected ascending aorta along with the intimal tear, restoring blood flow to the true lumen. This prevents rupture, retrograde progression, and usually resolves distal malperfusion syndromes. If malperfusion persists postoperatively, endovascular or open techniques to revascularization may then be undertaken.

Medical antihypertensive treatment should be initiated as soon as dissection is suspected. Agents that reduce the rate of rise of aortic pressure or dP/dt should be firstline, including beta blockers such as esmolol, metoprolol, labetolol, or propranolol. These are usually started as intermittent intravenous bolus or continuous infusion. This may be supplemented by calcium channel blockers such as nifedipine or nicardipine and sodium nitroprusside, as needed. The latter is a pure vasodilator that may increase aortic dP/dt, and should be used in conjunction with one of the other agents mentioned above. Finally, adequate pain control is ensured.

The patient is immediately brought to the operating room. The patient is placed under general endotracheal anesthesia. Standard monitoring devices including foley catheter, swan-ganz catheter, and arterial line are placed. Median sternotomy and deep hypothermic circulatory arrest are utilized to avoid crossclamping the dissected aorta and allow an "open" distal anastomosis such that the inside of the arch can be explored and any tears identified and repaired. Antegrade or retrograde cerebral perfusion is performed as described above for arch aneurysm repair. The ascending aorta is transected and the primary tear visualized. The aorta is resected from sinotubular junction to the innominate artery and the arch inspected for any tears which are repaired. The distal anastomosis is completed meticulously with 4-0 prolene, taking care to reapproximate the intima and adventitial layers. The tissue tends to be very thin and friable and hemostasis may be difficult to obtain. Systemic reperfusion via the axillary artery or via cannulation of the graft, depending on the method of cerebral perfusion, is initiated as described above and the proximal anastomosis completed. If the aortic valve commisures are detached by the dissection, they are resuspended to the graft and the proximal anastomosis completed as above. This is usually sufficient to resolve aortic regurgitation. If the aortic root is destroyed by the dissection, if significant aortic root aneurysm is present, or if the patient has Marfan syndrome or other connective tissue disease, the aortic root is replaced with techniques as described above. Similarly, if the aortic arch is involved beyond that repairable with a hemiarch repair, then total arch replacement is performed.

Postoperative Management

Postoperative management is similar to that described above for ascending aortic aneurysms with circulatory arrest. Neurologic and renal complications are more common and are thoroughly monitored for. Coagulopathy and postoperative hemorrhage are more common and require blood product transfusions and return to the operating room. Postoperative malperfusion syndromes are infrequent with adequate restoration of true lumen blood flow by ascending aortic replacement but must be searched for. Options include percutaneous stent grafting or fenestration of a descending aortic dissection flap or surgical fenestration or revascularization.

THORACOABDOMINAL ANEURYSMS

Introduction

Thoracoabdominal aneurysms involve varying lengths of the descending thoracic and abdominal aorta, from the left subclavian artery to the bifurcation of the abdominal aorta. Repair of these aneurysms is generally via the left chest and abdomen as needed, and entails several risks, including respiratory, cardiac, neurologic, and renal dysfunction, discussed below. Of these, spinal cord ischemia leading to paralysis is paramount in any discussion of thoracoabdominal aneurysm repair and postoperative management.

Classification

Thoracoabdominal aneurysms are classified according to their length of involvement into four extents. Extent I aneurysms begin in the proximal descending thoracic aorta above the sixth rib and extend to above the renal arteries, whereas Extent II aneurysms extend beyond the renal arteries. Extent III aneurysms begin in the distal descending thoracic aorta below the sixth rib and type IV aneurysms involve only the abdominal aorta. This classification scheme has prognostic significance with regards to the incidence of postoperative paralysis and the protective strategies employed to avoid this dreaded complication.

Etiology

The most common cause of thoracoabdominal aortic aneurysms is cystic medial necrosis. They are also strongly associated with connective tissue disorders. Progressive aneurysm formation is also commonly seen in the setting of chronic type B dissections. Less commonly, mycotic aneurysms, aortitis from inflammatory vasculitides, penetrating injury or blunt traumatic aortic rupture, and primary or recurrent aortic coarctation are the indication for thoracoabdominal aortic repair.

Presentation

Back pain is the most common symptom elicited from patients with thoracoabdominal aneurysms, and its presence is an ominous sign signifying an increased risk of rupture. Wheezing and dysphagia may be caused by bronchial and esophageal compression respectively. Hoarseness is seen in aneurysms involving the aortic arch from stretching of the left recurrent laryngeal nerve. Peripheral ischemia may be seen as a result of embolization of extensive atheromatous material frequently present in the aneurysm sac, resulting in "trash foot". Refractory hypertension may prompt a workup leading to the diagnosis of coarctation of the aorta, and frequently persists after surgery.

Preoperative Evaluation

Angiography has historically been the gold standard test for the diagnosis of thoracoabdominal aneurysms, although CTA and MRI have supplanted this, both because of the level of detail offered and their noninvasiveness. The aneurysm is assessed for its proximal and distal extent, size, presence of a dissection flap, and signs of rupture such as mediastinal hematoma or left pleural effusion. The presence of a cuff of uninvolved aorta distal to the left subclavian artery for clamping is of particular importance. Finally, in select cases the presence of significant intercostal vessels may be noted and reimplantation contemplated during aneurysm repair. Repair is recommended at 6cm for thoracoabdominal aneurysms, or at a growth rate of >5mm/6 months.

An extensive cardiac evaluation is crucial prior to thoracoabdominal aneurysm repair if time allows. Coronary artery disease is common and all patients undergo cardiac catheterization, with stenting or coronary artery bypass grafting preoperatively as needed. Bare metal stents are preferable to drug eluting stents as plavix can be discontinued after 30 days and surgery undertaken. In a study of 592 patients undergoing thoracic aneurysm repair, 44 (7.4%) underwent bare metal stenting preoperatively for single or double vessel disease with 4-6 weeks of antiplatelet therapy. No stent related complications occurred, no instances of aneurysm rupture occurred in the interval between stenting and surgery, and no instances of stent thrombosis, myocardial infarction, or mortality occurred postoperatively (Girardi, Rabotnikov, & Avgerinos, 2014). If coronary artery bypass grafting is pursued preoperatively, use of a pedicled left internal mammary artery should be avoided if the aneurysm involves the aortic arch or very proximal descending aorta in which case subclavian artery clamping is expected. Valvular disease, specifically aortic regurgitation, also must be ruled out or treated prior to aneurysm repair. Aortic crossclamping leads to an acute increase in afterload which, in the setting of significant aortic regurgitation, will lead to left ventricular distention, acute heart failure, and postoperative dysfunction. 3+ or greater aortic regurgitation should be treated with aortic valve replacement prior to aneurysm repair.

Tobacco use and coexisting pulmonary disease is not uncommon, and the risk of postoperative respiratory failure is a significant concern in this patient population undergoing thoracotomy for aneurysm repair. Room air arterial blood gas is performed on all patients and pulmonary function testing selectively performed in those with known pulmonary disease or blood gas abnormalities. A baseline carbon dioxide partial pressure above 45mmHg, room air oxygen partial pressure below 60mmHg, or a forced expiratory volume in 1 second of less than 1.2L/min is associated with an increased risk of postoperative respiratory failure. In a prospective study of respiratory failure after thoracoabdominal aneurysm repair, forced expiratory flow at 25% ($p = .03$) was an independent predictor of respiratory failure while forced expiratory volume in 1 second and carbon dioxide partial pressure were not (Svensson, Hess, Coselli, Safi, & Crawford 1991). In addition, the ability to clear secretions postoperatively is crucial to successful outcomes, and preoperative tobacco cessation can assist in this.

Operative Technique

Operative technique is focused on an expeditious repair that minimizes the risk of spinal cord ischemia and renal failure. Towards this end, certain adjuncts may be employed, including cerebrospinal fluid (CSF) drainage, left heart or full cardiopulmonary bypass, intercostal artery reimplantation, systemic cooling, and spinal motor evoked potential measurement.

A spinal catheter is placed in the awake patient at the level of L3-L4 for CSF drainage. The patient is then placed under general anesthesia via a double lumen endotracheal tube. Right radial arterial line, swan ganz catheter, and foley catheter are placed. A right femoral vein introducer is placed for rapid infuser access. The patient is placed in the right lateral decubitus position with the left chest up. The hips are rotated 45 degrees such that access to the left femoral vessels is available.

The decision of whether or not to employ left heart or full cardiopulmonary bypass is critical. Left heart bypass may utilize atriofemoral cannulation in which the left atrium is cannulated via the left inferior pulmonary vein for drainage and the left femoral artery is cannulated for return of blood, thus decompressing the left heart and perfusing the distal aorta. If the distal thoracic aorta is uninvolved with aneurysmal disease, this portion of the aorta maybe cannulated in lieu of the femoral artery for return of blood. In the setting of extensive aneurysms, such as extent II aneurysms, left heart bypass is recommended to reduce the risk of spinal cord ischemia. Similarly, its use is recommended in the setting of poor ventricular function or aortic regurgitation, as it allows for decompression of the left heart during the period of aortic crossclamping. If full cardiopulmonary bypass is utilized, as in the case of aneurysms involving the arch requiring circulatory arrest, the left femoral artery and vein are cannulated. The alternative to bypass is the "cut and sew" method, in which the proximal thoracic aorta is clamped and aneurysm is resected and replaced by a graft as fast as possible, with a period of low flow to the distal aorta. This method is appropriate in certain conditions such as coarctation in which significant collaterals have been formed or in short segment aneurysms.

If atriofemoral or full cardiopulmonary bypass is to be utilized, the left femoral vessels are dissected. Aortic repair is via a left thoracotomy for isolated descending thoracic aneurysms. For those extending into the abdomen, a thoracoabdominal approach is utilized in which the thoracotomy incision is extended inferiorly to an upper abdominal paramedian incision. The aorta to be resected is then exposed, dividing the diaphragm and utilizing a retroperitoneal dissection for exposure of the abdominal aorta. Systemic heparinization is then performed to an activated clotting time of 300 seconds. Bypass is initiated and the patient cooled to 34 degrees Celsius. If intrathecal papaverine is to be utilized, it is administered at this time.

The aorta is crossclamped proximal to the aneurysm. CSF drainage to gravity is commenced. If left heart bypass is utilized, a distal aortic clamp is placed and bypass initiated. The aneurysm is opened and intercostal vessels are inspected. Those that are briskly bleeding are likely well perfused via collateral flow and may be oversewn. Those that show no bleeding are likely thrombosed and may similarly be oversewn. Those that are weakly backbleeding likely are patent and dependent on forward flow and consideration is given to reimplantation of these. A rapid infuser system is used for returning large amounts of shed blood. The proximal anastomosis performed. In the setting of a known ascending aneurysm, the reverse elephant trunk technique may be employed for the proximal anastomosis, in which a length of graft is left folded onto itself for use during subsequent sternotomy and aortic arch replacement. If any intercostals are to be reimplanted into the graft, this is done at this time and the proximal clamp moved to the graft below the reimplanted intercostals to perfuse them. All relevant intercostals and visceral arteries are reimplanted and the clamp moved below each anastomosis in succession to perfuse the reimplanted vessel. Bypass is then terminated, the distal aortic crossclamp removed, and the distal anastomosis performed. The graft is deaired, unclamped, and hemostasis is ensured. The incision is closed in layers.

Spinal Cord Protection

Spinal cord ischemia and paralysis is one of the most dreaded complications of thoracoabdominal aneurysm repair. Neurologic deficits may occur intraoperatively or in a delayed fashion postoperatively. Neurologic deficits are caused by three main mechanisms: prolonged crossclamp time; interruption of important sources of blood flow to the spinal cord; and postoperative hemodynamic instability.

The duration of spinal cord ischemia is an important etiologic factor for neurologic deficits. The risk increases after 30 minutes of crossclamp time, but several additional factors play a role and may shift this curve. Conditions with less collateral blood supply to the spinal cord, such as acute dissections or traumatic rupture, have an increased risk for paralysis for a given crossclamp time than do those with greater established collateral blood supply, such as chronic aneurysms or coarctations.

The spinal cord derives blood supply from a single anterior spinal artery, formed by the branches of the vertebral arteries, and two posterolateral spinal arteries. The segmental intercostal and lumbar arteries arising from the aorta supply branches to these spinal arteries. A large such branch, the artery of Adamkiewicz, may arise between T7 and L2 to supply the lower spinal cord. Therefore, reattachment of intercostal arteries, specifically those in the lower thoracic and lumbar distributions, is crucial to prevent neurologic injury. Intercostal ischemia time has been shown to be a greater determinant of neurologic injury than aortic crossclamp time per se. Maneuvers which decrease intercostal ischemia time, such as intercostal reimplantation with successive repositioning of the clamp below each anastomosis to allow reperfusion of a given intercostal, as described above, reduce the risk of neurologic injury. However, in a study of 100 patients undergoing aneurysm repair without intercostal artery reimplantation, an average of eight segmental artery pairs were sacrificed. With the use of motor and somatosensory evoked potentials and hemodynamic manipulation as indicated by these modalities, postoperative paraplegia occurred in two patients (Etz et. al. 2006). The literature is conflicting with regards to intercostal reimpantation, and use of clinical judgement is recommended.

Left heart bypass, by maintaining perfusion pressure to the distal aorta and associated lumbar and intercostal branches, provides protection against neurologic injury. The alternative technique, "cut and sew", is reasonable in short segment aneurysms or coarctations in which crossclamp time is expected to be shorter, less intercostals will be sacrificed, and greater preexisting collateral blood flow to the spine exist, thus reducing the risk of spinal cord ischemia. However, in the setting of more extensive aneurysms or acute dissections, bypass is advisable.

Other intraoperative adjuncts to improve spinal cord protection include hypothermia, intrathecal papaverine, spinal motor evoked potentials, and CSF drainage. Intrathecal papaverine allows for vasodilation of local vessels supplying the spinal cord, while hypothermia reduces metabolic rate. Spinal cord perfusion pressure equals systemic pressure minus CSF pressure, and thus CSF drainage may increase spinal cord perfusion. CSF drainage has been shown to be beneficial in several retrospective and one prospective trial. One hundred forty-five patients undergoing extent I or II aneurysm repairs were prospectively randomized to CSF drainage ($n = 76$) or no CSF drainage ($n = 69$). The two groups were similar with regards to other preoperative and intraoperative variables. Paraplegia was more common in the no CSF drainage group (13% vs 2.6%, $p = .03$) and no patients in the CSF drainage group had immediate postoperative paraplegia (Coselli, LeMaire, Koksoy, Schmittling, & Curling 2002). In another study, 82 clinical series encompassing 15526 patients were analyzed. Expected rates of paraplegia were calculated based on logistic regression analysis of known associated variables. CSF drainage reduced the observed/expected risk of paraplegia both with (1.03 vs .24, p< .001) and without (.91 vs .23, p <.0013) the utilization of bypass (Archer &, Wynn 2009). Several other retrospective series demonstrated similar results (Estrera., Miller III, Huynh, Porat, & Safi 2001, Schepens, Heijmen, Ranschaert, Sonker, Morshuis 2009).

Spinal cord evoked potentials take advantage of the fact that the anterior horn motor neurons are more susceptible to ischemia than the posterior sensory pathways, thus explaining why neurologic deficits tend to present as paraplegia with variably intact sensation. The major setback is that muscle relaxant has to be titrated finely such that motor neuron action potentials are not completely abolished but overt movement is suppressed. Regardless, the degree to which its use will alter the operative course in terms of spinal protection is questionable.

Postoperative Management

Postoperatively, sedation is held immediately and neurologic status assessed hourly. Delayed neurologic deficits are most commonly associated with hemodynamic instability and respiratory dysfunction. Induced hypertension is protective, with vasoconstrictors administered to keep mean arterial pressure (MAP) between 85-90mmHg for the first 2-3 postoperative days, after which the goal MAP is slowly decreased. In the setting of aortic regurgitation where a low diastolic pressure may necessitate extremely high systolic pressures to maintain such MAP goals, vasoconstrictors may be titrated to a systolic blood pressure of 160mmHg. The importance of postoperative hemodynamics in the prevention of delayed paraplegia is difficult to overstate. In a study of 858 aneurysm repairs, ten patients developed delayed postoperative paraplegia despite intact spinal evoked potentials at the end of the operation and were compared to matched control patients who did not develop paraplegia. Patients with immediate postoperative paraplegia were excluded to evaluate only the effect of postoperative hemodynamics. Patients in the delayed postoperative paraplegia group had significantly higher central venous pressures (p = .03) and lower mean arterial pressure relative to their baseline arterial pressure (p = .03 [Etz et. al. 2008]). Every effort is made to avoid respiratory complications. Patients are extubated only after assuring optimal oxygenation and ventilation, and pulmonary toilet is rigorously employed with early ambulation, chest physiotherapy, and a low threshold for bronchoscopy. CSF drainage is maintained for 3 days postoperatively, with CSF pressure maintained below 12mmHg by drainage of no more than 25cc CSF per hour. If CSF pressures remain above 12mmHg despite reaching maximal drainage, the decision to continue drainage is based on neurologic exam. Headache during spinal drainage or after spinal drain removal warrants an assessment for CSF leak at the site of spinal drain skin entry and stitch placement if found. Additionally, head imaging should be performed to assess for subdural hematoma which may result from excessive negative pressure resulting in traction and bleeding from bridging subdural veins. In the setting of a delayed neurologic deficit, treatment consists of spinal drain replacement, induced hypertension, and return to a monitored setting. If treated expeditiously and aggressively, this is usually reversible.

Renal failure is another well described complication after thoracoabdominal aneurysm repair. Associated factors include preexisting renal insufficiency and crossclamp time. In the setting of infrarenal aneurysms requiring renal artery reimplantation, cold crystalloid solution is usually injected into the renal arteries during the ischemic period for protection. Postoperatively, a dopamine infusion and intravenous fluid infusion at a rate of 150-200cc/hr is used to maintain brisk urine output. Diuresis is instituted on postoperative day 2. Progressive renal failure postoperatively may require temporary or permanent hemodialysis.

In experienced hands, outcomes for descending thoracic aortic repair are excellent, with average paralysis rate of 3.4%, a stroke rate of 2.7%, a mortality rate of 4.8%, with five and ten year survival rates of 60% and 38%, respectively (Bavaria et. al. 2008).

DESCENDING AORTIC DISSECTION

Introduction

Type B dissections involve the descending aorta distal to the subclavian artery. They usually present with chest pain radiating to the back and abdomen, associated with hypertension. Management usually consists of medical therapy with antihypertensives, and serial imaging for detection of progressive aneurysm formation. However, acute complications, including malperfusion, rupture, or persistent pain may warrant intervention.

Classification

The classification scheme is described above for ascending aortic dissections.

Etiology

Type B dissection is most commonly a result of degeneration of the aortic media. An initial tear in the intima, usually located at the left subclavian artery and usually associated with hypertension, allows blood to track within the media, creating a false lumen. Propagation of the dissection usually occurs distally, but may extend retrograde to involve the arch and ascending aorta. The false lumen usually remains patent as a result of secondary tears or fenestrations in the distal flap that allow for blood reentry into the true lumen. If no reentry sites exist, the false lumen may thrombose. Branch vessels may become obstructed by progression of the dissection flap. If the dissection flap is fenestrated or sheared off at the site of a branch vessel, that vessel may become supplied by the false lumen. Hypertension and connective tissue disorders are commonly associated.

Presentation

The most common presenting symptom in type B dissection is severe, tearing chest or back pain, involving the interscapular area and radiating to the abdomen. Most patients are hypertensive at initial presentation. Hypotension is rare and should raise concern for rupture.

Malperfusion syndromes occur secondary to branch vessel involvement resulting in end-organ ischemia and dysfunction. Stroke is extremely uncommon. Paraplegia secondary to interruption of intercostal arteries, lower extremity ischemia with a peripheral pulse deficit, renal ischemia with oliguria or flank pain, and visceral ischemia presenting as pain out of proportion to physical exam may occur. In the chronic phase, type B dissections may progress to aneurysm formation, the management of which is as described above.

Preoperative Evaluation

Angiography has historically been the gold standard test for the diagnosis of type B dissections although CTA and MRI have supplanted this, both because of the level of detail offered and their noninvasiveness. MRI is less commonly used due to longer image acquisition time, limited patient access during the study, and limited availability. CTA has the disadvantage of requiring intravenous contrast but may delineate the extent of a dissection, branch vessel involvement, patency of the false lumen, presence of an IMH or PAU, and mediastinal hematoma or pleural effusion suggesting leak. When CTA is performed for suspected aortic dissection, the study should always include the chest, abdomen, and pelvis to include the proximal femoral arteries. Transesophageal echocardiography is also excellent for demonstrating type B dissections. Limitations include the need for sedation, potential hemodynamic fluctuations, user dependence, and inability to visualize branch vessel involvement below the diaphragm.

Management

The mainstay of therapy for type B dissection is with antihypertensive medical management, reserving surgery for those with persistent pain or complications such as rupture or malperfusion. The rationale behind this approach is that medical therapy is successful in the majority of patients while operative mortality is high. Medical treatment should be initiated as soon as dissection is suspected. Agents that reduce the rate of rise of aortic pressure or dP/dt should be firstline, including beta blockers such as esmolol, metoprolol, labetolol, or propranolol. These are usually started as intermittent intravenous bolus or continuous infusion. This may be supplemented by calcium channel blockers such as nifedipine or nicardipine and sodium nitroprusside, as needed. The latter is a pure vasodilator that may increase aortic dP/dt, and should be used in conjunction with one of the other agents mentioned above. Finally, adequate pain control is ensured.

An arterial line, foley catheter, and admission to an intensive care unit are recommended. Serial neurologic, abdominal, and peripheral vascular exams are performed. Serial monitoring of laboratory parameters of renal and hepatic function is performed as is chest radiography to assess for changes in the aortic contour or development of effusions which may suggest rupture. IMH and PAU are managed similarly.

Over the course of the hospitalization, intravenous antihypertensives are transitioned to oral agents including labetolol, metoprolol, or atenolol. Oral calcium channel blockers such as nifedipine, amlodipine, or verapamil and oral angiotensin-converting-enzyme inhibitors or angiotensin receptor blockers may be added. After discharge, rigorous follow-up with serial imaging is mandatory.

Operative Technique

Patients with complicated type B dissections will require more aggressive treatment than described above. Persistent pain, or malperfusion syndromes typically resulting in lower extremity, visceral, or renal ischemia are indications for surgical intervention, with the goal of resecting and replacing the segment of aorta with the primary tear, thus redirecting blood through the true lumen. In most cases this will reverse more distal malperfusion syndromes.

The operative management for acute type B dissections is similar to that of thoracoabdominal aneurysms described above with a few caveats. Spinal cord protection for acute dissections is critical due to the higher risk of spinal cord ischemia as sufficient time has not elapsed for the formation of collateral blood flow. Spinal cord protection is optimized with CSF drainage via a spinal catheter. General anesthesia via a double lumen endotracheal tube is employed. Radial arterial line, swan-ganz catheter, and foley catheter are placed. The patient is placed in the right lateral decubitus position with the left chest up.

Via a left thoracotomy, the descending thoracic aorta is exposed. The primary goal of the operation is to resect a small length of aorta including the primary tear, usually near the left subclavian artery. The "clamp and sew" technique as described above for thoracoabdominal aneurysms is infrequently used, as the risks of spinal cord ischemia are higher due to inadequate time for collateral formation. Left heart or full cardiopulmonary bypass with hypothermic circulatory arrest may be utilized, with the latter allowing an open technique where the proximal aorta is opened without clamping and any proximal extent of the dissection into the arch assessed. With any technique utilizing bypass, the arterial cannulation strategy has to be carefully thought out, with care taken to ensure the true lumen is cannulated. The femoral artery that is in continuity with the true lumen, usually the left, as assessed by preoperative CTA, may be cannulated. The proximal and distal anastomoses are performed with care taken to reapproximate the intima and adventitia such that blood flow is directed into the true lumen only.

In cases in which distal malperfusion syndromes do not resolve with replacement of the proximal tear site, additional options exist. Traditional treatment has been either surgical fenestration or bypass. Surgical fenestration of the distal dissection flap allows for decompression of the false lumen such that blood may more freely enter the true lumen to perfuse more distal branches. Bypass options may include extraanatomic bypass such as axillary femoral bypass or femoral femoral bypass, or bypass to the renal or mesenteric vessels as needed. In more recent times, endovascular options, including endovascular stent graft placement or percutaneous fenestration are more commonly utilized.

Postoperative Management

Postoperative management for acute type B dissections is again similar to thoracoabdominal aneurysms. Spinal cord protection is optimized with CSF drainage, induced hypertension, avoidance of respiratory complications, and frequent neurologic assessment. Dopamine infusions may be utilized to assist with diuresis.

FUTURE RESEARCH DIRECTIONS

Thoracic endovascular aortic repair (TEVAR) of the descending aorta for aneurysmal disease or dissection is a rapidly expanding field. As more data regarding early complications such as spinal cord ischemia and endoleak and long term results become available, this technology will likely have a role in the management of thoracic aortic disease. There are currently no randomized trials comparing TEVAR with surgical repair for chronic thoracic degenerative aneurysms. However, TEVAR has been demonstrated in multicenter, prospective, nonrandomized trials to be safe and efficacious for the treatment of degenerative aneurysmal disease of the thoracic aorta when compared to historical open controls. In the VALOR trial, TEVAR was performed with the Medtronic Talent device (Medtronic, Minneapolis, Minnesota) in 195 patients considered to be candidates for open surgery and compared to 189 historical control patients. TEVAR was associated with a 2.1% 30 day mortality rate, a 1.5% paraplegia rate, a 7.2% paraparesis rate, and a 3.6% stroke rate. At 12 months, TEVAR was associated with a 0.5% rate of conversion to open surgery, a 0.5% rate of rupture, a 12.2% rate of endoleak, and a 91.5% rate of stable or decreasing aneurysm diameter (Fairman et. al. 2008). The Medtronic Valiant device (Medtronic, Minneapolis, Minnesota), the Gore TAG device (W.L. Gore & Associates, Inc., Flagstaff, Arizona), and the Cook Zenith TX2 device (Cook Medical, Bloomington, Indiana) demonstrated similar results (Fairman, et. al.. 2012; Makaroun et. al. 2005; Matsumura et. al. 2008). As the midterm results of these studies suggest durable results over five years (Makaroun, Dillavou, Wheatley, & Cambria, 2008; Foley et. al. 2012), it is considered reasonable by many, to pursue TEVAR in patients at higher risk for conventional surgery (Bavaria et. al. 2008). However, long-term durability remains to be demonstrated, especially with regards to the presence of endoleak and aneurysm sac expansion. Furthermore, TEVAR has been utilized for complicated type B dissections, such as in the setting of rupture or malperfusion. Thirty day and one year mortality rates of 10.8% and 29.4%, respectively (White et. al. 2011) have been quoted in this extremely sick group of patients in whom surgical intervention would likely be poorly tolerated and medical management would be considered unacceptable. More recently, elective TEVAR has been demonstrated to be effective in the setting of acute dissection to prevent the sequelae of disease progression. In the INSTEAD-XL trial, 140 patients with stable type B aortic dissection were randomized to elective TEVAR in the acute/subacute setting (2-52 weeks) plus optimal medical treatment (n=72) or optimal medical treatment alone (n=68) and followed for five years. Elective TEVAR reduced all-cause mortality, aorta-specific mortality, progression of disease, and aorta-specific events. After an initial excess mortality in the TEVAR group attributed to periprocedural events, a significant decrease in mortality in the TEVAR group was seen at 2-5 years, resulting in an overall benefit of TEVAR at five years. This correlated with aortic remodeling in the TEVAR group observed on surveillance imaging, including true lumen expansion and false lumen thrombosis (Nienaber et. al. 2013). At this time, TEVAR for type B aortic dissection is only recommended in the setting of complications, with medical therapy considered optimal for uncomplicated type B dissections. In patients with arch disease, hybrid aortic arch debranching procedures in which the aortic arch great vessels are surgically reimplanted on the proximal ascending aorta allow for subsequent endovascular stenting of the remaining ascending aorta and arch as well as the descending aorta (Czerny et. al. 2007). The frozen elephant trunk procedure in which surgical type A dissection repair is performed with concomitant endovascular stenting of the descending aorta may prevent delayed aneurysmal dilatation of the descending aorta. Immediate and long term results of these and other methods of hybrid open and endovascular approaches to thoracic aortic disease remain to be seen.

CONCLUSION

Thoracic aortic disease represents a spectrum of clinical entities from acute dissection to chronic aneurysmal disease. Successful repair requires expedient surgical techniques that minimize bleeding complications and neurologic complications from prolonged spinal cord and brain ischemic times. Several adjuncts to reduce the neurologic injury rates have made these procedures standard of care in the current era. New and future techniques will incorporate endovascular approaches to stenting the descending aorta and aortic arch. Future studies will determine the long term results and applicability of these approaches.

REFERENCES

Archer, C. W., & Wynn, M. (2009). A modern theory of paraplegia in the treatment of aneurysms of the thoracoabdominal aorta: An analysis of technique specific observed/expected ratios for paralysis. *Journal of Vascular Surgery*, *49*(5), 1117–1124. doi:10.1016/j.jvs.2008.10.074 PMID:19394541

Bavaria, J. E., Coselli, J. S., Curi, M. A., Eggebrecht, H., Elefteriades, J. A., & Erbel, R. (2008). Expert consensus document on the treatment of descending thoracic aortic disease using endovascular stent-grafts. *The Annals of Thoracic Surgery*, *85*(1), S1–S41. doi:10.1016/j.athoracsur.2007.10.099 PMID:18083364

Cohn, L. H., Rizo, R. J., Adams, D. H., Aranki, S. F., Couper, G. S., Beckel, N., & Collins, J. J. (1996). Reduced mortality and morbidity for ascending aortic aneurysm resection regardless of cause. *The Annals of Thoracic Surgery*, *62*(2), 463–468. doi:10.1016/0003-4975(96)00280-9 PMID:8694606

Coselli, J. S., LeMaire, S. A., Koksoy, C., Schmittling, Z. C., & Curling, P. E. (2002). Cerebrospinal fluid drainage reduces paraplegia after thoracoabdominal aortic aneurysm repair: Results of a randomized clinical trial. *Journal of Vascular Surgery*, *35*(4), 631–639. doi:10.1067/mva.2002.122024 PMID:11932655

Czerny, M., Gottardi, R., Zimpfer, D., Schoder, M., Grabenwoger, M., Lammer, J., & Grimm, M. et al. (2007). Mid-ter.m results of supraaortic transpositions for extended endovascular repair of aortic arch pathologies *Europea.n. Journal of Cardiothoracic Surgery*, *31*(4), 623–627. doi:10.1016/j.ejcts.2006.12.030 PMID:17239613

Davies, R. R., Goldstein, L. J., Coady, M. A., Tittle, S. L., Rizzo, J. A., Kopf, G. S., & Elefteriades, J. A. (2002). Yearly rupture or dissection rates for thoracic aortic aneurysms: Simple prediction based on size. *The Annals of Thoracic Surgery*, *73*(1), 17–28. doi:10.1016/S0003-4975(01)03236-2 PMID:11834007

Estrera, A. L., Miller, C. C. III, Huynh, T. T., Porat, E., & Safi, H. J. (2001). Neurologic outcome after thoracic and thoracoabdominal aortic aneurysm repair. *The Annals of Thoracic Surgery*, *72*(4), 1225–1231. doi:10.1016/S0003-4975(01)02971-X PMID:11603441

Etz, C. D., Halstead, J. C., Spielvogel, D., Shahani, R., Lazala, R., Homann, T. M., & Griep, R. B. et al. (2006). Thoracic and thoracoabdominal aneurysm repair: Is reimplantation of spinal cord arteries a waste of time? *The Annals of Thoracic Surgery*, *82*(5), 1670–1678. doi:10.1016/j.athoracsur.2006.05.029 PMID:17062225

Etz, C. D., Luehr, M., Kari, F. A., Bodian, C. A., Smego, D., Plestis, K. A., & Griepp, R. B. (2008). Paraplegia after extensive thoracic and thoracoabdominal aortic aneurysm repair: Does critical spinal cord ischemia occur postoperatively? *The Journal of Thoracic and Cardiovascular Surgery*, *135*(2), 324–330. doi:10.1016/j.jtcvs.2007.11.002 PMID:18242262

Fairman, R. M., Criado, F., Farber, M., Kwolek, C., Mehta, M., White, R., & Tuchek, J. M. et al. (2008, September)..... Tuchek J.M. Pivotal results of the Medtronic Vascular Talent Thoracic Stent Graft System: The VALOR Trial. *Journal of Vascular Surgery*, *48*(3), 546–554. doi:10.1016/j.jvs.2008.03.061 PMID:18572352

Fairman, R. M., Tuchek, J. M., Lee, W. A., Karthikeshwar, K., White, R., Mehta, M., & Bavaria, J. et al. (2012). Pivotal. results for the Medtronic Valiant Thoracic Stent Graft System in the VALOR II trial. *Journal of Vascular Surgery*, *56*(5), 1222–1231. doi:10.1016/j.jvs.2012.04.062 PMID:22832267

Foley, P. J., Criado, F. J., Farber, M. A., Kwolek, C. J., Mehta, M., White, R. A., & Fairman, R. M. et al. (2012). Results with the Talent thoracic stent graft in the VALOR trial. *Journal of Vascular Surgery*, *56*(5), 1214–1221. doi:10.1016/j.jvs.2012.04.071 PMID:22925732

Girardi, L. N., Rabotnikov, Y., & Avgerinos, D. V. (2014). Preoperative percutaneous coronary intervention in patients undergoing open thoracoabdominal and descending thoracic aneurysm repair. *The Journal of Thoracic and Cardiovascular Surgery*, *147*(1), 163–168. doi:10.1016/j.jtcvs.2013.09.008 PMID:24176270

Girardi L.N., Shavladze S., Sedrakyan A., Neragi S. (2014). Safety and efficacy of retrograde cerebral perfusion as an adjunct for cerebral protection during surgery on the aortic arch. *The Journal of Thoracic and Cardiovascular Surgery,* Jul 30. pii: S0022-5223(14)00989-1. doi: . [Epub ahead of print].10.1016/j.jtcvs.2014.07.024

Lopes, R. J., Almeida, J., Dias, P. J., Pinho, P., & Maciel, M. J. (2009). Infectious thoracic aortitis: A literature review. *Clinical Cardiology*, *32*(9), 488–490. doi:10.1002/clc.20578 PMID:19743492

Makaroun, M. S., Dillaviy, E. D., Wheatley, G. H., & Cambria, R. P. (2008). Five year results of endovascular treatment with the Gore TAG device compared with open repair of thoracic aortic aneurysms. *Journal of Vascular Surgery*, *47*(5), 912–918. doi:10.1016/j.jvs.2007.12.006 PMID:18353605

Makaroun, M. S., Dillavou, E. D., Kee, S. T., Sicard, G., Chaikof, E., Bavaria, J., & Mitchell, R. S. et al. (2005). Endovas.cular treatment of thoracic aortic aneurysms: Results of the phase II multicenter trial of the GORE TAG thoracic endoprosthesis. *Journal of Vascular Surgery*, *41*(1), 1–9. doi:10.1016/j.jvs.2004.10.046 PMID:15696036

Matsumura, J. S., Cambria, R. P., Dake, M. D., Moore, R. D., Svensson, L. G., & Snyder, S. (2008). International controlled clinical trial of thoracic endovascular aneurysm repair with the Zenith TX2 endovascular graft: 1-year results. *Journal of Vascular Surgery*, *47*(2), 247–257. doi:10.1016/j.jvs.2007.10.032 PMID:18241743

Nienaber, C. A., Kische, S., Rosseau, H., Eggebrecht, H., Rehders, T. C., Kundt, G., & Ince, H. et al. (2013). Endovas.cular repair of type B aortic dissection: Long-term results of the randomized investigation of stent grafts in aortic dissection trial. *Circulation: Cardiovascular Interventions*, *6*(4), 407–416. doi:10.1161/CIRCINTERVENTIONS.113.000463 PMID:23922146

Pagni, S., Ganzel, B. L., Williams, M., Slater, A. D., & Trivedi, J. R. (2012). Inflammatory aneurysms of the ascending aorta: Diagnosis and surgical treatment. *Journal of Cardiac Surgery*, *27*(1), 70–74. doi:10.1111/j.1540-8191.2011.01335.x PMID:22103645

Pomianowski, P., & Elefteriades, J. A. (2013). The genetics and genomics of thoracic aortic disease. *Annals of Cardiothoracic Surgery*, *2*(3), 271–279. PMID:23977594

Schepens, M. A., Heijmen, R. H., Ranschaert, W., Sonker, U., & Morshuis, W. J. (2009). Thoracoabdominal aortic aneurysm repair: Results of conventional open surgery. *European Journal of Vascular and Endovascular Surgery*, *37*(6), 640–645. doi:10.1016/j.ejvs.2009.03.011 PMID:19362499

Svensson, L. G., Hess, K. R., Coselli, J. S., Safi, H. J., & Crawford, S. (1991). A prospective study of respiratory failure after high-risk surgery on the thoracoabdominal aorta. *Journal of Vascular Surgery*, *14*(3), 271–282. doi:10.1016/0741-5214(91)90077-8 PMID:1880835

Verma, S., & Siu, S. C. (2014). Aortic dilatation in patients with bicuspid aortic valve. *The New England Journal of Medicine*, *370*(20), 1920–1929. doi:10.1056/NEJMra1207059 PMID:24827036

White, R. A., Miller, D. C., Criado, F. J., Dake, M. D., Diethrich, E. B., Greenberg, R. K., & Siami, F. S. et al. (2011). Report on the results of thoracic endovascular aortic repair for acute, complicated, type B aortic dissection at 30 days and 1 year from a multidisciplinary subcommittee of the Society for Vascular Surgery Outcomes Committee. *Journal of Vascular Surgery*, *53*(4), 1082–1090. doi:10.1016/j.jvs.2010.11.124 PMID:21334174

ADDITIONAL READING

Bensley, R. P., Curran, T., Hurks, R., Lo, R. C., Wyers, M. C., Hamdan, A. D., & Schermerhorn, M. L. et al. (2013). Open repair of intact thoracoabdominal aortic aneurysms in the American College of Surgeons National Surgical Quality Improvement Program. *Journal of Vascular Surgery*, *58*(4), 894–900. doi:10.1016/j.jvs.2013.03.037 PMID:23642916

Canadas, V., Vilacosta, I., Bruna, U., & Fuster, V. (2010). Marfan syndrome. Part 1: Pathophysiology and diagnosis. *Nature Reviews. Cardiology*, *7*(5), 256–265. PMID:20351703

Cook, J. R., Carta, L., Galatioto, J., & Ramirez, F. (2014). Cardiovascular manifestations in Marfan syndrome and related diseases; multiple genes causing similar phenotypes. [Epub ahead of print]. *Clinical Genetics*. doi:10.1111/cge.12436 PMID:24867163

Coselli, J. S., Bozinovski, J., & LeMaire, S. A. (2007). Open surgical repair of 2286 thoracoabdominal aortic aneurysms. *The Annals of Thoracic Surgery*, *83*(2), S862–S864. doi:10.1016/j.athoracsur.2006.10.088 PMID:17257942

David, T. E. (2010). Surgery of the Aortic Root and Ascending Aorta. In Selke F.W., del Nido P.J., Swanson S.J. (Eds.) Sabiston and Spencer Surgery of the Chest (pp. 1021-1039). Philadelphia, PA. Elsiever/Saunders doi:10.1016/B978-1-4160-5225-8.00067-2

Demers, P., & Miller, D. C. (2010). Type A Aortic Dissection. In Selke F.W., del Nido P.J., Swanson S.J. (Eds.) Sabiston and Spencer Surgery of the Chest (pp. 1089-1114). Philadelphia, PA. Elsiever/Saunders

Demers, P., & Miller, D. C. (2010). Type B Aortic Dissection. In Selke F.W., del Nido P.J., Swanson S.J. (Eds.) Sabiston and Spencer Surgery of the Chest (pp. 1115-1126). Philadelphia, PA. Elsiever/Saunders

Desai, N. D., & Bavaria, J. E. (2012). Ascending Aortic Aneurysms. In L. H. Cohn (Ed.), *Cardiac Surgery in the Adult* (pp. 997–1028). New York, New York: McGraw-Hill Companies, Inc.

Elefteriades, J. A. (2002). Natural history of thoracic aortic aneurysms: Indications for surgery, and surgical versus nonsurgical risks. *The Annals of Thoracic Surgery*, *74*(5), S11877–S11880. doi:10.1016/S0003-4975(02)04147-4 PMID:12440685

Goldfinger, J. Z., Halperin, J. L., Marin, M. L., Stewart, A. S., Eagle, K. A., & Fuster, V. (2014, October). Thoracic aortic aneurysm and dissection. *Journal of the American College of Cardiology*, *64*(16), 1725–1739. doi:10.1016/j.jacc.2014.08.025 PMID:25323262

Hiratzka, L. F., Bakris, G. L., Beckman, J. A., Bersin, R. M., Carr, V. F., Casey, D. E. Jr, & Williams, D. M. et al. (2010). ACCF/AHA/AATS/ACR/ASA/SCA/SCAI/SIR/STS/SVM Guidelines for the diagnosis and management of patients with thoracic aortic disease. *Journal of the American College of Cardiology*, *55*(14), e27–e129. doi:10.1016/j.jacc.2010.02.015 PMID:20359588

Huh, J., LeMaire, S. A., & Coselli, J. S. (2012). Descending and Thoracoabdominal Aortic Aneurysms. In L. H. Cohn (Ed.), *Cardiac Surgery in the Adult* (pp. 997–1028). New York, New York: McGraw-Hill Companies, Inc.

Iba, Y., Minatoya, K., Matsuda, H., Sasaki, H., Tanaka, H., Morisaki, H., & Ogino, H. et al. (2012). Surgical experience with aggressive aortic pathologic process in Loeys-Dietz syndrome. *The Annals of Thoracic Surgery*, *94*(5), 1413–1417. doi:10.1016/j.athoracsur.2012.05.111 PMID:22921234

LeMaire, S. A., Price, M. D., Green, S. Y., Zarda, S., & Coselli, J. S. (2012). Results of open thoracoabdominal aortic aneurysm repair. *Annals of Cardiothoracic Surgery*, *1*(3), 286–292. PMID:23977510

Mery, C. M., Reece, T. B., & Kron, I. (2012). Aortic Dissection. In L. H. Cohn (Ed.), *Cardiac Surgery in the Adult* (pp. 997–1028). New York, New York: McGraw-Hill Companies, Inc.

Moffatt-Bruce, S. D., & Mitchell, R. S. (2012). Endovascular Therapy for the Treatment of Thoracic Aortic Disease. In L. H. Cohn (Ed.), *Cardiac Surgery in the Adult* (pp. 997–1028). New York, New York: McGraw-Hill Companies, Inc.

Patel, J. H., & Deeb, G. M. (2008). Ascending and arch aorta: Pathology, natural history, and treatment. *Circulation*, *118*(2), 188–195. doi:10.1161/CIRCULATIONAHA.107.690933 PMID:18606928

Romaniello F., Mazzaglia D., Pellegrino A., Grego S., Fiorito R., Ferlosio A.,…Orlandi A. (2014). Aortopathy in Marfan syndrome: an update. *Society for Cardiovascular Pathology*, pii: S1054-8807(14)00054-4. doi: . [Epub ahead of print]10.1016/j.carpath.2014.04.007

Sinha, A. C., & Cheung, A. T. (2010). Spinal cord protection and thoracic aortic surgery. *Current Opinion in Anaesthesiology*, *23*(1), 95–102. doi:10.1097/ACO.0b013e3283348975 PMID:19920758

Spielvogel, D., Mathur, M. N., & Griepp, R. B. (2012). Aneurysms of the Aortic Arch. In L. H. Cohn (Ed.), *Cardiac Surgery in the Adult* (pp. 997–1028). New York, New York: McGraw-Hill Companies, Inc.

Svensson, L. G. (2010). Surgery of the Aortic Arch. In Selke F.W., del Nido P.J., Swanson S.J. (Eds.) Sabiston and Spencer Surgery of the Chest (pp. 1041-1062). Philadelphia, PA. Elsiever/Saunders doi:10.1016/B978-1-4160-5225-8.00068-4

Svensson, L. G. (2010). Descending Thoracic and Thoracoabdominal Aortic Surgery. In Selke F.W., del Nido P.J., Swanson S.J. (Eds.) Sabiston and Spencer Surgery of the Chest (pp. 1063-1067). Philadelphia, PA. Elsiever/Saunders doi:10.1016/B978-1-4160-5225-8.00069-6

Svensson, L. G., Crawford, E. S., Hess, K. R., Coselli, J. S., & Safi, H. J. (1993). Experience with 1509 patients undergoing thoracoabdominal aortic operations. *Journal of Vascular Surgery*, *17*(2), 357–370. doi:10.1016/0741-5214(93)90421-H PMID:8433431

Wong, D. R., Coselli, J. S., Amerman, K., Bozinovski, J., Carter, S. A., Vaughn, W. K., & LeMaire, S. A. (2007). Delayed spinal cord deficits after thoracoabdominal aortic aneurysm repair. *The Annals of Thoracic Surgery*, *83*(4), 1345–1355. doi:10.1016/j.athoracsur.2006.11.035 PMID:17383338

KEY TERMS AND DEFINITIONS

Aneurysm: A localized, abnormal dilation of an artery, vein, or portion of the heart; arbitrarily defined by some as a dilation to twice the normal width.

Aortic Root: That portion of the aorta extending from the aortic valve to the sinotubular junction, containing the sinuses of Valsalva and the coronary ostia.

Cardiopulmonary Bypass: A procedure that circulates and oxygenates the blood while surgery is performed on the heart. With this process, blood is diverted from the heart and lungs through a heart-lung machine and oxygenated blood is returned to the aorta.

Deep Hypothermic Circulatory Arrest: A technique involving cooling the body of a patient and stopping circulation to allow operation on the aortic arch and certain brain aneurysms.

Dissection: A progressive tear in the wall of an artery such that the intima and media separate creating a false lumen in between that blood tracks through.

Malperfusion Syndrome: A complication of aortic dissection caused by branch vessel involvement resulting in end-organ ischemia and dysfunction.

Marfan Syndrome: An autosomal dominant disease caused by mutation of the gene encoding fibrillin-1, a glycoprotein component of the extracellular matrix, resulting in ophthalmologic, orthopedic, and cardiovascular manifestations.

Neurologic Protection: The act of reducing the risk of cerebral or spinal cord injury during periods of decreased or absent blood flow, as during surgery on the aortic arch or descending thoracic aorta.

Spinal Cord Ischemia: Decreased blood flow to the spinal cord, as occurs during surgery to the descending thoracic aorta.

Chapter 26
Heart Transplantation:
Surgical Techniques and Postoperative Concerns

Ahmed El-Eshmawi
Mount Sinai Medical Center, USA

Anelechi Anyanwu
Mount Sinai Medical Center, USA

ABSTRACT

Orthotopic heart transplantation (OHT) has evolved as the "gold standard" therapy for end stage cardiomyopathy, Advances in the fields of immunosuppression, infection prophylaxis and treatment, surgical techniques as well as intensice care management have transformed heart transplantation from what was once considered an experimental intervention into a standard therapy. This chapter focuses on the standard care for OHT including surgical techniques, perioperative management and management of common postoperative complications.

INTRODUCTION

Orthotopic heart transplantation (OHT) has evolved as the "gold standard" therapy for end stage cardiomyopathy, with median survival exceeding 10 years. Advances in the fields of immunosuppression, infection prophylaxis and treatment, as well as surgical techniques have transformed heart transplantation from what was once considered an experimental intervention into a standard therapy. Despite these advances, the annual number of transplants in most countries has been relatively static, or declining, over the last two decades due to paucity of donors. The lack of donors has led to increased use of marginal hearts from donors with traditional contraindications to heart donation, such as left ventricular hypertrophy, prolonged cardiac arrest, age > 60 years, active infections, amongst others. The paucity of donors has also lead to longer waiting times and widespread use of ventricular assist devices to bridge patients to transplant. Additionally, the successes of transplantation have led to expansion of the therapy to several

DOI: 10.4018/978-1-4666-8603-8.ch026

high risk recipient groups, who were previously not regarded as candidates for transplantation, such as patients aged > 70 years, patients with multiple prior operations and patients with multiple comorbidities. The net result has been that despite advances in therapy, patients coming to the intensive care unit after heart transplantation are paradoxically sicker than they were few decades ago and present unique challenge. The recipients tend to be more complex, the surgeries more complicated and the donor heart function less predictable.

This chapter focuses on the standard care for OHT including surgical techniques, perioperative management and management of common postoperative complications.

BACKGROUND

In the past decade, recipient demographics have shown dramatic changes. Because of advances in care of acute myocardial infarction, the leading indication for heart transplant shifted from ischemic cardiomyopathy to non-ischemic cardiomyopathy. Although the median age of an adult heart transplant recipient remained relatively static (about 54 years), a higher proportion of patients in their 60s and 70s have received a heart transplant during the last decade, compared to previous decades. The proportion of recipients with major comorbidities and patients sensitized to human leucocyte antigen (HLA) continue to increase. The number of patients bridged to transplant with mechanical circulatory support (MCS) devices has increased to more than 30%, and in some centers, such as the authors' over 90% of recipients are bridged with mechanical devices. In addition the paucity of donors has resulted in a universal trend toward transplanting urgent status recipients. It is becoming increasingly infrequent in many centers to transplant stable ambulatory patients who are not dependent on inotropes or mechanical devices. Also, the incidence of multiorgan transplantation, including heart–lung, heart–kidney and heart–liver, has risen steadily over the years (Taylor et al., 2008).

Subsequently, we are facing a complex heterogeneous heart transplant population with more challenging peri-transplant management necessitating involvement of a multidisciplinary team who are trained to handle general cardiac surgery patients with particular interest in OHT in order to achieve an excellent outcome.

Patient survival rate has improved to 93% at 3 months, 88% at 1 year, 73% at 5 years and 55% at 10 years. The median survival is currently 11 years. During the first year, graft failure, surgical complications, infection and acute rejection are the leading causes of death. After 5 years, malignancy and allograft vasculopathy are the leading causes (Stehlik et al., 2012).

PRETRANSPLANT MANAGEMENT

Indications for Cardiac Transplantation

Cardiac transplantation is reserved primarily for the treatment of patients with end-stage heart disease who have a reduced one-year expected survival despite optimal medical therapy. Patients should lack significant co-morbidities that might limit post-transplant survival.

Recipient Selection

Evaluation of patients with end stage heart failure and the selection of potential cardiac transplantation candidates is undertaken by a multidisciplinary team to ensure an equitable, objective and medically justified allocation of the limited donor organs.

The basic objective of the selection process is to identify those patients who would potentially resume a normal active life while maintaining compliance with a rigorous medical regimen after cardiac transplantation (Mehra et al., 2006; Hunt et al., 2009); (Table 1).

Alternate Listing

Alternate waiting lists allow patients denied transplantation under standard criteria to be considered for donor hearts that might otherwise be discarded. In so doing, this alternate list program hopes to expand both the donor and recipient pools.

Hearts from donors with relative (and sometimes absolute) contraindications to donor use (see *Donor selection* below) may selectively be considered for transplant to alternate list recipients. Alternate risk recipients include patients with single or multiple relative contraindications to listing (such as patients with HIV, patients aged > 70 years, severe diabetics etc.). Because the recipients and donors are highly selected, the results of alternate list transplants are comparable to that of standard donors of recipients, however, the complication rate and demands on peri-operative intensive care are predictably higher because of recipient complexity and marginal status of most such donors (Chen et al., 2005; Felker et al., 2005).

Donor Selection

The decision to accept a donor heart for a specific recipient is typically made by consensus between the transplant cardiologist and surgeon. Consideration is not limited to donor factors but also includes recipient and logistic factors that in combination may impact on outcome of transplantation. Sometimes the availability of intensive care resources to handle the perioperative care of a particular transplant can be a factor in deciding whether to proceed with a transplant.

Donors with a relative contraindication are considered marginal donors. Recipient factors will be considered to determine if such hearts are acceptable for a standard list recipient. Marginal hearts will generally be suitable for all alternate list recipients.

Donors with two or three relative contraindications are very-high risk donors and generally should only be considered for alternate list recipients or standard list recipients who are felt to have a very high probability of imminent death without transplant.

The presence of multiple relative contraindications usually implies an absolute contraindication for use of the donor (Zaroff et al., 2002). Table 2 lists the absolute and relative contraindications for donor selection.

Donor Harvest and Preservation

The brain death physiological environment predisposes the potential donor heart to profound metabolic and hemodynamic derangements including intensive vagal discharge with bradycardia and hypertension followed by a catecholamine storm; epinephrine and norepinephrine levels may increase more than 100-

Table 1.

Inclusion Criteria	
1.	End stage heart failure. Patients should meet following criteria d. NYHA Class III or IV heart failure despite optimal medical therapy e. Absence of correctable structural heart disease (unless myopathy is deemed minimally irreversible) f. Peak oxygen consumption (VO_2) <10 mL/kg/min, OR dependence on intravenous inotropic support or mechanical devices to maintain adequate organ perfusion, OR refractory cardiogenic shock.
2.	Malignant ventricular arrhythmias refractory to medical therapy.
3.	Congenital heart disease not amenable to further correction or repair.
4.	Hypertrophic cardiomyopathy with very high risk of sudden death despite implantable defibrillator.
5.	Localized, non-metastatic cardiac tumors.
6.	Inoperable structural heart disease.
Exclusion Criteria	
Absolute Contraindications	
1.	Severe pulmonary hypertension with an inability to reduce the Pulmonary Vascular Resistance (PVR) below 6 wood units
2.	Irreversible renal or hepatic dysfunction in patients considered for isolated OHT.
3.	Advanced lung disease
4.	Any major chronic disabling disease which significantly limits mid-term survival such that patient unlikely to survive two years beyond transplantation.
5.	Active or recent malignancy (within 5 years) excluding localized basal or squamous cell carcinoma of the skin; or localized renal or prostate carcinoma.
6.	Uncontrolled HIV infection
7.	Active tobacco use
8.	Active dependence upon alcohol or controlled substances
9.	Neurologic, psychological or social barriers that would preclude one's ability to reliably comply with medical therapy and follow-up examinations
Relative Contraindications	
1.	Age >70 years
2.	Diabetes with evidence of end-organ damage (retinopathy, nephropathy, vasculopathy) or uncontrolled DM (HbA1c > 7.5%)
3.	Chronic kidney disease with a glomerular filtration rate < 33 ml/min (combined heart/kidney transplantation may be a consideration for patients with GFR < 33 ml/min)
4.	Hepatic cirrhosis (Bilirubin >2.5 mg/dL, serum transaminases >3, international normalized ratio >1.5 off Warfarin or cirrhosis on biopsy). Combined heart/liver transplant is a consideration
5.	Pre-transplant BMI > 35 kg/m2 or percent ideal body weight (PIBW) >140%
6.	Cachexia (BMI < 18 kg/m2)
7.	Severe peripheral vascular or cerebrovascular disease not amenable to surgical or percutaneous therapy
8.	Chronic HIV infection, Chronic Hepatitis C infection with viremia, Active Hepatitis B infection with detectable HBV-DNA
9.	Active infection other than related to the heart or cardiac devices
10.	Dependence upon mechanical ventilation
11.	Active peptic ulcer disease
12.	Acute pulmonary thromboembolism

NYHA: New York Heart Association; **VO_2:** venous oxygen; **HIV:** human immunodeficiency virus; **DM:** diabetes mellitus; **HbA1c:** glycosylated hemoglobin; **GFR:** glomerular filtration rate; **HBV-DNA:** Hepatitis-B DNA (deoxyribonucleic acid); **BMI:** body mass index

Table 2.

Absolute Contraindications	
1.	Projected ischemia time > 5 hours
2.	Confirmed myocardial infarction with systolic dysfunction
3.	LVEF < 30% on most recent echocardiogram
4.	Structural cardiac disease not amenable to simple corrective surgery
5.	Active infection with transmissible pathogens including, but not limited to, HIV or hepatitis C virus
6.	Active bacterial infection with highly resistant bacteria
7.	Bacterial endocarditis
8.	Active or recent extracranial malignancy
9.	Penetrating cardiac trauma
10.	Prior cardiac surgery
11.	Severe left ventricular hypertrophy (wall thickness > 1.7cm)
12.	Left main coronary artery stenosis
13.	Critical coronary stenosis in two or more coronary vessels
Relative Contraindications	
1.	Donor - recipient height mismatch (donor may be no more than 6 inches shorter than recipient)
2.	Donor - recipient size mismatch (donor may weigh no more than 20% less than the recipient)
3.	Age > 60 years
4.	LVEF <45% or wall motion abnormality on rest echocardiography with minimal change on stress echocardiography
5.	High donor inotrope requirement which cannot be weaned (> 5 mcg/kg/min Dobutamine or equivalent)
6.	Prolonged cardiopulmonary resuscitation (>10 minutes) within 48 hours of procurement
7.	Male donors > 40 years and female donors > 45 years with cardiovascular risk factors and an inability to perform coronary angiography
8.	Active high risk behavior which increases the likelihood of viral hepatitis or HIV infection, including intravenous drug use or risky sexual activity
9.	Donor cardiovascular or respiratory instability
10.	Projected ischemia time 4 to 5 hours
11.	Left ventricular hypertrophy with wall thickness >1.4cm
12.	Bacteremia with positive blood cultures within 24 hours of procurement
13.	Carbon monoxide poisoning
14.	Major chest trauma with evidence of mediastinal injury
15.	Moderate valvular disease of donor heart including atrioventricular valve regurgitation and bicuspid aortic valve stenosis
16.	Non-obstructive coronary artery disease, or one vessel obstructive coronary artery disease amenable to surgical or percutaneous revascularization
17.	Active infection with HBS Ag+ serology

LVEF: Left ventricular ejection fraction; **HIV:** Human Immunodeficiency Virus; **HBS Ag:** Hepatitis B Surface Antigen fold and arterial blood pressure can rise substantially, with resultant coronary vasospasm. This may lead to subendocardial ischemia, necrosis, and myocardial depression with regional wall motion abnormalities.

Additionally, brain death leads to loss of central thermoregulation, central diabetes insipidus with hypovolemia, and frequent development of neurogenic pulmonary edema. Invasive monitoring and inotropic support might be required to maintain filling pressures as well as high inspired oxygen concentration and positive end-expiratory pressure ventilation.

Potential donors should be managed as aggressively in the intensive care units as any other critical patient with full hemodynamic monitoring to maintain adequate myocardial function, with aggressive volume resuscitation, avoiding of volume overload and maintaining normal electrolytes and acid base balance status, hemoglobin levels are kept above 10 gm with aggressive treatment of central diabetes insipidus (DI) as well as hormonal replacement therapy (free triiodothyroxin, steroids and insulin) while normothermia is maintained with standard ventilatory support.

Donor heart is harvested through a median sternotomy. After pericardiotomy, the heart is examined for any evidence of regional wall motion abnormalities, previous infarctions, myocardial contusion, and coronary calcifications. Donor is systemically heparinized. Great veins are ligated and heart exsanguinated by opening the inferior vena cava, additional venting is achieved by transection of the left superior pulmonary vein or opening the left atrial appendage in case of concurrent lung harvest. The ascending aorta is clamped just proximal to the innominate artery and the heart is arrested with crystalloid cardioplegia infused into the aortic root. Rapid cooling is facilitated by applying ice slush into the pericardial well. Assuring the competence of the aortic root while giving the cardioplegia, as well as maintaining completely flaccid non distended ventricles is of great importance to avoid subendocardial ischemia. Compromise in the procurement procedure can be a contributory factor to post-operative graft dysfunction.

Cold static preservation with crystalloid solutions is the current gold standard for donor heart myocardial protection. It allows safe overall ischemic time of up to 4 hours with a perioperative graft failure rate less than 20%; a wide variety of preservation solutions whether intracellular or extracellular are used with overall similar results.

Ischemic time for the donor heart starts with aortic cross-clamp during the harvest and ends with removal of the cross-clamp from the recipient aorta. In the situations when ischemic times longer than 4 hours are expected, caution should be taken in accepting hearts with other marginal characteristics (such as advanced donor age, ventricular hypertrophy and depressed ejection fraction).

The data from the ISHLT registry consistently shows a statistically significant increase in acute graft failure and in 1-year and 5-year mortality rates with ischemic times longer than 210 minutes (Wagner, 2011a; Stehlik et al., 2012) so, ideally, attempts should be made to avoid ischemic times that approach 4 hours.

Warm Blood Perfusion

In an effort to circumvent the length of cold ischemic time as a limiting factor, the Trans- Medics portable warm blood perfusion system, the Organ Care System (TransMedics,

Andover, Massachusetts), a transportable commercial system that allows warm preservation, has recently been developed.

The organ care system consists of a miniature pulsatile pump with an inline heater and oxygenator which allows the heart to beat and be continually perfused.

Proprietary solution for organ maintenance consists of a crystalloid part combined with oxygenated warm donor blood with hematocrit of 20% to 25%. This allows maintenance of the donor heart in a warm functioning beating state outside the body. The Organ Care System allows resuscitation of the allograft and continued functional evaluation. It also allows direct visual, biochemical and echocardiographic surveillance, and ex vivo coronary angiography of a donor heart.

Two phase-I trials, one in Europe and one in the United States, evaluated the Organ Care System in HT. Thirty-day patient survival rate was 93%. In both trials the cold ischemic time was reduced to approximately 60 to 80 minutes. In one case with perfusion time of 7 hours and 32 minutes, the Organ Care System allowed a transplant with excellent primary graft function (Yeter et al., 2011). This device remains under investigation in the United States.

OPERATIVE MANAGEMENT

Anesthetic and Perioperative Considerations

OHT occurs on an urgent or emergent basis, frequently during night hours. Timing of heart transplantation depends primarily on the timing of multiorgan donor procurement.

Preoperative evaluation and preparation of the recipient must be expeditious with quick history and examination for any updates with a new chest X-ray and full routine labs.

Preanesthetic evaluation includes a review of level of cardiovascular support (inotropic infusions, chronic medications for heart failure, and presence of LVAD), existing indwelling vascular catheters, and antiarrhythmic devices (pacemaker, ICD, CRT, or CRT-D). Recent chest radiographs and laboratory studies must be reviewed to assess pulmonary, hepatic, hematological, hemostatic and renal compromise associated with HF. Preoperative vitamin K injection administrated on admission for patients on warfarin is potentially helpful in reducing perioperative blood loss.

History of prior sternotomy, presence of LVAD, or history of difficult airway can increase recipient preparation time. Patients, particularly those with LVADs, should be reviewed for active and prior infections and perioperative antibiotic prophylaxis adjusted accordingly.

Evaluation of preoperative CT scans of the mediastinum is crucial in patients who had previous cardiac surgery to plan for sternal re-entry.

Antiarrhythmic devices need to be interrogated and reprogrammed to a mode that is not affected by electrocautery interference; this can be achieved in many devices by placement of a magnet. The perioperative team should be aware of implications and interactions of various medications on perioperative course and management. Patients with end-stage heart disease are frequently taking angiotensin-converting enzyme inhibitors which can increase the risk of vasoplegia, or chronically anticoagulated with warfarin that can increase the risk of bleeding. Vasopressin infusion can be beneficial for treatment of angiotensin-converting enzyme inhibitor-induced hypotension, and fresh frozen plasma or prothrombin complex concentrate should be ordered if the international normalized ratio is elevated.

Ideally, induction of anesthesia and recipient surgical incision begins after the harvesting team has examined the donor heart and made the final determination that the organ is acceptable. Optimally, the timing of donor excision and recipient surgery is aligned, such that the recipient is placed on cardiopulmonary bypass (CPB) and the heart is excised to coincide with arrival of the donor heart at the recipient hospital.

Large-bore intravenous access and arterial lines are placed before induction of general anesthesia. It is often helpful to have a central arterial monitoring catheter (axillary or femoral artery) because of abnormal pressure gradients that frequently develop between the radial artery and aorta.

Many anesthesiologists prefer continuous cardiac output – mixed venous oxygen saturation (MVO_2) pulmonary artery catheters placement before the induction for complete hemodynamic assessment. The pulmonary artery catheter needs to be withdrawn during the removal and implantation process. For this reason, it is important to ensure the sterile sheath encompasses at least 80 cm of the catheter when it is inserted. The catheter is typically removed to the 20 cm mark to ensure the scissors does not catch the tip during cardiectomy. The catheter can be advanced in to the pulmonary artery after weaning from bypass.

Adherence to sterile techniques is particularly important because of postoperative immunosuppression. In patients with prior sternotomy, the usual precautions and preparations include immediate availability of blood before sternotomy, multiple large-bore peripheral intravenous access or additional central catheter, application of external defibrillator pads, and preparation for peripheral cannulation by surgical team. The surgical team requests antibiotics specific to donor and recipient infection patterns and immunosuppressive medications. CMV-negative leucocyte depleted packed red blood cells are preferred.

Any prior bridging support such as inotropes, intra-aortic balloon pump (IABP) counterpulsation, and mechanical circulatory assistance have to be maintained during induction until the institution of CPB. Because of the emergent nature of these cases, it is common that patients have recently eaten, and rapid sequence induction may be necessary. The presence of LVAD is helpful in counteracting myocardial depression associated with general anesthesia. Instituting or increasing inotrope infusions can be beneficial in patients without LVAD support. Hypotension may not respond to ephedrine or phenylephrine, and rapidly escalating doses of inotropic support (epinephrine, norepinephrine, or Dobutamine) should be promptly instituted because most patients with end-stage heart disease have significant down-regulation of the beta receptors.

Antifibrinolytic drugs are usually started prior to the skin incision to minimize perioperative blood loss.

A comprehensive transesophageal echocardiographic examination (TEE) examination should be performed after anesthetic induction. The biventricular contractility of the native heart and regurgitant valvular lesions can be monitored before institution of CPB for changes. TEE guidance allows early detection of deterioration and facilitates rapid therapeutic intervention to maintain hemodynamic stability. The left atrium and left ventricle should be carefully examined for the presence of intracardiac thrombus. Manipulation of the heart is minimized before aortic cross-clamping if thrombus is noted or suspected. Absence of patent foramen ovale should be confirmed. The ascending aorta, aortic arch, and descending aorta are examined for presence of atheromatous plaque before aortic cannulation.

Operative Preparation of the Recipient

After confirming the donor suitability for procurement following visualization, median sternotomy is performed; the pericardium is opened. If the patient has had prior surgery, adhesions are carefully divided – this can sometimes take a few hours in patients with multiple prior surgeries or implantable circulatory devices. After systemic heparinization, cannulation of the aorta is performed high along the ascending aorta, near the aortic arch; the superior and inferior venae cavae (SVC, IVC) are cannulated individually and encircled with tourniquets, leaving the surgical field bloodless.

Recipient excision timing is at the discretion of the surgeon, who may choose to wait until the donor heart is in the operating room or until the donor team is 30 min away from the hospital.

The CPB is initiated and the patient is cooled to 34°C-32°C. Dissection of the heart and artificial device is completed at this point as required. The aorta is separated from the pulmonary artery (PA) and then the aorta is cross-clamped close to the aortic arch. Prior to resection of the native heart, the pulmonary artery catheter is withdrawn from the surgical field.

The aorta is divided just above the right coronary artery origin; the back wall of the aorta is dissected taking into consideration the right PA. The main PA just distal to the pulmonary valve is divided.

In preparation for bicaval technique, the right atrium is divided proximal to the SVC, leaving an atrial cuff on the proximal end of the cava. The right atrium is then divided just proximal to the IVC, with care to leave a long posterior cuff that tends to retract, following transection toward the diaphragm. The dome of the left atrium is then divided below the aorta, incision is then extended counterclockwise across the atrial septum, including the fossa ovalis, to the coronary sinus base, and the remaining of the left atrium is transected in a clockwise fashion, below the base of the left atrial appendage.

If the operation is a standard biatrial implantation, the right atrium is open across the atrioventricular groove, till the coronary sinus is encountered; the incision is then extended into the interatrial septum.

Hemostasis following explanation is extremely important; care is taken to cauterize the edges of the atria and the posterior pericardium.

Preparation of the Donor Heart for Transplantation

The donor heart is carefully inspected for abnormalities, particularly, patent foramen ovale (PFO), valvular abnormalities, and debris.

The SVC is identified and separated from the RPA with sharp dissection, the pulmonary veins openings are identified and connected, excess atrium is trimmed, the mitral valve is inspected for abnormalities, and excess aorta and PA are trimmed, a PFO, if present, is closed.

In preparation for biatrial procedure, the SVC is doubly ligated and the right atrium is opened from the lateral IVC toward the right atrial appendage, avoiding the sinus node.

If the tricuspid valve annulus was dilated particularly for patients with high PA pressures or at risk for right ventricular dysfunction, ex vivo tricuspid annuloplasty may be considered.

Implantation Techniques

Orthotopic Heart Transplantation (Figure 1)

There are 3 surgical techniques for orthotopic HT: the classic or biatrial approach, the bicaval approach, and the total transplantation technique.

Shumway and colleagues at Stanford University described the classic or biatrial method. The 4 anastomoses in biatrial technique include left and right atrial cuffs and end-to-end pulmonary artery and aortic anastomoses (Lower et al., 1961; Shumway et al., 1966).

In bicaval technique, recipient right atrium is totally excised and the donor right atrium attached directly to the inferior and superior vena cava requiring 5 anastomoses: left atrial cuff, individual end-to-end inferior vena cava and superior vena cava, and pulmonary artery and aorta. The bicaval approach was reported associated with better short-term results, such as perioperative mortality, preservation of sinus rhythm, less tricuspid and mitral regurgitation, and lower atrial pressures (Sievers et al., 1991; Schnoor et al., 2007).

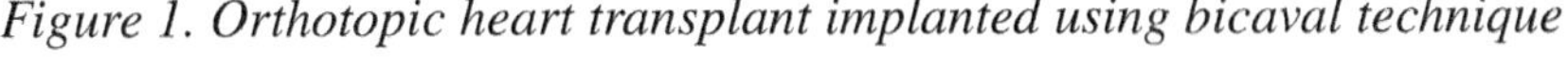

Figure 1. Orthotopic heart transplant implanted using bicaval technique

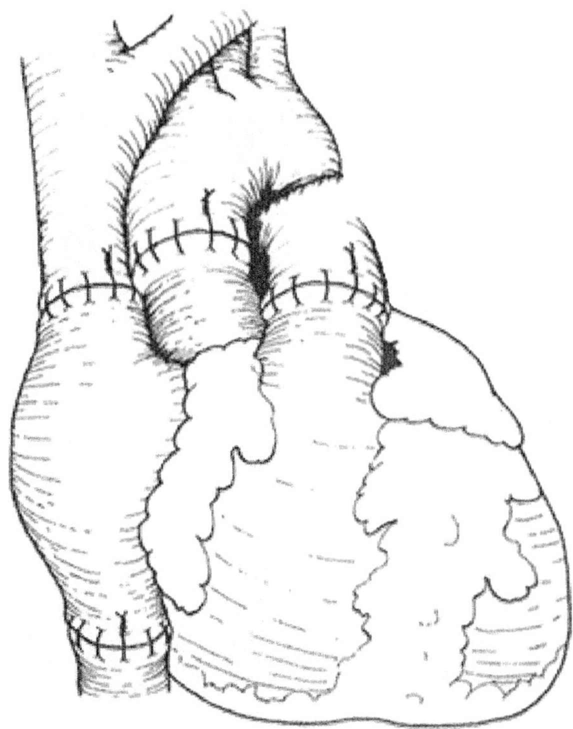

An analysis of the UNOS database found the use of the bicaval anastomosis the most commonly used technique today (62% in 2007) and associated with fewer pacemaker insertions and a small but significant survival advantage (Davies et al., 2010).

To decrease ischemic time for distant procurements, the additional surgical strategies include performing the left atrial anastomosis and the aortic anastomosis in a recipient first, followed by the releasing the cross-clamp to reperfuse the transplanted heart. The subsequent pulmonary artery and right atrial or bicaval anastomoses can be performed on a perfused and beating heart.

The total transplantation technique, involves total preservation of donor heart and 6 anastomoses: left and right pulmonary vein islands, separate inferior vena cava and superior vena cava, and pulmonary artery and aorta (Yacoub et al., 1990).

Heterotopic Heart Transplantation (Figure 2)

Heterotopic heart transplant in the left ventricular assist configuration. (LA = left atrium; LV = left ventricle; PA = pulmonary artery; RA = right atrium; RV = right ventricle; SVC = superior vena cava.)

Heterotopic HT is a largely historical operation. It involves preservation of recipient heart in orthotopic position and placement of donor heart in the right thorax attached in parallel with the native heart. Before the introduction of cyclosporine and mechanical circulatory support (MCS), heterotopic HT allowed a recipient to maintain some cardiac output if the allograft began to fail. It was also an option for HT recipients with pulmonary hypertension and high probability of postoperative donor right ventricular (RV)

Figure 2. Heterotopic heart transplantation

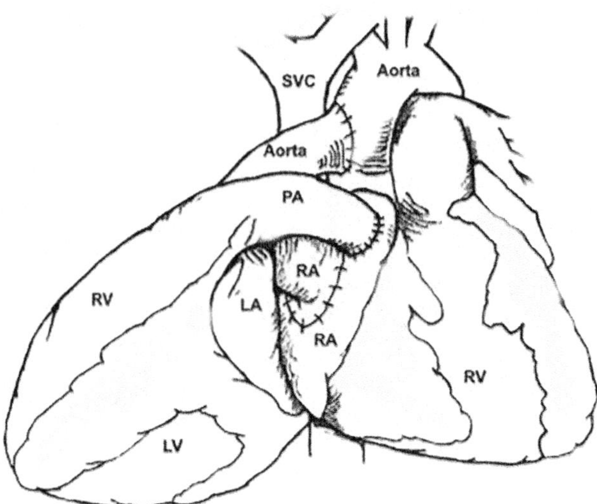

failure. Heterotopic transplantation was also indicated for pediatric transplant recipients with significant donor-to-recipient size mismatch as well as for patient with a potentially reversible causes as viral myocarditis with potential for recovery and recipients in need of very urgent transplantation may be served by a very small donor heart transplanted in a heterotopic fashion. With introduction of left ventricular assist device (LVAD) as a bridge to candidacy, the indications for heterotopic HT are probably limited to immunosuppressed patients with significant pulmonary hypertension requiring re-transplantation in whom LVAD represents high risk for infection.

Weaning from Cardiopulmonary Bypass

Intraoperative immunosuppression usually consists of mycophelonate or azothioprine (given sometimes preoperatively) and methylprednisone given just prior to reperfusion; weaning from CPB proceeds similarly to any other cardiac cases. The lungs are suctioned and ventilated with 100% oxygen; routine deairing maneuvers are performed. The heart is re-evaluated with TEE with attention to retention of air in the ostia of pulmonary veins, LV apex, intraventricular septum as well as the left atrium and left atrial appendage. A brief evaluation of ventricular and valvular function and confirmation of no intracardiac shunts should be performed as soon as a rhythm is present and there is some flow through the heart. Bradycardia and junctional rhythms may occur due to ischemic injury to sinus and atrioventricular nodes. Denervated donor heart lacks normal physiologic feedback loops controlling inotropy and chronotropy. Dobutamine or, less commonly, isoprenaline is used frequently for its direct effect on cardiac beta-receptors to increase heart rate. Use of temporary epicardial pacing should be initiated in the setting of relative bradycardia until the intravenous chronotropic agent has achieved the desired heart rate. Heart rate should be maintained within high normal range 90 to 110 beats per minute to augment cardiac output, increase RV contractility, and 'over-pace' possible arrhythmias. Temporary pacing wires are placed on donor right atrium and ventricle even if the initial rhythm is sinus. Most patients need temporary pacing in the immediate intraoperative and short-term postoperative period. However, 4% to 5% of patients require permanent pacemaker implantation due to the loss of sinus node function (Cantillon et al., 2009).

The heart is carefully loaded not to exceed central venous pressure more than 10 mm Hg to 12 mm Hg and CPB flow is slowly weaned while monitoring arterial and central venous pressure and biventricular function with TEE and direct observation of RV contractility in the surgical field, the rest of the surgery proceed routinely.

If primary allograft dysfunction is encountered, the first step is usually an extended period of reperfusion and cardiac 'rest'. During this time the surgeon should exclude any mechanical factors that could contribute to cardiac dysfunction, such as kinking of the pulmonary artery anastomosis. Consideration can be given for repair of tricuspid regurgitation. Inotropes are escalated. If the patient is not vasoplegic, a loading dose of milrinone may be administered. Inhaled Nitric Oxide may reduce afterload of the right ventricle. If the left ventricle is dysfunctional, an IABP is considered. Cardiopulmonary bypass is weaned slowly, sometimes over a period of up to 10 to 20 minutes with gradual reloading of the heart. Fluid boluses, including blood products should be administered with caution as excessive preload can lead to complete failure of the right ventricle. If hemodynamic stability cannot be maintained after repeat attempts at weaning, the patient is placed on mechanical support with ventricular assist device(s) or extracorporeal membrane oxygenation.

Absolute hemostasis is critical after a heart transplant operation. Sometimes this can take a few hours of packing and correction of coagulopathy. Persistent bleeding on return to the intensive care unit is associated with poor outcomes as the transplanted heart does not tolerate well massive volume transfusions (of blood products), tamponade and hemodynamic instability that arise from bleeding.

IMMEDIATE POSTTRANSPLANT MANAGEMENT

The transition from the operating room to the cardiothoracic intensive care (CTICU) defines the start of a critical time period for the newly transplanted graft; we will summarize the early CTICU management and the commonly encountered complications.

Postoperative Management and Potential Complications

The transplanted heart faces lots of physiological stresses, depletion of the myocardial catecholamine stores, ischemic-reperfusion injury, right ventricular dysfunction, sinoatrial nodal dysfunction, denervation related dependence on distal non cardiac catecholamines sources with associated delayed response to stress (hypoxia, hypovolemia, anemia), hypothermia, early vasoplegic shock, all contribute to the importance of critical graft monitoring and management in the early postoperative period.

Hemodynamic Management

An infusion of epinephrine, dopamine, dobutamine and/or milrinone is usually initiated in the operating room to provide inotropic support. Unlike other heart operations all transplanted hearts require inotropic support in the immediate post-operative period. Even if the function of the heart looks excellent to start with, there is almost invariably some compromise in right ventricular function due to ischemia-reperfusion injury, poor preservation, recipient factors such as high pulmonary artery resistance, size mismatch or operative factors. The transplanted heart may require escalating dose of inotropic support during the first several post-operative hours due to the reduced ventricular compliance and transient depression of the graft function. Abnormal atrial dynamics associated with midatrial anastomosis exacerbate the diastolic dysfunction on the non-compliant ventricles (this may be influenced by use of bicaval or total techniques). Milrinone (phosphodiaesterase-5 inhibitor) is a preferred drug to add either in the operating room or during the early postoperative period unless vasoplegia is predominant; it is a venodilator and pulmonary artery vasodilator and improves the right ventricular function particularly in patients with preoperative pulmonary hypertension.

Generally a taper of the vasoactive and inotropic drugs can be started 24-48 hours post-transplant. The taper of the inotropic support should be slow and we generally leave most patients on a low dose of milrinone that can be continued for few days and discontinued in the cardiac step down unit.

A pulmonary artery catheter aids hemodynamic management by allowing observation of the pulmonary arterial pressure, pulmonary wedge pressure, cardiac output and venous oxygen saturations. A direct left atrial pressure monitoring line is used occasionally and can help identify failing of the right (if the central venous pressure is much higher than the left atrial pressure) or left (if the left atrial pressure is elevated more than the right) ventricles. The ideal CVP for most transplant recipients is 8 to 12 mmHg. If the CVP is 15 mmHg or more, fluid boluses should be avoided as they can tip the allograft into severe right ventricular dysfunction. A rising CVP above 15 mmHg requires urgent attention with escalation of inotropes, institution of inhaled nitric oxide and consideration of echocardiography. A CVP above 20mmHg is a surgical emergency and requires immediate consultation with the cardiothoracic surgeon. Echocardiography is performed to exclude tamponade and assess right ventricular function. Tamponade mandates immediate re-exploration. If a severely hypokinetic right ventricle is seen then inotropic support is escalated further. Volume transfusions are limited to that necessary to deliver drugs. A persisting CVP above 20 mmHg despite these measures mandates return to the operating room for exploration to exclude tamponade and consideration of mechanical circulatory support.

Vasoplegic Shock

Post-bypass vasoplegia is a frequently encountered hemodynamic derangement particularly in the post-transplant period, due to preoperative use of vasodilators, pre-operative inflammatory states induced by ventricular assist devices, systemic inflammatory response induced by cytokine activation by the membrane oxygenator during the often prolonged periods on cardiopulmonary bypass, vasodilatory effect of some drugs as milrinone, in addition to depletion of the endogenous arginine vasopressin (AVP) in patients with decompensated heart failure.

Occasionally, vasoplegic shock is the dominant hemodynamic derangement post-bypass.

Vasoplegia is usually managed by avoiding drugs with vasodilator effects, optimizing the perioperative hematocrit by judicious use of packed red cells transfusion, liberal use of conventional hemofiltration on bypass and modified ultrafiltration post-bypass for hemoconcentration. However, in many instances, infusion of vasopressors is required. Low dose vasopressin in physiological doses of 2.4 U/hr is considered as an ideal vasopressor post-transplant as vasopressin receptors are lacking in the pulmonary vascular beds, thus avoiding exacerbation of pulmonary hypertension. Vasopressin also does not compromise the renal perfusion. However, vasopressor catecholamines - norepinephrine and epinephrine - remain the main stay of postcardiotomy vasodilatory shock; however their effectiveness can be limited by catecholamine resistance, worsening of pulmonary hypertension, splanchnic malperfusion and microcirculation hypoperfusion.

In transplanting patients with active device related infections, unexplained, refractory or delayed onset of vasoplegia can be an early sign of postoperative sepsis particularly with the initiation of immunosuppression. This should be promptly recognized and treated to prevent serious outcomes.

Right Ventricular Failure

Right ventricular failure is a common occurrence and a cause of morbidity and mortality after cardiac transplantation. Contemporary registry data from ISHLT indicate that approximately 20% of early deaths after cardiac transplantation are attributable to right ventricular failure (Stehlik et al., 2012).

Multiple factors predispose the RV to fail perioperatively including preoperative pulmonary hypertension, reactive pulmonary hypertension induced by cardiopulmonary bypass, transfusions, hypoxia or protamine, volume overload due to the use of blood products post bypass in coagulopathy patients, donor related issues as ischemia-reperfusion, poor myocardial preservation, prolonged ischemic times and donor receipt mismatch with transplanting a small donor heart in a big recipient predispose to right ventricular failure more then left ventricular dysfunction.

The donor right heart, especially when it is young and comparably small, is not accustomed to high pulmonary vascular resistance. The nonadapted thin-walled RV is able to maximally produce pressures of 45 mm Hg to 50 mm Hg after which it may fail acutely (Wagner, 2011b).

The onset of RV failure can be either intraoperative or early postoperative. Clinically, RV failure is evidenced by failure to wean a recipient from CPB and low cardiac output in the face of rising central venous pressure. The right heart can be seen in the surgical field to dilate and contract poorly. TEE shows a dilated, poorly contracting RV as evidenced by measurement of RV fractional area change in the midesophageal 4-chamber view and an underfilled vigorously contracting LV. Tricuspid regurgitation (TR) secondary to dilatation of the tricuspid valve annulus might also be seen.

RV failure can in turn cause a decrease in LV end-diastolic volume with septal shift to the left that further limits early diastolic LV filling. This vicious cycle results in a low cardiac output syndrome with hypotension and shock (Vlahakes, 2012).

Postoperatively, right ventricular failure should be differentiated from other causes of low cardiac output status with elevated filling pressures. Cardiac tamponade can often be excluded by TEE done at the bed side (though sometimes re-expoloration may still be required for definitive exclusion), and chest X-ray would also exclude any tension pneumothorax or large pleural collection that might mimic right ventricle failure clinically.

Therapy is directed at preventing a low cardiac output syndrome. The goal is to optimize RV preload, increase RV contractility, decrease RV afterload, and improve coronary perfusion. Mechanical circulatory support (MCS) should be considered early before secondary organ damage or profound metabolic acidosis occurs. Options include optimization of right ventricular coronary perfusion by implantation of intra-aortic balloon pump (Arafa et al., 2000), right ventricular assist devices (RVAD) or extracorporeal membrane oxygenator (ECMO).

Inotropic agents that can be used to augment RV function include isoproterenol, milrinone, dobutamine, and epinephrine. Systemic vasodilators with pulmonary vasodilating properties, including nitroglycerine and sodium nitroprusside, can be used in the absence of systemic hypotension. Selective inhaled pulmonary vasodilators, such as inhaled nitric oxide, prostaglandins (prostaglandin E1, alprostadil, and prostaglandin I2, epoprostenol/prostacyclin) can be used in the management of perioperative RV dysfunction with systemic hypotension.

Once inhaled therapy is initiated, it should not be weaned rapidly but slowly, typically over hours in an ICU setting. Rapid weaning of selective pulmonary vasodilators can occasionally precipitate life-threatening rebound pulmonary hypertension with acute RV failure.

Inhalation therapy provides ideal delivery method particularly if perfusion ventilation mismatch is an issue. In a recent clinical trial, use of oral sildenafil was proved an effective bridging strategy in the weaning of intravenous and inhaled pulmonary vasodilators after HT (Boffini et al., 2009; Rajek et al., 2000).

Use of vasopressin as the vasopressor of choice for treating systemic hypotension helps avoid the pulmonary vasopressor effect of catecholamines that might exacerbate the right ventricular dysfunction (Gold et al., 2000).

We liberally use modified ultrafiltration (MUF) post-bypass particularly in the context of coagulopathic post-bypass mediastinal bleeding and right ventricular dysfunction to avoid the inevitable volume overload associated with blood products transfusion.

Ex-vivo tricuspid annuloplasty can be done prophylactically for patients at risk for right ventricular failure due to preoperative recipient pulmonary hypertension.

Maintaining a fast sinus rhythm with atrial or atrioventricular pacing to a heart rate of 100 to 120 beats per minute increases RV output and is critical in the immediate postoperative phase. A high mean systemic arterial blood pressure improves the right ventricular perfusion; catecholamines should be used in this regard if necessary as the increased contractility due to improved RV perfusion outweighs the deleterious effects on increased pulmonary artery resistance (which can be counteracted to a degree with inhaled Nitric Oxide). Ventilation and oxygenation should be optimized as hypoxia and hypercarbia lead to pulmonary vasoconstriction. If necessary, patients should be heavily sedated to allow better ventilation. Other measures to optimize right ventricular function include tight acid-base balance management with tendency toward the alkalosis, sedation, draining of any pleural or pericardial effusion, and open chest management cautious fluid removal with continuous veno-venous hemofiltration (CVVH) particularly in the context of renal dysfunction and lack of adequate response to diuretics can help to unload the dysfunctional right ventricle.

Primary Allograft Dysfunction

Primary graft failure is defined as early post-transplant cardiac failure without an identifiable immunologic or anatomic etiology. The ISHLT reported >20% of deaths within 30 days of transplant were due to primary graft failure, making it the leading cause of perioperative mortality (Kirk et al., 2009).

Risk factors are long cross clamp time (particularly over 4 hours), poor myocardial preservation, ischemia-reperfusion injury and pre-existing donor heart dysfunction (Russo et al., 2010).

Acute myocardial dysfunction occurs in brain dead patients and in 20% precludes organ donation. Acute and hyperacute rejection are rare causes of acute graft failure, particularly in sensitized patients, however prospective cross match markedly reduces the likelihood of this possibility. In some instances where there is great concern for hyperacute rejection, plasmapheresis is undertaken on cardiopulmonary bypass to remove preformed antibodies.

Primary allograft dysfunction can happen in the operating room, precluding weaning off bypass or early in the postoperative course with signs of low cardiac output.

Allograft dysfunction manifests as severe biventricular dysfunction with hypotension, low cardiac output, and high filling pressures. Loss of QRS voltage on daily electrocardiograms can be a sign of acute rejection, while ST changes may indicate focal injury.

High dose inotropic support is usually required however MCS is often needed to allow weaning off the CPB. MCS may include an IABP, LVAD, RVAD, biventricular assist device (BIVAD) or ECMO. Patients who recover and wean eventually off MCS usually have a survival rate similar to the general post-transplant population, however prolonged support usually is associated with poor prognosis with multiorgan failure and mortality since these patients are generally not acceptable candidates for re-transplantation. Re-transplantation for primary graft dysfunction is associated with very poor survival and is generally not undertaken in the current era, except in very exceptional situations.

Hyperacute Rejection

Hyperacute rejection results from preformed donor specific antibodies (DSA) in the recipient or from inadvertent ABO mismatch; it is rarely seen in current era. The onset of hyperacute catastrophic rejection occurs within minutes to several hours after reperfusion. Gross inspection reveals a mottled or dark red, flaccid allograft, and histologic examination confirms the characteristic global interstitial hemorrhage and edema without lymphocytic infiltrate. Immunofluorescence techniques reveal deposits of immunoglobulins and complement on the vascular endothelium. Immediate plasmapheresis, intravenous immunoglobulin (IVIG), and mechanical support are instituted, but re-transplantation may be the only successful strategy to prevent patient death (Trento et al., 1988).

Mechanical Circulatory Support for Right Ventricular Failure and Primary Graft Failure

MCS is indicated for continuing or worsening hemodynamic deterioration, such as decreasing cardiac index or MvO_2 less than 50% refractory to medical management.

The choice of MCS modality depends on whether isolated RV failure versus biventricular failure is present, and on adequacy of lung function. In isolated RV failure, extracorporeal continuous flow RVADs, such as Thoratec CentriMag (Thoratec Corporation, Pleasanton, CA) can be used for temporary RV support.

Some investigators prefer the use of peripheral venoarterial ECMO in HT recipients with RV failure, reporting better in-hospital survival and graft survival rates compared to RVAD use (Taghavi et al., 2004).

In cases of Primary Graft Failure, the choice depends on the adequacy of lung function. Devices, such as TandemHeart (CardiacAssist, Inc Pittsburgh, PA) and Centrimag, can provide biventricular support (BiVAD). If lung function is also inadequate, venoarterial ECMO support is preferred. ECMO can be instituted from the peripheral vascular access, allowing sternal wound closure and obviating reopening the chest to remove support devices (Bittner, 2011). For patients who have had a complicated or turbulent operation, the CPB cannulas are simply connected to an ECMO circuit and the chest left open.

Postoperative bleeding is a major issue with ECMO because of obligatory need for systemic anticoagulation. Recent studies report in-hospital survival rates with the use of ECMO in the adults from 20% to 50% (Taghavi et al., 2004)

Typically most allografts will recover function within 4 to 7 days to allow weaning of mechanical support. The key aspect therefore of management in this period is to provide aggressive supportive care and maximize organ recovery and patient survival. Many patients will die of multiorgan failure in this period, but if patients can survive through the first few days without major organ dysfunction then the prognosis can be good with subsequent device explantation and relatively uneventful recovery thereafter. The prognosis is poor for patients in whom cardiac function has not returned within a week, as this often reflects permanent injury to the allograft.

Dysrhythmias

Sinus bradycardia is the commonest arrhythmia, commonly due to sinoatrial nodal ischemia, the use of bicaval technique significantly reduces the risk of sinus node dysfunction, historically isoprenaline was the preferred chronotropic agent however this has been replaced by atrioventricular pacing, we recommend pacing routinely at 100 bpm and keeping the pacing wires till all the chronotropic agents are weaned. Typically bradycardia usually resolves in 1-2 weeks; however the incidence of permanent pacemaker use remains at around 5%.

Atrial flutter/fibrillation is less common and can occasionally be a marker of acute graft rejection. Individual assessment of the risk:benefit ratio for anticoagulation therapy is necessary.

Supraventricular tachycardia in transplant patients should be treated with lower doses in the same manner as in nontransplant patients. Recurrent arrhythmias from reentry circuits or defined ectopic foci often can be cured by radiofrequency ablation. Sustained ventricular tachycardia and ventricular fibrillation presumably are responsible for a significant portion of the 10% of sudden and unexplained deaths in heart transplant patients (Patel et al., 1996).

Antiarrhythmic drugs such as amiodarone may be utilized but beta-blockers are generally avoided in the early post-operative period. Adenosine can cause profound atrioventricular block and is avoided.

Post-Transplant Renal Failure

Renal dysfunction is a frequent perioperative complication occurring in almost half of all heart transplant recipients, usually related to pre-existing nephropathy, pre-existing cardiorenal syndromes, perioperative hypotension, venous congestion, calcineurin inhibitors, aortic thromboemboli and other factors. Renal failure usually prolongs the hospitalization and increases overall post-transplant mortality. Most patients require diuretics after the first few post-operative days to achieve fluid balance. In some cases, mechanical fluid removal may be required (continuous veno-venous hemofiltration - CVVH). Some patients progress to dialysis dependency and require long-term indwelling catheters for dialysis – this greatly increases the risk of infection and reduces one-year survival. There seems no clear means of preventing onset of renal failure in susceptible patients. Some groups prefer to avoid early calcineurin inhibitors and instead rely on induction immunosuppression for the first few days post-transplant; however, this approach has not been demonstrated to result in superior outcomes.

Bleeding and Fluid Balance Management

Post-operative bleeding can be significant following heart transplantation. Causes are multi-factorial and include extensive dissection, cardiopulmonary bypass, multiple suture lines, pre-transplant anticoagulation, and poor pre-operative nutritional status. Platelet, cryoprecipitate, and fresh frozen plasma infusion should be used as necessary to control hemorrhage. Recombinant factor VII may be useful for refractory bleeding. Volume resuscitation with packed red blood cells is necessary, but should be administered judiciously, given the increased risk for allosensitization from transfused leukocytes which may express non-donor matched HLA antigens. Patients with refractory hemorrhage or those demonstrating clinical evidence of cardiac tamponade should be surgically explored.

Fluid management may be challenging. Care must be exercised to provide adequate cardiac filling without causing substantial overload to the already stressed right ventricle. Rapid volume loading should be avoided on weaning off cardiopulmonary bypass particularly as the extravascular fluid tends to shift intravascularly during the post-transplant period increasing the filling pressures of both the right and the left ventricles.

Immunosupression/Antimicrobial Prophylaxis Protocol (Costanzo et al., 2010; Kobashigawa et al., 1998; Kobashigawa et al., 2006)

Perioperative

Mycophenolate Mofetil (MMF, Cell Cept) 1500 mg PO or IV given intra-operatively and then continued at dose of 1500 mg twice a day. Alternatively Azathioprine may be used.

Methylprednisolone (Solumedrol) 1g is given intravenously prior to reperfusing the donor heart and continued at dose of 125 mg 8hrl for first 24 hours.

Post-Operative

Corticosteroids

Prednisone is started on day 1 and can be further weaned after each successive negative biopsy (< ISHLT 2R):

Calcineurin Inhibitors (CNI)

Tacrolimus (FK-506, Prograf) is our preferred calcineurin inhibitor. An initial 1.0 mg dose of tacrolimus may be given after the first twenty-four hours of transplant. Subsequent tacrolimus dosing is adjusted according to renal function and blood levels to achieve a target trough level of between 10 and 15 ng/ml by the seventh post-operative day. Oral or nasogastric tube administration is preferred over the intravenous route to minimize renal toxicity.

Cyclosporine

Cyclosporine (Neoral, Gengraf, Sandimmne) remains the CNI of choice in some institutions, but in many institutions is increasingly reserved for patients intolerant of tacrolimus Neoral, a microemulsion formulation of cyclosporine, is preferred because of its greater absorption and bioavailability. Neoral is given in two daily doses to achieve the trough levels below.

(0-6 weeks' time post-transplant 275 ng/ml -375 ng/ml cyclosporine level)

Anti-Proliferatives (Anti-Metabolites)

Mycophenolate mofetil (Cellcept) is given as a fixed dose of 1500 mg twice daily orally or intravenously. Dose reductions may be necessary in the setting of gastrointestinal upset or leukopenia.

Azathioprine (Imuran) is rarely used recently.

Proliferation Signal Inhibitors

Sirolimus (Rapamycin, Rapamune) is reserved for patients with cardiac allograft vasculopathy

Rescue Agents: Thymoglobulin.

It is a polyclonal antilymphocyte preparation which consists of rabbit gamma immune globulin. It is very effective in depleting circulating lymphocytes. It may be used as induction immunosuppression or for treatment of steroid resistant or hemodynamically significant allograft rejection. The dose of thymoglobulin is 1.5 mg/kg/day adjusted for WBC and administered over 5-10 days. A nurse or physician must be present during the first 30 minutes of the first infusion due to the risk of anaphylaxis.

OKT3 (Anti-CD3 Murine antibody).

It is a monoclonal antibody against T cell surface CD 3 receptors. It may be used as rescue for steroid-resistant allograft rejection. It is administered via IV push 3 mg – 5 mg for 5-7 days. Of note, anti- anaphylactic premedication is required one hour prior to OKT3 administration.

Antimicrobial Prophylaxis (Table 3)

The high incidence of acute rejection during the first postoperative months requiring addition immunosuppression results in an increased risk of infection.

During the initial hospital stay, bacteria are the most common origin of infection, while viral and fungal infections usually occur later. Our prophylactic protocol against early postoperative infections consists of contact isolation of the patient during the whole hospital stay. This includes protective clothing of all personnel and visitors entering the room (gloves, gown). In addition, antibiotic prophylaxis is administered during the first 24-48 postoperative hours (cephalosporin and vancomycin, as used prophylactically in other cardiac surgical patients). Antiviral and antiprotozoal and antifungal prophylaxis is commenced immediately, as appropriate, after the transplant procedure. Occasionally a longer course of antibiotic therapy is required for patients with drive line and or LVAD pocket infections particularly with positive intraoperative cultures. (Table 3)

Wound Infection

Wound infection is fortunately relatively rare after major cardiac surgery, including transplantation, but can, be potentially disastrous in the immunosuppressed patient. Its treatment in the transplant patient follows the guidelines for any patient who has undergone open-heart surgery. High index of suspicion is mandatory for patients with drive line/pocket or device related blood stream infection, usually prolonged course of intravenous antibiotics is recommended to prevent relapses on immunosuppression with associated high mortality and morbidity.

Table 3.

1.	*Bacterial prophylaxis*
	c. Cefazolin 750mg to 1.5 gm IV on induction of anesthesia and q 8h for 24 hours (dose size adjusted). d. Vancomycin 1gm IV on induction of anesthesia and q12 for 24 hours (dose renally adjusted).
2.	*CMV prophylaxis*
	e. CMV positive donor to negative recipient
	Ganciclovir 5 mg/kg IV bid until taking p/o then Valganciclovir 900 mg daily (dose adjusted for renal function) for 12 months (if tolerated). Surveillance screening with CMV PCR should be performed for one to three months if stopping valgancyclovir sooner than 12 months
	f. CMV positive recipient regardless of donor CMV status
	Valganciclovir 450 mg daily for 3 months (if tolerated)
	g. CMV negative donor to negative recipient
	Valacyclovir 500 mg daily for 3 months
	h. Reconsider duration of CMV prophylaxis in the setting of treated rejection
3.	*Hepatitis B prophylaxis*
	Patients lacking antibodies to hepatitis B will receive vaccination while awaiting heart transplantation as time allows
4.	*Influenza vaccination*
	All patients awaiting transplant as well as those more than 6 months post-transplantation will receive a yearly influenza vaccine
5.	*Pneumocystis jiroveci Pneumonia (PJP)/toxoplasmosis Prophylaxis*
	Trimethoprim-sulfamethoxazole (double strength qod or single strength qd) will be given for one year as prophylaxis against PJP. It should be restarted after one year for any patient receiving high dose steroids or a rescue agent Those patients who lack antibodies to toxoplasma and who receive a heart from a toxoplasma-positive donor will receive pyrimethamine 50 mg daily along with folinic acid 5 mg bid for 6 weeks. Bactrim (single strength daily) will be continued during this time Sulfa allergic patients will be given atovaquone (Mepron) 1500 mg daily
6.	*Fungal prophylaxis*
	Nystatin S&S 5 cc po QID for 3 months or Clotrimazole troche 1 tablet po QID for 3 months

IV: Intravenous; **CMV:** Cytomegalovirus; **PCR:** polymerase chain reaction

FUTURE CHALLENGES

In the future, novel approaches are needed to expand and optimize both the donor and recipient population. Institution based liberalization of marginal donor acceptance criteria needs to be evaluated. The efficacy and safety of third generation LVAD compared to heart transplantation, in specified subgroups of heart failure patients, needs to be determined by clinical studies; the hope is that LVAD therapy can provide a durable and safe option to transplantation in the future.

For sensitized patients, the utilization of the virtual cross-match could expand the available donor pool. A recent novel C1q assay to detect the ability of immunoglobulin G antibodies to fix complement is now available which can assess the functional significance of post-transplant alloantibodies.

Development of reliable, noninvasive diagnostic studies to assess allograft rejection and the untoward effects of immunosuppression will allow more precise control of complications.

Future improvements in organ preservation may permit a modest increase in the donor pool and better allocation of organs with respect to donor-recipient immunologic matching.

Improved immunosuppression with reduced side effects and the promising use of genomics assist in personalized therapy for specific patients based on pharmacogenetic polymorphisms.

Advances in mechanical assist device therapy, stem cell therapy, organ engineering and medical management in advanced heart failure patients may decrease or avoid the need for heart transplantation. However, progress on alternative therapies largely depends on our deeper understanding of the mechanisms of heart failure and how to prevent it (Kobashigawa, 2012).

CONCLUSION

There has been tremendous development recently in the medical therapy as well as catheter based procedures for patients with congestive heart failure that has dramatically decreased the mortality from end stage heart diseases. That has resulted in a steadily growing population with end stage heart failure who may benefit from advanced form of therapy, whether ventricular assist device therapy or cardiac transplantation. With an expanding use of bridging ventricular assist devices and total artificial hearts, the population of patients being transplanted is increasingly complex with greater demands on the Intensive Care resources. Awareness of the unique problems posed by this patient group and aggressive management of the numerous perioperative problems they face is critical to delivering good outcomes in this patient group.

ACKNOWLEDGMENT

We would like to thank Dimosthenis Pandis MD, MSc for his help in proof-reading and content editing of this chapter.

REFERENCES

Arafa, O. E., Geiran, O. R., Andersen, K., Fosse, E., Simonsen, S., & Svennevig, J. L. (2000). Intraaortic Balloon Pumping For Predominantly Right Ventricular Failure After Heart Transplantation. *The Annals of Thoracic Surgery, 70*(5), 1587-1593. from http://www.annalsthoracicsurgery.org/article/s0003-4975(00)01864-6/abstractRetrieved

Bittner, H. B. (2011). Extra-Corporeal Membrane Oxygenation Support In Cardiac Transplantation. *Applied Cardiopulmonary Pathophysiology, 15*, 272–277.

Boffini, M., Sansone, F., Ceresa, F., Ribezzo, M., Patanè, F., Comoglio, C., . . . Rinaldi, M. (2009). Role Of Oral Sildenafil In The Treatment Of Right Ventricular Dysfunction After Heart Transplantation. *Transplantation Proceedings, 41*(4), 1353-1356. Retrieved From http://www.transplantation-proceedings.org/article/s0041-1345(09)00473-4/abstract

Cantillon, D. J., Gorodeski, E. Z., Caccamo, M., Smedira, N. G., Wilkoff, B. L., Starling, R. C., & Saliba, W. (2009). Long-Term Outcomes And Clinical Predictors For Pacing After Cardiac Transplantation. *The Journal Of Heart And Lung Transplantation, 28*(8), 791-798. Retrieved From http://www.jhltonline.org/article/s1053-2498(09)00316-7/abstract

Chen, J. M., Russo, M. J., Hammond, K. M., Mancini, D. M., Kherani, A. R., & Fal, J. M. … Naka, Y. (2005). Alternate Waiting List Strategies For Heart Transplantation Maximize Donor Organ Utilization. *The Annals Of Thoracic Surgery, 80*(1), 224-228. Retrieved From http://www.annalsthoracicsurgery.org/article/s0003-4975(05)00030-5/abstract

Costanzo, M. R., Costanzo, M. R., Dipchand, A., Starling, R., Anderson, A., Chan, M. … Vanhaecke, J. (2010). The International Society Of Heart And Lung Transplantation Guidelines For The Care Of Heart Transplant Recipients. *The Journal Of Heart And Lung Transplantation, 29*(8), 914-956. Retrieved from http://www.jhltonline.org/article/s1053-2498(10)00358-x/abstract

Davies, R. R., Russo, M. J., Morgan, J. A., Sorabella, R. A., Naka, Y., & Chen, J. M. (2010). Standard Versus Bicaval Techniques For Orthotopic Heart Transplantation: An Analysis Of The United Network For Organ Sharing Database. *The Journal of Thoracic and Cardiovascular Surgery, 140*(3), 700-708. Retrieved from http://www.Jtcvsonline.Org/Article/S0022-5223(10)00435-6/Abstract

Felker, G. M., Milano, C. A., Yager, J. E. E., Hernandez, A. F., Blue, L., Higginbotham, M. B., . . . Russel, S. D. (2005). Outcomes With An Alternate List Strategy For Heart Transplantation. *The Journal Of Heart And Lung Transplantation, 24*(11), 1781-1786. Retrieved From http://www.jhltonline.org/article/s1053-2498(05)00198-1/abstract

Gold, J., Cullinane, S., Chen, J., Oz, M., Olover, J., & Landry, D. (2000). Vasopressin As An Alternative To Norepinephrine In The Treatment Of Milrinone-Induced Hypotension. *Critical Care Medicine, 28*(1), 249–252. doi:10.1097/00003246-200001000-00043 PMID:10667533

Hunt, S. A., Abraham, W. T., Chin, M. H., Feldman, A. M., Francis, G. S., Ganiats, T. G., . . . Yancy, C. W. (2009). 2009 Focused Update Incorporated Into The Acc/Aha 2005 Guidelines For The Diagnosis And Management Of Heart Failure In Adults: A Report Of The American College Of Cardiology Foundation/American Heart Association Task Force On Practice Guidelines Developed In Collaboration With The International Society For Heart And Lung Transplantation. *Journal Of The American College Of Cardiology, 53*(15), E1-E90. Retrieved from http://www.sciencedirect.com/science/article/pii/s0735109708038023

Kirk, R., Edwards, L. B., Aurora, P., Taylor, D. O., Christie, J. D., Dobbels, F., . . . Hertz, M. I. (2009). Registry Of The International Society For Heart And Lung Transplantation: Twelfth Official Pediatric Heart Transplantation Report–2009. *The Journal Of Heart And Lung Transplantation, 28*(10), 993-1006. Retrieved From http://www.jhltonline.org/article/s1053-2498(09)00634-2/abstract

Kobashigawa, J., Miller, L., Renlund, D., Mentzer, R., Alderman, E., Bourge, R., ... Valentine, H. The Mycophenolate Mofetil Investigators (1998). A Randomized Active-Controlled Trial Of Mycophenolate Mofetil In Heart Transplant Recipients. *Transplantation, 66*(4). Retrieved from http://journals.lww.com/transplantjournal/fulltext/1998/08270/a_randomized_active_controlled_trial_of.16.aspx

Kobashigawa, J. A. (2012). The Future Of Heart Transplantation. *American Journal Of Transplantation, 12*(11), 2875-2891. doi:10.1111/j.1600-6143.2012.04223.x

Kobashigawa, J. A., Miller, L. W., Russell, S. D., Ewald, G. A., Zucker, M. J., Goldberg, L. R., ... First, R. and the study Investigators (2006). Tacrolimus With Mycophenolate Mofetil (Mmf) Or Sirolimus Vs. Cyclosporine With Mmf In Cardiac Transplant Patients: 1-Year Report. *American Journal Of Transplantation, 6*(6), 1377-1386. doi:10.1111/j.1600-6143.2006.01290.x

Lower, R., Stofer, R., & Shumway, N. (1961). Homovital Transplantation Of The Heart. *The Journal of Thoracic and Cardiovascular Surgery, 41*, 196–204. PMID:13763849

Mehra, M. R., Kobashigawa, J., Starling, R., Russell, S., Uber, P. A., & Parameshwar, J. … Barr, M. (2006). Listing Criteria For Heart Transplantation: International Society For Heart And Lung Transplantation Guidelines For The Care Of Cardiac Transplant Candidates–2006. *The Journal Of Heart And Lung Transplantation, 25*(9), 1024-1042. Retrieved From http://www.jhltonline.org/article/s1053-2498(06)00460-8/abstract

Patel, V., Lim, M., Massin, E., Jonsyn, G., Ates, P., Abou-Awdi, N., . . . Frazier, O. H. (1996). Sudden Cardiac Death In Cardiac Transplant Recipients. *Circulation, 94*(9 Suppl) i273-Ii277. Retrieved From http://www.ncbi.nlm.nih.gov/pubmed/8901759

Rajek, A., Pernerstorfer, T., Kastner, J., Mares, P., Grabenwöger, M., Sessler, D. I., . . . Hiesmayr, M. (2000). Inhaled Nitric Oxide Reduces Pulmonary Vascular Resistance More Than Prostaglandin E1 During Heart Transplantation. *Anesthesia & Analgesia, 90*(3). Retrieved From http://journals.lww.com/anesthesia-analgesia/fulltext/2000/03000/inhaled_nitric_oxide_reduces_pulmonary_vascular.5.aspx

Russo, M. J., Iribarne, A., Hong, K. N., Ramlawi, B., Chen, J. M., Takayama, H., . . . Naka, Y. (2010). Factors Associated With Primary Graft Failure After Heart Transplantation. *Transplantation, 90*(4). Retrieved From http://journals.lww.com/transplantjournal/fulltext/2010/08270/factors_associated_with_primary_graft_failure.19.aspx

Schnoor, M., Schäfer, T., Lühmann, D., & Sievers, H. H. (2007). Bicaval Versus Standard Technique In Orthotopic Heart Transplantation: A Systematic Review And Meta-Analysis. *The Journal Of Thoracic And Cardiovascular Surgery, 134*(5), 1322-1331. Retrieved From http://www.jtcvsonline.org/article/s0022-5223(07)00935-x/abstract

Shumway, N., Lower, R., & Stofer, R. (1966). Transplantation Of The Heart. *Advances in Surgery, 2*, 265–284. PMID:5333297

Sievers, H. H., Weyand, M., Kraatz, G., & Bernhard, A. (1991). An Alternative Technique For Orthotopic Cardiac Transplantation, With Preservation Of The Normal Anatomy Of The Right Atrium. *The Thoracic and Cardiovascular Surgeon, 39*(02), 70–72. doi:10.1055/s-2007-1013934 PMID:1877054

Stehlik, J., Edwards, L. B., Kucheryavaya, A. Y., Benden, C., Christie, J. D., Dipchand, A. I., . . . Hertz, M. I. (2012). The Registry Of The International Society For Heart And Lung Transplantation: 29th Official Adult Heart Transplant Report–2012. *The Journal Of Heart And Lung Transplantation, 31*(10), 1052-1064. Retrieved From http://www.jhltonline.org/article/s1053-2498(12)01210-7/abstract

Taghavi, S., Zuckermann, A., Ankersmit, J., Wieselthaler, G., Rajek, A., Laufer, G., . . . Grimm, M. (2004). Extracorporeal Membrane Oxygenation Is Superior To Right Ventricular Assist Device For Acute Right Ventricular Failure After Heart Transplantation. *The Annals Of Thoracic Surgery, 78*(5), 1644-1649. Retrieved From http://www.annalsthoracicsurgery.org/article/S0003-4975(04)00997-X/abstract

Taylor, D. O., Edwards, L. B., Aurora, P., Christie, J. D., Dobbels, F., Kirk, R., . . . Hertz, M. I. (2008). Registry Of The International Society For Heart And Lung Transplantation: Twenty-Fifth Official Adult Heart Transplant Report-2008. *The Journal Of Heart And Lung Transplantation, 27*(9), 943-956. Retrieved From http://www.jhltonline.org/article/s1053-2498(08)00501-9/abstract

Trento, A., Hardesty, R., Griffith, B., Zerbe, T., Kormos, R., & Bahnson, H. (1988). Role Of The Antibody To Vascular Endothelial Cells In Hyperacute Rejection In Patients Undergoing Cardiac Transplantation. *The Journal of Thoracic and Cardiovascular Surgery*, *95*(1), 37–41. PMID:2447445

Vlahakes, G. J. (2012). Right Ventricular Failure After Cardiac Surgery. *Cardiology Clinics, 30*(2), 283-289. Retrieved From http://www.sciencedirect.com/science/article/pii/s073386511200029x

Wagner, F. M. (2011a). Donor Heart Preservation And Perfusion. *Applied Cardiopulmonary Pathophysiology*, *15*, 198–206.

Wagner, F. M. (2011b). Monitoring And Management Of Right Ventricular Function Following Cardiac Transplantation. *Applied Cardiopulmonary Pathophysiology*, *15*, 220–229.

Yacoub, M., Mankad, P., & Ledingham, S. (1990). Donor Procurement And Surgical Techniques For Cardiac Transplantation. *Seminars in Thoracic and Cardiovascular Surgery*, *2*(2), 153–161. PMID:2081225

Yeter, R., Hübler, M., Pasic, M., & Hetzer, R. (2011). Organ Preservation With The Organ Care System. *Applied Cardiopulmonary Pathophysiology*, *15*, 207–212.

Zaroff, J. G., Rosengard, B. R., Armstrong, W. F., Babcock, W. D., D'alessandro, A., Dec, G. W., . . . Young, J. B. (2002). Consensus Conference Report: Maximizing use of organs recovered from the cadaver donor: Cardiac recommendations: March 28–29, 2001, Crystal City, Va. *Circulation, 106*(7), 836-841. Retrieved From http://circ.ahajournals.org/content/106/7/836

Chapter 27
Lung Transplantation:
Post-Operative ICU Management

Aaron M. Cheng
University of Washington, USA

Michael S. Mulligan
University of Washington, USA

Kei Togashi
University of Washington, USA

ABSTRACT

Lung transplantation is a widely accepted surgical procedure for treatment of select patients suffering from end-stage lung disease. Recipients, however, require meticulous post-transplant care to preserve allograft lung function and to ensure optimal patient quality of life. In the post-operative period, these patients are predisposed to specific complications and pose unique considerations that clinicians caring for these patients in the intensive care setting should be familiar with managing. This chapter focuses on the early post-operative critical care management of the lung transplant recipient with specific emphasis on hemodynamic resuscitation; early lung graft dysfunction; and considerations regarding immunosuppression and infection. Non-pulmonary issues that affect the clinical care of these patients in the ICU setting are also discussed.

INTRODUCTION

Lung transplantation remains the primary treatment for qualified patients with non-malignant end-stage lung disease. The first single lung transplantation was successfully performed by Cooper and Patterson in Toronto in 1983, and in 1986, the first successful bilateral or double lung transplant procedure was performed.(Patterson, Cooper, Dark, & Jones, 1988; Patterson, Cooper, Goldman, et al., 1988; "Unilateral lung transplantation for pulmonary fibrosis. Toronto Lung Transplant Group," 1986) Since, there has been a steady increase in the number of lung transplants performed worldwide with recent statistics from 2013 indicating that over 3600 procedures were performed annually in adult patients with end-

DOI: 10.4018/978-1-4666-8603-8.ch027

stage lung disease.(Yusen et al., 2013) Nevertheless, due to organ donor shortage, the number of lung transplants performed remains proportionally small compared to the number of potential patients with end-stage lung disease who could benefit from transplantation.

The overwhelming majority of lung transplant recipients are adult patients in the age range of 50-65, although increasingly, select older patients (> 65) are being considered candidates for lung transplantation. (Abecassis et al., 2012; Mahidhara et al., 2008; Yusen et al., 2013) The procedure can be performed as single or double-lung transplants depending on the underlying lung disease and individual patient characteristics. For patients who have pulmonary sepsis, such as cystic fibrosis and bronchiectasis, bilateral lung transplantation is required due to concerns for recurrence of infectious pathogen if single lung transplant was to be selected. On the other hand, single lung transplantation can be successfully performed in patients with pulmonary fibrosis, chronic obstructive lung disease, and those with pulmonary hypertension. In most lung transplant centers, bilateral lung transplantation is performed when feasible, given its reported survival benefit over single lung transplantation.(Chang et al., 2007)

Overall, the median survival for patients who have undergone lung transplantation is 5.6 years with the median survival of those patients who survive beyond the first post-transplant year estimated to be 7.9 years (conditional median survival). The median survival for double lung transplant recipients is longer than those who receive single lung transplantation: 6.9 years vs. 4.6 years (conditional median survival, 9.6 years vs. 6.5 years).(Yusen et al., 2013) Despite the advances in care of transplant patients, however, survival after lung transplantation remains inferior to other solid organ transplantation due to the greater number of associated complications during the first year after transplantation. Consequently, meticulous attention to detail in the early post-operative phase is crucial to the success of the procedure and the long-term well-being of the recipient. This chapter focuses on aspects of critical care management of lung transplant recipients. A brief outline of the lung transplantation procedure will be introduced but the primary emphasis will be on critical care-related considerations in the early post-operative management of the lung allograft in these patients. Specific issues related to lung donor management and recipient-donor matching will not be covered.

OPERATIVE PROCEDURE

The lung transplant procedure can be performed through standard thoracic incisions. The contemporary double lung transplant procedure is performed through a bilateral transverse thoracosternotomy (clamshell incision), which provides the surgeon excellent exposure and access to the pulmonary hilum and both pleural spaces; bilateral anterior thoracotomies without dividing the sternum, or median sternotomy—the original double lung technique, have also been described and are currently applied. Single lung transplantation is usually performed through a posterolateral or anterolateral thoracotomy.

Cardiopulmonary bypass (CPB) is frequently utilized in the lung transplant procedure, and is usually performed through central cannulation, with the venous cannula inserted in the right atrium, and the arterial cannula inserted in the ascending artery, when required for double lung transplantation. The need for CPB depends upon intra-operative hemodynamic stability and oxygenation, and as such, patients with severe pulmonary hypertension and/or hypoxia are more likely to require CPB support.(de Hoyos et al., 1993; Szeto et al., 2002; Triantafillou et al., 1994) Pulmonary artery pressure will increase with hypoxia, hypercarbia, acidosis and when the pulmonary artery is clamped causing a dramatic decrease in the recipient's cardiac output due to increase in after load of the right ventricle, prompting the need for

CPB. Much caution and vigilance is required to prevent the pulmonary artery pressure from approaching a super systemic level. Frequently, single lung transplant procedures can be performed without CPB, but if required, can be conveniently performed via groin cannulation of femoral vessels. Once the native lung has been explanted, the donor lung is implanted with creation of the anastomoses in a posterior to anterior sequence: the bronchus, followed by the pulmonary vein-left atrial anastomosis, and the main pulmonary artery anastomosis. Upon completion of the vascular anastomoses on each lung graft, the pulmonary circulation is de-aired, and ventilation and perfusion is restored to the newly grafted lung. Much attention is required for possible changes in ECG waveform due to micro air embolization in the coronary arteries, more predominantly in the right coronary due to its anterior location, following this de-airing maneuver. Visualization of air entrapment in the cardiac chamber with a transesophageal echocardiogram (TEE) may be helpful under these circumstances. When double lung transplantation is undertaken, the preferred technique is to implant the lungs separately as bilateral sequential single lung transplants. Usually at least two chest tube are strategically positioned in each pleural space and carefully secured, and the incision is meticulously closed. Prior to leaving the operating room, bronchoscopy is performed to evaluate the freshly constructed bronchial anastomoses and to clear away any accumulated tracheobronchial secretions.

EARLY POSTOPERATIVE CRITICAL CARE

Patients routinely arrive intubated to the intensive care unit with inhaled pulmonary vasodilators attached to the respiratory circuit as necessary. Initial evaluation should focus on assessing the hemodynamic status of the patient and the function of the newly transplanted lung graft with specific management priorities in the ICU to include:

1. Fluid resuscitation and hemodynamic management
2. Assessment of lung graft function with mechanical ventilator support and weaning
3. Immunosuppression
4. Prophylaxis, prevention, and treatment of infection

Fluid Resuscitation and Hemodynamic Management

The transplant recipient usually requires a combination of judicious fluid administration and vasoactive medications (inotropes and vasopressors) to maintain an acceptable hemodynamic profile. It is prudent to avoid excessive volume of fluid administration which can aggravate existing graft lung injury. However, it is not unusual for the patient to become hypotensive upon arrival to the intensive care unit, and several common factors need to be considered: (1) hypovolemia; (2) vasodilation; (3) acute (often right-sided) ventricular dysfunction; and (4) elevated intra-thoracic pressures.

Intravascular hypovolemia in the immediate post-operative period is common. Lung transplant patients understandably receive limited intravenous fluid resuscitation by the anesthesiology team in the operating room to avoid hypoxia due to pulmonary edema, but these patients can sequester significant fluid volume into their interstitial tissue (third) space during the early (<12 hour) post-operative period and therefore will present with intravascular volume depletion. Those recipients who have chronic pulmonary infections for their end-stage lung disease are at increased post-operative risk to develop a vigorous systemic inflammatory response (SIRS) to the transplant procedure. This is can be profound also in those patients who have severe ischemia-reperfusion lung injury and a marked systemic inflammatory response can progress to significant whole-body edema from fluid sequestration into the interstitial tissues. Compounding this SIRS response with the known vasodilatory effects of CPB in those patients who require cardiopulmonary bypass to undergo lung transplantation, it is not surprising that many lung transplant recipients arrive post-operatively to the ICU hypotensive.

Bleeding is another common cause of hypovolemia and should always be considered in the differential for patients who are hypotensive after lung transplantation. Significant blood loss can occur intra-operatively during extraction of the native lungs.(Shigemura et al., 2014) The pleural space can present with dense pleural lung adhesions and pleural fibrosis that require tedious adhesiolysis intra-operatively.(Shigemura et al., 2012) Cystic fibrosis patients often have had a history of pneumothoraxes and may have undergone previous attempts to manage the pleural space, including chemical pleurodeses, which can significantly increase the technical difficulty of explanting the native lungs.(Curtis, Bourke, Dark, & Corris, 2005) Pleural hemorrhage is common in these cases, and CPB can further exacerbate the blood loss with the use of systemic anticoagulation. Although ongoing bleeding may not be present by the time the patient is transported to the intensive care unit, insufficient intra-operative replacement of blood volume can result in hypotension. Patients with ongoing bleeding are usually hemodynamically labile often associated with significant respiratory waveform variation of the arterial line waveform and low CVP (CVP < 8 mmHg), despite positive pressure ventilation. Echocardiography assessment may reveal, under filled cardiac ventricles and the patient will be notably fluid responsive.

Chest tube drainage should be measured accurately and frequently during the patient's initial post-operative course together with prompt review of the immediate post-operative chest radiograph. In addition to checking the chest x-ray for proper endotracheal tube and central line positions, one should evaluate for opacification of the pleural space and for a widened mediastinum. Evidence of accumulated fluid in the pleural space warrants attention, as this likely indicates a hemothorax from blood that has accumulated within the pleural space. Excessive bleeding from the chest tubes (> 200 ml/hr) and/or evidence of hemothorax on chest radiograph should be immediately communicated to the surgical team, as this may warrant re-exploration for a surgical source of bleeding and for evacuation of the retained hemothorax. Surgical bleeding from vascular anastomoses or the chest wall incision, originating from anatomy such as divided, un-ligated mammary vessel will inevitably lead to hemorrhagic shock, despite correction of abnormal coagulation results and will require urgent re-exploration.

Other common cause of post-operative hemorrhage is uncorrected coagulopathy. Therefore, appropriate coagulation laboratory studies should be obtained and abnormal parameters should be corrected with targeted blood products. If the patient has evidence of ongoing blood loss, it is crucial to aggres-

Table 1. Coagulopathy and bleeding: goal targets

Condition	Transfusion Target
Low hemogloblin/hematocrit	Hgb > 10 or HCT > 30
Thrombocytopenia	Plt > 100
Elevated INR	INR < 1.6
Elevated PTT	Normal PTT
Hypofibrinogenemia	Fibrinogen > 150

sively correct any abnormal coagulation parameters, targeting a normal PTT, an INR <1.6, fibrinogen levels > 150, and platelet counts over 100 (**Table 1**). Packed red blood cells should be transfused to try to maintain hematocrit target greater than 30, given the increased platelet dysfunction associated with anemia.(Valeri et al., 2001)

The optimal fluid choice in the post lung transplant period is unclear. Trials conducted on the choice of early fluid resuscitation in critical care are only available for septic patients and does not include lung transplantation.(Ernest, Belzberg, & Dodek, 1999; Finfer et al., 2004; Uhlig, Silva, Deckert, Schmitt, & de Abreu, 2014) In the immediate post-operative period, our practice at the University of Washington is to administer leukocyte-reduced packed red blood cells (pRBCs) to target a minimum hemoglobin level of 10 g/dl if there is evidence of ongoing bleeding in a hypotensive patient. In hypovolemic patients who remain hemodynamically stable, our preference for post-operative fluid resuscitation is crystalloid. The excessive use of normal saline (0.9% NaCl) for resuscitation fluid has been demonstrated to promote hyperchloremic metabolic acidosis and may contribute to acute kidney injury, and therefore, a balanced crystalloid such as lactated ringers should be selected.(A, Shaffer, & Schaefer, 2014; Hatherill et al., 2005; Raghunathan et al., 2014)

Although some transplant centers may prefer colloid over crystalloid, it is our practice to refrain from routine administration of albumin or other colloids in the post-operative period. Extrapolating from studies that have compared crystalloid to albumin administered to patients with acute respiratory failure and lung injury, albumin has not been demonstrated to be superior to crystalloid resuscitation.(Finfer et al., 2004; Uhlig et al., 2014) In addition, under conditions of severe SIRS and significant third-spacing of fluid, administration of excessive colloid will inevitably sequester longer in the lung interstitium from the associated pulmonary capillary leak and adversely affect gas exchange (Ernest et al., 1999). This is particularly relevant for patients who develop severe ischemia reperfusion injury of the allograft. The pulmonary edema resulting from ischemia-reperfusion injury of the lung occurs due to increased permeability and dysfunction of the alveolar-capillary barrier interface, which allows increased influx of plasma proteins across the barrier into the alveolar space.(Ware, Golden, Finkbeiner, & Matthay, 1999) Therefore, we advocate the primary usage of balanced crystalloid fluid and blood products for targeted resuscitation until more compelling data exists to guide practice consensus.

Defined hemodynamic targets for fluid resuscitation in the post-operative lung transplant patients have not been standardized. To help guide hemodynamic management of these patients, lung transplant recipients routinely receive PA catheters. In our institution, we target MAP ≥ 65 mmHg and cardiac index ≥ 2.2 L/min/m^2 and closely monitor serial lactate level and urine output to ensure hemodynamic resuscitation; nevertheless, the competing goals of administering sufficient fluid volume to maintain acceptable cardiac output and systemic blood pressure and the desire to avoid accumulation of excess lung water can be rather challenging in this group of patients. Because the amount of fluid resuscitation can affect lung function, intensivists should strategize combined fluid administration with vasopressor management to maintain these parameters. A retrospective study from Australia found that that high CVP (> 7mmHg) in the post lung transplant period were associated with longer duration on mechanical ventilation higher ICU mortality compared to lung transplant recipients with CVP (< 7 mmHg); the same group of investigators subsequently implemented hemodynamic management of guidelines for fluid and vasopressor management targeting CVP < 7 mmHg and showed less overall fluid administered was associated with reduced severity of primary graft dysfunction.(Currey et al., 2010; Pilcher et al., 2005) Collectively, these two studies suggest that a post-lung transplant management protocol prioritizing a low CVP results in better clinical outcomes in the ICU; however, it remains unclear whether the clinical improvement associated with lower CVPs can be attributed to less fluid administration or instead is a marker of less hemodynamic derangements post-operatively.

Acute post-operative myocardial systolic dysfunction can occur and contribute to early post-operative hypotension. Although appropriately selected recipients should have been evaluated for primary cardiac disease, older transplant recipients, patients with underlying pulmonary fibrosis, and those recipients with primary pulmonary hypertension often manifest impaired ventricular function and have a low cardiac index. When there is clinical evidence of acute systolic dysfunction, intravenous inotropic support, for example, using low dose epinephrine (0.01-0.05 µg/kg/min), in addition to appropriate fluid resuscitation, is required. Evaluation of these patients often reveals acutely impaired right ventricular systolic function due to the effects of acute and chronic pulmonary hypertension. Hypercarbia, hypoxemia, acidosis, and patient-ventilator dysynchrony will contribute to worsening right ventricular function and can lead to acute right ventricular failure; thus, such conditions should be aggressively corrected in the early post-operative period and often these patients benefit from administration of selective inhaled pulmonary vasodilators (nitric oxide or prostacyclin) to reduce the pulmonary vasculature afterload. Patients who have evidence of right ventricular hypertrophy due to primary or secondary pulmonary hypertension often require more generous fluid requirements than those without ventricular hypertrophy and the hemodynamic profile of these patients in the acute period can be quite labile and require longer time spent of the mechanical ventilator before weaning due to the instability. In these circumstances, echocardiogram assessments together with appropriate evaluation of pulmonary artery catheter measurements will be helpful as described by Denault et al.(Denault, Haddad, Jacobsohn, & Deschamps, 2013) On the right ventricular pressure waveform, a normal diastolic slope is typically horizontal under normal right ventricular compliance, as where in right ventricular dysfunction, a progressive change from horizontal to an oblique slope will be observed. As the right ventricular dysfunction deteriorates, it will change to a square root pattern. In cases where the patient has undergone CPB via central cannulation, one should have a low threshold to perform bedside echocardiography or focused cardiac ultrasound to evaluate ventricular function including cardiac filling. Focused cardiac ultrasound can also be used to better guide acute hemodynamic management if the patient remains hypotensive and unresponsive to fluid or blood product resuscitation.(Arntfield & Millington, 2012)

Elevated intra-thoracic pressures can occur due to pneumothorax and therefore noting the degree of air leaks from chest tubes upon the patient's arrival to the ICU and promptly reviewing the chest x-ray for radiographic evidence of pneumothoraces are mandatory. Although large air leaks are uncommon if the graft lung has been carefully handled, small air leaks due to small parenchymal lung injuries are often detectable in the setting of positive pressure ventilation. If a patient has not been adequately volume resuscitated, small pneumothoraces can have significant hemodynamic consequences resulting in hypotension. Therefore, we routinely examine the chest tubes to check for patency, to ensure that the proper amount of suction is being applied, and to note changes in air leaks during the immediate post-operative period. These exams should be done repeatedly.

When single lung transplantation has been performed in patients with end-stage COPD, hypotension can result from dynamic hyperinflation of the remaining native lung. In such circumstances the differential compliance between the graft lung and the native lung, leads to air trapping with the native lung causing increases in intra-thoracic pressure and thereby impairs venous return. When this acutely occurs, the patient's endotracheal tube should be promptly disconnected from the ventilator circuit to allow sufficient time for expiration. In such scenarios, the role of selective single lung ventilation strategies should be considered.

Once the patient has stabilized hemodynamically and remains normotensive, diuretic therapy is initiated. Most lung transplant patients, but particularly those who required CPB for the procedure, are often fluid overloaded and have a substantial weight increase. Diuretic therapy using a loop diuretic (e.g. furosemide) is administered intravenously and can be given as intermittent bolus dosing or as a continuous titrated drip. In general, we prefer administering diuretics as a continuous drip when patients have significant volume overload (e.g. increase in body weight over 10%) or when there is pre-existing evidence of protein calorie malnutrition. Diuresis should be carefully monitored and it is best to avoid overly aggressive daily fluid loss (>2 liters/day net negative fluid balance) given the adverse effects of pre-renal kidney injury in the setting of administering calcineurin inhibitor therapy required for immunosuppression.

Assessment of Lung Graft Function with Mechanical Ventilator Support and Weaning

Early routine post-operative care of lung transplanted patients requires cautious management of the transplanted lungs and vigilance paid to their respiratory status; all lung transplant recipients are at risk for developing acute respiratory failure from primary graft dysfunction (PGD), pulmonary edema from volume overload in the setting impaired lymphatic clearance, and respiratory infections. Primary graft dysfunction is a form of acute lung injury and remains the main cause of early morbidity and mortality in the lung transplanted recipients. PGD usually occurs within the first 72 hours after transplantation, and patients can have varying degrees of hypoxemia, depending upon the severity of PGD. The ISHLT Working Group on Primary Graft Dysfunction defined PGD as the presence of bilateral radiographic infiltrates with the acute onset of impaired oxygenation graded by radiographic findings and the ratio of arterial oxygen to fraction of inspired oxygen, PaO_2/FiO_2.(Shargall et al., 2005) This grading of PGD severity is similar to the original definitions used for ARDS (acute respiratory distress syndrome) and is shown in **Table 2**. Although nearly all lung transplant recipients will have some degree of hypoxemia

*Table 2. Definition: primary graft dysfunction**

Grade at T0, T24, T48, T72**	Presence of Radiographic Findings Consistent with Diffuse Pulmonary Edema	PaO_2 / FiO_2 (Ideally on Mech Vent PEEP 5, FiO_2=1.0)	Exceptions
0	No	Any	
1	Yes	>300	On nasal cannula or FiO_2 < 0.3, Grade as 0 or 1 based on radiographic findings
2	Yes	200-300	
3	Yes	<200	Any patient on ECMO or on inhaled pulmonary vasodilator with FiO_2 > 0.5 beyond T48

* ISHLT Working Group on Primary Graft Dysfunction

**T0: admission to the ICU; T24: 24 hrs after admission to the ICU; T48: 48 hrs after admission to the ICU; T72: 72 hrs after admission to the ICU immediately after the operation, the incidence of PGD has varied in published studies to range between 10-30%. Identifying definite risk factors for developing severe PGD has been challenging, but a recent multi-centered prospective cohort study sought to identify risk factors for PGD.(Diamond et al., 2013) Unfortunately, many of the risk factors are not easily modifiable in the post-operative period.

Given the significant deleterious effects associated with PGD, one should approach routine post-operative ventilator management of lung transplanted patients with a lung protective strategy. Our primary mechanical ventilator mode is Assist Control, either volume or pressure targeted. If the patient is able to maintain acceptable oxygenation on low FiO_2 (< 50%) with minimal PEEP, we target a tidal volume (V_t) of 7-8 ml/kg ideal body weight, while ensuring that plateau pressures remain less than 30 cm H_2O. If the patient requires higher levels of oxygenation support, we will increase the amount PEEP toward 10 mmHg and prefer to use a pressure targeted approach or lower the delivered V_t to 6 ml/kg, in accordance to the lung protective strategy recommended by the ARDS network study.("Ventilation with lower tidal volumes as compared with traditional tidal volumes for acute lung injury and the acute respiratory distress syndrome. The Acute Respiratory Distress Syndrome Network," 2000) Although there are no defining studies examining which ventilator mode is superior in managing hypoxemia from PGD, the similarities in lung injury between PGD and ARDS, should compel a lung protective strategy in severe PGD. When severe hypoxemia (PaO_2/FiO_2 < 200) persists despite increasing PEEP, inhaled pulmonary vasodilators, such as inhaled nitric oxide or nebulized prostacyclin (epoprostenol), which have been demonstrated to improve oxygenation in patients with ARDS, are appropriately initiated. Both inhaled nitric oxide and inhaled prostaglandins do have benefit in improving gas exchange in PGD as in their usage with ARDS, randomized studies to demonstrate the benefit on mortality have not been proven.(Fiser et al., 2001; Meade et al., 2003) Prone positioning also will improve oxygenation in patients with severe ARDS and therefore could be implemented in patients with severe hypoxemia from PGD. A recent randomized study has demonstrated that early prone positioning may lead to improved survival in ARDS patients; however, given the differences in institutional experience and the resource required to prone critically ill patients, there has not been universal consensus among intensivists on when to proceed with proning in those with severe ARDS, let alone an agreed upon proning strategy for lung transplant patients with severe PGD.(Guerin et al., 2013)

Extracorporeal membrane oxygenation (ECMO) support may be life-saving in lung transplanted patients who develop severe primary graft dysfunction (Grade 3) and do not respond to conventional respiratory support with mechanical ventilation and inhaled pulmonary vasodilators.(Bermudez et al., 2009; Fischer et al., 2007) Increasingly intensivists are implementing ECMO support for the management of acute refractory respiratory failure as the detrimental effect of ventilator-induced lung injury becomes more apparent and the safety and technology of ECLS has significantly improved.(Bittner et al., 2012; Hartwig, Walczak, Lin, & Davis, 2012; Oto et al., 2004) Universal indications on when to initiate ECMO still remain the subject of further investigation, but in general for severe ARDS, PaO_2/FiO_2 < 100 despite high FiO_2 > 70 and PEEP > 10 despite adjunctive support (e.g. iNO), have triggered ECMO therapy across different studies.(Davies et al., 2009; Morris et al., 1994; Peek et al., 2009)

Although there is variability among lung transplant centers in their criteria to consider ECLS initiation in acute post-transplant respiratory failure, what is evident, however, is that the benefit of ECLS support in patients with severe PGD comes from its early initiation (Wigfield, Lindsey, Steffens, Edwards, & Love, 2007). In general, venovenous-ECLS support in patient with acute respiratory failure is preferred unless there is concomitant need for hemodynamic support, which would then mandate venoarterial-

ECLS support. In addition to providing full respiratory support and allowing lung rest, VV-ECLS using a large diameter single bi-caval dual lumen cannula along with strategies to minimize patient sedation facilitates early mobilization and ambulation.

Immunosuppresion

Immunosuppression is arguably the most important aspect of post-operative management to ensure long term allograft lung function after transplantation, and the protocols for immunosuppression can be subdivided into induction therapy, and maintenance therapy, and therapy to treat acute graft rejection. In the early post-operative period, immunosuppressive management usually focuses on induction and maintenance therapy as hyperacute cellular rejection is rare with proper donor-recipient matching. Commonly used agents for induction and maintenance immunosuppression for lung transplantation are listed in **Table 3**. Acute cellular rejection occurs in up to one-third of lung transplant recipients in the first year, but this usually does not occur during the first couple of weeks after transplantation.(Kotloff & Thabut, 2011) Many transplant centers routinely administer induction therapy using rabbit anti-thymoctye globulin or interleukin-2 receptor blocking antibodies to reduce the initial T- cell response to the newly transplanted organ.(Sweet, 2013; Thompson, Flynn, & Clifford, 2013) Antibodies and high-dose corticosteroids are the mainstay of induction therapy, which seeks to rapidly achieve host immune suppression at the time of transplantation and in the first few days post-operatively. While the data for induction therapy remains controversial, recent data indicates that the majority of transplant centers administer some form of induction therapy. The benefit of induction therapy appears to reduce the frequency of episodes of early acute cellular graft rejection but with the potential risk of increasing infection in the immunosuppressed host.(Sweet, 2013)

Triple therapy using steroids, mycophenolate mofetil or azathioprine, and tacrolimus or cyclosporine are initiated usually within 24 hours and can be administered intravenously until the patient is able to take an oral diet well. However, we will routinely delay initiating the calcineurin inhibitor for a few days if there is clinical concern that the patient may have sustained acute kidney injury in the early post-operative period. We avoid using the mammalian target of rapamycin (mTOR) inhibitors, sirolimus or everolimus, due to the high risk of bronchial anastomotic wound dehiscence associated with their use in the early post-operative period.(Bhorade & Stern, 2009) It is crucial that if the mTOR inhibitors are to be administered, bronchial healing of the anastomoses has been well documented. At minimum, it takes about 6 weeks for the bronchial anastomosis to heal, and often it may be longer depending on the individual transplant recipient's circumstances.

Prophylaxis, Prevention, and Treatment of Infection

Infectious complications are a significant concern in the post-operative ICU period and remain a leading cause of early post-transplant morbidity and mortality. Lung transplant patients are at risk for nosocomial ICU-associated infections similar to other non-transplant critically ill patients in an intensive care unit. Bacterial pathogens remains the most likely cause of infection in the peri-operative period, but these immunosuppressed patients are also at risk for fungal and viral infections, which usually occur later. Broad spectrum antibiotic coverage is usually administered prophylactically during the peri-operative period, and includes coverage of any potential bacterial pathogens that have been isolated from obtained cultures from either the donor or the recipient. We customarily obtain intraoperative culture swabs from

Table 3. Commonly used immunosuppressive pharmacotherapy in lung transplantation

Induction Agent	Drug	Activity	Major Side Effects
IL-2 Receptor Antagonists (Chimeric or humanized monoclonal antibody)	Basiliximab	Interferes with IL-2 dependent T-cell activation by binding to CD25 on activate T-cells	Usually well-tolerated
Antithymocyte Globulin (Polyclonal antibody raised in horse or rabbit)	ATG Thymoglobulin® ATGAM®	Interacts with thymocyte surface proteins causing lysis and diminished function; prolonged T-cell depletion	Cytokine-release syndrome; cytopenia, serum sickness; anaphylaxis
Alemtuzumab (Monoclonal antibody against CD52)	Campath®	Binds to CD52 on circulating leukocytes, leads to cell lysis; prolonged leukocyte depletion	Cytokine-release syndrome; cytopenia; paroxysmal nocturnal hematuria

Maintenance Agent	Drug	Activity	Major Side Effects	Monitoring
Corticosteroid	Prednisone Methylprednisolone	Blocks synthesis of numerous cytokines, including IL-1, which activates T-cells	Decreases wound healing; hallucinations; muscle weakness; mood changes; edema	n/a
Calcineurin inhibitor	Tacrolimus Cyclosporine	Inhibits synthesis of IL-2	Nephrotoxicity; neurotoxicity	Serum trough: Tac 8-12 ng/mL Cyclo 200-250 ng/mL
T-cell proliferation inhibitor	Mycophenolate Azathioprine	Purine and DNA synthesis blockade	Diarrhea; nausea/ vomiting	n/a

the bronchial airways of the donor lungs during implantation, and will continue broad spectrum antibiotics until the culture results are finalized. If fungal species are identified, we will initiate fungal coverage with fluconazole for *Candida* species or voriconazole for Aspergillus, if there is clinical concern. Antibiotic therapy should be tailored according to culture results as soon as the microbiological culture data has been finalized. Patients who routinely are on chronic antibiotic regimens for colonization (e.g. cystic fibrosis, bronchiectasis patients) are usually continued on their specific antibiotic regimen with valuable input sought from the infectious disease specialists. The mandatory chronic immunosuppression required following lung transplantation places the recipient at risk for opportunistic infections and therefore routine solid organ transplant antimicrobial prophylaxes are also initiated.

OTHER POST-OPERATIVE CONSIDERATIONS AFTER LUNG TRANSPLANTATION

Operative Complications

Early technical complications associated with implantation of the donor lung are most often related to construction of the vascular anastomoses-- either the pulmonary arterial anastomoses or the pulmonary venous anastomoses. If a vascular anastomosis is misaligned, twisted, or kinked due to excessive length, poor blood flow will occur and the vessel can occasionally thrombose, resulting in a devastating outcome that must be promptly identified and treated with return to the operating room. Most often, such technical mishaps are readily recognized intra-operatively with correction of the problem. Post-operatively in the ICU setting, impeded blood flow through the pulmonary artery anastomosis with thrombosis can manifest as severely ischemic bronchial airway confirmed by bronchoscopy. If the airway mucosa appears well-vascularized, it is unlikely that significant pulmonary arterial thrombosis has occurred. TEE by an experienced operator also can be used to evaluate pulmonary artery blood flow, and echo findings will demonstrate increased right ventricular pressures and right ventricular dysfunction.

TEE also can diagnose problems with pulmonary venous return. Completely obstructed venous flow with resultant thrombosis of the pulmonary vein will rarely result in refractory pulmonary edema, and often time manifestations of impaired blood flow through the pulmonary vein are subtle. Thrombus formation can occur at the left atrial anastomotic suture line and carries the risk of systemic embolization and resultant embolic stroke. Pulmonary venous thrombosis often presents early in the post-operative course and those patients with evidence of pulmonary venous or left atrial clot can manifest increased hypoxemia, poor lung compliance due pulmonary edema, and bilateral radiographic infiltrates.(Gonzalez-Fernandez et al., 2009) These patients are at increased risk of early mortality. In general, if there is valid concern for the patency of any of the vascular anastomoses in the peri-operative period, prompt re-exploration in the operating room is warranted before irreversible lung damage occurs.

Early Airway Complications

Problems associated with the bronchial airway anastomoses usually do not occur in the immediate post-operative period; however, the airway anastomosis is the most vulnerable site for subsequent operative complications associated with lung transplantation, including anastomotic infection, necrosis, or dehiscence, which often develop within the first month following transplantation.(FitzSullivan et al., 2011; Murthy, Gildea, & Machuzak, 2010) It is thought that the increased risk for anastomotic complications is due to the relative ischemia to the site. The main bronchial anastomotic sites rely upon retrograde filling from the pulmonary arterial circulation as the normal systemic blood supply of the donor lung bronchial arteries are disrupted during the lung procedure. In general it takes several weeks before the bronchial anastomotic sites re-vascularize. Anastomotic infections are usually of bacterial or fungal etiology and not surprisingly are associated with subsequent early airway complications including anastomotic necrosis and dehiscence and later complications such as bronchial stenosis. Management of anastomotic infections include appropriate targeted antibiotics toward causative organism and serial bronchoscopic evaluation of the bronchial anastomosis for site necrosis and dehiscence.

Bronchial anastomotic necrosis and dehiscence ranges in spectrum of severity and grade (**Table 4**). Almost all patients will have some degree of anastomotic ischemia characterized by focal anastomotic

*Table 4. Grading: bronchial anastomotic necrosis and dehiscence**

GRADE I	Anastomosis healing well; no mucosal slough or necrosis evident
GRADE II	Any mucosal slough noted without any evidence of bronchial wall necrosis
GRADE III	Bronchial wall necrosis within 2 cm of the anastomosis
GRADE IV	Bronchial wall necrosis; extensive, beyond 2 cm of the anastomosis

* Murthy, S.C., T.R. Gildea, and M.S. Machuzak, *Anastomotic airway complications after lung transplantation.* Current opinion in organ transplantation, 2010. 15(5): p. 582-7.

mucosal erythema and sloughing in the first few days following lung transplantation, but these patients are asymptomatic. More extensive injury is thought to be related to ischemia reperfusion injury or early lung infection. These patients may present with increased dyspnea, difficulty weaning from the ventilator, and pneumothorax or pneumomediastinum. Plain chest radiographs may reveal pneumomediastinum or pneumothorax when there is severe anastomotic dehiscence, but should not be relied upon to make the diagnosis as this modality is too insensitive. Rather, fiberoptic bronchoscopy should be performed to identify bronchial necrosis and anastomotic dehiscence along with any associated pulmonary infection; high resolution CT scanning also is useful for detecting bronchial wall defects and luminal irregularities and any associated mediastinal or pleural fluid collections.

Management of anastomotic necrosis or dehiscence is usually conservative with antibiotic therapy, close bronchoscopic surveillance and aggressive pulmonary hygiene, avoidance of positive airway pressure as feasible, and placement of tube thoracostomy to aggressively treat any pleural space problems. Although some transplant centers advocate early uncovered metal stent placement for managing an anastomotic dehiscence(Mughal et al., 2005), this is not our practice, as we believe stent deployment in the early weeks following transplantation may enlarge the existing defect. Unfortunately, there are limited available options for the patient with extensive anastomotic necrosis and complete airway dehiscence. Direct surgical repair of the friable, necrotic tissue is often unrealistic, and often only pneumonectomy or urgent re-transplantation may be considered; these patients have very high associated morbidity and mortality. Other anastomotic complications including airway stenosis, formation of tissue granulation, and tracheobronchomalacia, usually develop beyond the critical care period and often as sequelae to early lung transplant complications. **Figure 1** provides a schematic timeline of complications that can occur during the early post-transplant period.

Respiratory Failure after Single Lung Transplantation: Independent Lung Ventilation (ILV)

Acute respiratory failure from primary graft dysfunction in the setting of singe lung transplantation can present unique challenges using mechanical ventilator support. Particularly, patients with end-stage lung disease due to chronic airflow obstruction (e.g. COPD, α_1-antitrypsin deficiency) who undergo single lung transplantation can be at risk for symptomatic acute native lung hyperinflation as each mechanical breath is preferentially distributed to the more compliant native emphysematous lung.(Angles et al., 2005; Yonan et al., 1998) Radiographically, this will manifest as mediastinal shift toward the new graft lung and diaphragmatic flattening of the native lung. In some circumstances, the overinflated lung will impede venous return and contribute to hypotension and hemodynamic instability. If the lung allograft is dysfunctional as from pulmonary edema, pneumonia, or primary graft dysfunction, native lung hyperinflation can potentially result in worsening V/Q matching. This results as preferential ventilation is distributed toward the more compliant native lung while pulmonary blood flow progressively is shunted toward the severely impaired functioning donor graft lung. If native lung hyperinflation is evident and the patient is unable to be weaned and separated from mechanical ventilation, ventilator settings should be adjusted to minimize tidal volume and PEEP, tolerating permissive hypercapnia, as initial management. However, in severe acute dysfunction of the graft lung, it is unlikely that this strategy of management will alone be adequate. Independent lung ventilation (ILV) has been successfully utilized in such situations and the primary purpose of establishing ILV is to avoid additional ventilator-associated lung injury to the dysfunctional single donor lung, to reduce the adverse hemodynamic effects of native lung

Figure 1. Timeline for complications after lung transplantation

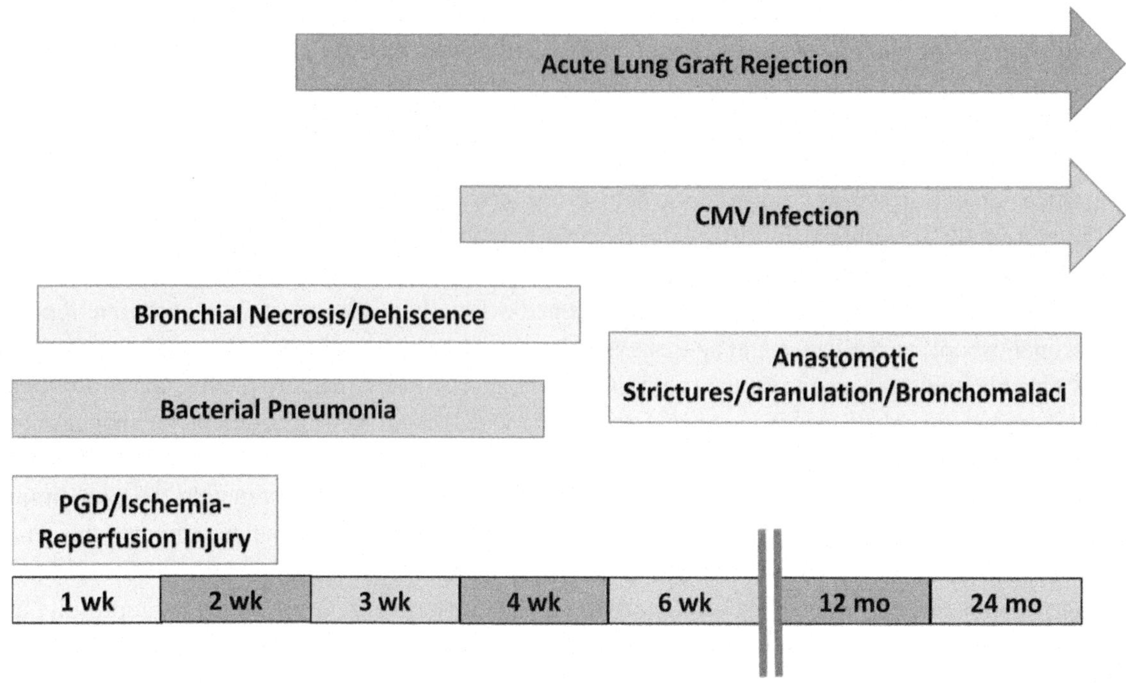

*Adapted from Chakinala MM, Khollef MH, Trulock EP, Critical Care Aspects of Lung Transplant Recipients. J Intensive Care Med 2002; 17:8-33.

hyperinflation and restore the mediastinum to midline, and to optimize overall oxygenation.(Mitchell, Shaw, Donald, & Farrimond, 2002; Smiley, Navedo, Kirby, & Schulman, 1991) These patients are usually already sedated and paralyzed, and independent lung ventilation requires placement of a double lumen endotracheal tube in order to establish the dual ventilator settings. Although a left-sided double lumen endotracheal is easier to properly position, a left-sided double lumen risks direct trauma and ischemic injury to the anastomosis with single left lung transplants; therefore, it is often preferable to place a double lumen endotracheal tube opposite the side of the single lung transplant. Lung protective ventilator settings with higher levels of PEEP can be applied to the donor graft lung in order to optimize gas exchange whereas the ventilator settings for the hyperinflated native lung should minimize PEEP (PEEP=0) and decrease the respiratory rate (Rate 3-5 breath/min) in order to decrease the extent of hyperinflation; often the set tidal volume applied to the native lung is intentionally low but with higher inspiratory flow rates to allow for the necessary prolonged expiratory time. If an acceptable hemodynamic profile and reasonable parameters for gas exchange cannot be achieved, it is usually necessary to promptly escalate to ECMO therapy.

Pleural Space Management

Pneumothoraces are commonly encountered during the early post-lung transplantation course. Most pneumothoraces are small and will resolve spontaneously. Prolonged pneumothorax (air leak > 10-14 days) can occur because the donor lungs are undersized relative to the recipient's thoracic cavity but these air leaks also usually resolve with conservative tube thoracostomy management. However, if bronchial anastomotic dehiscence is suspected for causing a persistent pneumothorax, video bronchoscopy should be performed to evaluate the integrity of the anastomoses; in these cases, prolonged thoracostomy tube management can be anticipated.

Early post-operative pleural effusions are very common after lung transplantation and are thought to occur from increased pulmonary capillary leak due to ischemia-reperfusion injury and the disruption of the donor lung lymphatic system. Other causes of early pleural effusions in the lung transplant patient, include retained hemothorax, infection, and chyle leak. Acute lung rejection, which can occur within the first month of transplantation (usually after 2 weeks) can also be associated with pleural effusions but often these present as new pleural effusions that do not resolve and continue to increase in size. Because of the long term complications that can result from inadequate management of pleural space problems in lung transplant recipients, it is imperative that post-operative pneumothoraces and pleural effusions are aggressively evaluated and managed. Chest tubes placed during the operative procedure are strategically placed to drain dependent fluid collections and also air leaks, and it is important to ensure that the chest tubes adequately drain the costophrenic recess.

Gastrointestinal and Intrabdominal Complications

Lung transplant recipients commonly present with gastrointestinal complaints during the post-operative period. The published literature varies in the rates of GI complications following lung transplantation, and these differences result from heterogeneity in the inclusion time periods after the lung transplant procedure and the variability used to define GI complications.(Hoekstra, Hawkins, de Boer, Rottier, & van der Bij, 2001; Lahon et al., 2011; Lubetkin et al., 1996; Miller et al., 2006; Paul et al., 2009; Timrott et al., 2014)

Cited GI complaints range from benign problems such as nausea, early satiety, constipation, and antibiotic-related diarrhea to more ominous findings of perforated bowel, bowel obstruction, *Clostridium difficile* colitis, cholycystitis, pancreatitis, ischemic bowel, and gastrointestinal bleeding ulcers.(Bravo et al., 2007; Hoekstra et al., 2001; Lubetkin et al., 1996; Paul et al., 2009; Smith et al., 1995) Morbidity and mortality are clearly increased in patients who develop severe GI complications, but their clinical presentation is frequently atypical, can be difficult to distinguish from other benign etiologies, and the subsequent management is often delayed. Immunosuppression with corticosteroids, opioid-induced constipation, and peri-operative bowel wall ischemia are thought to be risk factors for lung transplant patients to develop intra-abdominal complications, particularly colonic perforation.(Beaver et al., 1996; Lahon et al., 2011) In addition, pre-existing risk factors for GI complications is thought to be related to the recipient's underlying primary lung diagnosis, as patients transplanted for end-stage COPD or cystic fibrosis seem predisposed to early GI complications.(Paul et al., 2009)

The intensivists should maintain a low threshold to initiate evaluation and even vague abdominal symptoms in these patients should not be disregarded. Although abdominal radiographs may be useful to diagnosis bowel perforation if there is evidence of pneumoperitoneum or pneumatosis, radiographic findings are often non-specific. The CT scan is the preferred imaging modality and should be obtained if there is clinical suspicion for gastrointestinal pathology, even if abdominal X-rays are unrevealing. General surgical consultation should be obtained early, as frequently diagnostic laparotomy or laparoscopy is necessary and subsequent surgical intervention is required.

CONCLUSION/FUTURE DIRECTIONS FOR RESEARCH

The intensivists caring for lung transplant recipients in the early post-operative period must pay careful attention to details for the overall long-term success of the transplant procedure and use of this scarce organ resource. Optimal management of these patients requires specialist knowledge of the transplant procedure itself and its associated complications, particularly primary graft dysfunction. Primary goals of care are to stabilize the patient's hemodynamic and respiratory status, implement a tailored infection-prevention or treatment strategy, and initiate appropriate immunosuppression. Evidence-based advances in general critical care emphasizing early mobilization and rehabilitative therapy, sedation and analgesia management, and nutritional therapy also are pertinent, but specific ICU practice guidelines pertaining to this group of patients remain lacking. For example, management strategies for balancing fluid administration and use of vasoactive agents to restore early post-operative hemodynamic stability while minimizing lung injury are not agreed upon; the threshold to initiate extracorporeal respiratory support in primary graft dysfunction varies from institution to institution; and even consensus on the duration, extent, and need for antimicrobial coverage are not uniform. Similarly longitudinal research on how acute interventions in the post-operative period affect long term function of the transplanted lung and more importantly the quality of life of these recipients are scarce. Future collaborative studies to establish consensus guidelines to address such critical care management issues are necessary to ensure optimal outcomes in this challenging but unique population of ICU patients.

REFERENCES

A, V. D. L., Shaffer, C., & Schaefer, E. (2014). Early intensive care unit-acquired hypernatremia in severe sepsis patients receiving 0.9% saline fluid resuscitation. *Acta Anaesthesiologica Scandinavica*.

Abecassis, M., Bridges, N. D., Clancy, C. J., Dew, M. A., Eldadah, B., Englesbe, M. J., & High, K. P. et al. (2012). Solid-organ transplantation in older adults: Current status and future research. *American Journal of Transplantation*, *12*(10), 2608–2622. doi:10.1111/j.1600-6143.2012.04245.x

Angles, R., Tenorio, L., Roman, A., Soler, J., Rochera, M., & de Latorre, F. J. (2005). Lung transplantation for emphysema. Lung hyperinflation: Incidence and outcome. *Transplant International*, *17*(12), 810–814. doi:10.1111/j.1432-2277.2004.tb00515.x

Arntfield, R. T., & Millington, S. J. (2012). Point of care cardiac ultrasound applications in the emergency department and intensive care unit--a review. *Current Cardiology Reviews*, *8*(2), 98–108. doi:10.2174/157340312801784952

Beaver, T. M., Fullerton, D. A., Zamora, M. R., Badesch, D. B., Weill, D., Brown, J. M., & Grover, F. L. et al. (1996). Colon perforation after lung transplantation. *The Annals of Thoracic Surgery*, *62*(3), 839–843. doi:10.1016/S0003-4975(96)00393-1

Bermudez, C. A., Adusumilli, P. S., McCurry, K. R., Zaldonis, D., Crespo, M. M., Pilewski, J. M., & Toyoda, Y. (2009). Extracorporeal membrane oxygenation for primary graft dysfunction after lung transplantation: Long-term survival. *The Annals of Thoracic Surgery*, *87*(3), 854–860. doi:10.1016/j.athoracsur.2008.11.036

Bhorade, S. M., & Stern, E. (2009). Immunosuppression for lung transplantation. *Proceedings of the American Thoracic Society*, *6*(1), 47–53. doi:10.1513/pats.200808-096GO

Bittner, H. B., Lehmann, S., Rastan, A., Garbade, J., Binner, C., Mohr, F. W., & Barten, M. J. (2012). Outcome of extracorporeal membrane oxygenation as a bridge to lung transplantation and graft recovery. *The Annals of Thoracic Surgery*, *94*(3), 942–949. doi:10.1016/j.athoracsur.2012.05.006

Bravo, C., Gispert, P., Borro, J. M., de la Torre, M., Cifrian Martinez, J. M., Fernandez Rozas, S., & Group, M. S. et al. (2007). Prevalence and management of gastrointestinal complications in lung transplant patients: MITOS study group. *Transplantation Proceedings*, *39*(7), 2409–2412. doi:10.1016/j.transproceed.2007.07.054

Chang, A. C., Chan, K. M., Lonigro, R. J., Lau, C. L., Lama, V. N., Flaherty, K. R., & Orringer, M. B. et al. (2007). Surgical patient outcomes after the increased use of bilateral lung transplantation. *The Journal of Thoracic and Cardiovascular Surgery*, *133*(2), 532–540. doi:10.1016/j.jtcvs.2006.09.060

Currey, J., Pilcher, D. V., Davies, A., Scheinkestel, C., Botti, M., Bailey, M., & Snell, G. (2010). Implementation of a management guideline aimed at minimizing the severity of primary graft dysfunction after lung transplant. *The Journal of Thoracic and Cardiovascular Surgery*, *139*(1), 154–161. doi:10.1016/j.jtcvs.2009.08.031

Curtis, H. J., Bourke, S. J., Dark, J. H., & Corris, P. A. (2005). Lung transplantation outcome in cystic fibrosis patients with previous pneumothorax. *The Journal of Heart and Lung Transplantation*, *24*(7), 865–869. doi:10.1016/j.healun.2004.05.024

Davies, A., Jones, D., Bailey, M., Beca, J., Bellomo, R., Blackwell, N., & Ziegenfuss, M. et al. (2009). Extracorporeal Membrane Oxygenation for 2009 Influenza A(H1N1) Acute Respiratory Distress Syndrome. *Journal of the American Medical Association*, *302*(17), 1888–1895. doi:10.1001/jama.2009.1535

de Hoyos, A., Demajo, W., Snell, G., Miller, J., Winton, T., Maurer, J. R., & Patterson, G. A. (1993). Preoperative prediction for the use of cardiopulmonary bypass in lung transplantation. *The Journal of Thoracic and Cardiovascular Surgery*, *106*(5), 787–795.

Denault, A. Y., Haddad, F., Jacobsohn, E., & Deschamps, A. (2013). Perioperative right ventricular dysfunction. *Current Opinion in Anaesthesiology*, *26*(1), 71–81. doi:10.1097/ACO.0b013e32835b8be2

Diamond, J. M., Lee, J. C., Kawut, S. M., Shah, R. J., Localio, A. R., Bellamy, S. L., & Christie, J. D. et al. (2013). Clinical risk factors for primary graft dysfunction after lung transplantation. *American Journal of Respiratory and Critical Care Medicine*, *187*(5), 527–534. doi:10.1164/rccm.201210-1865OC

Ernest, D., Belzberg, A. S., & Dodek, P. M. (1999). Distribution of normal saline and 5% albumin infusions in septic patients. *Critical Care Medicine*, *27*(1), 46–50. doi:10.1097/00003246-199901000-00025

Finfer, S., Bellomo, R., Boyce, N., French, J., Myburgh, J., Norton, R., & Investigators, S. S. (2004). A comparison of albumin and saline for fluid resuscitation in the intensive care unit. *The New England Journal of Medicine*, *350*(22), 2247–2256. doi:10.1056/NEJMoa040232

Fischer, S., Bohn, D., Rycus, P., Pierre, A. F., de Perrot, M., Waddell, T. K., & Keshavjee, S. (2007). Extracorporeal membrane oxygenation for primary graft dysfunction after lung transplantation: Analysis of the Extracorporeal Life Support Organization (ELSO) registry. *The Journal of Heart and Lung Transplantation*, *26*(5), 472–477. doi:10.1016/j.healun.2007.01.031

Fiser, S. M., Cope, J. T., Kron, I. L., Kaza, A. K., Long, S. M., Kern, J. A., & Lowson, S. M. et al. (2001). Aerosolized prostacyclin (epoprostenol) as an alternative to inhaled nitric oxide for patients with reperfusion injury after lung transplantation. *The Journal of Thoracic and Cardiovascular Surgery*, *121*(5), 981–982. doi:10.1067/mtc.2001.115668

FitzSullivan, E., Gries, C. J., Phelan, P., Farjah, F., Gilbert, E., Keech, J. C., & Mulligan, M. S. et al. (2011). Reduction in airway complications after lung transplantation with novel anastomotic technique. *The Annals of Thoracic Surgery*, *92*(1), 309–315. doi:10.1016/j.athoracsur.2011.01.077

Gonzalez-Fernandez, C., Gonzalez-Castro, A., Rodriguez-Borregan, J. C., Lopez-Sanchez, M., Suberviola, B., Francisco Nistal, J., & Martin-Duran, R. (2009). Pulmonary venous obstruction after lung transplantation. Diagnostic advantages of transesophageal echocardiography. *Clinical Transplantation*, *23*(6), 975–980. doi:10.1111/j.1399-0012.2009.01078.x

Guerin, C., Reignier, J., Richard, J. C., Beuret, P., Gacouin, A., Boulain, T., & Ayzac, L. et al. (2013). Prone positioning in severe acute respiratory distress syndrome. *The New England Journal of Medicine*, *368*(23), 2159–2168. doi:10.1056/NEJMoa1214103

Hartwig, M. G., Walczak, R., Lin, S. S., & Davis, R. D. (2012). Improved survival but marginal allograft function in patients treated with extracorporeal membrane oxygenation after lung transplantation. *The Annals of Thoracic Surgery*, *93*(2), 366–371. doi:10.1016/j.athoracsur.2011.05.017

Hatherill, M., Salie, S., Waggie, Z., Lawrenson, J., Hewitson, J., Reynolds, L., & Argent, A. (2005). Hyperchloraemic metabolic acidosis following open cardiac surgery. *Archives of Disease in Childhood*, *90*(12), 1288–1292. doi:10.1136/adc.2005.078006

Hoekstra, H. J., Hawkins, K., de Boer, W. J., Rottier, K., & van der Bij, W. (2001). Gastrointestinal complications in lung transplant survivors that require surgical intervention. *British Journal of Surgery*, *88*(3), 433–438. doi:10.1046/j.1365-2168.2001.01693.x

Kotloff, R. M., & Thabut, G. (2011). Lung transplantation. *American Journal of Respiratory and Critical Care Medicine*, *184*(2), 159–171. doi:10.1164/rccm.201101-0134CI

Lahon, B., Mordant, P., Thabut, G., Georger, J. F., Dauriat, G., Mal, H., & Castier, Y. et al. (2011). Early severe digestive complications after lung transplantation. *European Journal of Cardio-Thoracic Surgery*, *40*(6), 1419–1424.

Lubetkin, E. I., Lipson, D. A., Palevsky, H. I., Kotloff, R., Morris, J., Berry, G. T., & Lichtenstein, G. R. et al. (1996). GI complications after orthotopic lung transplantation. *The American Journal of Gastroenterology*, *91*(11), 2382–2390.

Mahidhara, R., Bastani, S., Ross, D. J., Saggar, R., Lynch, J. III, Schnickel, G. T., & Ardehali, A. et al. (2008). Lung transplantation in older patients? *The Journal of Thoracic and Cardiovascular Surgery*, *135*(2), 412–420. doi:10.1016/j.jtcvs.2007.09.030

Meade, M. O., Granton, J. T., Matte-Martyn, A., McRae, K., Weaver, B., Cripps, P., & Keshavjee, S. H. (2003). A randomized trial of inhaled nitric oxide to prevent ischemia-reperfusion injury after lung transplantation. *American Journal of Respiratory and Critical Care Medicine*, *167*(11), 1483–1489. doi:10.1164/rccm.2203034

Miller, C. B., Malaisrie, S. C., Patel, J., Garrity, E., Vigneswaran, W. T., & Gamelli, R. L. (2006). Intraabdominal complications after lung transplantation. *Journal of the American College of Surgeons*, *203*(5), 653–660. doi:10.1016/j.jamcollsurg.2006.07.024

Mitchell, J. B., Shaw, A. D., Donald, S., & Farrimond, J. G. (2002). Differential lung ventilation after single-lung transplantation *Cardiothorac Vasc Anesth, 16*(4), 459-462.

Morris, A. H., Wallace, C. J., Menlove, R. L., Clemmer, T. P., Orme, J. F. Jr, Weaver, L. K., & Rasmusson, B. et al. (1994). Randomized clinical trial of pressure-controlled inverse ratio ventilation and extracorporeal CO2 removal for adult respiratory distress syndrome. *American Journal of Respiratory and Critical Care Medicine*, *149*(2 Pt 1), 295–305. doi:10.1164/ajrccm.149.2.8306022

Mughal, M. M., Gildea, T. R., Murthy, S., Pettersson, G., DeCamp, M., & Mehta, A. C. (2005). Short-term deployment of self-expanding metallic stents facilitates healing of bronchial dehiscence. *American Journal of Respiratory and Critical Care Medicine*, *172*(6), 768–771. doi:10.1164/rccm.200410-1388OC

Murthy, S. C., Gildea, T. R., & Machuzak, M. S. (2010). Anastomotic airway complications after lung transplantation. *Current Opinion in Organ Transplantation*, *15*(5), 582–587. doi:10.1097/MOT.0b013e32833e3e6e

Oto, T., Rosenfeldt, F., Rowland, M., Pick, A., Rabinov, M., Preovolos, A., & Esmore, D. et al. (2004). Extracorporeal membrane oxygenation after lung transplantation: Evolving technique improves outcomes. *The Annals of Thoracic Surgery*, *78*(4), 1230–1235. doi:10.1016/j.athoracsur.2004.03.095

Patterson, G. A., Cooper, J. D., Dark, J. H., & Jones, M. T. (1988). Experimental and clinical double lung transplantation. *The Journal of Thoracic and Cardiovascular Surgery*, *95*(1), 70–74.

Patterson, G. A., Cooper, J. D., Goldman, B., Weisel, R. D., Pearson, F. G., Waters, P. F., & Ginsberg, R. J. et al. (1988). Technique of successful clinical double-lung transplantation. *The Annals of Thoracic Surgery*, *45*(6), 626–633. doi:10.1016/S0003-4975(10)64763-7

Paul, S., Escareno, C. E., Clancy, K., Jaklitsch, M. T., Bueno, R., & Lautz, D. B. (2009). Gastrointestinal complications after lung transplantation. *The Journal of Heart and Lung Transplantation*, *28*(5), 475–479. doi:10.1016/j.healun.2009.02.011

Peek, G. J., Mugford, M., Tiruvoipati, R., Wilson, A., Allen, E., Thalanany, M. M., & Elbourne, D. et al. (2009). Efficacy and economic assessment of conventional ventilatory support versus extracorporeal membrane oxygenation for severe adult respiratory failure (CESAR): A multicentre randomised controlled trial. *Lancet*, *374*(9698), 1351–1363. doi:10.1016/S0140-6736(09)61069-2

Pilcher, D. V., Scheinkestel, C. D., Snell, G. I., Davey-Quinn, A., Bailey, M. J., & Williams, T. J. (2005). High central venous pressure is associated with prolonged mechanical ventilation and increased mortality after lung transplantation. *The Journal of Thoracic and Cardiovascular Surgery*, *129*(4), 912–918. doi:10.1016/j.jtcvs.2004.07.006

Raghunathan, K., Shaw, A., Nathanson, B., Sturmer, T., Brookhart, A., Stefan, M. S., & Lindenauer, P. K. et al. (2014). Association between the choice of IV crystalloid and in-hospital mortality among critically ill adults with sepsis. *Critical Care Medicine, 42*(7), 1585–1591. doi:10.1097/CCM.0000000000000305

Shargall, Y., Guenther, G., Ahya, V. N., Ardehali, A., Singhal, A., & Keshavjee, S. (2005). Report of the ISHLT Working Group on Primary Lung Graft Dysfunction part VI: Treatment. *The Journal of Heart and Lung Transplantation, 24*(10), 1489–1500. doi:10.1016/j.healun.2005.03.011

Shigemura, N., Bhama, J., Gries, C. J., Kawamura, T., Crespo, M., Johnson, B., & Bermudez, C. et al. (2012). Lung transplantation in patients with prior cardiothoracic surgical procedures. *American Journal of Transplantation, 12*(5), 1249–1255. doi:10.1111/j.1600-6143.2011.03946.x

Shigemura, N., Orhan, Y., Bhama, J. K., D'Cunha, J., Zaldonis, D., Pilewski, J. M., & Bermudez, C. A. et al. (2014). Delayed chest closure after lung transplantation: Techniques, outcomes, and strategies. *The Journal of Heart and Lung Transplantation, 33*(7), 741–748. doi:10.1016/j.healun.2014.03.003

Smiley, R. M., Navedo, A. T., Kirby, T., & Schulman, L. L. (1991). Postoperative independent lung ventilation in a single-lung transplant recipient. *Anesthesiology, 74*(6), 1144–1148. doi:10.1097/00000542-199106000-00026

Smith, P. C., Slaughter, M. S., Petty, M. G., Shumway, S. J., Kshettry, V. R., & Bolman, R. M. III. (1995). Abdominal complications after lung transplantation. *The Journal of Heart and Lung Transplantation, 14*(1 Pt 1), 44–51.

Sweet, S. C. (2013). Induction therapy in lung transplantation. *Transplant International, 26*(7), 696–703. doi:10.1111/tri.12115

Szeto, W. Y., Kreisel, D., Karakousis, G. C., Pochettino, A., Sterman, D. H., Kotloff, R. M., & Rosengard, B. R. et al. (2002). Cardiopulmonary bypass for bilateral sequential lung transplantation in patients with chronic obstructive pulmonary disease without adverse effect on lung function or clinical outcome. *The Journal of Thoracic and Cardiovascular Surgery, 124*(2), 241–249. doi:10.1067/mtc.2002.121303

The Acute Respiratory Distress Syndrome Network. (2000). Ventilation with lower tidal volumes as compared with traditional tidal volumes for acute lung injury and the acute respiratory distress syndrome. *New England Journal of Medicine, 342*(18), 1301-1308.

Thompson, M. L., Flynn, J. D., & Clifford, T. M. (2013). Pharmacotherapy of lung transplantation: An overview. *Journal of Pharmacy Practice, 26*(1), 5–13. doi:10.1177/0897190012466048

Timrott, K., Vondran, F. W., Kleine, M., Warnecke, G., Haverich, A., Lehner, F., & Klempnauer, J. (2014). The impact of abdominal complications on the outcome after thoracic transplantation-a single center experience. *Langenbeck's Archives of Surgery, 399*(6), 789–793. doi:10.1007/s00423-014-1193-7

Toronto Lung Transplant Group. (1986). Unilateral lung transplantation for pulmonary fibrosis. *New England Journal of Medicine, 314*(18), 1140-1145.

Triantafillou, A. N., Pasque, M. K., Huddleston, C. B., Pond, C. G., Cerza, R. F., Forstot, R. M., & Lappas, D. G. et al. (1994). Predictors, frequency, and indications for cardiopulmonary bypass during lung transplantation in adults. *The Annals of Thoracic Surgery*, *57*(5), 1248–1251. doi:10.1016/0003-4975(94)91367-6

Uhlig, C., Silva, P. L., Deckert, S., Schmitt, J., & de Abreu, M. G. (2014). Albumin versus crystalloid solutions in patients with the acute respiratory distress syndrome: A systematic review and meta-analysis. *Critical Care (London, England)*, *18*(2), R10. doi:10.1186/cc13187

Valeri, C. R., Cassidy, G., Pivacek, L. E., Ragno, G., Lieberthal, W., Crowley, J. P., & Loscalzo, J. et al. (2001). Anemia-induced increase in the bleeding time: Implications for treatment of nonsurgical blood loss. *Transfusion*, *41*(8), 977–983. doi:10.1046/j.1537-2995.2001.41080977.x

Ware, L. B., Golden, J. A., Finkbeiner, W. E., & Matthay, M. A. (1999). Alveolar epithelial fluid transport capacity in reperfusion lung injury after lung transplantation. *American Journal of Respiratory and Critical Care Medicine*, *159*(3), 980–988. doi:10.1164/ajrccm.159.3.9802105

Wigfield, C. H., Lindsey, J. D., Steffens, T. G., Edwards, N. M., & Love, R. B. (2007). Early institution of extracorporeal membrane oxygenation for primary graft dysfunction after lung transplantation improves outcome. *The Journal of Heart and Lung Transplantation*, *26*(4), 331–338. doi:10.1016/j.healun.2006.12.010

Yonan, N. A., el-Gamel, A., Egan, J., Kakadellis, J., Rahman, A., & Deiraniya, A. K. (1998). Single lung transplantation for emphysema: Predictors for native lung hyperinflation. *The Journal of Heart and Lung Transplantation*, *17*(2), 192–201.

Yusen, R. D., Christie, J. D., Edwards, L. B., Kucheryavaya, A. Y., Benden, C., Dipchand, A. I., & Stehlik, J. et al. (2013). The Registry of the International Society for Heart and Lung Transplantation: Thirtieth Adult Lung and Heart-Lung Transplant Report--2013; focus theme: age. *The Journal of Heart and Lung Transplantation*, *32*(10), 965–978. doi:10.1016/j.healun.2013.08.007

Chapter 28
Mechanical Circulatory Support

Dave Nagpal
Western University, Canada

ABSTRACT

An increasingly important component of the therapeutic armamentarium in the treatment of cardiac and cardiopulmonary pathology, utilization of mechanical circulatory support allows clinicians to help sicker patients with more advanced disease states. A plethora of options exist, each with multiple implant techniques and management strategies. To optimize patient care in a cost-conscious environment, one must understand the advantages and disadvantages of each permutation, and have an algorithmic approach for the selection and application of available technologies. This chapter aims to provide such an understanding by reviewing surgical implant techniques and peri-operative management strategies for a number of commonly used short-term and durable devices.

INTRODUCTION

Iterative refinements in cardiac surgical techniques and patient care have improved surgical outcomes in the preceding decades, which has led to sicker patients with more advanced disease states being submitted for cardiac surgical treatment. Patients with advanced cardiac and cardiopulmonary pathology, including ischemic and non-ischemic cardiomyopathies, advanced valvulopathy, de novo or failing congenital heart disease with treated or palliated lesions, pulmonary and pulmonary vascular disease, and multiple re-do cardiac surgical procedures are at an increased risk of cardiac and pulmonary failure in the peri-operative period. An understanding of Mechanical Circulatory Support (MCS) options provides cardiac surgeons and cardiac surgical intensivists a safety net with which to improve patient outcomes in such high-risk scenarios.

Many MCS techniques and management strategies have been described; each may have advantages and disadvantages, but all are expected to evolve over time with increasing collective experience and cumulative published data. Although consistent success is being achieved with the techniques and strategies described in this chapter, the constant progression of MCS options, surgical techniques, and post-operative management dictates that at some point in the future, this chapter will be obsolete. The latter notwithstanding, objectives for the reader of this chapter are to: (i) distinguish between a number

DOI: 10.4018/978-1-4666-8603-8.ch028

of common MCS options; (ii) rationalize a stepwise approach to the application of MCS options; (iii) review the most common surgical implant techniques; (iv) identify pertinent peri-operative management issues including weaning of MCS devices; and (v) recognize common complications of each device.

BACKGROUND

Historically, the advancement of cardiac surgery has paralleled the development of MCS. The earliest available device was ECMO, in the form of cardiopulmonary bypass, which allowed the development of safer surgical treatment of a wide range of cardiac pathology. Numerous heart and/or lung function replacement or assist devices have been developed over the past 60 years, which in turn has allowed the continual refinement of therapy in increasingly older and more sick patients.

Current common MCS devices may be categorized into cardiac and cardiopulmonary support systems, the latter comprised of ECMO. Cardiac support systems may be divided into short-term and durable devices, which may be further subcategorized by a number of characteristics including uni- or bi-ventricular assistance, partial or full support capability, and percutaneous or surgical implantation.

Device Selection

A step-wise, algorithmic approach for the selection of MCS based on the patient's physiologic derangement (i.e. expected time course of MCS requirement, level of support required, presence of oxygenation/ ventilation insufficiency, left and/or right ventricular failure), and anatomical considerations (if the patient has recently undergone a sternotomy / partial sternotomy or right anterior mini-thoractomy, this may support the selection of particular centrally cannulated devices; if the patient has had a mechanical aortic valve replacement, this renders the cardiac anatomy unsuitable for trans-aortic valve devices; if there is significant peripheral vascular disease, this makes peripherally inserted devices less attractive). In general, one selects the device most likely to optimize patient recovery. This seemingly obvious statement encompasses many factors, including not only the support requirements and the risk of implanting the MCS device, but also the ability to progress the patient in other domains while on MCS. As such, a cannulation strategy that potentially allows extubation and mobilization would be preferable if possible in a patient expected to require greater than 72 hours of support.

Institutional resources play a role in device selection. In centers mandating a perfusionist at the bedside for certain devices, one may lean against such devices in consideration of cost and/or elective cardiac surgery cancellation. Centers with larger MCS volume are able to train intensive care nurses or respiratory therapists to care for patients with their range of devices, allowing improved resource efficiency for the care of these sick patients.

As a general rule, our first tier of MCS for mild persistent hemodynamic instability or cardiogenic shock after pharmacologic optimization is an Intra-Aortic Balloon Pump (IABP). If greater hemodynamic support is required and is emergent, or if respiratory compromise exists or is expected, ECMO is placed. If not, a more nuanced approach for the selection of MCS is possible. Generally speaking, a post-cardiotomy patient still in the operating room will receive a centrally cannulated short-term uni- or bi-VAD. Other patients may be candidates for a peripherally cannulated trans-aortic valve LVAD. Before placing a durable VAD, consensus is required from our Advanced Heart Failure Program Committee.

The following sections will detail the most commonly used MCS devices, providing a brief overview, review insertion techniques and postoperative management strategies, and discuss issues, controversies, and problems of each device.

TEMPORARY MECHANICAL CIRCULATORY SUPPORT

Intra-Aortic Balloon Pump

After more than a decade of development, Dr. Kantrowitz published the first human experience with an IABP in 1968 (Kantrowitz et al., 1968). Further refinement, including the development of a percutaneous insertion platform in 1979, made IABP the most commonly used MCS device worldwide.

Overview of Physiology and Mechanics

The mechanism of IABP effect is that of rapid inflation of the intra-aortic balloon in diastole (hence the term counterpulsation), which increases diastolic blood pressure and coronary perfusion, and rapid deflation pre-systole, which reduces left ventricular afterload and myocardial oxygen consumption. The diastolic blood pressure augmentation depends on balloon size (aim for no more than 80-90% of aortic diameter), aortic and systemic vascular compliance, patient volume status, and heart rate. This augmentation improves right ventricular function as well, by improving right ventricular coronary perfusion pressure and optimizing LV factors relating to ventricular interdependence (Darrah, Sharpe, Guiraudon, & Neal, 1997). The IABP provides little support, an estimated 1 – 1.5 L/min of additional forward flow, but this is frequently adequate.

Insertion Techniques

Typically inserted percutaneously via the common femoral artery, with or without an arterial sheath, the IABP traverses the abdominal and thoracic descending aorta to an optimal position just distal to the left subclavian artery. Position can be confirmed real-time during placement by TEE or fluoroscopy, or following placement with estimation based on surface anatomy landmarks by chest radiography.

Occasionally one will encounter a patient with severe peripheral vascular disease, which either precludes femoral arterial placement or greatly increases the risk of atherosclerotic and embolic complications. Subclavian, axillary, and brachial arterial insertions of IABP have been described (Mayer 1978; Rubino, Onorati, Serraino, & Renzulli, 2009; Estep et al., 2013). For post-cardiotomy failure to wean from CPB in the severe vasculopath, intra-operative placement of trans-aortic IABP via an eight mm vascular graft tunneled trans-thoracic wall via the 2nd or 3rd right intercostal space is our preference, which allows for percutaneous removal in the ICU (see Figure 1). Various trans-aortic IABP strategies have been described (McGeehin, Sheikh, Donahoo, Lechman, & MacVaugh, 1987; Totkas, Yavuz, Eris, & Surer, 2014).

Figure 1. For cardiac surgical patients with severe peripheral vascular disease requiring minor hemodynamic support, ascending aortic insertion of IABP via 6 or 8 mm graft allows bedside percutaneous removal in the ICU

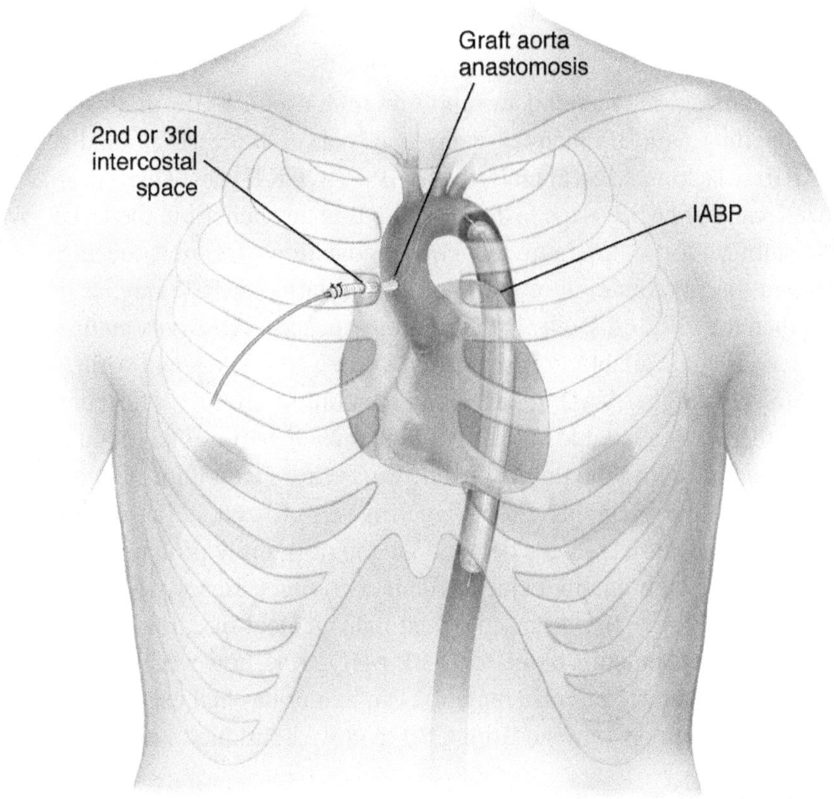

Post-Operative Management

Although optimal timing of intra-aortic balloon inflation and deflation is largely automatic with the current generation of IABP consoles, an understanding of the device is required for confident troubleshooting and optimization. Early or late inflation or deflation of the IABP results in suboptimal cardiac support, and in fact can even increase the cardiac workload and decrease cardiac output. These issues are exacerbated in arrythmia, when ECG-driven automatic IABP augmentation may not be most effective. The reader is referred to excellent resources available elsewhere (Hanlon-Pena & Quaal, 2011).

As with other MCS modalities, inotropic support should be weaned as able to take full advantage of the device. Peripheral vascular resistance is an important component of diastolic augmentation, and as such vasopressor support may remain an important component of therapy while using an IABP in vasoplegic patients. In the absence of complications of the device, we prefer to wean inotropic and vasopressor support to low doses or even off before removing the IABP.

Complications of IABP are related to vascular access (local bleeding, trauma / occlusion / atherosclerotic emboli leading to ischemia / infarction, infection) and trauma to the blood components with related cytopenia. We do not anticoagulate specifically for IABP, and therefore maintain full balloon augmentation at 1:1 counterpulsation whenever possible to minimize thromboembolic risk. Vigilant monitoring for complications, in particular ischemic and embolic complications, minimizes the potential morbidities associated with IABP.

Evidence, Issues, Controversies, Problems

Although theoretical and animal model data supporting the use of IABP in a variety of hemodynamic indications are compelling, as are the many case series and cohort studies, high-quality data demonstrating the efficacy of IABP are lacking. Most notably, the IABP-SHOCK II trial (Thiele et al., 2012), which is the largest randomized study of IABP usage to date, did not find any benefit in the IABP group with respect to hemodynamic stabilization or time on vasoactive medications, lactate concentration, renal function or renal replacement therapy, duration of mechanical ventilation or ICU stay, or re-infarction while in hospital. Of note, there was 10% crossover in the control arm, and a sensitivity analysis comparing groups by treatment received is not available. 5.5% of patients received a VAD, and while the authors state that there was a trend towards higher VAD utilization in the control group, no further information is available. Furthermore, there was a notable absence of higher average diastolic blood pressure in the IABP group, which seems at odds with the therapy itself; we are not given information about balloon sizing or augmentation strategy to explain this. ECG triggering was utilized; deflation at the R-wave is known to potentially increase myocardial oxygen demand via the transiently prolonged augmented afterload.

Despite the absence of high-quality evidence demonstrating efficacy, IABP use remains commonplace. One may reasonably rely on pharmacological management of cardiogenic shock in the general post-myocardial infarction population based on IABP-SHOCK II, however the post-cardiotomy population is sufficiently different that equipoise remains. Our center has had excellent results with IABP for patients requiring a little support to wean from CPB, and we continue to use IABP selectively for this and other indications.

Extra-Corporeal Membrane Oxygenation

Cardiopulmonary bypass was first used in cardiac surgery by Dr Gibbon in 1950 (Gibbon, 1978), but recognition of potential uses outside of the cardiac surgical operating theatres soon followed. Hill et al first reported successful use of ECMO in 1972 (Hill et al., 1972), but outcomes in that early era were limited by the technology of the time. Improvements in oxygenators, tubing, and blood pumps, which cause less inflammation and blood component trauma, allow milder anticoagulation routines, and suffer fewer mechanical failures, have all contributed to the remarkable safety of ECMO in the current era.

Overview of Physiology and Mechanics

Two basic configurations of ECMO are possible: (i) Veno-Arterial, or VA-ECMO, used for cardiopulmonary support; and (ii) Veno-Veno, or VV-ECMO, used for respiratory support. The focus of this section is VA-ECMO; the interested reader is referred to the growing body of literature for further information regarding respiratory VV-ECMO. The essential components of the VA-ECMO system are cannulae, tubing, a blood pump, an oxygenator, a filter, and a heat exchanger. Unlike cardiopulmonary bypass circuits used in cardiac surgical procedures, there is no reservoir; ECMO is a closed system without a blood-air interface. Nevertheless, there remains an inflammatory response of the blood-foreign body interface of the ECMO system components.

In current-era ECMO arrangements, blood is drawn into the circuit via the venous inflow cannula, propelled via a centrifugal pump, oxygenated and ventilated through a temperature-regulated polymethylpentene hollow-fiber oxygenator / heat exchanger, filtered, and returned to the patient via the arterial outflow cannula. Full cardiopulmonary support of up to 10 liters per minute can be achieved if adequate sized cannulae are used, allowing for luxurious organ perfusion.

Insertion Techniques

Cannulae placement for venous drainage and arterial inflow are only limited by vessel size and accessibility. Adult VA-ECMO in the arresting patient is generally placed via the femoral vessels given their relatively quick exposure and generally adequate size in patients without severe peripheral vascular disease. We prefer direct cannulation of the vessels through purse-string sutures with a distal superficial femoral artery cannula for leg perfusion because of problems with hyper-perfusion and ipsilateral limb edema / compartment syndrome when a 8 mm Dacron side- graft cannulation strategy is employed for prolonged periods.

In the post-cardiotomy patient, a central cannulation strategy is convenient simply because one can switch the circuit and leave the aortic and central venous cannulae in place or re-insert aortic and right atrial cannulae as per routine. However, if hemostasis allows, we prefer to expose and cannulate the axillary artery and use a percutaneous femoral venous cannula to close the chest in an effort to reduce wound healing complications. Compared with femoral arterial cannulation, a higher incidence of ipsilateral hyper-perfusion and compartment syndrome is noted with axillary side-graft perfusion (Chamogeorgakis et al, 2013), and we have therefore cannulated the artery directly by advancing a 17 or 19 french cannula through an 8 mm Dacron side-graft just into the artery proper.

Post-Operative Management

ECMO necessitates full anticoagulation. In the early post-cardiotomy setting, bleeding frequently prevents initiation of anticoagulation, and we therefore hold all anticoagulation until chest tube drainage is minimal. Unfractionated heparin by nomogram (no boluses after initial implantation bolus, aPTT target 50-65 initially, then 65-85 seconds when risk of bleeding is low) is our standard approach, reserving bivalirudin for patients with known or suspected Heparin-Induced Thrombocytopenia and Thrombosis. The incidence of oxygenator thrombus or early oxygenator failure has been very low in our experience despite this conservative anticoagulation strategy.

Once full ECMO flow has been achieved, all inotropic medications should be rapidly weaned, using only vasopressors to manage systemic vascular resistance. However, if the left ventricle does not eject, the risks of LV distension and cardiac thrombosis increase:

- LV distension results in failure to reduce LV wall tension, resulting in a failure to most effectively reduce myocardial oxygen demand, reducing the probability of myocardial recovery.
- Stasis of blood in the left-sided cardiac chambers risks cardiac thrombus and even cardiopulmonary thrombosis.

Therefore, when the LV is not ejecting adequately, inotropes +/- IABP or trans-aortic valve VAD +/- a left ventricular drainage vent are indicated. Petroni and colleagues have demostrated a significant hemodynamic effect of IABP in the setting of VA-ECMO (Petroni et al., 2014).

Volume management of patients on ECMO is nuanced. One must ensure adequate flows to perfuse, and to achieve adequate flow one must ensure sufficient intravascular volume and vascular tone. When the venous drainage line "chugs" or "kicks," it is generally indicative of inadequate intravenous volume for the level of venous line suction; the treatment is therefore either reduce venous suction (decrease ECMO flow) or improve venous return (add volume, or to a lesser degree, augment vasoconstriction). Crystalloid vs colloid volume and transfusion trigger thresholds are debatable; our usual strategy is crystalloid first, albumin (25% more often than 5%) if hypoalbuminemic, and red blood cell transfusion for hemoglobin < 70 g/L or any evidence of tissue malperfusion with hemoglobin < 90 g/L.

Close clinical and biochemical monitoring for potential complications is paramount to successful utilization of ECMO. Patients requiring ECMO support are among the most sick, typically suffer multi-organ dysfunction, and as such are at a high risk of further ECMO-related and non-ECMO-related complications. ECMO complications can be understood as some combination of circuit-related, access-related, and anti-coagulation / hematological issues. Circuit-related complications such as pump failure, circuit break with bleeding, or cavitation with air embolus are fortunately uncommon, but kinking of ECMO lines should be part of the primary survey of troubleshooting. Access-related complications include bleeding, vessel trauma / dissection and thromboembolism with distal ischemia, and hyper-perfusion (even compartment syndrome) if axillary or femoral artery side-graft inflow is utilized. Infection is also a concern. Anti-coagulation-related complications are remote bleeding due to anticoagulation, or thromboembolic phenomenon due to sub-optimal anticoagulation. Hematologic complications of hemolysis and thrombocytopenia are not usually clinically important problems. Routine care of the critically ill patient applies, including skin breakdown prophylaxis, gastrointestinal breakdown prophylaxis, enteral feeding, and passive joint range of motion.

Weaning from VA-ECMO requires a systematic approach for ongoing assessment of cardiac function using standard ICU monitors. Daily or twice daily reduction of ECMO flow to load the right and left ventricles is done at the bedside while observing changes and rates of change in systemic arterial pulse pressure, central venous pressure, pulmonary arterial systolic and diastolic pressures, heart rate and rhythm, and pulse oximetry. Short periods of low ECMO flow ~1 L/min are safe, however one must be cognizant of the exponential risk of oxygenator and circuit thrombus with low flows when inadequately anticoagulated. If the quick bedside test is adequately tolerated, a formal ECMO wean under echocardiographic guidance is performed after inotropic and vasopressor optimization and a bolus of intravenous heparin, gradually reducing flows by 0.5 L/min every 2-5 minutes to 0.5 -1 L/min; if tolerated for an adequate period of time, ECMO decannulation in the operating room is indicated.

Evidence, Issues, Controversies, Problems

ECMO is currently being utilized more frequently for a variety of indications, including respiratory insufficiency, cardiogenic shock, and septic shock. Evidence supporting non-respiratory failure ECMO is sparse, and cohort series looking at a septic and post-cardiotomy cardiogenic shock have reported poor outcomes (Huang, Tsai, Tsai, & Ko, 2013; Slottosch et al., 2013). Nevertheless, one does not wait for randomized trial evidence to support using parachutes when jumping out of airplanes; likewise, VA-

ECMO remains a reliable champion for Interagency Registry for Mechanically Assisted Circulatory Support (INTERMACS) profile 0 and 1 patients. When this context is taken into consideration, the reported dismal survival of post-cardiotomy VA-ECMO experience is better than the alternative, which is certain death. The question, then, is that of resource utilization and cost-efficiency in this moribund group.

We utilize VA-ECMO for acute post-cardiogenic shock in the CV-ICU, recognizing the poor prognosis these patients have. In an effort to limit wasted resources, we consent patients' families for short periods (72 hours) of ECMO support, and confront the difficult decision to withdraw support as soon as clinical circumstances dictate.

Temporary LVAD / RVAD / BiVAD

A number of temporary MCS devices are available, including CentriMag (Thoratec Corp, Pleasanton CA), Rotaflow (Maquet Holding B.V. & Co. KG, Rastatt Germany), Impella (Abiomed Inc., Danvers MA), and Tandem Heart (CardiacAssist Inc., Pittsburg PA). The selection of which device to use in which indication is far from clear; as mentioned in the Introduction and Device Selection sections above, there are many possible permutations which can lead to success. Temporary devices are useful in circumstances when native cardiac function is expected to improve ("Bridge To Recovery"), when a decision regarding appropriateness of more durable support requires more time or more information ("Bridge To Decision"), or when hemodynamic support is required until other advanced therapy can be instituted ("Bridge To Transplant" or "Bridge To Durable Device Implantation").

Overview of Physiology and Mechanics

Temporary MCS devices are designed to provide some degree of blood flow to support circulation and allow end-organ perfusion. The CentriMag and Rotaflow are both centrifugal pumps, able to provide maximum flow up to 10 L/min flow via surgically implanted inflow and outflow cannulae. The Impella family of products are intravascular microaxial pumps that sit across the aortic valve, propelling blood from the left ventricular inlet into the aortic outlet; a number of products are available, providing estimated maximum flows from 2.5 L/min to 5.0 L/min. The TandemHeart System also employs a centrifugal pump, which in theory provides up to 5 L/min when used with the supplied percutaneously placed trans-septal left atrial cannula and femoral artery cannula. These temporary MCS devices represent the current state-of-the-art in blood pump technology - previous pumps had higher incidences of hemolysis and thrombus due to greater shear stress, friction with heat generation, turbulent flow, and stasis. Newer designs have successfully reduced these problems: the Rotaflow pump is magnetically held on a sapphire bearing, with no shafts or seals, and a small prime volume of 32 mL; the CentriMag is completely magnetically levitated with no bearings, shafts or seals, and also has a small prime volume of 31 mL.

Appropriate selection of cannulae and cannulation strategy are critical for optimal application of temporary MCS. In accordance to Poiseuille's Equation, the resistance to blood flow in a tube (and resulting blood component trauma) is proportional to the length of the tube and the viscosity of the blood (the hematocrit), and inversely proportional to the fourth power of the radius of the tube. Therefore, the diameter of the cannulae and tubing is paramount for achieving high blood flow with low hemolytic complications. Central cannulation affords short, large-bore cannulae, while peripheral cannulation typically requires smaller and longer cannulae. Various coatings have been developed to improve tube performance, for example Carmeda BioActive Surface Coating to reduce initial anticoagulation requirements and potentially reduce blood component activation, but none have been shown to improve clinical outcomes in practice.

Insertion Techniques

Our MCS cannulation strategy emphasizes early mobilization, and as such, we commonly route most cannulae trans-thoracic through the lateral chest wall when possible. Insertion techniques for the Rotaflow and CentriMag systems are identical, differing only in the external pump and controls at the other end of the tubing. For a centrally cannulated LVAD, we place a 21 – 24 french arterial cannula through two pledget-reinforced purse-string sutures in the mid-ascending aorta, and a 22 – 26 french single stage malleable venous cannula through two pledget-reinforced purse-string sutures at the right superior pulmonary vein / left atrial confluence in Sondergaard's groove to avoid potential future pulmonary vein stenosis, tunneled through the 5th-7th right intercostal space at the anterior axillary line (see Figure 2). For

Figure 2. Centrally-cannulated temporary MCS tunneled through the right lateral chest wall allows for mobilization

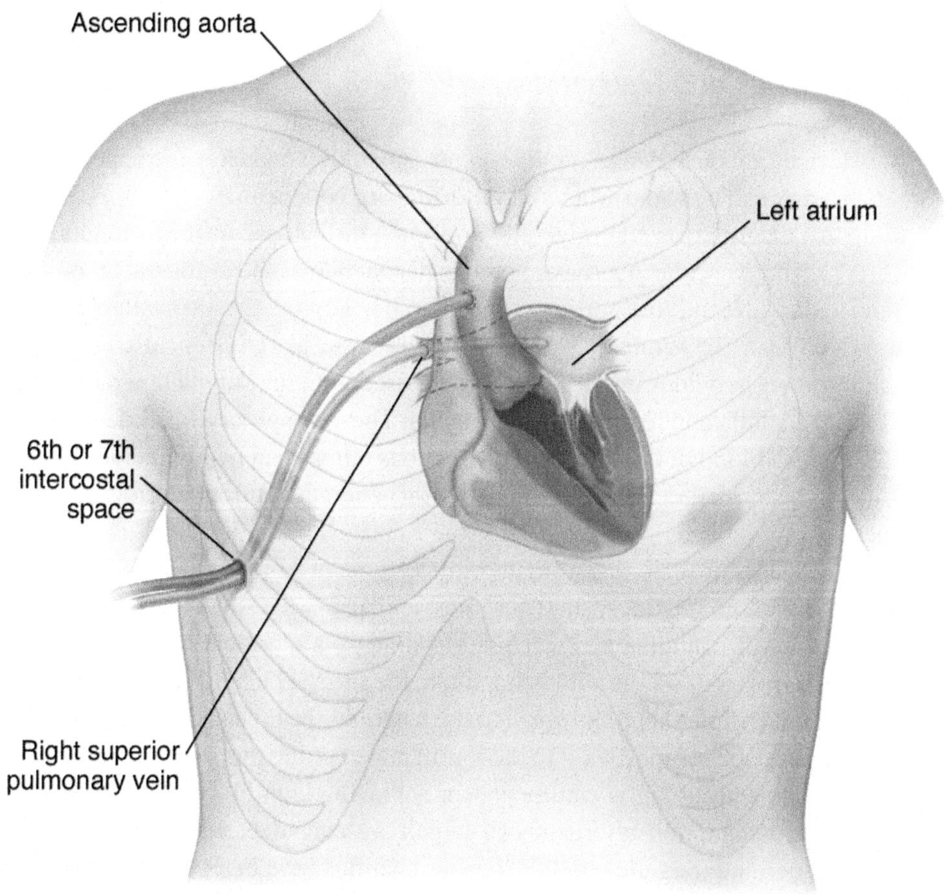

a centrally cannulated RVAD, we place a 21 french arterial cannula though a ten millimetre graft which is anastamosed to the distal main pulmonary artery, and a 24 – 28 french malleable / curved metal tip cannula either though two pledget-reinforced purse-string sutures or a ten millimeter graft on the right atrial free wall, and tunnel through the 2nd – 5th right intercostal space – cannula position for optimal drainage of right atrium determines exit location. We utilize grafts in cases of isolated temporary RVAD to allow percutaneous removal of the device. Of note, when using grafts, we advance the cannulae up to the anastamosis to eliminate the risk of graft kinking. We place the Impella 5.0 through an eight millimetre graft sewn to the left (or alternatively the right) subclavian artery, and tunnel the graft externally approximately 2 centimetres lateral to the subclavian exposure incision (see Figure 3).

Post-Operative Management

Although anticoagulation is essential for all temporary MCS, anticoagulation requirements are less than that of ECMO given the absence of an oxygenator. As such, we routinely hold all anticoagulation until surgical hemostasis and coagulopathic bleeding issues resolve. We then utilize our standard unfraction-

Figure 3. Impella 5.0 implanted via 8 mm graft on the left subclavian artery allows for mobilization

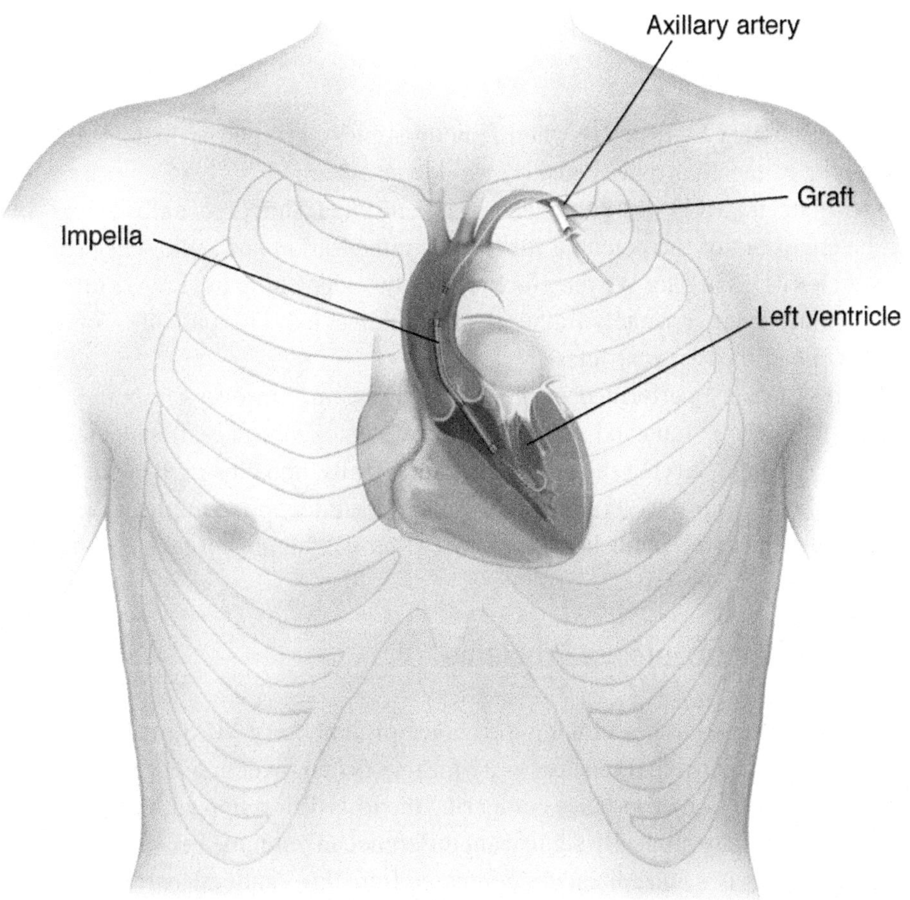

ated heparin nomogram (no initial bolus, start infusion at 500 – 750 units / hour, aPTT target 50-65 initially, then 65-85 seconds when risk of bleeding is low), reserving bivalirudin for patients with known or suspected Heparin-Induced Thrombocytopenia and Thrombosis (HITT). In patients with adequate renal function, we have recently begun utilizing low molecular weight heparin (dalteparin) in patients stable on heparin infusions for at least 48 hours, as this helps with mobilization, decreases venous access and laboratory work requirements, and is associated with a lower risk of HITT. We follow standard manufacturer's protocols and recommendations for Impella pumps.

Unlike ECMO or Total Artificial Heart (TAH) implants, inotropic support might still be required for temporary univentricular MCS given the unsupported ventricle. In cases of biventricular support, all inotropic medications are rapidly weaned, using vasopressors to manage afterload / peripheral vascular resistance. As with all critically ill patients, ensuring adequate intravascular volume is important for flow and tissue perfusion, but de-resuscitation and limiting volume administration can be equally important after the initial resuscitation. We routinely use a multi-modality assessment of volume status including invasive hemodynamics, ultrasonography, and physical examination of the patient.

Routine care of these patients mirrors that of other cardiac surgery patients, in particular weaning sedation and extubation as hemostatic, metabolic, respiratory, and hemodynamic parameters dictate. As discussed above in the postoperative care of ECMO patients, clinical and biochemical monitoring of these sicker patients for both device-related and non-related complications and issues, and routine care for the critically ill patient is essential for a successful outcome. Unless the duration of MCS requirement is expected to be less than 72 hours, we prefer to extubate and mobilize these patients. The CentriMag and Rotaflow pumps fit well on a walker with a modified basket below the seat, facilitating convenient assisted mobilization.

Weaning from temporary MCS begins when hemodynamics and organ perfusion are stable on minimal / no intropic support. Rather than quick bedside turn-downs as with ECMO, we rely on echocardiographic and clinical assessment for MCS weaning. Weaning biventricular support usually occurs simultaneously, but one must be cognizant of the potential for LV decompensation and pulmonary edema with LVAD weaning when an RVAD is in situ. We therefore relatively under-pump the RVAD in this setting. Often, BiVAD weaning must occur separately (rather than simultaneously) for patients requiring significantly more support for one of the two ventricles.

Decannulation is usually performed in the operating room, however temporary RVAD cannulae placed through grafts may be removed at the bedside by sterilizing the graft exit site, ligating the graft after removing the cannula, burying the graft intra-thoracically, and closing the exit site after thorough irrigation. We have not seen any bleeding, thromboembolic, or infectious complications with this strategy, which is consistent with others' published experience (Shafii, Chamogeorgakis, Mountis, & Gonzalez-Stawinski, 2012).

Evidence, Issues, Controversies, Problems

There is a growing evidence base examining the choice of temporary MCS in a variety of settings, but thus far there is no consistent signal of superiority for one system over another. Palanzo and colleagues reported their single-institution experience comparing the Rotaflow pump with a CentriMag pump in an ECLS circuit, not finding any clinically significant difference in outcome between the systems (Palanzo et al., 2013). Chamogeorgakis and colleagues compared Impella / TandemHeart with ECMO in patients with cardiogenic shock, not finding significant differences between groups (Chamogeorgakis et al., 2013). Interestingly, both of these papers comment on the significant cost reduction when utilizing a Rotaflow-based system as compared with the other systems.

Early mobilization is becoming increasingly recognized as an important strategy for improving outcomes in critically ill patients, and patients requiring temporary MCS are no exception (Marrone et al.,1996; Perme, Southard, Joyce, Noon, & Loebe, 2006). Significant barriers to implementation of an early mobilization program which includes patients who are mechanically ventilated and dependent on extracorporeal temporary MCS may be encountered; we found it best to start with lower acuity patients in the Intensive Care Unit, and gradually progress to include these more complicated patients with multiple lines and tubes, ensuring that nursing, physiotherapy, and perfusion are prepared and comfortable with mobilization.

DURABLE MECHANICAL CIRCULATORY SUPPORT

Continuous Flow Left Ventricular Assist Devices: HeartMate 2 / HeartWare LVAD

Implantable mechanical circulatory support, initially in the form of total artificial hearts (TAH), and more recently uni- and bi-ventricular assist devices, have been in clinical use for over 60 years with varying success. Continuous flow LVADs have significantly altered the treatment of advanced heart failure in the last decade owing to favourable results in large trials (Slaughter et al., 2009; Strueber et al., 2011). Given the resource intensity of implantation and care of patients with these devices, we require multidisciplinary committee consensus before implantation. Typical indications for a durable device in the setting of end-stage heart failure may be optimization pre-transplant (bridge to transplant, or BTT), optimization for the assessment regarding transplant candidacy (bridge to candidacy, or BTC), or as a stand-alone treatment strategy (destination therapy, or DT) in patients who are not transplant candidates or wish not to receive a heart transplant.

Overview of Physiology and Mechanics

Durable continuous flow LVADs are axial flow (e.g. HeartMate II, Thoratec Corp., Pleasanton CA; HeartWare MVAD, HeartWare International Inc., Framingham MA), and centrifugal flow (e.g. HeartWare HVAD, HeartWare International Inc., Framingham MA; HeartMate III, Thoratec Corp., Pleasanton CA). A comprehensive review of the similarities and differences between axial and centrifugal flow devices is presented by Moazami and colleagues (Moazami et al., 2013). For the purposes of this chapter, a few clinically important differences between these two categories of devices include a greater pulsatility and afterload sensitivity of centrifugal flow LVADs, and higher inflow suction (especially at low flow) and potentially greater LV size reduction with axial flow LVADs.

Insertion Techniques

Standard insertion of both HeartMate II and HeartWare LVADs is via median sternotomy incision, utilizing cardiopulmonary bypass for placement on the beating heart. Routine cannulation includes a dual stage venous cannula, unless the tricuspid valve needs an intervention. Our strategy has been to repair moderate or more tricuspid regurgitation, being more aggressive in cases of any clinically significant right heart failure. We have adopted a modified Park Stitch (Park, Liao, Segurola, Madhu, & Miller, 2004) for aortic insufficiency greater than trace/mild. Typical LV inflow cannula insertion point is anterolateral to the anatomical LV apex. For HeartMate II implantation, the pre-peritoneal pump pocket is created in such a manner that the diaphram is divided anteriorly and lateral enough to point the cannula posteromedially, and the pump body is held in position by anchoring sutures to the abdominal wall, if required, to optimize positioning.

One of the goals of the LVAD implant operation is to facilitate re-entry for pump exchange or heart transplantation, and thus we preserve as many native tissue planes as possible, closing with an expanded polytetrafluoroethylene neo-pericardium to cover the pump, outflow bend-relief / graft, and anterior heart. Many centres have described alternative approaches, including left thoracotomy and left sub-costal sternotomy-sparing incisions. The HeartWare device may be particularly suited for alternative approaches given the smaller device size and intra-pericardial placement without the need for a pre-peritoneal pump pocket. Many institutions have described minimal-access left mini-thoracotomy for HeartWare implantation at the LV apex without the use of cardiopulmonary bypass, and placing the outflow graft on the ascending aorta via a mini-sternotomy or mini-right anterior thoracotomy, or alternatively on the left subclavian artery or descending aorta.

We have a moderately low threshold for placement of temporary CentriMag RVADs in the setting of LVAD implant, finding that pharmacologic optimization of the RV is adequate in the majority of cases. A number of RV failure risk prediction scores have been developed (REFs), and although no single score or scoring system has proved infallible, we have found RV stroke work index and PA systolic / CVP ratio to be helpful. When required, the temporary RVAD is placed as described above in Temporary MCS section, utilizing grafts to avoid sternal re-entry for decannulation. For the rare case of persistent RV failure on temporary RVAD support refractory to pharmacologic optimization, we prefer to implant an RV to PA HeartWare rather than a paracorporeal RVAD to facilitate discharge from the acute care hospital setting.

Post-Operative Management

Optimization of RV function is paramount in the immediate post-implant care of the LVAD patient, beginning in the operating room and continuing in the cardiac surgical recovery unit. Our usual pharmacologic strategy includes milrinone, inhaled nitric oxide (other inhaled pulmonary vasodilators may be similarly effective), and maintenance of an adequate MAP to perfuse the RV. To reduce RV distension, we promote tachycardia (target heart rate 110-120 by dopamine / beta agonism / pacing) and are conservative with fluid administration. Limiting hypoxia and acidemia, and minimizing blood product administration are also important factors in optimizing pulmonary vascular resistance. Similar to all post-operative patients, we strive for early weaning and extubation as hemostatic, metabolic, respiratory, and hemodynamic parameters allow.

Besides the routine use of invasive hemodynamic monitoring including a pulmonary artery catheter in these patients, both the HeartMate II and Heartware devices themselves offer valuable hemodynamic and pump function information. The pulsatility index (PI, the difference between systolic and diastolic flow divided by mean flow) displayed with the HeartMate II and the pulsatile flow waveform displayed with the HeartWare reflects LV preload, contractility, and afterload. A lower PI / flattened flow waveform is associated with decreased LV preload (e.g. hypovolemia, tamponade, RV dysfunction), decreased contractility, or increased systemic mean arterial pressure; conversely, a higher PI / flow waveform is associated with an inadequately unloaded LV, greater contractility, and decreased afterload. Ventricular suck-down, or a "PI event," is more likely when PI is low / waveform is flattened. Generally, PI may be useful as a trending tool and as an aid in diagnosing circulatory issues in the context of other findings. As a reflection of post-operative physiology, a slight increase in PI at the 48-72 hour mark would be typical, in keeping with interstitial fluid shifting back into the vascular compartment as peri-operative tissue edema begins to resolve. Pump power is a measurement of the power required to spin the device at the set RPM; this value is useful to identify isolated spikes as well as trends over time. Early isolated power spikes may reflect normal post-implant findings of uncertain significance, while later spikes in power or persistently increased power may reflect pump thrombus or dysfunction. Estimated pump flow is also displayed on the system monitors and the device controllers; we do not use this number, relying instead on clinical assessment of end-organ perfusion along with echocardiographic findings to adjust pump speed. In general, we lean towards lower RPM settings in the peri-operative period.

Anticoagulation of durable continuous flow LVADs is a dynamic decision. Immediate post-operative hemostasis takes precedence to reduce the risk for bleeding and/or tamponade requiring surgical exploration, and reduce the need for blood and blood product transfusion. However, early anticoagulation may be important in reducing late pump thrombus, and therefore low-dose heparin infusion is initiated when hemostasis and chest tube drainage is deemed adequate. We typically administer 500-750 units of unfractionated heparin / hour starting at 12 hours postoperatively, gradually increasing the infusion until aPTT reaches 50-65 seconds; we target an aPTT of 65-80 seconds after 24 hours if hemostasis remains secure. ASA (81mg for HeartMate II and 325mg for HeartWare) and Warfarin (target INR 2.0 – 2.5 for HeartMate II and 2.0 – 3.0 for HeartWare) is initiated on the first postoperative day. For patients with suspected or confirmed HITT, a bivalirudin infusion provides safe and stable anticoagulation. Bleeding complications, in particular arterio-venous malformation (AVM) gastrointestinal bleeding, is seen in patients with continuous-flow LVADs, and is thought to be exacerbated by an acquired von Willebrand's syndrome (Klovaite, Gustafsson, Mortensen, Sander, & Nielsen, 2009).

Ventricular arrhythmia may be encountered in the durable LVAD patient as a consequence of the underlying cardiomyopathy, the LV apical incision for the inflow cannula, or ventricular suck-down events. Ventricular arrhythmia can be very well tolerated in patients supported by an LVAD, however LV filling may be compromised by the loss of RV function in the setting of elevated pulmonary vascular resistance. As per usual management of ventricular arrhythmia, cardioversion may be required for hemodynamically significant episodes, keeping in mind that a fluid bolus may be the only required treatment if a low PI / ventricular suck-down is the cause of the arrhythmia.

The risks and benefits of CPR for catastrophic pump dysfunction and cardiac arrest have been debated. Our policy is to administer CPR, as we believe that the risk of pump / cannula dislodgement is low, while the risk to life without CPR in the setting of true circulatory arrest is very high. Circulatory arrest in the first week after LVAD implantation should have open cardiac massage if pump function / return of spontaneous circulation cannot be achieved in 10 – 15 minutes. Importantly, a non-functional LVAD should not be restarted unless it is explicitly known that the maximum time at risk for pump thrombus generation is less than 5 minutes (less if not known to be therapeutically anticoagulated).

Evidence, Issues, Controversies, Problems

The HeartMate II and HeartWare LVADs are by far the dominant devices on the market. Clinical outcomes for the two devices are similar (Topkara et al., 2014), although some have reported differences in outcomes and possible differences in cost-effectiveness between the two devices (Lalonde et al., 2013; Pulikottil-Jacob et al., 2014). There remains little debate on the survival and functional status benefit of these LVADs in selected patients, but the cost per quality-adjusted life years gained remains above usual accepted thresholds. However, outcomes will improve with iterative refinements in post-operative care, destination therapy patients will accumulate more years per device, and device pricing will decrease with greater competition and technological advancement - one can expect a demonstration of improved cost-effectiveness in the near future.

An increased incidence of pump thrombosis was identified in a few major LVAD centres (Starling et al., 2014), which lead to some speculation regarding the root cause of this problem. Some believe that lax anticoagulation strategies played the most important role, others believe that manufacturing changes were at least in part responsible, while most believe that the etiology is multifactorial. As a result of this experience, most centres are now strictly enforcing the anticoagulation parameters discussed above.

Although the field of durable LVAD therapy has progressed remarkably in the past 10 years, there remain many unanswered questions with respect to pre-, peri-, and post-LVAD implant management decisions. Pre-implant patient selection and optimization strategies have evolved, with many centres now using temporary MCS for patients who are INTERMACS 1-2 and reserving durable devices for INTERMACS 2-3; current work is investigating whether LVAD implantation in less advanced heart failure patients (INTERMACS 4-7, non-inotrope-dependant) can lead to improved survival and quality of life (Baldwin & Mann, 2010). Peri-operative decisions regarding need for tricuspid valvular intervention, threshold for temporary RVAD implantation, replace or occlude mechanical aortic valve, and other nuanced issues are receiving more attention in the published literature. Post-implant decisions regarding optimal level of LVAD support / LV decompression / AV opening, safest anticoagulation routines, infection prophylaxis, and the feasibility / durability of LV recovery in the LVAD patient are only a few examples of current debate. These and other issues are gradually achieving some more clarity as a result of dedicated clinicians, researchers, and industry partners generating and sharing new information and current best practices.

Total Artificial Heart

Development of a Total Artificial Heart (TAH) solution for advanced heart failure has followed a storied past with many cardiothoracic surgical giants making significant contributions (Debakey, 2000; Cooley, 2013). A number of devices have been developed and utilized, however the most implanted TAH device today is the SynCardia TAH (TAH-t). To date, over 1,100 patients have been supported by the TAH-t, with the longest duration of support being 3.75 years (Copeland, 2013). Increased interest is developing for this device in many centres in part due to the availability of a smaller portable driver, which potentially allows discharge from the acute care hospital setting.

Overview of Physiology and Mechanics

The TAH-t consists of two polyurethane ventricles with pneumatically-driven diaphragms providing pulsatile flow through four Medtronic-Hall tilting disc mechanical valves. The device typically provides an output of 6 – 8 L/min and a maximum output of 10 L/min, with stroke volumes of approximately 70mL per ejection (beat), and 100 – 130 ejections/min. Higher ejection rates and percentage time in systole may reduce blood stasis and risk of thromboembolic complications. Cardiac output is modulated via an intrinsic Starling-like mechanism, whereby increased atrial pressure will further stretch the ipsilateral diaphragm, increasing ejection volume, and therefore increasing cardiac output.

An external driver moves air in and out of the device to move the diaphrams via two large-bore percutaneously tunneled tubes. Previously, only 36 in-hospital drivers were available to service the entire world market (affectionately called "Big Blue" given the size and 418 pound weight), but more recently an improved 55 pound in-hospital console was developed, and the 13 pound backpack-sized "Freedom Driver" is now FDA approved for use.

Insertion Techniques

Minor modifications of the insertion technique have made implantation of the TAH-t more efficient and hemostatic (Arabia, Copeland, Pavie, & Smith, 1999). In brief, after tunneling the drivelines, the patient is heparinized and cardiopulmonary bypass is initiated with snared bicaval venous drainage. Biventriculectomy is carried out, and the cuffs are reinforced with a sandwich technique using mitral / tricuspid valve tissue and a felt strip. The atrial connectors and great vessel conduits are sized, anastamosed, and tested for leaks. The ventricles are connected, de-aired, and the device is initiated. De-airing and weaning from cardiopulmonary bypass are followed by securing absolute hemostasis. Space permitting, a sterile saline implant is placed in the apex of the pericardial sac to prevent possible transplanted heart fitment problems related to mediastinal fibrosis, then the entire device (including posteriorly) is covered with expanded polytetrafluoroethylene to facilitate re-entry and device removal.

Post-Operative Management

All inotropes and anti-arrhythmics are stopped, usually only requiring vasodilators to maintain hemodynamics and tissue perfusion. Initial and early postoperative TAH-t settings usually approximate left drive pressure 180-200 mmHg, right drive pressure 30-60 mmHg, ejection rate 100-130 / minute, 50-55% systole, and vacuum 10-15 mmHg. Careful attention to balancing pulmonary and systemic drive pressure and circulation is required to prevent pulmonary edema, particularly in the immediate postoperative phase in the setting of chronic pulmonary hypertension.

Bivalirudin infusion is initiated at 0.005 mg/kg/h when chest tube drainage is minimal, usually 12 – 24 hours postoperatively; 81 mg of aspirin and 50 mg of dipyridamole daily are started on the first postoperative day. When stable, warfarin is started, and bivalirudin is weaned when the INR is at target of 2 – 3. Nesiritide infusion (0.005 mcg/kg/min) is utilized when urine output is inadequate.

Similar to all postoperative cardiac surgery patients, early mobilization and physiotherapy are emphasized. However, TAH-t patients tend to be more sick with multi-organ dysfunction, and hence a more concerted effort is required for optimal convalescence.

Evidence, Issues, Controversies, Problems

Although adequate outcomes are being achieved with current-generation TAH, there is debate regarding optimal MCS management of severe biventricular dysfunction. Laforte and colleagues reported their experience comparing TAH or initial permanent BiVAD implantation with LVAD with initial temporary RVAD implantation, finding similar hospital and 6-month survival in both groups, however the majority of patients (65% vs. 6.5%) were able to be discharged without a permanent RVAD (HeartWare was utilized in this setting) (Laforte et al., 2013). There is a clear need for a current-generation TAH solution, which would be expected to provide improved device implant / durability / anticoagulation-related complication profile, and have a more user-friendly controller and interface. One such example is the Cleveland Clinic Total Artificial Heart (CC-TAH), which is currently progressing well in animal models (Kobayashi et al., 2012). This continuous-flow TAH has a single rotating assembly that passively balances biventricular pre- and afterload, and has been shown to have a good response in a wide range of hemodynamic milieu. We await further development of this and other TAH solutions.

FUTURE RESEARCH DIRECTIONS

No longer in its infancy, MCS technology continues to mature with ongoing innovation and iterative improvements in technology and peri-operative / long-term management strategies. This incredible pace of advancement is derived from the pace of research and development, and requires ongoing research in all aspects of MCS utilization for continued improvement in patient outcomes.

Much of the early LVAD implant experience was characterized by salvage and even moribund patients, but clinicians soon developed a comfort and trust with the devices, and more moderately-sick patients are now referred for VAD consideration. As MCS devices continue to become more cost-efficient with a lower morbidity profile, and implantable with lesser invasive approaches, this technology will potentially become increasingly attractive and useful in both ends of the heart failure spectrum of less sick (INTERMACS 4-7) and more sick (INTERMACS 0-1) patients. It is in these areas that continued clinical investigation will define optimal management for these circumstances, and work is already underway in selected subgroups of interest (Baldwin & Mann, 2010; Rogers et al., 2014; Sabashnikov et al., 2014).

Further investigation into virtually all aspects of peri-operative critical care management has the potential to further optimize care in this relatively sick and resource-intensive patient population. Thus far, the vast majority of published investigation is in the form of retrospective cohort comparisons with varying degrees of statistical compensation to allow a closer understanding of the truth. Because individual implant centers are typically unable to adequately power randomized clinical trial designs in this patient population, multi-centre trials will be required. Key areas for further investigation in the post-implant critical care realm include elucidation of optimal LV decompression / LVAD flow, threshold for temporary RVAD implantation, optimal early anticoagulation strategy, timing of nutritional support, and definition of optimal antimicrobial prophylaxis, among many, many other topics.

CONCLUSION

Over the last 10 years, utilization of mechanical circulatory support for the advanced heart failure patient has increased exponentially with generally excellent results. The pace of technological advancement and regulatory approval is all that holds back further advancements in available devices, while laboratory and clinical investigation continues to optimize postoperative management strategies and patient outcomes. The most common MCS devices and peri-operative management strategies as discussed in this chapter are relevant today, but are expected to evolve over time with cumulative experience and scientific investigation. Optimal care of the post-cardiac surgical patient with significant cardiopulmonary dysfunction requires the cardiac surgical intensivist to have an understanding of various MCS options and management algorithms, working closely with cardiovascular surgeons and heart failure specialists to continue to achieve excellent outcomes for our patients.

REFERENCES

Arabia, F., Copeland, J. G., Pavie, A., & Smith, R. G. (1999). Implantation technique for the CardioWest total artificial heart. *The Annals of Thoracic Surgery*, *68*(2), 698–704. doi:10.1016/S0003-4975(99)00540-8 PMID:10475474

Baldwin, J. T., & Mann, D. L. (2010). NHLBI's program for VAD therapy for moderately advanced heart failure: The REVIVE-IT pilot trial. *Journal of Cardiac Failure*, *16*(11), 855–858. doi:10.1016/j.cardfail.2010.06.414 PMID:21055648

Chamogeorgakis, T., Lima, B., Shafii, A. E., Nagpal, D., Pokersnik, J. A., Navia, J. L., & Gonzalez-Stawinski, G. V. et al. (2013). Outcomes of axillary artery side graft cannulation for extracorporeal membrane oxygenation. *The Journal of Thoracic and Cardiovascular Surgery*, *145*(4), 1088–1092. doi:10.1016/j.jtcvs.2012.08.070 PMID:22999514

Chamogeorgakis, T., Rafael, A., Shafii, A. E., Nagpal, D., Pokersnik, J. A., & Gonzalez-Stawinski, G. V. (2013). Which Is Better: A Miniaturized Percutaneous Ventricular Assist Device or Extracorporeal Membrane Oxygenation for Patients With Cardiogenic Shock? *ASAIO Journal (American Society for Artificial Internal Organs)*, *59*(6), 607–611. doi:10.1097/MAT.0b013e3182a8baf7 PMID:24088905

Cooley, D. A. (2013). Some thoughts about the historic events that led to the first clinical implantation of a total artificial heart. *Texas Heart Institute Journal*, *40*(2), 117–119. PMID:23678207

Copeland, J. G. (2013). SynCardia Total Artificial Heart: Update and Future. *Texas Heart Institute Journal*, *40*(5), 587–588. PMID:24391330

Darrah, W. C., Sharpe, M. D., Guiraudon, G. M., & Neal, A. (1997). Intraaortic balloon counterpulsation improves right ventricular failure resulting from pressure overload. *The Annals of Thoracic Surgery*, *64*(6), 1718–1723. doi:10.1016/S0003-4975(97)01102-8 PMID:9436561

Debakey, M. E. (2000). The odyssey of the artificial heart. *Artificial Organs*, *24*(6), 405–411. doi:10.1046/j.1525-1594.2000.06635.x PMID:10886056

Estep, J. D., Cordero-Reyes, A. M., Bhimaraj, A., Trachtenberg, B., Khalil, N., Loebe, M., & Torre-Amione, G. et al. (2013). Percutaneous placement of an intra-aortic balloon pump in the left axillary/subclavian position provides safe, ambulatory long-term support as bridge to heart transplantation. *JACC Heart Failure*, *1*(5), 382–388. doi:10.1016/j.jchf.2013.06.002 PMID:24621970

Gibbon, J. H. Jr. (1978). The development of the heart-lung apparatus. *American Journal of Surgery*, *135*(5), 608–619. doi:10.1016/0002-9610(78)90119-8 PMID:347960

Hanlon-Pena, M., & Quaal, S. J. (2011). Intra-Aortic Balloon Pump: Review of evidence supporting current practice. *American Journal of Critical Care*, *10*(4), 323–334. doi:10.4037/ajcc2011542 PMID:21724636

Hill, J. D., O'Brien, T. G., Murray, J. J., Dontigny, L., Bramson, M. L., Osborn, J. J., & Gerbode, F. (1972). Extracorporeal oxygenation for acute post-traumatic respiratory failure (shock-lung syndrome): Use of the Bramson membrane lung. *The New England Journal of Medicine*, *286*, 629–634. doi:10.1056/NEJM197203232861204 PMID:5060491

Huang, C. T., Tsai, Y. J., Tsai, P. R., & Ko, W. J. (2013). Extracorporeal membrane oxygenation resuscitation in adult patients with refractory septic shock. *The Journal of Thoracic and Cardiovascular Surgery*, *146*(5), 1041–1046. doi:10.1016/j.jtcvs.2012.08.022 PMID:22959322

Kantrowitz, A., Tjonneland, S., Freed, P. S., Phillips, S. J., Butner, A. N., & Sherman, J. L. (1968). Initial clinical experience with intraaortic balloon pumping in cardiogenic shock. *Journal of the American Medical Association*, *203*(2), 113–118. doi:10.1001/jama.1968.03140020041011 PMID:5694059

Klovaite, J., Gustafsson, F., Mortensen, S. A., Sander, K., & Nielsen, L. B. (2009). Severely impaired von Willebrand factor-dependent platelet aggregation in patients with a continuous-flow left ventricular assist device (HeartMate II). *Journal of the American College of Cardiology*, *53*(23), 2162–2167. doi:10.1016/j.jacc.2009.02.048 PMID:19497443

Kobayashi, M., Horvath, D. J., Mielke, N., Shiose, A., Kuban, B., Goodin, M., & Golding, L. A. et al. (2012). Progress on the design and development of the continuous-flow total artificial heart. *Artificial Organs*, *36*(8), 705–713. doi:10.1111/j.1525-1594.2012.01489.x PMID:22747979

Lalonde, S. D., Alba, A. C., Rigobon, A., Ross, H. J., Delgado, D. H., Billia, F., & Rao, V. et al. (2013). Clinical differences between continuous flow ventricular assist devices: A comparison between HeartMate II and HeartWare HVAD. *Journal of Cardiac Surgery*, *28*(5), 604–610. doi:10.1111/jocs.12158 PMID:23844652

Loforte, A., Stepanenko, A., Potapov, E. V., Musumeci, F., Dranishnikov, N., Schweiger, M., & Hetzer, R. et al. (2013). Temporary right ventricular mechanical support in high-risk left ventricular assist device recipients versus permanent biventricular or total artificial heart support. *Artificial Organs*, *37*(6), 523–530. doi:10.1111/aor.12038 PMID:23550592

Mayer, J. (1978). Subclavian artery approach for insertion of intraaortic balloon. *The Journal of Thoracic and Cardiovascular Surgery*, *76*, 61–63. PMID:661368

McGeehin, W., Sheikh, F., Donahoo, J. S., Lechman, M. J., & MacVaugh, H. III. (1987). Transthoracic intraaortic balloon pump support: Experience in 39 patients. *The Annals of Thoracic Surgery*, *44*(1), 26–30. doi:10.1016/S0003-4975(10)62350-8 PMID:3606257

Moazami, N., Fukamachi, K., Kobayashi, M., Smedira, N. G., Hoercher, K. J., Massiello, A., & Starling, R. C. et al. (2013). Axial and centrifugal continuous-flow rotary pumps: A translation from pump mechanics to clinical practice. *The Journal of Heart and Lung Transplantation*, *32*(1), 1–11. doi:10.1016/j.healun.2012.10.001 PMID:23260699

Morrone, T. M., Buck, L. A., Catanese, K. A., Goldsmith, R. L., Cahalin, L. P., Oz, M. C., & Levin, H. R. (1996). Early progressive mobilization of patients with left ventricular assist devices is safe and optimizes recovery before heart transplantation. *The Journal of Heart and Lung Transplantation*, *15*(4), 423–429. PMID:8732603

Palanzo, D. A., El-Banayosy, A., Stephenson, E., Brehm, C., Kunselman, A., & Pae, W. E. (2013). Comparison of hemolysis between CentriMag and RotaFlow rotary blood pumps during extracorporeal membrane oxygenation. *Artificial Organs*, *37*(9), E162–E166. PMID:23981131

Park, S. J., Liao, K. K., Segurola, R., Madhu, K. P., & Miller, L. W. (2004). Management of aortic insufficiency in patients with left ventricular assist devices: A simple coaptation stitch method (Park's stitch). *The Journal of Thoracic and Cardiovascular Surgery*, *127*(1), 264–266. doi:10.1016/S0022-5223(03)01301-1 PMID:14752440

Perme, C. S., Southard, R. E., Joyce, D. L., Noon, G. P., & Loebe, M. (2006). Early mobilization of LVAD recipients who require prolonged mechanical ventilation. *Texas Heart Institute Journal*, *33*(2), 130–133. PMID:16878612

Petroni, T., Harrois, A., Amour, J., Lebreton, G., Brechot, N., Tanaka, S., & Combes, A. et al. (2014). Intra-aortic balloon pump effects on macrocirculation and microcirculation in cardiogenic shock patients supported by venoarterial extracorporeal membrane oxygenation. *Critical Care Medicine*, *42*(9), 2075–2082. doi:10.1097/CCM.0000000000000410 PMID:24810530

Pulikottil-Jacob, R., Suri, G., Connock, M., Kandala, N. B., Sutcliffe, P., Maheswaran, H., & Clarke, A. et al. (2014). Comparative cost-effectiveness of the HeartWare versus HeartMate II left ventricular assist devices used in the United Kingdom National Health Service bridge-to-transplant program for patients with heart failure. *The Journal of Heart and Lung Transplantation*, *33*(4), 350–358. doi:10.1016/j.healun.2014.01.003 PMID:24582838

Rogers, J.G., Boyle, A.J., O'Connell, J.B., Horstmanshof, D.A., Haas, D.C., Slaughter, M.S., … Starling, R.C. (2014). Risk Assessment and Comparative Effectiveness of Left Ventricular Assist Device and Medical Management in Ambulatory Heart Failure Patients: Design and Rationale of the ROADMAP Clinical Trial. *American Heart Journal*. DOI:10.1016/j.ahj.2014.11.004

Rubino, A. S., Onorati, F., Serraino, F., & Renzulli, A. (2009). Safety and efficacy of transbrachial intra-aortic balloon pumping with the use of 7-Fr catheters in patients undergoing coronary bypass surgery. *Interactive Cardiovascular and Thoracic Surgery*, *9*(1), 135–137. doi:10.1510/icvts.2009.205823 PMID:19383637

Sabashnikov, A., Popov, A. F., Bowles, C. T., Mohite, P. N., Weymann, A., Hards, R., & Simon, A. R. et al. (2014). Outcomes after implantation of partial-support left ventricular assist devices in inotropic-dependent patients: Do we still need full-support assist devices? *The Journal of Thoracic and Cardiovascular Surgery*, *148*(3), 1115–1121, discussion 1021–1022. doi:10.1016/j.jtcvs.2014.05.063 PMID:25129605

Shafii, A. E., Chamogeorgakis, T., Mountis, M., & Gonzalez-Stawinski, G. (2012). Fate of retained right ventricular assist device outflow grafts after right ventricular recovery. *The Journal of Heart and Lung Transplantation*, *31*(6), 672–673. doi:10.1016/j.healun.2012.02.028 PMID:22483411

Slaughter, M. S., Rogers, J. G., Milano, C. A., Russell, S. D., Conte, J. V., Feldman, D., & Frazier, O. H. et al. (2009). Advanced heart failure treated with continuous-flow left ventricular assist device. *The New England Journal of Medicine*, *361*(23), 2241–2251. doi:10.1056/NEJMoa0909938 PMID:19920051

Slottosch, I., Liakopoulos, O., Kuhn, E., Deppe, A. C., Scherner, M., Madershahian, N., & Wahlers, T. et al. (2013). Outcomes after peripheral extracorporeal membrane oxygenation therapy for postcardiotomy cardiogenic shock: A single-center experience. *The Journal of Surgical Research*, *181*(2), e47–e55. doi:10.1016/j.jss.2012.07.030 PMID:22878151

Starling, R. C., Moazami, N., Silvestry, S. C., Ewald, G., Rogers, J. G., Milano, C. A., & Smedira, N. G. et al. (2014). Unexpected abrupt increase in left ventricular assist device thrombosis. *The New England Journal of Medicine*, *370*(1), 33–40. doi:10.1056/NEJMoa1313385 PMID:24283197

Strueber, M., O'Driscoll, G., Jansz, P., Khaghani, A., Levy, W. C., & Wieselthaler, G. M. (2011). Multicenter evaluation of an intrapericardial left ventricular assist system. *Journal of the American College of Cardiology*, *57*(12), 1375–1382. doi:10.1016/j.jacc.2010.10.040 PMID:21414534

Thiele, H., Zeymer, U., Neumann, F. J., Ferenc, M., Olbrich, H. G., Hausleiter, J., & Werdan, K. et al. (2012). Intraaortic balloon support for myocardial infarction with cardiogenic shock. *The New England Journal of Medicine*, *367*(14), 1287–1296. doi:10.1056/NEJMoa1208410 PMID:22920912

Toktas, F., Yavuz, S., Eris, C., & Surer, S. (2014). Transaortic intra-aortic balloon pump catheter insertion through a separate saphenous vein graft in patients with severe aortoiliac disease. *TheScientificWorldJournal*, *247803*. doi:10.1155/2014/247803 PMID:24516360

Topkara, V. K., O'Neill, J. K., Carlisle, A., Novak, E., Silvestry, S. C., & Ewald, G. A. (2014). HeartWare and HeartMate II left ventricular assist devices as bridge to transplantation: A comparative analysis. *The Annals of Thoracic Surgery*, *97*(2), 506–512. doi:10.1016/j.athoracsur.2013.08.048 PMID:24140211

ADDITIONAL READING

Abrams, D., Combes, A., & Brodie, D. (2014). Extracorporeal membrane oxygenation in cardiopulmonary disease in adults. *Journal of the American College of Cardiology*, *63*(2525 Pt A), 2769–2778. doi:10.1016/j.jacc.2014.03.046 PMID:24814488

Ahmad, T., Patel, C. B., Milano, C. A., & Rogers, J. G. (2012). When the heart runs out of heartbeats: Treatment options for refractory end-stage heart failure. *Circulation*, *125*(23), 2948–2955. doi:10.1161/CIRCULATIONAHA.112.097337 PMID:22689932

Ambardekar, A. V., & Buttrick, P. M. (2011). Reverse remodeling with left ventricular assist devices: A review of clinical, cellular, and molecular effects. *Circulation: Heart Failure*, *4*(2), 224–233. doi:10.1161/CIRCHEARTFAILURE.110.959684 PMID:21406678

Bermudez, C. A., Rocha, R. V., Toyoda, Y., Zaldonis, D., Sappington, P. L., Mulukutla, S., & Kormos, R. L. et al. (2011). Extracorporeal membrane oxygenation for advanced refractory shock in acute and chronic cardiomyopathy. *The Annals of Thoracic Surgery*, *92*(6), 2125–2131. doi:10.1016/j.athoracsur.2011.07.029 PMID:21982150

Birks, E. J., George, R. S., Hedger, M., Bahrami, T., Wilton, P., Bowles, C. T., & Khaghani, A. et al. (2011). Reversal of severe heart failure with a continuous-flow left ventricular assist device and pharmacological therapy: A prospective study. *Circulation*, *123*(4), 381–390. doi:10.1161/CIRCULATIONAHA.109.933960 PMID:21242487

Feldman, D., Pamboukian, S. V., Teuteberg, J. J., Birks, E., Lietz, K., Moore, S. A., & Rogers, J. et al. (2013). The 2013 International Society for Heart and Lung Transplantation Guidelines for mechanical circulatory support: Executive summary. *The Journal of Heart and Lung Transplantation*, *32*(2), 157–187. doi:10.1016/j.healun.2012.09.013 PMID:23352391

John, R., Liao, K., Lietz, K., Kamdar, F., Colvin-Adams, M., Boyle, A., & Joyce, L. et al. (2007). Experience with the Levitronix CentriMag circulatory support system as a bridge to decision in patients with refractory acute cardiogenic shock and multisystem organ failure. *The Journal of Thoracic and Cardiovascular Surgery*, *134*(2), 351–358. doi:10.1016/j.jtcvs.2007.01.085 PMID:17662772

Kirklin, J. K., Naftel, D. C., Pagani, F. D., Kormos, R. L., Stevenson, L., Miller, M., & Young, J. B. (2012). Long-term mechanical circulatory support (destination therapy): On track to compete with heart transplantation? *The Journal of Thoracic and Cardiovascular Surgery*, *144*(3), 584–603, discussion 597–598. doi:10.1016/j.jtcvs.2012.05.044 PMID:22795459

Maltais, S., Tchantchaleishvili, V., Schaff, H. V., Daly, R. C., Suri, R. M., Dearani, J. A., & Park, S. J. et al. (2014). Management of severe ischemic cardiomyopathy: Left ventricular assist device as destination therapy versus conventional bypass and mitral valve surgery. *The Journal of Thoracic and Cardiovascular Surgery*, *147*(4), 1246–1250. doi:10.1016/j.jtcvs.2013.04.012 PMID:23764411

Marasco, S. F., Vale, M., Pellegrino, V., Preovolos, A., Leet, A., Kras, A., & Esmore, D. S. et al. (2010). Extracorporeal membrane oxygenation in primary graft failure after heart transplantation. *The Annals of Thoracic Surgery*, *90*(5), 1541–1546. doi:10.1016/j.athoracsur.2010.05.066 PMID:20971259

Moazami, N., Fukamachi, K., Kobayashi, M., Smedira, N. G., Hoercher, K. J., Massiello, A., & Starling, R. C. et al. (2013). Axial and centrifugal continuous-flow rotary pumps: A translation from pump mechanics to clinical practice. *The Journal of Heart and Lung Transplantation*, *32*(1), 1–11. doi:10.1016/j.healun.2012.10.001 PMID:23260699

Pratt, A. K., Shah, N. S., & Boyce, S. W. (2014). Left ventricular assist device management in the ICU. *Critical Care Medicine*, *42*(1), 158–168. doi:10.1097/01.ccm.0000435675.91305.76 PMID:24240731

Rose, E. A., Gelijns, A. C., Moskowitz, A. J., Heitjan, D. F., Stevenson, L. W., Dembitsky, W., & Meier, P. et al. (2001). Long-term use of a left ventricular assist device for end-stage heart failure. *The New England Journal of Medicine*, *345*(20), 1435–1443. doi:10.1056/NEJMoa012175 PMID:11794191

Sayer, G. T., Baker, J. N., & Parks, K. A. (2012). Heart rescue: The role of mechanical circulatory support in the management of severe refractory cardiogenic shock. *Current Opinion in Critical Care*, *18*(5), 409–416. doi:10.1097/MCC.0b013e328357f1e6 PMID:22895213

Slaughter, M. S., Pagani, F. D., Rogers, J. G., Miller, L. W., Sun, B., Russell, S. D., & Farrar, D. J. et al. (2010). Clinical management of continuous-flow left ventricular assist devices in advanced heart failure. *The Journal of Heart and Lung Transplantation*, *29*(4Suppl), S1–S39. doi:10.1016/j.healun.2010.01.011 PMID:20181499

Slaughter, M. S., Rogers, J. G., Milano, C. A., Russell, S. D., Conte, J. V., Feldman, D., & Frazier, O. H. et al. (2009). Advanced heart failure treated with continuous-flow left ventricular assist device. *The New England Journal of Medicine*, *361*(23), 2241–2251. doi:10.1056/NEJMoa0909938 PMID:19920051

Stevenson, L. W., Pagani, F. D., Young, J. B., Jessup, M., Miller, L., Kormos, R. L., & Kirklin, J. K. et al. (2009). INTERMACS profiles of advanced heart failure: The current picture. *The Journal of Heart and Lung Transplantation*, *28*(6), 535–541. doi:10.1016/j.healun.2009.02.015 PMID:19481012

Strueber, M., O'Driscoll, G., Jansz, P., Khaghani, A., Levy, W. C., & Wieselthaler, G. M. (2011). Multicenter evaluation of an intrapericardial left ventricular assist system. *Journal of the American College of Cardiology*, *57*(12), 1375–1382. doi:10.1016/j.jacc.2010.10.040 PMID:21414534

Takayama, H., Soni, L., Kalesan, B., Truby, L. K., Ota, T., Cedola, S., & Naka, Y. et al. (2014). Bridge-to-decision therapy with a continuous-flow external ventricular assist device in refractory cardiogenic shock of various causes. *Circulation: Heart Failure*, *7*(5), 799–806. doi:10.1161/CIRCHEARTFAILURE.113.000271 PMID:25027874

Tang, G. H., Malekan, R., Kai, M., Lansman, S. L., & Spielvogel, D. (2013). Peripheral venoarterial extracorporeal membrane oxygenation improves survival in myocardial infarction with cardiogenic shock. *The Journal of Thoracic and Cardiovascular Surgery*, *145*(3), e32–e33. doi:10.1016/j.jtcvs.2012.12.038 PMID:23312972

Trivedi, J. R., Cheng, A., Singh, R., Williams, M. L., & Slaughter, M. S. (2014). Survival on the heart transplant waiting list: Impact of continuous flow left ventricular assist device as bridge to transplant. *The Annals of Thoracic Surgery*, *98*(3), 830–834. doi:10.1016/j.athoracsur.2014.05.019 PMID:25087934

Uriel, N., Morrison, K. A., Garan, A. R., Kato, T. S., Yuzefpolskaya, M., Latif, F., & Jorde, U. P. et al. (2012). Development of a novel echocardiography ramp test for speed optimization and diagnosis of device thrombosis in continuous-flow left ventricular assist devices: The Columbia ramp study. *Journal of the American College of Cardiology*, *60*(18), 1764–1775. doi:10.1016/j.jacc.2012.07.052 PMID:23040584

Wever-Pinzon, O., Stehlik, J., Kfoury, A. G., Terrovitis, J. V., Diakos, N. A., Charitos, C., & Drakos, S. G. et al. (2012). Ventricular assist devices: Pharmacological aspects of a mechanical therapy. *Pharmacology & Therapeutics*, *134*(2), 189–199. doi:10.1016/j.pharmthera.2012.01.003 PMID:22281238

Wozniak, C. J., Stehlik, J., Baird, B. C., McKellar, S. H., Song, H. K., Drakos, S. G., & Selzman, C. H. (2014). Ventricular assist devices or inotropic agents in status 1A patients? Survival analysis of the United Network of Organ Sharing database. *The Annals of Thoracic Surgery*, *97*(4), 1364–1371, discussion 1371–1372. doi:10.1016/j.athoracsur.2013.10.077 PMID:24424016

KEY TERMS AND DEFINITIONS

Axial-Flow VAD: In reference to continuous-flow VADs, axial-flow devices are considered to be second-generation devices, and have a single inflow – rotor – outflow axis. The current generation axial-flow VADs require higher RPMs to achieve target flow. These devices are less afterload sensitive, and generate higher inlet suction, which increases the risk of ventricular suck-down events.

Centrifugal-Flow VAD: In reference to continuous-flow VADs, centrifugal-flow devices are considered to be third-generation devices, and have an outflow that is perpendicular to the inflow axis. These devices are more afterload sensitive, and with less inlet suction at low flow, are less likely to generate ventricular suck-down events.

Continuous-Flow VAD: In reference to durable VADs, continuous-flow technology refers to the pattern of constant blood propulsion via an axial or centrifugal design. Broadly speaking, this technology is smaller and utilizes fewer moving parts compared with pulsatile VADs, resulting in a more durable device.

Durable Mechanical Circulatory Support: A circulatory assist device that allows discharge from the acute care hospital setting. These pumps are usually implantable, tethered only by a percutaneous driveline.

INTERMACS: The Interagency Registry for Mechanically Assisted Circulatory Support was born out of collaboration between the National Heart, Lung and Blood Institute (NHLBI), the Centers for Medicare and Medicaid Services (CMS), and the Food and Drug Administration (FDA), with involvement of clinicians, scientists and industry. The registry prospectively collects data, which provides an important resource for continuous quality improvement / assurance and some testing of research hypotheses.

Pulsatile-Flow VAD: In reference to durable VADs, pulsatile-flow technology refers to the rhythmic propulsion of blood via moving pusher-plates or diaphragms on a chamber of blood. This technology was the first generation of VAD design, and has been entirely supplanted by continuous-flow technology in the LVAD setting due to well-documented improved outcomes.

Temporary Mechanical Circulatory Support: A circulatory assist device that requires the patient remain in an acute care hospital setting. These pumps are frequently used for prolonged periods of time, even up to 2-3 months, despite much shorter FDA approval usage times.

Chapter 29
Critical Care of the Thoracic Surgical Patient

Madhuri Rao
Mount Sinai Hospital, USA

Dong-Seok Daniel Lee
Mount Sinai Hospital, USA

ABSTRACT

Patients having major general thoracic surgery constitute an integral part of any cardiothoracic intensive care unit. Pulmonary or esophageal resection especially in a patient who has cardiopulmonary issues at baseline demands close monitoring by a critical care team postoperatively. This chapter aims to cover the important aspects of the perioperative care involved with these patients. In addition, procedures requiring an intensive care unit postoeratively such as, pneumonectomy, esophagectomy, thymectomy are dealt with in some detail where key technical aspects and care and complications specific to each are discussed.

INTRODUCTION

Thoracic surgical patients are potentially high risk patients given the nature of the surgery, anesthesia and the prevalent co-morbidities such as long smoking history and the intrinsic lung pathology. The goal of pre-operative evaluation is careful patient selection and pre-operative optimization. Post-operative care should be directed at prevention of complications and early recognition and management of complications when they do occur. This chapter will address the important aspects in perioperative evaluation and care of general thoracic patients with emphasis on post-operative management of those procedures that routinely demand critical care management.

DOI: 10.4018/978-1-4666-8603-8.ch029

PRE-OPERATIVE ASSESSMENT

Pulmonary Function Testing/Assessment

Functional Residual Capacity and Closing Volume: Functional Residual Capacity (FRC) is the lung volume at the end of normal expiration and is the most important lung volume measurement that affects development of pulmonary complications. The closing volume (CV) is the volume of lung at which airflow from dependent parts of the lung stops during expiration owing to airway closure. Decreased FRC (from factors that increase intra-abdominal pressure) or increased CV (from advancing age, fluid overload, bronchospasm, etc.) will result in premature airway closure and atelectasis (Alexander, Hamilton, Parikh, Spence, & Stewart, 1972).

Spirometry: Forced Expiratory Volume in 1 second (FEV1) is one of the best predictors of risk for major lung surgery. An FEV1 < 2 liters is indicative of increased risk and the guidelines recommend additional physiological studies. A post-operative predicted FEV1 of 800ml to 1 liter is considered by many surgeons to be a precluding factor for lung resection. Spirometric values are more valuable when expressed as a percentage of predicted normal value based on age, sex and body height. Several authors have suggested a post-operative predicted value for FEV1 of 40% of normal as a cut off for selecting high risk patients (Pate, Tenholder, Griffin, Eastridge, & Weiman, 1996; Schuurmans, Diacon, & Bolliger, 2002).

Quantitative perfusion scan: The functional contribution of the different segments of the lung can be measured by split perfusion scanning using technetium or by quantitative CT scanning.

DL_{CO}: Diffusing Capacity of the Lung is a measurement of the gas exchange function of the lung at the alveolar-capillary interface. It provides a measure of lung parenchymal disease. A preoperative DL_{CO} of < 45% of the predicted value is associated with a higher mortality and pulmonary morbidity rate in patients undergoing pulmonary resection (Win et al., 2005).

Exercise testing: Preoperative exercise testing include tests such as the shuttle walk, the 6 minute walk, exercise oximetry, and oxygen consumption during maximum exercise ($VO_{2\,max}$). Exercise testing is the best determinant of functional capacity. By generally agreed standards, a $VO_{2\,max}$ < 10ml/kg/minute puts a patient in an extremely high risk category for major lung resection and a $VO_{2\,max}$ > 15ml/kg/minute is indicative of an average risk patient (Benzo, Kelley, Recchi, Hofman, & Sciurba, 2007; Bolliger et al., 1995).

The evaluation algorithm proposed by the ACCP consensus guidelines is presented below in Figure 1 (Colice, Shafazand, Griffin, 2007).

Age and performance status: Both advancing age and performance status have been shown to be independent predictors of increased post-operative mortality (Dales, Dionne, Leech, Lunau, & Schweitzer, 1993; Kohman, Meyer, Ikins, & Oates, 1986; Harpole et al., 1999). The decision to operate or not should not be based on age alone and the functional status of the patient should be taken into consideration.

Cardiac Evaluation

All patients undergoing major pulmonary resection should have at a minimum, a pre-operative electrocardiogram. Any abnormalities should prompt an echocardiogram. As per the American Heart Association, non-cardiac surgery is acceptable 6 weeks after a myocardial infarction. Patients with major risk predictors should be considered for revascularization or valve surgery prior to pulmonary resection. Some

Figure 1. Evaluation algorithm for preoperative pulmonary function testing as proposed by the ACCP consensus guidelines

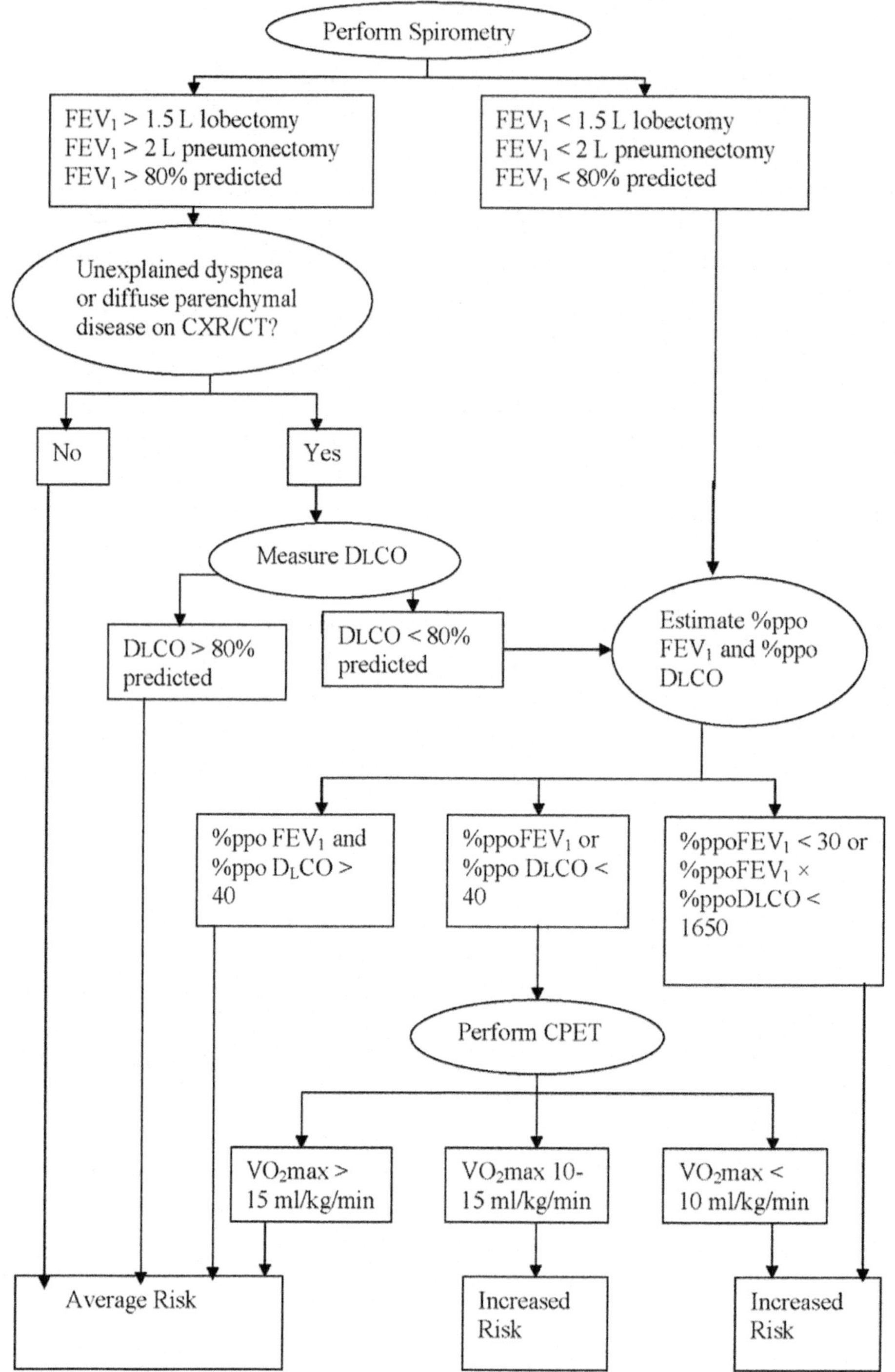

of the major risk predictors include unstable coronary syndromes, decompensated congestive cardiac failure, severe valvular disease and significant arrhythmias. Mild angina, compensated heart failure and previous myocardial infarction are all considered intermediate predictors. Findings such as abnormal electrocardiogram, history of stroke, uncontrolled hypertension, etc., are minor risk factors.

If cardiac surgery is needed, it may be possible to perform lung resection at the same time.

Incisions and Their Significance

Thoracotomy: It is the operative approach associated with highest risk for pulmonary complications. A thoracotomy incision results in a precipitous drop in ventilatory parameters post operatively on day 1. Recovery can take between 2 weeks to 3 months. Although thoracoscopic operations affect the pulmonary function to a lesser degree in the first post-operative week, the long-term outcomes of both approaches are similar.

Sternotomy: The post-operative chest wall mechanics alter to result in a restrictive ventilatory defect. This is attributed to structural alterations and decreased blood flow to intercostal muscles.

Upper abdominal laparotomy: Open upper abdominal incisions affect the functions of the diaphragm and lungs. FRC is reduced by 30%. The cause for the diaphragmatic and ventilatory dysfunction has been attributed to inhibition of phrenic nerve output in some studies. (Dureuil, Vires, Cantineau, Aubier, & Desmonts, 1986)

GENERAL POST-OPERATIVE CARE

Post-operative monitoring in an intensive care unit or step-down unit is warranted for patients with significant cardiac or respiratory comorbidities and/or after major pulmonary or esophageal resection.

Pulmonary Care

Pulmonary care of these patients involves an aggressive approach towards early extubation. Most patients will require some supplemental oxygen in the immediate post-operative period. The most common complication after thoracic surgery is pulmonary complications like atelectasis and pneumonia. Pulmonary toilet measures including chest physiotherapy, the appropriate use of incentive spirometry, chest percussion and vibration, postural drainage and early ambulation should be implemented as soon after surgery as possible. If the patient cannot clear his or her own secretions for some reason, a bronchoscopy and lavage should be performed.

An immediate post-operative chest x-ray is obtained to confirm position of lines and tubes and to visualize adequate lung expansion.

Pain Control

Effective analgesia is extremely important to help with pulmonary toilet, to reduce risk of myocardial ischemia by decreasing sympathetic stimulation, to encourage mobility and decrease risk of venous thromboembolism. Thoracic epidural analgesia is one of the more commonly used means of pain control and it has been shown to decrease post-operative pulmonary complications (Licker et al., 2002,

Pennefather & Russell, 2004) . The side effect of blockade of the thoracic and cervical sympathetic nerves is hypotension and bradycardia, and this is more pronounced in the presence of hypovolemia. If the catheter is inadvertently placed in the subarachnoid space, it could result in a "total spinal" with profound hypotension, apnea, and loss of consciousness.

Other methods include paravertebral analgesia, extra-pleural analgesia, intercostal nerve block, intravenous patient-controlled analgesia

Fluid Management

The incidence of post operative pulmonary edema after thoracic surgery is in the range of 12-15% (Jordan, Mitchell, Quinlan, Goldstraw, & Evans, 2000). It is extremely important to maintain a restrictive approach towards post operative fluids after lung surgery. Crystalloid maintainance with target urine output of 0.5-1 ml/kg/hr is usually sufficient. Pulmonary, thymic, or benign esophageal surgery is not associated with large postoperative fluid shifts. The factors contributing to pulmonary edema after lung surgery include lung manipulation and single lung ventilation which could impair alveolar-capillary membrane permeability lymphatic drainage.Excessive fluids can also result in decreased alveolar gas permeability, decreased pulmonary compliance, atelectasis, and hypoxia.

The fluid restriction after a pneumonectomy or lung volume reduction surgery is even more critical . Fluid administered with medications, creatinine level, nephrotoxic medications such as NSAIDs are all to be closely monitored.

Postoperative acute lung injury (ALI) occurs in about 7% of patients after a pulmonary resection and can be primary (within 3 days of surgery) or secondary (more than 3 days after surgery) where it is because of another cause such as pneumonia or aspiration . There is evidence to show that increased perioperative fluid administration increases the incidence of ALI (Alam et al., 2007).

Chest Tube Management

A patient that has had a thoracic surgery will post-operatively usually have one to three chest tubes depending on the procedure. These are connected to an underwater seal which is connected to low pressure suction. After a pneumonectomy, however, there is either no drain or a drain left to water seal alone with no suction. Suctioning a pneumonectomy space will cause mediastinal shift to the operative side resulting in cardiovascular compromise. Chest tubes are removed when there is minimal output and no air leak. Daily chest x-rays should be obtained for the duration that the tubes are present.

If postoperatively the patient has a massive air leak or worsening subcutaneous emphysema, the tubes should be checked to make sure they are not clogged. The tubes are placed to a higher negative suction. Sometimes, an additional tube may be necessary to drain the chest cavity adequately.

Cardiac Care

Arrhythmias: Atrial fibrillation and supraventricular tachycardia are the most common cardiac arrhythmias. The incidence of AF after pulmonary and esophageal resection is 12-14% (Roselli et al., 2005; Irshad et al., 2002) and >50% of patients will have a transient arrhythmia. The recommendations for AF prophylaxis after general thoracic surgical procedures as per the Society of Thoracic Surgeons and American Association for Thoracic Surgery guidelines (Frendl et al., 2014; Fernando et al., 2011) are:

- Beta blockers are continued in those pts taking them pre operatively
- In intermediate and high risk patients not taking beta blockers, diltiazem prophylaxis should be considered

The management of hemodynamically stable post-operative atrial fibrillation is summarized below in Figure 2.

Myocardial infarction: The incidence of MI in patients undergoing non cardiac surgery is about 5%. Only about 14% of these patients actually complain of chest pain (Devereaux et al., 2005). Beta-blockers, in these patients, decrease myocardial oxygen requirement by decreasing the heart rate. Post-operative pain and fever can contribute significantly to increased oxygen demand and it is important to have adequate pain control. intravascular Volume status of the postoperative patient must be maintained, because increased filling pressures can cause increased oxygen demand and lead to increased catecholamine levels . In general the indications for coronary angiography are similar to those in the nonoperative setting.

Nutrition

Enteral feeding is the best form of nutrition and oral diet can be initiated as early as 12 hours after most general thoracic procedures. The patient should be hemodynamically stable, have no nausea and there should be no risk of aspiration. After esophageal resection and anastomosis, a swallow study is mandated prior to enteral feeding.

For patients that have had prolonged fasting or have baseline nutritional deficiencies and cannot resume oral diet soon after surgery, nutritional support with alternate means of enteral or parenteral nutrition should be considered.

Neurological Issues

Delerium: Postoperative delerium is associated with a higher morbidity and mortality rate after thoracic surgery. Non cardiac thoracic surgery is a risk factor in itself for the development of postoperative delerium. Other independent predictors include age greater than 70 years, alcohol abuse, poor cognitive status, poor functional status, and markedly abnormal preoperative serum sodium, potassium, or glucose levels (Marcantonio et al., 1994; Yıldızeli et al., 2005).

PROCEDURES REQUIRING ICU CARE

Pneumonectomy

Most common indication is for a lung cancer that cannot be removed by a lesser resection. A right pneumonectomy is associated with higher morbidity and mortality as it results in more physiological alterations

Key Surgical Steps

The most common incision is a posterolateral thoracotomy although occasionally a median sternotomy can be used by some surgeons. Dissection of the hilum involves identifying the pulmonary artery and

Figure 2. 2014 AATS guidelines for the prevention and management of perioperative atrial fibrillation and flutter for thoracic surgical procedures

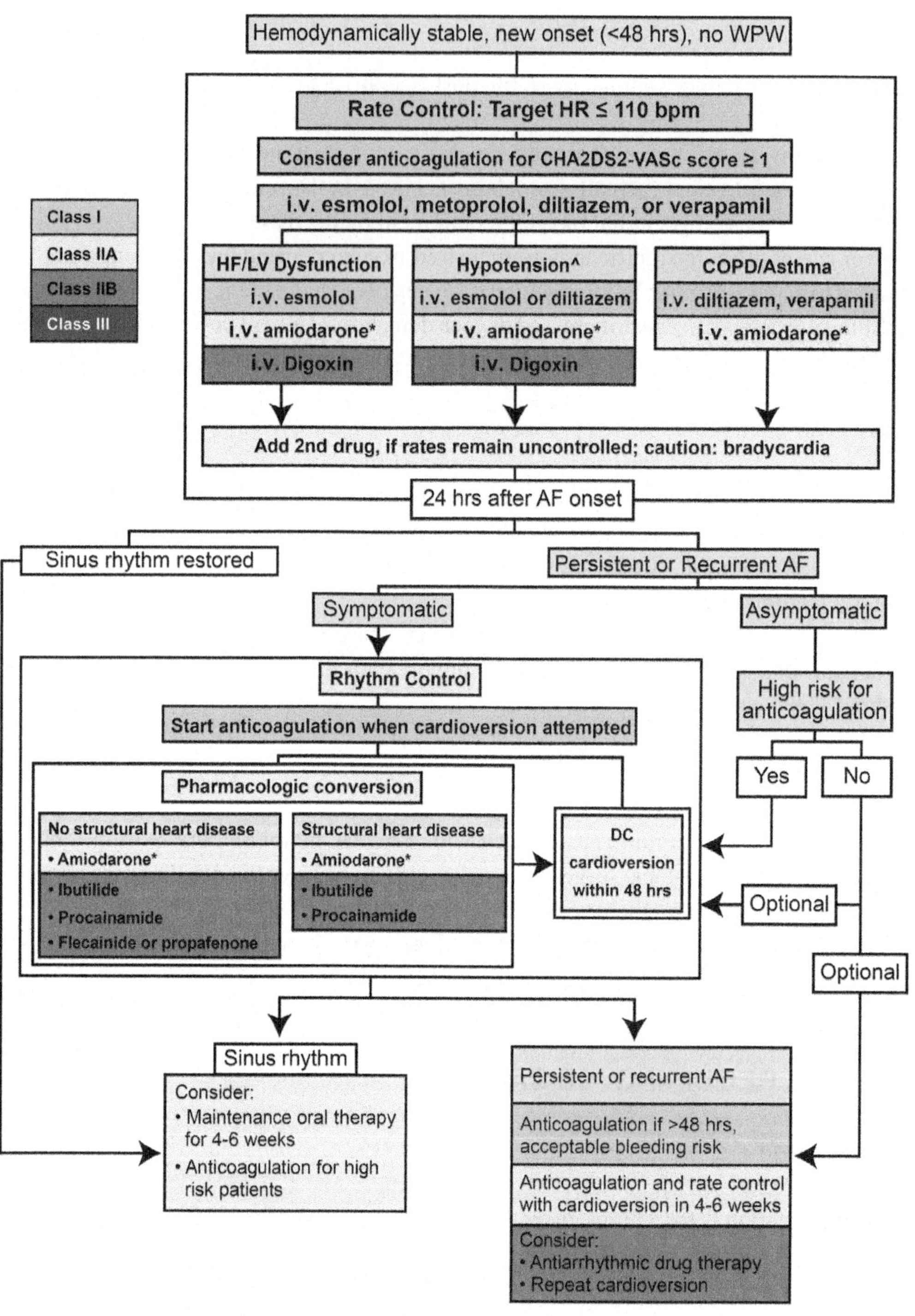

*Caution should be exercised and a TEE considered if amiodarone is used after 48 hours after the onset of AF, as there is a possibility that the rhythm could convert with risk of thromboembolism.

^Esmolol or diltiazem first line depending on degree of hypotension pulmonary veins to assess resectability followed by dissection of the bronchus. Once resectability is confirmed, the hilar structures are divided. Sometimes, intrapericardial dissection may be necessary to get a good margin. The division of the bronchus is done as proximal to the origin as possible to avoid a long stump. . A large pericardial defect may need to be patched to prevent cardiac herniation The bronchial stump may be patched with neighboring vascularized tissue such as pleura, pericardium, pericardial fat or an intercostal bundle.

Drainage of Post Pneumonectomy Space

Several options exist to drain the post pneumonectomy space and prevent mediastinal shift. There are commercially available 'balanced' mediastinal drainage systems. A regular 28-Fr chest tube or a drain can be left in for about 24 hours then removed. Absolutely no suction should be used on these tubes. An intrapleural catheter with a 3-way stop cock can be used to evacuate or insert air as needed based on post-operative chest x-rays and mediastinal position. Some surgeons may not even leave a chest drain. They aspirate the cavity soon after the surgery and close the chest. A postoperative chest X-ray is extremely important in making sure that there is no significant mediastinal shift.

Post-Operative Management

Patients need to be closely monitored for the first 24-48 hours. Antibiotic prophylaxis is per guidelines for clean surgical cases. There is no need for prolonged antibiotic coverage. Strict fluid restriction to no more than 1000ml/day should be adhered to. Patients are kept NPO the day of surgery and allowed to eat and ambulate the following day if there are no critical issues and no aspiration risk.

The rate of atrial arrhythmias after pneumonectomy is as high as 20%. Risk factors are age greater than 65 years, right pneumonectomy, male gender, clamshell incision, intrapericardial pneumonectomy, preexisting coronary artery disease, and hypertension. (Foroulis et al., 2003; Roselli et al., 2005). As previously discussed, although there is some evidence to state that pharmacological prophylaxis does help decrease the rate of atrial fibrillation, it hasn't been widely practiced. Most surgeons avoid amiodarone for fear of the associated pulmonary toxicity

Respiratory care involves adequate pain management as with any other major pulmonary resection, incentive spirometry, and chest physiotherapy. Bedside bronchoscopy should be used to assist with pulmonary toilet if the patient is not optimally clearing tracheobronchial secretions.

Daily chest x-rays are obtained to assess gradual filling of the post pneumonectomy space with fluid. An early white out of the hemithorax should alert the clinician to the possibility of bleeding. A sudden drop in the air-fluid level is suggestive of a bronchopleural fistula and should be appropriately evaluated by flexible bronchoscopy by the surgeon.

Venous thromboembolism prophylaxis is as per established guidelines for surgical patients. Venous thromboembolism can complicate upto 7% of pneumonectomy cases. The origin for a pulmonary embolus after a pneumonectomy is usually the lower extremities, but, rarely can be the pulmonary artery stump itself, specially in a right pneumonectomy.

The other rare but potentially life- threatening complication post operatively is cardiac herniation. The heart can herniate through a pericardial defect into the empty pneumonectomy space. It is usually triggered by coughing or vomiting and symptoms include sudden hypotension, cyanosis, superior vena cava syndrome and chest pain. A chest X-ray can aid in diagnosis. The treatment is immediate return to the operating room to reposition the heart repair the defect

Esophagectomy

Controversy exists regarding the management of esophageal cancer based on stage and cell type. Esophageal resection when performed is usually as a part of combined modality treatment with chemotherapy and radiation and is intended to be curative.

Esophagectomy as the first line of treatment is appropriate for patients with a T1 or clinical T2 lesion (in some centers) with no nodal or distant metastasis. Neoadjuvant chemoradiation followed by surgical resection is the choice in patients with thoracic or esophagogastric junction tumors and full-thickness (T3) involvement of the esophagus with/without nodal disease and in selected patients with T4 disease where en bloc resection is considered possible. Metastasis to a distant site or other solid organs makes the patient unresectable (Hirst, Smithers, Gotley, Thomas, & Barbour, 2011; Miyata et al., 2011; Van Hagen et al., 2012).

In this section we will discuss the most common surgical approaches to performing an esophagectomy, general post-operative care and care specific, if any to the different approaches. The extent of lymph node dissection and the nature of associated complications varies with these approaches and is another area of constant debate in the management of esophageal cancer.

Technical Aspects

Transhiatal esophagectomy: This approach, popularized by Orringer, involves an upper midline laparotomy and a cervical incision. Gastric mobilization and a pyloric drainage procedure followed by blunt lower esophageal mobilization through the esophageal hiatus is performed through the laparotomy. The cervical incision is used to complete the upper portion of the esophageal mobilization and resection. A cervical esophagogastric anastomosis is then performed. The advantages of this approach include a lower incidence of pulmonary complications, an ability to achieve good vertical resection margins. However there is limited peri-esophageal and perigastric lymph node clearance. The anastomotic leak rate has been quoted from 7-15% (Hulscher et al., 2002).

Transthoracic esophagectomy: The most common transthoracic approach is the Ivor-Lewis esophagectomy which involves an upper midline laparotomy and a right thoracotomy with an intrathoracic anastomosis. A left thoracoabdominal incision can be used for tumors in the gastroesophageal junction or lower third of the esophagus. The extent of lymph node dissection via this approach will include a more complete mediastinal dissection with clearance of peri-esophageal, perigastric and cardial nodes. Some studies quote a higher pulmonary complication rate with transthoracic esophagectomy but a more recent prospective cohort study comparing TTE to THE found similar rates of pulmonary complications in both groups (Avendano, Flume, Silvestri, King, & Reed, 2002; Connors, Reuben, Neumayer, & Bull, 2007). The anastomotic leak rate and local recurrence rate is much lower.

The 3 incision esophagogastrectomy, also known as the McKeown esophagogastrectomy, involves a right thoracotomy for thoracic esophageal immobilization, laparotomy for abdominal exploration and gastric mobilization and a left cervical incision for anastomosis. This approach gives the oncological benefits similar to Ivor-Lewis procedure together with a neck anastomosis which is easier to manage in the event of a leak.

Minimally invasive techniques: A combination of laparoscopy and thoracoscopy or laparotomy and thoracoscopy have been used for mobilization and dissection. The robotic technique can be performed during the thoracic dissection of the esophagus, gastric mobilization, and intrathoracic anastomosis. It can also be performed in combination with laparoscopic, hand-assisted laparoscopic, or thoracoscopic approaches.

Conduits: A tubularized gastric conduit is most commonly used as the esophageal substitute post resection. The gastric conduit is based off the right gastroepiploic artery and the right gastric artery is also preserved in most cases. The next most common option is a colonic interposition where an iso-peristalitic long segment of colon based on a reliable vascular pedicle is used to replace the resected esophagus . The colon is used when the stomach is not available or, when gastrointestinal continuity has to be re-established via an extrathoracic or substernal route. Sometimes a jejunal interposition or a jejunal free flap may need to be utilized.

Overall morbidity of an esophagectomy is in the range of 30-50%.

Post Operative Care

These patients are usually monitored in an intensive care or step down unit for the first 24-48 hours. Although traditionally, patients after an esophagectomy were kept intubated overnight as a standard protocol, several studies have proved that early extubation i.e. immediately post operatively to less than 12 hours after, is safe and associated with shorter ICU length of stay (Lanuti et al., 2006; Yap, Chan, & Joynt, 2000). Some patients may require ventilatory support for a few hours postoperatively if the surgery is prolonged with significant fluid shifts and technical difficulties. But otherwise, every attempt should be made to extubate the patient as soon as tolerated.

Reintubation if needed should be done preferably with glidescope or bronchoscopic assistance, especially if there is a cervical anastomosis to avoid inadvertently disrupting the fresh anastomosis.

A nasogastric or nasojejunal tube that goes across the anastomosis is usually secured in place after its position has been confirmed by direct visualization and palpation intraoperatively. Hence, if these are unintentionally removed, the surgical team should be made aware immediately and replacement if deemed necessary at the time should be done preferably with fluoroscopy. If the surgical approach involved a thoracotomy or thoracoscopy, the patient will have one or two chest tubes. These can be to underwaterseal drains and not necessarily to suction. The tubes usually are left in until oral diet is initiated to detect any chyle leaks or anastomotic leaks where there is an intrathoracic anastomosis.

A chest radiograph is obtained on arrival to the ICU to confirm position of tubes and lines.

An esophagectomy is associated with significant third space fluid losses. Fluid resuscitation should be liberal enough to maintain intravascular volume status and adequate perfusion to the anastomosis. Maintainance fluids at the rate of 100-150cc / hr of crystalloid is usually adequate.

Adequate pain relief preferably via thoracic epidural analgesia is recommended to minimize cardiopulmonary complications.

Bear in mind to avoid the neck on the side of the anastomosis for intravenous access.

A contrast study to evaluate the integrity of the anastomosis is performed on postoperative day 5-7. Presence of aspiration and adequacy of gastric emptying is also examined at this time and oral diet is initiated if there is no leak or aspiration. Patients with esophageal cancer tend to be malnourished. The options for nutritional supplementation while awaiting the swallow study in a patient with severe nutritional deficiencies preoperatively, include parenteral nutrition with TPN or enteral nutrition. Enteral nutrition can be instituted as early as day 1 via a jejunal feeding tube if one has been placed during surgery or feeding can be delayed until the contrast study . Early enteral nutrition has been associated with a reduced rate of life threatening complications (Fujita, Daiko, & Nishimura, 2012) .It has also been shown, however, that routine placement of feeding jejunostomy tubes is not indicated (Fenton, Bergeron, Coello, Welsh, & Chmielewski, 2011).

Complications

The most feared complication is an anastomotic leak. It is important to have a high index of suspicion for a leak in a patient who is not following the anticipated path to recovery. Presentaton may range from tachycardia and other signs of a systemic inflammatory response syndrome in the early stages to fulminant sepsis and septic shock if not detected in a timely fashion. Other signs include change in the quantity and quality of chest tube drainage, subcutaneous emphysema, drainage from the neck wound in case of a cervical anastomosis, multiple organ failure etc.

Diagnosis is confirmed with an esophogram . A CT scan of the chest can add to the information to make a decision on whether the chest tubes are adequately draining the leak or if there is a need to re-open the chest for control of sepsis. In case of a cervical anastomosis, the neck wound is opened up to facilitate drainage . A more extensive procedure may be required though depending on the extent of tracking through the fascial planes. The mortality rate from an intrathoracic anastomosis can be as high as 35-40% (Alanezi & Urschel, 2004).

As with any other major pulmonary or upper gastrointestinal surgery, respiratory failure from atelectasis pneumonia, ARDS can occur.

Other significant complications include aspiration from recurrent laryngeal nerve palsy, chylothorax,and esophageal conduit necrosis. Gastric conduits have the lowest incidence of necrosis. Symptoms include unexplained tachycardia, leukocytosis, respiratory failure, or evidence of a leak. A contrast esophagography or endoscopy can diagnose conduit ischemia necrosis. Management involves conduit takedown with proximal esophageal diversion and feeding tube placement (Wormuth & Heitmiller 2006).

Mediastinal Tumors/Thymectomy for Myasthenia Gravis

Indications for Thymectomy with Myasthenia

Thymectomy in myasthenia is believed to be beneficial in patients that have a thymoma or thymic hyperplasia and for those that have generalized myasthenia and acetylcholine receptor antibodies. There are no randomized controlled trials proving the effectiveness of a thymectomy in a patient with MG without a thymoma. However, available evidence does suggest benefit in these patients and it has been shown that surgical treatment was two times more likely to result in medication- free remission (Gronseth & Barohn, 2000).

Preoperative Preparation

It is best to get the patient as medically optimized as possible prior to the surgery. Usually the anticholinesterase agents are continued into the time of surgery but it must be attempted to taper and wean off the steroids prior to surgery to help minimize post operative complications including wound healing.

Patients with generalized symptoms or respiratory or bulbar symptoms may need plasmapheresis prior to surgery (Nagayasu et al., 2005).

Technical Aspects

The operative approaches used for a thymectomy are:

- Transsternal – This approach is the preferred approach for patients with a known thymoma and MG. It allows for a full exploration and complete removal of all thymic tissue and fat.
- Trancervical – A simple transcervical incision is usually not adequate to completely clear all thymic tissue. An extended cervical thymectomy involving a manubrial retractor to help visualize and remove all mediastinal thymic tissue and fat may be a better approach.
- Combined transcervical and transsternal – A cervical incision with a partial median sternotomy gives good exposure to the anterior mediastinum.
- Minimally invasive (videoscopic, robot-assisted)

The aim of the surgery is to resect all thymic tissue including both inferior and superior horns and all associated fat without injuring the phrenic nerves, left vagus and recurrent nerves and the innominate vessels.

Postoperative Considerations

Majority of patients are extubated in the operating room soon after surgery. Most institutions follow an anesthetic protocol where neuromuscular blocking agents are avoided and only inhalational anesthetics are used with a very small dose of non-depolarizing agent.

There are several preoperative factors that are associated with post operative worsening of myasthenic symtpoms and the need for prolonged mechanical ventilation (Loach, Young, Spalding, & Smith, 1975; Gracey, Divertie, Howard, & Payne, 1984; Younger, Braun, Jaretzki, Penn, & Lovelace, 1984; Watanabe et al., 2004). These include,

- Pre operative expiratory weakness
- Preoperative vital capacity < 2.0L
- Preoperative bulbar symptoms
- History of preoperative myasthenic crisis
- Preoperative acetylcholine receptor antibody serum level of greater than 100nmol/L
- Intraoperative blood loss greater than 1000ml

The patient is closely monitored in a critical care unit postoperatively with a multidisciplinary team weighing in on various aspects of care. Inspiratory-expiratory pressures and vital capacity are measured every 6 hrs. Perioperative steroids and plasmapheresis may need to be used to help control symptoms. Cholinergics do not help control acute symtpoms.

Tracheal Resection and Reconstruction

Tracheal surgery involving resection and reconstruction may be required for both benign and malignant conditions such as tracheal stenosis both idiopathic and post-intubation, and primary tracheal tumors.

Technical Aspects

Surgical approaches: Lesions in the upper half of the trachea and benign lesions are approached via a cervical or cervicomediastinal incision with a sternal split as needed. Neoplastic lesions of the lower half of the trachea will need a right posterolateral thoracotomy in a higher space. If a postoperative tracheostomy is planned, the incision is made away from the potential tracheostomy site.

Key Steps

It must be attempted to wean the patient off steroids preoperatively. Once the involved portion of the trachea is exposed with a collar incision, it is circumferentially mobilized taking care not to disrupt the lateral blood supply. Distal resection is performed first so that a sterile endotracheal tube can then be passed into the distal airway and the patient can be ventilated for the rest of the case as shown in *Figure 3*. After resection of the desired length, a tension-free anastomosis is created using absorbable interrupted sutures. There are various tracheal release techniques that add extra length for a tension free repair. A pedicled muscle flap is made to protect the anastomosis and buttress it from the neighboring structures (innominate, esophagus etc.)

A chin stich is placed at the end of the procedure to remind the patient to keep the neck flexed to avoid tension on the anastomosis.

Postoperative Care

Every attempt should be made to extubate the patient in the operating room. A flexible bronchoscopy pre-extubation helps assess the anastomosis and clear secretions. It may also be required post operatively to assist with pulmonary toilet.

Measures to prevent laryngeal edema include racemic epinephrine, judicious use of intravenous fluids, head of bed elevation, minimizing talking and maintaining the neck in flexion. Some surgeons use steroids to control the edema but it is not mandated.

On day 7, flexible bronchoscopy is performed with topical anesthesia in the operating room to assess the anastomosis and if satisfactory, the chin stich is removed

Figure 3. Technique of tracheal resection (Reproduced with permission from Pearson's Thoracic and Esophageal Surgery, Third Edition, Elsevier, 2008)

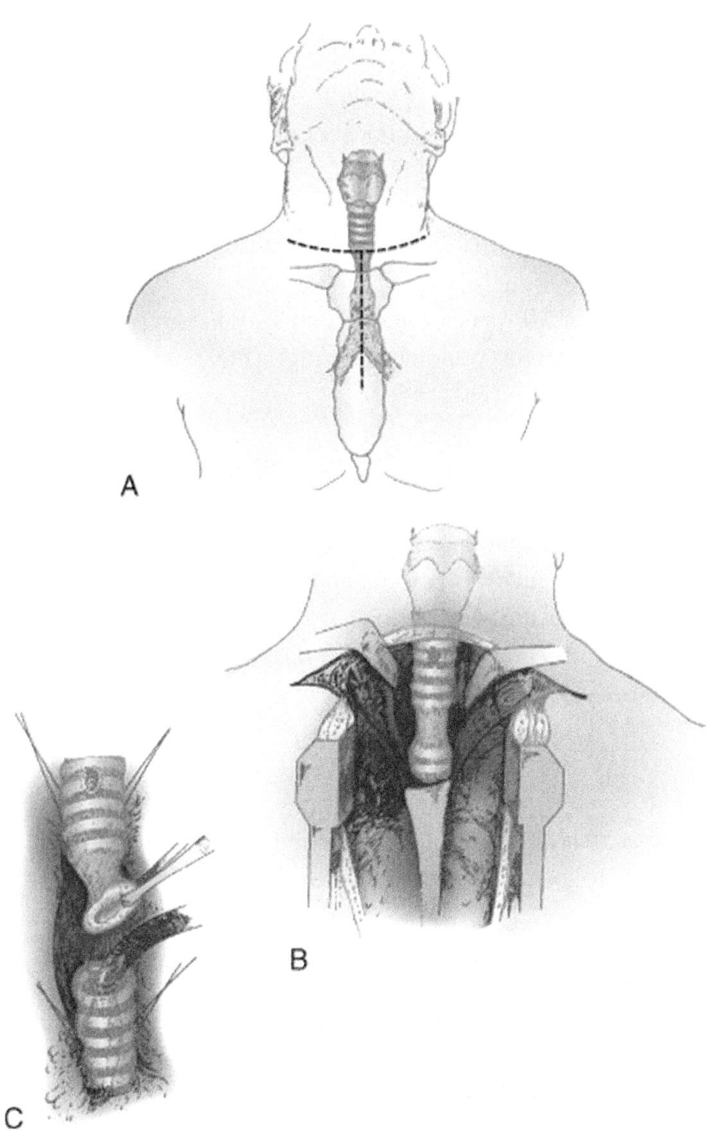

Complications

The most worrisome complication after a tracheal resection/ reconstruction is anastomotic dehiscence. Predictors of anastomotic complications include

- Diabetes
- Long resections (>4cm)
- Laryngotracheal resection

- Age <17yrs
- Need for pre-operative tracheostomy
- Steroid use

Other complications specific to this surgery include granulation tissue, laryngeal dysfunction, hemorrhage, edema tracheoinnominate fistula and tracheoesophageal fistula (Grillo, Donahue, Mathisen, Wain, & Wright, 1995)

Surgical Management of Malignant Pleural Mesothelioma

The role of definitive surgery in MPM is a topic of debate. The surgical options include extrapleural pneumonectomy (EPP) and pleurectomy and decortication (P/D)

Technical Aspects

Extrapleural pneumonectomy involves en-bloc resection of the parietal and visceral pleura with the ipsilateral lung, pericardium and diaphragm.

Pleurectomy and decortication involves parietal and visceral pleurectomy to remove all gross tumor with or without diaphragm or pericardial resection.

There are no randomized trials comparing EPP vs. P/D. However several retrospective analyses have suggested similar outcomes. (Flores et al., 2008)

Post-Operative Care

Care after EPP is similar to that of a patient after a standard pneumonectomy. In addition, particular attention must be paid to the following in patients undergoing EPP or P/D:

- Careful fluid management with a more restrictive strategy
- Transfusion may need to be initiated intraoperatively as guided by blood loss to prevent post-operative hypotension
- Massive fluid shifts and intravascular equilibration may cause the patient to become hypotensive in the first 24-48 hours. Blood transfusion and low-dose vasopressors may be needed to support the patient.
- Arrhythmia prophylaxis
- P/D patients can have prolonged air leaks. Chest tube management may involve leaving the tube to underwater seal drainage for prolonged periods and sometimes even discharge with a Heimlich valve.

CONCLUSION

The above mentioned procedures are the most common operations requiring an intensive care unit for immediate post-operative monitoring and management. The list however is not exhaustive. Even a 'minor' thoracic surgical procedure such as a lung biopsy or a wedge resection in a patient with poor cardiopulmonary reserve can warrant critical care management. It is thus important for the intensivist taking care of these patients in the ICU to have a general sense of what the different operations entail including the post-operative care and complications specific to each of them.

REFERENCES

Alam, N., Park, B., Wilton, A., Seshan, V., Bains, M., Downey, R., & Amar, D. et al. (2007). Incidence and Risk Factors for Lung Injury After Lung Cancer Resection. *The Annals of Thoracic Surgery*, *84*(4), 1085–1091. doi:10.1016/j.athoracsur.2007.05.053 PMID:17888952

Alanezi, K., & Urschel, J. (2004). Mortality secondary to esophageal anastomotic leak. *Annals of Thoracic and Cardiovascular Surgery*, *10*(2). PMID:15209546

Alexander, J., Hamilton, W., Parikh, R., Spence, A., & Stewart, B. (1972). Further studies on the role of airways closure in postoperative hypoxaemia. *British Journal of Anaesthesia*, *44*(8), 905–906. PMID:5083032

Avendano, C., Flume, P., Silvestri, G., King, L., & Reed, C. (2002). Pulmonary complications after esophagectomy. *The Annals of Thoracic Surgery*, *73*(3), 922–926. doi:10.1016/S0003-4975(01)03584-6 PMID:11899202

Benzo, R., Kelley, G., Recchi, L., Hofman, A., & Sciurba, F. (2007). Complications of lung resection and exercise capacity: A meta-analysis. *Respiratory Medicine*, *101*(8), 1790–1797. doi:10.1016/j.rmed.2007.02.012 PMID:17408941

Bolliger, C., Jordan, P., Solèr, M., Stulz, P., Grädel, E., Skarvan, K., & Tamm, M. et al. (1995). Exercise capacity as a predictor of postoperative complications in lung resection candidates. *American Journal of Respiratory and Critical Care Medicine*, *151*(5), 1472–1480. doi:10.1164/ajrccm.151.5.7735602 PMID:7735602

Brunelli, A., Kim, A., Berger, K., & Addrizzo-Harris, D. (2013). Physiologic evaluation of the patient with lung cancer being considered for resectional surgery: Diagnosis and management of lung cancer, 3rd ed: American College of Chest Physicians evidence-based clinical practice guidelines. Chest, 143(5 Suppl), E166S-90S.

Connors, R., Reuben, B., Neumayer, L., & Bull, D. (2007). Comparing Outcomes after Transthoracic and Transhiatal Esophagectomy: A 5-Year Prospective Cohort of 17,395 Patients. *Journal of the American College of Surgeons*, *205*(6), 735–740. doi:10.1016/j.jamcollsurg.2007.07.001 PMID:18035255

Dales, R., Dionne, G., Leech, J., Lunau, M., & Schweitzer, I. (1993). Preoperative prediction of pulmonary complications following thoracic surgery. *Chest*, *104*(1), 155–159. doi:10.1378/chest.104.1.155 PMID:8325061

Devereaux, P., Goldman, L., Yusuf, S., Gilbert, K., Leslie, K., & Guyatt, G. (2005). Surveillance and prevention of major perioperative ischemic cardiac events in patients undergoing noncardiac surgery: A review. *Canadian Medical Association Journal*, *173*(7), 779–788. doi:10.1503/cmaj.050316 PMID:16186585

Dureuil, B., Vires, N., Cantineau, J., Aubier, M., & Desmonts, J. (1986). Diaphragmatic contractility after upper abdominal surgery. *Journal of Applied Physiology*, *61*(5), 1775–1780. PMID:3781987

Fenton, J., Bergeron, E., Coello, M., Welsh, R., & Chmielewski, G. (2011). Feeding Jejunostomy Tubes Placed During Esophagectomy: Are They Necessary? *The Annals of Thoracic Surgery*, *92*(2), 504–512. doi:10.1016/j.athoracsur.2011.03.101 PMID:21704294

Fernando, H., Jaklitsch, M., Walsh, G., Tisdale, J., Bridges, C., Mitchell, J., & Shrager, J. (2011). The Society of Thoracic Surgeons Practice Guideline on the Prophylaxis and Management of Atrial Fibrillation Associated With General Thoracic Surgery: Executive Summary. *The Annals of Thoracic Surgery*, *92*(3), 1144–1152. doi:10.1016/j.athoracsur.2011.06.104 PMID:21871327

Flores, R., Pass, H., Seshan, V., Dycoco, J., Zakowski, M., Carbone, M., ... Rusch, V. (2008). Extrapleural pneumonectomy versus pleurectomy/decortication in the surgical management of malignant pleural mesothelioma: Results in 663 patients. *The Journal of Thoracic and Cardiovascular Surgery, 135*(3), 620-626, 626.e1-3.

Foroulis, C., Kotoulas, C., Lachanas, H., Lazopoulos, G., Konstantinou, M., & Lioulias, A. (2003). Factors associated with cardiac rhythm disturbances in the early post-pneumonectomy period: A study on 259 pneumonectomies. *European Journal of Cardio-Thoracic Surgery*, *23*(3), 384–389. doi:10.1016/s1010-7940(02)00797-2 PMID:12614811

Frendl, G., Sodickson, A., Chung, M., Waldo, A., Gersh, B., Tisdale, J., & Adler, D. et al. (2014). 2014 AATS guidelines for the prevention and management of perioperative atrial fibrillation and flutter for thoracic surgical procedures. *The Journal of Thoracic and Cardiovascular Surgery*, *148*(3), E153–E193. doi:10.1016/j.jtcvs.2014.06.036 PMID:25129609

Fujita, T., Daiko, H., & Nishimura, M. (2012). Early Enteral Nutrition Reduces the Rate of Life-Threatening Complications after Thoracic Esophagectomy in Patients with Esophageal Cancer. *European Surgical Research*, *48*(2), 79–84. doi:10.1159/000336574 PMID:22377820

Gracey, D., Divertie, M., Howard, F., & Payne, W. (1984). Postoperative respiratory care after transsternal thymectomy in myasthenia gravis. A 3-year experience in 53 patients. *Chest*, *86*(1), 67–71. doi:10.1378/chest.86.1.67 PMID:6734295

Grillo, H., Donahue, D., Mathisen, D., Wain, J., & Wright, C. (1995). Postintubation tracheal stenosis. Treatment and results. *The Journal of Thoracic and Cardiovascular Surgery*, *109*(3), 486–492. doi:10.1016/S0022-5223(95)70279-2 PMID:7877309

Gronseth, G., & Barohn, R. (2000). Practice parameter: thymectomy for autoimmune myasthenia gravis (an evidence-based review): report of the Quality Standards Subcommittee of the American Academy of Neurology. *Neurology*, *55*(1), 7–15. doi:10.1212/WNL.55.1.7 PMID:10891896

Harpole, D. Jr, Decamp, M. Jr, Daley, J., Hur, K., Oprian, C., Henderson, W., & Khuri, S. (1999). Prognostic models of thirty-day mortality and morbidity after major pulmonary resection. *The Journal of Thoracic and Cardiovascular Surgery*, *117*(5), 969–979. doi:10.1016/S0022-5223(99)70378-8 PMID:10220692

Hirst, J., Smithers, B., Gotley, D., Thomas, J., & Barbour, A. (2011). Defining Cure for Esophageal Cancer: Analysis of Actual 5-Year Survivors Following Esophagectomy. *Annals of Surgical Oncology*, *18*(6), 1766–1774. doi:10.1245/s10434-010-1508-z PMID:21213056

Hulscher, J., Sandick, J., Boer, A., Wijnhoven, B., Tijssen, J., Fockens, P., & Lanschot, J. et al. (2002). Extended Transthoracic Resection Compared with Limited Transhiatal Resection for Adenocarcinoma of the Esophagus. *The New England Journal of Medicine*, *347*(21), 1662–1669. doi:10.1056/NEJMoa022343 PMID:12444180

Irshad, K., Feldman, L., Chu, V., Dorval, J., Baslaim, G., & Morin, J. (2002). Causes of increased length of hospitalization on a general thoracic surgery service: A prospective observational study. *Canadian Journal of Surgery*, *45*(4), 264–268. PMID:12174980

Jordan, S., Mitchell, J., Quinlan, G., Goldstraw, P., & Evans, T. (2000). The pathogenesis of lung injury following pulmonary resection. *The European Respiratory Journal*, *15*(4), 790–799. doi:10.1034/j.1399-3003.2000.15d26.x PMID:10780775

Kohman, L., Meyer, J., Ikins, P., & Oates, R. (1986). Random versus predictable risks of mortality after thoracotomy for lung cancer. *The Journal of Thoracic and Cardiovascular Surgery*, *91*(4). PMID:3959574

Lanuti, M., Delva, P., Maher, A., Wright, C., Gaissert, H., Wain, J., & Mathisen, D. et al. (2006). Feasibility and Outcomes of an Early Extubation Policy After Esophagectomy. *The Annals of Thoracic Surgery*, *82*(6), 2037–2041. doi:10.1016/j.athoracsur.2006.07.024 PMID:17126107

Licker, M., Spiliopoulos, A., Frey, J., Robert, J., Hohn, L., De Perrot, M., & Tschopp, J. (2002). Risk Factors for Early Mortality and Major Complications Following Pneumonectomy for Non-small Cell Carcinoma of the Lung. *Chest*, *121*(6), 1890–1897. doi:10.1378/chest.121.6.1890 PMID:12065354

Loach, A., Young, A., Spalding, J., & Smith, A. (1975). Postoperative management after thymectomy. *British Medical Journal*, *1*(5953), 309–312. doi:10.1136/bmj.1.5953.309 PMID:1111793

Marcantonio, E., Goldman, L., Mangione, C., Ludwig, L., Muraca, B., Haslauer, C., & Lee, T. et al. (1994). A Clinical Prediction Rule for Delirium After Elective Noncardiac Surgery. *Journal of the American Medical Association*, *271*(2), 134–139. doi:10.1001/jama.1994.03510260066030 PMID:8264068

Miyata, H., Yamasaki, M., Kurokawa, Y., Takiguchi, S., Nakajima, K., Fujiwara, Y., & Doki, Y. et al. (2011). Multimodal treatment for resectable esophageal cancer. *General Thoracic and Cardiovascular Surgery*, *59*(7), 461–466. doi:10.1007/s11748-011-0780-6 PMID:21751104

Nagayasu, T., Yamayoshi, T., Matsumoto, K., Ide, N., Hashizume, S., Nomura, M., & Oka, T. et al. (2005). Beneficial effects of plasmapheresis before thymectomy on the outcome in myasthenia gravis. *Japanese Journal of Thoracic and Cardiovascular Surgery*, *53*(1), 2–7. doi:10.1007/s11748-005-1001-y PMID:15724495

Pate, P., Tenholder, M., Griffin, J., Eastridge, C., & Weiman, D. (1996). Preoperative assessment of the high-risk patient for lung resection. *The Annals of Thoracic Surgery*, *61*(5), 1494–1500. doi:10.1016/0003-4975(96)00087-2 PMID:8633965

Pennefather, S., & Russell, G. (2004). Postthoracotomy analgesia: Recent advances and future directions. In *Progress in Thoracic Anesthesia* (pp. 163–185). Baltimore: Lippincott Williams & Wilkins.

Roselli, E., Murthy, S., Rice, T., Houghtaling, P., Pierce, C., Karchmer, D., & Blackstone, E. (2005). Atrial fibrillation complicating lung cancer resection. *The Journal of Thoracic and Cardiovascular Surgery*, *130*(2), 438.e1–438.e9. doi:10.1016/j.jtcvs.2005.02.010 PMID:16077410

Roselli, E., Murthy, S., Rice, T., Houghtaling, P., Pierce, C., Karchmer, D., & Blackstone, E. (2005). Atrial fibrillation complicating lung cancer resection. *The Journal of Thoracic and Cardiovascular Surgery*, *130*(2), 438.e1–438.e9. doi:10.1016/j.jtcvs.2005.02.010 PMID:16077410

Schuurmans, M., Diacon, A., & Bolliger, C. (2002). Functional evaluation before lung resection. *Clinics in Chest Medicine*, *23*(1), 159–172. doi:10.1016/S0272-5231(03)00066-2 PMID:11901909

Van Hagen, P., Hulshof, M., Van Lanschot, J., Steyerberg, E., Van Berge Henegouwen, M., Wijnhoven, B., & Van der Gaast, A. (2012). Preoperative chemoradiotherapy for esophageal or junctional cancer. *The New England Journal of Medicine*, *366*(22), 2074–2084. doi:10.1056/NEJMoa1112088 PMID:22646630

Watanabe, A., Watanabe, T., Obama, T., Mawatari, T., Ohsawa, H., Ichimiya, Y., & Abe, T. et al. (2004). Prognostic factors for myasthenic crisis after transsternal thymectomy in patients with myasthenia gravis. *The Journal of Thoracic and Cardiovascular Surgery*, *127*(3), 868–876. doi:10.1016/j.jtcvs.2003.07.036 PMID:15001919

Win, T., Jackson, A., Sharples, L., Groves, A., Wells, F., Ritchie, A., & Laroche, C. (2005). Relationship between pulmonary function and lung cancer surgical outcome. *The European Respiratory Journal*, *25*(4), 594–599. doi:10.1183/09031936.05.00077504 PMID:15802330

Wormuth, J., & Heitmiller, R. (2006). Esophageal Conduit Necrosis. *Thoracic Surgery Clinics*, *16*(1), 11–22. doi:10.1016/j.thorsurg.2006.01.003 PMID:16696279

Yap, F., Chan, A., & Joynt, G. (2000). Timing of extubation after esophagectomy. *Critical Care (London, England)*, *4*(Suppl 1), 101–101. doi:10.1186/cc821

Yıldızeli, B., Özyurtkan, M., Batırel, H., Kuşcu, K., Bekiroğlu, N., & Yüksel, M. (2005). Factors Associated With Postoperative Delirium After Thoracic Surgery. *The Annals of Thoracic Surgery*, *79*(3), 1004–1009. doi:10.1016/j.athoracsur.2004.06.022 PMID:15734423

Younger, D., Braun, N., Jaretzki, A., Penn, A., & Lovelace, R. (1984). Myasthenia gravis: Determinants for independent ventilation after transsternal thymectomy. *Neurology*, *34*(3), 336–336. doi:10.1212/WNL.34.3.336 PMID:6538272

Section 6

Monitoring the Postoperative Cardiac Patient

Chapter 30
Physiologic Monitoring

James Osorio
New York Presbyterian Hospital, USA & Weill Cornell Medical College, USA

Christopher Tam
New York Presbyterian Hospital, USA & Weill Cornell Medical College, USA

ABSTRACT

This chapter will provide a review of modern concepts of cardiovascular monitoring with emphasis on essential hemodynamic variables in the early post cardiac surgery patient. When defining circulatory function, importance of the entire circulatory system is underscored. This includes the function and interaction of the heart, blood vessels and circulatory blood volume to deliver sufficient amount of oxygenated blood to tissue beds. In post cardiac surgery patients, the pulmonary artery catheter remains the most widely used technology to assess cardiac function. This chapter highlights the importance of validation of less invasive and noninvasive hemodynamic monitors for the management of critically ill patients and early post cardiac surgery patients. In addition, this chapter describes the evolution of monitoring of post cardiac surgery and critically ill patients, examines different monitoring technologies and address controversial questions in modern practice as well as future directions.

INTRODUCTION

Hemodynamic monitoring is fundamental to early post cardiac surgery care and patient recovery after cardiac surgery. Historically, the pulmonary artery catheter (PAC) has been the principal hemodynamic monitor for intraoperative and early post cardiac surgery patient management. In the last two decades, technological developments, in particular the development of less invasive and noninvasive methodologies for hemodynamic monitoring, contributed to the establishment of controversial opinions in this rapidly developing field. Although the PAC remains the most widely used technology for decision making in early post cardiac surgery monitoring, potential for complications and diagnostic limitations have laid the foundations for the development of other ways to monitor and care for early post cardiac surgery patients.

This chapter will review the exciting history of cardiac output monitoring. It will examine the established surrogates of organ and tissue perfusion monitored by the bedside physician in respect to available

DOI: 10.4018/978-1-4666-8603-8.ch030

published studies. This chapter will give a review of different methods and therefore relatively new monitors for cardiac output and hemodynamic monitoring with emphasis on method validation and associated clinical trials. This chapter will further attempt to address future directions in this rapidly growing field.

BACKGROUND

The success of a cardiac operation is determined by the events in the operating room and in the postoperative period. Hemodynamic monitoring of the early post cardiac surgery patient is of great importance during normal and complicated convalescence. Determination of adequate blood flow to meet metabolic demands is essential in the early post-cardiac surgery period.

Surrogates of Adequate Tissue Perfusion in the Postoperative Cardiac Surgery Patient

Monitoring post cardiac surgery patients includes: Continuous telemetry, invasive continuous blood pressure monitoring, monitoring of cardiac performance, laboratory and radiology assessment central laboratory and point-of care analysis, (e.g. blood gas analysis), temperature monitoring and close observation for postoperative blood loss.

In the early postoperative period it is essential to ensure adequate blood flow to meet organ and tissue metabolic demands.

Commonly used surrogates to assess adequate tissue perfusion are:

1. Arterial blood pressure
2. Urine output
3. Mental status
4. Cardiac output and cardiac index
5. Mixed venous oxygen saturation
6. Lactic Acid

Arterial Blood Pressure, Urine Output, and Mental Status

Arterial blood pressure, urine output and a mental status change can all provide information about organ and tissue perfusion. Arterial blood pressure is an insensitive measure of adequate blood flow and perfusion. Similarly, urine output and mental status change can be late signs of inadequate perfusion and cannot be used alone to guide resuscitation, titration of vasopressors and inotropes in the early post cardiac surgery period and in critically ill patients.

IMPORTANCE OF ARTERIAL WAVEFORM INTERPRETATION

Careful observation of pressure tracing characteristics can provide useful diagnostic information. Interpretation of invasive pressure tracings requires an understanding of dampening and natural frequency of pressure waveforms. The shape, timing and changes with respiration should not be overlooked. Pressure tracing from different sites of the arterial tree will have different morphologies as the pressure wave travels from the aorta to small arterioles. Distal arterial pressure wave measured away from the aorta, such as the radial or femoral artery has a higher and steeper systolic peak. The dicrotic notch also appears later and the diastolic wave is more prominent. This effect has been referred to as distal pulse amplification. The systolic pressure measured from the radial or femoral artery is higher than the aorta. (Figure 1.)

The (MAP) mean arterial pressure from the aorta and radial artery are more closely correlated suggesting (MAP) being a more relevant target for therapy guidance. In distal arterial branches, there is a substantial increase in vascular resistance that further augments the arterial systolic pulse. In elderly increased arterial stiffness results in a greater systolic peak (wide pulse pressure), explained by rapid return of the propagated wave during systole. (Figure 2.)

Systolic pressure variation predicts hypovolemia in acute blood loss (Ornstein 1998). This was an important observation that led to further research and enhanced our understanding of fluid responsiveness, a target for fluid resuscitation.

Interpreting the influence of positive pressure ventilation on the arterial pressure waveform - pulse pressure variation, can provide information about cardiopulmonary interactions applied in the assessment of cardiac preload.

Positive pressure inspiration rapidly increases left atrium and therefore left ventricular filling from the pulmonary veins. During positive pressure inspiration left ventricular afterload also decreases. This transient increase in preload and decrease in afterload accounts for a transient increase in stroke volume. The stroke volume and therefore measured pulse pressure variation is exaggerated with hypovolemia (Michard 2005). (Figure 3.)

Figure 1. This figure Illustrates the differences in the arterial waveform in the aortic arch compared to peripheral recorded tracing's in the radial or femoral artery. The peripheral femoral artery waveform tracing shows a wider pulse pressure, a delayed upstroke a delayed, slurred dicrotic notch and a more prominent diastolic wave.
(From Mark JB: Atlas of Cardiovascular Monitoring. New York, Churchill Livingstone, 1998: Fig. 8–4.)

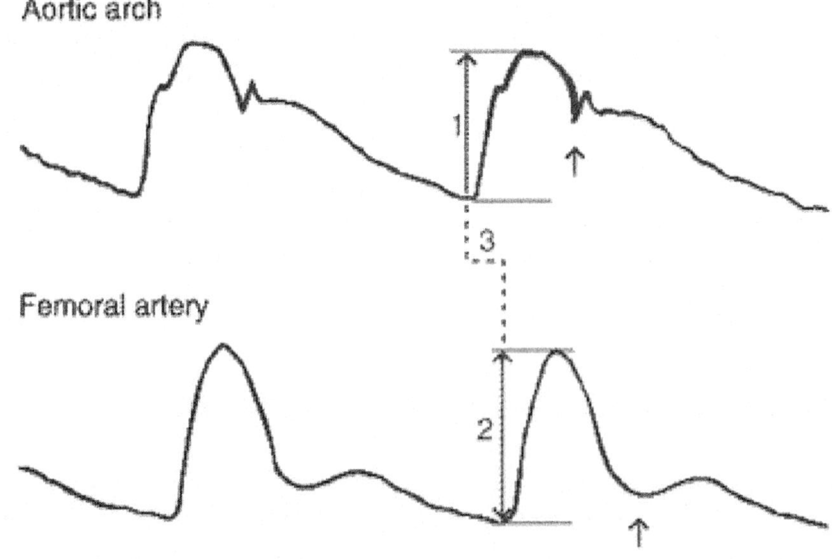

Figure 2. The reflected wave augments the diastolic pressure. (See left tracing) When the reflected pressure wave returns early it augments the systolic blood pressure. This is typically seen in elderly patients with stiff vessels. (See right tracing). This can have an impact on oxygen balance in elderly. Myocardial oxygen demand is increased in systole while oxygen supply is reduced in diastole.
(From Mark JB: Atlas of Cardiovascular Monitoring. New York, Churchill Livingstone, 1998: Fig. 8–4.)

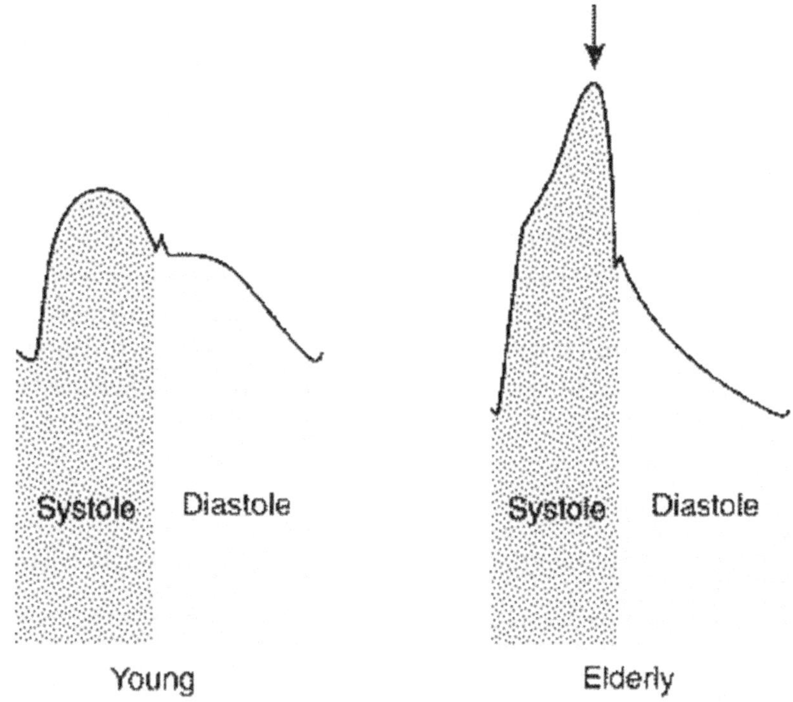

Figure 3. A systolic pressure down-slope during inspiration (Δ down) and upslope during expiration (Δ up) or systolic pressure variation (SPV), is an effect of positive pressure ventilation on the arterial pressure waveform in hypovolemia.
(From Mark JB: Atlas of Cardiovascular Monitoring. New York, Churchill Livingstone, 1998: Figs. 18–10C, and 16–16.)

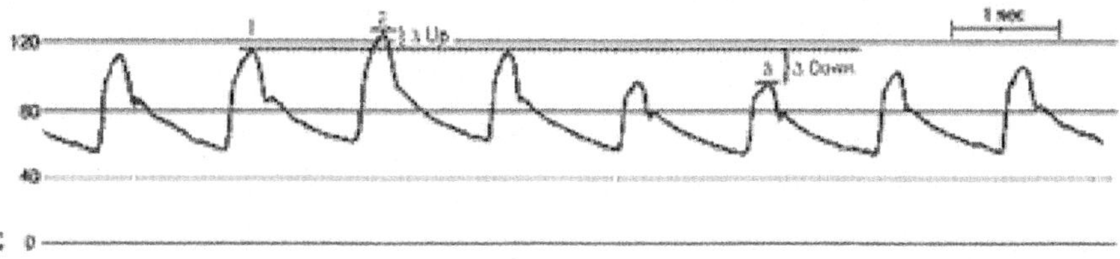

A recent meta-analysis was performed where the authors addressed the question if (PPV) positive pressure ventilation predicted fluid responsiveness in critically ill patients. The study conclusions were that PPV predicted fluid responsiveness in mechanically ventilated patients treated with relatively large tidal volumes, without spontaneous breathing or without cardiac arrhythmias (Xiaobo 2014).

Characteristic arterial waveform tracings are observed in certain disease states. Pulsus Alternans represents alternating strong and weak beats seen in congestive heart failure. Pulsus Paradoxus is an exaggerated decrease (greater than 10 mmHg) in SBP and wave amplitude during inspiration in Cardiac Tamponade. Pulsus Bisferiens or Biphasic Pulse is a palpated double peak pulse seen in aortic insufficiency, waveform in Hypertrophic Cardiomyopathy shows a peculiar "spike-and-dome" configuration and Pulsus Parvus et Tardus is a slow rising pulse in aortic stenosis. (Figures 4-8.)

Beneficial effects of pulsatile blood flow have been debated for decades. In today's world of ECMO and LVAD assist devices; long-term consequences of non-pulsatile flow can be studied. It has been reported that muscle sympathetic nerve activity in non-pulsatile patients was significantly increased compared to patients supported with pulsatile LVADs and healthy controls during head-up tilting. This finding was attributed to unloading of the baroreceptors from absence of arterial pulsatility (Markham 2013).

The importance of measuring pressure accurately with invasive and non-invasive technology has added additional challenges to postoperative and outpatient management of LVAD patients (HeartMate II). BP target is a MAP between 70-80mmHg and not above 90 mmHg. High afterload may compromise unloading of the left ventricle. The rate of strokes has been shown to be as high as 19% with hypertension in patients with LVAD (HeartMate II) assist devices (Slaughter, 2009). In a recent study addressed an important question of non-invasive BP measuring method in LVAD HeartMate II patients. Doppler method has been the gold standard for non-invasive measurement in LVAD patients with non-pulsatile flow. Knowing whether Doppler measures more closely SBP or MAP is important for clinical decision-making.

Figure 4. Pulsus Alternans, represents alternating strong and weak beats seen in congestive heart failure

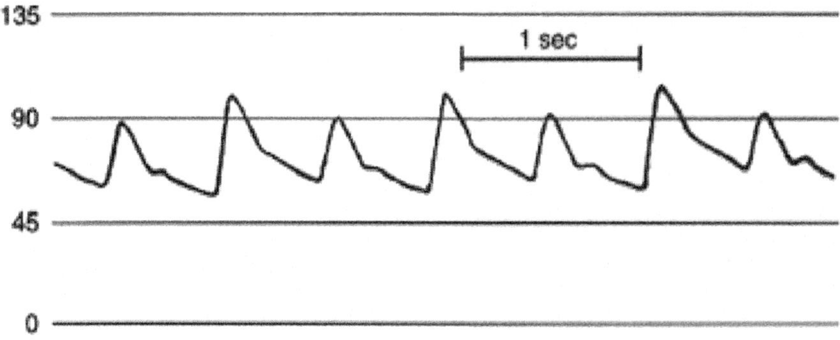

Figure 5. Pulsus Paradoxus is an exaggerated decrease (greater than 10 mmHg) in SBP and wave amplitude during inspiration in Cardiac Tamponade

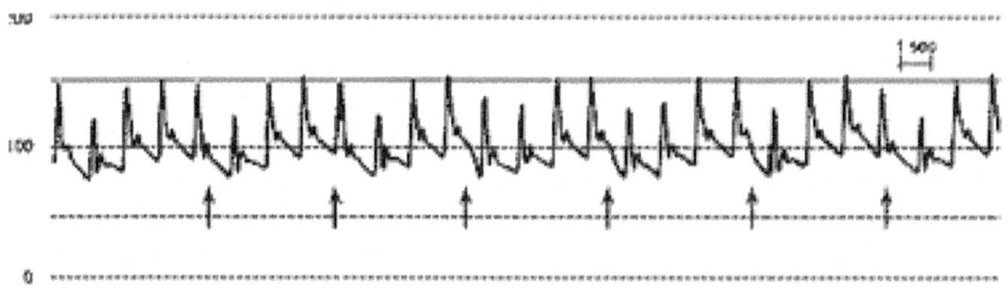

Figure 6. (Left Image) Pulsus Bisferiens tracing observed in aortic insufficiency. (Right Image) shows a peculiar "spike-and-dome" waveform seen in Hypertrophic Cardiomyopathy

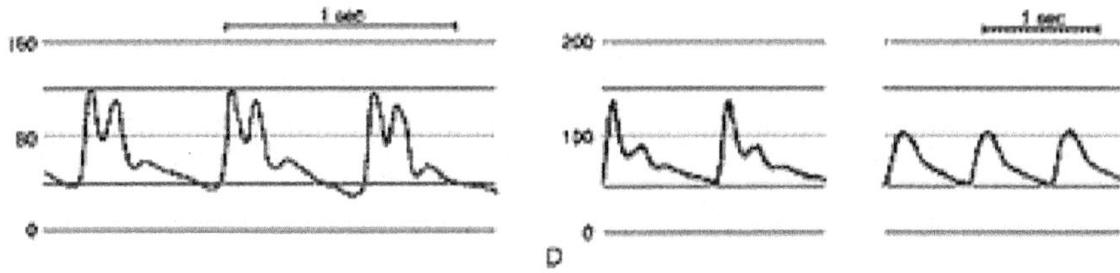

Figure 7. Left tracing represents a normal arterial and pulmonary artery tracing. The right arterial tracing is a tracing of a patient with aortic stenosis. The arterial waveform is distorted. Characteristic feature is the slurred upstroke and delayed systolic peak

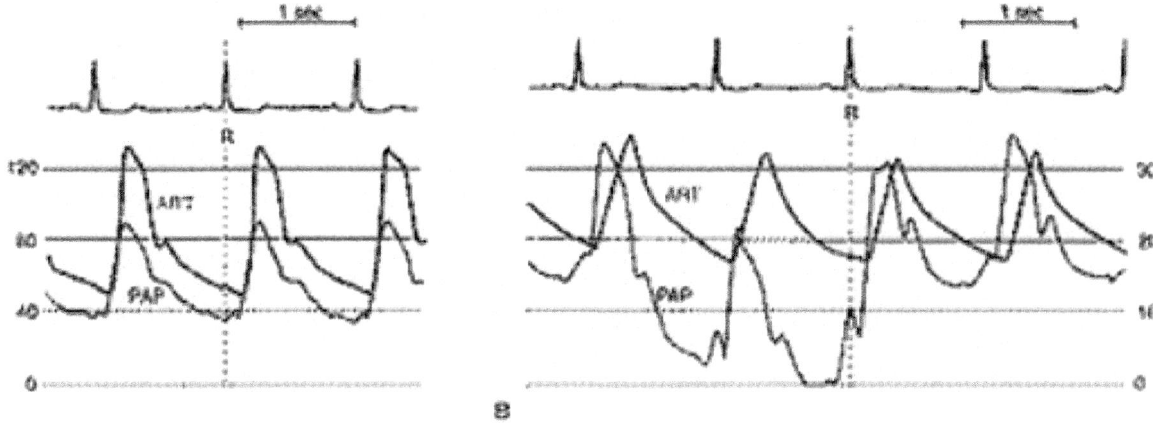

In this study Doppler underestimated SBP by 4.1 +/- 1.5 mmHg and overestimated MAP by 9.5 +/- 1.9-mmHg suggesting that it better reflected SBP. A further observation was that Doppler SBP measurements were not significantly affected by pulsatile flow, in LVAD patients with pulsatility. This finding was judged to be relevant because the Doppler method could lead to over treatment of presumed hypertension and development of symptoms, dizziness and syncope. Slow cuff deflation device-Terumo Elemano showed to correlate better to arterial line measurements than standard automated BP monitor-GE CARESCAPETM V100 or Doppler measurements in LVAD patients (Lanier 2013).

CARDIAC OUTPUT AND OUTCOME AFTER CARDIAC SURGERY

Close monitoring of cardiac output has been essential practice in the early post cardiac surgery period to ensure adequate cardiac performance. Postoperative low cardiac output is associated with higher mortality. Back in 1969 the relationship between cardiac index and survival was studied in adults. A cardiac

Figure 8. LVOT VTI- Left Ventricular Outflow Time Velocity Integral

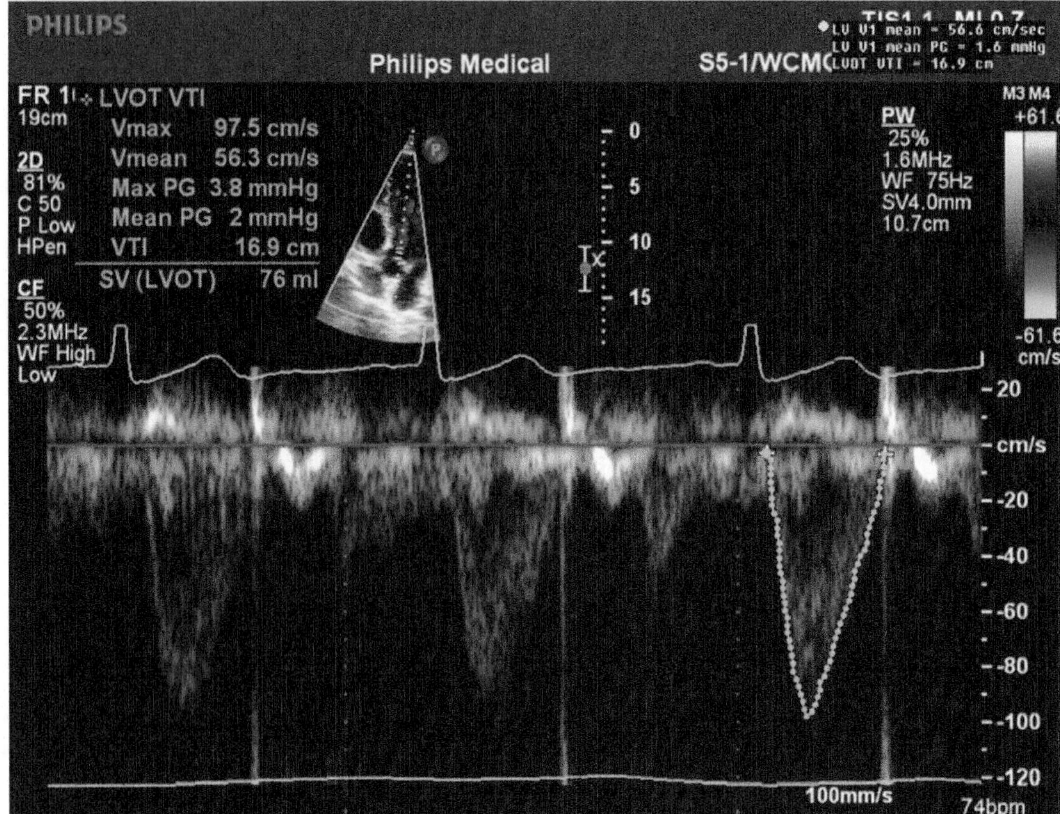

index of at least 2.0 lit /min/m2 during the first few hours of ICU admission were required for normal recovery. Cardiac indexes bellow these levels were reported to be inadequate for early postoperative recovery and were associated with an increase probability of hospital death (Dietzman 1969).

Risk factors associated with low cardiac output syndrome (LCOS) after cardiac surgery are patient specific and related to the procedure.

MIXED VENOUS OXYGEN TENSION AND MIXED VENOUS OXYGEN SATURATION

Mixed venous oxygen saturation is the oxygen saturation in the blood after oxygen has been extracted from the entire body, including the heart with its contribution via the coronary sinus. Mixed venous oxygen saturation (SvO2) is a global measure of oxygen balance in the body and not regional or organ specific. SvO2 is dependent on arterial oxygen saturation, hemoglobin concentration, cardiac output, and tissue oxygen consumption. A decrease in SvO2 may imply anemia, arterial oxygen desaturation and/or inadequate cardiac output. However, high values are measured in states of decreased oxygen extraction, such as advanced shock. SvO2 can be measured by obtaining a blood sample from the pulmonary artery with the use of a pulmonary artery catheter (PAC). Although PAC and information obtained from its use has not shown to improve patient outcome, SVO2 when available can help guide therapy in addition to other relevant clinical information.

At a time when there was limited monitoring for adequate tissue perfusion in children, venous partial pressure was studied as a surrogate of cardiac output. A study in infants and young children showed that when the venous partial pressure of oxygen was less than 30 mmHg, the cardiac output was likely insufficient and when below 23 mmHg it was associated with an increased probability of death (Parr 1975).

LACTIC ACIDOSIS AND CARDIAC SURGERY

Lactic acid forms in tissues as a result of anaerobic metabolism due to negative oxygen balance. Elevated serum lactate levels after cardiac surgery shown to be an indicator of systemic hypoperfusion and tissue hypoxia (Cerovic 2003). Furthermore, persistent elevation serum lactate and base deficit were predictors of mortality and morbidity after cardiac surgery (Husain 2003).

Serum lactate was studied as a prognostic factor after coronary artery bypass graft operations. Study results showed a significantly higher serum lactate level in ABG samples post cardiopulmonary bypass (2.84 ± 1.68) and on ICU admission (4.33 ± 2.56) in patients with a poor outcome ($p<0.001$). ABG lactate levels did not correlate with the magnitude of intra-operative bleeding or volume of packed cell transfusion ($p>0.05$). The pH of ABG samples did not generally correlate with the ABG lactate concentration ($r=0.116, p=0.68$). The increased lactate concentration was reliably associated with patient hemodynamic parameters, inotrope dosage, pump time and aorta cross clamp time (Jabbari 2013).

HISTORY OF CARDIAC OUTPUT MEASUREMENT

Cardiac output is the amount of blood that the heart ejects in one minute and can be determined by multiplying stroke volume with the heart rate. Cardiac output represents a measure of blood flow provided from the heart to tissues. Whereas, the Cardiac index is the cardiac output adjusted for body surface area. Fick understood the importance to measure cardiac output and was first to postulate in 1870 that blood flow to an organ can be calculated by using a marker substance.

The Fick Principle, cardiac output measurement is based on conservation of mass.

The total uptake of (or release of) a substance by the peripheral tissues is equal to the product of the blood flow to the peripheral tissues and the arterial-venous concentration difference (gradient) of the substance. (A.E. Fick – 1870)

Fick equation:

VO2= (CO – CaO2) – (CO – CvO2)
CO – Cardiac Output in lit/min.
VO2 – Oxygen Consumption in ml's/min
CaO2 – Arterial Oxygen Content ml'/lit
CvO2 – Venous Oxygen Content ml's/lit

By rearranging the formula:

CO = VO2/Ca – Cv

It wasn't until the late 1930's that measurement of oxygen saturation, oxygen partial tension and oxygen consumption made it possible to prove Fick's principle accurate.

The Fick principle has been adopted and continues to be routinely used for measuring cardiac output in the catheterization laboratory with right heart catheterization to this day. A limitation of the Fick method is that the measurement of oxygen uptake takes at least 5-10 minutes. This may affect accuracy of the Fick method in a patient with rapidly changing hemodynamics. Based on the Fick principle, later investigators developed cardiac output monitors that have been introduced into practice. (NICO), partial CO2 re-breathing is an example of a noninvasive cardiac output monitor that uses CO2 as a marker substance, after applying the Fick principle, cardiac output is calculated.

Since Fick, there have been a number of methods developed for cardiac output measurement. These methods have become the basis for hemodynamic monitors that have been developed and introduced into practice that can also provide a comprehensive assessment of circulatory variables in critically ill patients. Hemodynamic monitoring in the early post cardiac surgery period has proven essential to early postoperative recovery. In adults, the pulmonary artery catheter has been the preferred monitoring technology to determine cardiac function. Other validated less invasive devices have subsequently been introduced into clinical practice based on methods developed in the last century with the ability to measure cardiac output. It is important to know how they work, how they have been validated and to review the clinical trials in order to define their role.

METHODS FOR CARDIAC OUTPUT MEASUREMENT

Cardiac Output Measurement Based on the Arterial Contour Analysis

Sagawa, published a translation of Otto Frank's 1899 original paper, description of the circulation in terms of the "Windkessel Air Chamber Model". The original two-component model had a capacitance and resistor. Based on this model, blood ejected from the heart into the aorta and elastic arteries exceeds that leaving the aorta due to the effect of peripheral resistance. There is a net storage of blood during systole in large elastic arteries, which discharges during diastole. Therefore large elastic arteries likened to a capacitor. This effect helps dampen the fluctuation in blood pressure (pulse pressure) over the cardiac cycle and assists in the maintenance of organ perfusion during diastole when cardiac ejection ceases (Sagawa 1990).

In 1904, Erlenger and Hooker hypothesized that cardiac output was proportional to arterial pulse pressure. This hypothesis was the foundation for the development of cardiac output monitors based on usage of the contour arterial waveform. Historical improvements in this method included: calibration, pulse pressure correction for arterial compliance and addition of a mathematical correction factor to the systolic area by adopting the 3-element Windekessel model.

Further refining of the pulse contour analysis mathematical algorithm was the basis for measurement of cardiac output used in the devices such as Flotrack sensor, pulse contour analysis of the PICCO catheter and contour analysis of the LIDCO technology.

A simplified formula that represents the basis for cardiac output derived from arterial contour analysis.

$SV = SD_{AP} * X$

SD_{AP} - standard deviation of arterial pressure
Factor X is the conversion factor of arterial compliance
Computation of these two values generates SV.

Cardiac Output Measurement Based on Electrical Bio-Impedance

Thoracic bio-impedance cardiography is a noninvasive and indirect method for measuring stroke volume and therefore, calculation of cardiac output. Impedance cardiography is based on measurement of thoracic electrical resistance change synchronous with cardiac rhythm. In 1931, Atzler and Lehmann provided the first description of this method and later in 1940, Nyboer developed the first mathematical formula for stroke volume calculation.

$$SV = Q \times L^2 \times \Delta Z / Z_0^2$$

SV – Stroke volume
Q - Specific resistivity of blood (ohm)
L - Distance between two inner electrodes (cm)
Z_0 - Base impedance between both inner electrodes (ohm)
ΔZ – Impedance change during systole (ohm)

Kubicek in 1966, as part of the NASA project, significantly improved the method. To the Nyboer's formula he introduced the ventricular ejection time (T) and first derivative of the impedance change, dZ/dt.

$$SV = Q \times L^2 \times T \times dZ/dt / Z_0^2$$

Despite successful early clinical trials on healthy volunteers, widespread use in clinical practice was not achieved. In the 1980's ECG electrodes were introduced instead of the band electrodes that improved the quality of the signal. In addition, individual patient data were incorporated into the software, modifying the formula (Sramek 1980). In 1991, results of the first generation of a electrical bio-impedance monitor were published (Klocke 1991). This first generation had good agreement tested by Bland Altman. However a number of limitations were realized.

The introduction of bio-reactance advanced the development of a monitor that could perform well in patients receiving vasopressors, inotropes as well as with arrhythmias. Bio-reactance is a time delay, or phase shift, which occurs when an alternating electrical current (AC) is passed through the thorax. More detail on this technology will be described in more detail later in the chapter. Based on the Bio-reactance technology, the (NICOM) cardiac output monitor was developed that performed well in patients receiving vasopressors, inotropes as well as with arrhythmias.

INDICATOR DILUTION METHOD FOR CARDIAC OUTPUT MEASUREMENT

Hamilton, described the indicator dilution method for measuring cardiac output (Hamilton 1932). Indocyanine green dye (2 - 4 mg) was injected rapidly as a marker substance into a vein and was continuously sampled from the arterial blood through a constant withdrawal syringe and the integral concentration curve over time assayed by a photo-densitometer. Cardiac output was estimated based on the amount of indicator injected divided by its average concentration in the arterial blood after a circulation through the heart. This method assumes that the rate at which the indicator was diluted reflected flow. This method is used to measure cardiac output in the LiDCO technology for calibration.

Cardiac output was calculated based on the formula:

$$CO = \text{Amount of dye Injected} / \int^{\infty} \mathrm{oc}\ (t)\ dt$$

$$\int^{\infty} \mathrm{oc}\ (t)\ DT = \text{Integral concentration change of injected dye over time}$$

THERMODILUTION CARDIAC OUTPUT MEASUREMENT

Stewart and Hamilton developed the thermo dilution method to measure cardiac output. Cardiac output based on the "Stewart-Hamilton" equation is estimated by measurement of an integral temperature change over time curve of a fixed volume, 10 ml's of cold crystalloid solution mixing with blood until the blood temperature reaches baseline temperature. Factors affecting measurement are: volume and temperature of injectate and blood, density factor and computation coefficient. This method is the basis for cardiac output measurement with the pulmonary artery catheter (PAC) and thermo dilution cardiac output measurement with PiCCO.

Cardiac output was calculated based on the formula:

$$CO = Vi(TB - Ti)\ K1\ X\ K2 / (dTb/dt)$$

Vi = Volume of Injectate (ml)
TB = Initial blood temperature ('C)
TI = initial Injectate temperature ('C)
K1 = Density factor
K2 = Computation constant
dTb/dt = Integral temperature change over time

ECHO TECHNOLOGY FOR CARDIAC OUTPUT MEASUREMENT

There are two echo methods for stroke volume measurement and therefore cardiac output calculation: Volumetric and Doppler method.

With the volumetric method, stroke volume can be measured using two-dimensional (2D) and three-dimensional (3D) echocardiography. The volumetric stroke volume measurement is calculated by subtracting end diastolic and end systolic volume.

SV = EDV – ESV

EDV - End Diastolic Volume
ESV - End Systolic Volume

Doppler stroke volume can be estimated by applying the "area length formula for tubular structures". This method is the basis for cardiac output measurement with the Esophageal Doppler cardiac output monitor.

SV = Area X VTI

Area of a circle = D^2 X 0785
D - Diameter of the LVOT
VTI - Time Velocity Integral

Stroke volume and therefore cardiac output can be measured at the bedside noninvasively using Transthoracic Echocardiography (TTE). The pulsed wave Doppler signature (VTI) is obtained in the apical 5-chamber view. The Echo pulsed wave signal is received by the echo probe crystals after hitting RBC's, as the RBC's travel away from the emitted Echo pulsed wave. For accuracy of this method, it is important to sample the Echo pulsed wave parallel to blood flow. A pulsed wave velocity signature over time is created and a time velocity integral calculated (VTI). (Picture number 1.) The LVOT diameter is measured in the parasternal long axis view. (Picture 2.) By obtaining these measurements, stroke volume can be calculated from the above formula.

THE IDEAL CARDIAC OUTPUT MONITOR

The ideal cardiac output (CO) monitor needs to be accurate, validated, needs to be reproducible, reliable and perform under a number of different physiologic conditions, such as shock states. Furthermore, it should be continuous and improve patient outcome with clinical trials. The most frequently used analytic method for validating CO monitoring devices is the Bland-Altman method, by plotting the bias against the mean CO and determining the limits of agreement (LOAs). The proposed percentage error calculated as the ratio of 2 standard deviations (SDs) of the bias (LOA) to the mean CO, is considered to be clinically acceptable if it is below 30% (Critchley & Critchley 1999).

Figure 9. Green line Indicates LVOT Diameter in cm

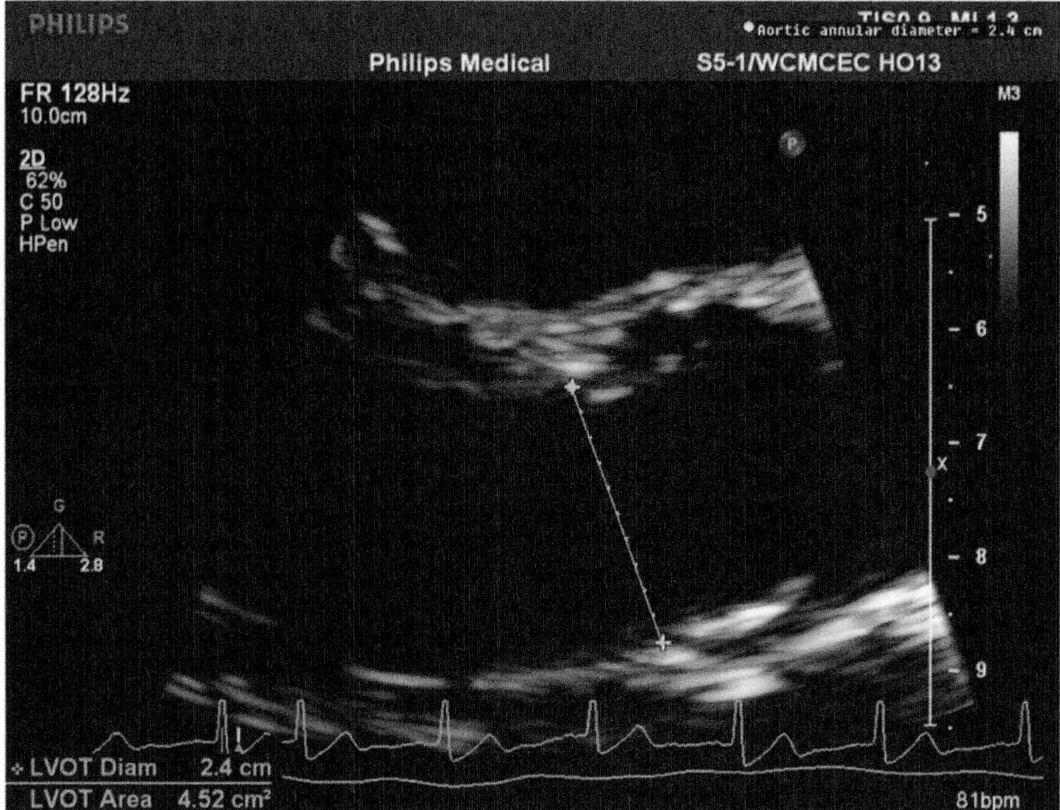

The Bland-Altman method addresses how well the method of CO monitoring being evaluated agrees with the compared gold standard method for cardiac output measurement. However, the Bland-Altman method fails to show whether the test method reliably detects changes in CO. Although the accuracy of noninvasive CO devices to measure trends in CO has not been standardized, a number of methods have been described in the literature. These methods include the use of the correlation coefficient, the 4-quadrant plot, and receiver-operator characteristic (ROC) curve analysis.

CIRCULATORY MONITORING IN THE POST CARDIAC SURGERY PATIENT

The early postoperative period can be associated with a number of changes in intravascular volume (cardiac preload), cardiac afterload and cardiac performance (systolic and diastolic function). Historically, adult hemodynamic monitoring of post cardiac surgery patients has been performed with the pulmonary artery catheter. Originally introduced in 1970 by Drs. HJ Swan and W Ganz, this monitor has been the mainstay in the management of intraoperative and post cardiac surgery patients for almost half a century. Widespread use was adopted in cardiac surgery and critically ill patients at a time without clinical trials supporting its use. It wasn't until the late seventies that David M. Eddy suggested using clinical trials to gather evidence in order to make recommendations for practice and practice change. Despite the lack of outcome data in adult cardiac surgery patients, the pulmonary artery catheter remains the most commonly used technology for hemodynamic monitoring.

The Swan-Ganz (Pulmonary-artery) catheter is floated through a large bore central venous access port through the right atrium, followed by the right ventricle and into the pulmonary artery to measure "filling" pressures of the right side of the heart: (CVP) central venous pressure, (PAS/PAD) pulmonary systolic and diastolic pressures, (PCWP) pulmonary capillary wedge pressure and (CO) cardiac output. Blood samples from the catheter tip located in the pulmonary artery can provide a measurement of the (SVO2), mixed venous oxygen saturation. PAC measures cardiac output by thermodilution described earlier in this chapter. Technological advancements enabled the development of catheters that provide a measurement of continuous (SVO2) mixed venous oxygen saturation and/or frequent automatic sampling for cardiac output measurements.

The PAC enables continuously (CVP) central venous pressure monitoring. Intravascular volume, venous tone, right ventricular function and thoracic pressures influence CVP. Traditional pressure waveform teaching is interpretation of CVP tracing morphology. Normal CVP waveform consists of an *a*, *c* and *v* wave, a systolic *x* descent and *a* diastolic *y* descent. Components of the CVP wave overlap corresponding phases of ECG tracing. The *a* wave and *c* wave result from atrial and ventricular contraction. The (v) wave results from right atrial filling. For clinical interpretation, the normal CVP tracing has 3 systolic components, *c* wave, *x* descent and the *v* wave and 2 diastolic components, the *y* descent and the *a* wave. (Figure 10.)

Figure 10. This figure illustrates a normal central venous pressure waveform with the timing to the electrocardiogram. Note the 3 systolic components (c wave, x descent, v wave) and 2 diastolic components (y descent, a wave). Wave component identification is timed by the R wave on the ECG.
(From Mark JB: Atlas of Cardiovascular Monitoring. New York, Churchill Livingstone, 1998: Fig. 2–5.)

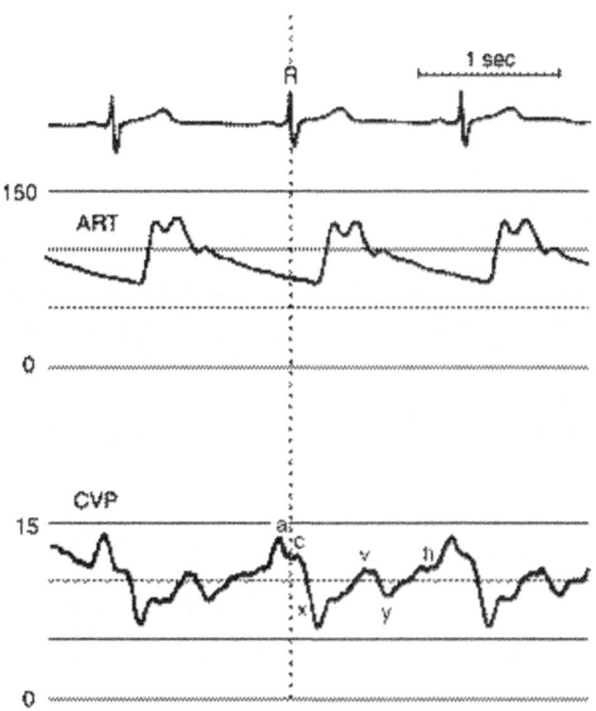

An abnormally tall *a* wave, called cannon *a* wave is observed with atrial contraction during a closed tricuspid valve. This is classically seen in patients with a junctional rhythm. In atrial fibrillation, *a* wave is absent, and in tricuspid stenosis, there is a prominent *a* wave and an attenuated *y* descent resulting from obstruction to right atrial emptying. In tricuspid regurgitation, retrograde filling of the atrium in systole result in fusion of *c* and *v* wave, creating a large, fused regurgitant *cv* wave with loss of the *x* descent. (Figures 11 and 12)

Interpretation and reading of CVP tracing provides understanding of cardiac physiology in normal and pathological conditions. One can argue that due to widespread use of point-of-care sonography, the need for clinical CVP tracing interpretation has decreased. In addition, value of the use of a CVP target in goal – directed – resuscitation has also become less valuable for fluid status assessment in modern practice due to a number of methods shown to accurately predict fluid responsiveness, such as - changes in IVC diameter observed with 2D echo (sniff test), pulse pressure and stroke volume variation with passive leg raise, measured with Doppler echocardiography and less invasive monitors discussed later in this chapter.

Placement of the PAC is not without risks. Potential complications include the following: Atrial and or ventricular arrhythmias (>20%), RBBB and complete heart block (0.3%-3.8%), injury during placement of central venous access (pneumothorax, air embolism, injury to nerves- occurring in less than 3.6%), pulmonary artery rupture, infarction, venous thrombosis (0.03% to 3%) and death (0.02% to 1.5%) (Sandham 2003).

In Cochrane Review of thirteen randomized controlled trials, a total of 5686 patients were evaluated that included a mix of medical and surgical ICU patients, who were either randomized in the PAC group or control group. Overall, this meta-analysis showed that the PAC group did not have a greater

Figure 11. Left panel illustrates a normal CVP tracing. Right panel (Atrioventricular dissociation) shows an early systolic cannon a wave. Atrial contraction occurs during ventricular systole when the tricuspid valve is closed. Decrease in arterial blood pressure can follow decreased ventricular filling.

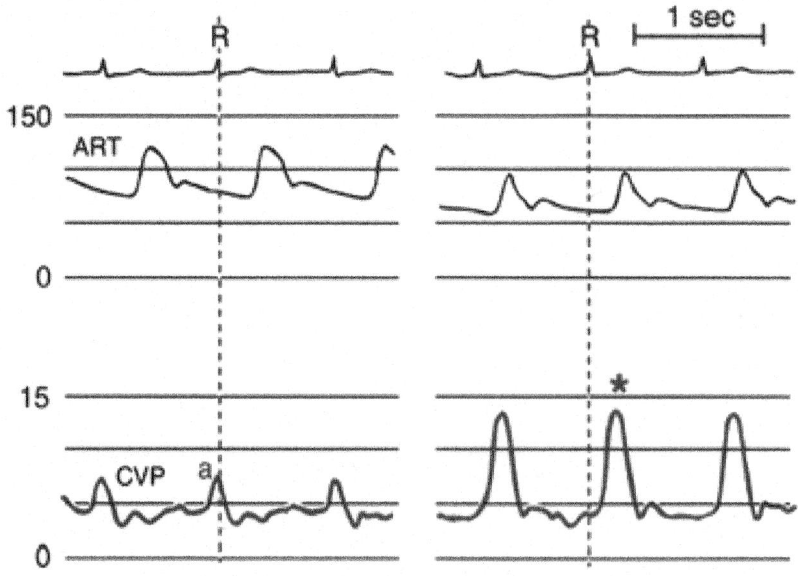

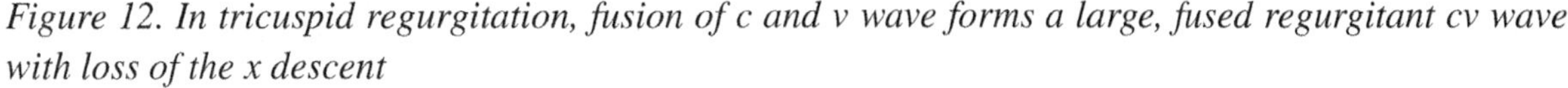

Figure 12. In tricuspid regurgitation, fusion of c and v wave forms a large, fused regurgitant cv wave with loss of the x descent

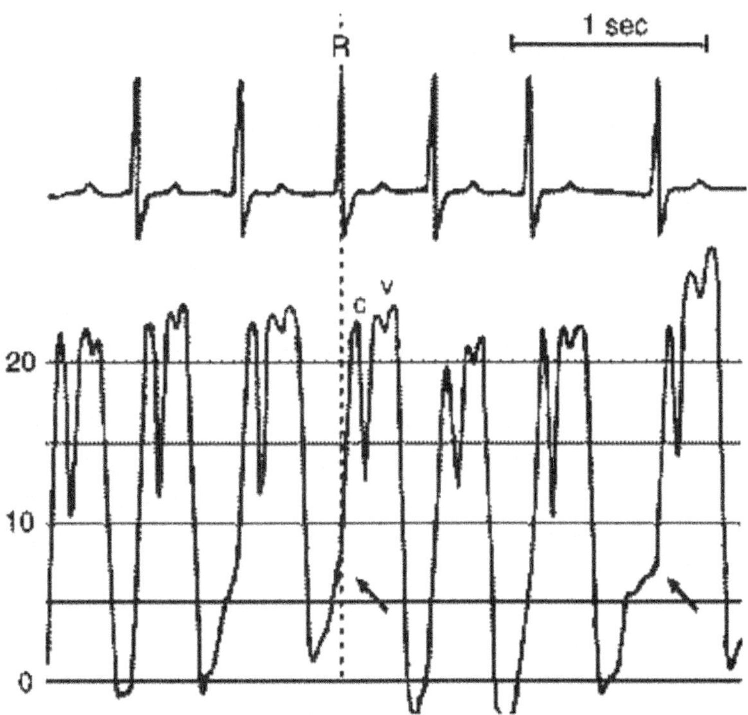

mortality rate, hospital length of stay and or cost of care when compared to the control group in both medical as well as surgical ICU patient populations. The authors concluded that the PAC could be used as a diagnostic tool and guide for treatment in selected patients (Rajaram 2013).

Despite widespread use in cardiac surgery patients, information obtained from the PAC must be accurately interpreted in order to deliver appropriate treatment. Thermodilution cardiac output has been shown inaccurate in situations where there are rapid changes in temperature, blood density. Accuracy of cardiac output measurement has been shown to be affected by intra cardiac shunts and tricuspid regurgitation.

While interpreting information obtained from a pulmonary artery catheter to assess intravascular volume, the assumption is that measured pressures such as CVP, PAS/PAD and PCWP reflect intravascular volume. However, in post cardiac surgery patients this is not always the case. For example, patients with high intra-thoracic pressures commonly seen with postoperative pleural effusions, with a tension pneumothorax or with advanced valvular disease and diastolic dysfunction will all have high filling pressures measured, that does not accurately reflect their intravascular volume status. On the other hand, the pulmonary artery catheter is the only method available to continuously measure pulmonary artery pressures. In the early post cardiac surgery period this can be helpful for managing right heart failure and titration of selective pulmonary artery vasodilators. In patients with severe pulmonary hypertension undergoing cardiac surgery, some advocate that monitoring with a PAC be enhanced with a left atrial pressure line (LA line), as measurements obtained from an LA line are more representative of the left ventricular end diastolic pressure and end diastolic volume. Lastly, Trans Esophageal (TEE) and Transthoracic (TTE) Echocardiography complement diagnostic information obtained by a central line or PAC in the early postoperative period.

PiCCO FOR MEASUREMENT OF CARDIAC OUTPUT AND HEMODYNAMIC MONITORING

PiCCO technology is widely used in Europe for hemodynamic monitoring of critically ill and high-risk surgical patients. This technology requires a central venous catheter and a femoral or axillary arterial line for calibration. The PiCCO technology intermittently measures cardiac output via trans-pulmonary thermodilution (TPTD) and also performs a pulse contour analysis to measure cardiac output continuously. Using the TPTD technique, the PiCCO device calibrates its arterial pressure driven pulse contour cardiac output method. Radial artery catheterization is not sufficient, as the damped waveform that can occur in particular with the use of vasopressors or changes in SVR, has shown to invalidate contour analysis CO measurements. PICCO technology also measures (SV) stroke volume and (SVV) stroke volume variation continuously, (ITBV) intrathoracic blood volume derived from (GEDV) global and (EVLW) extravascular lung water intermittently. Of note, a comparison study suggested that increased cardiac preload is more reliably predicted by measuring ITBV rather than CVP or PCWP (Wiesenack 2001). The PiCCO technology has been studied in a wide variety of patients. It has been validated to accurately measure cardiac output and also reliably serve for intravascular volume assessment in critically ill patients. However, in cardiac surgery patients with hemodynamic instability, with arrhythmias and patients with reduced myocardial function, the PiCCO catheter may have decreased accuracy (see next section).

Validation Studies

Contour analysis cardiac output demonstrated good agreement with thermodilution CO in a wide range of surgical and critically ill patients. In patients undergoing CABG surgery bias ranged from 0.04 to 0.3 L/min (Button 2007). However, findings in patients with hemodynamic instability, demonstrated that the PiCCO system was not as accurate, reporting bias of 0.68 L/min and limits of agreement of 1.94 L/min (Compton 2008). In post cardiac surgery patients, continuous pulse contour cardiac output measurement may be of limited value because irregular heart rates (atrial fibrillation) are fairly common in cardiac surgery patients. Based on these findings, there is a need in the above-mentioned clinical situations, to use the intermittent TPTD cardiac output measurements obtained by the PiCCO catheter and disregard the continuously measured cardiac output by pressure contour analysis. Frequency of recalibration of the contour analysis cardiac output measurement is another valid question with this technology. De Wilde also reported that measurement of global end diastolic volume (GEDV) is of limited value in predicting fluid responsiveness in patients with reduced myocardial function (De Wilde 2008).

Clinical Trials

Cardiac patients were studied with a goal directed fluid management strategy. The results showed a reduction in vasopressor and catecholamine use in the study group (Goepfert 2007).

A direct comparison, multinational prospective epidemiological study was performed where PiCCO technology was compared to the PAC (Pulmonary artery catheter) for monitoring outcome in critically ill patients. A total of 331 critically ill patients were enrolled in the study. 192 patients received a PiCCO catheter and 150 patients a PAC for monitoring. In this study patients that received a PAC were older, (68 vs 64 years of age; $p=0, 0037$) received more inotropes, (37.3% vs 13%; $p<0.001$) and had an average lower cardiac index (2.6 vs 3.2 lit/mi/m^2; $p<0.001$). The mean daily fluid balance was greater in the PiCCO treated group (+ 659 vs + 350 mls/day; p=0.017) and ventilator free days were fewer in the PiCCO treated group (12 for PiCCO vs 21 for PAC; p=0.045). However, after a multiple regression analysis was performed, no significant difference in monitoring technique was found for mean daily fluid balance or ventilator free days in the two study groups. The study conclusions were that the choice of monitor PiCCO or PAC did not influence major outcomes (Uchino 2006).

LiDCO FOR MEASUREMENT OF CARDIAC OUTPUT AND HEMODYNAMIC MONITORING

LiDCO hemodynamic device was developed based on pulse contour analysis and lithium dilution to measure cardiac output. It is considered a less invasive technique that provides a continuous measurement of the (SV) stroke volume, (SVV) stroke volume variation and essentially fluid responsiveness. Calibration is achieved by injection of a small dose of lithium into a peripheral or central vein. Following a lithium injection, concentration of lithium is measured by the arterial line sensor and concentration-curve over time created to estimate a cardiac output (Indicator dilution method). Once calibration is performed of the arterial pulse contour, recalibration has been shown to be unnecessary for up to 8 hours unless changes in the arterial line tracing occurs that may compromise the pulse contour analysis (Hamilton et al. 2002). LiDCO technology has been studied in critically ill and cardiac surgery patients with good agreement by Bland-Altman analysis.

Validation Studies

In a validation study, cardiac output measured by thermodilution through a PAC was compared with the lithium dilution (LiDCO) and Pulse-CO method in 20 patients who had undergone coronary artery bypass grafting. A Wilcoxon paired rank test and Bland-Altman analysis were performed for direct method comparison. Good correlation was observed between all methods based on concordance correlations Pulse-CO versus Thermo, r (correlation coefficient) 0.86; LiDCO versus Thermo, r 0.86; and Pulse-CO versus LiDCO, r 0.99. Bland-Altman plots demonstrated good agreement between values obtained by Pulse- CO and Thermo for all data collected at post coronary artery bypass grafting hours 0, 2, 4, 6, and 8. These data suggested that Pulse-CO measurements of cardiac output were reliable in patients for at least 8 hours after cardiac operations, despite the potential inherent fluctuations in the arterial pressure waveform caused by temperature changes, use of vasopressors, inotropic agents, vasodilators or use of the arterial line for blood sampling (Hamilton 2002).

Missant et al, performed a comparison study where CO measured by pulse contour was compared to CO by thermodilution in off –pump coronary bypass patients. This study showed a bias ± limits of agreement of -0.03 ± 1.30 L min^{-1} (mean error 29%). Pulse contour cardiac output was concluded to be an acceptable technique to measure cardiac output less invasively in off-pump coronary bypass patients (Missant 2008).

Mora et al., studied 30 post-cardiac surgery patients with LVEF <40% and on multiple vasopressors and inotropes. Study results showed that the LiDCO technology had good correlation (correlation coefficient 0.82), marginal bias (0.28 l.min^{-1}) and acceptable percentage error (27%) when compared to the PAC thermodilution technique (Mora 2011).

Results from wide range of studies showed good limits of agreement, within 2 standard deviation, LiDCO CO pulse contour cardiac output compared to thermodilution cardiac output tested by Bland Altman with acceptable percentage error below 30%, as proposed by Critchley and Critchley.

These studies included: critically ill general surgical patients, hyperdynamic liver transplantation patients, post pediatric heart transplantation patients, post-operative care patients, pre-eclampsia patients, patients in congestive heart failure and medical patients receiving treatment general intensive care (Hamilton 2002; Heller 2002; Pitman 2005; Smith 2005; Kim 2006; Costa 2007; Kemps 2008; Mills et al. 2010; Cecconi 2010; Brass 2011: and Dyer 2011).

Clinical Trials

In the recently conducted OPTIMISE multicenter trial, 734 patients were randomized to receive either: peri-operative hemodynamic therapy using a LiDCO derived algorithm, LiDCO guided fluid resuscitation and dopexamine or standard of care in high-risk patients undergoing major gastrointestinal surgery. The study failed to show statistical significant improvement in 30day mortality. The primary outcome occurred in 36.6% of intervention and 43.4% of usual care participants (relative risk [RR], 0.84 [95% CI, 0.71-1.01]; absolute risk reduction, 6.8% [95% CI, −0.3% to 13.9%]; $P=.07$). However, after inclusion of these data in an updated meta-analysis, patients in the intervention group had a reduction in complication rates (4.9% vs. 6.5% intervention and control group respectively, RR 0.82 [95% CI, 0.67-1.01] and mortality at longest follow-up (8.3%vs.10.3% intervention and control group respectively, RR, 0.86 [95% CI, 0.74-1.00]. The authors concluded from this study that the intervention group had fewer complications (Pearce 2014).

FLOTRAC FOR CARDIAC OUTPUT MEASUREMENT AND HEMODYNAMIC MONITORING

Flotrack sensor arterial contour analysis requires patient demographic and physical characteristics for arterial impedance estimation. Cardiac output measurement is based on the equation:

$SV= SD_{AP} * X.$

(SD_{AP} -Standard deviation of arterial pressure)
(X – Conversion factor)

Standard deviation of arterial pressure is determined from the arterial line waveform, which is sampled every 20 seconds at 100 Hz to generate a total of 2,000 data points. The standard deviation of these data points reflects pulse pressure. Factor X is a conversion factor of arterial compliance that influences stroke volume measurement. Biometric factors including sex, height, age and weight, are taken into account in the calculation of the conversion factor (Langewouters 1979). Computation of these two values generates SV and therefore cardiac output. The Flotrac sensor can be used with the vigilleo or EV1000 platform monitoring system. Besides cardiac output, SV and SVV can be measured with this technology. The Flotrac sensor underwent a number changes over the last decade as validation studies have shown lack of accuracy. One of the differences of the Flotrac algorithm compared to the PiCCO and LiDCO technologies is that the Flotrac sensor is not calibrated by thermodilution as in the case of PiCCO or indicator dilution method as with the LiDCO. Stroke volume derived from the Flotrac sensor is exclusively based on contour analysis and mathematical correction.

Validation Studies

The Flotrac system has been studied extensively in the perioperative period and post-cardiac surgery patients. This device demonstrated a lack of accuracy when compared with PAC intermittent thermodilution in multiple validation studies.

Camporata demonstrated that Flotrac/Vigileo overestimated CO in patients with significant aortic regurgitation and CO was underestimated in high-output, vasodilatory states (Camporata 2010). Furthermore the Flotrac sensor has shown to be inaccurate during IABP counter pulsation. With rapidly changing hemodynamics, the Vigileo/Flotrac sensor and thermodilution may not simultaneously show changes in cardiac output (Sander 2006). In a study of cardiac surgery patients, where measurements were obtained immediately after cardiopulmonary, Flotrac CO measurements showed poor agreement with PAC intermittent thermodilution (ITD) measurements (Senn 2007). Of note in this setting, PAC thermodilution cardiac output measurements may be inaccurate immediately post cardio-pulmonary bypass. This may be a result of temperature changes of the patient's blood and the sample crystalloid injectate used for ITD measurement. Computation coefficient calibration problems and density changes of blood can also occur at this stage of the operation. All of these factors can affect accuracy of PAC (ITD) measurements, gold standard used for cardiac output comparison.

Monnet demonstrated that during hemodynamic instability or in extreme conditions of vasodilation or vasoconstriction, the Flotrac system measured CO may diverge from an independent bolus indicator dilution measurement, particularly if a peripheral artery is used (Monnet 2012).

Clinical Trials

Kapoor conducted a randomized trial in immediately post cardiopulmonary bypass, cardiac surgery patients to receive either early goal-directed therapy (EGDT) or standardized care. All subjects received standardized care. In the study EGTD group, in addition to standard monitors, cardiac index was measured using FloTrac™ and a continuous central venous oxygen saturation using PreSep™.

Targets used for the control group were: central venous pressure 6-8 mmHg, mean arterial pressure 90-105 mmHg, normal arterial blood gas analysis values, pulse oximetry above 95%, hematocrit value above 30% and urine output more than 1 ml/kg/h.

Goal directed targets for the study group, were the control group parameters as described, cardiac index at 2.5-4.2 l/min/m^2, stroke volume index 30-65 ml/beat/m^2, systemic vascular resistance index 1500-2500 dynes/s/cm ^{5} /m ^{2}, oxygen delivery index 450-600 ml/min/m ^{2}, continuous central venous oximetry more than 70%, and stroke volume variation less than 10%. Subjects in the EGDT group demonstrated shorter duration of ventilation, and ICU LOS in moderate to high-risk cardiac surgery patients. In this study, Flotrack proved to be useful in early resuscitation by using an early goal directed therapy resuscitation strategy (Kapoor 2008).

NICOM FOR CARDIAC OUTPUT MEASUREMENT AND HEMODYNAMIC MONITORING

NICOM is a non-invasive monitor used to measure cardiac output and assess volume status. This technology measures bio-reactance that represents a time delay, or phase shift that occurs when an alternating electrical current (AC) is passed through the thorax. The NICOM sensor delivers a signal at a frequency of 75 kHz into the thorax. The sensors compare the received signal to what was delivered. There have been a number of factors documented to contribute to flow. This includes - pressure, volumetric flow, resistance, capacitance, compliance, velocity, and viscosity. Factors of pulsatile flow cause a shift in the signal called "phase shift" or "time delay". The amount of blood that leaves the aorta to cause that specific time delay represents the stroke volume. With estimation of stroke volume, ECG leads built into the sensors provides the heart rate needed to calculate cardiac output. Four dual electrode stickers are placed on the chest, and two are placed on each side of the body. Each electrode has both, a high-frequency current generator and a voltage input amplifier. Cardiac output is generated from each side of the body and an average cardiac output is used. Besides cardiac output measurement, SV and SVV are also measured.

Stroke volume is estimated through the formula:

$$SV = C \times VET \times d\varphi/dt_{max}$$

C – Constant of Proportionality
VET - Ventricular Ejection Time
$d\varphi/dtmax$- Peak rate of change

Maximum flow is measured by obtaining the maximum point of the peak rate of change ($d\varphi/dtmax$). The Ventricular Ejection Time (VET) is measured from the first zero crossing to the second zero crossing. Stroke volume is proportional to the product of the peak rate of change and ventricular ejection time, which result in an approximation of the positive area of the NICOM signal.

Bio-reactance based CO measurement does not use static impedance (Zo) for stroke volume calculations. Therefore, it does not depend on the distance between the electrodes.

NICOM averages the signal over 1 minute, which may improve accuracy in determination of CO in patients with arrhythmias. (Figure 13.)

Figure 13 shows that pulsatile changes in thoracic volume induce phase shifts that are detected continuously by the NICOM's phase-detection mechanism and captured in the form of the recorded signal. Based this signature, the peak rate of change and ventricular ejection time is determined in calculating the cardiac output.

Validation Studies

Squara conducted a validation study where the NICOM system was compared to the PAC measured CO in 110 patients after cardiac surgery for accuracy, precision, responsiveness, and reliability of NICOM in detecting cardiac output changes. A total of 65,888 pairs of cardiac output measurements were collected. Mean reference values for cardiac output ranged from 2.79 to 9.27 l/min. During periods of stable PAC-CCO (slope $< \pm 10\%$, 2 SD/mean $< 20\%$), the correlation between NICOM and thermodilution

Figure 13.
Source: Noninvasive Cardiac Output Monitors: A State-of the-Art Review. Paul E. Marik, Journal of Cardiothoracic and Vascular Anesthesia, Vol 27, No 1 (February), 2013: pp. 121-134 121

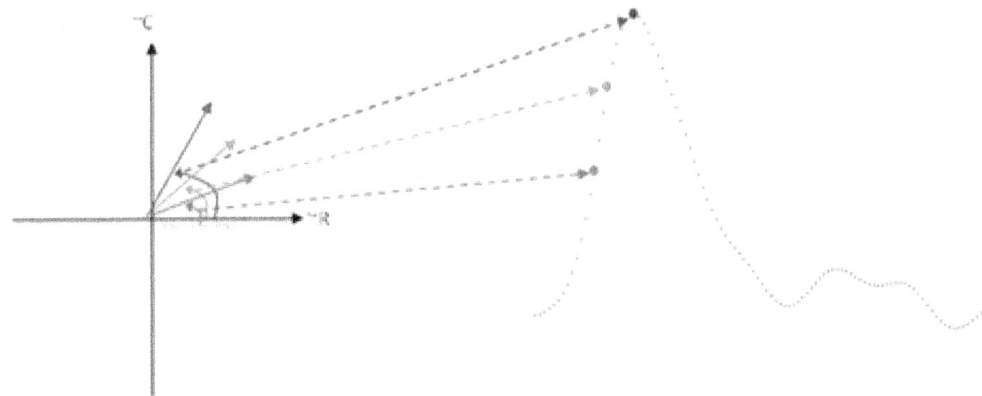

was $R = 0.82$; bias (+0.16 ± 0.52 l/min (+4.0 ± 11.3%), and relative error 9.1% ± 7.8%. In 85% of patients the relative error was < 20%. During periods of increasing output, slopes were similar with the two methods in 96% of patients and intra-class correlation was positive in 96%. Corresponding values during periods of decreasing output were 90% and 84%, respectively. Sensitivity of the NICOM for detecting significant directional changes was 93% and specificity was 93%. The study conclusions were that cardiac output measured by NICOM had most often acceptable accuracy, precision, and responsiveness in a wide range of circulatory situations (Squara 2007).

In a study of 75 post-cardiac surgery patients, bio-reactance technology demonstrated that a change in cardiac output with fluid resuscitation correlated with changes noted with SV and passive leg raise (Benomar 2010).

In a recent study by Marik, NICOM showed to predict fluid responsiveness with a change in SVI>10% via passive leg raise in 49 hemodynamically unstable critically ill patients (Marik 2013).

ESOPHAGEAL DOPPLER MONITOR FOR CARDIAC OUTPUT MEASUREMENT AND HEMODYNAMIC MONITORING

The Esophageal Doppler monitor (EDM) was developed in the 1970's as a less-invasive method for measuring aortic blood flow (CO) based on pulsed wave Doppler methodology. The probe is inserted into the esophagus of a mechanically ventilated patient. The transducer is rotated so the transducer echo crystals are facing the descending aorta, parallel to flow. The aorta is assumed to be of cylindrical shape and flow is measured by multiplying the cross-sectional area (area of a circle –aorta on short axis) by the time velocity integral over time graph dV/dT.

SV = Cross Sectional Area X VTI
CO = HR X SV
SV-Stroke volume; VTI-Time velocity integral; CO-Cardiac output

One advantage of the EDM is the ability to leave the probe in position for an extended period of time as an oral-gastric tube, lying close to the aorta, with ease for obtaining repeated measurements. EDM can also measure a corrected flow time (FTc) that represents a measure of cardiac preload. The corrected flow time is the time measured from the beginning of the aortic pulsed waveform upstroke to the return to baseline. In the calculation FTc is corrected for a HR of 60 bpm. There are a few limitations of this technology. Because this monitor only measures aortic blood flow in the descending aorta and excludes flow to aortic arch vessels, there is an assumption that a fixed cardiac output is delivered to the head and descending aorta. The cross-sectional area of the aorta is not fixed, rather it is in flux with changes in pulse pressure, vascular tone, aortic compliance, volume status and vasopressor use. Therefore, minute changes in the radius of the aorta can significantly affect cardiac output and FTc measurements. Furthermore, the placement and positioning of the Esophageal Doppler probe is operator dependent. Correct placement is essential in providing accurate data for calculation. The probe must be within 20 degrees of axial flow to measure aortic blood flow.

Validation Studies

Several studies have been conducted to validate of the EDM cardiac output measurement.

In a comparison study the (FTc) measurement obtained with the EDM showed good correlation with the (PCWP) pulmonary artery occlusion pressure for volume assessment (Hartz 1999).

In a meta-analysis performed 2004, the authors evaluated 11 EDM validation papers that showed a high validity, median bias of 0.19 L/min for cardiac output and clinical agreement of 86%. However, the majority of the studies evaluated in this meta-analysis were performed in a small set of patients, with lack of blinding and therefore there is a possibility of systemic bias (Dark 2004).

Bundgaard-Nielson et al., studied fluid optimization with SV as a guide for fluid administration versus FTc in patients undergoing radical prostatectomy. Fluid optimization was more consistent with SV for fluid administration guidance than FTc (Bundgaard-Nielson 2007).

Clinical Trials

Mythen et al., showed a statistically significant decrease in gut mucosal hypoperfusion, major complications, hospital and ICU stay in a goal directed resuscitation study, with the use of Esophageal Doppler monitor in elective cardiac surgery patients (Mythen 1995). Similar studies by others demonstrated a decrease in ICU and hospital length of stay with Esophageal Doppler goal directed fluid resuscitation therapy in postsurgical patients (Sinclair 1997; Venn 2002; Gan 2002).

A study performed on postoperative colorectal patients that received Goal Directed Fluid Therapy guided by either the NICOM or by the EDM showed that the NICOM performed similarly to the EDM. The authors concluded that the NICOM, may serve as a viable alternative to guide fluid administration (Waldron 2012).

FUTURE RESEARCH DIRECTIONS

Earlier in the chapter the pros-and cons for each monitor was discussed. In the coming years, we will see an increase in the use of less invasive and noninvasive monitors as studies further define their role in postoperative care. We have learned that there are limitations to every available method. Echocardiography modality is an attractive diagnostic tool that has established its role in the post cardiac surgery period when other monitors fail to provide enough information. However, more studies are needed to define the role of bedside echocardiography. A goal directed approach to fluid management and vasoactive substance titration in the perioperative period has shown to decrease morbidity, length of ICU stay and length of hospital stay. To date no hemodynamic monitor has shown to decrease patient mortality. In the future we may expect to see a change in practice when it comes to volume status assessment and resuscitation guidance in post cardiac surgery patients. New technologies are adopting volume responsiveness methodology rather than the use of filling pressures to guide fluid resuscitation. We may also see a change in how we assess cardiac function and measure cardiac output by means of less invasive and noninvasive methods. However, more studies are needed, likely in a "multimodal approach", to demonstrate that use of these type monitors have an impact on patient outcome.

CONCLUSION

The pulmonary artery catheter has been the most widely used technology to monitor cardiac surgery patients in the early postoperative period. In this chapter we reviewed the vibrant development of less invasive and noninvasive hemodynamic monitors for the management of critically ill patients and in early post cardiac surgery patients. Studies to date have not shown improvement in patient mortality with any particular technology for hemodynamic monitoring. However, validated less invasive and noninvasive technologies for the purpose of perioperative resuscitation have shown a decrease in ICU and hospital length of stay as well as a decrease in postoperative complications in selected postsurgical patients. Institutional culture and "team" familiarity are certainly an important factor in choosing a hemodynamic monitor for patient care. Despite greater complication risk, the use of the PAC may not be entirely replaced by other hemodynamic monitors. It remains the only monitor that continuously measures pulmonary artery pressures and remains the monitor of choice for selected patients with advanced pulmonary hypertension, while managing right heart failure and titrating selective pulmonary vasodilators.

Based on the current literature, there is growing interest among physicians in the use of less invasive and noninvasive hemodynamic monitors in post cardiac surgery and in critically ill patients. It is, therefore, fair to say that we can expect an increased use of less invasive and noninvasive hemodynamic monitors in post cardiac surgery patients in the future.

REFERENCES

Benomar, B., Ouattara, A., Estagnasie, P., Brusset, A., & Squara, P. (2010). Fluid responsiveness predicted by noninvasive bioreactance-based passive leg raise test. *Intensive Care Medicine*, *11*(11), 1875–1881. doi:10.1007/s00134-010-1990-6 PMID:20665001

Button, D., Weibel, L., Reuthebuch, O., Genoni, M., Zollinger, A., & Hofer, C. K. (2007). Clinical evaluation of the FloTrac/Vigileo system and two established continuous cardiac-output monitoring devices in patients undergoing cardiac surgery. *British Journal of Anaesthesia*, *99*(3), 329–336. doi:10.1093/bja/aem188 PMID:17631509

Camporata, L. (2010). Pitfalls in haemodynamic monitoring based on the arterial pressure waveform. *Critical Care (London, England)*, *14*(2), 124. doi:10.1186/cc8845 PMID:20236463

Cerovic, O., Golubović, V., Špec-Marn, A., Kremžar, B., & Vidmar, G. (2003). Relationship between injury severity and lactate levels in severely injured patients. *Intensive Care Medicine*, *29*(8), 1300–1305. doi:10.1007/s00134-003-1753-8 PMID:12904861

Compton, F. D., Zukunft, B., Hoffmann, C., Zidek, W., & Schaefer, J.-H. (2008). Performance of a minimally invasive uncalibrated cardiac output monitoring system (Flotrac/Vigileo) in haemodynamically unstable patients. *British Journal of Anaesthesia*, *100*(4), 451–456. doi:10.1093/bja/aem409 PMID:18256056

Critchley, L. A., & Critchley, J. A. (1999). A meta-analysis of studies using bias and precision statistics to compare cardiac output measurement techniques. *Journal of Clinical Monitoring and Computing*, *15*(2), 85–91. doi:10.1023/A:1009982611386 PMID:12578081

Dark, P. M., & Singer, M. (2004). Trans-esohphageal Doppler ultrasonography as a measure of cardiac output in critically ill adults. *Intensive Care Medicine*, *30*(11), 2060–2066. doi:10.1007/s00134-004-2430-2 PMID:15368037

de Wilde, R. B. P. (2008). Review of the PiCCO device; our experience in the ICU. *The Netherlands Journal of Critical Care*, *12*, 60–64.

Dietzman. (1969). Low cardiac output syndrome: Recognition and treatment. *The Journal of Thoracic and Cardiovascular Surgery*, *57*, 137.

Gan, T. J., Soppitt, A., Maroof, M., El-Moalem, H., Robertson, K. M., Moretti, E., & Glass, P. S. A. et al. (2002). Goal-directed intraoperative fluid administration reduces length of hospital stay after major surgery. *Anesthesiology*, *97*(4), 820–826. doi:10.1097/00000542-200210000-00012 PMID:12357146

Goepfert. (2007). Goal-directed fluid management reduces vasopressor and catecholamine use in cardiac surgery patients. *Intensive Care Medicine*, *33*, 96–103.

Hamilton, T. T., Huber, L. M., & Jessen, M. E. (2002). PulseCO: A Less-Invasive Method to Monitor Cardiac Output from Arterial Pressure after Cardiac Surgery. *The Annals of Thoracic Surgery*, *74*(4), S1408–S1412. doi:10.1016/S0003-4975(02)04059-6 PMID:12400827

Hamilton, W. F. (1932). Studies on the circulation IV. Further analysis of the injection methods and of changes in hemodynamics under physiological conditions. *The American Journal of Physiology*, *99*, 534–551.

Hartz, R. S. et al.. (1999). Esophageal Doppler ultrasound monitor versus Pulmonary artery catheter in hemodynamic management of critically ill surgical patients. *Journal of Trauma and Acute Care Surgery*, *46*(4), 607–611. doi:10.1097/00005373-199904000-00008 PMID:10217222

Hofer, C. K. (2007). Clinical evaluation of the FloTrac/Vigileo system and two established continuous cardiac output monitoring devices in patients undergoing cardiac surgery. *British Journal of Anaesthesia*, *99*(3), 329–336. doi:10.1093/bja/aem188 PMID:17631509

Husain, F. A., Martin, M. J., Mullenix, P. S., Steele, S. R., & Elliott, D. C. (2003). Serum lactate and base deficit as predictors of mortality and morbidity. *American Journal of Surgery*, *185*(5), 485–491. doi:10.1016/S0002-9610(03)00044-8 PMID:12727572

Jabbari, A. (2013). Serum lactate as a prognostic factor in coronary artery bypass graft operation by on pump method. *Caspian Journal of Internal Medicine*, *4*(2), 662–666. PMID:24009956

Kapoor, P. M., Kakani, M., Chowdhury, U., Choudhury, M., Lakshmy, R., & Kiran, U. (2008). Early goal-directed therapy in moderate to high-risk cardiac surgery patients. *Annals of Cardiac Anaesthesia*, *11*(1), 27–34. doi:10.4103/0971-9784.38446 PMID:18182756

Keren, H. (2007). Evaluation of a noninvasive continuous cardiac output monitoring system based on thoracic bioreactance. *The American Journal of Physiology*, *293*, H583–H589. PMID:17384132

Klocke. (1991). Thoracic Electrical Bioimpedance Alternative or Complement in Cardio-pulmonary Exercise Testing? *Computerized Cardiopulmonary Exercise Testing*, 63-70.

Langewouters, et al.. (1979). Computing the total arterial compliance of the arterial system from its input impedance. *Medical & Biological Engineering & Computing*, *17*(5), 623–628. doi:10.1007/BF02440907 PMID:316077

Lanier, G., Orlanes, K., Hayashi, Y., Murphy, J., Flannery, M., Te-Frey, R., & Colombo, P. C. et al. (2013). Validity and reliability of a novel slow cuff-deflation system for noninvasive blood pressure monitoring in patients with continuous-flow left ventricular assist device. *Circulation: Heart Failure*, *6*(5), 1005–1012. doi:10.1161/CIRCHEARTFAILURE.112.000186 PMID:23811966

Lorsomradee, S., Lorsomradee, S., Cromheecke, S., & De Hert, S. G. (2007). Uncalibrated arterial pulse contour analysis versus continuous thermodilution technique: Effects of alterations in arterial waveform. *Journal of Cardiothoracic and Vascular Anesthesia*, *21*(5), 636–643. doi:10.1053/j.jvca.2007.02.003 PMID:17905266

Marik, P., Monnet, X., & Teboul, J.-L. (2011). Hemodynamic parameters to guide fluid therapy. *Annals of Intensive Care*, *1*(1), 1. doi:10.1186/2110-5820-1-1 PMID:21906322

Marik, P. E., Levitov, A., Young, A., & Andrews, L. (2013). The use of bioreactance and carotid Doppler to determine volume responsiveness and blood flow redistribution following passive leg raising in hemodynamically unstable patients. *Chest*, *143*(2), 364–370. doi:10.1378/chest.12-1274 PMID:22910834

Markham, D. (2013). Sympathetic neural and hemodynamic responses to upright tilt in patients with pulsatile and non-pulsatile left ventricular assist devices. *Circulation: Heart Failure*, *6*, 293–299. PMID:23250982

Medin, D. L., Brown, D. T., Wesley, R., Cunnion, R. E., & Ognibene, F. F. (1998). Validation of continuous thermodilution cardiac output in critically ill patients with analysis of systematic errors. *Journal of Critical Care*, *13*(4), 184–189. doi:10.1016/S0883-9441(98)90004-1 PMID:9869545

Metzelder, S., Coburn, M., Fries, M., Reinges, M., Reich, S., Rossaint, R., & Rex, S. et al. (2011). Performance of cardiac output measurement derived from arterial pressure waveform analysis in patients requiring high-dose vasopressor therapy. *British Journal of Anaesthesia*, *106*(6), 776–784. doi:10.1093/bja/aer066 PMID:21441548

Michard, F. (2005). Changes in arterial pressure during mechanical ventilation. *Anesthesiology, 103*(2), 419–428. doi:10.1097/00000542-200508000-00026 PMID:16052125

Missant, C., Rex, S., & Wouters, P. F. (2008). Accuracy of cardiac output measurements with pulse contour analysis (PulseCO) and Doppler echocardiography during off-pump coronary artery bypass grafting. *European Journal of Anaesthesiology, 25*(3), 243–24. doi:10.1017/S0265021507002979 PMID:17996125

Monnet, X., Anguel, N., Jozwiak, M., Richard, C., & Teboul, J.-L. (2012). Third-generation FloTrac/Vigileo does not reliably track changes in cardiac output induced by norepinephrine in critically ill patients. *British Journal of Anaesthesia, 108*(4), 615–622. doi:10.1093/bja/aer491 PMID:22265900

Mora, B., Ince, I., Birkenberg, B., Skhirtladze, K., Pernicka, E., Ankersmit, H. J., & Dworschak, M. (2011). Validation of cardiac output measurement with the LiDCO™ pulse contour system in patients with impaired left ventricular function after cardiac surgery. *Anaesthesia, 66*(8), 675–681. doi:10.1111/j.1365-2044.2011.06754.x PMID:21564044

Mythen, M. (1995). Perioperative plasma volume expansion reduces the incidence of gut mucosal hypoperfusion during cardiac surgery. *Archives of Surgery, 130*(4), 423–429. doi:10.1001/archsurg.1995.01430040085019 PMID:7535996

Ornstein, E. (1998). Systolic pressure variation predicts the response to acute blood loss. *Journal of Clinical Anesthesia, 10*, 137–140. doi:10.1016/S0952-8180(97)00257-2 PMID:9524899

Parr. (1975). Cardiac performance and early mortality after cardiac surgery in infants and young children. *Circulation, 51*, 867.

Pearse, R., Dawson, D., Fawcett, J., Rhodes, A., Grounds, R. M., & Bennett, E. D. (2005). Early goal-directed therapy after major surgery reduces complications and duration of hospital stay. A randomised, controlled trial. *Critical Care (London, England), 9*(6), R687–R693. doi:10.1186/cc3887 PMID:16356219

Pearse, R. M., Harrison, D. A., MacDonald, N., Gillies, M. A., Blunt, M., Ackland, G., & Rowan, K. et al. (2014). Effect of a perioperative, cardiac output-guided hemodynamic therapy algorithm on outcomes following major gastrointestinal surgery: A randomized clinical trial and systematic review. *Journal of the American Medical Association, 311*(21), 2181–2190. doi:10.1001/jama.2014.5305 PMID:24842135

Phan, T. D. (2011). A comparison of three minimally invasive cardiac output devices with thermodilution in elective cardiac surgery. *Anaesthesia and Intensive Care Journal, 39*, 1014–1021. PMID:22165352

Sagawa, K. (1990). "Translation of Otto Frank's Paper" Otto Frank. (1899). "Die Grundform des Arteriellen Pulses" Zeitschriftfür Biologie, 37, 483-526. *Journal of Molecular and Cellular Cardiology, 22*(3), 253–254. doi:10.1016/0022-2828(90)91459-K PMID:2192068

Sakka, S. G., Kozieras, J., Thuemer, O., & van Hout, N. (2007). Measurement of cardiac output: A comparison between transpulmonary thermodilution and uncalibrated pulse contour analysis. *British Journal of Anaesthesia, 99*(3), 337–342. doi:10.1093/bja/aem177 PMID:17611251

Sander, M., Spies, C. D., Grubitzsch, H., Foer, A., Müller, M., & von Heymann, C. (2006). Comparison of uncalibrated arterial waveform analysis in cardiac surgery patients with thermodilution cardiac output measurements. *Critical Care (London, England), 10*(6), R164. doi:10.1186/cc5103 PMID:17118186

Sandham. (2003). Randomized, Controlled Trial of the Use of Pulmonary-Artery Catheters in High-Risk Surgical Patients. *The New England Journal of Medicine, 348*, 5-14.

Senn, A., Button, D., Zollinger, A., & Hofer, C. K. (2007). Assessment of the cardiac output changes using a modified FloTrac/Vigileo Algorithm in cardiac surgery patients. *Critical Care (London, England), 13*(2), R32. doi:10.1186/cc7739 PMID:19261180

Sinclair. (1997). Intraoperative intravascular volume optimization and length of hospital stay after repair of proximal femoral fracture: randomized controlled trial. *The BMJ, 315*, 909–12.

Slaughter, M. S., Rogers, J. G., Milano, C. A., Russell, S. D., Conte, J. V., Feldman, D., & Frazier, O. H. et al. (2009). HeartMate II Investigators. Advanced heart failure treated with continuous-flow left ventricular assist device. *The New England Journal of Medicine, 361*(23), 2241–2251. doi:10.1056/NEJMoa0909938 PMID:19920051

Squara, P., Denjean, D., Estagnasie, P., Brusset, A., Dib, J. C., & Dubois, C. (2007). Noninvasive cardiac output monitoring (NICOM): A clinical validation. *Intensive Care Medicine, 33*(7), 1191–1194. doi:10.1007/s00134-007-0640-0 PMID:17458538

Uchino S, et al., (2006). Pulmonary artery catheter versus pulse contour analysis: a prospective epidemiological study. *Critical Care, 10*(6), R 174.

Venn, R. (2002). Randomized controlled trial to investigate influence of the fluid challenge on duration of hospital stay and perioperative morbidity in patients with hip fractures. *British Journal of Anaesthesia, 88*(1), 65–67. doi:10.1093/bja/88.1.65 PMID:11881887

Wakeling, H. G., Barclay, G. R., & Fleming, S. C. (2005). Intraoperative Oesophageal Doppler guided fluid management shortens postoperative hospital stay after major bowel surgery. *British Journal of Anaesthesia, 95*(5), 634–642. doi:10.1093/bja/aei223 PMID:16155038

Waldron, N. (2012). *A Prospective Comparison of Outcomes in NICOM- Versus EDM-Guided Goal Directed Fluid Therapy*. Duke Anesthesia Celebration of Research.

Weisenack, C. et al.. (2001). Assessment of intrathoracic blood volume as an indicator of cardiac preload: Single transpulmonary thermodilution technique vs assessment of pressure preloadparameters derived from a pulmonary artery catheter. *Journal of Cardiothoracic and Vascular Anesthesia, 15*(5), 584–588. doi:10.1053/jcan.2001.26536 PMID:11687999

Xiaobo, Y. (2014). Does pulse pressure variation predict fluid responsiveness in critically ill patients? A systematic review and meta-analysis. *Critical Care (London, England), 18*(6), 650. doi:10.1186/s13054-014-0650-6 PMID:25427970

ADDITIONAL READING

Funk, M., Moretti, E. W., & Gan, T. J. (2009). Minimally invasive cardiac output monitoring in the perioperative setting. *Anesthesia and Analgesia, 108*(3), 887–897. doi:10.1213/ane.0b013e31818ffd99 PMID:19224798

Pittman, J. A. L., Ping, J. S., & Mark, J. B.Pittman & Mark. (2004). Arterial and Central Venous Pressure Monitoring. *International Anesthesiology Clinics*, *42*(1), 13–30. doi:10.1097/00004311-200404210-00004 PMID:14716195

Sandham. (2003). Randomized, Controlled Trial of the Use of Pulmonary-Artery Catheters in High-Risk Surgical Patients. *The New England Journal of Medicine, 348*, 5-14.

KEY TERMS AND DEFINITIONS

Cardiac Output (CO): Cardiac output is the amount of blood that the heart ejects in one minute and can be determined by multiplying stroke volume with the heart rate.

Mixed Venous Oxygen Saturation (SVO2): Mixed venous oxygen saturation is the oxygen saturation in the blood after oxygen has been extracted from the entire body, including the heart with its contribution via the coronary sinus.

Pulsus Alternans: Represents alternating strong and weak beats seen in congestive heart failure.

Pulsus Bisferens: Is a bi-phasic tracing observed in aortic insufficiency. It also can be palpated as a double peak pulse.

Pulsus Paradoxus: Is an exaggerated decrease (greater than 10 mmHg) in SBP and wave amplitude during inspiration in Cardiac Tamponade.

Systolic Pressure (SBP) and Stroke Volume Variation (SVV): Positive pressure inspiration rapidly increases left atrium and therefore left ventricular filling from the pulmonary veins. During positive pressure inspiration left ventricular afterload also decreases. This transient increase in preload and decrease in afterload accounts for a transient increase in stroke volume. The stroke volume and therefore measured pulse pressure variation is exaggerated with hypovolemia.

Chapter 31
Management of Bleeding in the Postoperative Cardiac Patient

Nadia Hensley
Johns Hopkins University School of Medicine, USA

Marc Sussman
Johns Hopkins University School of Medicine, USA

ABSTRACT

Bleeding in the postoperative cardiac surgical patient can be multifactorial. This chapter examines the preoperative and intraoperative risk factors for having significant postoperative bleeding. It also discuss the advantages and disadvantages of standard laboratory testing as well as point-of-care tests, such as thromboelastography (TEG) and thromboelastometry (ROTEM), in their diagnostic capabilities. Finally, we conclude with different treatment strategies in this challenging patient population along with diagnostic criteria of clinically significant postoperative bleeding and when to return to the operating room for re-exploration.

DIAGNOSING THE COAGULOPATHY

Preoperative Coagulopathy Risk Factors in the Cardiac Surgery Patient

The cardiac surgical patient may have many reasons for having a coagulopathy prior to surgery and a complete history and physical examination preoperatively should reveal these risk factors. These include known coagulation factor deficiencies that are congenital or acquired, pharmacotherapy, concurrent systemic disease such as renal failure or severe liver compromise and rarely, infection causing disseminated intravascular coagulopathy (DIC).

The most common of these is pharmacotherapy since many of these patients have had recent non-ST elevated myocardial infarctions (NSTEMI) or ST elevated myocardial infarctions (STEMI) and had a loading dose of either thienopyridines, such as Plavix, or glycoprotein IIb/IIIa inhibitors, i.e., tirofiban. In acute coronary syndromes, atherosclerotic plaque is disrupted and activates platelet aggregation and intracoronary thrombus formation which can subsequently lead to further myocardial infarction territory

DOI: 10.4018/978-1-4666-8603-8.ch031

and death (Boersma et al., 2002). Thienopyridines inhibit P2Y12 receptors on platelets and given with aspirin, which inhibits cyclooxygenase-1 enzyme, constitutes the standard of care of dual antiplatelet therapy (Silvain et al., 2011). Dual antiplatelet therapy is recommended by the American College of Cardiology, American Heart Association, American College of Chest Physicians and European Society of Cardiology for patients undergoing percutaneous coronary interventions (PCI) with STEMI or with unstable angina/NSTEMI(Hirsh et al., 2008).

Other pharmacotherapies that may interfere with a balanced coagulation system prior to cardiac surgery are vitamin K antagonists, such as warfarin, direct IIa (thrombin) inhibitors, i.e. dabigatran or direct Xa inhibitors, i.e. rivaroxaban. These drugs can be used to prevent stroke in those patients with atrial fibrillation. Unfractionated heparin is a class I recommended treatment after the diagnosis of unstable angina/NSTEMI or STEMI is made (Jneid et al., 2012). Heparin exerts its effect by accelerating the action of antithrombin, a proteolytic enzyme that inactivates IIa (thrombin), IXa and Xa. The use of unfractionated heparin can lead to an acquired factor deficiency or heparin resistance.

A final category of drugs that potentially interferes with normal clotting mechanisms are the herbal supplements and vitamins. These have become increasingly popular in recent decades, from 22% in the 1990s to approximately 60% currently (Eisenberg et al., 1998; Heller et al., 2006). Fish oil is one of the leading vitamins due to its beneficial effects in preventing cardiovascular diseases. Decreased thromboxane A2 production, prolonged bleeding time, and attenuated platelet aggregation have been demonstrated to be a dose-dependent complication of fish oil (Marsh & Coombes, 2006; Schmidt, Varming, Ernst, Madsen, & Dyerberg, 1990). Even though these effects on the hemostatic pathway are known, the controversy lies in if these mechanisms cause clinically significant bleeding. Two recent studies in patients undergoing lumbar decompression surgery demonstrated no increase in intraoperative and postoperative bleeding (Kepler, Huang, Meredith, Kim, & Sharma, 2012; Meredith et al., 2012). Other popular herbal and vitamin supplements that may increase bleeding in the surgical patient are garlic, ginkgo biloba, ginseng, saw palmetto, chrondroitin and glucosamine, and vitamin E (Wong, Gabriel, Maxwell, & Gupta, 2012).

Uremia due to renal failure can cause a coagulopathy that is multifactorial and includes intrinsic platelet defects as well as abnormal platelet-endothelial interaction (Weigert & Schafer, 1998). Most importantly is platelet dysfunction which is due to both decreased platelet aggregation and impaired platelet adhesiveness. Diminished platelet adhesiveness is most likely caused by intrinsic dysfunction of glycoprotein IIa/IIIb in uremia, a platelet membrane glycoprotein which actions include platelet aggregation and adhesion by its interaction with fibrinogen and von Willebrand factor (Gawaz et al., 1994). Severe liver disease can cause most coagulation factors to be present in decreased quantity. Liver dysfunction also results in additional sialic acid residues on fibrinogen and other factors that impair coagulation. Splenomegaly, in these patients, can cause thrombocytopenia. Impaired clearance of endogenous plasminogen activators accentuates fibrinolysis and decreased levels of coagulation inhibitors induce a consumptive coagulopathy in cirrhotic patients (Marengo-Rowe AJ, 1988). In patients suffering from endocarditis, a coagulopathy can occur in the preoperative period due to low coagulation factors. Low coagulation factors may be caused by DIC, as well as by loss of plasma and impaired hepatic synthesis in the course of sepsis (Levi, Toh, Thachil, & Watson, 2009).

The preoperative cardiac surgical patient may have congenital or acquired coagulation factor deficiencies. von Willebrand disease is the most common inherited coagulopathy since it is an autosomal dominant disorder with variable expressivity. It has an incident rate of 1.4 to 5 cases per 1000 population (B. D. Spiess,,, Jay Horrow, Joel A. Kaplan 2011). Heyde's syndrome has recently been recognized as a type IIa, acquired von Willebrand disorder, due to a deficiency of high-molecular-weight von Willebrand factor (vWF) multimers in patients with severe aortic stenosis(Loscalzo, 2012). Blood flow through the stenotic aortic valves alters the conformation of the high-molecular-weight (HMW) vWF multimers and therefore, they are reduced in size and hemostatically less competent.

The cardiac surgical patient may have one or more of these risk factors and mitigation of hemorrhage intraoperatively and postoperatively can occur through conducting a thorough history and physical examination which will reveal these hazards.

Intraoperative Coagulopathy Risk Factors in the Cardiac Surgery Patient

Just as there are numerous risk factors for bleeding preoperatively for the cardiac surgical patient, there are several intraoperatively as well. Cardiopulmonary bypass (CPB), hypothermia and the surgical dissection, itself, are all risk factors intraoperatively that can impair coagulation postoperatively. Exposure of blood to the CPB circuit leads to activation of both the contact activation pathway (intrinsic) and tissue factor (extrinsic) pathway. This activation results in excessive thrombin and fibrinolytic activity, which can lead to a consumptive coagulopathy of platelets and clotting factors (G. Despotis, Eby, & Lublin, 2008).

Thrombocytopenia during CPB occurs as a result of hypothermia-induced splenic sequestration of platelets, hemodilution, and platelet destruction by cardiotomy suction and filters (. Spiess, Horrow, & Kaplan, 2011). Platelet factor 4 (PF4) is a cytokine and β-thromboglobulin (β-TG) is a platelet-specific protein released from alpha-granules of activated platelets (Kehara, Takano, Ohashi, Terasaki, & Amano, 2014). Several studies that used CPB circuits and cardiotomy suction and reservoir have shown significantly higher PF4 and βTG concentrations at the end of CPB than before (Izuha et al., 2005; Morgan, Codispoti, Sanger, & Mankad, 1998). However, Kehara et al., recently found in their study of roller pumps versus centrifugal pumps that they did not have significantly higher concentrations of PF4 or βTG when they did not utilize cardiotomy suction and reservoir(Kehara et al., 2014). Fibrinogen and fibrin, which adhere to artificial surfaces of the CPB circuit, activate platelet adhesion and aggregation. CPB down-regulates glycoprotein (GP)1b and GP IIb/IIIa receptors and decreases platelet responsiveness to thrombin and adenosine diphosphate (ADP)(Gelb et al., 1996; Maquelin et al., 1998; Rinder et al., 1991).

Activation of the fibrinolytic system at the onset of CPB is mainly limited to the intrinsic coagulation pathway due to blood contact with the foreign CPB surface. Fibrinolysis then becomes extrinsically activated by release of tissue plasminogen activator (t-PA) from vascular walls during bypass (Paparella, Brister, & Buchanan, 2004). Activation of the fibrinolytic system may contribute to platelet dysfunction. Formation of plasmin affects platelet membrane receptors (Adelman, Rizk, & Hanners, 1988). Fibrinolysis during bypass is also associated with increases in D-dimer, t-PA-plasminogen activator inhibitor-1 (PAI-1) complexes and a decrease in PAI-1 levels. PAI-1 is a serine protease that inhibits t-PA and other components of the fibrinolytic system (Paparella et al., 2004).

Hypothermia can effect coagulation by many mechanisms. As previously mentioned, platelet sequestration occurs in the spleen as result of hypothermia (Spiess, Horrow, & Kaplan, 2011). Hypothermia also causes decreased creation of thromboxane A2 by inhibition of thromboxane synthetase; thromboxane A2 is necessary for platelet activation and aggregation (Valeri et al., 1987). Hypothermia most likely promotes pathologic platelet aggregation in the presence of enhanced platelet activators (Faraday & Rosenfeld, 1998). Cold core body temperatures inhibit thrombin and thromboxane-induced platelet aggregation, increase in platelet surface expression of P-selectin (reflecting alpha granule secretion), and decrease in platelet surface expression of glycoprotein GP1b-IX complex (vWF receptor)(Michelson, 1994). Hypothermia slows the enzymatic cleavage of clotting zymogens (inactive coagulation factors) to serine proteases (active coagulation factors).

DIAGNOSING THE COAGULOPATHY POSTOPERATIVELY BY STANDARD LABORATORY OR POINT-OF-CARE TESTING

Traditional laboratory testing such as prothrombin time (PT), activated partial thromboplastin time (aPTT), fibrinogen and platelet count are significantly helpful to the clinician in guiding transfusion management of the postoperative bleeding cardiac surgical patient. However, the deficiencies are: 1) time in obtaining results; 2) quantitative measurements of platelets do not assess qualitative function; 3) PT and PTT provide information only on the initiation of clot formation not the strength or stability of the clot (Whiting & DiNardo, 2014). Point- of- care tests (POCTs) such as activated clotting time (ACT), thromboelastography (TEG) or rotational thromboelastometry (ROTEM), and platelet function POCTs, such as PlateletWorks®, can aid in establishing the diagnosis of clotting factor or platelet deficiency or unneutralized heparin quickly. After CPB, the ACT should normalize or return to the patient's baseline, which demonstrates sufficient neutralization of heparin with protamine. The ACT measures the time until fibrin is formed and it correlates with the partial thromboplastin time(B. D. Spiess et al., 1987). Because the PT and aPTT usually are prolonged by several seconds after CPB, only values more than 1.5 times control are concerning for need for replacement or consideration of remaining circulating heparin.

Both ROTEM and TEG assess clot formation/lysis kinetics and strength by measuring the amount of a continuously applied rotational force that is imparted to an electromechanical transduction system by developing clot(Whiting & DiNardo, 2014). TEG utilizes a cylindrical cup containing the whole blood sample that oscillates through 4° 45' every 5 seconds and a pin on a torsion wire is suspended in the blood. As the viscoelastic strength increases in the clot, more tension is applied to the wire and this is transmitted to the electromagnetic transducer (Fig 1)(Whiting & DiNardo, 2014). ROTEM uses a fixed cup of whole blood while the pin suspended on a ball bearing mechanism oscillates through 4° 75' every 6 seconds through application of a constant force. As the viscoelastic strength increases, the pin rotation is hindered and is detected optically using a charge coupled device image sensor system (Fig 2). Figures 3 and 4 demonstrate the graphic display for ROTEM and TEG, respectively.

Standard TEG may be sensitive to many causes of platelet dysfunction, however, it is insensitive to most drug-induced causes of platelet damage. This is due to the presence of thrombin in standard TEG cups. Standard TEG is insensitive to antiplatelet effects of COX-1 inhibitors (aspirin and other NSAIDS) and P2Y12 antagonists (ticlopidine and clopidogrel). However, it is sensitive to GP IIb/IIIa inhibitors since they have a thrombin independent pathway of platelet impairment(Gibbs, 2009).

In the ICHOR PlateletWorks® (Helena Laboratories, Beaumont, TX, USA), the platelet count in a 'control' ethylenediamine tetra-acetic blood sample is compared to platelet count in a similar 'test' sample that has been exposed to a platelet agonist. In patients with normal platelets, the platelet agonist reduces the platelet count to almost zero due to aggregation. The platelet count in the 'control' is not affected since there is no agonist. However, in the abnormal platelets there will be an attenuated effect of the agonist and a diminished ratio of 'test' to 'control' platelet counts(Gibbs, 2009).

Another POC platelet function test is whole blood impedance aggregometry which was introduced by Cardinal and Flower(Cardinal & Flower, 1980). It is based on attachment of platelets on 2 platinum electrodes resulting in an increase of electrical resistance between the electrodes. The change in resistance (impedance) is recorded and is proportional to amount of platelets sticking to electrodes. There is the ability to have 4 electrodes per test cell with the multiple electrode aggregometry (MEA) analyzer or Multiplate®. Platelet dysfunction mediated by antiplatelet drugs like aspirin, nonsteroidal anti-inflammatory

Figure 1. A depiction of a TEG device in which a pin suspended from a torsion wire is immersed in a cup of whole blood. The cup is held in a heating block and continually oscillates through 4° 45' every 5 sec. Changes in viscoelastic strength are directly transmitted to the torsion wire and detected by an electromechanical transducer.
Used with permission by Whiting, D. & Dinardo, J.A. TEG and ROTEM: Technology and clinical applications. Am J Hematol. 2013;89:228-232.

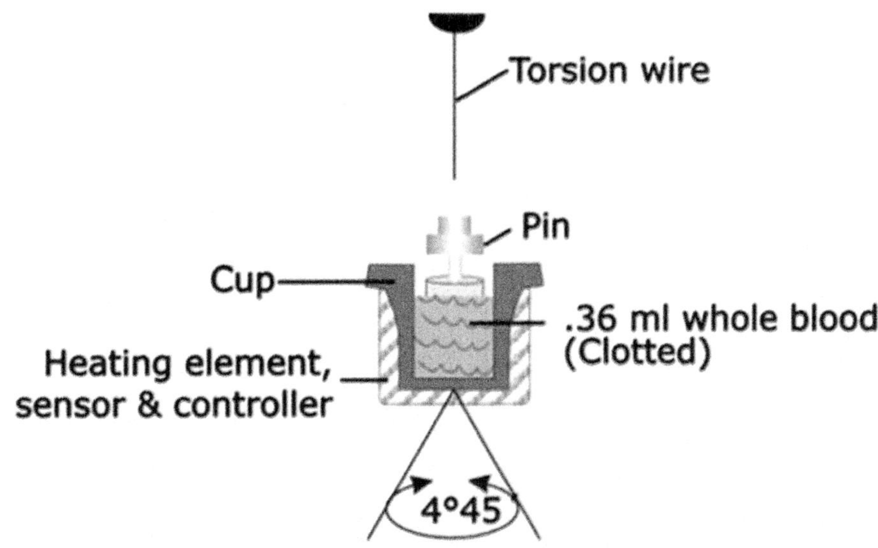

drugs, platelet P2Y12 receptor antagonists, glycoprotein IIb/IIIa receptor antagonists, or by CPB itself can be detected by whole blood impedance(Kozek-Langenecker, 2010; Velik-Salchner et al., 2009).

TREATMENT STRATEGIES FOR COAGULOPATHY IN THE POST-CARDIAC SURGICAL PATIENT

Several prospective studies have demonstrated reduced transfusion of allogeneic blood products utilizing a TEG-based algorithm in deciding how to treat post-bypass coagulopathy. Shore-Lesserson et al. demonstrated that by utilizing a TEG-based algorithm to treat post-bypass bleeding in a randomized, blinded, prospective trial, that there were significantly fewer postoperative and total transfusions (Shore-Lesserson et al., 1999). Ak et al. performed a prospective randomized trial looking at two groups (Ak et al., 2009). The 1st group was transfused by clinician discretion and standard lab tests and the 2nd group was transfused by TEG-based algorithm (Table 1)(Ak et al., 2009; Royston & von Kier, 2001). The 2nd group had significantly lower median units of FFP and platelets compared with the other group, as well as total allogeneic units and transexamic acid(Ak et al., 2009). Royston et al. also demonstrated that the amount of allogeneic products given in the TEG-algorithm group was significantly less that that given in the clinician "wishes" group(Royston & von Kier, 2001).

Figure 2. A depiction of a ROTEM device in which a cup of whole blood remains fixed in a heating block while a pin suspended on a ball bearing mechanism initially oscillates through 4° 75' every 6 sec. The subsequent rotation of the pin is inversely related to the viscoelastic clot strength and detected optically using a charge coupled device (CDD) image sensor system.
Used with permission by Whiting, D. & Dinardo, J.A. TEG and ROTEM: Technology and clinical applications. Am J Hematol. 2013; 89:228-232.

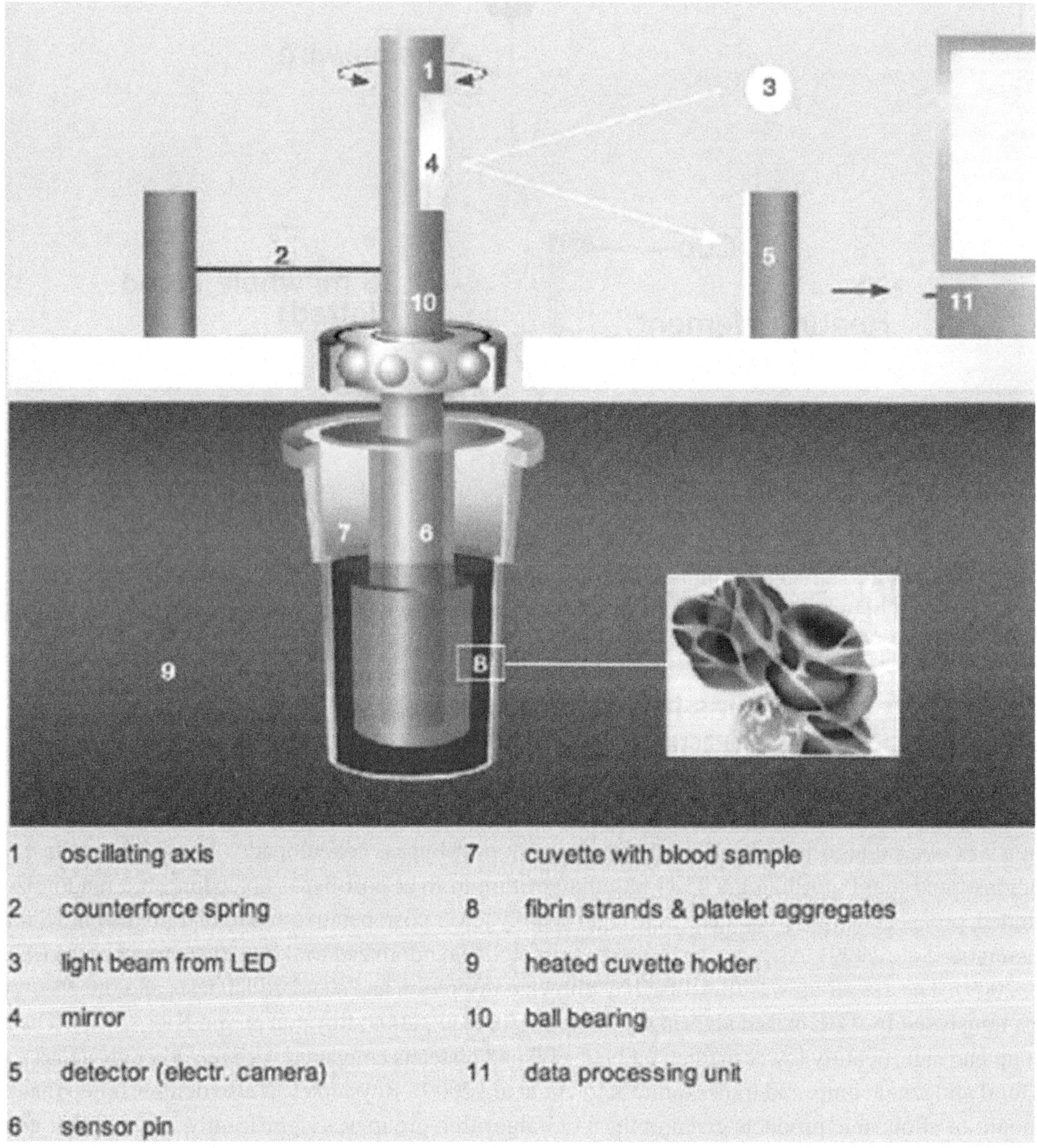

Figure 3. (a) A depiction of a ROTEM output demonstrating clot initiation, propagation, stabilization, and lysis. (b) A depiction of a TEG output demonstrating clot initiation, propagation, stabilization, and lysis. Used with permission by Whiting, D. & Dinardo, J.A. TEG and ROTEM: Technology and clinical applications. Am J Hematol. 2013;89:228-232.

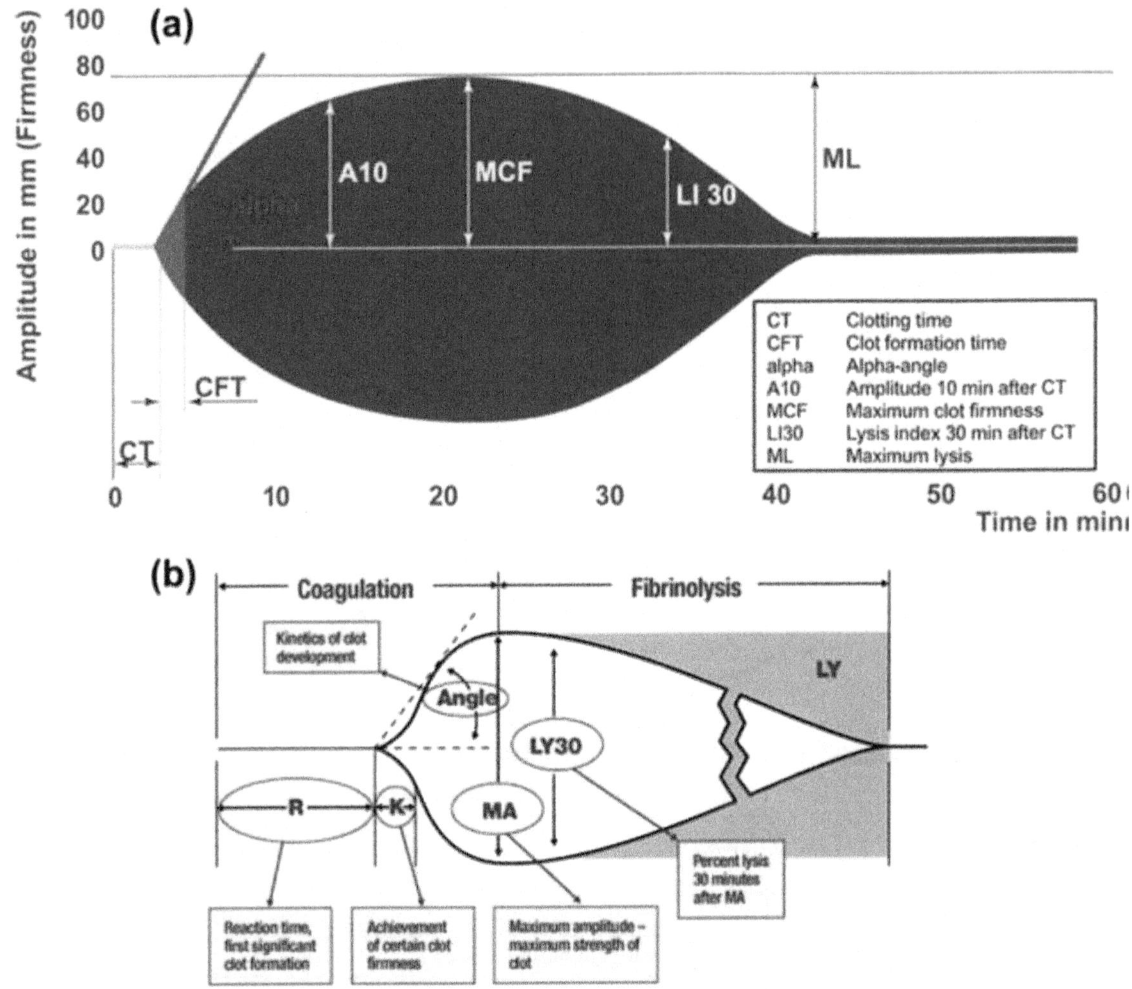

Similarly, ROTEM-based algorithms have been developed to treat post-cardiac surgical bleeding. In a retrospective cohort study including 3,865 patients, a coagulation management algorithm based on first line therapy with specific coagulation factor concentrates combined with ROTEM results was associated with significantly and substantially decreased allogeneic blood transfusion (primary end point) as well as decreased incidence of thrombotic and thromboembolic events (Gorlinger et al., 2011). It also must be kept in mind that most of these studies are small, single institution, randomized studies with different control arms, with and without POC platelet function analysis. Recently a systematic review with meta-analyses of randomized clinical trials (RCTs) of TEG/ROTEM-based algorithm compared with standard treatment in bleeding patients with the primary outcome being all-cause mortality(Wikkelsoe, Afshari, Wetterslev, Brok, & Moeller, 2011). It found that ROTEM and TEG-based treatment algorithms

Figure 4. The relationship between a normal TEG output and standard tests of coagulation, the PT, and PTT, is depicted. Note that PT and PTT provide information only on the initiation of clot formation; information similar to that provided by the R of the TEG. R=reaction rate= time in minutes it takes for the trace to reach an amplitude of 2 mm. K=kinetics time= time necessary for clot amplitude to increase from 2 to 20 mm. α°=angle=determined by creating a tangent line from the point of clot initiation (R) to the slope of the developing curve. MA=maximum amplitude=peak amplitude (strength) of the clot. A30/A60= Lysis 30 and Lysis 60= the percent reductions in the area under the TEG curve, assuming MA remains constant, that occur 30 and 60 min after MA is reached.

Used with permission by Whiting, D. & Dinardo, J.A. TEG and ROTEM: Technology and clinical applications. Am J Hematol. 2013;89:228-232.

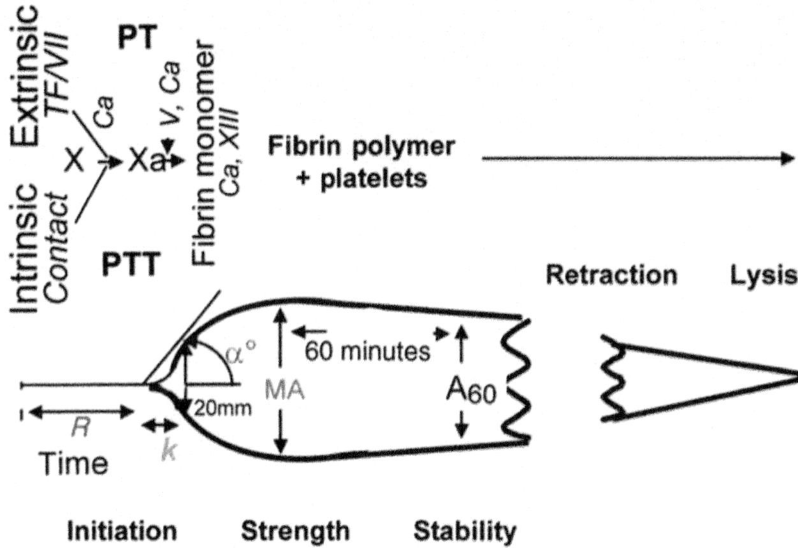

Table 1. Modified version of the TEG-based transfusion algorithm proposed by Royston and Kier

TEG Parameter		Treatment
14< r < 21 (mm)	Mild deficiency in coagulation factors*	1 unit FFP
21≤ r < 28 (mm)	Moderate deficiency in coagulation factors*	2 units FFP
r ≥ 28 (mm)	Severe deficiency in coagulation factors*	4 units FFP
40 ≤ MA < 48 (mm)	Moderate deficiency in the number/ function of platelets	1 unit platelets+
MA < 40 (mm)	Severe deficiency in the number/function of platelets	2 units platelets
LY30 > 7.5 (%)	Exaggerated fibrinolysis	TA

FFP=fresh frozen plasma; TA=tranexamic acid *=If the r time on the heparinase TEG was less than one-half of the nonheparinase r time. + represents single-donor platelets obtained by apheresis are the equivalent of approximately six platelet concentrates. Obtained by permission from Ak, K. et al. J Card Surg 2009;24:404-410.

may reduce the amount of blood loss in patients requiring massive transfusion with no evidence that this results in an attenuation of transfused blood or either morbidity or mortality.

Fibrinogen is vitally important in the clotting process, as it is both a precursor to fibrin and a cofactor that enhances platelet aggregation (Lowe, Rumley, & Mackie, 2004). It induces platelet activation and aggregation by binding to the platelet fibrinogen receptor glycoprotein IIb/IIIa (Mosesson, 2005). Additionally, as the substrate of clot formation, fibrinogen represents greater than 90% of all plasmatic coagulation factors by weight (Gorlinger et al., 2013). Fibrinogen is only available in the vascular space and therefore, there are no reserves that can be mobilized in case of severe bleeding. It is the first to drop below a critical level in large volume bleeding, whereas other coagulation factors and platelets remain at acceptable values for a longer time.

Cryoprecipitate is one of the blood products administered that can replenish fibrinogen. It is formed by careful thawing of plasma in order to precipitate the high molecular weight proteins, such as vWF, factor VIII and fibrinogen. The precipitated proteins are separated by centrifugation, re-suspended in small volumes of plasma and stored frozen (Franchini & Lippi, 2012). Most transfusion guidelines recommend treating with cryoprecipitate once the fibrinogen level reaches 0.8-1.0 g/L(American Society of Anesthesiologists Task Force on Perioperative Blood & Adjuvant, 2006). However, these recommendations are based primarily on expert opinion and may need to be revised in order to reflect the need in current practice.

Toronto General recently reported on a retrospective observational study of 4,606 cardiac surgical patients and the relationship between post-CPB fibrinogen level with large volume transfusion (Karkouti et al., 2013). The cubic spline function graphs suggested the probability of large amount of transfusion increased when fibrinogen levels decreased below 2.0 g/L. They categorized patients into either normal fibrinogen (≥2.0 g/L) or low fibrinogen (<2.0 g/L) groups to assess the independent relationship between low fibrinogen levels and large volume red cell transfusion. Even though the 2 groups had very similar bleeding risk scores, the low fibrinogen group received significantly more transfusions that the normal fibrinogen group (Karkouti et al., 2013). This retrospective observational study suggests we need a more aggressive approach to replacement of fibrinogen than earlier recommendations.

The disadvantages for utilizing cryoprecipitate to replace fibrinogen include: 1) it is necessary to perform blood group matching; 2) time to thaw; 3) a risk of viral transmission similar to FFP. Fibrinogen concentrate is produced from pooled human plasma using the Cohn/Oncley cryoprecipitation procedure (Rahe-Meyer & Sorensen, 2011). The concentration of fibrinogen is standardized (unlike cryoprecipitate) and the product is stored as a lyophilized powder at room temperature that can be reconstituted quickly with sterile water.

Prothrombin Complex Concentrate (PCC) are a group of coagulation factor concentrates that have significant variability in their composition (Kalina, Bickhard, & Schulte, 2008). The 4-factor PCCs used in Europe seem to have well-balanced contents with factors II, VII, IX and X and inhibitors (proteins C and S). However, the 3-factor PCC's utilized in the United States contain only very small amounts of factor VII and proteins C and S(Gorlinger et al., 2013). There is a concern regarding the efficacy and safety of these products (3-factor PCC's) in the setting of coagulopathic perioperative bleeding(Holland et al., 2009).

Gorlinger et al. published a single-center, retrospective cohort study examining first-line therapy with coagulation factor concentrates combined with point-of-care (POC) coagulation testing(Gorlinger et al., 2011). Incidence of any allogeneic blood transfusion (52.5 vs. 42.2%; $p<0.0001$), packed red blood cells (49.7 vs. 40.4%; $p<0.0001$), and fresh frozen plasma (19.4 vs. 1.1%; $p<0.0001$) decreased, whereas platelet transfusion increased (10.1 vs. 13.0%; p=0.004). Their POC methods included activated clotting time (ACT), thromboelastrometry (ROTEM) and multiple electrode aggregometry (MEA). The decrease in transfusion was seen in both study periods of with aprotinin and after aprotinin was replaced by tranexamic acid. Their rationale for using fibrinogen concentrate is due to evidence that it has been very effective in decreasing blood loss and transfusions in cardiac surgery without increased incidence of thromboembolic events(Karlsson et al., 2009; Rahe-Meyer, Pichlmaier, et al., 2009; Rahe-Meyer, Solomon, et al., 2009).

Many studies have also noted the length of cardiopulmonary bypass (CPB) and attenuation of all elements of coagulation. Despotis et al. found an association between CPB duration and increased hemostatic transfusion (G. J. Despotis et al., 1996). Other studies have reported CPB duration has a direct impact on bleeding time measured 2 hours after discontinuation of bypass and attributed mainly to platelet dysfunction due to cardiotomy suction (Khuri et al., 1992). Increased CBP duration also results in more hypothermic time which can affect enzymatic reactions of coagulation assessed by *in vitro* assays(Rohrer & Natale, 1992).

DIAGNOSTIC CRITERIA FOR SIGNIFICANT BLEEDING IN THE POSTOPERATIVE CARDIAC PATIENT

The amount of bleeding occurring in the operating room prior to placement of chest tubes is largely a qualitative estimate. Amongst the factors considered include the amount of blood being collected in suction canisters, and the rapidity with which sponges become saturated. Once chest tubes have been placed and the chest is either closed or covered with an occlusive dressing, the amount of blood loss is easier to measure; however, greater or lesser amounts of blood may be sequestered in the mediastinal or pleural spaces. There is not a generally recognized amount of bleeding that is deemed excessive, although many surgeons would consider greater than 100-150ml/hr in the first few hours after surgery cause for concern. The lack of coordination in this area is highlighted by the fact that the STS Database deals with bleeding, not by amount, but only with take backs for bleeding (STS Data Collection Form). The amount of bleeding to be expected will vary with the preoperative integrity of the elements of hemostasis, as well as the complexity of the surgery (See Table 2). The surgeon has an effect on the amount of bleeding as well (Dixon et al., 2014). Recently a group was formed that proposed a "Universal Definition of Perioperative Bleeding". This is summarized in Table 3 for characterizing postoperative bleeding (Dyke et al., 2014). When this was evaluated in a test population, greater amounts of bleeding were associated with higher mortality.

Decisions about when to leave the operating room when a patient is still bleeding and when and whether to return to the operating room if the patient continues to bleed are primarily based on the surgeon's experience. Meticulous hemostasis has been a dictum since the advent of modern surgery. However, this cannot be achieved in the face of a severe coagulopathy. Furthermore, diffuse bleeding due to coagulopathy will tend to obscure discrete sources of bleeding. Rather than persist, most surgeons will close, or at least cover the wound with a sterile dressing and proceed to the ICU to continue resuscitation. Closing the wound may allow pressure of surrounding tissues to aid in hemostasis and will diminish the heat loss from an open wound.

Management of continued bleeding in the ICU follows the same algorithms as in the OR to replete those components of the hemostasis cascades that are diminished or dysfunctional. In addition, atten-

Table 2. Common causes of postoperative bleeding, diagnostic tests, and treatment strategy

Common Causes for Postoperative Bleeding	Diagnostic Tests	Treatment Strategy
Inadequate platelet number/platelet dysfunction	CBC/TEG/PlateletWorks®/ whole blood impedance aggregometry	Platelet transfusion
Inadequate Coagulation Factor Quantity	INR/Fibrinogen concentration/TEG	FFP/cryoprecipitate/fibrinogen concentrate/ Prothrombin Complex Concentrate
Residual anticoagulant (heparin)	aPTT/TEG	Protamine
Excessive fibrinolysis	TEG	Amicar/tranexamic acid

CBC=complete blood count; TEG=thromboelastography; FFP=fresh frozen plasma; aPTT=activated partial thromboplastin time

Table 3. Universal definition for perioperative bleeding

Bleeding Definition	Sternal Closure Delayed	Postoperative Chest Tube Blood Loss within 12 Hours (mL)	pRBC (Units)	FFP (Units)	PLT (Units)	Cryoprecipitate	PCCs	RFVIIa	Reexploration/ Tamponade
Class 0 (insignificant)	No	<600	0*	0	0	No	No	No	No
Class 1 (mild)	No	601-800	1	0	0	No	No	No	No
Class 2 (moderate)	No	801-1000	2-4	2-4	Yes	Yes	Yes	No	No
Class 3 (severe)	Yes	1001-2000	5-10	5-10	N/A	N/A	N/A	No	Yes
Class 4 (massive)	N/A	>2000	>10	>10	N/A	N/A	N/A	Yes	N/A

pRBC=packed red blood cells; FFP=fresh frozen plasma; PLT= platelet concentrates; PCCs= prothrombin complex concentrates; rVIIa=recombinant factor VII; N/A=not applicable. *Correction of preoperative anemia or hemodilution only; the number of pRBCs used should only be considered in the universal definition for perioperative bleeding when accompanied by other signs of perioperative bleeding.

Used by permission from Dyke et al. (Dyke et al., 2014)

tion is turned to maintaining normothermia. Utilizing point- of- care testing in the ICU maybe more difficult than it is in the operating room. In particular, for many ICUs it will be difficult to maintain a cadre of staff to run the tests and maintain the devices, including quality control, when they are used infrequently. Although point- of- care testing has shown benefits, it remains to be seen if similar results can be obtained with improved protocols using lab- based testing (Thiele & Raphael, 2014).

Like many of the other issues discussed, the decision to re-open the wound is by and large not based on definitive numbers or hard science. The one principle almost universally agreed upon is if the patient shows signs of tamponade, which usually manifests as falling perfusion in the face of rising filling pressures. In this case, re-exploration is mandatory. Frequently, this is carried out at the bedside rather than transporting an unstable patient to the operating room.

The timing of re-exploration for continued bleeding is also the subject of competing pressures. If possible, re-exploration should be avoided since it carries an increased risk of wound complications and infection (Lu, Grayson, Jha, Srinivasan, & Fabri, 2003). However delay, especially beyond 12 hours, is associated with an increase in adverse outcomes(Karthik, Grayson, McCarron, Pullan, & Desmond, 2004). Most surgeons would agree that if excessive bleeding continues despite correction of coagulopathy and platelet dysfunction, then re-exploration is warranted. Some authors have advocated accomplishing this in the ICU, rather than returning to the operating room.

REFERENCES

Adelman, B., Rizk, A., & Hanners, E. (1988). Plasminogen interactions with platelets in plasma. *Blood, 72*(5), 1530–1535. PMID:3179439

Ak, K., Isbir, C. S., Tetik, S., Atalan, N., Tekeli, A., Aljodi, M., & Arsan, S. et al. (2009). Thromboelastography-based transfusion algorithm reduces blood product use after elective CABG: A prospective randomized study. *Journal of Cardiac Surgery, 24*(4), 404–410. doi:10.1111/j.1540-8191.2009.00840.x PMID:19583608

American Society of Anesthesiologists Task Force on Perioperative Blood, T., & Adjuvant, T. (2006). Practice guidelines for perioperative blood transfusion and adjuvant therapies: An updated report by the American Society of Anesthesiologists Task Force on Perioperative Blood Transfusion and Adjuvant Therapies. *Anesthesiology, 105*(1), 198–208. doi:10.1097/00000542-200607000-00030 PMID:16810012

Boersma, E., Harrington, R. A., Moliterno, D. J., White, H., Theroux, P., Van de Werf, F., & Simoons, M. L. et al. (2002). Platelet glycoprotein IIb/IIIa inhibitors in acute coronary syndromes: A meta-analysis of all major randomised clinical trials. *Lancet, 359*(9302), 189–198. doi:10.1016/S0140-6736(02)07442-1 PMID:11812552

Cardinal, D. C., & Flower, R. J. (1980). The electronic aggregometer: A novel device for assessing platelet behavior in blood. *Journal of Pharmacological Methods, 3*(2), 135–158. doi:10.1016/0160-5402(80)90024-8 PMID:7392654

Despotis, G., Eby, C., & Lublin, D. M. (2008). A review of transfusion risks and optimal management of perioperative bleeding with cardiac surgery. *Transfusion, 48*(1Suppl), 2S–30S. doi:10.1111/j.1537-2995.2007.01573.x PMID:18302579

Despotis, G. J., Filos, K. S., Zoys, T. N., Hogue, C. W. Jr, Spitznagel, E., & Lappas, D. G. (1996). Factors associated with excessive postoperative blood loss and hemostatic transfusion requirements: A multivariate analysis in cardiac surgical patients. *Anesthesia and Analgesia, 82*(1), 13–21. PMID:8712388

Dixon, B., Reid, D., Collins, M., Newcomb, A. E., Rosalion, A., Yap, C. H., & Campbell, D. J. et al. (2014). The operating surgeon is an independent predictor of chest tube drainage following cardiac surgery. *Journal of Cardiothoracic and Vascular Anesthesia, 28*(2), 242–246. doi:10.1053/j.jvca.2013.09.010 PMID:24439890

Dyke, C., Aronson, S., Dietrich, W., Hofmann, A., Karkouti, K., Levi, M., . . . Ranucci, M. (2014). Universal definition of perioperative bleeding in adult cardiac surgery. *J Thorac Cardiovasc Surg, 147*(5), 1458-1463 e1451. doi: 10.1016/j.jtcvs.2013.10.070

Eisenberg, D. M., Davis, R. B., Ettner, S. L., Appel, S., Wilkey, S., Van Rompay, M., & Kessler, R. C. (1998). Trends in alternative medicine use in the United States, 1990-1997: Results of a follow-up national survey. *Journal of the American Medical Association, 280*(18), 1569–1575. doi:10.1001/jama.280.18.1569 PMID:9820257

Faraday, N., & Rosenfeld, B. A. (1998). In vitro hypothermia enhances platelet GPIIb-IIIa activation and P-selectin expression. *Anesthesiology, 88*(6), 1579–1585. doi:10.1097/00000542-199806000-00022 PMID:9637652

Franchini, M., & Lippi, G. (2012). Fibrinogen replacement therapy: A critical review of the literature. *Blood Transfusion*, *10*(1), 23–27. doi:10.2450/2011.0015-11 PMID:22153684

Gawaz, M. P., Dobos, G., Spath, M., Schollmeyer, P., Gurland, H. J., & Mujais, S. K. (1994). Impaired function of platelet membrane glycoprotein IIb-IIIa in end-stage renal disease. *Journal of the American Society of Nephrology*, *5*(1), 36–46. PMID:7524718

Gelb, A. B., Roth, R. I., Levin, J., London, M. J., Noall, R. A., Hauck, W. W., & Mangano, D. T. et al. (1996). Changes in blood coagulation during and following cardiopulmonary bypass: Lack of correlation with clinical bleeding. *American Journal of Clinical Pathology*, *106*(1), 87–99. PMID:8701939

Gibbs, N. M. (2009). Point-of-care assessment of antiplatelet agents in the perioperative period: A review. *Anaesthesia and Intensive Care*, *37*(3), 354–369. PMID:19499855

Gorlinger, K., Dirkmann, D., Hanke, A. A., Kamler, M., Kottenberg, E., Thielmann, M., & Peters, J. et al. (2011). First-line therapy with coagulation factor concentrates combined with point-of-care coagulation testing is associated with decreased allogeneic blood transfusion in cardiovascular surgery: A retrospective, single-center cohort study. *Anesthesiology*, *115*(6), 1179–1191. doi:10.1097/ALN.0b013e31823497dd PMID:21970887

Gorlinger, K., Shore-Lesserson, L., Dirkmann, D., Hanke, A. A., Rahe-Meyer, N., & Tanaka, K. A. (2013). Management of hemorrhage in cardiothoracic surgery. *Journal of Cardiothoracic and Vascular Anesthesia*, *27*(4Suppl), S20–S34. doi:10.1053/j.jvca.2013.05.014 PMID:23910533

Heller, J., Gabbay, J. S., Ghadjar, K., Jourabchi, M., O'Hara, C., Heller, M., & Bradley, J. P. (2006). Top-10 list of herbal and supplemental medicines used by cosmetic patients: what the plastic surgeon needs to know. *Plast Reconstr Surg, 117*(2), 436-445; discussion 446-437. doi: 10.1097/01.prs.0000197217.46219.a7

Hirsh, J., Guyatt, G., Albers, G. W., Harrington, R., Schunemann, H. J., & American College of Chest, P. (2008). Antithrombotic and thrombolytic therapy: American College of Chest Physicians Evidence-Based Clinical Practice Guidelines (8th Edition). *Chest, 133*(6 Suppl), 110S-112S. doi: 10.1378/chest.08-0652

Holland, L., Warkentin, T. E., Refaai, M., Crowther, M. A., Johnston, M. A., & Sarode, R. (2009). Suboptimal effect of a three-factor prothrombin complex concentrate (Profilnine-SD) in correcting supratherapeutic international normalized ratio due to warfarin overdose. *Transfusion*, *49*(6), 1171–1177. doi:10.1111/j.1537-2995.2008.02080.x PMID:19210325

Izuha, H., Hattori, M., Igari, T., Wakamatsu, D., Watanabe, M., & Yokoyama, H. (2005). Changes in platelet aggregation during cardiopulmonary bypass: Comparison of poly-2-methoxyethylacrylate and heparin as a circuit coating material. *Journal of Artificial Organs*, *8*(1), 41–46. doi:10.1007/s10047-004-0280-x PMID:15951979

Jneid, H., Anderson, J. L., Wright, R. S., Adams, C. D., Bridges, C. R., Casey, D. E. Jr, & Zidar, J. P. et al. (2012). 2012 ACCF/AHA focused update of the guideline for the management of patients with unstable angina/non-ST-elevation myocardial infarction (updating the 2007 guideline and replacing the 2011 focused update): A report of the American College of Cardiology Foundation/American Heart Association Task Force on Practice Guidelines. *Journal of the American College of Cardiology*, *60*(7), 645–681. doi:10.1016/j.jacc.2012.06.004 PMID:22809746

Kalina, U., Bickhard, H., & Schulte, S. (2008). Biochemical comparison of seven commercially available prothrombin complex concentrates. *International Journal of Clinical Practice*, *62*(10), 1614–1622. doi:10.1111/j.1742-1241.2008.01859.x PMID:18691229

Karkouti, K., Callum, J., Crowther, M. A., McCluskey, S. A., Pendergrast, J., Tait, G., & Beattie, W. S. et al. (2013). The relationship between fibrinogen levels after cardiopulmonary bypass and large volume red cell transfusion in cardiac surgery: An observational study. *Anesthesia and Analgesia*, *117*(1), 14–22. doi:10.1213/ANE.0b013e318292efa4 PMID:23687229

Karlsson, M., Ternstrom, L., Hyllner, M., Baghaei, F., Flinck, A., Skrtic, S., & Jeppsson, A. (2009). Prophylactic fibrinogen infusion reduces bleeding after coronary artery bypass surgery. A prospective randomised pilot study. *Thrombosis and Haemostasis*, *102*(1), 137–144. doi:10.1160/TH08-09-0587 PMID:19572078

Karthik, S., Grayson, A. D., McCarron, E. E., Pullan, D. M., & Desmond, M. J. (2004). Reexploration for bleeding after coronary artery bypass surgery: Risk factors, outcomes, and the effect of time delay. *The Annals of Thoracic Surgery*, *78*(2), 527–534, discussion 534. doi:10.1016/j.athoracsur.2004.02.088 PMID:15276512

Kehara, H., Takano, T., Ohashi, N., Terasaki, T., & Amano, J. (2014). Platelet Function During Cardiopulmonary Bypass Using Multiple Electrode Aggregometry: Comparison of Centrifugal and Roller Pumps. *Artificial Organs*, *38*(11), 924–930. doi:10.1111/aor.12299 PMID:24720284

Kepler, C. K., Huang, R. C., Meredith, D., Kim, J. H., & Sharma, A. K. (2012). Omega-3 and fish oil supplements do not cause increased bleeding during spinal decompression surgery. *Journal of Spinal Disorders & Techniques*, *25*(3), 129–132. doi:10.1097/BSD.0b013e3182120227 PMID:21423055

Khuri, S. F., Wolfe, J. A., Josa, M., Axford, T. C., Szymanski, I., & Assousa, S. et al.. (1992). Hematologic changes during and after cardiopulmonary bypass and their relationship to the bleeding time and nonsurgical blood loss. *The Journal of Thoracic and Cardiovascular Surgery*, *104*(1), 94–107. PMID:1614220

Kozek-Langenecker, S. A. (2010). Perioperative coagulation monitoring. *Best Practice & Research. Clinical Anaesthesiology*, *24*(1), 27–40. doi:10.1016/j.bpa.2009.09.009 PMID:20402168

Levi, M., Toh, C. H., Thachil, J., & Watson, H. G. (2009). Guidelines for the diagnosis and management of disseminated intravascular coagulation. British Committee for Standards in Haematology. *British Journal of Haematology*, *145*(1), 24–33. doi:10.1111/j.1365-2141.2009.07600.x PMID:19222477

Loscalzo, J. (2012). From clinical observation to mechanism--Heyde's syndrome. *The New England Journal of Medicine*, *367*(20), 1954–1956. doi:10.1056/NEJMcibr1205363 PMID:23150964

Lowe, G. D., Rumley, A., & Mackie, I. J. (2004). Plasma fibrinogen. *Annals of Clinical Biochemistry*, *41*(Pt 6), 430–440. doi:10.1258/0004563042466884 PMID:15588432

Lu, J. C., Grayson, A. D., Jha, P., Srinivasan, A. K., & Fabri, B. M. (2003). Risk factors for sternal wound infection and mid-term survival following coronary artery bypass surgery. *European Journal of Cardio-Thoracic Surgery*, *23*(6), 943–949. doi:10.1016/S1010-7940(03)00137-4 PMID:12829070

Maquelin, K. N., Berckmans, R. J., Nieuwland, R., Schaap, M. C., ten Have, K., Eijsman, L., & Sturk, A. (1998). Disappearance of glycoprotein Ib from the platelet surface in pericardial blood during cardiopulmonary bypass. *The Journal of Thoracic and Cardiovascular Surgery*, *115*(5), 1160–1165. doi:10.1016/S0022-5223(98)70416-7 PMID:9605086

Marengo-Rowe, A. J. J. L. (1988). Fibrinolysis: A frequent cause of bleeding (N. Ellison, D.R. Jobes Ed.). Philadelphia: WB Saunders.

Marsh, S. A., & Coombes, J. S. (2006). Vitamin E and alpha-lipoic acid supplementation increase bleeding tendency via an intrinsic coagulation pathway. *Clinical and Applied Thrombosis/Hemostasis*, *12*(2), 169–173. doi:10.1177/107602960601200204 PMID:16708118

Meredith, D. S., Kepler, C. K., Huang, R. C., Hirsch, B., Nguyen, J., Farmer, J. C., & Cammisa, F. P. et al. (2012). The effect of omega-3 fatty-acid supplements on perioperative bleeding following posterior spinal arthrodesis. *European Spine Journal*, *21*(12), 2659–2663. doi:10.1007/s00586-012-2365-1 PMID:22581258

Michelson, A. D. (1994). Platelet activation by thrombin can be directly measured in whole blood through the use of the peptide GPRP and flow cytometry: Methods and clinical applications. *Blood Coagulation & Fibrinolysis*, *5*(1), 121–131. doi:10.1097/00001721-199402000-00014 PMID:8180332

Morgan, I. S., Codispoti, M., Sanger, K., & Mankad, P. S. (1998). Superiority of centrifugal pump over roller pump in paediatric cardiac surgery: Prospective randomised trial. *European Journal of Cardio-Thoracic Surgery*, *13*(5), 526–532. doi:10.1016/S1010-7940(98)00067-0 PMID:9663533

Mosesson, M. W. (2005). Fibrinogen and fibrin structure and functions. *Journal of Thrombosis and Haemostasis*, *3*(8), 1894–1904. doi:10.1111/j.1538-7836.2005.01365.x PMID:16102057

Paparella, D., Brister, S. J., & Buchanan, M. R. (2004). Coagulation disorders of cardiopulmonary bypass: A review. *Intensive Care Medicine*, *30*(10), 1873–1881. doi:10.1007/s00134-004-2388-0 PMID:15278267

Rahe-Meyer, N., Pichlmaier, M., Haverich, A., Solomon, C., Winterhalter, M., Piepenbrock, S., & Tanaka, K. A. (2009). Bleeding management with fibrinogen concentrate targeting a high-normal plasma fibrinogen level: A pilot study. *British Journal of Anaesthesia*, *102*(6), 785–792. doi:10.1093/bja/aep089 PMID:19411671

Rahe-Meyer, N., Solomon, C., Winterhalter, M., Piepenbrock, S., Tanaka, K., Haverich, A., & Pichlmaier, M. (2009). Thromboelastometry-guided administration of fibrinogen concentrate for the treatment of excessive intraoperative bleeding in thoracoabdominal aortic aneurysm surgery. *The Journal of Thoracic and Cardiovascular Surgery*, *138*(3), 694–702. doi:10.1016/j.jtcvs.2008.11.065 PMID:19698858

Rahe-Meyer, N., & Sorensen, B. (2011). For: Fibrinogen concentrate for management of bleeding. *Journal of Thrombosis and Haemostasis*, *9*(1), 1–5. doi:10.1111/j.1538-7836.2010.04099.x PMID:20946151

Rinder, C. S., Bohnert, J., Rinder, H. M., Mitchell, J., Ault, K., & Hillman, R. (1991). Platelet activation and aggregation during cardiopulmonary bypass. *Anesthesiology*, *75*(3), 388–393. doi:10.1097/00000542-199109000-00002 PMID:1716077

Rohrer, M. J., & Natale, A. M. (1992). Effect of hypothermia on the coagulation cascade. *Critical Care Medicine*, *20*(10), 1402–1405. doi:10.1097/00003246-199210000-00007 PMID:1395660

Royston, D., & von Kier, S. (2001). Reduced haemostatic factor transfusion using heparinase-modified thrombelastography during cardiopulmonary bypass. *British Journal of Anaesthesia*, *86*(4), 575–578. doi:10.1093/bja/86.4.575 PMID:11573637

Schmidt, E. B., Varming, K., Ernst, E., Madsen, P., & Dyerberg, J. (1990). Dose-response studies on the effect of n-3 polyunsaturated fatty acids on lipids and haemostasis. *Thrombosis and Haemostasis*, *63*(1), 1–5. PMID:2339345

Shore-Lesserson, L., Manspeizer, H. E., DePerio, M., Francis, S., Vela-Cantos, F., & Ergin, M. A. (1999). Thromboelastography-guided transfusion algorithm reduces transfusions in complex cardiac surgery. *Anesthesia and Analgesia*, *88*(2), 312–319. PMID:9972747

Silvain, J., Bellemain-Appaix, A., Barthelemy, O., Beygui, F., Collet, J. P., & Montalescot, G. (2011). Optimal use of thienopyridines in non-ST-elevation acute coronary syndrome following CURRENT-OASIS 7. *Circulation: Cardiovascular Interventions*, *4*(1), 95–103. doi:10.1161/CIRCINTERVENTIONS.109.910406 PMID:21325198

Spiess, B. D., Horrow, J., & Kaplan, J. A. (2011). Kaplan's Cardiac Anesthesia (D. L. R. Joel A. Kaplan, Joseph S. Savino Ed. 6th edition ed.). St. Louis, MO: Elsevier Saunders.

Spiess, B. D., Tuman, K. J., McCarthy, R. J., DeLaria, G. A., Schillo, R., & Ivankovich, A. D. (1987). Thromboelastography as an indicator of post-cardiopulmonary bypass coagulopathies. *Journal of Clinical Monitoring*, *3*(1), 25–30. doi:10.1007/BF00770880 PMID:3819793

Thiele, R. H., & Raphael, J. (2014). A 2014 Update on Coagulation Management for Cardiopulmonary Bypass. *Seminars in Cardiothoracic and Vascular Anesthesia*, *18*(2), 177–189. doi:10.1177/1089253214534782 PMID:24876232

Valeri, C. R., Feingold, H., Cassidy, G., Ragno, G., Khuri, S., & Altschule, M. D. (1987). Hypothermia-induced reversible platelet dysfunction. *Annals of Surgery*, *205*(2), 175–181. doi:10.1097/00000658-198702000-00012 PMID:3813688

Velik-Salchner, C., Maier, S., Innerhofer, P., Kolbitsch, C., Streif, W., Mittermayr, M., & Fries, D. et al. (2009). An assessment of cardiopulmonary bypass-induced changes in platelet function using whole blood and classical light transmission aggregometry: The results of a pilot study. *Anesthesia and Analgesia*, *108*(6), 1747–1754. doi:10.1213/ane.0b013e3181a198ac PMID:19448196

Weigert, A. L., & Schafer, A. I. (1998). Uremic bleeding: Pathogenesis and therapy. *The American Journal of the Medical Sciences*, *316*(2), 94–104. doi:10.1097/00000441-199808000-00005 PMID:9704663

Whiting, D., & DiNardo, J. A. (2014). TEG and ROTEM: Technology and clinical applications. *American Journal of Hematology*, *89*(2), 228–232. doi:10.1002/ajh.23599 PMID:24123050

Wikkelsoe, A. J., Afshari, A., Wetterslev, J., Brok, J., & Moeller, A. M. (2011). Monitoring patients at risk of massive transfusion with Thrombelastography or Thromboelastometry: A systematic review. *Acta Anaesthesiologica Scandinavica*, *55*(10), 1174–1189. doi:10.1111/j.1399-6576.2011.02534.x PMID:22092122

Wong, W. W., Gabriel, A., Maxwell, G. P., & Gupta, S. C. (2012). Bleeding risks of herbal, homeopathic, and dietary supplements: A hidden nightmare for plastic surgeons? *Aesthetic Surgery Journal*, *32*(3), 332–346. doi:10.1177/1090820X12438913 PMID:22395325

Chapter 32
Echocardiography and Ultrasound in the Intensive Care Unit

Pranav R. Shah
Vanderbilt University Medical Center, USA

Chad Wagner
Vanderbilt University Medical Center, USA

Andrew Shaw
Vanderbilt University Medical Center, USA

ABSTRACT

Sonography in the intensive care unit is a rapidly emerging point-of-care diagnostic tool. Literature supports the use of sonography for the evaluation of lung pathology, protocol based focused cardiac evaluation, and abdominal pathology, as well as identifying deep venous thrombosis. There is also evidence that ultrasound guided procedures such as venous access, thoracentesis, and paracentesis may decrease complications compared to a landmark based technique. However, there is ambiguity in the literature regarding definition, scope, and training in this modality as used by intensivists. The purpose of this chapter is to provide a broad overview of the role of ultrasound in the ICU and data supporting the use of point-of-care protocols. This chapter does not provide instruction on how to perform a complete transthoracic or transesophageal exam, nor does it provide a library of images of various pathologies since a reader seeking such depth would be better served by a full textbook on echocardiography.

INTRODUCTION

Sonography is emerging as a versatile tool for rapid assessment of the critically ill patient. Key factors in this trend include convenience and an intuitive understanding that visualizing the structure of interest is more accurate than surrogate measures of its function. For example, Rugolotto et al. found major differences in assessment of cardiovascular status via a physical exam performed by second year cardiology fellows versus an exam using a portable hand-held ultrasound (Rugolotto, Chang, Hu, Schnittger, &

DOI: 10.4018/978-1-4666-8603-8.ch032

Liang, 2002). Kobal and colleagues showed a similar phenomenon when comparing medical students with ultrasound training and a cardiologist's physical examination when assessing valvular and non-valvular cardiac pathology (Kobal et al., 2005).

Ultrasound in the cardiac intensive care unit can be used in multiple ways. It is a useful in assisting in procedures such as central venous access. It can also provide rapid, goal directed assessment of the lungs, heart, abdominal cavity, and lower extremity veins. Of note, this chapter will not cover the FAST exam for rapid evaluation of the trauma patient as a trauma patient is unlikely to be admitted to the cardiac intensive care unit.

The objective of this chapter is to briefly discuss ultrasound-guided procedures in the ICU, and to more thoroughly discuss lung ultrasound, focused cardiac ultrasound, and ultrasound training. The reader is encouraged to consult a formal textbook in sonography in order to see a library of sonographic normal and abnormal findings, or learn to perform full transthoracic (TTE) or transesophageal (TEE) exams with various Doppler modalities or 3D examination. At the end of this chapter, Table 1 provides a summary of common point-of-care views and their uses, and Figure 1 shows images acquired with a point-of-care ultrasound machine.

SONOGRAPHY FOR PROCEDURES

Central Venous Cannulation

There are numerous articles dealing with ultrasound guidance for central venous cannulation in the intensive care unit. The reader is encouraged to refer to the American Society of Echocardiography (ASE) and Society of Cardiovascular Anesthesiologists (SCA) joint guideline, published in 2011, for recommendations for vascular cannulation. For internal jugular vein cannulation, the guideline recommends that properly trained individuals use real-time ultrasound based on Level 1 evidence. For the subclavian vein, it states that the use of ultrasound for routine cannulation is not supported by literature, but for high-risk individuals, ultrasound to assess location and patency of the vein may be beneficial. For the femoral vein, the guideline states that the scientific evidence does not support routine use of ultrasound (Troianos et al., 2011).

As an aside, ultrasound techniques have been well described for femoral vein and internal jugular vein cannulation. Both static and real-time ultrasound guided cannulation techniques have also been described for the subclavian vein though they are more technically difficult. Fragou and colleagues reported on a comparison between real-time ultrasound guided cannulation and a landmark technique for subclavian vein and found the real-time technique to be superior in terms of complication rates. Their technique utilized the identification of the axillary vein between 1st and 2nd rib in the infraclavicular region in a long-axis (longitudinal) view, and watching the needle enter the vein (Fragou et al., 2011).

Arterial Cannulation

Though there are no Level 1 recommendations on the role of sonography in arterial cannulation, there are a fraction of patients in the cardiac ICU who have mechanical devices that reduce native arterial pulsatility. In this patient population, ultrasound is very useful in locating an arterial vessel and guiding cannulation.

Thoracentesis and Paracentesis

Ultrasound can be used to identify and guide drainage of pleural and ascites fluid. In a study with 52 spontaneously breathing patients with a documented pleural effusion obliterating over half of the hemi-diaphragm, patients were randomized to thoracentesis with sonography guidance using needle based drainage, a landmark based technique with needle based drainage, and landmark based technique with needle and catheter inserted for drainage. Pneumothorax was observed in 0/19 patients with sonography technique, 3/15 with needle only technique, and 7/18 with needle plus catheter technique. Of note, the non-catheter groups used a 20-gauge needle, and the catheter arm used a 14G-gauge needle through which a 16-gauge catheter was inserted. Moreover, radiology residents performed the sonography based technique, and medical residents performed the landmark based techniques (Grogan et al., 1990). Patel and colleagues performed a retrospective analysis based on the Premier hospital database using ICD-9 and CPT codes for thoracentesis and ultrasound use. In their analysis of 19,339 procedures performed in 2008, of which 46% were done using ultrasound, there was a reduced risk of pneumothorax by 16.3%, and reduction in risk of hemorrhage by 38.7% when ultrasound was used to guide the procedure. The absolute risk of pneumothorax was 3.9% with ultrasound vs. 4.6% without it (Patel, Ernst, & Gunnarsson, 2012).

A similar analysis performed in the Premier database for thoracentesis and paracentesis done in 2007-2008 led to a comparable conclusion. There were 61,261 thoracentesis and 69,859 paracentesis procedures done of which 45% utilized sonography. Ultrasound reduced the risk of pneumothorax by 19% (2.26% vs 3.09%) in thoracentesis, and bleeding by 69% (0.27% vs 1.25%) for paracentesis (Mercaldi & Lanes, 2013). Hence, the data show that sonographic guidance can reduce major complications from thoracentesis and paracentesis.

SONOGRAPHY AS A TOOL FOR PATIENT ASSESSMENT: LUNG

Lung ultrasound can be used to detect a pneumothorax, pulmonary edema, pleural effusion, and consolidation. It is typically performed with either a 5-7 MHz or 3-5 MHz ultrasound probe. Lung sonography has its own nomenclature for findings. Normal lungs have "lung sliding" which is generally defined as the movement of pleura underneath the ribs due to respiratory motion. "B-line" or "comet-tails" are types of reverberations. They start at the pleural surface and go to end of the screen away from the transducer. In a normal lung, there are a few (2-3) in each sonography window in dependent lung regions. "Lung point" is the point at which lung sliding is no longer seen and is seen at the edge of where the pneumothorax prevents contact of the lung with the pleura. "A line" refers to multiple horizontal reverberations and are typically suggestive of a pneumothorax at that location. Each sonographic finding adds to a picture of the lung as normal or abnormal. For example, the differential diagnosis for lack of lung sliding includes acute respiratory distress syndrome, pneumonia, pleural adhesions, apnea, atelectasis as well as a pneumothorax (Bouhemad, Zhang, Lu, & Rouby, 2007; Shostak, Brylka, Krepp, Pua, & Sanders, 2013). Typically, each side of the chest is scanned in multiple cranial-caudal and anterior-posterior locations. A common sonography pattern divides the lung into two cranial-caudal regions (upper & lower) and three anterior-posterior regions - anterior to anterior axillary line, between the anterior and posterior axillary line, and posterior to the posterior axillary line (patient may need to be turned or placed lateral). Hence, six regions per lung. Morbid obesity may impair the quality of the sonographic image, as can subcutaneous air (Bouhemad et al., 2007; Cortellaro, Colombo, Coen, & Duca, 2012; Manno et al., 2012).

Common patterns of lung pathologies are as follows:

- Normal lung has pleural sliding, and less than 2-3 B-lines in the dependent regions. In the non-dependent regions, there should be even fewer B-lines.
- Pulmonary edema is generally associated with multiple closely spaced B-lines due to thickening of the sub-pleural septa causing acoustic artifacts.
- Consolidation is demonstrated by small punctate hyperechoic regions in the lung, dynamic air bronchograms, and is generally surrounded by a pleural effusion.
- Hyperechoic regions are usually a manifestation of air trapped in the small airways.
- Pleural effusion lacks pleural sliding and has a dark region underneath the rib.
- Pneumothorax lacks pleural siding and B-lines, and typically has lung points. The presence of B-lines rules out a pneumothorax

Of note, when there is loss of lung aeration and increased lung tissue-water, ultrasound penetration increases and ultrasound shows deeper structures (such as the heart or the great vessels) (Bouhemad et al., 2007; D. A. Lichtenstein et al., 2005; Daniel Lichtenstein, Mezière, & Seitz, 2009; D Lichtenstein, Mezière, Biderman, & Gepner, 1999; D Lichtenstein, Mézière, Biderman, Gepner, & Barré, 1997; Shostak et al., 2013; Soldati et al., 2008).

Shostak et al. used chest x-ray as a gold standard, and investigated the utility of ultrasound for identification of post-procedural pneumothorax after thoracentesis, transbronchial biopsies, and CT guided lung biopsies. They defined a pneumothorax as the loss of both lung sliding and comet tails, along with identification of lung point. The patients were scanned both pre- and post-procedure, and in multiple rib spaces in multiple anterior-posterior locations on both sides. The criteria for an adequate scan were when "the pleural surface was imaged in at least 3 consecutive intercostal spaces on each line of scanning … and if B-lines of lung sliding were present on a pre-procedure scan." Using this criteria, 7/8 pneumothoraces were detected with sonography resulting in a sensitivity of 88% and specificity of 97% (Shostak et al., 2013). Lung ultrasound was also accurate in detecting occult traumatic pneumothorax. One hundred and nine spontaneously breathing trauma patients who were hemodynamically stable underwent a lung sonogram by emergency room physicians with greater than 1 year experience. Diagnostic criteria for pneumothorax were lack of lung sliding, presence of lung points, and absence of B lines. Using a CT scan as gold standard, 25/218 hemi-thoraces had a pneumothorax. Of these 13/25 were detected on AP supine chest x-ray, and 23/25 by ultrasound. Of note, the two missed pneumothoraces by ultrasound were "miniscule," and located in the left paracardiac region. In 20/25 cases, sonography also accurately predicted the extent of the pneumothorax compared to a CT scan. Ultrasound did have one false positive. Overall, ultrasound was 92% sensitive, 99.4% specific, and the examination took less than three minutes (Soldati et al., 2008).

Additionally, lung ultrasound has been used to provide radiologic evidence for pneumonia. In an adult emergency room in Italy, in patients with a clinical suspicion of pneumonia, lung ultrasound was compared to a chest x-ray with the gold standard being either a CT scan obtained after admission, or a discharge diagnosis of pneumonia. In this setting, the initial chest x-ray accurately diagnosed 54/81 patients with pneumonia, and 33/39 who did not have pneumonia. Comparatively, lung ultrasound was 80/81 for true positive rate, and 37/39 for true negative rate. All the patients had adequate windows, and sonography time was less than five minutes. This study also utilized six scanning regions (upper & lower divided by the third interspace, and three anterior-posterior regions) per lung. Of note, sonography was done by a single operator, and pneumonia was defined as a subpleural lung consolidation. Hence, in this study, the lung ultrasound was more sensitive and specific compared to chest x-ray (Cortellaro et al., 2012).

Lichtenstein et al. studied the diagnostic accuracy of a lung ultrasound protocol - "BLUE Protocol" - in an observational study of 260 dyspneic patients. Using lung ultrasound with a 5MHz, convex probe, and scanning in six lung regions per thorax, they identified patterns of lung pathology that were 90.5% accurate with clinical diagnosis. Specially, COPD and asthma had similar patterns (n=49 & n= 34) consisting of lung sliding plus A-lines (89% sensitive, 97% specific). Pulmonary edema pattern was multiple anterior diffuse B-lines (n=64, 97% sensitive, 95% specific). The pneumothorax pattern was absent anterior lung sliding, with A lines and presence of a lung point (n=9, 81% sensitive, 100% specific). This study was most notable for a comprehensive, and systematic use of ultrasonography for evaluation of dyspnea (D. A. Lichtenstein & Mezière, 2008).

SONOGRAPHY AS A TOOL FOR PATIENT ASSESSMENT: FOCUSED CARDIAC EXAMINATION

The cardiothoracic critical care unit is, by its nature of dealing with care of patients post cardiac surgery, a place where patients are not only undergoing dynamic change in cardiac filling pressures, but also in cardiac performance as they recover from cardiopulmonary bypass and aortic cross clamping. The ability to visualize the heart is a powerful diagnostic ability in these patients. In general, there are two overarching echocardiographic modalities - transthoracic (TTE), and transesophageal (TEE). Transthoracic echo is non-invasive and has been evaluated in the acute care focused sonography literature more thoroughly. Moreover, it can be done on intubated and extubated patients easily. However, the location of chest tubes - in the mediastinum, and pleura - along with their exit sites and dressings often limit the locations from which the typical TTE views are obtained. Conceptually, there is also recognition that a *focused* assessment using TTE or TEE is different from a comprehensive examination performed by a consultant (cardiologist, or cardiac anesthesiologist). Generally, a focused assessment is limited in some manner. This is discussed further in the training section. We generally discuss the role of focused cardiac examination in this section, and will not generally discuss role of Doppler modalities, 3D echocardiography, or diagnosis of valvular disease.

Transthoracic Ultrasound

Faris, Veltman, and Royse provide a framework for a focused TTE assessment of these patients. The purpose of a focused exam is to answer specific questions: Is there significant right or left ventricular dysfunction? Is there pericardial fluid in a clinical setting compatible with tamponade? Are the ventricles empty, or full? Among these questions, one should also consider whether a focused exam is adequate, or if the clinical setting requires a comprehensive echocardiographic exam by a consultant (ie. in the setting of bacteremia and a concern for endocarditis) (Faris, Veltman, & Royse, 2009). Common indications to trigger a focused exam include persistent inadequate cardiac output or hypoperfusion state, hypotension, clinical suspicion of right heart failure, or suspicion of tamponade (Geisen, Spray, & Nicholas Fletcher, 2013).

Focused TTE allows for monitoring for various cardiac parameters. A combination of parasternal short and long axis views, apical views, and subcostal views are used. Ventricular contractility is visually estimated in a qualitative continuum (normal, mild, moderate, or severely depressed) for right and left ventricles. Relating to this, ventricular size (empty, normal, dilated) is assessed. Ventricular size has implications for volume status and fluid responsiveness. For example, in the setting of normal right ventricular (RV) function, "kissing papillary muscles" or low end-systolic area (ESA) of the left ventricle (LV) in a short-axis view generally implies hypovolemia or vasodilation. If the LV end diastolic area (EDA) is also small, it is hypovolemia, and fluid administration will lead to increased cardiac output. However, in the same LV, if the right ventricle was dilated, then the left ventricle is likely under-filled not from inadequate intravascular volume, but due to RV dysfunction. Similarly, clinical suspicion of tamponade is further supported if pericardial fluid is noted. However, in a post cardiac surgery setting, a focal hematoma behind the atria may cause tamponade and may not be visible on TTE (Geisen et al., 2013). Likewise, there is often clot present behind the right atrium, and this is not necessarily an automatic indication to return to the operating room. An assessment of the clot's functional impact is required before that decision can be made.

Orme et al. asked whether echocardiography changes management. They retrospectively reviewed all TEE and TTE studies ordered in a mixed medical and surgical ICU patient population. These were comprehensive studies performed by a consultant. In their population, adequate images to answer the clinical question were obtained in 84% of patients. Fifty one percent of the studies changed management (Orme, Oram, & McKinstry, 2009). Vignon et al. demonstrated the feasibility of training residents in critical care TTE. Six residents in the medical ICU were given a twelve-hour training session composed of didactics, case presentation, and hands-on examination on 10-12 patients. They were trained to assess global LV function (normal, increased, EF 30-50%, or <30%), and recognize dilated LV, RV, or IVC, and pericardial effusions. TTE views included parasternal long & short axis, apical four chamber, subcostal, and subcostal-IVC. This was done as part of a prospective, observational study. The trigger for an exam was a request from the intensivist. During the study, 201 patients being mechanically ventilated underwent the focused TTE. The most common reasons for requesting an exam were acute circulatory or respiratory failure. During the study, the trainees were able to accurately identify the pathology (Philippe Vignon et al., 2011).

In a feasibility study involving 210 patients in a medical-surgical ICU, a focused TTE exam was conducted if the patient was "not making clinical progress after cardiopulmonary evaluation based on conventional monitoring." They utilized the FATE sequence (Focus Assessed Transthoracic Echocardiography) involving subcostal, parasternal, and apical views. They assessed the size and contractility of the right and left ventricles, and whether or not there was an effusion in the pleural or pericardial space. A TEE was performed if the TTE inconclusive. They performed a total of 233 TTE and 4 TEE examinations in their population, of which over 50% of the patients studied were post-cardiac surgery. 97% of the exams had usable images - 58% of subcostal views were of acceptable quality, 80% apical, and 69% parasternal. All three windows were obtained in 34% patients, only two in 41%, and only one in 23% of patients. The results of the echocardiography provided "decisive" information in 24.5% of exams, "supplemental" in 37%, and "supportive" in 35% (Jensen, Sloth, Larsen, & Schmidt, 2004).

Numerous sequences of cardiac sonography have been developed to evaluate the critically ill patient. For example, a focused TTE protocol was proposed by Perera called the Rapid Ultrasound in Shock (RUSH) to evaluate patients in shock. It is composed of evaluation of the pump (cardiac function in the parasternal long & short views, subcostal, and apical views), "tank" or preload (IVC collapsibility) and pipes or large vessels (ascending, thoracic, and abdominal aorta, along with lower extremities for DVT).

Their goal was to use the information to classify shock more definitively as hypovolemic, cardiogenic, obstructive, or distributive (Perera, Mailhot, Riley, & Mandavia, 2010).

Transesophageal Ultrasound

A proportion of post-cardiac surgery patients need information from echocardiography, but may have poor quality images from transthoracic windows. In these patients, a formal TEE may be done. However, in the same light as a focused TTE, a small 72-hour disposable TEE probe with 2D and color Doppler capability is available (Imacor Inc, Uniondale, NY, USA). Most of the literature regarding miniature TEE probe involves the Imacor device. In a pilot study with 94 patients, Vieillard-Baron et al. evaluated the feasibility of using this device in mechanically ventilated patients. Eighty-six percent of patients had respiratory or circulatory failure (70% due to sepsis). They sought to obtain three views: upper esophageal SVC, mid-esophageal four chamber (ME4C), and transgastric short-axis (TGSAX). Their goal was to evaluate SVC respiratory variation, LV function, RV size, septal motion, tamponade, and massive valvular regurgitation. Their results showed 100% insertion rate (though in 17% the NG tube had to be removed), with greater than 90% success in achieving each of the three views. The average duration of monitoring was 32 hours, and over 50% of the exams had a direct therapeutic impact. Complications included two lip ulcerations, and two self-limited GI bleeds. Their patient population was very ill with an ICU mortality of 49%. Of key importance, these exams were carried out by "highly trained intensivists with expertise in critical care echocardiography" (Vieillard-Baron et al., 2013).

Our institution has also investigated the role of the miniaturized TEE probe. Maltais et al. enrolled a series of unstable cardiac surgery patients in whom the attending intensivist placed the probe. Indications for insertion included persistent systolic blood pressure < 100 mmHg, cardiac index of less than 2.2 L/min/m2, SvO2 < 60%, suspected tamponade physiology, hypoperfusion state (base deficit > 8 mEq/L or lactate > 5 mg/dL), concern for RV failure, or tamponade. In that study 20 of 21 patient were post-operative, and one patient was admitted for preoperative workup for endocarditis. The most common findings were RV dysfunction in 33%, and hypovolemia in 57%. Interestingly, there was a 66% discordance rate between the hemodynamic monitoring, and TEE findings.

The role of episodic monoplane TEE monitoring has also been investigated in patients with mechanical support. Haglund and colleagues conducted a retrospective review of hemodynamic TEE monitoring in 100 consecutive patients who had a continuous flow left ventricular device (CF-LVAD) placed. Key evaluation points with the exam included RV function, ventricular filling as assessed via the position of the interatrial and intraventricular septum, and focal or circumferential tamponade. The probe was inserted at the discretion of the intensivist though common triggers included acute hemodynamic changes (MAP < 60 mmHg with a norepinephrine infusion at greater than 10 mcg/min, unclear volume status, persistent CI < 2.2 L/min/m^2, SvO_2 < 60% on inotropic therapy, suspected pericardial effusion). Of the 100 patients with CF-LVAD, 41 were enrolled, but only 33/41 were included in analysis due to lack of all study data points. All patients also had a PA catheter placed in the operating room. The most common indications for placement of a TEE probe were hypotension (60%), questions regarding volume status (24%), and concern for RV function (12%). Not surprisingly, the patients with a TEE probe were sicker, as defined by higher blood product requirements, and a larger fraction of patients whose chest was left open. In this population, echocardiography changed management in over 72% of patients. The individuals who performed the echo in this complex patient population were either board certified echocardiographers, or anesthesiologists with over two months of training on miniature TEE system and credentialed by the ICU medical director (Haglund et al., 2014). Similarly, Cavarocchi et al investigated the impact of a miniTEE system in patients undergoing veno-arterial extracorporeal membrane oxygenation (VA ECMO) for cardiogenic shock. They sought to use the TEE data to predict ability to wean from VA ECMO. Once the patients were afebrile, euvolemic, had resolution of pulmonary edema on chest x-ray, and end-organ dysfunction had recovered to baseline, a four-step weaning protocol was carried out under TEE: 1) ventricular function evaluated on full VA ECMO flow; 2) VA ECMO flows decreased by 0.5 L/min while watching for ventricular distension or hypotension; 3) at 1.2-1.5 L/min of VA ECMO flow, the heart was volume challenged with up to 10 cc/kg of colloid (5% albumin) until preload was deemed adequate; 4) Inotropes started (milrinone or dobutamine) and ventricular function re-evaluated. Of 21 patients, 6/21 had biventricular recovery after revascularization or therapy for ischemia, 7/21 were deemed non-recoverable, and 8/21 had RV recovery and were bridged to LVAD. They concluded that mini-TEE can predict weaning success of patients on VA ECMO using the above protocol. (Cavarocchi et al., 2013).

SONOGRAPHY AS A TOOL FOR PATIENT ASSESSMENT: DEEP VENOUS THROMBOSIS (DVT)

Kory and colleagues have investigated the accuracy of critical care sonography in the diagnosis of DVT. In a retrospective, multicenter study of 128 patients, the Intensivist exam had 86% sensitivity, and 96% specificity for detecting a DVT. The gold standard was a formal lower extremity Doppler conducted after the bedside study. A total of 18 fellows performed the exams. They received one hour of didactic training, and two hours of hands on training on life models, along with one hour of training on the interpretation of normal and abnormal findings. Their protocol involved obtaining 2D views in transverse planes (no color flow), and doing three compressions along the course of the common femoral vein, two along the popliteal vein, and one on the superficial femoral vein in 2 cm increments. A DVT was defined as the inability to compress a vein segment. The average time for an exam was 12.5 minutes. Overall, with an approximate 20% prevalence rate, they reported 6 false positives, and 3 false negatives (Kory et al., 2011)

TRAINING FOR CRITICAL CARE ULTRASOUND

As ultrasound is gaining a foothold in the ICU, several groups have made recommendations for training in this area. Among the key questions in this field is the one relating to training and demonstration of competence as this ties into the question of certification, documentation, billing, and credentialing. Patients can reasonably expect a physician who is doing any procedure or examination to have qualifications and experience with that modality (Huang & McLean, 2012; Oxorn & Pearlman, 2012). A pyramid of competence has been proposed, in which the emergency echo level is acute care ultrasound, level 1 is the ability to acquire all standard views & diagnose common abnormalities, level 2 is a comprehensive TTE and TEE examination and diagnosis of all abnormalities, and level 3 being specialist examination (Oxorn & Pearlman, 2012; Spencer et al., 2013). By limiting the questions being asked and answered with basic sonographic techniques, one can lower the threshold for training and use, while at the same time identifying major findings affecting patient care (P Vignon, 2012).

As a reference, the international consensus conference on FAST examination stated the majority viewpoint was that during training for FAST examination, 4 hours of theoretical instruction, and 4 hours of practical instruction are necessary. They also stated that the minimum number of supervised examinations during training were 200 (Scalea et al., 1999). The American College of Chest Physicans in conjunction with La Société de Réanimation de Langue Française published a statement on critical care sonography. They divided sonography into general critical care ultrasound (GCCUS) consisting of thoracic, abdominal, vascular access, and DVT portions, and critical care echocardiography (CCE). CCE was then subdivided into basic and advanced. Basic exam could be done via TTE or TEE but was limited to a 2D examination and attempted to answer questions of hypovolemia, LV/RV failure, tamponade, and massive left sided valvular regurgitation. They also provided a curriculum, but did not provide an opinion on how to measure competency (Mayo et al., 2009).

The Consensus Recommendations from the Council of Emergency Medicine Residency Directors provide some discrete values regarding training. They recommend sonographic training for evaluation of multiple organ systems including FAST examination, emergency cardiac imaging, AAA evaluation, early uterine pregnancy, and procedural guidance. An educational program is recommended to include a one-day orientation course, 80 hours of dedicated time for ultrasonography, an additional 20 hours of scheduled educational sessions, and a minimum of 150 examinations. They also recommend an assessment of image acquisition skills via an examination, and image interpretation skills focused on clinical application (Akhtar et al., 2009).

The ASE has issued recommendations regarding Focused Cardiac Ultrasound (FCU). They differentiated a limited TTE and FCU. FCU is defined as "a focused examination of the cardiovascular system performed by a physician using ultrasound as an adjunct to the physical examination to recognize specific ultrasonic signs that represent a narrow list of potential diagnoses in specific clinical settings." They go on to state that a physician trained in FCU does not have expertise to evaluate a full symptomatic cardiac patient, and give an example of a patient with dyspnea. FCU would be able to rule out large pericardial effusion or significant LV dysfunction, but the patient would need a comprehensive TTE to rule out other cardiac causes of dyspnea. They also recommend a three component based educational curriculum involving didactic education, hands-on image acquisition, and image interpretation. However, they also do not give details on how to demonstrate competence (Spencer et al., 2013)

Recently, the Society of Critical Care Anesthesiologists has drafted an opinion position paper on critical care ultrasound (CCUS). They state that it incorporates vascular ultrasound (venous and arterial access, DVT study), abdominal ultrasound (paracentesis guidance, FAST exam), thoracic ultrasound (thoracentesis, and lung ultrasound), and cardiac ultrasound (studies to evaluate shock, sepsis, hypotension, as well as diastology, and severe valvular dysfunction). They recommend a didactic program of greater than 10 hours, and 30-50 independent exams with supervision of image quality (Fagley et al., 2015)

There is a definite continuum in skill, and technology between critical care sonography and consultant level comprehensive echocardiography. This becomes clear in the example of valvular dysfunction. Some literature on focused TTE only uses the 2D and M-mode functionality due to limitation in training (Philippe Vignon et al., 2011). In other words, when more functionality is used during an echo exam, more knowledge is necessary in order to properly understand the limitations of the method and its proper application. Some protocols use poor cusp separation of the aortic valve to identify severe aortic stenosis, and use that finding as a trigger to order a comprehensive exam. Others use color flow Doppler and train sonographers to identify severe valvular disease (versus not severe). Similarly, some TTE protocols will consider use of trans-mitral flows and variations in their pattern to further support diagnosis of tamponade post cardiac surgery even if fluid is not seen (Geisen et al., 2013). Clearly, the more ultrasound modalities one wishes to use, the longer duration and depth of training required. To further define the role of focused cardiac ultrasound, the American Society of Echocardiography (ASE) and the American College of Emergency Physicians (ACEP) published a consensus statement on this topic. The specified role of the focused cardiac ultrasound was defined as "the time sensitive assessment of the symptomatic patient." Goals of the exam were for assessment of pericardial effusion, global LV systolic function, identification of RV or LV enlargement, intravascular volume assessment, guidance of pericardiocentesis, and confirmation of transvenous pacing wire placement. Note, all these can be evaluated with a simple 2D-based exam. They further noted that application of this bedside exam included cardiac trauma (often in conjunction with a FAST exam), in cardiac arrest with PEA or asystolic rhythms only (VT/VF require immediate defibrillation), and hypotension or shock. They pointed out that dyspnea or chest pain are class I indications for comprehensive assessment (Labovitz et al., 2010)

SONOGRAPHY IN CARDIOVASCULAR ICU: COMPREHENSIVE APPROACH

There are many tools available in the intensive care unit for assessment of the patient. Some are non-invasive such as the physical exam, vital signs, and chest x-ray. Others are invasive such as an arterial line, central venous line, pulmonary artery catheter and so on. All these are part of the armamentarium available to the intensivist and all these need interpretation in context of the clinical situation. Echocardiography is another tool. It has tremendous potential; it is rapid, readily available, can help reduce the diagnostic uncertainty, and monitor the effect of a treatment.

There have been multiple studies regarding sonography focused on a particular organ system. Manno and colleagues created a comprehensive critical care sonography protocol, the "ICU Sound" protocol, and assessed its utility in 125 general ICU patients. The protocol involved three probes and involved the following locations: optic nerve, chest (six locations per hemithorax), heart (six views - parasternal short & long view, apical two, four & five chamber views, subcostal view), abdomen (six views incorporating some from the FAST exam), venous exam (lower & upper limb vessels, and neck vessels). Clearly this was a thorough exam, and the median time to complete it was 19.5 minutes. The exam had notable findings in the CNS in 3.1% of patients, pulmonary in 36.7%, cardiovascular in 48%, abdominal in 9.6%, and venous in 1.5% of patients. Overall these findings modified the admitting diagnosis in 25.6% of patients, and confirmed it in 58.4%. The sonographic findings lead to further testing in 18.4% of patients, changed medical therapy in 17.6%, and led to an invasive procedure in 21.6% of patients. This protocol was meticulous, and sonography made an impact on the care of these patients (Manno et al., 2012).

Overall the last several years, in our cardiovascular intensive care unit (CVICU) at Vanderbilt University Medical Center, the role of sonography in ICU, and training of fellows in it have evolved. Training for critical care fellows currently involves training in use of ultrasound in arterial and venous access, as well as for thoracentesis and paracentesis. Fellows are trained in lung examination particularly for presence of pleural effusions, and post procedure pneumothorax. Training in use of lung ultrasound for consolidation and lung water is evolving. For cardiac sonography, fellows spend time with sonographers in the cardiology echo laboratory to pick up basic technical skills in acquiring images necessary for the FATE protocol, and use of 2D imaging and M-mode. Fellows are expected to use sonography (FATE protocol) in evaluation of the hemodynamically unstable patient. Fellows are also expected to place a minature TEE probe in patients meeting criteria for the probe, and acquire mid-esophageal four chamber, and transgastric short-axis 2D images. Fellows are also encouraged to scan lower extremities for DVT, and perform a FAST examination to build up their own library of normal and pathologic images. We are now also archiving point-of-care examinations for regular review and QA/QI, as well as expecting fellows to write point-of-care sonography notes with their findings in the medical record.

Staffing in our CVICU is a mix of anesthesiologist intensivists, and cardiac anesthesiologist intensivists. Patients having central line placement for internal jugular vein or femoral access will have ultrasound guided vascular access. In patients with reduced pulsatility, arterial access will be generally ultrasound or hand-held Doppler guided. Patients with minor hemodynamic instability post procedure will have an initial focused TTE examination. As a side note, patients will have a wedge placed underneath their right side to facilitate improved imaging windows. If based on the results of the examination, a new plan of care does not lead to clinical improvement, a TEE probe is placed. If the clinical question is to rule out a particular etiology to facilitate surgical decision-making (i.e. single exam to rule our pulmonary vein stenosis post lung transplant, cardiac tamponade, acute new ventricular dysfunction, concern for VAD cannula position), then a comprehensive TEE examination is performed. If the patient's course is expected to be challenging for greater than twelve hours such as requiring titration of multiple pressors, particularly in an individual who has mechanical support device, a minature TEE probe is placed to facilitate multiple serial examinations to monitor treatment effect. Similarly, in patients who are having inotropes titrated post procedure, and in whom clinical variables (cardiac index, stroke volume, lactate clearance, mixed venous saturations) are discordant, a focused TTE examination is done. Another common use of focused TTE examination is for determination of volume status and plan for volume management. In a patient with rising creatinine, if the focused examination supports the clinical determination that the patient has adequate cardiac output (ie. adequate ventricular function, and adequate ventricular size), the patient is diuresed. If there is significant discordance between clinical impression and focused sonographic examination, then other parameters are used to create a unifying picture. For example, if patient is found be clinically in a low cardiac state, but the right ventricle is dilated with interventricular septum D shaped in diastole, the patient is still diuresed in concert with support for the right ventricle.

In patients with ventricular assist devices, serial focused TTE examination is done to evaluate right ventricular function, right ventricular size, and left ventricular size. The decision to change VAD speed is generally based on clinical impression, or formal TTE examination done as part of a ramp study. In patients with ECMO, echocardiography is also commonly used. In our VV ECMO patients, we used either TTE, or TEE to guide cannula position. Placement is generally done with a comprehensive TEE guidance though recently we have used focused TTE from the subcostal position to help VV ECMO cannulation. In our VA ECMO patients, a comprehensive TEE is used to help cannulation, and make management decisions about LV decompression.

SUMMARY

Overall, there is a consistent signal in the literature that focused echocardiography done by the intensive care team can provide rapid and relevant information to aid in diagnosis and management. The ability to visualize structures of interest both directly and non-invasively, as well as rapidly at the bedside provides a rationale for their growing use. Lung, heart, abdominal structures, and lower extremity veins are readily assessed. All this needs to be tempered with the knowledge that this is a monitoring tool. It improves diagnosis, but the management and outcomes are still dependent on the ability of the physician to properly interpret the values (or images in this case) provided by the monitor. It is also a tool with complex design, physics, and multiple investigative modalities beyond simply 2D echo. One must be aware that just because the structure looks "normal" on 2D, it may not do so on other echocardiographic modalities. However, an appropriate note of caution should be exercised in patients in the cardiac intensive care where position of surgical dressings and tubes may impair TTE views, and in whom cardiac function can be much more dynamic, and in whom and mechanical devices may affect interpretation. As stated by Maltais et al. specifically regarding the application of the FCU to the post-operative cardiac patient, "while the debate rages on the national stage, it is important to appreciate the complexity of post-operative cardiac surgery patients, and echocardiography of this patient population requires substantive knowledge that cannot be gained in 1-2 courses or 1-2 months" (Maltais et al., 2013).

Table 1. Suggested critical care ultrasound assisted organ system examination

	Views	Pathology Identified
Lung (based on BLUE protocol	Anterior Chest Wall Upper & Lower Lateral Chest Wall Upper& Lower Posterolateral Chest Wall Upper & Lower	Pneumothorax; Pleural Effusion, Consolidation, Pulmonary Edema
Heart (based on FATE protocol)	Subcostal View Apical (Four Chamber) View Parasternal Short-axis, Mid-papillary View Parasternal Long-axis view	Gross biventricular systolic function Gross biventricular dilation Pericardial Tamponade
Abdomen (based on FAST protocol)	Right Coronal View Left Coronal View Pelvic Longitudinal and Transverse Views	Intraabdominal free fluid
DVT (based on Kory et. al.)	Common femoral vein x 3 per leg Popliteal Vein x 2 per leg Superficial Femoral vein course per leg	Lower extremity DVT

Figure 1. Common critical care ultrasound views. (A) Right Anterior Chest. Thin white line is pleural line. On real-time imaging, clear sliding movement is seen in normal lung. (B) Parasternal long-axis view (C) Parasternal short-axis view (D) Apical 4 Chamber view (E) Apical 2 Chamber view (F) Subcostal view.

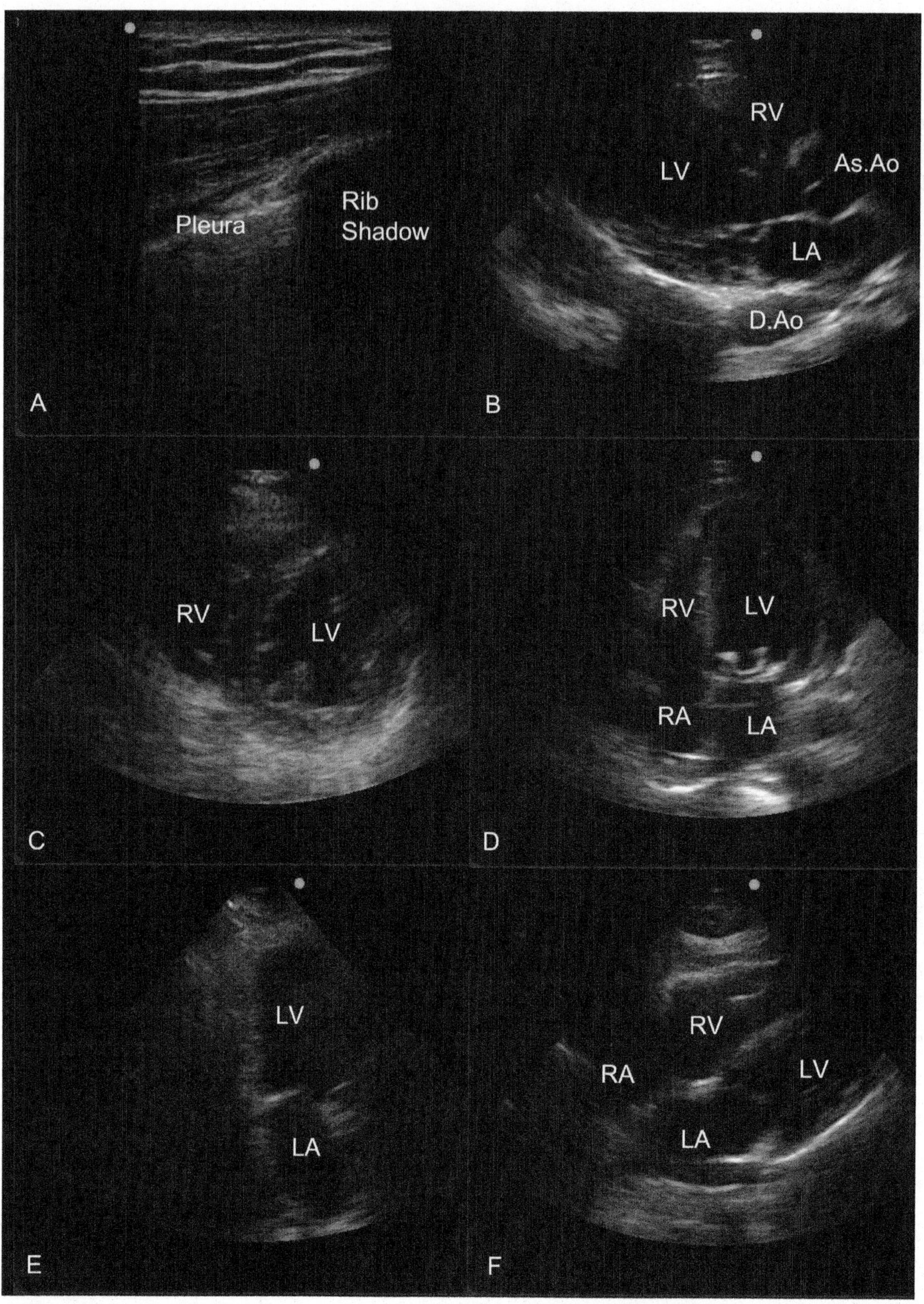

Figure 2. (G) Subcostal IVC view (H) IVC view from probe placed slightly lateral to mid-clavicular line underneath ribs aimed towards midline. This transhepatic IVC view is useful in individuals who have midline incision. (I) Right Coronal View (J) Left Coronal View. RV (Right ventricle), RA (Right Atrium), LV (Left Ventricle), LA (Left Atrium), As.Ao (Ascending Aorta), D.Ao (Descending Aorta), IVC (Inferior Vena Cava). Images acquired using Sonosite(R) S series ultrasound machine. For (A) higher frequency L25 13-6 MHz probe was used. For the rest, P21 5-1 MHz probe used.

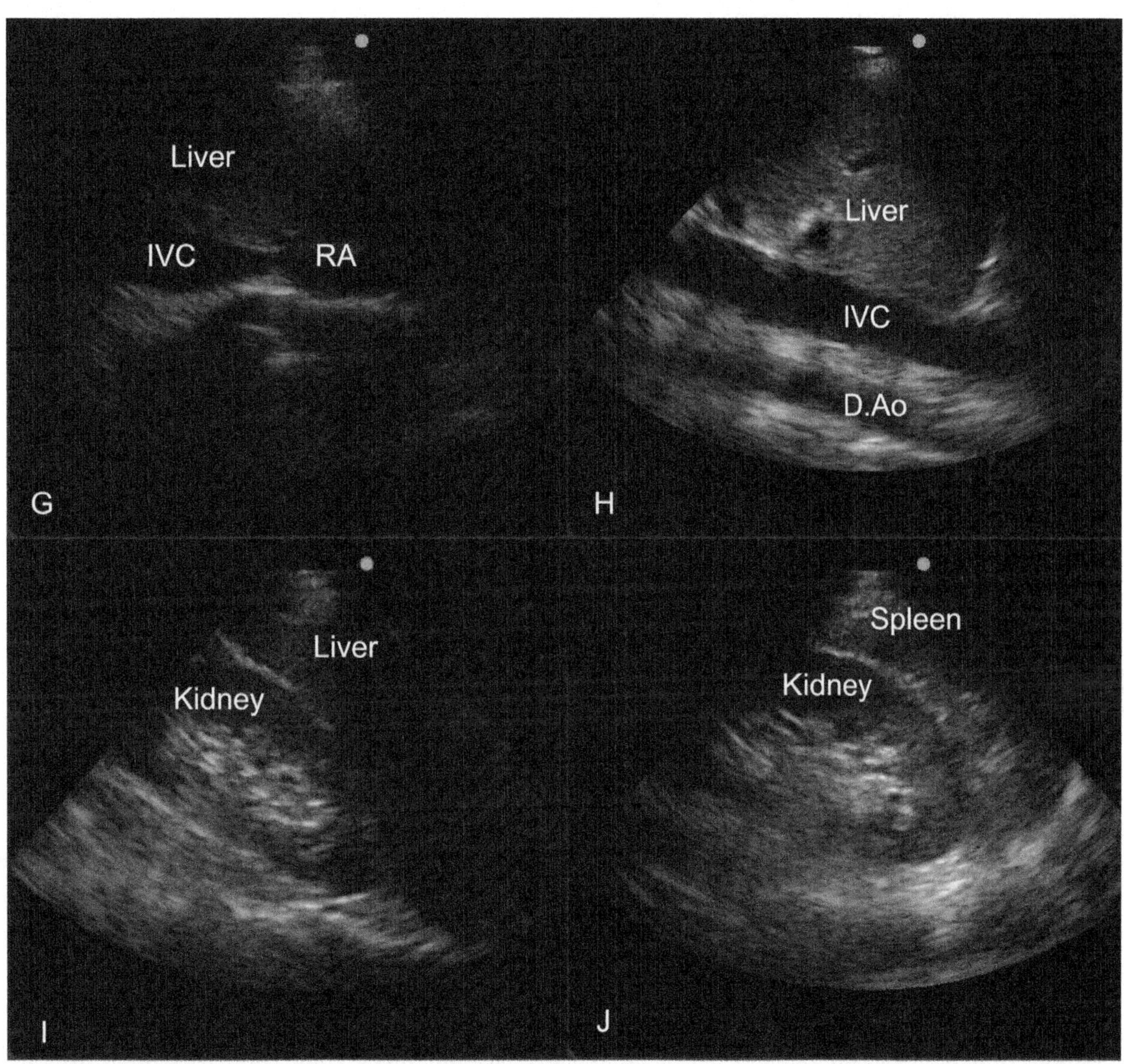

REFERENCES

Akhtar, S., Theodoro, D., Gaspari, R., Tayal, V., Sierzenski, P., Lamantia, J., & Raio, C. et al. (2009). Resident training in emergency ultrasound: Consensus recommendations from the 2008 Council of Emergency Medicine Residency Directors Conference. *Academic Emergency Medicine: Official Journal of the Society for Academic Emergency Medicine*, *16*(Suppl 2), S32–S36. doi:10.1111/j.1553-2712.2009.00589.x PMID:20053207

Bouhemad, B., Zhang, M., Lu, Q., & Rouby, J.-J. (2007). Clinical review: Bedside lung ultrasound in critical care practice. *Critical Care (London, England)*, *11*(1), 205. doi:10.1186/cc5668 PMID:17316468

Cavarocchi, N. C., Pitcher, H. T., Yang, Q., Karbowski, P., Miessau, J., Hastings, H. M., & Hirose, H. (2013). Weaning of extracorporeal membrane oxygenation using continuous hemodynamic transesophageal echocardiography. *The Journal of Thoracic and Cardiovascular Surgery*, *146*(6), 1474–1479. doi:10.1016/j.jtcvs.2013.06.055 PMID:23993027

Cortellaro, F., Colombo, S., Coen, D., & Duca, P. G. (2012). Lung ultrasound is an accurate diagnostic tool for the diagnosis of pneumonia in the emergency department. *Emergency Medicine Journal: EMJ*, *29*(1), 19–23. doi:10.1136/emj.2010.101584 PMID:21030550

Fagley, R. E., Haney, M. F., Beraud, A.-S., Comfere, T., Kohl, B. A., Merkel, M. J., & Wall, M. H. et al. (2015). Critical care basic ultrasound learning goals for american anesthesiology critical care trainees: Recommendations from an expert group. *Anesthesia and Analgesia*, *120*(5), 1041–1053. doi:10.1213/ANE.0000000000000652 PMID:25899271

Faris, J. G., Veltman, M. G., & Royse, C. F. (2009). Limited transthoracic echocardiography assessment in anaesthesia and critical care. *Best Practice & Research. Clinical Anaesthesiology*, *23*(3), 285–298. doi:10.1016/j.bpa.2009.02.008 PMID:19862888

Fragou, M., Gravvanis, A., Dimitriou, V., Papalois, A., Kouraklis, G., Karabinis, A., & Karakitsos, D. et al. (2011). Real-time ultrasound-guided subclavian vein cannulation versus the landmark method in critical care patients: A prospective randomized study. *Critical Care Medicine*, *39*(7), 1607–1612. doi:10.1097/CCM.0b013e318218a1ae PMID:21494105

Geisen, M., Spray, D., & Nicholas Fletcher, S. (2013). Echocardiography-Based Hemodynamic Management in the Cardiac Surgical Intensive Care Unit. *Journal of Cardiothoracic and Vascular Anesthesia*. Retrieved from http://linkinghub.elsevier.com/retrieve/pii/S1053077013004801

Grogan, D. R., Irwin, R. S., Channick, R., Raptopoulos, V., Curley, F. J., Bartter, T., & Corwin, R. W. (1990). Complications associated with thoracentesis. A prospective, randomized study comparing three different methods. *Archives of Internal Medicine*, *150*(4), 873–877. doi:10.1001/archinte.1990.00390160119023 PMID:2183735

Haglund, N. A., Maltais, S., Bick, J. S., Costello, W., Keebler, M., Davis, M. E., & Wagner, C. E. et al. (2014). Hemodynamic transesophageal echocardiography after left ventricular assist device implantation. *Journal of Cardiothoracic and Vascular Anesthesia*, *28*(5), 1184–1190. doi:10.1053/j.jvca.2014.02.012 PMID:25104081

Huang, S. J., & McLean, A. S. (2012). Appreciating the Strengths and Weaknesses of Transthoracic Echocardiography in Hemodynamic Assessments. *Cardiology Research and Practice*, *2012*, 1–7. doi:10.1155/2012/894308 PMID:22454777

Jensen, M. B., Sloth, E., Larsen, K. M., & Schmidt, M. B. (2004). Transthoracic echocardiography for cardiopulmonary monitoring in intensive care. *European Journal of Anaesthesiology*, *21*(9), 700–707. doi:10.1097/00003643-200409000-00006 PMID:15595582

Kobal, S. L., Trento, L., Baharami, S., Tolstrup, K., Naqvi, T. Z., Cercek, B., & Siegel, R. J. et al. (2005). Comparison of effectiveness of hand-carried ultrasound to bedside cardiovascular physical examination. *The American Journal of Cardiology*, *96*(7), 1002–1006. doi:10.1016/j.amjcard.2005.05.060 PMID:16188532

Kory, P. D., Pellecchia, C. M., Shiloh, A. L., Mayo, P. H., DiBello, C., & Koenig, S. (2011). Accuracy of ultrasonography performed by critical care physicians for the diagnosis of DVT. *Chest*, *139*(3), 538–542. doi:10.1378/chest.10-1479 PMID:21030490

Labovitz, A. J., Noble, V. E., Bierig, M., Goldstein, S. A., Jones, R., Kort, S., & Wei, K. et al. (2010). Focused Cardiac Ultrasound in the Emergent Setting: A Consensus Statement of the American Society of Echocardiography and American College of Emergency Physicians. *Journal of the American Society of Echocardiography*, *23*(12), 1225–1230. doi:10.1016/j.echo.2010.10.005 PMID:21111923

Lichtenstein, D., Mezière, G., Biderman, P., & Gepner, A. (1999). The comet-tail artifact: An ultrasound sign ruling out pneumothorax. *Intensive Care Medicine*, *25*(4), 383–388. doi:10.1007/s001340050862 PMID:10342512

Lichtenstein, D., Mézière, G., Biderman, P., Gepner, A., & Barré, O. (1997). The comet-tail artifact. An ultrasound sign of alveolar-interstitial syndrome. *American Journal of Respiratory and Critical Care Medicine*, *156*(5), 1640–1646. doi:10.1164/ajrccm.156.5.96-07096 PMID:9372688

Lichtenstein, D., Mezière, G., & Seitz, J. (2009). The dynamic air bronchogram. A lung ultrasound sign of alveolar consolidation ruling out atelectasis. *Chest*, *135*(6), 1421–1425. doi:10.1378/chest.08-2281 PMID:19225063

Lichtenstein, D. A., Mezière, G., Lascols, N., Biderman, P., Courret, J.-P., Gepner, A., & Tenoudji-Cohen, M. et al. (2005). Ultrasound diagnosis of occult pneumothorax*. *Critical Care Medicine*, *33*(6), 1231–1238. doi:10.1097/01.CCM.0000164542.86954.B4 PMID:15942336

Lichtenstein, D. A., & Mezière, G. A. (2008). Relevance of lung ultrasound in the diagnosis of acute respiratory failure: The BLUE protocol. *Chest*, *134*(1), 117–125. doi:10.1378/chest.07-2800 PMID:18403664

Maltais, S., Costello, W. T., Billings, F. T. IV, Bick, J. S., Byrne, J. G., Ahmad, R. M., & Wagner, C. E. (2013). Episodic Monoplane Transesophageal Echocardiography Impacts Postoperative Management of the Cardiac Surgery Patient. *Journal of Cardiothoracic and Vascular Anesthesia*, *27*(4), 665–669. doi:10.1053/j.jvca.2013.02.012 PMID:23849522

Manno, E., Navarra, M., Faccio, L., Motevallian, M., Bertolaccini, L., Mfochivè, A., & Evangelista, A. et al. (2012). Deep impact of ultrasound in the intensive care unit: The "ICU-sound" protocol. *Anesthesiology*, *117*(4), 801–809. doi:10.1097/ALN.0b013e318264c621 PMID:22990179

Mayo, P. H., Beaulieu, Y., Doelken, P., Feller-Kopman, D., Harrod, C., Kaplan, A., & Lichtenstein, D. et al. (2009). American College of Chest Physicians/La Société de Réanimation de Langue Française statement on competence in critical care ultrasonography. *CHEST Journal*, *135*(4), 1050–1060. doi:10.1378/chest.08-2305 PMID:19188546

Mercaldi, C. J., & Lanes, S. F. (2013). Ultrasound guidance decreases complications and improves the cost of care among patients undergoing thoracentesis and paracentesis. *Chest*, *143*(2), 532–538. doi:10.1378/chest.12-0447 PMID:23381318

Orme, R. M. L., Oram, M. P., & McKinstry, C. E. (2009). Impact of echocardiography on patient management in the intensive care unit: An audit of district general hospital practice. *British Journal of Anaesthesia*, *102*(3), 340–344. doi:10.1093/bja/aen378 PMID:19151420

Oxorn, D., & Pearlman, A. (2012). CON: physician-performed ultrasound: the time has come for routine use in acute care medicine. *Anesthesia and Analgesia*, *115*(5), 1004–1006. doi:10.1213/ANE.0b013e31826a118a PMID:23093582

Patel, P. A., Ernst, F. R., & Gunnarsson, C. L. (2012). Ultrasonography guidance reduces complications and costs associated with thoracentesis procedures. *Journal of Clinical Ultrasound: JCU*, *40*(3), 135–141. doi:10.1002/jcu.20884 PMID:21994047

Perera, P., Mailhot, T., Riley, D., & Mandavia, D. (2010). The RUSH exam: Rapid Ultrasound in SHock in the evaluation of the critically lll. [vii.]. *Emergency Medicine Clinics of North America*, *28*(1), 29–56. doi:10.1016/j.emc.2009.09.010 PMID:19945597

Rugolotto, M., Chang, C.-P., Hu, B., Schnittger, I., & Liang, D. H. (2002). Clinical use of cardiac ultrasound performed with a hand-carried device in patients admitted for acute cardiac care. *The American Journal of Cardiology*, *90*(9), 1040–1042. doi:10.1016/S0002-9149(02)02700-5 PMID:12398985

Scalea, T. M., Rodriguez, A., Chiu, W. C., Brenneman, F. D., Fallon, W. F. Jr, Kato, K., & Yoshii, H. et al. (1999). Focused Assessment with Sonography for Trauma (FAST): Results from an international consensus conference. *The Journal of Trauma*, *46*(3), 466–472. doi:10.1097/00005373-199903000-00022 PMID:10088853

Shostak, E., Brylka, D., Krepp, J., Pua, B., & Sanders, A. (2013). Bedside sonography for detection of postprocedure pneumothorax. *Journal of Ultrasound in Medicine: Official Journal of the American Institute of Ultrasound in Medicine*, *32*(6), 1003–1009. doi:10.7863/ultra.32.6.1003 PMID:23716522

Soldati, G., Testa, A., Sher, S., Pignataro, G., La Sala, M., & Silveri, N. G. (2008). Occult traumatic pneumothorax: Diagnostic accuracy of lung ultrasonography in the emergency department. *Chest*, *133*(1), 204–211. doi:10.1378/chest.07-1595 PMID:17925411

Spencer, K. T., Kimura, B. J., Korcarz, C. E., Pellikka, P. A., Rahko, P. S., & Siegel, R. J. (2013). Focused Cardiac Ultrasound: Recommendations from the American Society of Echocardiography. *Journal of the American Society of Echocardiography*, *26*(6), 567–581. doi:10.1016/j.echo.2013.04.001 PMID:23711341

Troianos, C. A., Hartman, G. S., Glas, K. E., Skubas, N. J., Eberhardt, R. T., Walker, J. D., & Reeves, S. T. (2011). Guidelines for Performing Ultrasound Guided Vascular Cannulation: Recommendations of the American Society of Echocardiography and the Society of Cardiovascular Anesthesiologists. *Journal of the American Society of Echocardiography*, *24*(12), 1291–1318. doi:10.1016/j.echo.2011.09.021 PMID:22115322

Vieillard-Baron, A., Slama, M., Mayo, P., Charron, C., Amiel, J.-B., Esterez, C., & Vignon, P. et al. (2013). A pilot study on safety and clinical utility of a single-use 72-hour indwelling transesophageal echocardiography probe. *Intensive Care Medicine*, *39*(4), 629–635. doi:10.1007/s00134-012-2797-4 PMID:23287876

Vignon, P. (2012). PRO: physician-performed ultrasound: the time has come for routine use in acute care medicine. *Anesthesia and Analgesia*, *115*(5), 999–1003. doi:10.1213/ANE.0b013e31826bfa7d PMID:23093581

Vignon, P., Mücke, F., Bellec, F., Marin, B., Croce, J., Brouqui, T., & Amiel, J.-B. et al. (2011). Basic critical care echocardiography: Validation of a curriculum dedicated to noncardiologist residents*. *Critical Care Medicine*, *39*(4), 636–642. doi:10.1097/CCM.0b013e318206c1e4 PMID:21221001

KEY TERMS AND DEFINITIONS

FAST: Focused Assessment with Sonography for Trauma.
FCU: Focused Cardiac Ultrasound.
CCUS: Critical Care Sonography.

Compilation of References

A, V. D. L., Shaffer, C., & Schaefer, E. (2014). Early intensive care unit-acquired hypernatremia in severe sepsis patients receiving 0.9% saline fluid resuscitation. *Acta Anaesthesiologica Scandinavica.*

Aaronson, K., Schwartz, J., Chen, T., Wong, K., Goin, J., & Mancini, D. (1997). Development and prospective validation of a clinical index to predict survival in ambulatory patients referred for cardiac transplant evaluation. *Circulation, 95*(12), 2660–2667. doi:10.1161/01.CIR.95.12.2660 PMID:9193435

Aarts, M. A., Hancock, J. N., Heyland, D., McLeod, R. S., & Marshall, J. C. (2008). Empiric antibiotic therapy for suspected ventilator-associated pneumonia: A systematic review and meta-analysis of randomized trials. *Critical Care Medicine, 36*(1), 108–117. doi:10.1097/01.CCM.0000297956.27474.9D PMID:18007262

Abboud, B., Daher, R., Sleilaty, G., Madi-Jebara, S., El Asmar, B., Achouch, R., & Jebara, V. (2008). Is prompt exploratory laparotomy the best attitude for mesenteric ischemia after cardiac surgery? *Interactive Cardiovascular and Thoracic Surgery, 7*(6), 1079–1083. doi:10.1510/icvts.2008.176271 PMID:18815161

Abecassis, M., Bridges, N. D., Clancy, C. J., Dew, M. A., Eldadah, B., Englesbe, M. J., & High, K. P. et al. (2012). Solid-organ transplantation in older adults: Current status and future research. *American Journal of Transplantation, 12*(10), 2608–2622. doi:10.1111/j.1600-6143.2012.04245.x

Abraham, W. T., Adams, K. F., Fonarow, G. C., Costanzo, M. R., Berkowitz, R. L., LeJemtel, T. H., & Wynne, J. et al. (2005). In-hospital mortality in patients with acute decompensated heart failure requiring intravenous vasoactive medications: An Analysis from the Acute Decompensated Heart Failure National Registry (ADHERE). *Journal of the American College of Cardiology, 46*(1), 57–64. doi:10.1016/j.jacc.2005.03.051 PMID:15992636

Abrams, D. C., Prager, K., Blinderman, C. D., Burkart, K. M., & Brodie, D. (2014). Ethical dilemmas encountered with the use of extracorporeal membrane oxygenation in adults. *Chest, 145*(4), 876–882. doi:10.1378/chest.13-1138 PMID:24687709

Abu-Salah, T., & Dhand, R. (2011). Inhaled antibiotic therapy for ventilator-associated tracheobronchitis and ventilator-associated pneumonia: An update. *Advances in Therapy, 28*(9), 728–747. doi:10.1007/s12325-011-0051-z PMID:21833701

Acar, C., Jebara, V. A., Portoghese, M., Beyssen, B., Pagny, J. Y., & Grare, P. … Guermonprez, J. L. (1992). Revival of the radial artery for coronary artery bypass grafting. *The Annals of Thoracic Surgery, 54*(4), 652–9; discussion 659–60. Retrieved from http://www.ncbi.nlm.nih.gov/pubmed/1358040

Accreditation Council for Graduate Medical Education. (2013). *Common Program Requirements.* Retrieved May 9, 2014 from https://www.acgme.org/acgmeweb/Portals/0/PFAssets/ProgramRequirements/CPRs2013.pdf

Accreditation Council for Graduate Medical Education. (2014). *Program Requirements for Graduate Medical Education in Anesthesiology Critical Care Medicine.* Retrieved May 9, 2014, from http://www.acgme.org/acgmeweb/Portals/0/PFAssets/ProgramRequirements/045_critical_care_anes_07012014_1-YR.pdf

Achneck, H. E., Sileshi, B., Parikh, A., Milano, C. A., Welsby, I. J., & Lawson, J. H. (2010). Pathophysiology of bleeding and clotting in the cardiac surgery patient: From vascular endothelium to circulatory assist device surface. *Circulation*, *122*(20), 2068–2077. doi:10.1161/CIRCULATIONAHA.110.936773 PMID:21098468

Achouh, P., & Acar, C. (2013). Twenty-year fate of the radial artery graft. *Annals of Cardiothoracic Surgery*, *2*(4), 481–484. doi:10.3978/j.issn.2225-319X.2013.07.13 PMID:23977626

Achouh, P., Isselmou, K. O., Boutekadjirt, R., D'Alessandro, C., Pagny, J.-Y., Fouquet, R., & Acar, C. et al. (2012). Reappraisal of a 20-year experience with the radial artery as a conduit for coronary bypass grafting. *European Journal of Cardio-Thoracic Surgery : Official Journal of the European Association for Cardio-Thoracic Surgery*, *41*(1), 87–92. doi:10.1016/j.ejcts.2011.05.027 PMID:21900019

Adabag, A. S., Ishani, A., Bloomfield, H. E., Ngo, A. K., & Wilt, T. J. (2009). Efficacy of N-acetylcysteine in preventing renal injury after heart surgery: A systematic review of randomized trials. *European Heart Journal*, *30*(15), 1910–1917. doi:10.1093/eurheartj/ehp053 PMID:19282300

Adams, D. H., Popma, J. J., Reardon, M. J., Yakubov, S. J., Coselli, J. S., Deeb, G. M., & Oh, J. K. et al. (2014). Transcatheter aortic-valve replacement with a self-expanding prosthesis. *The New England Journal of Medicine*, *370*(19), 1790–1798. doi:10.1056/NEJMoa1400590 PMID:24678937

Adams, H. P. Jr, del Zoppo, G., Alberts, M. J., Bhatt, D. L., Brass, L., Furlan, A., & Wijdicks, E. F. M. et al. (2007). Guidelines for the early management of adults with ischemic stroke: a guideline from the American Heart Association/American Stroke Association Stroke Council, Clinical Cardiology Council, Cardiovascular Radiology and Intervention Council, and the Atherosclerotic Peripheral Vascular Disease and Quality of Care Outcomes in Research Interdisciplinary Working Groups: The American Academy of Neurology affirms the value of this guideline as an educational tool for neurologists. *Circulation*, *115*(20), e478–e534. doi:10.1161/CIRCULATIONAHA.107.181486 PMID:17515473

Adams, S. D., & Mercer, D. W. (2007). Fulminant Clostridium difficile colitis. *Current Opinion in Critical Care*, *13*(4), 450–455. doi:10.1097/MCC.0b013e3282638879 PMID:17599017

Adelman, B., Rizk, A., & Hanners, E. (1988). Plasminogen interactions with platelets in plasma. *Blood*, *72*(5), 1530–1535. PMID:3179439

Adhikari, N., Burns, K. E., Friedrich, J. O., Granton, J. T., Cook, D. J., & Meade, M. O. (2007). Effect of nitric oxide on oxygenation and mortality in acute lung injury: Systematic review and meta-analysis. *British Medical Journal*, *334*(7597), 779. doi:10.1136/bmj.39139.716794.55 PMID:17383982

Adler, S. M., & Wartofsky, L. (2007). The nonthyroidal illness syndrome. *Endocrinology and Metabolism Clinics of North America*, *36*(3), 657–672. doi:10.1016/j.ecl.2007.04.007 PMID:17673123

Afilalo, J., Mottillo, S., Eisenberg, M. J., Alexander, K. P., Noiseux, N., Perrault, L. P., & Bergman, H. et al. (2012). Addition of frailty and disability to cardiac surgery risk scores identifies elderly patients at high risk of mortality or major morbidity. *Circulation: Cardiovascular Quality and Outcomes*, *5*(2), 222–228. doi:10.1161/CIRCOUTCOMES.111.963157 PMID:22396586

Agerstrand, C. L., Bacchetta, M. D., & Brodie, D. (2014). ECMO for adult respiratory failure: Current use and evolving applications. *ASAIO Journal (American Society for Artificial Internal Organs)*, *60*(3), 255–262. doi:10.1097/MAT.0000000000000062 PMID:24625534

Ahlers, S. J. G. M., van Gulik, L., van der Veen, A. M., van Dongen, H. P. A., Bruins, P., Belitser, S. V., & Knibbe, C. A. J. et al. (2007). Comparison of different pain scoring systems in critically ill patients in a general ICU. *Critical Care (London, England)*, *12*(1), R15. doi:10.1186/cc6789 PMID:18279522

Akhtar, S., Theodoro, D., Gaspari, R., Tayal, V., Sierzenski, P., Lamantia, J., & Raio, C. et al. (2009). Resident training in emergency ultrasound: Consensus recommendations from the 2008 Council of Emergency Medicine Residency Directors Conference. *Academic Emergency Medicine: Official Journal of the Society for Academic Emergency Medicine*, *16*(Suppl 2), S32–S36. doi:10.1111/j.1553-2712.2009.00589.x PMID:20053207

Akins, C. W. (1984). Noncardioplegic myocardial preservation for coronary revascularization. *The Journal of Thoracic and Cardiovascular Surgery*, *88*(2), 174–181. Retrieved from http://www.ncbi.nlm.nih.gov/pubmed/6611456 PMID:6611456

Ak, K., Isbir, C. S., Tetik, S., Atalan, N., Tekeli, A., Aljodi, M., & Arsan, S. et al. (2009). Thromboelastography-based transfusion algorithm reduces blood product use after elective CABG: A prospective randomized study. *Journal of Cardiac Surgery*, *24*(4), 404–410. doi:10.1111/j.1540-8191.2009.00840.x PMID:19583608

Akoumianaki, E., Maggiore, S. M., Valenza, F., Bellani, G., Jubran, A., Loring, S. H., & Brochard, L. et al. (2014). The application of esophageal pressure measurement in patients with respiratory failure. *American Journal of Respiratory and Critical Care Medicine*, *189*(5), 520–531. doi:10.1164/rccm.201312-2193CI PMID:24467647

Akram, M. R., Chan, T., McAuliffe, S., & Chenzbraun, A. (2008). Non-rheumatic annular mitral stenosis: Prevalence and characteristics. *European Journal of Echocardiography*, *10*(1), 103–105. doi:10.1093/ejechocard/jen179 PMID:18579487

Alam, N., Park, B., Wilton, A., Seshan, V., Bains, M., Downey, R., & Amar, D. et al. (2007). Incidence and Risk Factors for Lung Injury After Lung Cancer Resection. *The Annals of Thoracic Surgery*, *84*(4), 1085–1091. doi:10.1016/j.athoracsur.2007.05.053 PMID:17888952

Alanezi, K., & Urschel, J. (2004). Mortality secondary to esophageal anastomotic leak. *Annals of Thoracic and Cardiovascular Surgery*, *10*(2). PMID:15209546

Al-Bahrani, A. Z., Abid, G. H., Sahgal, E., O'shea, S., Lee, S., & Ammori, B. J. (2007). A prospective evaluation of CT features predictive of intra-abdominal hypertension and abdominal compartment syndrome in critically ill surgical patients. *Clinical Radiology*, *62*(7), 676–682. doi:10.1016/j.crad.2006.11.006 PMID:17556037

Alexander, J., Hamilton, W., Parikh, R., Spence, A., & Stewart, B. (1972). Further studies on the role of airways closure in postoperative hypoxaemia. *British Journal of Anaesthesia*, *44*(8), 905–906. PMID:5083032

Alexander, J., Lopes, R., James, S., Kilaru, R., He, Y., Mohan, P., & Atar, D. et al. (2011). Apixaban with Antiplatelet Therapy after Acute Coronary Syndrome. *The New England Journal of Medicine*, *365*(8), 699–708. doi:10.1056/NEJMoa1105819 PMID:21780946

Alexiou, V. G., Ierodiakonou, V., Dimopoulos, G., & Falagas, M. E. (2009). Impact of patient position on the incidence of ventilator-associated pneumonia: A meta-analysis of randomized controlled trials. *Journal of Critical Care*, *24*(4), 515–522. doi:10.1016/j.jcrc.2008.09.003 PMID:19327314

Algarni, K. D., Elhenawy, A. M., Maganti, M., Collins, S., & Yau, T. M. (2012). Decreasing prevalence but increasing importance of left ventricular dysfunction and reoperative surgery in prediction of mortality in coronary artery bypass surgery: trends over 18 years. *The Journal of Thoracic and Cardiovascular Surgery*, *144*(2), 340–6– 346.e1. doi:10.1016/j.jtcvs.2011.06.043

Algarni, K. D., Maganti, M., & Yau, T. M. (2011). Predictors of Low Cardiac Output Syndrome After Isolated Coronary Artery Bypass Surgery: Trends Over 20 Years. *Ats*, *92*(5), 1678–1684. doi:10.1016/j.athoracsur.2011.06.017 PMID:21939957

Alghamdi, A. A., Albanna, M. J., Guru, V., & Brister, S. J. (2006a). Does the use of erythropoietin reduce the risk of exposure to allogeneic blood transfusion in cardiac surgery? A systematic review and meta-analysis. *Journal of Cardiac Surgery*, *21*(3), 320–326. doi:10.1111/j.1540-8191.2006.00241.x PMID:16684074

Alghamdi, A. A., Davis, A., Brister, S., Corey, P., & Logan, A. (2006b). Development and validation of Transfusion Risk Understanding Scoring Tool (TRUST) to stratify cardiac surgery patients according to their blood transfusion needs. *Transfusion*, *46*(7), 1120–1129. doi:10.1111/j.1537-2995.2006.00860.x PMID:16836558

Alhashemi, J. A., Sharpe, M. D., Harris, C. L., Sherman, V., & Boyd, D. (2000). Effect of subarachnoid morphine administration on extubation time after coronary artery bypass graft surgery. *Journal of Cardiothoracic and Vascular Anesthesia*, *14*(6), 639–644. doi:10.1053/jcan.2000.18300 PMID:11139101

Alhazzani, W., Alenezi, F., Jaeschke, R. Z., Moayyedi, P., & Cook, D. J. (2013). Proton pump inhibitors versus histamine 2 receptor antagonists for stress ulcer prophylaxis in critically ill patients: A systematic review and meta-analysis. *Critical Care Medicine*, *41*(3), 693–705. doi:10.1097/CCM.0b013e3182758734 PMID:23318494

Allen, D. J., & Chae-Kim, S. H. (2002). Risks and complications of neuraxial anesthesia and the use of anticoagulation in the surgical patient. ... *(Baylor University Medical* .... Allen, G. A., Hoffman, M., Roberts, H. R., & Monroe, D. M. (2002). Recombinant activated factor VII: Its mechanism of action and role in the control of hemorrhage. *Canadian Journal of Anaesthesia*, *49*(10), S7–S14. PMID:12546000

Allen, L. A., Fonarow, G. C., Grau-Sepulveda, M. V., Hernandez, A. F., Peterson, P. N., Partovian, C., & Krumholz, H. M. et al. (2014). Hospital variation in intravenous inotrope use for patients hospitalized with heart failure: Insights from Get With The Guidelines. *Circulation: Heart Failure*, *7*(2), 251–260. doi:10.1161/CIRCHEARTFAILURE.113.000761 PMID:24488983

Allou, N., Bronchard, R., Guglielminotti, J., Dilly, M. P., Provenchere, S., Lucet, J. C., & Montravers, P. et al. (2014). Risk factors for postoperative pneumonia after cardiac surgery and development of a preoperative risk score*. *Critical Care Medicine*, *42*(5), 1150–1156. doi:10.1097/CCM.0000000000000143 PMID:24351376

Allsop, P., Taylor, M. B., Grounds, R. M., & Morgan, M. (1988). Ventilatory effects of a propofol infusion using a method to rapidly achieve steady-state equilibrium. *European Journal of Anaesthesiology*, *5*, 293–303. PMID:3065083

Alqahtani, A. A. R. (2010). Atrial fibrillation post cardiac surgery trends towards management. *Heart Views*, *11*(2), 57–63. doi:10.4103/1995-705X.73212 PMID:21187998

Alsolamy, S. (2014). Islamic views on artificial nutrition and hydration in terminally ill patients. *Bioethics*, *28*(2), 96–99. doi:10.1111/j.1467-8519.2012.01996.x PMID:22845721

Althouse, L. A., Stritter, F. T., & Steiner, B. D. (1999). Attitudes and Approaches of Influential Role Models in Clinical Education. *Advances in Health Sciences Education: Theory and Practice*, *4*(2), 111–122. doi:10.1023/A:1009768526142 PMID:12386424

Amarenco, P., Cohen, A., & Tzouirio, C. (1994). Atherosclerotic disease of the aortic arch and the risk of ischemic stroke. *The New England Journal of Medicine*, *331*(22), 1474–1479. doi:10.1056/NEJM199412013312202 PMID:7969297

America, A. T. S. I. D. S. (2005). Guidelines for the management of adults with hospital-acquired, ventilator-associated, and healthcare-associated pneumonia. *American Journal of Respiratory and Critical Care Medicine*, *171*(4), 388–416. doi:10.1164/rccm.200405-644ST PMID:15699079

American Heart Association. (2014). AHA Statistical Update: Heart Disease and Stroke Statistics - 2014 Update. *Circulation*, *129*, e28–e292. doi:10.1161/01.cir.0000441139.02102.80 PMID:24352519

American Society of Anesthesiologists Task Force on Perioperative Blood, T., & Adjuvant, T. (2006). Practice guidelines for perioperative blood transfusion and adjuvant therapies: An updated report by the American Society of Anesthesiologists Task Force on Perioperative Blood Transfusion and Adjuvant Therapies. *Anesthesiology*, *105*(1), 198–208. doi:10.1097/00000542-200607000-00030 PMID:16810012

Amin, S., Morrow, D., Braunwald, E., Sloan, S., Contant, C., Murphy, S., & Antman, E. (2013). Dynamic TIMI risk score for STEMI. *Journal of the American Heart Association*, *2*(1), e003269. doi:10.1161/JAHA.112.003269 PMID:23525425

Amiodarone Trials Meta-Analysis Investigators. (1997). Effect of prophylactic amiodarone on mortality after acute myocardial infaction and in congestive heart failure: Meta-analysis of individual data from 6500 patients in randomized trials. *Lancet*, *350*(9089), 1417–1424. doi:10.1016/S0140-6736(97)05281-1 PMID:9371164

Anderson, B. J. (2008). Paracetamol (acetaminophen): Mechanisms of action. *Paediatric Anaesthesia*, *18*(10), 915–921. doi:10.1111/j.1460-9592.2008.02764.x PMID:18811827

Anderson, C. A., Filsoufi, F., Aklog, L., Farivar, R. S., Byrne, J. G., & Adams, D. H. (2002). Liberal use of delayed sternal closure for postcardiotomy hemodynamic instability. *Ats*, *73*(5), 1484–1488. PMID:12022537

Anderson, J., Adams, C., Antman, E., Bridges, C., Califf, R., Casey, D. E., & Wright, R. S. et al. (2007). ACC/AHA 2007 guidelines for the Management of Patients With Unstable Angina/Non-ST-Elevation Myocardial Infarction. *Circulation*, *116*(7), e148–e304. doi:10.1161/CIRCULATIONAHA.107.181940 PMID:17679616

Anderson, L. W., Krathwohl, D. R., & Bloom, B. S. (2001). *A taxonomy for learning, teaching, and assessing*. New York: Longman.

Anderson, R. E., Brismar, K., Barr, G., & Ivert, T. (2005). Effects of cardiopulmonary bypass on glucose homestasis after coronary artery bypass surgery. *European Journal of Cardio-Thoracic Surgery*, *28*(3), 425–430. doi:10.1016/j.ejcts.2005.05.025 PMID:16054822

Andrews, P. J. D., Avenell, A., Noble, D. W., Campbell, M. K., Croal, B. L., Simpson, W. G., … Cook, J. A. (2011). Randomised trial of glutamine, selenium, or both, to supplement parenteral nutrition for critically ill patients. *British Medical Journal*, *342*, d1542.

An, G., & West, M. A. (2008). Abdominal compartment syndrome: A concise clinical review. *Critical Care Medicine*, *36*(4), 1304–1310. doi:10.1097/CCM.0b013e31816929f4 PMID:18379259

Angelini, G. D., Taylor, F. C., Reeves, B. C., & Ascione, R. (2002). Early and midterm outcome after off-pump and on-pump surgery in Beating Heart Against Cardioplegic Arrest Studies (BHACAS 1 and 2): A pooled analysis of two randomised controlled trials. *Lancet*, *359*(9313), 1194–1199. doi:10.1016/S0140-6736(02)08216-8 PMID:11955537

Angiolillo, D., Firstenberg, M., Price, M., Tummala, P., Hutyra, M., Welsby, I., & Topol, E. et al. (2012). Bridging Antiplatelet Therapy With Cangrelor in Patients Undergoing Cardiac Surgery. *Journal of the American Medical Association*, *307*(3), 265–274. doi:10.1001/jama.2011.2002 PMID:22253393

Angles, R., Tenorio, L., Roman, A., Soler, J., Rochera, M., & de Latorre, F. J. (2005). Lung transplantation for emphysema. Lung hyperinflation: Incidence and outcome. *Transplant International*, *17*(12), 810–814. doi:10.1111/j.1432-2277.2004.tb00515.x

Angst, M. S., Koppert, W., Pahl, I., Clark, D. J., & Schmelz, M. (2003). Short-term infusion of the mu-opioid agonist remifentanil in humans causes hyperalgesia during withdrawal. *Pain*, *106*(1), 49–57. doi:10.1016/S0304-3959(03)00276-8 PMID:14581110

Ankeny, R. A., Clifford, R., Jordens, C. F. C., Kerridge, I. H., & Benson, R. (2005). Religious perspectives on withdrawal of treatment from patients with multiple organ failure. *The Medical Journal of Australia*, *183*, 616–621. PMID:16336148

Annane, D., Maxime, V., Ibrahim, F., Alvarez, J. C., Abe, E., & Boudou, P. (2006). Diagnosis of adrenal insufficiency in severe sepsis and septic shock. *American Journal of Respiratory and Critical Care Medicine*, *174*(12), 1319–1326. doi:10.1164/rccm.200509-1369OC PMID:16973979

Annane, D., Sebille, V., Charpentier, C., Bollaert, P. E., Francois, B., Korach, J. M., & Bellissant, E. et al. (2002). Effect of treatment with low doses of hydrocortisone and fludrocortisone on mortality in patients with septic shock. *Journal of the American Medical Association*, *288*(7), 862–871. doi:10.1001/jama.288.7.862 PMID:12186604

Annane, D., Sebille, V., Troche, G., Raphael, J. C., Gajdos, P., & Bellissant, E. (2000). A 3-level prognostic classification in septic shock based on cortisol levels and cortisol response to corticotropin. *Journal of the American Medical Association*, *283*(8), 1038–1045. doi:10.1001/jama.283.8.1038 PMID:10697064

Annane, D., Vignon, P., Renault, A., Bollaert, P., Charpentier, C., Martin, C., & Bellissant, E. et al. (2007). Norepinephrine plus dobutamine versus epinephrine alone for management of septic shock: A randomised trial. *Lancet*, *370*(9588), 676–684. doi:10.1016/S0140-6736(07)61344-0 PMID:17720019

Anthi, A., Tzelepis, G. E., Alivizatos, P., Michalis, A., Palatianos, G. M., & Geroulanos, S. (1998). Unexpected cardiac arrest after cardiac surgery: Incidence, predisposing causes, and outcome of open chest cardiopulmonary resuscitation. *Chest*, *113*(1), 15–19. http://www.ncbi.nlm.nih.gov/pubmed/9440561 doi:10.1378/chest.113.1.15 PMID:9440561

Antman, E. M., Cohen, M., Bernink, P., McCabe, C. H., Horacek, T., Papuchis, G., & Braunwald, E. et al. (2000). The TIMI Risk Score for Unstable Angina / Non-ST Elevation MI. *Journal of the American Medical Association*, *284*(7), 835–842. doi:10.1001/jama.284.7.835 PMID:10938172

Anyanwu, A. C., Chikwe, J., & Adams, D. H. (2008). Tricuspid valve repair for treatment and prevention of secondary tricuspid regurgitation in patients undergoing mitral valve surgery. *Current Cardiology Reports*, *10*(2), 110–117. doi:10.1007/s11886-008-0020-6 PMID:18417011

Anyanwu, A. C., Filsoufi, F., Salzberg, S. P., Bronster, D. J., & Adams, D. H. (2007). Epidemiology of stroke after cardiac surgery in the current era. *The Journal of Thoracic and Cardiovascular Surgery*, *134*(5), 1121–1127. doi:10.1016/j.jtcvs.2007.06.031 PMID:17976438

Apisarnthanarak, A., Rutjanawech, S., Wichansawakun, S., Ratanabunjerdkul, H., Patthranitima, P., Thongphubeth, K., & Fraser, V. J. et al. (2007). Initial inappropriate urinary catheters use in a tertiary-care center: Incidence, risk factors, and outcomes. *American Journal of Infection Control*, *35*(9), 594–599. doi:10.1016/j.ajic.2006.11.007 PMID:17980238

Apostolakis, E. E., Baikoussis, N. G., Parissis, H., Siminelakis, S. N., & Papadopoulos, G. S. (2009). Left ventricular diastolic dysfunction of the cardiac surgery patient; a point of view for the cardiac surgeon and cardio-anesthesiologist. *Journal of Cardiothoracic Surgery*, *4*(1), 67. doi:10.1186/1749-8090-4-67 PMID:19930694

Applebaum, P. S. (2007). Assessment of Patients' Competence to Consent to Treatment. *The New England Journal of Medicine*, *357*(18), 1834–1840. doi:10.1056/NEJMcp074045 PMID:17978292

Appoo, J. J., Augoustides, J. G., Pochettino, A., Savino, J. S., McGarvey, M. L., Cowie, D. C., & Bavaria, J. E. et al. (2006). Perioperative outcome in adults undergoing elective deep hypothermic circulatory arrest with retrograde cerebral perfusion in proximal aortic arch repair: Evaluation of protocol-based care. *Journal of Cardiothoracic and Vascular Anesthesia*, *20*(1), 3–7. doi:10.1053/j.jvca.2005.08.005 PMID:16458205

APPRAISE Steering Committee and Investigators. (2009). Apixaban, an oral, direct, selective factor Xa inhibitor, in combination with antiplatelet therapy after acute coronary syndrome: Results of the Apixaban for Prevention of Acute Ischemic and Safety Events (APPRAISE) trial. *Circulation*, *119*(22), 2877–2885. doi:10.1161/CIRCULATIONAHA.108.832139 PMID:19470889

Apter, A., Metzger, R., & Glassroth, J. (1988). Residents' perceptions of their role as teachers. *Journal of Medical Education*, *63*(12), 900–905. PMID:3199418

Arabia, F., Copeland, J. G., Pavie, A., & Smith, R. G. (1999). Implantation technique for the CardioWest total artificial heart. *The Annals of Thoracic Surgery*, *68*(2), 698–704. doi:10.1016/S0003-4975(99)00540-8 PMID:10475474

Arafa, O. E., Geiran, O. R., Andersen, K., Fosse, E., Simonsen, S., & Svennevig, J. L. (2000). Intraaortic Balloon Pumping For Predominantly Right Ventricular Failure After Heart Transplantation. *The Annals of Thoracic Surgery, 70*(5), 1587-1593. from http://www.annalsthoracicsurgery.org/article/s0003-4975(00)01864-6/abstractRetrieved

Arai, N., Matsumoto, A., Nishikawa, N., Yonekura, K., Eto, Y., Kuwada, Y., & Aoyahi, T. et al. (2001). Beta-blocker therapy improved symptoms and exercise capacity in a patient with dynamic intra-right ventricular obstruction an atypical form of double-chambered right ventricle. *Journal of the American Society of Echocardiography*, *14*(6), 650–653. doi:10.1067/mje.2001.110782 PMID:11391298

Aranki, S., Shaw, D., Adams, D., Rizzo, R., Couper, G., VanderVliet, M., & Burstin, H. R. et al. (1996). Predictors of Atrial Fibrillation After Coronary Artery Surgery: Current Trends and Impact on Hospital Resources. *Circulation*, *94*(3), 390–397. doi:10.1161/01.CIR.94.3.390 PMID:8759081

Arcasoy, S. M., Christie, J. D., Ferrari, V. A., Sutton, M. S., Zisman, D. A., Blumenthal, N. P., & Kotloff, R. M. et al. (2003). Echocardiographic assessment of pulmonary hypertension in patients with advanced lung disease. *American Journal of Respiratory and Critical Care Medicine*, *167*(5), 735–740. doi:10.1164/rccm.200210-1130OC PMID:12480614

Archer, C. W., & Wynn, M. (2009). A modern theory of paraplegia in the treatment of aneurysms of the thoracoabdominal aorta: An analysis of technique specific observed/expected ratios for paralysis. *Journal of Vascular Surgery*, *49*(5), 1117–1124. doi:10.1016/j.jvs.2008.10.074 PMID:19394541

Archer, S. L., Weir, E. K., & Wilkins, M. R. (2010). Basic Science of Pulmonary Arterial Hypertension for Clinicians. *Circulation*, *12*(18), 2045–2066. doi:10.1161/CIRCULATIONAHA.108.847707 PMID:20458021

Arends, D., & Kilcher, A. (2010). *Teaching for Student Learning*. New York: Routledge.

Arenson, B. G., MacDonald, L. A., Grocott, H. P., Hiebert, B. M., & Arora, R. C. (2013). Effect of intensive care unit environment on in-hospital delirium after cardiac surgery. *The Journal of Thoracic and Cardiovascular Surgery*, *146*(1), 172–178. doi:10.1016/j.jtcvs.2012.12.042 PMID:23317943

Argenziano, M., Choudhri, A. F., Oz, M. C., Rose, E. A., Smith, C. R., & Landry, D. W. (1997). A prospective randomized trial of arginine vasopressin in the treatment of vasodilatory shock after left ventricular assist device placement. *Circulation*, *96*(9suppl), II-286–II-290. PMID:9386112

Arias, C. A., Torres, H. A., Singh, K. V., Panesso, D., Moore, J., Wanger, A., & Murray, B. (2007). Failure of daptomycin monotherapy for endocarditis caused by an Enterococcus faecium strain with vancomycin-resistant and vancomycin-susceptible subpopulations and evidence of in vivo loss of the vanA gene cluster. *Clinical Infectious Diseases*, *45*(10), 1343–1346. doi:10.1086/522656 PMID:17968832

Arntfield, R. T., & Millington, S. J. (2012). Point of care cardiac ultrasound applications in the emergency department and intensive care unit--a review. *Current Cardiology Reviews*, *8*(2), 98–108. doi:10.2174/157340312801784952

Aronson, S., Phillips-Bute, B., Stafford-Smith, M., Fontes, M., Gaca, J., Mathew, J. P., & Newman, M. F. (2013). The Association of Postcardiac Surgery Acute Kidney Injury with Intraoperative Systolic Blood Pressure Hypotension. *Anesthesiology Research and Practice*, *2013*, 1–7. doi:10.1155/2013/174091 PMID:24324489

Arozullah, A. M., Daley, J., Henderson, W. G., & Khuri, S. F. (2000). Multifactorial risk index for predicting postoperative respiratory failure in men after major noncardiac surgery. The National Veterans Administration Surgical Quality Improvement Program. *Annals of Surgery*, *232*(2), 242–253. doi:10.1097/00000658-200008000-00015 PMID:10903604

Arrowsmith, J. E., Grocott, H. P., Reves, J. G., & Newman, M. F. (2000). Central nervous system complications of cardiac surgery. *British Journal of Anaesthesia*, *84*(3), 378–393. doi:10.1093/oxfordjournals.bja.a013444 PMID:10793601

Artang, R., Galloway, G., & Nielsen, J. D. (2014). Monitoring novel anticoagulants dabigatran, rivaroxaban and apixabain using thrombelastography. *Journal of the American College of Cardiology*, *63*(12), A439. doi:10.1016/S0735-1097(14)60439-3

Arzt, M., Floras, J., Logan, A., Kimoff, J., Series, F., Morrison, D., & Bradley, D. et al. (2007). Suppression of central sleep apnea by continuous positive airway pressure and transplant-free survival in heart failure: A post hoc analysis of the Canadian Continuous Positive Airway Pressure for Patients with Central Sleep Apnea and Heart Failure Trial (CANPAP). *Circulation*, *115*(25), 3173–3180. doi:10.1161/CIRCULATIONAHA.106.683482 PMID:17562959

Ascione, R., Ghosh, A., Rogers, C. A., Cohen, A., Monk, C., & Angelini, G. D. (2005). In-hospital patients exposed to clopidogrel before coronary artery bypass graft surgery: A word of caution. *The Annals of Thoracic Surgery*, *79*(4), 1210–1216. doi:10.1016/j.athoracsur.2004.09.046 PMID:15797051

Askar, F. Z., Kocabas, S., Yucel, S., Samancilar, O., Cetin, H., & Uyar, M. (2007). The efficacy of intrathecal morphine in post-thoracotomy pain management. *The Journal of International Medical Research*, *35*(3), 314–322. doi:10.1177/147323000703500305 PMID:17593859

Aslakson, R. A., Wyskiel, R., Shaeffer, D., Zyra, M., Ahuja, N., Nelson, J. E., & Pronovost, P. J. (2010). Surgical intensive care unit clinician estimates of the adequacy of communication regarding patient prognosis. *Critical Care (London, England)*, *14*(6), R218. doi:10.1186/cc9346 PMID:21114837

Aslakson, R. A., Wyskiel, R., Thornton, I., Copley, C., Shaffer, D., Zyra, M., & Pronovost, P. J. et al. (2012). Nurse-perceived barriers to effective communication regarding prognosis and optimal end-of-life care for surgical ICU patients: A qualitative exploration. *Journal of Palliative Medicine*, *15*(8), 910–915. doi:10.1089/jpm.2011.0481 PMID:22676315

Athan, E., Chu, V. H., Tattevin, P., Selton-Suty, C., Jones, P., & Naber, C. (2012). Clinical characteristics and outcome of infective endocarditis involving implantable cardiac devices. *Journal of the American Medical Association*, *307*(16), 1727–1735. doi:10.1001/jama.2012.497 PMID:22535857

Athappan, G., Gajulapalli, R. D., Sengodan, P., Bhardwaj, A., Ellis, S. G., Svensson, L., & Kapadia, S. R. et al. (2014). Influence of transcatheter aortic valve replacement strategy and valve design on stroke after transcatheter aortic valve replacement: A meta-analysis and systematic review of literature. *Journal of the American College of Cardiology*, *63*(20), 2101–2110. doi:10.1016/j.jacc.2014.02.540 PMID:24632286

Attaran, S., John, L., & El-Gamel, A. (2008). Clinical and potential use of pharmacological agents to reduce radial artery spasm in coronary artery surgery. *The Annals of Thoracic Surgery*, *85*(4), 1483–1489. doi:10.1016/j.athoracsur.2007.10.042 PMID:18355566

Augoustides, J. G. T. (2012). The inflammatory response to cardiac surgery with cardiopulmonary bypass: Should steroid prophylaxis be routine? *Journal of Cardiothoracic and Vascular Anesthesia*, *26*(5), 952–958. doi:10.1053/j.jvca.2012.05.001 PMID:22765991

Avecilla, S. T., Ferrell, C., Chandler, W. L., & Reyes, M. (2012). Plasma diluted thrombin time to measure dabigatran etexilate therapy. *American Journal of Clinical Pathology*, *137*, 572–574. doi:10.1309/AJCPAU7OQM0SRPZQ PMID:22431533

Avendano, C., Flume, P., Silvestri, G., King, L., & Reed, C. (2002). Pulmonary complications after esophagectomy. *The Annals of Thoracic Surgery*, *73*(3), 922–926. doi:10.1016/S0003-4975(01)03584-6 PMID:11899202

Avgerinos, D. V., Debois, W., & Salemi, A. (2014). Blood conservation strategies in cardiac surgery: More is better. *European Journal of Cardio-Thoracic Surgery*, *46*(5), 865–870. doi:10.1093/ejcts/ezt661 PMID:24482391

Aviado, D. M. Jr, & Schmidt, C. F. (1957). Effects of sympathomimetic drugs on pulmonary circulation: With special reference to a new pulmonary vasodilator. *The Journal of Pharmacology and Experimental Therapeutics*, *120*(4), 512–527. PMID:13476376

Avidan, M. S., Alcock, E. L., Da Fonseca, J., Ponte, J., Desai, J. B., Despotis, G. J., & Hunt, B. J. (2004). Comparison of structured use of routine laboratory tests or near-patient assessment with clinical judgement in the management of bleeding after cardiac surgery. *British Journal of Anaesthesia*, *92*(2), 178–186. doi:10.1093/bja/aeh037 PMID:14722166

Awtry, E. H., & Loscalzo, J. (2000). Aspirin. *Circulation*, *101*(10), 1206–1218. doi:10.1161/01.CIR.101.10.1206 PMID:10715270

Backman, C., Zoutman, D. E., & Marck, P. B. (2008). An integrative review of the current evidence on the relationship between hand hygiene interventions and the incidence of healthcare-associated infections. *American Journal of Infection Control*, *36*(5), 33–48. doi:10.1016/j.ajic.2007.08.007 PMID:18241734

Baddour, L. M., Epstein, A. E., Erickson, C. C., Knight, B. P., Levison, M. E., Lockhart, P. B., & Taubert, K. A. et al. (2010). Update on cardiovascular implantable electronic device infections and their management: A scientific statement from the American Heart Association. *Circulation*, *121*(3), 458–477. doi:10.1161/CIRCULATIONAHA.109.192665 PMID:20048212

Baddour, L. M., Wilson, W. R., Bayer, A. S., Fowler, V. G. Jr, Bolger, A. F., Levison, M. E., & Taubert, K. A. et al. (2005). Infective endocarditis: Diagnosis, antimicrobial therapy, and management of complications: A statement for healthcare professionals from the Committee on Rheumatic Fever, Emdocarditis, and Kawasaki Disease, Council on Cardiovascular Disease in the Young, and the Councils on Clinical Cardiology, Stroke, and Cardiovascular Surgery and Anesthesia, American Heart Association: Endorsed by the Infectious Disease Society of America. *Circulation*, *111*(23), e394–e434. doi:10.1161/CIRCULATIONAHA.105.165564 PMID:15956145

Badhwar, V., Ofenloch, J. C., Rovin, J. D., van Gelder, H. M., & Jacobs, J. P. (2012). Noninferiority of closely monitored mechanical valves to bioprostheses overshadowed by early mortality benefit in younger patients. *The Annals of Thoracic Surgery*, *93*(3), 748–753. doi:10.1016/j.athoracsur.2011.12.032 PMID:22364968

Baeke, G., Wils, J. P., & Broeckaert, B. (2005). 'There is a time to be born and a time to die' (Ecclesiastes 3:2a): Jewish perspectives on euthanasia. *Journal of Religion and Health*, *50*(4), 778–795. doi:10.1007/s10943-011-9465-9 PMID:21253848

Bagshaw, S. M., Cruz, D. N., Gibney, R. N., & Ronco, C. (2009). A proposed algorithm for initiation of renal replacement therapy in adult critically ill patients. *Critical Care (London, England)*, *13*(6), 317. doi:10.1186/cc8037 PMID:19909493

Bagshaw, S. M., & Gibney, R. T. N. (2008). Conventional markers of kidney function. *Critical Care Medicine*, *36*(4Suppl), S152–S158. doi:10.1097/CCM.0b013e318168c613 PMID:18382187

Baim, D. S. (1989). Effect of phosphodiesterase inhibition on myocardial oxygen consumption and coronary blood flow. *The American Journal of Cardiology*, *63*(2), 23A–26A. doi:10.1016/0002-9149(89)90388-3 PMID:2521267

Baird, T. A., Parsons, M. W., Phan, T., Butcher, K. S., Desmond, P. M., Tress, B. M., & Davis, S. M. et al. (2003). Persistent poststroke hyperglycemia is independently associated with infarct expansion and worse clinical outcome. *Stroke*, *34*(9), 2208–2214. doi:10.1161/01.STR.0000085087.41330.FF PMID:12893952

Baisden, C. E., Greenwald, L. V., & Symbas, P. N. (1984). Occult rib fractures and brachial plexus injury following median sternotomy for open-heart operations. *The Annals of Thoracic Surgery*, *38*(3), 192–194. doi:10.1016/S0003-4975(10)62235-7 PMID:6332585

Baker, D. P., Beaubien, M. J., Holtzman, A., Salas, E., & Barach, P. (2004). Medical team training: An initial assessment and future directions. Presented at the 19th annual meeting of the Society for Industrial and Organizational Psychology, Chicago.

Baker, D., Gustafson, S., Beaubian, J., Salas, E., & Barach, P. (2005, July). Medical Teamwork and Patient Safety. *Agency for Health Care Research and Quality*. Rockville. Retrieved May 12, 2014, from http://www.ahrq.gov/research/findings/final-reports/medteam/index.html

Baldini, G., Bagry, H., Aprikian, A., & Carli, F. (2009). Postoperative urinary retention. Anesthetic and perioperative considerations. *Anesthesiology*, *110*(5), 1139–1157. doi:10.1097/ALN.0b013e31819f7aea PMID:19352147

Baldwin, J. T., & Mann, D. L. (2010). NHLBI's program for VAD therapy for moderately advanced heart failure: The REVIVE-IT pilot trial. *Journal of Cardiac Failure*, *16*(11), 855–858. doi:10.1016/j.cardfail.2010.06.414 PMID:21055648

Baldwin, M. R., Wunsch, H., Reyfman, P. A., Narain, W. R., Blinderman, C. D., Schluger, N. W., & Bach, P. (2013). *High Burden of Palliative Needs among Older ICU Survivors Transferred to Post-Acute Care Facilities: A Single Center Study*. Ann Am Thorac Soc. doi:10.1513/AnnalsATS.201303-039OC

Ballantyne, J. C., Carr, D. B., deFerranti, S., Suarez, T., Lau, J., Chalmers, T. C., & Mosteller, F. et al. (1998). The comparative effects of postoperative analgesic therapies on pulmonary outcome: Cumulative meta-analyses of randomized, controlled trials. *Anesthesia and Analgesia*, *86*, 598–612. PMID:9495424

Balogh, Z., Jones, F., D'Amours, S., Parr, M., & Sugrue, M. (2004). Continuous intra-abdominal pressure measurement technique. *American Journal of Surgery*, *188*(6), 679–684. doi:10.1016/j.amjsurg.2004.08.052 PMID:15619483

Balogh, Z., McKinley, B. A., Holcomb, J. B., Miller, C. C., Cocanour, C. S., Kozar, R. A., & Moore, F. A. et al. (2003). Both primary and secondary abdominal compartment syndrome can be predicted early and are harbingers of multiple organ failure. *The Journal of Trauma*, *54*(5), 848–859. doi:10.1097/01.TA.0000070166.29649.F3 PMID:12777898

Bannay, A., Hoen, B., Duval, X., Obadia, J., Selton-Suty, C., Le Moing, V., & Alla, F. et al.AEPEI Study Group. (2011). The impact of valve surgery on short- and long-term mortality in left-sided infective endocarditis: Do differences in methodological approaches explain previous conflicting results? *European Heart Journal*, *32*(16), 2003–2015. doi:10.1093/eurheartj/ehp008 PMID:19208650

Bansal, S. (2012). Post-surgical acute kidney injury. *Clinical Queries: Nephrology*, *1*(1), 50–57. doi:10.1016/S2211-9477(11)70008-5

Bansilal, S., Farkouh, M. E., Hueb, W., Ogdie, M., Dangas, G., Lansky, A. J., & Fuster, V. et al. (2012). The Future REvascularization Evaluation in patients with Diabetes mellitus: optimal management of Multivessel disease (FREEDOM) trial: clinical and angiographic profile at study entry. *American Heart Journal*, *164*(4), 591–599. doi:10.1016/j.ahj.2012.06.012 PMID:23067919

Bao, S., Oiknine, R., & Fisher, S. J. (2012). Differentiating nonthyroidal illness syndrome from central hypothyroidism in the acutely ill hospitalized patient. *Endocrine*, *42*(3), 758–760. doi:10.1007/s12020-012-9685-0 PMID:22562722

Baram, D., & Richman, P. (2010). Mechanical Ventilation in the Cardiac Care Unit. In A. Jeremias & D. L. Brown (Eds.), *Cardiac Intensive Care* (2nd ed., pp. 632–643). Philadelphia: Saunders Elsevier. doi:10.1016/B978-1-4160-3773-6.10050-3

Barazangi, N., Wintermark, M., Lease, K., Rao, R., Smith, W., & Josephson, S. A. (2011). Comparison of computed tomography angiography and transesophageal echocardiography for evaluating aortic arch disease. *Journal of Stroke and Cerebrovascular Diseases*, *20*(5), 436–442. doi:10.1016/j.jstrokecerebrovasdis.2010.02.016 PMID:20813553

Barbash, I. M., Ben-Dor, I., Dvir, D., Maluenda, G., Xue, Z., Torguson, R., & Waksman, R. et al. (2012). Incidence and predictors of acute kidney injury after transcatheter aortic valve replacement. *American Heart Journal*, *163*(6), 1031–1036. doi:10.1016/j.ahj.2012.01.009 PMID:22709757

Bardy, G., Lee, K., Mark, D., Poole, J., Packer, D., Boineau, R., & Ip, J. et al. (2005). Amiodarone or an Implantable Cardioverter–Defibrillator for Congestive Heart Failure. *The New England Journal of Medicine*, *352*(3), 225–237. doi:10.1056/NEJMoa043399 PMID:15659722

Barker, J., Martino, R., Reichardt, B., Hickey, E. J., & Ralph-Edwards, A. (2009). Incidence and impact of dysphagia in patients receiving prolonged endotracheal intubation after cardiac surgery. *Canadian Journal of Surgery*, *52*(2), 119–124. PMID:19399206

Barletta, J. F., El-Ibiary, S. Y., Davis, L. E., Nguyen, B., & Raney, C. R. (2013). Proton pump inhibitors and the risk for hospital-acquired Clostridium difficile infection. *Mayo Clinic Proceedings*, *88*(10), 1085–1090. doi:10.1016/j.mayocp.2013.07.004 PMID:24012413

Barletta, J. F., & Sclar, D. A. (2014). Use of proton pump inhibitors for the provision of stress ulcer prophylaxis: Clinical and economic consequences. *PharmacoEconomics*, *32*(1), 5–13. doi:10.1007/s40273-013-0119-5 PMID:24271943

Barnett, R. (1994). *The Limits of Competence*. Buckingham, UK: Open University Press.

Barquist, E., & Kirton, O. (1997). Adrenal insufficiency in the surgical intensive care unit patient. *Journal of Trauma and Acute Care Surgery*, *42*(1), 27–31. doi:10.1097/00005373-199701000-00006 PMID:9003254

Barr, R. G., Rowe, B. H., & Camargo, C. A. (2003). Methylxanthines for exacerbations of chronic obstructive pulmonary disease. *Cochrane Database of Systematic Reviews,* (2), CD002168. doi: 10.1002/14651858.CD002168

Barrientos-Vega, R., Mar Sanchez-Soria, M., Morales-Garcia, C., Robas-Gomez, A., Cuena-Boy, R., & Ayensa-Rincon, A. (1997). Prolonged sedation of critically ill patients with midazolam or propofol: Impact on weaning and costs. *Critical Care Medicine*, *25*(1), 33–40. doi:10.1097/00003246-199701000-00009 PMID:8989173

Barr, J., Fraser, G. L., Puntillo, K., Ely, E. W., Gelinas, C., Dasta, J. F., & Jaeschke, R. et al. (2013). Clinical practice guidelines for the management of pain, agitation and delirium in adult patients in the intensive care unit. *Critical Care Medicine*, *41*(1), 263–306. doi:10.1097/CCM.0b013e3182783b72 PMID:23269131

Barst, R. J., Gibbs, J. S., Ghofrani, H. A., Hoeper, M. M., McLaughlin, V. V., Rubin, L. J., & Galiè, N. et al. (2009). Updated Evidence-Based Treatment Algorithm in Pulmonary Arterial Hypertension. *Journal of the American College of Cardiology*, *54*(1), S78–S84. doi:10.1016/j.jacc.2009.04.017 PMID:19555861

Barsuk, J. H., McGaghie, W. C., Cohen, E. R., O'Leary, K. J., & Wayne, D. B. (2009). Simulation-based mastery learning reduces complications during central venous catheter insertion in a medical intensive care unit. *Critical Care Medicine*, *37*(10), 2697–2701. doi:10.1097/CCM.0b013e3181a57bc1 PMID:19885989

Basbaum, A. I., & Fields, H. L. (2004). Endogenous pain control mechanisms: Review and hypothesis. *Annals of Neurology*, *4*(5), 451–462. doi:10.1002/ana.410040511 PMID:216303

Bass, N. M., Mullen, K. D., Sanyal, A., Poordad, F., Neff, G., Leevy, C. B., & Forbes, W. P. et al. (2010). Rifaximin treatment in hepatic encephalopathy. *The New England Journal of Medicine*, *362*(12), 1071–1081. doi:10.1056/NEJMoa0907893 PMID:20335583

Bastin, A. J., Ostermann, M., Slack, A. J., Diller, G. P., Finney, S. J., & Evans, T. W. (2013). Acute kidney injury after cardiac surgery according to Risk/Injury/Failure/Loss/End-stage, Acute Kidney Injury Network, and Kidney Disease: Improving Global Outcomes classifications. *Journal of Critical Care*, *28*(4), 389–396. doi:10.1016/j.jcrc.2012.12.008 PMID:23743540

Bates, S. M., & Weitz, J. I. (2005). Coagulation assays. *Circulation*, *112*(4), e53–e60. doi:10.1161/CIRCULATIONAHA.104.478222 PMID:16043649

Baud, F. J., Barriot, P., Toffis, V., Riou, B., Vicaut, E., Lecarpentier, Y., & Bismuth, C. et al. (1991). Elevated blood CN concentrations in victims of smoke inhalation. *The New England Journal of Medicine*, *325*(25), 1761–1766. doi:10.1056/NEJM199112193252502 PMID:1944484

Baud, F. J., Borron, S. W., Mégarbane, B., Trout, H., Lapostolle, F., Vicaut, E., & Bismuth, C. et al. (2002). Value of lactic acidosis in the assessment of the severity of acute CN poisoning. *Critical Care Medicine*, *30*(9), 2044–2050. doi:10.1097/00003246-200209000-00015 PMID:12352039

Baumann, M. H., & Sahn, S. A. (1990). Medical management and therapy of bronchopleural fistulas in the mechanically ventilated patient. *Chest Journal*, *97*(3), 721–728. doi:10.1378/chest.97.3.721 PMID:2407455

Bavaria, J. E., Coselli, J. S., Curi, M. A., Eggebrecht, H., Elefteriades, J. A., & Erbel, R. (2008). Expert consensus document on the treatment of descending thoracic aortic disease using endovascular stent-grafts. *The Annals of Thoracic Surgery*, *85*(1), S1–S41. doi:10.1016/j.athoracsur.2007.10.099 PMID:18083364

Beachamp, T. L., & Childress, J. F. (1979). *Principles of Biomedical Ethics*. New York, NY: Oxford University Press, Incorporated.

Beane, A. L. (1997). A teaching model that promotes commitment, accountability, and responsibility. *Educational Horizons*, *76*(1), 45–52.

Beaver, T. M., Fullerton, D. A., Zamora, M. R., Badesch, D. B., Weill, D., Brown, J. M., & Grover, F. L. et al. (1996). Colon perforation after lung transplantation. *The Annals of Thoracic Surgery*, *62*(3), 839–843. doi:10.1016/S0003-4975(96)00393-1

Beck, A. H. (2004). The Flexner report and the standardization of American medical education. *Journal of the American Medical Association*, *291*(17), 2139–2140. doi:10.1001/jama.291.17.2139 PMID:15126445

Beck, C. S. (1935). The development of a new blood supply to the heart by operation. *Annals of Surgery*, *102*(5), 801–813. doi:10.1097/00000658-193511000-00001 PMID:17856670

Beiderlinden, M., Treschan, T. A., Gorlinger, K., & Peters, J. (2007). Argatroban anticoagulation in critically ill patients. *The Annals of Pharmacotherapy*, *41*(5), 749–754. doi:10.1345/aph.1H569 PMID:17440009

Bell, D. D., Ostryzniuk, T., Verhoff, B., Spanier, A., & Roberts, D. E. (1998). Postoperative laboratory and imaging investigations in intensive care units following coronary artery bypass grafting: A comparison of two Canadian hospitals. *The Canadian Journal of Cardiology*, *14*(3), 379–384. PMID:9551032

Bell, D. S., Fonarow, G. C., Hays, R. D., & Mangione, C. M. (2000). Self-study from web-based and printed guideline materials. A randomized, controlled trial among resident physicians. *Annals of Internal Medicine*, *132*(12), 938–946. doi:10.7326/0003-4819-132-12-200006200-00003 PMID:10858176

Bello, G., Pennisi, M. A., Maviglia, R., Maggiore, S. M., Bocci, M. G., Montini, L., & Antonelli, M. (2005). Online vs live methods for teaching difficult airway management to anesthesiology residents. *Intensive Care Medicine*, *31*(4), 547–552. doi:10.1007/s00134-005-2561-0 PMID:15754200

Bellomo, R., Ronco, C., Kellum, J. A., Mehta, R. L., & Palevsky, P. (2004). Acute renal failure - definition, outcome measures, animal models, fluid therapy and information technology needs: the Second International Consensus Conference of the Acute Dialysis Quality Initiative (ADQI) Group. *Critical Care (London, England), 8*(4), R204–12. doi:10.1186/cc2872

Bellomo, R., Chapman, M., Finfer, S., Hickling, K., & Myburgh, J. (2000). Low-dose dopamine in patients with early renal dysfunction: A placebo-controlled randomised trial. Australian and New Zealand Intensive Care Society (ANZICS) Clinical Trials Group. *Lancet, 356*(9248), 2139–2143. doi:10.1016/S0140-6736(00)03495-4 PMID:11191541

Bellomo, R., Kellum, J., & Ronco, C. (2007). Defining and classifying acute renal failure: From advocacy to consensus and validation of the RIFLE criteria. *Intensive Care Medicine, 33*(3), 409–413. doi:10.1007/s00134-006-0478-x PMID:17165018

Bellomo, R., & Ronco, C. (2000). Continuous haemofiltration in the intensive care unit. *Critical Care (London, England), 4*(6), 339–345. doi:10.1186/cc718 PMID:11123877

Bell, R. F., Dahl, J. B., Moore, R. A., & Kalso, E. (2006). Perioperative ketamine for acute postoperative pain. *Cochrane Database of Systematic Reviews, 1*, 1–43. PMID:16437490

Beloucif, S., & Paven, D. (1998). A European Survey of the use of inhaled nitric oxide in the ICU. Working group on inhaled NO in ICU of the European Society of Intensive Care Medicine. *Intensive Care Medicine, 24*(8), 864–877. doi:10.1007/s001340050679 PMID:9757934

Ben Morrison, T., Horst, B., Brown, M., Bell, M., & Daniels, P. (2012). Bridging with glycoprotein IIb/IIIa inhibitors for periprocedural management of antiplatelet therapy in patients with drug eluting stents. *Catheterization and Cardiovascular Interventions, 79*(4), 575–582. doi:10.1002/ccd.23172 PMID:22448399

Ben-David, B., & Stahl, S. (1997). Prognosis of intraoperative brachial plexus injury: A review of 22 cases. *British Journal of Anaesthesia, 79*(4), 440–445. doi:10.1093/bja/79.4.440 PMID:9389259

Benedetto, U., Angeloni, E., Luciani, R., Refice, S., Stefanelli, M., Comito, C., & Sinatra, R. et al. (2010). Acute kidney injury after coronary artery bypass grafting: Does rhabdomyolysis play a role? *The Journal of Thoracic and Cardiovascular Surgery, 140*(2), 464–470. doi:10.1016/j.jtcvs.2010.03.028 PMID:20416892

Benhamou, D., Girault, C., Faure, C., Portier, F., & Muir, J. F. (1992). Nasal mask ventilation in acute respiratory failure. Experience in elderly patients. *Chest Journal, 102*(3), 912–917. doi:10.1378/chest.102.3.912 PMID:1516421

Benner, P. (2004). Using the Dreyfus model of skill acquisition to describe and interpret skill acquisition and clinical judgment in nursing practice and education. *Bulletin of Science, Technology & Society, 24*(3), 188–199. doi:10.1177/0270467604265061

Bennett-Guerrero, E., Ferguson, T.B. Jr, Lin, M., Garg, J., Mark, D.B., & Scavo, V.A. Jr, … Corey, G.R., for the SWIPE-1 Trial Group. (2010). Effect of an implantable gentamicin-collagen sponge on sternal wound infections following cardiac surgery. A randomized trial. *Journal of the American Medical Association, 304*, 755–762. doi:10.1001/jama.2010.1152 PMID:20716738

Bennett-Guerrero, E., Zhao, Y., O'Brien, S. M., Ferguson, T. B., Peterson, E. D., Gammie, J. S., & Song, H. K. (2010). Variation in use of blood transfusion in coronary artery bypass graft surgery. *Journal of the American Medical Association, 304*(14), 1568–1575. doi:10.1001/jama.2010.1406 PMID:20940382

Benomar, B., Ouattara, A., Estagnasie, P., Brusset, A., & Squara, P. (2010). Fluid responsiveness predicted by noninvasive bioreactance-based passive leg raise test. *Intensive Care Medicine, 11*(11), 1875–1881. doi:10.1007/s00134-010-1990-6 PMID:20665001

Benotti, P., Wood, G., Winegar, D., Petrick, A., Still, C., Argyropoulos, G., & Gerhard, G. (2014). Risk Factors Associated With Mortality After Roux-en-Y Gastric Bypass Surgery. *Annals of Surgery*, *259*(1), 123–130. doi:10.1097/SLA.0b013e31828a0ee4 PMID:23470583

Bensinger, L. D., Meah, Y. S., & Smith, L. G. (2005). Resident as teacher: The Mount Sinai experience and a review of the literature. *Mount Sinai Journal of Medicine: a Journal of Translational and Personalized Medicine*, *72*(5), 307–311. PMID:16184293

Benumof, J. L., & Wahrenbrock, E. A. (1975). Local effects of anesthetics on regional hypoxic pulmonary vasoconstriction. *Anesthesiology*, *43*(5), 525–532. doi:10.1097/00000542-197511000-00008 PMID:1190522

Benza, R., Tapson, V. F., Gomberg-Maitland, M., Poms, A., Barst, R. J., & McLaughlin, V. V. (2013). One-year Experience with Intravenous Treprostinil for Pulmonary Arterial Hypertension. *The Journal of Heart and Lung Transplantation*, *32*(9), 889–896. doi:10.1016/j.healun.2013.06.008 PMID:23953817

Benzo, R., Kelley, G., Recchi, L., Hofman, A., & Sciurba, F. (2007). Complications of lung resection and exercise capacity: A meta-analysis. *Respiratory Medicine*, *101*(8), 1790–1797. doi:10.1016/j.rmed.2007.02.012 PMID:17408941

Berenholtz, S. M., Pronovost, P. J., Lipsett, P. A., Hobson, D., Earsing, K., Farley, J. E., & Perl, T. M. et al. (2004). Eliminating catheter-related bloodstream infections in the intensive care unit. *Critical Care Medicine*, *32*(10), 2014–2020. doi:10.1097/01.CCM.0000142399.70913.2F PMID:15483409

Berger, J., Sallum, R., Katona, B., Maya, J., Ranganathan, G., Xu, Y., & Mwamburi, M. (2012). Is there an association between aspirin dosing and cardiac and bleeding events after treatment of acute coronary syndrome? A systematic review of the literature. *American Heart Journal*, *164*(2), 153–162. doi:10.1016/j.ahj.2012.04.001 PMID:22877800

Berger, M. M., & Mechanick, J. I. (2010). Continuing controversy in the intensive care unit: Why tight glycemic control, nutrition support, and nutritional pharmacology are each necessary therapeutic considerations. *Current Opinion in Clinical Nutrition and Metabolic Care*, *13*(2), 167–169. doi:10.1097/MCO.0b013e328335f2e0 PMID:20075721

Bergeron, N., Dubois, M. J., Dumont, M., Dial, S., & Skrobik, Y. (2001). Intensive Care Delirium Screening Checklist: Evaluation of a new screening tool. *Intensive Care Medicine*, *27*(5), 859–864. doi:10.1007/s001340100909 PMID:11430542

Bergh, C. H., Andersson, B., Dahlström, U., Forfang, K., Kivikko, M., Sarapohja, T., & Wikström, G. et al. (2010). Intravenous levosimendan vs. dobutamine in acute decompensated heart failure patients on beta-blockers. *European Journal of Heart Failure*, *12*(4), 404–410. doi:10.1093/eurjhf/hfq032 PMID:20335355

Bermudez, C. A., Adusumilli, P. S., McCurry, K. R., Zaldonis, D., Crespo, M. M., Pilewski, J. M., & Toyoda, Y. (2009). Extracorporeal membrane oxygenation for primary graft dysfunction after lung transplantation: Long-term survival. *The Annals of Thoracic Surgery*, *87*(3), 854–860. doi:10.1016/j.athoracsur.2008.11.036

Bernard, S. A., Gray, T. W., Buist, M. D., Jones, B. M., Silvester, W., Gutteridge, G., & Smith, K. (2002). Treatment of comatose survivors of out-of-hospital cardiac arrest with induced hypothermia. *The New England Journal of Medicine*, *346*(8), 557–563. doi:10.1056/NEJMoa003289 PMID:11856794

Berne, J. D., Norwood, S. H., McAuley, C. E., Vallina, V. L., Villareal, D., Weston, J., & McClarty, J. (2002). Erythromycin reduces delayed gastric emptying in critically ill trauma patients: A randomized, controlled trial. *The Journal of Trauma*, *53*(3), 422–425. doi:10.1097/00005373-200209000-00004 PMID:12352474

Berriel-Cass, D., Adkins, F. W., Jones, P., & Fakih, M. G. (2006). Eliminating nosocomial infections at Ascension Health. *Joint Commission Journal on Quality and Patient Safety*, *32*(11), 612–620. PMID:17120920

Best, M., & Neuhauser, D. (2004). Avedis Donabedian: Father of quality assurance and poet. *Quality & Safety in Health Care*, *13*(6), 472–473. doi:10.1136/qshc.2004.012591 PMID:15576711

Bhagat, K., Hingorani, A. D., Palacios, M., Charles, I. G., & Vallance, P. (1999). Cytokine-induced venodilation in humans in vivo: eNOS masquerading as iNOS. *Cardiovascular Research*, *41*(3), 754–764. doi:10.1016/S0008-6363(98)00249-1 PMID:10435048

Bhakta, B., Tennant, A., Horton, M., Lawton, G., & Andrich, D. (2005). Using item response theory to explore the psychometric properties of extended matching questions examination in undergraduate medical education. *BMC Medical Education*, *5*(1), 9. doi:10.1186/1472-6920-5-9 PMID:15752421

Bhaskar, B., Dulhunty, J., Mullany, D. V., & Fraser, J. F. (2012). Impact of blood product transfusion on short and long-term survival after cardiac surgery: More evidence. *The Annals of Thoracic Surgery*, *94*(2), 460–467. doi:10.1016/j.athoracsur.2012.04.005 PMID:22626751

Bhat, M., Larocque, M., Amorim, M., Herba, K., Martel, M., De Varennes, B., & Barkun, A. (2012). Prediction and prevention of upper gastrointestinal bleeding after cardiac surgery: A case control study. *Chinese Journal of Gastroenterology and Hepatology*, *26*(6), 340–344. PMID:22720275

Bhatt, D. L., Lincoff, A. M., Gibson, C. M., Stone, G. W., McNulty, S., Montalescot, G., & Mahaffey, K. W. et al. (2009). Intravenous platelet blockade with cangrelor during PCI. *The New England Journal of Medicine*, *361*(24), 2330–2341. doi:10.1056/NEJMoa0908629 PMID:19915222

Bhatt, D. L., Stone, G. W., Mahaffey, K. W., Gibson, C. M., Steg, P. G., Hamm, C. W., & Radke, P. W. et al. (2013). Effect of Platelet Inhibition with Cangrelor during PCI on Ischemic Events. *The New England Journal of Medicine*, *368*(14), 1303–1313. PMID:23473369

Bhorade, S. M., & Stern, E. (2009). Immunosuppression for lung transplantation. *Proceedings of the American Thoracic Society*, *6*(1), 47–53. doi:10.1513/pats.200808-096GO

Biancari, F., Catania, A., & D'Andrea, V. (2011). Elective endovascular vs. open repair for abdominal aortic aneurysm in patients aged 80 years and older: Systematic review and meta-analysis. *European Journal of Vascular and Endovascular Surgery*, *42*(5), 571–576. doi:10.1016/j.ejvs.2011.07.011 PMID:21820922

Bigelow, W. G., Lindsay, W. K., & Greenwood, W. F. (1950). Hypothermia It's possible role in cardiac surgery: An investigation of factors governing survival in dogs at low body temperatures. *Annals of Surgery*, *132*, 849–866. doi:10.1097/00000658-195011000-00001 PMID:14771796

Bilgin, Y. M., van de Watering, L. M. G., Eijsman, L., Versteegh, M. I. M., van Oers, M. H. J., & Brand, A. (2007). Is increased mortality associated with post-operative infections after leukocytes containing red blood cell transfusions in cardiac surgery? An extended analysis. *Transfusion Medicine (Oxford, England)*, *17*(4), 304–311. doi:10.1111/j.1365-3148.2007.00746.x PMID:17680957

Billings, F. T., Pretorius, M., Schildcrout, J. S., Mercaldo, N. D., Byrne, J. G., Ikizler, T. A., & Brown, N. J. (2012). Obesity and Oxidative Stress Predict AKI after Cardiac Surgery. *Journal of the American Society of Nephrology*, *23*(7), 1221–1228. doi:10.1681/ASN.2011090940 PMID:22626819

Bilotta, F., Doronzio, A., Stazi, E., Titi, L., Zeppa, I. O., Cianchi, A., & Lumb, P. et al. (2011). Early postoperative cognitive dysfunction and postoperative delirium after anaesthesia with various hypnotics: Study protocol for a randomised controlled trial--the PINOCCHIO trial. *Trials*, *12*(1), 170. doi:10.1186/1745-6215-12-170 PMID:21733178

Bilotta, F., & Rosa, G. (2012). Glycemia management in critical care patients. *World Journal of Diabetes*, *3*(7), 130–134. doi:10.4239/wjd.v3.i7.130 PMID:22816025

Birdi, I., Chaudhuri, N., Lenthall, K., Reddy, S., & Nashef, S. A. (2000). Emergency reinstitution of cardiopulmonary bypass following cardiac surgery: Outcome justifies the cost. *European Journal of Cardio-Thoracic Surgery : Official Journal of the European Association for Cardio-Thoracic Surgery*, *17*(6), 743–746. http://www.ncbi.nlm.nih.gov/pubmed/10856870 doi:10.1016/S1010-7940(00)00453-X PMID:10856870

Birgand, G., Radu, C., Alkhoder, S., Al Attar, N., Raffoul, R., Dilly, M., & Lucet, J. et al. (2013). Does a gentamicin-impregnated collagen sponge reduce sternal wound infections in high-risk cardiac surgery patients? *Interactive Cardiovascular and Thoracic Surgery*, *16*(2), 134–142. doi:10.1093/icvts/ivs449 PMID:23115102

Bishop, M. J., Benson, M. S., & Pierson, D. J. (1987). Carbon dioxide excretion via bronchopleural fistulas in adult respiratory distress syndrome. *Chest Journal*, *91*(3), 400–402. doi:10.1378/chest.91.3.400 PMID:3102170

Bittner, H. B. (2011). Extra-Corporeal Membrane Oxygenation Support In Cardiac Transplantation. *Applied Cardiopulmonary Pathophysiology*, *15*, 272–277.

Bittner, H. B., Lehmann, S., Rastan, A., Garbade, J., Binner, C., Mohr, F. W., & Barten, M. J. (2012). Outcome of extracorporeal membrane oxygenation as a bridge to lung transplantation and graft recovery. *The Annals of Thoracic Surgery*, *94*(3), 942–949. doi:10.1016/j.athoracsur.2012.05.006

Bittner, H. B., & Savitt, M. A. (2001). Management of porcelain aorta and calcified great vessels in coronary artery bypass grafting with off-pump and no-touch technology. *The Annals of Thoracic Surgery*, *72*(4), 1378–1380. http://www.ncbi.nlm.nih.gov/pubmed/11603471 doi:10.1016/S0003-4975(01)02568-1 PMID:11603471

Bjork, I., & Lindahl, U. (1982). Mechanism of the anticoagulant action of heparin. *Molecular and Cellular Biology*, *48*(3), 161–182. PMID:6757715

Bjursten, H., Dardashti, A., Ederoth, P., Brondén, B., & Algotsson, L. (2013). Increased long-term mortality with plasma transfusion after coronary artery bypass surgery. *Intensive Care Medicine*, *39*(3), 437–444. doi:10.1007/s00134-012-2723-9 PMID:23052960

Blacker, A. B., Oertel, M. D., & Valgus, J. M. (2008). Fondaparinux and the management of heparin-induced thrombocytopenia: The journey continues. *The Annals of Pharmacotherapy*, *43*(1), 1636–1646. PMID:19737996

Black, I. W., Hopkins, A. P., Lee, L. C. L., & Walsh, W. F. (1993). Evaluation of transoesophageal echocardiography before cardioversion of atrial fibrillation and flutter in nonanticoagulated patients. *American Heart Journal*, *126*(2), 375–381. doi:10.1016/0002-8703(93)91054-I PMID:8338008

Black, P., Harrison, C., Lee, C., Marshall, B., & Wiliam, D. (2004). Working Inside the Black Box: Assessment for Learning in the Classroom. *Phi Delta Kappan*, *86*(1), 8–21. doi:10.1177/003172170408600105

Black, P., & Wiliam, D. (1998). Assessment and Classroom Learning. *Assessment in Education: Principles, Policy & Practice*, *5*(1), 7–74. doi:10.1080/0969595980050102

Blackstone, E. H., Cosgrove, D. M., Jamieson, W. R., Birkmeyer, N. J., Lemmer, J. H. Jr, Miller, D. C., & Chai, A. et al. (2003). Prosthesis size and long-term survival after aortic valve replacement. *The Journal of Thoracic and Cardiovascular Surgery*, *126*(3), 783–796. doi:10.1016/S0022-5223(03)00591-9 PMID:14502155

Blais, C., Dumesnil, J. G., Baillot, R., Simard, S., Doyle, D., & Pibarot, P. (2003). Impact of valve prosthesis-patient mismatch on short-term mortality after aortic valve replacement. *Circulation*, *108*(8), 983–988. doi:10.1161/01.CIR.0000085167.67105.32 PMID:12912812

Blalock, A., & Taussig, H. B. (1945). The surgical treatment of malformations of the heart in which there is pulmonary stenosis or pulmonary atresia. *Journal of the American Medical Association*, *128*(3), 189–202. doi:10.1001/jama.1945.02860200029009 PMID:6368878

Blamoun, J., Alfakir, M., Rella, M. E., Wojcik, J. M., Solis, R. A., Anees Khan, M., & DeBari, V. A. (2009). Efficacy of an expanded ventilator bundle for the reduction of ventilator-associated pneumonia in the medical intensive care unit. *American Journal of Infection Control*, *37*(2), 172–175. doi:10.1016/j.ajic.2008.05.010 PMID:18945515

Blenkharn, A., Faughnan, S., & Morgan, A. (2002). Developing a pain assessment tool for use by nurses in an adult intensive care unit. *Intensive & Critical Care Nursing*, *1*(6), 332–341. doi:10.1016/S0964-3397(02)00071-X PMID:12526871

Blog. (n.d.). Blog. *Merriam-Webster.com*. Retrieved May 11, 2014, from http://www.merriam-webster.com/dictionary/blog

Blondet, J. J., & Beilman, G. J. (2007). Glycemic control and prevention of perioperative infection. *Current Opinion in Critical Care*, *13*(4), 421–427. doi:10.1097/MCC.0b013e32826388a1 PMID:17599013

Bloom, B. S., Engelhart, M. D., Furst, E. J., & Hill, W. H. (1956). *Taxonomy of educational objectives: Handbook I: Cognitive domain*. New York: David.

Bloom, S. W. (1989). The medical school as a social organization: The sources of resistance to change. *Medical Education*, *23*(3), 228–241. doi:10.1111/j.1365-2923.1989.tb01538.x PMID:2725360

Bloor, B. C., Ward, D. S., Belleville, J. P., & Maze, M. (1992). Effects of intravenous dexmedetomidine in humans- II: Hemodynamic changes. *Anesthesiology*, *77*(6), 1134–1142. doi:10.1097/00000542-199212000-00014 PMID:1361311

Blot, F., Nitenberg, G., Chachaty, E., Raynard, B., Germann, N., Antoun, S., & Tancrède, C. et al. (1999). Diagnosis of catheter-related bacteraemia: A prospective comparison of the time to positivity of hub-blood versus peripheral-blood cultures. *Lancet*, *354*(9184), 1071–1077. doi:10.1016/S0140-6736(98)11134-0 PMID:10509498

Blot, F., Schmidt, E., Nitenberg, G., Tancrède, C., Leclercq, B., Laplanche, A., & Andremont, A. (1998). Earlier positivity of central-venous- versus peripheral-blood cultures is highly predictive of catheter-related sepsis. *Journal of Clinical Microbiology*, *36*, 105–109. PMID:9431930

Bock, J. S., & Gottlieb, S. S. (2010). Cardiorenal Syndrome: New Perspectives. *Circulation*, *121*(23), 2592–2600. doi:10.1161/CIRCULATIONAHA.109.886473 PMID:20547939

Boersma, E., Harrington, R. A., Moliterno, D. J., White, H., Theroux, P., Van de Werf, F., & Simoons, M. L. et al. (2002). Platelet glycoprotein IIb/IIIa inhibitors in acute coronary syndromes: A meta-analysis of all major randomised clinical trials. *Lancet*, *359*(9302), 189–198. doi:10.1016/S0140-6736(02)07442-1 PMID:11812552

Boersma, E., Pieper, K. S., Steyerberg, E. W., Wilcox, R. G., Chang, W.-C., Lee, K. L., & Simoons, M. L. et al. (2000). Predictors of Outcome in Patients With Acute Coronary Syndromes Without Persistent ST-Segment Elevation. *Circulation*, *101*(22), 2557–2567. doi:10.1161/01.CIR.101.22.2557 PMID:10840005

Boffini, M., Sansone, F., Ceresa, F., Ribezzo, M., Patanè, F., Comoglio, C., . . . Rinaldi, M. (2009). Role Of Oral Sildenafil In The Treatment Of Right Ventricular Dysfunction After Heart Transplantation. *Transplantation Proceedings*, *41*(4), 1353-1356. Retrieved From http://www.transplantation-proceedings.org/article/s0041-1345(09)00473-4/abstract

Bog'a, M., Islamog'lu, F., Badak, I., Cikirikçiog'lu, M., Bakalim, T., Yag'di, T., & Hamulu, A. et al. (2000). The effects of modified hemofiltration on inflammatory mediators and cardiac performance in coronary artery bypass grafting. *Perfusion*, *15*(2), 143–150. doi:10.1177/026765910001500209 PMID:10789569

Bojar, R. M. (2011). Respiratory Management. In R. M. Bojar (Ed.), Manual of perioperative care in adult cardiac surgery (5th ed.). Wiley-Blackwell.

Bojar, R. M. (2011). *Manual of Perioperative Care in Adult Cardiac Surgery*. John Wiley & Sons.

Bokhari, F., Newman, D., Greene, M., Korley, V., Mangat, I., & Dorian, P. (2004). Long-term comparison of the implantable cardioverter defibrillator versus amiodarone: Eleven year follow-up of a subset of patients in the Canadian Implantable Defibrillator Study (CIDS). *Circulation*, *110*(2), 112–116. doi:10.1161/01.CIR.0000134957.51747.6E PMID:15238454

Boles, J. M., Bion, J., Connors, A., Herridge, M., Marsh, B., Melot, C., & Welte, T. et al. (2007). Weaning from mechanical ventilation. *The European Respiratory Journal*, *29*(5), 1033–1056. doi:10.1183/09031936.00010206 PMID:17470624

Bolesta, S., Uhrin, L. M., & Guzek, J. R. (2011). Preoperative Statins and Acute Kidney Injury After Cardiac Surgery: Utilization of a Consensus Definition of Acute Kidney Injury. *The Annals of Pharmacotherapy*, *45*(1), 23–30. doi:10.1345/aph.1P384 PMID:21205946

Bolliger, C., Jordan, P., Solèr, M., Stulz, P., Grädel, E., Skarvan, K., & Tamm, M. et al. (1995). Exercise capacity as a predictor of postoperative complications in lung resection candidates. *American Journal of Respiratory and Critical Care Medicine*, *151*(5), 1472–1480. doi:10.1164/ajrccm.151.5.7735602 PMID:7735602

Bolon, M. K., Morlote, M., Weber, S. G., Koplan, B., Carmeli, Y., & Wright, S. B. (2004). Glycopeptides are no more effective than β-lactam agents for prevention of surgical site infection after cardiac surgery: A meta-analysis. *Clinical Infectious Diseases*, *38*(10), 1357–1363. doi:10.1086/383318 PMID:15156470

Bolz, S. S., & Pohl, U. (1997). Indomethacin enhances endothelial NO release: Evidence for a role of PGI2 in the autocrine control of calcium-dependent autacoid production. *Cardiovascular Research*, *36*(3), 437–444. doi:10.1016/S0008-6363(97)00197-1 PMID:9534864

Bond, C. A., & Raehl, C. L. (2007). Clinical pharmacy services, pharmacy staffing, and hospital mortality rates. *Pharmacotherapy*, *27*(4), 481–493. doi:10.1592/phco.27.4.481 PMID:17381374

Bonow, R. O., Carabello, B. A., Chatterjee, K., de Leon, A. C. Jr, Faxon, D. P., & Freed, M. D. et al. American College of Cardiology/American Heart Association Task, F. (2008). (2008). Focused update incorporated into the ACC/AHA 2006 guidelines for the management of patients with valvular heart disease: a report of the American College of Cardiology/American Heart Association Task Force on Practice Guidelines (Writing Committee to Revise the 1998 Guidelines for the Management of Patients With Valvular Heart Disease): endorsed by the Society of Cardiovascular Anesthesiologists, Society for Cardiovascular Angiography and Interventions, and Society of Thoracic Surgeons. *Circulation*, *118*(15), e523–e661. doi:10.1161/CIRCULATIONAHA.108.190748 PMID:18820172

Boon, A., Cheriex, E., Lodder, J., & Kessels, F. (1997). Cardiac valve calcification: Characteristics of patients with calcification of the mitral annulus or aortic valve. *Heart (British Cardiac Society)*, *78*(5), 472–474. doi:10.1136/hrt.78.5.472 PMID:9415006

Boonen, E., & Van den Berghe, G. (2014). Endocrine responses to critical illness: Novel insights and therapeutic implications.[Epub ahead of print]. *The Journal of Clinical Endocrinology and Metabolism*, jc20134115. PMID:24517153

Boonen, E., Vervenne, H., Meersseman, P., Andrew, R., Mortier, L., Declercq, P. E., & Van den Berghe, G. et al. (2013). Reduced cortisol metabolism during critical illness. *The New England Journal of Medicine*, *368*(16), 1477–1488. doi:10.1056/NEJMoa1214969 PMID:23506003

Boon, N. A., & Bloomfield, P. (2002). The medical management of valvar heart disease. *Heart (British Cardiac Society)*, *87*(4), 395–400. doi:10.1136/heart.87.4.395 PMID:11907022

Bornstein, S. R., Engeland, W. C., Ehrhart-Bornstein, M., & Herman, J. P. (2008). Dissociation of ACTH and glucocorticoids. *Trends in Endocrinology and Metabolism*, *19*(5), 175–180. doi:10.1016/j.tem.2008.01.009 PMID:18394919

Bortman, G., Sellanes, M., Odell, D., Ring, W., & Olivari, M. (1994). Discrepancy between pre- and post-transplant diagnosis of end-stage dilated cardiomyopathy. *The American Journal of Cardiology*, *74*(9), 921–924. doi:10.1016/0002-9149(94)90587-8 PMID:7977122

Botelho-Nevers, E., Thuny, F., Casalta, J. P., Richet, H., Gouriet, F., Collart, F., & Raoult, D. et al. (2009). Dramatic reduction in infective endocarditis-related mortality with a management-based approach. *Archives of Internal Medicine*, *169*(14), 1290–1298. doi:10.1001/archinternmed.2009.192 PMID:19636030

Bottiger, B. A., Esper, S. A., & Stafford-Smith, M. (2014). Pain management strategies for thoracotomy and thoracic pain syndromes. *Seminars in Cardiothoracic and Vascular Anesthesia*, *18*(1), 45–56. doi:10.1177/1089253213514484 PMID:24336691

Boucher, H., Miller, L. G., & Razonable, R. R. (2010). Serious infections caused by methicillin-resistant Staphylococcus aureus. *Clinical Infectious Diseases*, *15*(S2), S183–S197. doi:10.1086/653519 PMID:20731576

Bouhemad, B., Zhang, M., Lu, Q., & Rouby, J.-J. (2007). Clinical review: Bedside lung ultrasound in critical care practice. *Critical Care (London, England)*, *11*(1), 205. doi:10.1186/cc5668 PMID:17316468

Bould, M. D., Crabtree, N. A., & Naik, V. N. (2009). Assessment of procedural skills in anaesthesia, *103*(4), 472–483. doi:10.1093/bja/aep241

Bouri, S., Shun-Shin, M. J., Cole, G. D., Mayet, J., & Francis, D. P. (2014). Meta-analysis of secure randomised controlled trials of beta-blockade to prevent perioperative death in non-cardiac surgery. *Heart (British Cardiac Society)*, *100*(6), 456–464. doi:10.1136/heartjnl-2013-304262 PMID:23904357

Bouza, E., Alvarado, N., Alcalá, L., Pérez, M. J., Rincón, C., & Muñoz, P. (2007). A randomized and prospective study of 3 procedures for the diagnosis of catheter-related bloodstream infection without catheter withdrawal. *Clinical Infectious Diseases*, *44*(6), 820–826. doi:10.1086/511865 PMID:17304454

Bouza, E., Pérez, M. J., Muñoz, P., Rincón, C., Barrio, J. M., & Hortal, J. (2008). Continuous aspiration of subglottic secretions in the prevention of ventilator-associated pneumonia in the postoperative period of major heart surgery. *Chest*, *134*(5), 938–946. doi:10.1378/chest.08-0103 PMID:18641114

Bouzas, B., Kilner, P. J., & Gatzoulis, M. A. (2005). Pulmonary regurgitation: Not a benign lesion. *European Heart Journal*, *26*(5), 433–439. doi:10.1093/eurheartj/ehi091 PMID:15640261

Boyce, J. M., Ligi, C., Kohan, C., Dumigan, D., & Havill, N. L. (2006). Lack of association between the increased incidence of Clostridium difficile-associated disease and the increasing use of alcohol-based hand scrubs. *Infection Control and Hospital Epidemiology*, *27*(5), 479–483. doi:10.1086/504362 PMID:16671029

Boyd, E. A., Lo, B., Evans, L. R., Malvar, G., Apatira, L., Luce, J. M., & White, D. B. (2010). "It's not just what the doctor tells me:" factors that influence surrogate decision-makers' perceptions of prognosis. *Critical Care Medicine*, *38*(5), 1270–1275. doi:10.1097/CCM.0b013e3181d8a217 PMID:20228686

Boyle, A., Ascheim, D., Russo, M., Kormos, R., John, R., Naka, Y., & Teuteberg, J. et al. (2011). Clinical outcomes for continuous-flow left ventricular assist device patients stratified by pre-operative INTERMACS classification. *The Journal of Heart and Lung Transplantation*, *30*(4), 402–407. doi:10.1016/j.healun.2010.10.016 PMID:21168346

Bradley, C. T., Brasel, K. J., & Schwarze, M. L. (2010b). Physician attitudes regarding advance directives for high-risk surgical patients: A qualitative analysis. *Surgery*, *148*(2), 209–216. doi:10.1016/j.surg.2010.05.020 PMID:20580048

Bradley, C., Weaver, J., & Brasel, K. (2010a). Addressing access to palliative care services in the surgical intensive care unit. *Surgery*, *147*(6), 871–877. doi:10.1016/j.surg.2009.11.005 PMID:20097397

Bradley, D., Creswell, L. L., Hogue, C. W., Epstein, A. E., Prystowsky, E. N., & Daoud, E. G.American College of Chest Physicians. (2005). Pharmacologic prophylaxis: American College of Chest Physicians guidelines for the prevention and management of postoperative atrial fibrillation after cardiac surgery. *Chest*, *128*(2Suppl), 39S–47S. doi:10.1378/chest.128.2_suppl.39S PMID:16167664

Bradley, P. (2006). The history of simulation in medical education and possible future directions. *Medical Education*, *40*(3), 254–262. doi:10.1111/j.1365-2929.2006.02394.x PMID:16483328

Brady, K., Joshi, B., Zweifel, C., Smielewski, P., Czosnyka, M., Easley, R. B., & Hogue, C. W. Jr. (2010). Real-time continuous monitoring of cerebral blood flow autoregulation using near-infrared spectroscopy in patients undergoing cardiopulmonary bypass. *Stroke*, *41*(9), 1951–1956. doi:10.1161/STROKEAHA.109.575159 PMID:20651274

Branson, R. D., & Johannigman, J. A. (2004). What is the evidence base for the newer ventilation modes? *Respiratory Care*, *49*(7), 742–760. PMID:15222907

Brasel, K. J., & Weissman, D. E. (2004). Palliative care education for surgeons. *Journal of the American College of Surgeons*, *199*(3), 495–499. doi:10.1016/j.jamcollsurg.2004.06.004 PMID:15325621

Bratzler, D. W., & Hunt, D. R. (2006). The surgical infection prevention and surgical care improvement projects: National initiatives to improve outcomes for patients having surgery. *Clinical Infectious Diseases*, *43*(3), 322–330. doi:10.1086/505220 PMID:16804848

Braunschweig, C. L., Levy, P., Sheean, P. M., & Wang, X. (2001). Enteral compared with parenteral nutrition: A meta-analysis. *The American Journal of Clinical Nutrition*, *74*(4), 534–542. PMID:11566654

Bravo, C., Gispert, P., Borro, J. M., de la Torre, M., Cifrian Martinez, J. M., Fernandez Rozas, S., & Group, M. S. et al. (2007). Prevalence and management of gastrointestinal complications in lung transplant patients: MITOS study group. *Transplantation Proceedings*, *39*(7), 2409–2412. doi:10.1016/j.transproceed.2007.07.054

Breet, N. J., van Werkum, J. W., Bouman, H. J., Kelder, J. C., Ruven, H. J. T., Bal, E. T., & ten Berg, J. M. et al. (2010). Comparison of platelet function tests in predicting clinical outcomes in patients undergoing coronary stent implantation. *Journal of the American Medical Association*, *303*(8), 754–762. doi:10.1001/jama.2010.181 PMID:20179285

Brener, S. J., Duffy, C. I., Thomas, J. D., & Stewart, W. J. (1995). Progression of aortic stenosis in 394 patients: Relation to changes in myocardial and mitral valve dysfunction. *Journal of the American College of Cardiology*, *25*(2), 305–310. doi:10.1016/0735-1097(94)00406-G PMID:7829781

Brener, S. J., Lytle, B. W., Casserly, I. P., Schneider, J. P., Topol, E. J., & Lauer, M. S. (2004). Propensity analysis of long-term survival after surgical or percutaneous revascularization in patients with multivessel coronary artery disease and high-risk features. *Circulation*, *109*(19), 2290–2295. doi:10.1161/01.CIR.0000126826.58526.14 PMID:15117846

Brenner, A. M., Mathai, S., Jain, S., & Mohl, P. C. (2010). Can we predict "problem residents"? *Academic Medicine*, *85*(7), 1147–1151. doi:10.1097/ACM.0b013e3181e1a85d PMID:20592510

Brenner, D. S. (2002). *Embracing life & facing death: a Jewish guide to palliative care*. New York, NY: CLAL.

Brims, F. J., Lansley, S. M., Waterer, G. W., & Lee, Y. C. (2010). Empyema thoracis. New insights into an old disease. *European Respiratory Review*, *19*(117), 220–228. doi:10.1183/09059180.00005610 PMID:20956197

Brisard, L., Le Gouge, A., Lascarrou, J.-B., Dupont, H., Asfar, P., Sirodot, M., & Reignier, J. et al. (2014). Impact of early enteral versus parenteral nutrition on mortality in patients requiring mechanical ventilation and catecholamines: Study protocol for a randomized controlled trial (NUTRIREA-2). *Trials*, *15*(1), 507. doi:10.1186/1745-6215-15-507 PMID:25539571

Brister, S. J., Ofosu, F. A., & Buchanan, M. R. (1993). Thrombin generation during cardiac surgery: Is heparin the ideal anticoagulant? *Thrombosis and Haemostasis*, *70*(2), 259–262. PMID:8236131

Bristow, M. R., Shakar, S. F., Linseman, J. V., & Lowes, B. D. (2001). Inotropes and β-blockers: Is there a need for new guidelines? *Journal of Cardiac Failure*, *7*(2Suppl 1), 8–12. doi:10.1054/jcaf.2001.26655 PMID:11605160

Bristow, M., Gilbert, E., Abraham, W., Fowler, M., Hershberger, R., Kubo, S., & Shusterman, N. et al. (1996). Carvedilol produces dose-related improvements in left ventricular function and survival in subjects with chronic heart failure. MOCHA Investigators. *Circulation*, *94*(11), 2807–2816. doi:10.1161/01.CIR.94.11.2807 PMID:8941106

Britt, R. C., Novosel, T. J., Britt, L. D., & Sullivan, M. (2009). The impact of central line simulation before the ICU experience. *American Journal of Surgery*, *197*(4), 533–536. doi:10.1016/j.amjsurg.2008.11.016 PMID:19249739

Brochard, L., Isabey, D., Piquet, J., Amaro, P., Mancebo, J., Messadi, A. A., & Harf, A. et al. (1990). Reversal of acute exacerbations of chronic obstructive lung disease by inspiratory assistance with a face mask. *The New England Journal of Medicine*, *323*(22), 1523–1530. doi:10.1056/NEJM199011293232204 PMID:2122253

Bromage, P. R. (1975). Mechanism of action of extradural analgesia. *British Journal of Anaesthesia*, *47*, 199–211. PMID:1096918

Bronicki, R. A., & Anas, N. G. (2009). Cardiopulmonary interaction. *Pediatric Critical Care Medicine*, *10*(3), 313–322. doi:10.1097/PCC.0b013e31819887f0 PMID:19307810

Brown, J. M., O'Brien, S. M., Wu, C., Sikora, J. A., Griffith, B. P., & Gammie, J. S. (2009). Isolated aortic valve replacement in North America comprising 108,687 patients in 10 years: changes in risks, valve types, and outcomes in the Society of Thoracic Surgeons National Database. *Journal of Thoracic and Cardiovascular Surgery*, *137*(1), 82-90. doi: S0022-5223(08)01409-8 [pii] 10.1016/j.jtcvs.2008.08.015

Brown, J. R., Cochran, R. P., Mackenzie, T. A., Furnary, A. P., Kunzelman, K. S., Ross, C. S., & O'Connor, G. T. et al. (2008). Long-Term Survival After Cardiac Surgery is Predicted by Estimated Glomerular Filtration Rate. *The Annals of Thoracic Surgery*, *86*(1), 4–11. doi:10.1016/j.athoracsur.2008.03.006 PMID:18573389

Brown, J. R., Kramer, R. S., Coca, S. G., & Parikh, C. R. (2010). Duration of Acute Kidney Injury Impacts Long-Term Survival After Cardiac Surgery. *The Annals of Thoracic Surgery*, *90*(4), 1142–1148. doi:10.1016/j.athoracsur.2010.04.039 PMID:20868804

Bruce, D., & Nokes, T. J. C. (2008). Prothrombin complex concentrate (Beriplex P/N) in severe bleeding: Experience in a large tertiary hospital. *Critical Care (London, England)*, *12*(4), R105. doi:10.1186/cc6987 PMID:18706082

Bruggemans, E. F. (2013). Cognitive dysfunction after cardiac surgery: Pathophysiological mechanisms and preventive strategies. *Netherlands Heart Journal; Monthly Journal of the Netherlands Society of Cardiology and the Netherlands Heart Foundation*, *21*(2), 70–73. doi:10.1007/s12471-012-0347-x PMID:23184600

Brunelli, A., Kim, A., Berger, K., & Addrizzo-Harris, D. (2013). Physiologic evaluation of the patient with lung cancer being considered for resectional surgery: Diagnosis and management of lung cancer, 3rd ed: American College of Chest Physicians evidence-based clinical practice guidelines. Chest, 143(5 Suppl), E166S-90S.

Brush, S., Budge, D., Alharethi, R., McCormick, A. J., MacPherson, J. E., Reid, B. B., & Kfoury, A. G. et al. (2010). End-of-life decision making and implementation in recipients of a destination left ventricular assist device. *The Journal of Heart and Lung Transplantation*, *29*(12), 1337–1341. doi:10.1016/j.healun.2010.07.001 PMID:20817564

Bryson, G. L., Wyand, A., Wozny, D., Rees, L., Taljaard, M., & Nathan, H. (2011). A prospective cohort study evaluating associations among delirium, postoperative cognitive dysfunction, and apolipoprotein E genotype following open aortic repair. *Canadian Journal of Anaesthesia*, *58*(3), 246–255. doi:10.1007/s12630-010-9446-6 PMID:21222188

Bucerius, J., Gummert, J. F., Borger, M. A., Walther, T., Doll, N., Onnasch, J. F., & Mohr, F. W. et al. (2003). Stroke after cardiac surgery: A risk factor analysis of 16,184 consecutive adult patients. *The Annals of Thoracic Surgery*, *75*(2), 472–478. doi:10.1016/S0003-4975(02)04370-9 PMID:12607656

Buckley, D., & Gillham, M. (2007). Invasive Respiratory Support. In D. Sidebotham, A. McKee, M. Gillham, & J. H. Levy (Eds.), *Cardiothoracic Critical Care*. Philadelphia: Butterworth Heinemann Elsevier. doi:10.1016/B978-075067572-7.50032-1

Buckley, S. G., Coleman, J., Davison, I., Khan, K. S., Zamora, J., Malick, S., & Sayers, J. et al. (2009). The educational effects of portfolios on undergraduate student learning: A Best Evidence Medical Education (BEME) systematic review. BEME Guide No. 11. *Medical Teacher*, *31*(4), 340–355. doi:10.1080/01421590902889897 PMID:19404891

Buendgens, L., Bruensing, J., Matthes, M., Dückers, H., Luedde, T., Trautwein, C., & Koch, A. et al. (2014). Administration of proton pump inhibitors in critically ill medical patients is associated with increased risk of developing Clostridium difficile-associated diarrhea. *Journal of Critical Care*, *29*(4), 696.e11–696.e15. doi:10.1016/j.jcrc.2014.03.002 PMID:24674763

Bunte, M. C., Blackstone, E. H., Thuita, L., Fowler, J., Joseph, L., Ozaki, A., & Mountis, M. M. et al. (2013). Major bleeding during heartmate II support. *Journal of the American College of Cardiology*, *62*(23), 2188–2196. doi:10.1016/j.jacc.2013.05.089 PMID:23994419

Burch, J. W., Stanford, N., & Majerus, P. W. (1979). Inhibition of platelet prostaglandin synthase by oral aspirin. *The Journal of Clinical Investigation*, *61*(2), 314–319. doi:10.1172/JCI108941 PMID:413839

Burden, A. R., Torjman, M. C., Dy, G. E., Jaffe, J. D., Littman, J. J., Nawar, F., & Reboli, A. C. et al. (2012). Prevention of central venous catheter-related bloodstream infections: Is it time to add simulation training to the prevention bundle? *Journal of Clinical Anesthesia*, *24*(7), 555–560. doi:10.1016/j.jclinane.2012.04.006 PMID:23101770

Burke, J. P. (2003). Infection control – A problem for patient safety. *The New England Journal of Medicine*, *348*(7), 651–656. doi:10.1056/NEJMhpr020557 PMID:12584377

Burry, L., Rose, L., McCullagh, I.J., Fergusson, D.A., Ferguson, N.D., & Mehta, S. (2014). Daily sedation interruption versus no daily sedation interruption for critically ill adult patients requiring invasive mechanical ventilation. *Cochrane Database of Systematic Reviews, Jul 9*, 7:CD009176.

Burry, L., Little, A., Hallett, D., & Mehta, S. (2013). Detection of critical illness-related corticosteroid insufficiency using a 1 μg adrenocorticotropic hormone test. *Shock (Augusta, Ga.)*, *39*(2), 144–148. PMID:23324883

Busari, J. O., & Scherpbier, A. J. (2004). Why residents should teach: A literature review. *Journal of Postgraduate Medicine*, *50*(3), 205–210. PMID:15377808

Busari, J. O., Scherpbier, A. J. J. A., Van Der Vleuten, C. P. M., & Essed, G. E. (2000). Residents' perception of their role in teaching undergraduate students in the clinical setting. *Medical Teacher*, *22*(4), 348–353. doi:10.1080/014215900409438

Buszman, P. E., Kiesz, S. R., Bochenek, A., Peszek-Przybyla, E., Szkrobka, I., Debinski, M., & Tendera, M. et al. (2008). Acute and late outcomes of unprotected left main stenting in comparison with surgical revascularization. *Journal of the American College of Cardiology*, *51*(5), 538–545. doi:10.1016/j.jacc.2007.09.054 PMID:18237682

Buth, K. J., Gainer, R. A., Legare, J. F., & Hirsch, G. M. (2014). The changing face of cardiac surgery: Practice patterns and outcomes 2001-2010. *The Canadian Journal of Cardiology*, *30*(2), 224–230. doi:10.1016/j.cjca.2013.10.020 PMID:24373760

Butterworth, J. F. t., Legault, C., Royster, R. L., & Hammon, J. W. Jr. (1998). Factors that predict the use of positive inotropic drug support after cardiac valve surgery. *Anesthesia and Analgesia*, *86*(3), 461–467. PMID:9495394

Butterworth, J. F. IV, Prielipp, R. C., Royster, R. L., Spray, B. J., Kon, N. D., Wallenhaupt, S. L., & Zaloga, G. P. (1992). Dobutamine increases heart rate more than epinephrine in patients recovering from aortocoronary bypass surgery. *Journal of Cardiothoracic and Vascular Anesthesia*, *6*(5), 535–541. doi:10.1016/1053-0770(92)90095-O PMID:1421064

Button, D., Weibel, L., Reuthebuch, O., Genoni, M., Zollinger, A., & Hofer, C. K. (2007). Clinical evaluation of the FloTrac/Vigileo system and two established continuous cardiac-output monitoring devices in patients undergoing cardiac surgery. *British Journal of Anaesthesia*, *99*(3), 329–336. doi:10.1093/bja/aem188 PMID:17631509

Buxton, B. F., Hayward, P., Newcomb, A. E., Moten, S., Seevanayagam, S., & Gordon, I. (2009). Choice of conduits for coronary artery bypass grafting: Craft or science? *European Journal of Cardio-Thoracic Surgery : Official Journal of the European Association for Cardio-Thoracic Surgery*, *35*(4), 658–670. doi:10.1016/j.ejcts.2008.10.058 PMID:19231230

Bybee, K. A., Powell, B. D., Valeti, U., Rosales, A. G., Kopecky, S. L., Mullany, C., & Wright, R. S. (2005). Preoperative Aspirin Therapy Is Associated With Improved Postoperative Outcomes in Patients Undergoing Coronary Artery Bypass Grafting. *Circulation*, *112*(9suppl), I-286–I292. PMID:16159833

Byrne, J. G., Rezai, K., Sanchez, J. A., Bernstein, R. A., Okum, E., Leacche, M., & Higgins, R. S. D. et al. (2011). Surgical management of endocarditis: The Society of Thoracic Surgeons clinical practice guideline. *The Annals of Thoracic Surgery*, *91*(6), 2012–2019. doi:10.1016/j.athoracsur.2011.01.106 PMID:21620012

Byszewski, A., Hendelman, W., McGuinty, C., & Moineau, G. V. (2012). Wanted: Role models - medical students' perceptions of professionalism. *BMC Medical Education*, *12*(1), 1–1. doi:10.1186/1472-6920-12-115 PMID:23153359

Cabell, C. H., Jollis, J. G., Peterson, G. E., Corey, G. R., Anderson, D. J., Sexton, D. J., & Fowler, V. G. et al. (2002). Changing patient characteristics and the effect on mortality in endocarditis. *Archives of Internal Medicine*, *162*(1), 90–94. doi:10.1001/archinte.162.1.90 PMID:11784225

Cabrini, L., Plumari, V. P., Nobile, L., Olper, L., Pasin, S., Bocchino, S., & Zangrillo, A. et al. (2013). Non-invasive ventilation in cardiac surgery: A concise review. *Heart. Lung and Vessels*, *5*, 137–141. PMID:24364004

Cade, C. H. (2008). Clinical tools for the assessment of pain in sedated critically ill adults. *Nursing in Critical Care*, *13*(6), 288–297. doi:10.1111/j.1478-5153.2008.00294.x PMID:19128312

Cady, R. F. (2008). "Becoming a high reliability organization-operational advice for hospital leaders" report. *JONA'S Healthcare Law, Ethics and Regulation*, *10*, 33. doi:10.1097/01.NHL.0000300780.65358.e0 PMID:18525400

Caine, N., Sharples, L. D., & Wallwork, J. (1999). Prospective study of health related quality of life before and after coronary artery bypass grafting: Outcomes at five years. *Heart (British Cardiac Society)*, *81*(4), 357–361. doi:10.1136/hrt.81.4.347 PMID:10092558

Calafiore, a M., Giammarco, G. D., Teodori, G., Bosco, G., D'Annunzio, E., Barsotti, a, … Contini, M. (1996). Left anterior descending coronary artery grafting via left anterior small thoracotomy without cardiopulmonary bypass. *The Annals of Thoracic Surgery*, *61*(6), 1658–63; discussion 1664–5. Retrieved from http://www.ncbi.nlm.nih.gov/pubmed/8651765

Campbell, M. L., & Guzman, J. A. (2003). Impact of a proactive approach to improve end-of-life care in a medical ICU. *Chest*, *123*(1), 266–271. doi:10.1378/chest.123.1.266 PMID:12527629

Campeau, L., Enjalbert, M., Lespérance, J., Bourassa, M. G., Kwiterovich, P. Jr, Wacholder, S., & Sniderman, A. (1984). The relation of risk factors to the development of atherosclerosis in saphenous-vein bypass grafts and the progression of disease in the native circulation. A study 10 years after aortocoronary bypass surgery. *The New England Journal of Medicine*, *311*(21), 1329–1332. doi:10.1056/NEJM198411223112101 PMID:6333635

Camporata, L. (2010). Pitfalls in haemodynamic monitoring based on the arterial pressure waveform. *Critical Care (London, England)*, *14*(2), 124. doi:10.1186/cc8845 PMID:20236463

Campos, J., & Parekh, K. R. (2011). Thoracic Imaging. In P. D. Slinger (Ed.), *Principles and practice of anesthesia for thoracic surgery* (pp. 35–48). New York: Elsevier. doi:10.1007/978-1-4419-0184-2_3

Čanádyová, J., Zmeko, D., & Mokráček, A. (2012). Re-exploration for bleeding or tamponade after cardiac operation. *Interactive Cardiovascular and Thoracic Surgery*, *14*(6), 704–707. doi:10.1093/icvts/ivs087 PMID:22434857

Canbaz, S., Turgut, N., Halici, U., Sunar, H., Balci, K., & Duran, E. (2005). Brachial plexus injury during open heart surgery--controlled prospective study. *The Thoracic and Cardiovascular Surgeon*, *53*(5), 295–299. doi:10.1055/s-2005-865672 PMID:16208616

Cannegieter, S. C., Rosendaal, F. R., & Briet, E. (1994). Thromboembolic and bleeding complications in patients with mechanical heart valve prostheses. *Circulation*, *89*(2), 635–641. doi:10.1161/01.CIR.89.2.635 PMID:8313552

Cannon, C. P., Braunwald, E., McCabe, C. H., Rader, D. J., Rouleau, J. L., Belder, R., & Skene, A. M. et al. (2004). Intensive versus Moderate Lipid Lowering with Statins after Acute Coronary Syndromes. *The New England Journal of Medicine*, *350*(15), 1495–1504. doi:10.1056/NEJMoa040583 PMID:15007110

Cantillon, D. J., Gorodeski, E. Z., Caccamo, M., Smedira, N. G., Wilkoff, B. L., Starling, R. C., & Saliba, W. (2009). Long-Term Outcomes And Clinical Predictors For Pacing After Cardiac Transplantation. *The Journal Of Heart And Lung Transplantation*, *28*(8), 791-798. Retrieved From http://www.jhltonline.org/article/s1053-2498(09)00316-7/abstract

Capanni, F., & Checkley, W. (2013). Differences in hospital mortality by ICU staffing models: You cannot always get what you want, but sometimes you get what you need. *Critical Care Medicine*, *41*(10), 2433–2434. doi:10.1097/CCM.0b013e31829cb0aa PMID:24060770

Carabello, B. A. (2005). Modern management of mitral stenosis. *Circulation*, *112*(3), 432–437. doi:10.1161/CIRCULATIONAHA.104.532498 PMID:16027271

Carabello, B. A., & Paulus, W. J. (2009). Aortic stenosis. *Lancet*, *373*(9667), 956–966. doi:10.1016/S0140-6736(09)60211-7 PMID:19232707

Carchman, E. H., Peitzman, A. B., Simmons, R. L., & Zuckerbraun, B. S. (2012). The role of acute care surgery in the treatment of severe, complicated Clostridium difficile-associated disease. *Journal of Trauma and Acute Care Surgery*, *73*(4), 789–800. doi:10.1097/TA.0b013e318265d19f PMID:23026914

Cardarelli, M. G., Young, A. J., & Griffith, B. (2009). Use of extracorporeal membrane oxygenation for adults in cardiac arrest (E-CPR): a meta-analysis of observational studies. *ASAIO Journal (American Society for Artificial Internal Organs: 1992)*, *55*(6), 581–586. doi:10.1097/MAT.0b013e3181bad907

Cardinal, D. C., & Flower, R. J. (1980). The electronic aggregometer: A novel device for assessing platelet behavior in blood. *Journal of Pharmacological Methods*, *3*(2), 135–158. doi:10.1016/0160-5402(80)90024-8 PMID:7392654

Cargill, R. I., & Lipworth, B. J. (1996). Lisinopril attenuates acute hypoxic pulmonary vasoconstriction in humans. *Chest Journal*, *109*(2), 424–429. doi:10.1378/chest.109.2.424 PMID:8620717

Carling, P. C., Parry, M. F., & Von Beheren, S. M.Healthcare Environmental Hygiene Study Group. (2008). Identifying opportunities to enhance environmental cleaning in 23 acute care hospitals. *Infection Control and Hospital Epidemiology, 29*(1), 1–7. doi:10.1086/524329 PMID:18171180

Carpentier, A., Adams, D. H., & Filsoufi, F. (2010). *Carpentier's Reconstructive Valve Surgery*. Saunders Elsevier.

Carpentier, A., Guermonprez, J. L., Deloche, A., Frechette, C., & DuBost, C. (1973). The aorta-to-coronary radial artery bypass graft. A technique avoiding pathological changes in grafts. *The Annals of Thoracic Surgery, 16*(2), 111–121. http://www.ncbi.nlm.nih.gov/pubmed/4582222 doi:10.1016/S0003-4975(10)65825-0 PMID:4582222

Carraccio, C., & Englander, R. (2004). Evaluating competence using a portfolio: A literature review and web-based application to the ACGME competencies. *Teaching and Learning in Medicine, 16*(4), 381–387. doi:10.1207/s15328015tlm1604_13 PMID:15582877

Carraccio, C., Wolfsthal, S. D., Englander, R., Ferentz, K., & Martin, C. (2002). Shifting paradigms: From Flexner to competencies. *Academic Medicine, 77*(5), 361–367. doi:10.1097/00001888-200205000-00003 PMID:12010689

Carrascal, Y., Guerrero, A. L., Blanco, M., Valenzuela, H., Pareja, P., & Laguna, G. (2014). Postoperative stroke related to cardiac surgery in octogenarians. *Interactive Cardiovascular and Thoracic Surgery, 18*(5), 596–601. doi:10.1093/icvts/ivu022 PMID:24556446

Carrel, T. P., Eisinger, E., Vogt, M., & Turina, M. I. (2001). Pneumonia after cardiac surgery is predictable by tracheal aspirates but cannot be prevented by prolonged antibiotic prophylaxis. *The Annals of Thoracic Surgery, 72*(1), 143–148. doi:10.1016/S0003-4975(01)02669-8 PMID:11465169

Carretta, A., Zannini, P., Chiesa, G., Altese, R., Melloni, G., & Grossi, A. (1996). Efficacy of ketorolac tromethamine and extrapleural intercostal nerve block on post-thoracotomy pain: A prospective, randomized study. *International Surgery, 81*, 224–228. PMID:9028977

Carson, J. L., Terrin, M. L., Noveck, H., Sanders, D. W., Chaitman, B. R., & Rhoads, G. G. et al.. (2011). Liberal or Restrictive Transfusion in High-Risk Patients after Hip Surgery. *The New England Journal of Medicine*, 111214140020001. PMID:22168590

Carson, J., Scholz, P., Chen, A., Peterson, E., Gold, J., & Schneider, S. (2002). Diabetes mellitus increases short-term mortality and morbidity in patients undergoing coronary artery bypass graft surgery. *Journal of the American College of Cardiology, 40*(3), 418–423. doi:10.1016/S0735-1097(02)01969-1 PMID:12142105

Carson, P., Ziesche, S., Johnson, G., & Cohn, J. (1999). Racial differences in response to therapy for heart failure: analysis of the vasodilator-heart failure trials: Vasodilator-Heart Failure Trial Study Group. *Journal of Cardiac Failure, 5*(3), 178–187. doi:10.1016/S1071-9164(99)90001-5 PMID:10496190

Cartwright, P. D., & Pingel, S. M. (2007). Midazolam and diazepam in ketamine anesthesia. *Anaesthesia, 39*(5), 439–442. doi:10.1111/j.1365-2044.1984.tb07312.x PMID:6731772

Casaer, M. P., Mesotten, D., Hermans, G., Wouters, P. J., Schetz, M., Meyfroidt, G., & Van den Berghe, G. et al. (2011). Early versus late parenteral nutrition in critically ill adults. *The New England Journal of Medicine, 365*(6), 506–517. doi:10.1056/NEJMoa1102662 PMID:21714640

Casaer, M. P., & Van den Berghe, G. (2014). Nutrition in the Acute Phase of Critical Illness. *The New England Journal of Medicine, 370*(13), 1227–1236. doi:10.1056/NEJMra1304623 PMID:24670169

Casaer, M. P., Wilmer, A., & Van den Berghe, G. (2013). Supplemental parenteral nutrition in critically ill patients. *Lancet, 381*(9879), 1715. doi:10.1016/S0140-6736(13)61068-5 PMID:23683628

Casey, A. L., Mermel, L. A., Nightingale, P., & Elliott, T. S. (2008). Antimicrobial central venous catheters in adults: A systematic review and meta-analysis. *The Lancet Infectious Diseases*, *8*(12), 763–776. doi:10.1016/S1473-3099(08)70280-9 PMID:19022192

Casthely, P. A., Lear, S., Cottrell, J. E., & Lear, E. (1982). Intrapulmonary shunting during induced hypotension. *Anesthesia and Analgesia*, *61*(3), 231–235. doi:10.1213/00000539-198203000-00002 PMID:6802027

Castillo, J., Leira, R., Garcia, M. M., Serena, J., Blanco, M., & Davalos, A. (2004). Blood pressure decrease during the acute phase of ischemic stroke is associated with brain injury and poor stroke outcome. *Stroke*, *35*(2), 520–526. doi:10.1161/01.STR.0000109769.22917.B0 PMID:14726553

Cavarocchi, N. C., Pitcher, H. T., Yang, Q., Karbowski, P., Miessau, J., Hastings, H. M., & Hirose, H. (2013). Weaning of extracorporeal membrane oxygenation using continuous hemodynamic transesophageal echocardiography. *The Journal of Thoracic and Cardiovascular Surgery*, *146*(6), 1474–1479. doi:10.1016/j.jtcvs.2013.06.055 PMID:23993027

Cecconi, M., Johnston, E., & Rhodes, A. (2006). What role does the right side of the heart play in circulation? *Critical Care (London, England)*, *10 Suppl 3*(Suppl 3), S5. doi:10.1186/cc4832

Cerfolio, R. J., Bass, C., & Katholi, C. R. (2001). Prospective randomized trial compares suction versus water seal for air leaks. *The Annals of Thoracic Surgery*, *71*(5), 1613–1617. doi:10.1016/S0003-4975(01)02474-2 PMID:11383809

Cerfolio, R. J., & Bryant, A. S. (2008). Results of a prospective algorithm to remove chest tubes after pulmonary resection with high output. *The Journal of Thoracic and Cardiovascular Surgery*, *135*(2), 269–273. doi:10.1016/j.jtcvs.2007.08.066 PMID:18242249

Cerfolio, R. J., Bryant, A. S., Singh, S., Bass, C. S., & Bartolucci, A. A. (2005). The management of chest tubes in patients with a pneumothorax and an air leak after pulmonary resection. *Chest Journal*, *128*(2), 816–820. doi:10.1378/chest.128.2.816 PMID:16100173

Cerovic, O., Golubović, V., Špec-Marn, A., Kremžar, B., & Vidmar, G. (2003). Relationship between injury severity and lactate levels in severely injured patients. *Intensive Care Medicine*, *29*(8), 1300–1305. doi:10.1007/s00134-003-1753-8 PMID:12904861

Chahoud, J., Kanafani, Z. A., & Kanj, S. S. (2013). Management of candidaemia and invasive candidiasis in critically ill patients. *International Journal of Antimicrobial Agents*, *42S*, S29–S35. doi:10.1016/j.ijantimicag.2013.04.008 PMID:23664579

Chaicharoen, P., & Ratanakul, P. (1998). Letting-Go or Killing: Thai Buddhist Perspectives on Euthanasia. *Journal of Asian and International Bioethics*, *8*, 37–40.

Chaitman, B. R., Alderman, E. L., Sheffield, L. T., Tong, T., Fisher, L., & Mock, M. B. … Killip, T. (1983). Use of survival analysis to determine the clinical significance of new Q waves after coronary bypass surgery. *Circulation*, *67*(2), 302–9. Retrieved from http://www.ncbi.nlm.nih.gov/pubmed/6600217

Chalaby, M. P. J. (2010). Acute Respiratory Failure. In A. Jeremias & D. L. Brown (Eds.), *Cardiac Intensive Care* (2nd ed., pp. 388–397). Philadelphia, PA: Saunders/Elsevier. doi:10.1016/B978-1-4160-3773-6.10031-X

Chalk, K., Meisel, C., Spies, C., Volk, T., Thuenemann, K., Linneweber, J., & Sander, M. et al. (2013). Dysfunction of alveolar macrophages after cardiac surgery: Predisposing factor for the development of postoperative pneumonia? – An observational study. *Critical Care (London, England)*, *17*, R285. doi:10.1186/cc13148 PMID:24321282

Chalmers, J. D., Rother, C., Salih, W., & Ewig, S. (2014). Healthcare-associated pneumonia does not accurately identify potentially resistant pathogens: A systematic review and meta-analysis. *Clinical Infectious Diseases*, *58*(3), 330–339. doi:10.1093/cid/cit734 PMID:24270053

Chambers, A., Routledge, T., Dunning, J., & Scarci, M. (2010). Is video-assisted thoracoscopic surgical decortication superior to open surgery in the management of adults with primary empyema? *Interactive Cardiovascular and Thoracic Surgery*, *11*(2), 171–177. doi:10.1510/icvts.2010.240408 PMID:20439299

Chambers, H. F., Miller, R. T., & Newman, M. D. (1988). Right-sided Staphylococcus aureus endocarditis in intravenous drug abusers: Two-week combination therapy. *Annals of Internal Medicine*, *109*(8), 619–624. doi:10.7326/0003-4819-109-8-619 PMID:3421575

Chambers, S. T., Murdoch, D., Morris, A., Holland, D., Pappas, P., Almela, M., & Chu, V. H. et al. (2013). HACEK infective endocarditis: Characteristics and outcomes from a large, mulit-national cohort. *PLoS ONE*, *8*(5), e63181. doi:10.1371/journal.pone.0063181 PMID:23690995

Chamogeorgakis, T., Lima, B., Shafii, A. E., Nagpal, D., Pokersnik, J. A., Navia, J. L., & Gonzalez-Stawinski, G. V. et al. (2013). Outcomes of axillary artery side graft cannulation for extracorporeal membrane oxygenation. *The Journal of Thoracic and Cardiovascular Surgery*, *145*(4), 1088–1092. doi:10.1016/j.jtcvs.2012.08.070 PMID:22999514

Chamogeorgakis, T., Rafael, A., Shafii, A. E., Nagpal, D., Pokersnik, J. A., & Gonzalez-Stawinski, G. V. (2013). Which Is Better: A Miniaturized Percutaneous Ventricular Assist Device or Extracorporeal Membrane Oxygenation for Patients With Cardiogenic Shock? *ASAIO Journal (American Society for Artificial Internal Organs)*, *59*(6), 607–611. doi:10.1097/MAT.0b013e3182a8baf7 PMID:24088905

Chanda, J., Brichkov, I., & Canver, C. C. (2000). Prevention of radial artery graft vasospasm after coronary bypass. *The Annals of Thoracic Surgery*, *70*(6), 2070–2074. http://www.ncbi.nlm.nih.gov/pubmed/11156122 doi:10.1016/S0003-4975(00)02001-4 PMID:11156122

Chaney, M. A. (2002). Corticosteroids and cardiopulmonary bypass: A review of clinical investigations. *Chest*, *121*(3), 921–931. doi:10.1378/chest.121.3.921 PMID:11888978

Chaney, M. A., Furry, P. A., Fluder, E. M., & Slogoff, S. (1997). Intrathecal morphine for coronary artery bypass grafting and early extubation. *Anesthesia and Analgesia*, *84*, 241–248. PMID:9024009

Chang, A. C., Chan, K. M., Lonigro, R. J., Lau, C. L., Lama, V. N., Flaherty, K. R., & Orringer, M. B. et al. (2007). Surgical patient outcomes after the increased use of bilateral lung transplantation. *The Journal of Thoracic and Cardiovascular Surgery*, *133*(2), 532–540. doi:10.1016/j.jtcvs.2006.09.060

Chang, H. R., & Bistrian, B. (1998). The role of cytokines in the catabolic consequences of infection and injury. *Journal of Parenteral and Enteral Nutrition*, *22*(3), 156–166. doi:10.1177/0148607198022003156 PMID:9586794

Chang, R., Greene, M. T., Chenoweth, C. E., Kuhn, L., Shuman, E., Rogers, M. A. M., & Saint, S. (2011). Epidemiology of hospital-acquired urinary tract-related bloodstream infection at a university hospital. *Infection Control and Hospital Epidemiology*, *32*(11), 1127–1129. doi:10.1086/662378 PMID:22011543

Chang, S.-J., & Huang, H.-H. (2013). Diarrhea in enterally fed patients: Blame the diet? *Current Opinion in Clinical Nutrition and Metabolic Care*, *16*(5), 588–594. doi:10.1097/MCO.0b013e328363bcaf PMID:23799327

Chan, K. L., Teo, K., Dumesnil, J. G., Ni, A., & Tam, J. (2010). Effect of lipid lowering with rosuvastatin on progression of aortic stenosis. *Circulation*, *121*(2), 306–314. doi:10.1161/CIRCULATIONAHA.109.900027 PMID:20048204

Channick, R. N., Voswinckel, R., Rubin, L. J., & Vultaggio, . (2012). Inhaled Treprostinil: A therapeutic review. *Drug Design. Development and Therapy*, *6*, 19–28. doi:10.2147/DDDT.S19281

Chan, R. W., & Hegney, D. (2012). Buddhism and medical futility. *Bioethical Inquiry*, *9*(4), 433–438. doi:10.1007/s11673-012-9392-9 PMID:23188402

Charlin, B., Roy, L., Brailovsky, C., Goulet, F., & van der Vleuten, C. (2000). The Script Concordance test: A tool to assess the reflective clinician. *Teaching and Learning in Medicine*, *12*(4), 189–195. doi:10.1207/S15328015TLM1204_5 PMID:11273368

Chastre, J., & Fagon, J.-Y. (2002). Ventilator-associated pneumonia. *American Journal of Respiratory and Critical Care Medicine*, *165*(7), 867–903. doi:10.1164/ajrccm.165.7.2105078 PMID:11934711

Chastre, J., Wolff, M., Fagon, J.-Y., Chevret, S., Thomas, F., Wermert, D., & Group, P. T. et al. (2003). Comparison of 8 vs 15 days of antibiotic therapy for ventilator-associated pneumonia in adults: A randomized trial. *Journal of the American Medical Association*, *290*(19), 2588–2598. doi:10.1001/jama.290.19.2588 PMID:14625336

Chatterjee, S., Chaudhuri, D., Vedanthan, R., Fuster, V., Ibanez, B., & Sripal Bangalore, D. M. (2013). Early intravenous beta-blockers in patients with acute coronary syndrome - A meta-analysis of randomized trials. *International Journal of Cardiology*, *168*(2), 915–921. doi:10.1016/j.ijcard.2012.10.050 PMID:23168009

Chatzinikolaou, I., Hanna, H., Hachem, R., Alakech, B., Tarrand, J., & Raad, I. (2004). Differental quantitative blood cultures for the diagnosis of catheter-related bloodstream infections associated with short- and long-term catheters: A prospective study. *Diagnostic Microbiology and Infectious Disease*, *50*(3), 167–172. doi:10.1016/j.diagmicrobio.2004.07.007 PMID:15541601

Chaumais, M. C., Jobard, M., Huertas, A., Vignand-Courtin, C., Humbert, M., Sitbon, O., & Montani, D. et al. (2010). Pharmacokinetic Evaluation of Continuous Intravenous Epoprostenol. *Expert Opinion on Drug Metabolism & Toxicology*, *6*(12), 1587–1598. doi:10.1517/17425255.2010.534458 PMID:21077785

Chawla, L. S., Zhao, Y., Lough, F. C., Schroeder, E., Seneff, M. G., & Brennan, J. M. (2012). Off-Pump versus On-Pump Coronary Artery Bypass Grafting Outcomes Stratified by Preoperative Renal Function. *Journal of the American Society of Nephrology*, *23*(8), 1389–1397. doi:10.1681/ASN.2012020122 PMID:22595302

Cheatham, M. L., Malbrain, M. L. N. G., Kirkpatrick, A., Sugrue, M., Parr, M., De Waele, J., & Wilmer, A. et al. (2007). Results from the international conference of experts on intra-abdominal hypertension and abdominal compartment syndrome. II. *Recommendations. Intensive Care Med*, *33*(6), 951–962. doi:10.1007/s00134-007-0592-4 PMID:17377769

Cheitlin, M. D., Gertz, E. W., Brundage, B. H., Carlson, C. J., Quash, J. A., & Bode, R. S. Jr. (1979). Rate of progression of severity of valvular aortic stenosis in the adult. *American Heart Journal*, *98*(6), 689–700. doi:10.1016/0002-8703(79)90465-4 PMID:495418

Chen, J. M., Russo, M. J., Hammond, K. M., Mancini, D. M., Kherani, A. R., & Fal, J. M. … Naka, Y. (2005). Alternate Waiting List Strategies For Heart Transplantation Maximize Donor Organ Utilization. *The Annals Of Thoracic Surgery*, *80*(1), 224-228. Retrieved From http://www.annalsthoracicsurgery.org/article/s0003-4975(05)00030-5/abstract

Cheng, A., & Slaughter, M. S. (2013). How I choose conduits and configure grafts for my patients-rationales and practices. *Annals of Cardiothoracic Surgery*, *2*(4), 527–532. doi:10.3978/j.issn.2225-319X.2013.07.17 PMID:23977632

Cheng, D. C., Bainbridge, D., Martin, J. E., & Novick, R. J. (2005). Does off-pump coronary artery bypass reduce mortality, morbidity, and resource utilization when compared with conventional coronary artery bypass? A meta-analysis of randomized trials. *Anesthesiology*, *102*(1), 188–203. doi:10.1097/00000542-200501000-00028 PMID:15618803

Cheng, D. C., Karski, J., Peniston, C., Raveendran, G., Asokumar, B., Carroll, J., & Sandler, A. et al. (1996). Early tracheal extubation after coronary artery bypass graft surgery reduces costs and improves resource use. A prospective, randomized, controlled trial. *Anesthesiology*, *85*(6), 1300–1310. doi:10.1097/00000542-199612000-00011 PMID:8968177

Chen, H. H., Anstrom, K. J., Givertz, M. M., Stevenson, L. W., Semigran, M. J., Goldsmith, S. R., & Redfield, M. M. et al. (2013). Low-dose dopamine or low-dose nesiritide in acute heart failure with renal dysfunction: The ROSE acute heart failure randomized trial. *Journal of the American Medical Association*, *310*(23), 2533–2543. doi:10.1001/jama.2013.282190 PMID:24247300

Chenoweth, C., & Saint, S. (2013). Preventing catheter-associated urinary tract infections in the intensive care unit. *Critical Care Clinics*, *29*(1), 19–32. doi:10.1016/j.ccc.2012.10.005 PMID:23182525

Chertow, G. M., Lazarus, J. M., Christiansen, C. L., Cook, E. F., Hammermeister, K. E., Grover, F., & Daley, J. (1997). Preoperative renal risk stratification. *Circulation*, *95*(4), 878–884. http://www.ncbi.nlm.nih.gov/pubmed/9054745 doi:10.1161/01.CIR.95.4.878 PMID:9054745

Chevernak, J., McCullough, L. B., & Chevernak, F. A. (2014). Surgery Without Consent or Miscommunication? A New Look at a Landmark Legal Case. *American Journal of Obstetrics and Gynecology*, *212*(5), 586–590. doi:10.1016/j.ajog.2014.06.062 PMID:24995772

Childs, S., Blenkinsopp, E., Hall, A., & Walton, G. (2005). Effective e-learning for health professionals and students--barriers and their solutions. A systematic review of the literature--findings from the HeXL project. *Health Information and Libraries Journal*, *22*(s2Suppl 2), 20–32. doi:10.1111/j.1470-3327.2005.00614.x PMID:16279973

Chiles, C., Guthaner, D. F., Jamieson, S. W., Stinson, E. B., Oyer, P. E., & Silverman, J. F. (1985). Heart-lung transplantation: The postoperative chest radiograph. *Radiology*, *154*(2), 299–304. doi:10.1148/radiology.154.2.3917571 PMID:3917571

Chirouze, C., Athan, E., Alla, F., Chu, V. H., Corey, G. R., & Selton-Suty, C. (2013). Enterococcal endocarditis in the beginning of the 21st century: An analysis from the International Collaboration on Endocarditis – Prospective cohort study. *Clinical Microbiology and Infection*, *19*(12), 1140–1147. doi:10.1111/1469-0691.12166 PMID:23517406

Chiumello, D., Cressoni, M., Carlesso, E., Caspani, M. L., Marino, A., Gallazzi, E., & Gattinoni, L. et al. (2014). Bedside selection of positive end-expiratory pressure in mild, moderate, and severe acute respiratory distress syndrome. *Critical Care Medicine*, *42*(2), 252–264. doi:10.1097/CCM.0b013e3182a6384f PMID:24196193

Chlebicki, M. P., & Safdar, N. (2007). Topical chlorhexidine for the prevention of ventilator-associated pneumonia: A meta-analysis. *Critical Care Medicine*, *35*(2), 595–602. doi:10.1097/01.CCM.0000253395.70708.AC PMID:17205028

Choi, B. W., Bacharach, S. L., Barbour, D. J., Leon, M. B., McCarthy, K. E., & Bonow, R. O. (1995). Left ventricular systolic dysfunction diastolic filling characteristics and exercise cardiac reserve in mitral stenosis. *The American Journal of Cardiology*, *75*(7), 526–529. doi:10.1016/S0002-9149(99)80599-2 PMID:7864006

Choi, W. S., & Samman, N. (2008). Risks and benefits of deliberate hypotension in anesthesia: A systematic review. *International Journal of Oral and Maxillofacial Surgery*, *37*(8), 687–703. doi:10.1016/j.ijom.2008.03.011 PMID:18511238

Choi, Y. S., Shim, J. K., Kim, J. C., Kang, K., Seo, Y. H., Ahn, K., & Kwak, Y. L. (2011). Effect of remote ischemic preconditioning on renal dysfunction after complex valvular heart surgery: A randomized controlled trial. *The Journal of Thoracic and Cardiovascular Surgery*, *142*(1), 148–154. doi:10.1016/j.jtcvs.2010.11.018 PMID:21272897

Choong, C. K., Gerrard, C., Goldsmith, K. A., Dunningham, H., & Vuylsteke, A. (2007). Delayed re-exploration for bleeding after coronary artery bypass surgery results in adverse outcomes. *European Journal of Cardio-Thoracic Surgery*, *31*(5), 834–838. doi:10.1016/j.ejcts.2007.02.001 PMID:17360191

Chopra, V., O'Horo, J. C., Rogers, M. A. M., Maki, D. G., & Safdar, N. (2013). The risk of bloodstream infection associated with peripherally inserted central catheters compared with central venous catheters in adults: A systematic review and meta-analysis. *Infection Control and Hospital Epidemiology*, *34*(9), 908–918. doi:10.1086/671737 PMID:23917904

Choules, A. P. (2007). The use of elearning in medical education: A review of the current situation. *Postgraduate Medical Journal*, *83*(978), 212–216. doi:10.1136/pgmj.2006.054189 PMID:17403945

Christensen, M. C., Dziewior, F., Kempel, A., & von Heymann, C. (2012). Increased chest tube drainage is independently associated with adverse outcome after cardiac surgery. *Journal of Cardiothoracic and Vascular Anesthesia*, *26*(1), 46–51. doi:10.1053/j.jvca.2011.09.021 PMID:22100857

Christrup, L. L. (1997). Morphine metabolites. *Acta Anaesthesiologica Scandinavica*, *41*(1), 116–122. doi:10.1111/j.1399-6576.1997.tb04625.x PMID:9061094

Chung, J. H., Gikakis, N., Rao, A. K., Drake, T. A., Colman, R. W., & Edmunds, L. H. (1996). Pericardial blood activates the extrinsic coagulation pathway during clinical cardiopulmonary bypass. *Circulation*, *93*(11), 2014–2018. doi:10.1161/01.CIR.93.11.2014 PMID:8640976

Chung, J. W., Ryu, S. H., Jo, J. H., Park, J. Y., Lee, S., Park, S. W., & Chung, J. B. et al.J.W. (2013). Clinical implications and risk factors of acute pancreatitis after cardiac valve surgery. *Yonsei Medical Journal*, *54*(1), 154–159. doi:10.3349/ymj.2013.54.1.154 PMID:23225812

Chung, M. K. (2000). Cardiac surgery: Postoperative arrhythmias. *Critical Care Medicine*, *28*(10Suppl), N136–N144. doi:10.1097/00003246-200010001-00005 PMID:11055682

Chu, V. H., Cabell, C. H., Benjamin, D. K. Jr, Kuniholm, E. F., Fowler, V. G. Jr, Engemann, J., & Wang, A. et al. (2004). Early predictors of in-hospital death in infective endocarditis. *Circulation*, *109*(14), 1745–1749. doi:10.1161/01.CIR.0000124719.61827.7F PMID:15037538

Chu, V. H., Miro, J. M., Hoen, B., Cabell, C. H., Pappas, P. A., Jones, P., & Fowler, V. G. et al. (2009). Coagulase-negative staphylococcal prosthetic valve endocarditis – A contemporary update based on the International Collaboration on Endocarditis: Prospective cohort study. *Heart (British Cardiac Society)*, *95*(7), 570–576. doi:10.1136/hrt.2008.152975 PMID:18952633

Çilingiroğlu M, Akkuş N, Sethi S, Modi KA. (2014). Large pericardial effusion induced by minoxidil. *Türk Kardiyoloji Derneği arşivi: Türk Kardiyoloji Derneğinin yayın organıdı, 40*(3), 255.

Cirillo, M., Messina, A., Dalla Tomba, M., Brunelli, F., Mhagna, Z., Villa, E., & Troise, G. et al. (2009). A new no-touch aorta technique for arterial-source, off-pump coronary surgery. *The Annals of Thoracic Surgery*, *88*(4), e46–e47. doi:10.1016/j.athoracsur.2009.07.045 PMID:19766780

Clark, R. E., & Estes, F. (1996). Cognitive task analysis for training. *International Journal of Educational Research*, *25*(5), 403–417. doi:10.1016/S0883-0355(97)81235-9

Clark, S. C. (2006). Lung injury after cardiopulmonary bypass. *Perfusion*, *21*(4), 225–228. doi:10.1191/0267659106pf872oa PMID:16939116

Coca, S. G., Garg, A. X., Swaminathan, M., Garwood, S., Hong, K., Thiessen-Philbrook, H., & Parikh, C. R. et al. TRIBE-AKI Consortium. (2013). Preoperative angiotensin-converting enzyme inhibitors and angiotensin receptor blocker use and acute kidney injury in patients undergoing cardiac surgery. *Nephrology, Dialysis, Transplantation*, *28*(11), 2787–2799. PMID:24081864

Cochran, A., Edelman, L. S., Morris, S. E., & Saffle, J. R. (2008). Learner satisfaction with Web-based learning as an adjunct to clinical experience in burn surgery. *Journal of Burn Care & Research; Official Publication of the American Burn Association, 29*(1), 222–226. doi:10.1097/BCR.0b013e31815ff2ac PMID:18182926

Cogan, J. (2010). Pain management after cardiac surgery. *Seminars in Cardiothoracic and Vascular Anesthesia, 14*(3), 201–204. doi:10.1177/1089253210378401 PMID:20705642

Cohen, J. (2002). The immunopathogenesis of sepsis. *Nature, 420*(6917), 885–891. doi:10.1038/nature01326 PMID:12490963

Cohen, J. J. (2007). Viewpoint: linking professionalism to humanism: what it means, why it matters. *Academic Medicine, 82*(11), 1029–1032. doi:10.1097/01.ACM.0000285307.17430.74 PMID:17971686

Cohen, S. H., Gerding, D. N., Johnson, S., Kelly, C. P., Loo, V. G., McDonald, L. C., & Wilcox, M. H. et al. (2010). Clinical practice guidelines for Clostridium difficile infection in adults: 2010 update by the society for healthcare epidemiology of America (SHEA) and the infectious diseases society of America (IDSA). *Infection Control and Hospital Epidemiology, 31*(5), 431–455. doi:10.1086/651706 PMID:20307191

Cohn, L. H., Rizo, R. J., Adams, D. H., Aranki, S. F., Couper, G. S., Beckel, N., & Collins, J. J. (1996). Reduced mortality and morbidity for ascending aortic aneurysm resection regardless of cause. *The Annals of Thoracic Surgery, 62*(2), 463–468. doi:10.1016/0003-4975(96)00280-9 PMID:8694606

Collins, N., Miller, R., Kapu, A., Martin, R., Morton, M., Forrester, M., & Wilkinson, L. et al. (2014). Outcomes of adding acute care nurse practitioners to a Level I trauma service with the goal of decreased length of stay and improved physician and nursing satisfaction. *J Trauma Acute Care Surg, 76*(2), 353–357. doi:10.1097/TA.0000000000000097 PMID:24398767

Collins, P., Webb, C. M., Chong, C. F., & Moat, N. E. (2008). Radial artery versus saphenous vein patency randomized trial: Five-year angiographic follow-up. *Circulation, 117*(22), 2859–2864. doi:10.1161/CIRCULATIONAHA.107.736215 PMID:18506009

Colucci, W. S., Wright, R. F., Jaski, B. E., Fifer, M. A., & Braunwald, E. (1986). Milrinone and dobutamine in severe heart failure: Differing hemodynamic effects and individual patient responsiveness. *Circulation, 73*(3 Pt 2), III175–III183. PMID:3510774

Colvin-Adams, M., Smith, J. M., Heubner, B. M., Skeans, M. A., Edwards, L. B., Waller, C., & Kasiske, B. L. et al. (2013). OPTN/SRTR 2011 Annual Data Report: Heart. *American Journal of Transplantation, 13*(suppl 1), 119–148. doi:10.1111/ajt.12023 PMID:23237699

Comparison of coronary bypass surgery with angioplasty in patients with multivessel disease. The Bypass Angioplasty Revascularization Investigation (BARI) Investigators. (1996). *The New England Journal of Medicine, 335*(4), 217–25. doi:10.1056/NEJM199607253350401

Compton, F. D., Zukunft, B., Hoffmann, C., Zidek, W., & Schaefer, J.-H. (2008). Performance of a minimally invasive uncalibrated cardiac output monitoring system (Flotrac/Vigileo) in haemodynamically unstable patients. *British Journal of Anaesthesia, 100*(4), 451–456. doi:10.1093/bja/aem409 PMID:18256056

Confalonieri, M., Garuti, G., Cattaruzza, M. S., Osborn, J. F., Antonelli, M., & Conti, G. et al.. (2005). A chart of failure risk for noninvasive ventilation in patients with COPD exacerbation. *The European Respiratory Journal, 25*(2), 348–355. doi:10.1183/09031936.05.00085304 PMID:15684302

Connolly, S. J., Ezekowitz, M. D., Yusuf, S., Eikelboom, J., Oldgren, J., Parekh, A., & Wallentin, L. et al. (2009). Dabigatran versus warfarin in patients with atrial fibrillation. *The New England Journal of Medicine*, *361*(12), 1139–1151. doi:10.1056/NEJMoa0905561 PMID:19717844

Connors, R., Reuben, B., Neumayer, L., & Bull, D. (2007). Comparing Outcomes after Transthoracic and Transhiatal Esophagectomy: A 5-Year Prospective Cohort of 17,395 Patients. *Journal of the American College of Surgeons*, *205*(6), 735–740. doi:10.1016/j.jamcollsurg.2007.07.001 PMID:18035255

Conolly, S. A. J., klein AA. (2010). Deep hypothermic circulatory arrest. *Continuing Education in Anaesthesia, Critical Care & Pain, 10*(5).

Conolly, S., Arrowsmith, J. E., & Klein, A. A. (2010). Deep hypothermic circulatory arrest. *Continuing Education in Anaesthesia. Critical Care & Pain*, *10*(5), 138–142. doi:10.1093/bjaceaccp/mkq024

Consales, G., Chelazzi, C., Rinaldi, S., & De Gaudio, A. R. (2006). Bispectral index compared to Ramsay score for sedation monitoring in intensive care units. *Minerva Anestesiologica*, *72*, 329–336. PMID:16675941

Conway Morris, A., Anderson, N., Brittan, M., Wilkinson, T. S., McAuley, D. F., Antonelli, J., & Simpson, A. J. et al. (2013). Combined dysfunctions of immune cells predict nosocomial infection in critically ill patients. *British Journal of Anaesthesia*, *111*(5), 778–787. doi:10.1093/bja/aet205 PMID:23756248

Cook, D. A. (2005). The Research We Still Are Not Doing: An Agenda for the Study of Computer-Based Learning. *Academic Medicine*, *80*(6), 541–548. doi:10.1097/00001888-200506000-00005 PMID:15917356

Cook, D. A. (2007). Web-based learning: Pros, cons and controversies. *Clinical Medicine*, *7*(1), 37–42. doi:10.7861/clinmedicine.7-1-37 PMID:17348573

Cook, D. A., Dupras, D. M., Thompson, W. G., & Pankratz, V. S. (2005). Web-based learning in residents' continuity clinics: A randomized, controlled trial. *Academic Medicine*, *80*(1), 90–97. doi:10.1097/00001888-200501000-00022 PMID:15618102

Cook, D. A., & McDonald, F. S. (2008). E-learning: Is there anything special about the "E"? *Perspectives in Biology and Medicine*, *51*(1), 5–21. doi:10.1353/pbm.2008.0007 PMID:18192762

Cook, D. J., Fuller, H. D., Guyatt, G. H., Marshall, J. C., Leasa, D., Hall, R., & Willan, A. et al. (1994). Risk factors for gastrointestinal bleeding in critically ill patients. Canadian Critical Care Trials Group. *The New England Journal of Medicine*, *330*(6), 377–381. doi:10.1056/NEJM199402103300601 PMID:8284001

Cook, D. J., Griffith, L. E., Walter, S. D., Guyatt, G. H., Meade, M. O., Heyland, D. K., & Tryba, M. et al. (2001). The attributable mortality and length of intensive care unit stay of clinically important gastrointestinal bleeding in critically ill patients. *Critical Care (London, England)*, *5*(6), 368–375. doi:10.1186/cc1071 PMID:11737927

Cook, D. J., Witt, L. G., Cook, R. J., & Guyatt, G. H. (1991). Stress ulcer prophylaxis in the critically ill: A meta-analysis. *The American Journal of Medicine*, *91*(5), 519–527. doi:10.1016/0002-9343(91)90189-5 PMID:1835294

Cook, D., Guyatt, G., Marshall, J., Leasa, D., Fuller, H., Hall, R., & Kirby, A. et al. (1998). A comparison of sucralfate and ranitidine for the prevention of upper gastrointestinal bleeding in patients requiring mechanical ventilation. Canadian Critical Care Trials Group. *The New England Journal of Medicine*, *338*(12), 791–797. doi:10.1056/NEJM199803193381203 PMID:9504939

Cooley, D. A. (2013). Some thoughts about the historic events that led to the first clinical implantation of a total artificial heart. *Texas Heart Institute Journal*, *40*(2), 117–119. PMID:23678207

Cooper, M. S., & Stewart, P. M. (2003). Corticosteroid insufficiency in acutely ill patients. *The New England Journal of Medicine*, *348*(8), 727–734. doi:10.1056/NEJMra020529 PMID:12594318

Copeland, J. G. (2013). SynCardia Total Artificial Heart: Update and Future. *Texas Heart Institute Journal*, *40*(5), 587–588. PMID:24391330

Cope, M., Cevallos, M. E., Cadle, R. M., Darouiche, R. O., Musher, D. M., & Trautner, B. W. (2009). Inappropriate treatment of catheter-associated asymptomatic bacteriuria in a tertiary care hospital. *Clinical Infectious Diseases*, *48*(9), 1182–1188. doi:10.1086/597403 PMID:19292664

Cornia, P. B., Amory, J. K., Fraser, S., Saint, S., & Lipsky, B. A. (2003). Computer-based order entry decreased duration of indwelling urinary catheterization in hospitalized patients. *The American Journal of Medicine*, *114*(5), 404–407. doi:10.1016/S0002-9343(02)01568-1 PMID:12714131

Cortellaro, F., Colombo, S., Coen, D., & Duca, P. G. (2012). Lung ultrasound is an accurate diagnostic tool for the diagnosis of pneumonia in the emergency department. *Emergency Medicine Journal: EMJ*, *29*(1), 19–23. doi:10.1136/emj.2010.101584 PMID:21030550

Coselli, J. S., LeMaire, S. A., Koksoy, C., Schmittling, Z. C., & Curling, P. E. (2002). Cerebrospinal fluid drainage reduces paraplegia after thoracoabdominal aortic aneurysm repair: Results of a randomized clinical trial. *Journal of Vascular Surgery*, *35*(4), 631–639. doi:10.1067/mva.2002.122024 PMID:11932655

Costa, D. K., Wallace, D. J., Barnato, A. E., & Kahn, J. M. (2014). Nurse practitioner/physician assistant staffing and critical care mortality. *Chest*, *146*(6), 1566–1573. doi:10.1378/chest.14-0566 PMID:25167081

Costanzo, M. R., Costanzo, M. R., Dipchand, A., Starling, R., Anderson, A., Chan, M. … Vanhaecke, J. (2010). The International Society Of Heart And Lung Transplantation Guidelines For The Care Of Heart Transplant Recipients. *The Journal Of Heart And Lung Transplantation*, *29*(8), 914-956. Retrieved from http://www.jhltonline.org/article/s1053-2498(10)00358-x/abstract

Costanzo, L. (2014). *Physiology* (5th ed.). Philadelphia: Saunders Elsevier.

Coulehan, J., & Williams, P. C. (2000). Professional Ethics and Social Activism. In D. Wear & J. Bickel (Eds.), *Educating For Professionalism: Creating A Culture Of Humanism In Medical Education*. Iowa City: University of Iowa Press.

Coulehan, J., & Williams, P. C. (2001). Vanquishing virtue: The impact of medical education. *Academic Medicine*, *76*(6), 598–605. doi:10.1097/00001888-200106000-00008 PMID:11401802

Coutinho, G. F., Correia, P. M., Pauperio, G., de Oliveira, F., & Antunes, M. J. (2011). Aortic root enlargement does not increase the surgical risk and short-term patient outcome? *European Journal of Cardio-Thoracic Surgery*, *40*(2), 441–447. doi:10.1016/j.ejcts.2010.11.064 PMID:21236693

Cove, M. E., Maclaren, G., Federspiel, W. J., & Kellum, J. A. (2012). Bench to bedside review: Extracorporeal carbon dioxide removal, past present and future. *Critical Care (London, England)*, *16*(5), 232. doi:10.1186/cc11356 PMID:23014710

Cowell, S. J., Newby, D. E., Prescott, R. J., Bloomfield, P., Reid, J., Northridge, D. B., & Boon, N. A.Lipid Lowering Trial, Impact on Regression Investigators. (2005). A randomized trial of intensive lipid-lowering therapy in calcific aortic stenosis. *The New England Journal of Medicine*, *352*(23), 2389–2397. doi:10.1056/NEJMoa043876 PMID:15944423

Cox, M., Irby, D. M., & Epstein, R. M. (2007). Assessment in Medical Education. *The New England Journal of Medicine*, *356*(4), 387–396. doi:10.1056/NEJMra054784 PMID:17251535

Craven, D. E., Lei, Y., Ruthazer, R., Sarwar, A., & Hudcova, J. (2013). Incidence and outcomes of ventilator-associated tracheobronchitis and pneumonia. *The American Journal of Medicine*, *126*(6), 542–549. doi:10.1016/j.amjmed.2012.12.012 PMID:23561632

Crawford, M. H., Souchek, J., Oprian, C. A., Miller, D. C., Rahimtoola, S., Giacomini, J. C., & Hammermeister, K. E. et al.Department of Veterans Affairs Cooperative Study on Valvular Heart Disease. (1990). Determinants of survival and left ventricular performance after mitral surgery. *Circulation*, *81*(4), 1173–1181. doi:10.1161/01.CIR.81.4.1173 PMID:2317900

Critchley, L. A., & Critchley, J. A. (1999). A meta-analysis of studies using bias and precision statistics to compare cardiac output measurement techniques. *Journal of Clinical Monitoring and Computing*, *15*(2), 85–91. doi:10.1023/A:1009982611386 PMID:12578081

Croce, M. A., Swanson, J. M., Magnotti, L. J., Claridge, J. A., Weinberg, J. A., Wood, G. C., & Fabian, T. C. et al. (2006). The futility of the clinical pulmonary infections score in trauma patients. *The Journal of Trauma*, *60*(3), 523–527. doi:10.1097/01.ta.0000204033.78125.1b PMID:16531849

Cronin, L., Cook, D. J., Carlet, J., Heyland, D. K., King, D., Lansang, M. A., & Fisher, C. J. Jr. (1995). Corticosteroid treatment for sepsis: A critical appraisal and meta-analysis of the literature. *Critical Care Medicine*, *23*(8), 1430–1439. doi:10.1097/00003246-199508000-00019 PMID:7634816

Crossley, J., Marriott, J., Purdie, H., & Beard, J. D. (2011). Prospective observational study to evaluate NOTSS (Non-Technical Skills for Surgeons) for assessing trainees' non-technical performance in the operating theatre. *British Journal of Surgery*, *98*(7), 1010–1020. doi:10.1002/bjs.7478 PMID:21480195

Crouzet, J., Bertrand, X., Venier, A. G., Badoz, M., Husson, C., & Talon, D. (2007). Control of the duration of urinary catheterization: Impact on catheter-associated urinary tract infection. *The Journal of Hospital Infection*, *67*(3), 253–257. doi:10.1016/j.jhin.2007.08.014 PMID:17949851

Cruess, S. R., & Cruess, R. L. (2012). Teaching professionalism - Why, What and How. *Facts. Views & Vision in ObGyn*, *4*(4), 259–265.

Cruickshank, M. K., Levine, M. N., Hirsh, J., Roberts, R., & Siguenza, M. (1991). A standard heparin nomogram for the management of heparin therapy. *Archives of Internal Medicine*, *151*(2), 333–337. doi:10.1001/archinte.1991.00400020085018 PMID:1789820

Cruz, D. N., Ricci, Z., & Ronco, C. (2009). Clinical review: RIFLE and AKIN – time for reappraisal. *Critical Care (London, England)*, *13*(3), 211. doi:10.1186/cc7759 PMID:19638179

Cuffe, M.S., Califf, R.M., Adams, K.F. Jr, Benza, R., Bourge, R., & Colucci, W.S., … Outcomes of a Prospective Trial of Intravenous Milrinone for Exacerbations of Chronic Heart Failure (OPTIME-CHF) Investigators. (2002). Outcomes of a Prospective Trial of Intravenous Milrinone for Exacerbations of Chronic Heart Failure I. Short-term intravenous milrinone for acute exacerbation of chronic heart failure: A randomized controlled trial. *Journal of the American Medical Association*, *287*(12), 1541–1547. doi:10.1001/jama.287.12.1541 PMID:11911756

Cuisset, T., Frere, C., Quilici, J., Morange, P.-E., Nait-Saidi, L., Carvajal, J., & Aless, M.-C. et al. (2006). Benefit of a 600-mg Loading Dose of Clopidogrel on Platelet Reactivity and Clinical Outcomes in Patients With Non–ST-Segment Elevation Acute Coronary Syndrome Undergoing Coronary Stenting. *Journal of the American College of Cardiology*, *48*(7), 1339–1345. doi:10.1016/j.jacc.2006.06.049 PMID:17010792

Cujec, B., Polasek, P., Mayers, I., & Johnson, D. (1993). Positive end-expiratory pressure increases the right-to-left shunt in mechanically ventilated patients with patent foramen ovale. *Annals of Internal Medicine*, *119*(9), 887–894. doi:10.7326/0003-4819-119-9-199311010-00004 PMID:8215000

Cullen, L., Mueller, C., Parsonage, W., Wildi, K., Greenslade, J., Twerenbold, R., & Mosimann, T. et al. (2013). Validation of high-sensitivity troponin I in a 2-hour diagnostic strategy to assess 30-day outcomes in emergency department patients with possible acute coronary syndrome. *Journal of the American College of Cardiology*, *62*(14), 1242–1249. doi:10.1016/j.jacc.2013.02.078 PMID:23583250

Culliford, A. T., Colvin, S. B., Rohrer, K., Baumann, F. G., & Spencer, F. C. (1986). The atherosclerotic ascending aorta and transverse arch: a new technique to prevent cerebral injury during bypass: experience with 13 patients. *The Annals of Thoracic Surgery*, *41*(1), 27–35. http://www.ncbi.nlm.nih.gov/pubmed/3942429 doi:10.1016/S0003-4975(10)64492-X PMID:3942429

Currey, J., Pilcher, D. V., Davies, A., Scheinkestel, C., Botti, M., Bailey, M., & Snell, G. (2010). Implementation of a management guideline aimed at minimizing the severity of primary graft dysfunction after lung transplant. *The Journal of Thoracic and Cardiovascular Surgery*, *139*(1), 154–161. doi:10.1016/j.jtcvs.2009.08.031

Curtis, A., Worley, S., Adamson, P., Chung, E., Niazi, I., Sherfesee, L., & Sutton, M. et al. (2013). Biventricular pacing for atrioventricular block and systolic dysfunction. *The New England Journal of Medicine*, *368*(17), 1585–1593. doi:10.1056/NEJMoa1210356 PMID:23614585

Curtis, H. J., Bourke, S. J., Dark, J. H., & Corris, P. A. (2005). Lung transplantation outcome in cystic fibrosis patients with previous pneumothorax. *The Journal of Heart and Lung Transplantation*, *24*(7), 865–869. doi:10.1016/j.healun.2004.05.024

Czerny, M., Gottardi, R., Zimpfer, D., Schoder, M., Grabenwoger, M., Lammer, J., & Grimm, M. et al. (2007). Mid-ter.m results of supraaortic transpositions for extended endovascular repair of aortic arch pathologies E*uropea.n. Journal of Cardiothoracic Surgery*, *31*(4), 623–627. doi:10.1016/j.ejcts.2006.12.030 PMID:17239613

D'Ancona, G., Baillot, R., Poirier, B., Dagenais, F., de Ibarra, J. I. S., Bauset, R., & Doyle, D. et al. (2003a). Determinants of gastrointestinal complications in cardiac surgery. *Texas Heart Institute Journal*, *30*(4), 280–285. PMID:14677737

Dacey, L. J., Likosky, D. S., Leavitt, B. J., Lahey, S. J., Quinn, R. D., & Hernandez, F. Jr et al. Northern New England Cardiovascular Disease Study, G. (2005). Perioperative stroke and long-term survival after coronary bypass graft surgery. *The Annals of Thoracic Surgery*, *79*(2), 532–536, discussion 537. doi:10.1016/j.athoracsur.2004.07.027 PMID:15680829

Dahan, A., Aarts, L., & Smith, T. W. (2010). Incidence, reversal, and prevention of opioid-induced respiratory depression. *Anesthesiology*, *112*(1), 226–238. doi:10.1097/ALN.0b013e3181c38c25 PMID:20010421

Dales, R. E., Dionne, G., Leech, J. A., Lunau, M., & Schweitzer, I. (1993). Preoperative prediction of pulmonary complications following thoracic surgery. *Chest Journal*, *104*(1), 155–159. doi:10.1378/chest.104.1.155 PMID:8325061

Daley, R. J., Rebuck, J. A., Welage, L. S., & Rogers, F. B. (2004). Prevention of stress ulceration: Current trends in critical care. *Critical Care Medicine*, *32*(10), 2008–2013. doi:10.1097/01.CCM.0000142398.73762.20 PMID:15483408

Dantas, A. M., & Kemm, R. E. (2008). A blended approach to active learning in a physiology laboratory-based subject facilitated by an e-learning component. *AJP: Advances in Physiology Education*, *32*(1), 65–75. doi:10.1152/advan.00006.2007 PMID:18334571

Dardashti, A., Ederoth, P., Algotsson, L., Brondén, B., & Bjursten, H. (2013). Incidence, dynamics, and prognostic value of acute kidney injury for death after cardiac surgery. *The Journal of Thoracic and Cardiovascular Surgery*, *147*(2), 800–807. doi:10.1016/j.jtcvs.2013.07.073 PMID:24100099

Dark, P. M., & Singer, M. (2004). Trans-esohphageal Doppler ultrasonography as a measure of cardiac output in critically ill adults. *Intensive Care Medicine*, *30*(11), 2060–2066. doi:10.1007/s00134-004-2430-2 PMID:15368037

Darrah, W. C., Sharpe, M. D., Guiraudon, G. M., & Neal, A. (1997). Intraaortic balloon counterpulsation improves right ventricular failure resulting from pressure overload. *The Annals of Thoracic Surgery*, *64*(6), 1718–1723. doi:10.1016/S0003-4975(97)01102-8 PMID:9436561

Dasta, J. F., Kane-Gill, S. L., Durtschi, A. J., Pathak, D. S., & Kellum, J. A. (2008). Costs and outcomes of acute kidney injury (AKI) following cardiac surgery. *Nephrology, Dialysis, Transplantation*, *23*(6), 1970–1974. doi:10.1093/ndt/gfm908 PMID:18178605

Dave, D. H. (1970). Psychomotor levels. In R. J. Armstrong (Ed.), *Developing and writing educational objectives* (pp. 33–34). Tucson: Educational Innovators Press.

Davie, E. W., & Ratnoff, O. D. (1964). Waterfall sequence for intrinsic blood clotting. *Science*, *145*(3638), 1310–1312. doi:10.1126/science.145.3638.1310 PMID:14173416

Davies, R. R., Russo, M. J., Morgan, J. A., Sorabella, R. A., Naka, Y., & Chen, J. M. (2010). Standard Versus Bicaval Techniques For Orthotopic Heart Transplantation: An Analysis Of The United Network For Organ Sharing Database. *The Journal of Thoracic and Cardiovascular Surgery, 140*(3), 700-708. Retrieved from http://www.Jtcvsonline.Org/Article/S0022-5223(10)00435-6/Abstract

Davies, A., Jones, D., Bailey, M., Beca, J., Bellomo, R., Blackwell, N., & Ziegenfuss, M. et al. (2009). Extracorporeal Membrane Oxygenation for 2009 Influenza A(H1N1) Acute Respiratory Distress Syndrome. *Journal of the American Medical Association*, *302*(17), 1888–1895. doi:10.1001/jama.2009.1535

Davies, C. W., Kearney, S. E., Gleeson, F. V., & Davies, R. J. (1999). Predictors of outcome and long-term survival in patients with pleural infections. *American Journal of Respiratory and Critical Care Medicine*, *160*(5), 1682–1687. doi:10.1164/ajrccm.160.5.9903002 PMID:10556140

Davies, E., Moxham, T., Rees, K., Singh, S., Coats, A., Ebrahim, S., & Taylor, S. et al. (2010). Exercise training for systolic heart failure: Cochrane systematic review and meta-analysis. *European Journal of Heart Failure*, *12*(7), 706–715. doi:10.1093/eurjhf/hfq056 PMID:20494922

Davies, R. R., Goldstein, L. J., Coady, M. A., Tittle, S. L., Rizzo, J. A., Kopf, G. S., & Elefteriades, J. A. (2002). Yearly rupture or dissection rates for thoracic aortic aneurysms: Simple prediction based on size. *The Annals of Thoracic Surgery*, *73*(1), 17–28. doi:10.1016/S0003-4975(01)03236-2 PMID:11834007

Davies, R., & Morrell, N. W. (2008). Molecular Mechanisms of Pulmonary Arterial Hypertension: Role of Mutations in the Bone Morphogenetic Protein Type II Receptor. *Chest*, *134*(6), 1271–1277. doi:10.1378/chest.08-1341 PMID:19059957

Davies, S. W., Gershlick, A. H., & Balcon, R. (1991). Progression of valvar aortic stenosis: A long-term retrospective study. *European Heart Journal*, *12*(1), 10–14. PMID:2009886

Davydow, D. S., Gifford, J. M., Desai, S. V., Needham, D. M., & Bienvenu, O. J. (2008). Posttraumatic stress disorder in general intensive care unit survivors: A systematic review. *General Hospital Psychiatry*, *30*(5), 421–434. doi:10.1016/j.genhosppsych.2008.05.006 PMID:18774425

Day, N. P., Phu, N. H., Bethell, D. P., Mai, N. T., Chau, T. T., Hien, T. T., & White, N. J. (1996). The effects of dopamine and adrenaline infusions on acid-base balance and systemic haemodynamics in severe infection. *Lancet*, *348*(9022), 219–223. doi:10.1016/S0140-6736(96)09096-4 PMID:8684198

De Backer, D., Aldecoa, C., Njimi, H., & Vincent, J. L. (2012). Dopamine versus norepinephrine in the treatment of septic shock: A meta-analysis*. *Critical Care Medicine*, *40*(3), 725–730. doi:10.1097/CCM.0b013e31823778ee PMID:22036860

De Backer, D., Biston, P., Devriendt, J., Madl, C., Chochrad, D., Aldecoa, C., & Vincent, J.-L. et al. (2010). Comparison of dopamine and norepinephrine in the treatment of shock. *The New England Journal of Medicine*, *362*(9), 779–789. doi:10.1056/NEJMoa0907118 PMID:20200382

De Bonis, M., Maisano, F., La Canna, G., & Alfieri, O. (2012). Treatment and management of mitral regurgitation. *Nature Reviews. Cardiology*, *9*(3), 133–144. doi:10.1038/nrcardio.2011.169 PMID:22105677

De Bono, S., Heling, G., & Borg, M. A. (2014). Organizational culture and its implications for infection prevention and control in healthcare institutions. *The Journal of Hospital Infection*, *86*(1), 1–6. doi:10.1016/j.jhin.2013.10.007 PMID:24309419

De Groot, L. (2006). Non-thyroidal illness syndrome is a manifestation of hypothalamic-pituitary dysfunction, and in view of current evidence, should be treated with appropriate replacement therapies. *Critical Care Clinics*, *22*(1), 57–86. doi:10.1016/j.ccc.2005.10.001 PMID:16399020

de Hoyos, A., Demajo, W., Snell, G., Miller, J., Winton, T., Maurer, J. R., & Patterson, G. A. (1993). Preoperative prediction for the use of cardiopulmonary bypass in lung transplantation. *The Journal of Thoracic and Cardiovascular Surgery*, *106*(5), 787–795.

De Jonghe, B., Bastuji-Garin, S., Durand, M.-C., Malissin, I., Rodrigues, P., Cerf, C., & Sharshar, T. et al. (2007). Respiratory weakness is associated with limb weakness and delayed weaning in critical illness. *Critical Care Medicine*, *35*(9), 2007–2015. doi:10.1097/01.ccm.0000281450.01881.d8 PMID:17855814

de Jong, R., Houtgraff, J., Samiei, S., Boersma, E., & Duckers, H. (2014). Intracoronary stem cell infusion after acute myocardial infarction: A meta-analysis and update on clinical trials. *Circulation: Cardiovascular Interventions*, *7*(2), 156–167. doi:10.1161/CIRCINTERVENTIONS.113.001009 PMID:24668227

De Lange, S., Van Aken, H., & Burchardi, H. (2002). European Society of Intensive Care Medicine statement: Intensive care medicine in Europe--structure, organisation and training guidelines of the Multidisciplinary Joint Committee of Intensive Care Medicine (MJCICM) of the European Union of Medical Specialists (UEMS). *Intensive Care Medicine*, *28*(11), 1505–1511. doi:10.1007/s00134-002-1504-2 PMID:12583367

De Smet, A. M. G. A., Kluytmans, J. A. J. W., Cooper, B. S., Mascini, E. M., Benus, R. F. J., van der Werf, T. S., & Bonten, M. J. M. et al. (2009). Decontamination of the digestive tract and oropharynx in ICU patients. *The New England Journal of Medicine*, *360*(1), 20–31. doi:10.1056/NEJMoa0800394 PMID:19118302

de Wilde, R. B. P. (2008). Review of the PiCCO device; our experience in the ICU. *The Netherlands Journal of Critical Care*, *12*, 60–64.

Debakey, M. E. (2000). The odyssey of the artificial heart. *Artificial Organs*, *24*(6), 405–411. doi:10.1046/j.1525-1594.2000.06635.x PMID:10886056

Deb, S., Cohen, E., Singh, S. K., Une, D., Laupacis, A., & Fremes, S. E. (2012). Radial artery and saphenous vein patency more than 5 years after coronary artery bypass surgery: Results from RAPS (Radial Artery Patency Study). *Journal of the American College of Cardiology*, *60*(1), 28–35. doi:10.1016/j.jacc.2012.03.037 PMID:22742399

Deb, S., Wijeysunera, H. C., Ko, D. T., Tsubota, H., Hill, S., & Fremes, S. E. (2013). Coronary Artery Bypass Graft Surgery vs. Percutaneous Interventions in Coronary Revascularization: A Systematic Review. *Journal of the American Medical Association*, *310*(19), 2086–2095. doi:10.1001/jama.2013.281718 PMID:24240936

DeFoe, G. R., Krumholz, C. F., DioDato, C. P., Ross, C. S., Olmstead, E. M., Groom, R. C., & O'Connor, G. T. et al. (2003). Lowest core body temperature and adverse outcomes associated with coronary artery bypass surgery. *Perfusion, 18*(2), 127–133. doi:10.1191/0267659103pf660oa PMID:12868791

Delgado-Guay, M. O., Parsons, H. A., Li, Z., Palmer, L. J., & Bruera, E. (2009). Symptom distress, interventions, and outcomes of intensive care unit cancer patients referred to a palliative care consult team. *Cancer, 115*(2), 437–445. doi:10.1002/cncr.24017 PMID:19107768

Dellinger, E. P., Hausmann, S. M., Bratzler, D. W., Johnson, R. M., Daniel, D. M., Bunt, K. M., & Sugarman, J. R. et al. (2005). Hospitals collaborate to decrease surgical site infections. *American Journal of Surgery, 190*(1), 9–15. doi:10.1016/j.amjsurg.2004.12.001 PMID:15972163

Dellinger, R. P., Levy, M. M., Rhodes, A., Annane, D., Gerlach, H., Opal, S. M., & Moreno, R. et al. (2013). Surviving sepsis campaign: international guidelines for management of severe sepsis and septic shock: 2012. *Critical Care Medicine, 41*(2), 580–637. doi:10.1097/CCM.0b013e31827e83af PMID:23353941

Delva, M. D., Kirby, J., Schultz, K., & Godwin, M. (2004). Assessing the relationship of learning approaches to workplace climate in clerkship and residency. *Academic Medicine, 79*(11), 1120–1126. doi:10.1097/00001888-200411000-00025 PMID:15504785

Denault, A. Y., Haddad, F., Jacobsohn, E., & Deschamps, A. (2013). Perioperative right ventricular dysfunction. *Current Opinion in Anaesthesiology, 26*(1), 71–81. doi:10.1097/ACO.0b013e32835b8be2

Denault, A., Deschamps, A., & Murkin, J. M. (2007). A proposed algorithm for the intraoperative use of cerebral near-infrared spectroscopy. *Seminars in Cardiothoracic and Vascular Anesthesia, 11*(4), 274–281. doi:10.1177/1089253207311685 PMID:18270192

Dennis, B. M., Eckert, M. J., Gunter, O. L., Morris, J. A., Jr., & May, A. K. (2013). Safety of bedside percutaneous tracheostomy in the critically ill: evaluation of more than 3,000 procedures.*Journal of American College of Surgeons, 216*(4), 858-865; discussion 865-857. doi: 10.1016/j.jamcollsurg.2012.12.017

Desai, N. D., Cohen, E. A., Naylor, C. D., & Fremes, S. E. (2004). A randomized comparison of radial-artery and saphenous-vein coronary bypass grafts. *The New England Journal of Medicine, 351*(22), 2302–2309. doi:10.1056/NEJMoa040982 PMID:15564545

Desai, N. D., Naylor, C. D., Kiss, A., Cohen, E., Feder-Elituv, R., Miwa, S., & Fremes, S. E. et al. (2007). Impact of patient and target-vessel characteristics on arterial and venous bypass graft patency: Insight from a randomized trial. *Circulation, 115*(6), 684–691. doi:10.1161/CIRCULATIONAHA.105.567495 PMID:17283268

Deschka, H., Erler, S., El-Ayoubi, L., Vogel, C., Vöhringer, L., & Wimmer-Greinecker, G. (2013). Suction-irrigation drainage: An underestimated therapeutic option for surgical treatment of deep sternal wound infections. *Interactive Cardiovascular and Thoracic Surgery, 17*(1), 85–89. doi:10.1093/icvts/ivt078 PMID:23529753

Deshpande, K. S., Hatem, C., Ulrich, H. L., Currie, B. P., Aldrich, T. K., Bryan-Brown, C. W., & Kvetan, V. (2005). The incidence of infectious complications of central venous catheters at the subclavian, internal jugular, and femoral sites in an intensive care unit population. *Critical Care Medicine, 33*(1), 13–20. doi:10.1097/01.CCM.0000149838.47048.60 PMID:15644643

Desimone, D. C., Tleyjeh, I. M., Correa de Sa, D. D., Anavekar, N. S., Lahr, B. D., Sohail, M. R., & Baddour, L. M. et al. (2012). Incidence of infective endocarditis caused by viridans group streptococci before and after publication of the 2007 American Heart Association's endocarditis prevention guidelines. *Circulation, 126*(1), 60–64. doi:10.1161/CIRCULATIONAHA.112.095281 PMID:22689929

Desmonts, J. M., & Marty, J. (1984). Anesthetic management of patients with pheochromocytoma. *British Journal of Anaesthesia*, *56*(7), 781–789. doi:10.1093/bja/56.7.781 PMID:6375708

Despotis, G. J., Filos, K. S., Zoys, T. N., Hogue, C. W., Spitznagel, E., & Lappas, D. G. (1996). Factors associated with excessive postoperative blood loss and hemostatic transfusion requirements: A multivariate analysis in cardiac surgical patients. *Anesthesia and Analgesia*, *82*(1), 13–21. PMID:8712388

Despotis, G. J., & Goodnough, L. T. (2000). Management approaches to platelet-related microvascular bleeding in cardiothoracic surgery. *The Annals of Thoracic Surgery*, *70*(2), S20–S32. doi:10.1016/S0003-4975(00)01604-0 PMID:10966007

Despotis, G., Eby, C., & Lublin, D. M. (2008). A review of transfusion risks and optimal management of perioperative bleeding with cardiac surgery. *Transfusion*, *48*(1 Suppl), 2S–30S. doi:10.1111/j.1537-2995.2007.01573.x PMID:18302579

Detre, K., Murphy, M. L., & Hultgren, H. (1977). Effect of coronary bypass surgery on longevity in high and low risk patients. Report from the VA Cooperative Coronary Surgery Study. *Lancet*, *2*(8051), 1243–1245. doi:10.1016/S0140-6736(77)92659-9 PMID:73949

Deverall, P. B., Olley, P. M., Smith, D. R., Watson, D. A., & Whitaker, W. (1968). Incidence of systemic embolism before and after mitral valvotomy. *Thorax*, *23*(5), 530–536. doi:10.1136/thx.23.5.530 PMID:5680237

Devereaux, P. J., Chan, M. T. V., Alonso-Coello, P., Walsh, M., Berwanger, O., Villar, J. C., & Yusuf, S. et al. (2012). Association between postoperative troponin levels and 30-day mortality among patients undergoing noncardiac surgery. *Journal of the American Medical Association*, *307*(21), 2295–2304. doi:10.1001/jama.2012.5502 PMID:22706835

Devereaux, P., Goldman, L., Yusuf, S., Gilbert, K., Leslie, K., & Guyatt, G. (2005). Surveillance and prevention of major perioperative ischemic cardiac events in patients undergoing noncardiac surgery: A review. *Canadian Medical Association Journal*, *173*(7), 779–788. doi:10.1503/cmaj.050316 PMID:16186585

Deviri, E., Sareli, P., Wisenbaugh, T., & Cronje, S. L. (1991). Obstruction of mechanical heart valve prostheses: Clinical aspect and surgical management. *Journal of the American College of Cardiology*, *17*(3), 646–650. doi:10.1016/S0735-1097(10)80178-0 PMID:1993782

Devlin, J. W., Roberts, R. J., Fong, J. J., Skrobik, Y., Riker, R. R., Hill, N. S., & Garpestad, E. et al. (2010). Efficacy and safety of quetiapine in critically ill patients with delirium: A prospective, multicenter, randomized, double-blind, placebo-controlled pilot study. *Critical Care Medicine*, *38*(2), 419–427. doi:10.1097/CCM.0b013e3181b9e302 PMID:19915454

Dewan, N. A., Gayasaddin, M., Angelillo, V. A., O'Donohue, W. J., & Mohiuddin, S. (1986). Persistent hypoxemia due to patent foramen ovale in a patient with adult respiratory distress syndrome. *Chest Journal*, *89*(4), 611–613. doi:10.1378/chest.89.4.611 PMID:3514169

Dhareshwar, J., Sundt, T. M. III, Dearani, J. A., Schaff, H. V., Cook, D. J., & Orszulak, T. A. (2007). Aortic root enlargement: What are the operative risks? *The Journal of Thoracic and Cardiovascular Surgery*, *134*(4), 916–924. doi:10.1016/j.jtcvs.2007.01.097 PMID:17903507

Di Lorenzo, L., De Pergola, G., Zocchetti, C., L'Abbate, N., Basso, A., Pannacciulli, N., & Soleo, L. et al. (2003). Effect of shift work on body mass index: Results of a study performed in 319 glucose-tolerant men working in a Southern Italian industry. *International Journal of Obesity and Related Metabolic Disorders*, *27*(11), 1353–1358. doi:10.1038/sj.ijo.0802419 PMID:14574346

Diamond, J. M., Lee, J. C., Kawut, S. M., Shah, R. J., Localio, A. R., Bellamy, S. L., & Christie, J. D. et al. (2013). Clinical risk factors for primary graft dysfunction after lung transplantation. *American Journal of Respiratory and Critical Care Medicine*, *187*(5), 527–534. doi:10.1164/rccm.201210-1865OC

Dickerman, S. A., Abrutyn, E., Barsic, B., Bouza, E., Cecchi, E., Moreno, A., & Cabell, C. H. et al. (2007). The relationship between the initiation of antimicrobial therapy and the incidence of stroke in infective endocarditis: An analysis from the ICE Prospective Cohort Study (ICE-PCS). *American Heart Journal, 154*(6), 1086–1094. doi:10.1016/j.ahj.2007.07.023 PMID:18035080

Dickerman, S.A., Abrutyn, E., Barsic, B., Bouza, E., Cecchi, E., & Moreno, A., … Cabell, C.H., for the ICE Investigators. (2007). The relationship between the initiation of antimicrobial therapy and the incidence of stroke in infective endocarditis: An analysis from the ICE Prospective Cohort Study Group (ICE-PCS). *American Heart Journal, 154*, 1086–1094. PMID:18035080

Dickerson, R. N., & Melnik, G. (1988). Osmolality of oral drug solutions and suspensions. *American Journal of Health-System Pharmacy, 45*(4), 832–834. PMID:3376967

Diegeler, A., Borgermann, J., Kappert, U., Breuer, M., Boning, A., Ursulescu, A., & Group, G. S. et al. (2013). Off-pump versus on-pump coronary-artery bypass grafting in elderly patients. *The New England Journal of Medicine, 368*(13), 1189–1198. doi:10.1056/NEJMoa1211666 PMID:23477657

Dieleman, J. M., Nierich, A. P., Rosseel, P. M., van der Maaten, J. M., Hofland, J., & Diephuis, J. C. (2012). Intraoperative high-dose dexamethasone for cardiac surgery. A randomized controlled trial. *Journal of the American Medical Association, 308*(17), 1761–1767. doi:10.1001/jama.2012.14144 PMID:23117776

Dieleman, J. M., van Paassen, J., van Dijk, D., Arbous, M., Kalkman, C. J., Vandenbroucke, J. P., & Dekkers, O. M. et al. (2011). Prophylactic corticosteroids for cardiopulmonary bypass in adults. *Cochrane Database of Systematic Reviews*, CD005566. PMID:21563145

Dietzman. (1969). Low cardiac output syndrome: Recognition and treatment. *The Journal of Thoracic and Cardiovascular Surgery, 57*, 137.

Diez, C., Koch, D., Kuss, O., Silber, R., Friedrich, I., & Boergermann, J. (2007). Risk factors for mediastinitis after cardiac surgery – A retrospective analysis of 1700 patients. *Journal of Cardiothoracic Surgery, 2*(1), 23. doi:10.1186/1749-8090-2-23 PMID:17511885

Dimick, J. B., Pelz, R. K., Consunji, R., Swoboda, S. M., Hendrix, C. W., & Lipsett, P. A. (2001). Increased resource use associated with catheter-related bloodstream infection in the surgical intensive care unit. *Archives of Surgery, 136*(2), 229–234. doi:10.1001/archsurg.136.2.229 PMID:11177147

Dimopoulos, G., Poulakou, G., Pneumatikos, I. A., Armaganidis, A., Kollef, M. H., & Matthaiou, D. K. (2013). Short- vs long-duration antibiotic regimens for ventilator-associated pneumonia. A systematic review and meta-analysis. *Chest, 144*(6), 1759–1767. doi:10.1378/chest.13-0076 PMID:23788274

Dimopoulou, I., Anthi, A., Michalis, A., & Tzelepis, G. E. (2001). Functional status and quality of life in long-term survivors of cardiac arrest after cardiac surgery. *Critical Care Medicine, 29*(7), 1408–1411. doi:10.1097/00003246-200107000-00018 PMID:11445698

Ding, X., Jin, S., Niu, X., Ren, H., Fu, S., & Li, Q. (2014). A comparison of the analgesia efficacy and side effects of paravertebral compared with epidural blockade for thoracotomy: An updated meta-analysis. *PLoS ONE, 9*(5), e96233. doi:10.1371/journal.pone.0096233 PMID:24797238

Dirkes, S., & Hodge, K. (2007). Continuous Renal Replacement Therapy in the Adult Intensive Care Unit. *Critical Care Nurse, 27*(2), 61–80. PMID:17389414

Dirocco, D. P., Bisi, J., Roberts, P., Strum, J., Wong, K., Sharpless, N., & Humphreys, B. D. (2014). CDK4/6 inhibition induces epithelial cell cycle arrest and ameliorates acute kidney injury. *AJP: Renal Physiology*, *306*(4), F379–F388. PMID:24338822

Dismore, J., & Dib, N. (2010). Stem Cell Therapy for the Treatment of Acute Myocardial Infarction. *Cardiology Clinics*, *28*(1), 127–138. doi:10.1016/j.ccl.2009.09.004 PMID:19962054

Dixon, B., Reid, D., Collins, M., Newcomb, A. E., Rosalion, A., Yap, C. H., & Campbell, D. J. et al. (2014). The operating surgeon is an independent predictor of chest tube drainage following cardiac surgery. *Journal of Cardiothoracic and Vascular Anesthesia*, *28*(2), 242–246. doi:10.1053/j.jvca.2013.09.010 PMID:24439890

Djaiani, G., Ali, M., Borger, M. A., Woo, A., Carroll, J., Feindel, C., & Rakowski, H. et al. (2008). Epiaortic scanning modifies planned intraoperative surgical management but not cerebral embolic load during coronary artery bypass surgery. *Anesthesia and Analgesia*, *106*(6), 1611–1618. doi:10.1213/ane.0b013e318172b044 PMID:18499587

Dobesh, P. P., & Olsen, K. M. (2014). Statins role in the prevention and treatment of sepsis. *Pharmacological Research*, *88*, 31–40. doi:10.1016/j.phrs.2014.04.010 PMID:24794878

Dobler, C. C., & Waterer, G. (2013). Healthcare-associated pneumonia: A US disease or relevant to the Asia Pacific, too? *Respirology (Carlton, Vic.)*, *18*(6), 923–932. doi:10.1111/resp.12132 PMID:23714303

Dodek, P. M. (2012). Ventilator-associated pneumonia--in the eyes of the beholder. *Critical Care Medicine*, *40*(1), 352–353. doi:10.1097/CCM.0b013e318232665b PMID:22179380

Doenst, T., Wijeysundera, D., Karkouti, K., Zechner, C., Maganti, M., Rao, V., & Borger, M. A. (2005). Hyperglycemia during cardiopulmonary bypass is an independent risk factor for mortality in patients undergoing cardiac surgery. *The Journal of Thoracic and Cardiovascular Surgery*, *130*(4), 1144–1149. doi:10.1016/j.jtcvs.2005.05.049 PMID:16214532

Doig, G. S., Heighes, P. T., Simpson, F., Sweetman, E. A., & Davies, A. R. (2009). Early enteral nutrition, provided within 24 h of injury or intensive care unit admission, significantly reduces mortality in critically ill patients: A meta-analysis of randomised controlled trials. *Intensive Care Medicine*, *35*(12), 2018–2027. doi:10.1007/s00134-009-1664-4 PMID:19777207

Doig, G. S., Simpson, F., Finfer, S., Delaney, A., Davies, A. R., Mitchell, I., & Dobb, G. (2008). Effect of evidence-based feeding guidelines on mortality of critically ill adults: A cluster randomized controlled trial. *Journal of the American Medical Association*, *300*(23), 2731–2741. doi:10.1001/jama.2008.826 PMID:19088351

Doig, G. S., Simpson, F., & Sweetman, E. (2013). Early parenteral nutrition in critically ill patients with short-term relative contraindications to early enteral nutrition: A randomized controlled trial. *Journal of the American Medical Association*, *309*(20), 2130–2138. doi:10.1001/jama.2013.5124 PMID:23689848

Dolman, R. M., Bentley, K. C., Head, T. W., & English, M. (2000). The effect of hypotensive anesthesia on blood loss and operative time during Lefort 1 osteotomies. *Journal of Oral and Maxillofacial Surgery*, *58*(8), 834–839. doi:10.1053/joms.2000.8194 PMID:10935580

Domanski, M. J., Mahaffey, K., Hasselblad, V., Brener, S. J., Smith, P. K., & Hillis, G. et al.. (2011). Association of myocardial enzyme elevation and survival following coronary artery bypass graft surgery. *Journal of the American Medical Association*, *305*(6), 585–591. doi:10.1001/jama.2011.99 PMID:21304084

Domkowski, P. W., Smith, M. L., Gonyon, D. L. Jr, Drye, C., Wooten, M. K., Levin, L. S., & Wolfe, W. G. (2003). Evaluation of vacuum-assisted closure in the treatment of poststernotomy mediastinitis. *The Journal of Thoracic and Cardiovascular Surgery*, *126*(2), 386–390. doi:10.1016/S0022-5223(03)00352-0 PMID:12928634

Donabedian, A. (1966). Evaluating the quality of medical care. *The Milbank Memorial Fund Quarterly*, *44*(3Suppl), 166–206. doi:10.2307/3348969 PMID:5338568

Dong, G., Liu, C., Xu, B., Jing, H., Li, D., & Wu, H. (2012). Postoperative abdominal complications after cardiopulmonary bypass. *Journal of Cardiothoracic Surgery*, *7*(1), 108. doi:10.1186/1749-8090-7-108 PMID:23046511

Donovan, G. K. (1997). Decisions at the end of life: Catholic tradition. *Christ.*, *3*(3), 188–203. doi:10.1093/cb/3.3.188 PMID:11655313

Doorenbos, A. Z., Starks, H., Bourget, E., McMullan, D. M., Lewis-Newby, M., Rue, T. C., & Wilfond, B. S. et al. (2013). Examining palliative care team involvement in automatic consultations for children on extracorporeal life support in the pediatric intensive care unit. *Journal of Palliative Medicine*, *16*(5), 492–495. doi:10.1089/jpm.2012.0536 PMID:23540309

Dorian, P., Cass, D., Schwartz, B., Cooper, R., Gelaznikas, R., & Barr, A. (2002). Amiodarone as compared with lidocaine for shock-resistant ventricular fibrillation. *The New England Journal of Medicine*, *346*(12), 884–890. doi:10.1056/NEJMoa013029 PMID:11907287

Dorman, T., Angood, P. B., Angus, D. C., Clemmer, T. P., Cohen, N. H., Durbin, C. G. Jr, & Napolitano, L. M. et al. (2004). Guidelines for critical care medicine training and continuing medical education. *Critical Care Medicine*, *32*(1), 263–272. doi:10.1097/01.CCM.0000104916.33769.9A PMID:14707590

Douglas, S., Cartmill, R., Brown, R., Hoonakker, P., Slagle, J., Schultz Van Roy, K., & Carayon, P. et al. (2013). The work of adult and pediatric intensive care unit nurses. *Nursing Research*, *62*(1), 50–58. doi:10.1097/NNR.0b013e318270714b PMID:23222843

Dowd, N. P., Cheng, D. C., Karski, J. M., Wong, D. T., Munro, J. A., & Sandler, A. N. (1998). Intraoperative awareness in fast-track cardiac anesthesia. *Anesthesiology, 89*(5), 1068-1073; discussion 1069A.

Drakulovic, M. B., Torres, A., Bauer, T. T., Nicolas, J. M., Nogue, S., & Ferrer, M. (1999). Supine body position as a risk factor for nosocomial pneumonia in mechanically ventilated patients: A randomised trial. *Lancet*, *354*(9193), 1851–1858. doi:10.1016/S0140-6736(98)12251-1 PMID:10584721

Draper, H. M., & Eppert, J. A. (2008). Association of pharmacist presence on compliance with advanced cardiac life support guidelines during in-hospital cardiac arrest. *The Annals of Pharmacotherapy*, *42*(4), 469–474. doi:10.1345/aph.1K475 PMID:18349308

Dreifaldt, M., Mannion, J. D., Bodin, L., Olsson, H., Zagozdzon, L., & Souza, D. (2013). The no-touch saphenous vein as the preferred second conduit for coronary artery bypass grafting. *The Annals of Thoracic Surgery*, *96*(1), 105–111. doi:10.1016/j.athoracsur.2013.01.102 PMID:23684156

Dreyfus, G. D., Corbi, P. J., Chan, K. M., & Bahrami, T. (2005). Secondary tricuspid regurgitation or dilatation: Which should be the criteria for surgical repair? *The Annals of Thoracic Surgery*, *79*(1), 127–132. doi:10.1016/j.athoracsur.2004.06.057 PMID:15620928

Dreyfus, H. L., & Dreyfus, S. E. (1986). *Mind over Machine: the power of human intuition and expertise in the age of the computer*. Oxford: Basil Blackwell.

Dua, A., Dang, P., Shaker, R., Varadarajan, P., & Pai, R. G. (2011). Barriers to surgery in severe aortic stenosis patients with Class I indications for aortic valve replacement. *The Journal of Heart Valve Disease*, *20*(4), 396–400. PMID:21863651

Dua, A., Desai, S. S., Seabrook, G. R., Brown, K. R., Lewis, B. D., Rossi, P. J., & Lee, C. J. et al. (2014). The effect of Surgical Care Improvement Project measures on national trends on surgical site infections in open vascular procedures. *Journal of Vascular Surgery*, *60*(6), 1635–1639. doi:10.1016/j.jvs.2014.08.072 PMID:25454105

Duckro, A. N., Blom, D. W., Lyle, E. A., Weinstein, R. A., & Hayden, M. K. (2005). Transfer of vancomycin-resistant enterococci via health care worker hands. *Archives of Internal Medicine*, *165*(3), 302–307. doi:10.1001/archinte.165.3.302 PMID:15710793

Dueck, M. H., Oberthuer, A., Wedekind, C., Paul, M., & Boerner, U. (2003). Propofol impairs the central but not the peripheral part of the motor system. *Anesthesia and Analgesia*, *96*, 449–455. PMID:12538195

Duncan, A. E., Abd-Elsayed, A., Maheshwari, A., Xu, M., Soltesz, E., & Koch, C. G. (2010). Role of intraoperative and postoperative blood glucose concentrations in predicting outcomes after cardiac surgery. *Anesthesiology*, *112*(4), 860–871. doi:10.1097/ALN.0b013e3181d3d4b4 PMID:20216389

Dungan, K. M., Braithwaite, S. S., & Preiser, J. C. (2009). Stress hyperglycemia. *Lancet*, *373*(9677), 1798–1807. doi:10.1016/S0140-6736(09)60553-5 PMID:19465235

Dungan, K., Hall, C., Schuster, D., & Osei, K. (2011). Comparison of 3 algorithms for basal insulin in transitioning from intravenous to subcutaneous insulin in stable patients after cardiothoracic surgery. *Endocrine Practice*, *17*(5), 753–758. doi:10.4158/EP11027.OR PMID:21550950

Dunning, J., Fabbri, A., Kolh, P. H., Levine, A., Lockowandt, U., Mackay, J., et al. (2009, July). Guideline for resuscitation in cardiac arrest after cardiac surgery. *European Journal of Cardio-Thoracic Surgery: Official Journal of the European Association for Cardio-Thoracic Surgery*. Oxford University Press. doi:10.1016/j.ejcts.2009.01.033

Dunning, J., Nandi, J., Ariffin, S., Jerstice, J., Danitsch, D., & Levine, A. (2006). The Cardiac Surgery Advanced Life Support Course (CALS): Delivering significant improvements in emergency cardiothoracic care. *The Annals of Thoracic Surgery*, *81*(5), 1767–1772. doi:10.1016/j.athoracsur.2005.12.012 PMID:16631670

Duplaga, B. A., Rivers, C. W., & Nutescu, E. (2001). Dosing and monitoring of low-molecular-weight heparins in special populations. *Pharmacotherapy*, *21*(2), 218–234. doi:10.1592/phco.21.2.218.34112 PMID:11213859

Dupras, D. M., Edson, R. S., Halvorsen, A. J., Hopkins, R. H. Jr, & McDonald, F. S. (2012). "Problem residents": Prevalence, problems and remediation in the era of core competencies. *The American Journal of Medicine*, *125*(4), 421–425. doi:10.1016/j.amjmed.2011.12.008 PMID:22444106

Durack, D. T. (1995). Prevention of infective endocarditis. *The New England Journal of Medicine*, *332*(1), 38–44. doi:10.1056/NEJM199501053320107 PMID:7990863

Durack, D. T., Lukes, A. S., & Bright, D. K.Duke Endocarditis Service. (1994). New criteria for diagnosis of infective endocarditis: Utilization of specific echocardiographic findings. *The American Journal of Medicine*, *96*(3), 200–209. doi:10.1016/0002-9343(94)90143-0 PMID:8154507

Dureuil, B., Vires, N., Cantineau, J., Aubier, M., & Desmonts, J. (1986). Diaphragmatic contractility after upper abdominal surgery. *Journal of Applied Physiology*, *61*(5), 1775–1780. PMID:3781987

Duval, X., Iung, B., Klein, I., Brochet, E., Thabut, G., Arnoult, F., & Leport, C. et al. (2010). Effect of early cerebral magnetic resonance imaging on clinical decisions in infective endocarditis: A prospective study. *Annals of Internal Medicine*, *152*(8), 497–504. doi:10.7326/0003-4819-152-8-201004200-00006 PMID:20404380

Dybdahl, B., Wahba, A., Lien, E., Flo, T. H., Waage, A., Qureshi, N., & Sundan, A. et al. (2002). Inflammatory response after open heart surgery: Release of heat-shock protein 70 and signaling through toll-like receptor-4. *Circulation*, *105*(6), 685–690. doi:10.1161/hc0602.103617 PMID:11839622

Dyke, C., Aronson, S., Dietrich, W., Hofmann, A., Karkouti, K., Levi, M., . . . Ranucci, M. (2014). Universal definition of perioperative bleeding in adult cardiac surgery. *J Thorac Cardiovasc Surg, 147*(5), 1458-1463 e1451. doi: 10.1016/j.jtcvs.2013.10.070

Dyke, C. M., Aldea, G., Koster, A., Smedira, N., Avery, E., Aronson, S., & Lincoff, A. M. et al. (2007). Off-pump coronary artery bypass with bivalirudin for patients with heparin-induced thrombocytopenia or antiplatelet factor four/heparin antibodies. *The Annals of Thoracic Surgery, 84*(3), 836–839. doi:10.1016/j.athoracsur.2007.04.007 PMID:17720385

Eagle, K. A., Guyton, R. A., Davidoff, R., Ewy, G., Fonger, J., Gardner, T. J., & Yusuf, S. et al. (1999). ACC/AHA guidelines for coronary artery bypass surgery: Executive summary and recommendations. *Circulation, 100*, 1464–1480. doi:10.1161/01.CIR.100.13.1464 PMID:10500052

Eagle, K., Lim, M., Dabbous, O., Pieper, K., Goldberg, R., VandeWerf, F., & Fox, K. et al.for the GRACE Investigators. (2004). A Validated Prediction Model for All Forms of Acute Coronary Syndrome. *Journal of the American Medical Association, 291*(22), 2727–2733. doi:10.1001/jama.291.22.2727 PMID:15187054

Echahidi, N., Pibarot, P., O'Hara, G., & Mathieu, P. (2008). Mechanisms, prevention, and treatment of atrial fibrillation after cardiac surgery. *Journal of the American College of Cardiology, 51*(8), 793–801. doi:10.1016/j.jacc.2007.10.043 PMID:18294562

Edmonds, H. L. (2002). Multi-modality neurophysiologic monitoring for cardiac surgery. *The Heart Surgery Forum, 5*, 225–228. PMID:12538134

Edmunds, S., & Brown, G. (2010). Effective small group learning: AMEE Guide No. 48. *Medical Teacher, 32*(9), 715–726. doi:10.3109/0142159X.2010.505454 PMID:20795801

Edwards, F. H., Engelman, R. M., Houck, P., Shahian, D. M., & Bridges, C. R. (2006). The Society of Thoracic Surgeons Practice Guideline Series: Antibiotic Prophylaxis in Cardiac Surgery, Part I: Duration. *The Annals of Thoracic Surgery, 81*(1), 397–404. doi:10.1016/j.athoracsur.2005.06.034 PMID:16368422

Egan, T. D., Lemmens, H. J., Fiset, P., Hermann, D. J., Muir, K. T., Stanski, D. R., & Shafer, S. L. (1998). The pharmacokinetics of the new short-acting opioid remifentanil (GI87084B) in healthy adult male volunteers. *Anesthesiology, 79*(5), 881–892. doi:10.1097/00000542-199311000-00004 PMID:7902032

Eggebrecht, H., Schmermund, A., Voigtlander, T., Kahlert, P., Erbel, R., & Mehta, R. H. (2012). Risk of stroke after transcatheter aortic valve implantation (TAVI): A meta-analysis of 10,037 published patients. *EuroIntervention, 8*(1), 129–138. doi:10.4244/EIJV8I1A20 PMID:22391581

Eggimann, P., & Revelly, J. (2006). Should antibiotic combinations be used to treat ventilator-associated pneumonia? *Seminars in Respiratory and Critical Care Medicine, 27*(01), 68–81. doi:10.1055/s-2006-933675 PMID:16508883

Egi, M., Bellomo, R., Stachowski, E., French, C. J., Hart, G. K., Taori, G., & Bailey, M. et al. (2011). The interaction of chronic and acute glycemia with mortality in critically ill patients with diabetes. *Critical Care Medicine, 39*(1), 105–111. doi:10.1097/CCM.0b013e3181feb5ea PMID:20975552

Egleston, C. V, Wood, a E., Gorey, T. F., & McGovern, E. M. (1993). Gastrointestinal complications after cardiac surgery. *Annals of the Royal College of Surgeons of England, 75*(1), 52–56. PMID:8422146

Eichhorn, E. J., Konstam, M. A., Weiland, D. S., Roberts, D. J., Martin, T. T., Stransky, N. B., & Salem, D. N. (1987). Differential effects of milrinone and dobutamine on right ventricular preload, afterload and systolic performance in congestive heart failure secondary to ischemic or idiopathic dilated cardiomyopathy. *The American Journal of Cardiology, 60*(16), 1329–1333. doi:10.1016/0002-9149(87)90616-3 PMID:3687783

Eichler, P., Friesen, H. J., Lubenow, N., Jaeger, B., & Greinacher, A. (2000). Antihirudin antibodies in patients with heparin-induced thrombocytopenia treated with lepirudin: Incidence, effects on aPTT, and clinical relevance. *Blood, 96*(7), 2373–2378. PMID:11001886

Eifert, S., Reichenspurner, H., Pfefferkorn, T., Baur, B., von Schlippenbach, C., Mayer, T. E., & Reichart, B. et al. (2003). Neurological and neuropsychological examination and outcome after use of an intra-aortic filter device during cardiac surgery. *Perfusion, 18*(1), 55–60. doi:10.1191/0267659103pf628oa PMID:12708766

Eikelboom, J. W., Connolly, S. J., Brueckmann, M., Granger, C. B., Kappetein, A. P., Mack, M. J., & Van de Werf, F. et al. (2013). Dabigatran versus warfarin in patients with mechanical heart vales. *The New England Journal of Medicine, 369*(13), 1206–1214. doi:10.1056/NEJMoa1300615 PMID:23991661

Eisenberg, D. M., Davis, R. B., Ettner, S. L., Appel, S., Wilkey, S., Van Rompay, M., & Kessler, R. C. (1998). Trends in alternative medicine use in the United States, 1990-1997: Results of a follow-up national survey. *Journal of the American Medical Association, 280*(18), 1569–1575. doi:10.1001/jama.280.18.1569 PMID:9820257

El Solh, A. A., Bhora, M., Pineda, L., & Dhillon, R. (2006). Nosocomial pneumonia in elderly patients following cardiac surgery. *Respiratory Medicine, 100*(4), 729–736. doi:10.1016/j.rmed.2005.07.011 PMID:16126381

Elahi, M., Asopa, S., Pflueger, A., Hakim, N., & Matata, B. (2009). Acute kidney injury following cardiac surgery: Impact of early versus late haemofiltration on morbidity and mortality. *European Journal of Cardio-Thoracic Surgery, 35*(5), 854–863. doi:10.1016/j.ejcts.2008.12.019 PMID:19216088

el-Banayosy, A., Brehm, C., Kizner, L., Hartmann, D., Körtke, H., Körner, M. M., … Körfer, R. (1998). Cardiopulmonary resuscitation after cardiac surgery: a two-year study. *Journal of Cardiothoracic and Vascular Anesthesia, 12*(4), 390–2. Retrieved from http://www.ncbi.nlm.nih.gov/pubmed/9713724

Elie, M., Cole, M. G., Primeau, F. J., & Bellavance, F. (1998). Delirium risk factors in elderly hospitalized patients. *Journal of General Internal Medicine, 13*(3), 204–212. doi:10.1046/j.1525-1497.1998.00047.x PMID:9541379

Ellaway, R., & Masters, K. (2008). AMEE Guide 32: e-Learning in medical education Part 1: Learning, teaching and assessment. *Medical Teacher, 30*(5), 455–473. doi:10.1080/01421590802108331 PMID:18576185

Ellis, L. B., & Harken, D. E. (1961). Arterial embolization in relation to mitral valvuloplasty. *American Heart Journal, 62*(5), 611–620. doi:10.1016/0002-8703(61)90369-6 PMID:13889996

Ellis, M. E., Al-Abdely, H., Sandridge, A., Greer, W., & Ventura, W. (2001). Fungal endocarditis: Evidence in the world literature, 1965-1995. *Clinical Infectious Diseases, 32*(1), 50–62. doi:10.1086/317550 PMID:11118386

Ely, E. W., Margolin, R., Francis, J., May, L., Truman, B., Dittus, R., … Inouye, S. K. (2001). Evaluation of delirium in critically ill patients: Validation of the Confusion Assessment Method for the Intensive Care Unit (CAM-ICU), *29*(7).

Ely, E. W., Inouye, S. K., Bernard, G. R., Gordon, S., Francis, J., May, L., & Dittus, R. et al. (2001). Delirium in mechanically ventilated patients validity and reliabilty os the confusion assessment method for the intensive care unit. *Journal of the American Medical Association, 286*(21), 2703–2710. doi:10.1001/jama.286.21.2703 PMID:11730446

Ely, E. W., Margolin, R., Francis, J., May, L., Truman, B., Dittus, R., & Inouye, S. K. et al. (2001). Evaluation of delirium in critically ill patients: Validation of the Confusion Assessment Method for the Intensive Care Unit (CAM-ICU). *Critical Care Medicine, 29*(7), 1370–1379. doi:10.1097/00003246-200107000-00012 PMID:11445689

Ely, E. W., Shintani, A., Truman, B., Speroff, T., Gordon, S. M., Harrell, F. E. Jr, & Dittus, R. S. et al. (2004). Delirium as a predictor of mortality in mechanically ventilated patients in the intensive care unit. *Journal of the American Medical Association, 291*(14), 1753–1762. doi:10.1001/jama.291.14.1753 PMID:15082703

Emazabel-Yunta, I., Casado-Campo, I., Telletxea-Benguira, S., Torre-Mollinedo, F., Largo, L. F. O., & Maguregui, A. A. (2008). Subarachnoid hematoma following spinal anesthesia. *Ambulatory Surgery*, *14*, 49–52.

Ende, J. (1983). Feedback in clinical medical education. *Journal of the American Medical Association*, *250*(6), 777–781. doi:10.1001/jama.1983.03340060055026 PMID:6876333

Endre, Z. H., Walker, R. J., Pickering, J. W., Shaw, G. M., Frampton, C. M., Henderson, S. J., & George, P. M. et al. (2010). Early intervention with erythropoietin does not affect the outcome of acute kidney injury (the EARLYARF trial). *Kidney International*, *77*(11), 1020–1030. doi:10.1038/ki.2010.25 PMID:20164823

Engelmann, B. (2006). Initiation of coagulation by tissue factor carriers in blood. *Blood Cells, Molecules & Diseases*, *36*(2), 188–190. doi:10.1016/j.bcmd.2005.12.020 PMID:16473535

Engelman, R., Shahian, D., Shemin, R., Guy, T. S., Bratzler, D., Edwards, F., & Bridges, C. et al. (2007). The Society of Thoracic Surgeons practice guideline series: Antibiotic prophylaxis in cardiac surgery, part II: Antibiotic choice. *The Annals of Thoracic Surgery*, *83*(4), 1569–1576. doi:10.1016/j.athoracsur.2006.09.046 PMID:17383396

Englehart, M. S., & Schreiber, M. A. (2006). Measurement of acid-base resuscitation endpoints: Lactate, base deficit, bicarbonate or what? *Current Opinion in Critical Care*, *12*(6), 569–574. doi:10.1097/MCC.0b013e328010ba4f PMID:17077689

Engoren, M., Hadaway, J., Schwann, T. A., & Habib, R. H. (2011). Ketorolac improves graft patency after coronary artery bypass grafting: A propensity-matched analysis. *The Annals of Thoracic Surgery*, *92*(2), 603–609. doi:10.1016/j.athoracsur.2011.04.050 PMID:21801915

Enriquez-Sarano, M., Tajik, A. J., Schaff, H. V., Orszulak, T. A., Bailey, K. R., & Frye, R. L. (1994). Echocardiographic prediction of survival after surgical correction of organic mitral regurgitation. *Circulation*, *90*(2), 830–837. doi:10.1161/01.CIR.90.2.830 PMID:8044955

Eom, J. S., Lee, M., Chun, H., Choi, H. J., Jung, S., Kim, Y., & Lee, J. S. et al. (2014). The impact of a ventilator bundle on preventing ventilator-associated pneumonia: A multicenter study. *American Journal of Infection Control*, *42*(1), 34–37. doi:10.1016/j.ajic.2013.06.023 PMID:24189326

Epstein, A., Abraham, W., Bianco, N., Kern, K., Mirro, M., Rao, S., & Szymkiewicz, S. et al. (2013). Wearable Cardioverter-Defibrillator Use in Patients Perceived to Be at High Risk Early Post-Myocardial Infarction. *Journal of the American College of Cardiology*, *62*(21), 2000–2007. doi:10.1016/j.jacc.2013.05.086 PMID:23916930

Epstein, A., DiMarco, J., Ellenbogen, K., Estes, N., Freedman, R., Gettes, L., & Sweeney, M. et al. (2013). 2012 ACCF/AHA/HRS Focused Update Incorporated Into the ACCF/AHA/HRS 2008 Guidelines for Device-Based Therapy of Cardiac Rhythm Abnormalities. *Journal of the American College of Cardiology*, 6–e75. PMID:23265327

Epstein, R. M., & Hundert, E. M. (2002). Defining and assessing professional competence. *Journal of the American Medical Association*, *287*(2), 226–235. doi:10.1001/jama.287.2.226 PMID:11779266

Erb, S., Frei, R., Schregenberger, K., Dangel, M., Nogarth, D., & Widmer, A. F. (2014). Sonication for diagnosis of catheter-related infection is not better than traditional roll-plate culture: A prospective cohort study with 975 central venous catheters. *Clinical Infectious Diseases*, *59*(4), 541–544. doi:10.1093/cid/ciu352 PMID:24825872

Erdei, N., Papp, Z., Pollesello, P., Edes, I., & Bagi, Z. (2006). The levosimendan metabolite OR-1896 elicits vasodilation by activating the K(ATP) and BK(Ca) channels in rat isolated arterioles. *British Journal of Pharmacology*, *148*(5), 696–702. doi:10.1038/sj.bjp.0706781 PMID:16715115

Eris, C., Yavuz, S., Yalcinkaya, S., Gucu, A., Toktas, F., & Yumun, G. (2013). … Ozyazıcıoglu, A. (2013). Acute mesenteric ischemia after cardiac surgery: An analysis of 52 patients. *TheScientificWorldJournal*, 631534. PMID:24288499

Erkapic, D., De Rosa, S., Kelava, A., Lehmann, R., Fichtlscherer, S., & Hohnloser, S. H. (2012). Risk for permanent pacemaker after transcatheter aortic valve implantation: A comprehensive analysis of the literature. *Journal of Cardiovascular Electrophysiology*, *23*(4), 391–397. doi:10.1111/j.1540-8167.2011.02211.x PMID:22050112

Ernest, D., Belzberg, A. S., & Dodek, P. M. (1999). Distribution of normal saline and 5% albumin infusions in septic patients. *Critical Care Medicine*, *27*(1), 46–50. doi:10.1097/00003246-199901000-00025

Erniquez-Sarano, M., Akins, C. W., & Vahanian, A. (2009). Mitral regurgitation. *Lancet*, *373*(9672), 1382–1394. doi:10.1016/S0140-6736(09)60692-9 PMID:19356795

Eshaghian, S., Horwich, T., & Fonarow, G. (2006). Relation of Loop Diuretic Dose to Mortality in Advanced Heart Failure. *The American Journal of Cardiology*, *97*(12), 1759–1764. doi:10.1016/j.amjcard.2005.12.072 PMID:16765130

Estep, J. D., Cordero-Reyes, A. M., Bhimaraj, A., Trachtenberg, B., Khalil, N., Loebe, M., & Torre-Amione, G. et al. (2013). Percutaneous placement of an intra-aortic balloon pump in the left axillary/subclavian position provides safe, ambulatory long-term support as bridge to heart transplantation. *JACC Heart Failure*, *1*(5), 382–388. doi:10.1016/j.jchf.2013.06.002 PMID:24621970

Estrera, A. L., Miller, C. C. III, Huynh, T. T., Porat, E., & Safi, H. J. (2001). Neurologic outcome after thoracic and thoracoabdominal aortic aneurysm repair. *The Annals of Thoracic Surgery*, *72*(4), 1225–1231. doi:10.1016/S0003-4975(01)02971-X PMID:11603441

Etz, C. D., Halstead, J. C., Spielvogel, D., Shahani, R., Lazala, R., Homann, T. M., & Griep, R. B. et al. (2006). Thoracic and thoracoabdominal aneurysm repair: Is reimplantation of spinal cord arteries a waste of time? *The Annals of Thoracic Surgery*, *82*(5), 1670–1678. doi:10.1016/j.athoracsur.2006.05.029 PMID:17062225

Etz, C. D., Luehr, M., Kari, F. A., Bodian, C. A., Smego, D., Plestis, K. A., & Griepp, R. B. (2008). Paraplegia after extensive thoracic and thoracoabdominal aortic aneurysm repair: Does critical spinal cord ischemia occur postoperatively? *The Journal of Thoracic and Cardiovascular Surgery*, *135*(2), 324–330. doi:10.1016/j.jtcvs.2007.11.002 PMID:18242262

European Coronary Surgery Study Group. (1979). Coronary-artery bypass surgery in stable angina pectoris: Survival at two years. *Lancet*, *1*, 889–893. PMID:86665

Evangelista, A., Tornos, P., Sambola, A., Permanyer-Miralda, G., & Soler-Soler, J. (2005). Long-term vasodilator therapy in patients with severe aortic regurgitation. *The New England Journal of Medicine*, *353*(13), 1342–1349. doi:10.1056/NEJMoa050666 PMID:16192479

Eveborn, G. W., Schirmer, H., Heggelund, G., Lunde, P., & Rasmussen, K. (2013). The evolving epidemiology of valvular aortic stenosis. the Tromso study. *Heart (British Cardiac Society)*, *99*(6), 396–400. doi:10.1136/heartjnl-2012-302265 PMID:22942293

Ewig, S., Welte, T., & Torres, A. (2012). Is healthcare-associated pneumonia a distinct entity needing specific therapy? *Current Opinion in Infectious Diseases*, *25*(2), 166–175. doi:10.1097/QCO.0b013e32835023fb PMID:22248977

Exadactylos, N., Sugrue, D. D., & Oakley, C. M. (1984). Prevalence of coronary artery disease in patients with isolated aortic stenosis. *British Heart Journal*, *51*(2), 121–124. doi:10.1136/hrt.51.2.121 PMID:6691863

Exadaktylos, A. K., Buggy, D. J., Moriarty, D. C., Mascha, E., & Sessler, D. I. (2006). Can anesthetic technique for primary breast cancer surgery affect recurrence or metastasis? *Anesthesiology*, *105*(4), 660–664. doi:10.1097/00000542-200610000-00008 PMID:17006061

Eyer, S., Brummitt, C., Crossley, K., Siegel, R., & Cerra, F. (1990). Catheter-related sepsis: Prospective, randomized study of three methods of long-term catheter maintenance. *Critical Care Medicine, 18*(10), 1073–1079. doi:10.1097/00003246-199010000-00005 PMID:2209033

Fagan, R. P., Edwards, J. R., Park, B. J., Fridkin, S. K., & Magill, S. S. (2013). Incidence trends in pathogen-specific central line-associated bloodstream infections in US intensive care units, 1990-2010. *Infection Control and Hospital Epidemiology, 34*(9), 893–899. doi:10.1086/671724 PMID:23917902

Fagley, R. E., Haney, M. F., Beraud, A.-S., Comfere, T., Kohl, B. A., Merkel, M. J., & Wall, M. H. et al. (2015). Critical care basic ultrasound learning goals for american anesthesiology critical care trainees: Recommendations from an expert group. *Anesthesia and Analgesia, 120*(5), 1041–1053. doi:10.1213/ANE.0000000000000652 PMID:25899271

Fahmy, N. R. (1985). Nitroprusside vs a nitroprusside trimethaphan mixture for induced hypotension: Hemodynamic effects and CN release. *Clinical Pharmacology and Therapeutics, 37*(3), 264–270. doi:10.1038/clpt.1985.38 PMID:3971651

Fairbairn, T. A., Mather, A. N., Bijsterveld, P., Worthy, G., Currie, S., Goddard, A. J., & Greenwood, J. P. et al. (2012). Diffusion-weighted MRI determined cerebral embolic infarction following transcatheter aortic valve implantation: Assessment of predictive risk factors and the relationship to subsequent health status. *Heart (British Cardiac Society), 98*(1), 18–23. doi:10.1136/heartjnl-2011-300065 PMID:21737581

Fairman, R. M., Criado, F., Farber, M., Kwolek, C., Mehta, M., White, R., & Tuchek, J. M. et al. (2008, September)..... Tuchek J.M. Pivotal results of the Medtronic Vascular Talent Thoracic Stent Graft System: The VALOR Trial. *Journal of Vascular Surgery, 48*(3), 546–554. doi:10.1016/j.jvs.2008.03.061 PMID:18572352

Fairman, R. M., Tuchek, J. M., Lee, W. A., Karthikeshwar, K., White, R., Mehta, M., & Bavaria, J. et al. (2012). Pivotal. results for the Medtronic Valiant Thoracic Stent Graft System in the VALOR II trial. *Journal of Vascular Surgery, 56*(5), 1222–1231. doi:10.1016/j.jvs.2012.04.062 PMID:22832267

Faisy, C., Guerot, E., Diehl, J. L., Iftimovici, E., & Fagon, J. Y. (2003). Clinically significant gastrointestinal bleeding in critically ill patients with and without stress-ulcer prophylaxis. *Intensive Care Medicine, 29*(8), 1306–1313. doi:10.1007/s00134-003-1863-3 PMID:12830375

Fakhry, S. M. (2000). Billing, coding, and documentation in the critical care environment. *The Surgical Clinics of North America, 80*(3), 1067–1083. doi:10.1016/S0039-6109(05)70114-6 PMID:10897279

Fakih, M. G., Dueweke, C., Meisner, S., Berriel-Cass, D., Savoy-Moore, R., Brach, N., & Saravolatz, L. D. et al. (2008). Effect of nurse-led multidisciplinary roundson reducing the unnecessary use of urinary catheterization in hospitalized patients. *Infection Control and Hospital Epidemiology, 29*(9), 815–819. doi:10.1086/589584 PMID:18700831

Faraday, N., & Rosenfeld, B. A. (1998). In vitro hypothermia enhances platelet GPIIb-IIIa activation and P-selectin expression. *Anesthesiology, 88*(6), 1579–1585. doi:10.1097/00000542-199806000-00022 PMID:9637652

Faris, J. G., Veltman, M. G., & Royse, C. F. (2009). Limited transthoracic echocardiography assessment in anaesthesia and critical care. *Best Practice & Research. Clinical Anaesthesiology, 23*(3), 285–298. doi:10.1016/j.bpa.2009.02.008 PMID:19862888

Farkouh, M. E., Dangas, G., Leon, M. B., Smith, C., Nesto, R., Buse, J. B., & Fuster, V. et al. (2008). Design of the Future REvascularization Evaluation in patients with Diabetes mellitus: Optimal management of Multivessel disease (FREEDOM) Trial. *American Heart Journal, 155*(2), 215–223. doi:10.1016/j.ahj.2007.10.012 PMID:18215589

Farkouh, M., Domanski, M., Sleeper, L., Siami, F., Dangas, G., Mack, M., & Fuster, V. et al. (2011). Strategies for multivessel revascularization in patients with diabetes. *The New England Journal of Medicine, 367*(25), 2375–2384. doi:10.1056/NEJMoa1211585 PMID:23121323

Farnan, J. M., Petty, L. A., Georgitis, E., Martin, S., Chiu, E., Prochaska, M., & Arora, V. M. (2012). A systematic review: The effect of clinical supervision on patient and residency education outcomes. *Academic Medicine: Journal of the Association of American Medical Colleges*, *87*(4), 428–442. doi:10.1097/ACM.0b013e31824822cc PMID:22361801

Favaloro, R. G. (1968). Saphenous vein autograft replacement of severe segmental coronary artery occlusion: Operative technique. *The Annals of Thoracic Surgery*, *5*(4), 334–339. http://www.ncbi.nlm.nih.gov/pubmed/5647919 doi:10.1016/S0003-4975(10)66351-5 PMID:5647919

Favaloro, R. G. (1969). Saphenous vein graft in the surgical treatment of coronary artery disease. Operative technique. *The Journal of Thoracic and Cardiovascular Surgery*, *58*, 178–185. PMID:5798222

Fayaz, M. K., Abel, R. J., Pugh, S. C., Hall, J. E., Djaiani, G., & Mecklenburgh, J. S. (2004). Opioid-sparing effects of diclofenac and paracetamol lead to improved outcomes after cardiac surgery. *Journal of Cardiothoracic and Vascular Anesthesia*, *18*(6), 742–747. doi:10.1053/j.jvca.2004.08.012 PMID:15650984

Feiner, H. (1976). Pancreatitis after cardiac surgery. *American Journal of Surgery*, *131*(6), 684–688. doi:10.1016/0002-9610(76)90178-1 PMID:937646

Felden, L., Walter, C., Harder, S., Treede, R. D., Kayser, H., Drover, D., & Lotsch, J. et al. (2011). Comparative clinical effects of hydromorphone and morphine: A meta-analysis. *British Journal of Anaesthesia*, *107*(3), 319–328. doi:10.1093/bja/aer232 PMID:21841049

Felker, G. M., Milano, C. A., Yager, J. E. E., Hernandez, A. F., Blue, L., Higginbotham, M. B., . . . Russel, S. D. (2005). Outcomes With An Alternate List Strategy For Heart Transplantation. *The Journal Of Heart And Lung Transplantation*, *24*(11), 1781-1786. Retrieved From http://www.jhltonline.org/article/s1053-2498(05)00198-1/abstract

Fellahi, J. L., Parienti, J. J., Hanouz, J. L., Plaud, B., Riou, B., & Ouattara, A. (2008). Perioperative use of dobutamine in cardiac surgery and adverse cardiac outcome: Propensity-adjusted analyses. *Anesthesiology*, *108*(6), 979–987. doi:10.1097/ALN.0b013e318173026f PMID:18497597

Fenollar, F., & Raoult, D. (2007). Molecular diagnosis of bloodstream infections caused by non cultivable bacteria. *International Journal of Antimicrobial Agents*, *30*(suppl 1), S7–S15. doi:10.1016/j.ijantimicag.2007.06.024 PMID:17707613

Fenton, J., Bergeron, E., Coello, M., Welsh, R., & Chmielewski, G. (2011). Feeding Jejunostomy Tubes Placed During Esophagectomy: Are They Necessary? *The Annals of Thoracic Surgery*, *92*(2), 504–512. doi:10.1016/j.athoracsur.2011.03.101 PMID:21704294

Fenyvesi, T., Jorg, I., & Harenber, J. (2002). Monitoring anticoagulant effects of direct thrombin inhibitors. *Seminars in Thrombosis and Hemostasis*, *28*(4), 361–368. doi:10.1055/s-2002-34305 PMID:12244483

Ferguson, T. B. Jr. (2012). Mortality in coronary artery bypass grafting: What's next? *Circulation*, *125*(20), 2409–2411. doi:10.1161/CIRCULATIONAHA.112.106856 PMID:22547672

Fergusson, D. A., Hebert, P. C., Mazer, C. D., Fremes, S. E., MacAdams, C., Murkin, J. M., & Pretorius, R. et al. (2008). A comparison of Aprotinin and Lysine analogues in high-risk cardiac surgery. *The New England Journal of Medicine*, *358*(22), 2319–2331. doi:10.1056/NEJMoa0802395 PMID:18480196

Fernandez-del Castillo, C., Harringer, W., Warshaw, A., Vlahakes, G. J., Koski, G., Zaslavsky, A. M., & Rattner, D. W. (1991). Risk factors for pancreatic cellular injury after cardiopulmonary bypass. *The New England Journal of Medicine*, *325*(6), 382–387. doi:10.1056/NEJM199108083250602 PMID:1712076

Fernández-Hidalgo, N., Almirante, B., Gavaldà, J., Gurgui, M., Peña, C., de Alarcón, A., & Pahissa, A. et al. (2013). Ampicillin plus ceftriaxone is as effective as ampicillin plus gentamycin for treating Enterococcus faecalis infective endocarditis. *Clinical Infectious Diseases*, *56*(9), 1261–1268. doi:10.1093/cid/cit052 PMID:23392394

Fernando, H., Jaklitsch, M., Walsh, G., Tisdale, J., Bridges, C., Mitchell, J., & Shrager, J. (2011). The Society of Thoracic Surgeons Practice Guideline on the Prophylaxis and Management of Atrial Fibrillation Associated With General Thoracic Surgery: Executive Summary. *The Annals of Thoracic Surgery*, *92*(3), 1144–1152. doi:10.1016/j.athoracsur.2011.06.104 PMID:21871327

Ferraris, V., Brown, J. R., Despotis, G. J., Hammon, J. W., Reece, T. B., Saha, S. P., … Shann, K. G. (2011). 2011 update to the Society of Thoracic Surgeons and the Society of Cardiovascular Anesthesiologists blood conservation clinical practice guidelines. *The Annals of Thoracic Surgery, 91*(3), 944–82. doi:10.1016/j.athoracsur.2010.11.078

Ferraris, V. A., Brown, J. R., Despotis, G. J., Hammon, J. W., Reece, T. B., & Saha, S. P. et al.. (2011). 2011 update to the Society of Thoracic Surgeons and the Society of Cardiovascular Anesthesiologists blood conservation clinical practice guidelines. *The Annals of Thoracic Surgery*, *91*(3), 944–982. PMID:21353044

Ferraris, V. A., & Ferraris, S. P. (1995). Limiting excessive postoperative blood transfusion after cardiac procedures. A review. *Texas Heart Institute Journal*, *22*(3), 216–230. PMID:7580359

Ferreira, A. C., Peter, A., Salerno, T., Bolooki, H., & de Marchena, E. (2003). Clinical impact of drug-eluting stents in changing referral practices for coronary surgical revascularization in a tertiary care center. *The Annals of Thoracic Surgery, 75*(2), 485–9. Retrieved from http://www.ncbi.nlm.nih.gov/pubmed/12607658

Feuchtner, G. M., Stolzmann, P., Dichtl, W., Schertler, T., Bonatti, J., Scheffel, H., & Alkadhi, H. et al. (2009). Multislice computed tomography in infective endocarditis: Comparison with transesophageal echocardiography and intraoperative findings. *Journal of the American College of Cardiology*, *53*(5), 436–444. doi:10.1016/j.jacc.2008.01.077 PMID:19179202

Field, J. M., Hazinski, M. F., Sayre, M. R., Chameides, L., Schexnayder, S. M., Hemphill, R., & Vanden Hoek, T. L. et al. (2010). Part 1: executive summary: 2010 American Heart Association Guidelines for Cardiopulmonary Resuscitation and Emergency Cardiovascular Care. *Circulation*, *122*(18Suppl 3), S640–S656. doi:10.1161/CIRCULATIONAHA.110.970889 PMID:20956217

Filsoufi, F., Castillo, J. G., Rahmanian, P. B., Broumand, S. R., Silvay, G., Carpentier, A., & Adams, D. H. (2009). Epidemiology of deep sternal wound infection in cardiac surgery. *Journal of Cardiothoracic and Vascular Anesthesia*, *23*(4), 488–494. doi:10.1053/j.jvca.2009.02.007 PMID:19376733

Filsoufi, F., Rahmanian, P. B., Castillo, J. G., Scurlock, C., Legnani, P. E., & Adams, D. H. (2007). Predictors and outcome of gastrointestinal complications in patients undergoing cardiac surgery. *Annals of Surgery*, *246*(2), 323–329. doi:10.1097/SLA.0b013e3180603010 PMID:17667513

Finfer, S., Bellomo, R., Boyce, N., French, J., Myburgh, J., Norton, R., & Investigators, S. S. (2004). A comparison of albumin and saline for fluid resuscitation in the intensive care unit. *The New England Journal of Medicine*, *350*(22), 2247–2256. doi:10.1056/NEJMoa040232

Finkel, M. S., Oddis, C. V., Jacob, T. D., Watkins, S. C., Hattler, B. G., & Simmons, R. L. (1992). Negative inotropic effects of cytokines on the heart mediated by nitric oxide. *Science*, *257*(5068), 387–389. doi:10.1126/science.1631560 PMID:1631560

Fiore, G., Brienza, N., Cicala, P., Tunzi, P., Marraudino, N., Schinosa, L., & Fiore, T. (2006). Superior mesenteric artery blood flow modifications during off-pump coronary surgery. *The Annals of Thoracic Surgery*, *82*(1), 62–67. doi:10.1016/j.athoracsur.2006.02.012 PMID:16798189

Fischer, G. W., & Levin, M. A. (2010). Vasoplegia during cardiac surgery: Current concepts and management. *Seminars in Thoracic and Cardiovascular Surgery*, *22*(2), 140–144. doi:10.1053/j.semtcvs.2010.09.007 PMID:21092891

Fischer, S., Bohn, D., Rycus, P., Pierre, A. F., de Perrot, M., Waddell, T. K., & Keshavjee, S. (2007). Extracorporeal membrane oxygenation for primary graft dysfunction after lung transplantation: Analysis of the Extracorporeal Life Support Organization (ELSO) registry. *The Journal of Heart and Lung Transplantation*, *26*(5), 472–477. doi:10.1016/j.healun.2007.01.031

Fiser, S. M., Cope, J. T., Kron, I. L., Kaza, A. K., Long, S. M., Kern, J. A., & Lowson, S. M. et al. (2001). Aerosolized prostacyclin (epoprostenol) as an alternative to inhaled nitric oxide for patients with reperfusion injury after lung transplantation. *The Journal of Thoracic and Cardiovascular Surgery*, *121*(5), 981–982. doi:10.1067/mtc.2001.115668

Fish, D., & Coles, C. (2005). Clarifying curriculum aims: the practice of education, its nature and expertise. In *Medical Education: Developing A Curriculum For Practice*. Maidenhead: Open University Press.

Fitch, Z. W., & Whitman, G. J. R. (2014). Incidence, risk, and prevention of ventilator-associated pneumonia in adult cardiac surgery patients: A systematic review. *Journal of Cardiac Surgery*, *29*(2), 196–203. doi:10.1111/jocs.12260 PMID:24304223

Fitzgibbon, G. M., Kafka, H. P., Leach, A. J., Keon, W. J., Hooper, G. D., & Burton, J. R. (1996). Coronary bypass graft fate and patient outcome: Angiographic follow-up of 5,065 grafts related to survival and reoperation in 1,388 patients during 25 years. *Journal of the American College of Cardiology*, *28*(3), 616–626. http://www.ncbi.nlm.nih.gov/pubmed/8772748 doi:10.1016/0735-1097(96)00206-9 PMID:8772748

FitzSullivan, E., Gries, C. J., Phelan, P., Farjah, F., Gilbert, E., Keech, J. C., & Mulligan, M. S. et al. (2011). Reduction in airway complications after lung transplantation with novel anastomotic technique. *The Annals of Thoracic Surgery*, *92*(1), 309–315. doi:10.1016/j.athoracsur.2011.01.077

Flaker, G. C., Barolozzi, J., Davis, V., McCabe, C., & Cannon, C. P. (1994). Use of a standardized heparin nomogram to achieve therapeutic anticoagulation after thrombolytic therapy in myocardial infarction. TIMI 4 investigators. *Archives of Internal Medicine*, *154*(13), 1492–1496. doi:10.1001/archinte.1994.00420130084011 PMID:8018004

Fleming, G. A., Murray, K. T., Yu, C., Byrne, J. G., Greelish, J. P., Petracek, M. R., & Pretorius, M. et al. (2008). Milrinone use is associated with postoperative atrial fibrillation after cardiac surgery. *Circulation*, *118*(16), 1619–1625. doi:10.1161/CIRCULATIONAHA.108.790162 PMID:18824641

Fletcher, G., Flin, R., McGeorge, P., Glavin, R., Maran, N., & Patey, R. (2003). Anaesthetists' Non-Technical Skills (ANTS): Evaluation of a behavioural marker system. *British Journal of Anaesthesia*, *90*(5), 580–588. doi:10.1093/bja/aeg112 PMID:12697584

Flier, S., Concepcion, A. N., Versteeg, D., Kappen, T. H., Hoefer, I. E., de Lange, D. W., & Buhre, W. F. et al. (2014). Monocyte hyporesponsiveness and toll-like receptor expression profiles in coronary artery bypass grafting and its clinical implications for postoperative inflammatory response and pneumonia. *European Journal of Anaesthesiology*, *31*, 1–12. PMID:24225728

Flinders, D. J., & Thornton, S. J. (2004). *The Curriculum Studies Reader*. Psychology Press.

Flin, R. H., O'Connor, P., & Crichton, M. (2008). *Safety at the sharp end: a guide to non-technical skills*. Aldershot: Ashgate Publishing, Ltd.

Flin, R., Patey, R., Glavin, R., & Maran, N. (2010). Anaesthetists' non-technical skills. *British Journal of Anaesthesia*, *105*(1), 38–44. doi:10.1093/bja/aeq134 PMID:20522911

Flint, K., Matlock, D., Lindenfeld, J., & Allen, L. (2012). Frailty and the Selection of Patients for Destination Therapy Left Ventricular Assist Device. *Circulation: Heart Failure*, *5*(2), 286–293. doi:10.1161/CIRCHEARTFAILURE.111.963215 PMID:22438521

Flores, R., Pass, H., Seshan, V., Dycoco, J., Zakowski, M., Carbone, M., ... Rusch, V. (2008). Extrapleural pneumonectomy versus pleurectomy/decortication in the surgical management of malignant pleural mesothelioma: Results in 663 patients. *The Journal of Thoracic and Cardiovascular Surgery, 135*(3), 620-626, 626.e1-3.

Floros, P., Sawhney, R., Vrtik, M., Hinton-Bayre, A., Weimers, P., Senewiratne, S., & Shah, P. et al. (2011). Risk factors and management approach for deep sternal wound infection after cardiac surgery at a tertiary medical centre. *Heart Lung and Circulation*, *20*(11), 712–717. doi:10.1016/j.hlc.2011.08.001 PMID:21906999

Foley, P. J., Criado, F. J., Farber, M. A., Kwolek, C. J., Mehta, M., White, R. A., & Fairman, R. M. et al. (2012). Results with the Talent thoracic stent graft in the VALOR trial. *Journal of Vascular Surgery*, *56*(5), 1214–1221. doi:10.1016/j.jvs.2012.04.071 PMID:22925732

Fonarow, G. C., Saver, J. L., Smith, E. E., Broderick, J. P., Kleindorfer, D. O., Sacco, R. L., & Schwamm, L. H. et al. (2012). Relationship of national institutes of health stroke scale to 30-day mortality in medicare beneficiaries with acute ischemic stroke. *J Am Heart Assoc*, *1*(1), 42–50. doi:10.1161/JAHA.111.000034 PMID:23130117

Fonarow, G. C., Wright, R. S., Spencer, F. A., Fredrick, P. D., Dong, W., Every, N., & French, W. J. (2005). Effect of statin use within the first 24 hours of admission for acute myocardial infarction on early morbidity and mortality. *The American Journal of Cardiology*, *96*(5), 611–616. doi:10.1016/j.amjcard.2005.04.029 PMID:16125480

Force, A. D. T., Ranieri, V. M., Rubenfeld, G. D., Thompson, B. T., Ferguson, N. D., Caldwell, E., & Slutsky, A. S. et al. (2012). Acute respiratory distress syndrome: The Berlin Definition. *Journal of the American Medical Medical Association*, *307*(23), 2526–2533. doi:10.1001/jama.2012.5669 PMID:22797452

Foroulis, C., Kotoulas, C., Lachanas, H., Lazopoulos, G., Konstantinou, M., & Lioulias, A. (2003). Factors associated with cardiac rhythm disturbances in the early post-pneumonectomy period: A study on 259 pneumonectomies. *European Journal of Cardio-Thoracic Surgery*, *23*(3), 384–389. doi:10.1016/s1010-7940(02)00797-2 PMID:12614811

Forster, A., Gardaz, J. P., Suter, P. M., & Gemperle, M. (1980). Respiratory depression by midazolam and diazepam. *Anesthesiology*, *53*(6), 494–497. doi:10.1097/00000542-198012000-00010 PMID:7457966

Forte, D. N., Vincent, J. L., Velasco, I. T., & Park, M. (2012). Association between education in EOL care and variability in EOL practice: A survey of ICU physicians. *Intensive Care Medicine*, *38*(3), 404–412. doi:10.1007/s00134-011-2400-4 PMID:22222566

Fournier, P. E., Drancourt, M., Colson, P., Rolain, J. M., La Scola, B., & Raoult, D. (2013). Modern clinical microbiology: New challenges and solutions. *Nature Reviews. Microbiology*, *11*(8), 574–585. doi:10.1038/nrmicro3068 PMID:24020074

Fowler, M. B., Alderman, E. L., Oesterle, S. N., Derby, G., Daughters, G. T., Stinson, E. B., & Miller, D. C. et al. (1984). Dobutamine and dopamine after cardiac surgery: Greater augmentation of myocardial blood flow with dobutamine. *Circulation*, *70*(3 Pt 2), I103–I111. PMID:6744557

Fowler, V. G. Jr, Boucher, H. W., Corey, R. G., Abrutyn, E., Karchmer, A. W., Rupp, M. E., & Cosgrove, S. E. et al. (2006). Daptomycin versus standard therapy for bacteremia and endocarditis caused by Staphylococcus aureus. *The New England Journal of Medicine*, *355*(7), 653–665. doi:10.1056/NEJMoa053783 PMID:16914701

Fowler, V. G. Jr, O'Brien, S. M., Muhlbaier, L. H., Corey, G. R., Ferguson, T. B., & Peterson, E. D. (2005). Clinical predictors of major infections after cardiac surgery. *Circulation*, *112*, I-358–I-365. PMID:16159846

Fox, C., Liu, H., & Kaye, A. D. (2011). Antianxiety agents. In Manchikanti, L., Trescot, A.M., and Christo, P.J. (Eds.), Clinical Aspects of Pain Medicine and Interventional Pain Management: A Comprehensive Review (pp. 543-552). Paducah, KY: ASIP Publishing.

Fox, R. C., & Swazey, J. P. (2002). The courage to fail: a social view of organ transplants and dialysis (New ed.). New Brunswick, NJ: Transaction Publishers.

Fox, D. L., Stream, A. R., & Bull, T. (2014). Perioperative Management of the Patient With Pulmonary Hypertension. *Seminars in Cardiothoracic and Vascular Anesthesia*, *18*(4), 310–318. doi:10.1177/1089253214534780 PMID:24828282

Fragou, M., Gravvanis, A., Dimitriou, V., Papalois, A., Kouraklis, G., Karabinis, A., & Karakitsos, D. et al. (2011). Real-time ultrasound-guided subclavian vein cannulation versus the landmark method in critical care patients: A prospective randomized study. *Critical Care Medicine*, *39*(7), 1607–1612. doi:10.1097/CCM.0b013e318218a1ae PMID:21494105

Franchini, M., & Lippi, G. (2012). Fibrinogen replacement therapy: A critical review of the literature. *Blood Transfusion*, *10*(1), 23–27. doi:10.2450/2011.0015-11 PMID:22153684

Francioli, P., Ruch, W., & Stamboulian, D. (1995). Treatment of streptococcal endocarditis with a single daily dose of ceftriaxone and netilmicin for 14 days: A prospective multicenter study. *Clinical Infectious Diseases*, *21*(6), 1406–1410. doi:10.1093/clinids/21.6.1406 PMID:8749624

Francis, G. S., Bartos, J. A., & Adatya, S. (2014). Inotropes. *Journal of the American College of Cardiology*, *63*(20), 2069–2078. doi:10.1016/j.jacc.2014.01.016 PMID:24530672

Francois, C., Schiebler, M., & Reeder, S. (2010). Cardiac MRI evaluation of nonischemic cardiomyopathies. *Journal of Magnetic Resonance Imaging*, *31*(3), 518–530. doi:10.1002/jmri.22030 PMID:20187194

Frankenfield, D. C., & Ashcraft, C. M. (2011). Estimating energy needs in nutrition support patients. *Journal of Parenteral and Enteral Nutrition*, *35*(5), 563–570. doi:10.1177/0148607111415859 PMID:21832143

Frank, J. R., Snell, L. S., Cate, O. T., Holmboe, E. S., Carraccio, C., Swing, S. R., & Harris, K. A. et al. (2010). Competency-based medical education: Theory to practice. *Medical Teacher*, *32*(8), 638–645. doi:10.3109/0142159X.2010.501190 PMID:20662574

Fransen, E., Maessen, J., Dentener, M., Senden, N., & Buurman, W. (1999). Impact of blood transfusions on inflammatory mediator release in patients undergoing cardiac surgery. *Chest*, *116*(5), 1233–1239. doi:10.1378/chest.116.5.1233 PMID:10559080

Fraser, G. L., Devlin, J. W., Worby, C. P., Alhazzani, W., Barr, J., Dasta, J. F., & Spencer, F. A. et al. (2013). Benzodiazepine versus nonbenzodiazepine-based sedation for mechanically ventilated, critically ill adults: A systematic review and meta-analysis of randomized trials. *Critical Care Medicine*, *41*, S30–S38. doi:10.1097/CCM.0b013e3182a16898 PMID:23989093

Fredriksson, P., Jaakkola, N., & Jaakkola, J. J. K. (2007). Management and outcomes of small bowel obstruction in older adult patients: A prospective cohort study. *Canadian Journal of Surgery*, *57*(6), 1–7.

Freed, B. H., Sugeng, L., Furlong, K., Mor-Avi, V., Raman, J., Jeevanandam, V., & Lang, R. M. (2010). Reasons for nonadherence to guidelines for aortic valve replacement in patients with severe aortic stenosis and potential solutions. *The American Journal of Cardiology*, *105*(9), 1339–1342. doi:10.1016/j.amjcard.2009.12.056 PMID:20403489

Freedman, L. R. (1987). The pathogenesis of infective endocarditis. *The Journal of Antimicrobial Chemotherapy*, *20*(Suppl A), 1–6. doi:10.1093/jac/20.suppl_A.1 PMID:3316154

Freeman, B. D., & Morris, P. E. (2012). Tracheostomy practice in adults with acute respiratory failure. *Critical Care Medicine*, *40*(10), 2890–2896. doi:10.1097/CCM.0b013e31825bc948 PMID:22824938

Frendl, G., Sodickson, A.C., Chung, M.K., Waldo, A.L., Gersh, B.J., & Tisdale, J.E., ...American Association for Thoracic Surgery. (2014). (2014). AATS guidelines for the prevention and management of perioperative atrial fibrillation and flutter for thoracic surgical procedures. *The Journal of Thoracic and Cardiovascular Surgery*, *148*(3), e153–e193.

Frendl, G., Sodickson, A., Chung, M., Waldo, A., Gersh, B., Tisdale, J., & Adler, D. et al. (2014). 2014 AATS guidelines for the prevention and management of perioperative atrial fibrillation and flutter for thoracic surgical procedures. *The Journal of Thoracic and Cardiovascular Surgery*, *148*(3), E153–E193. doi:10.1016/j.jtcvs.2014.06.036 PMID:25129609

Freund, Y., Jabre, P., Mourad, J., Lapostolle, F., Reuter, P. G., Woimant, M., & Adnet, F. et al. (2014). Relative adrenal insufficiency in critically ill patient after rapid sequence intubation: KETASED ancillary study. *Journal of Critical Care*; epub ahead of print. PMID:24508204

Friedenberg, A. S., Levy, M. M., Ross, S., & Evans, L. E. (2012). Barriers to end-of-life care in the intensive care unit: Perceptions vary by level of training, discipline, and institution. *Journal of Palliative Medicine*, *15*(4), 404–411. doi:10.1089/jpm.2011.0261 PMID:22468773

Friederich, J. A., & Butterworth, J. F. (1995). Sodium Nitroprusside: Twenty years and counting. *Anesthesia and Analgesia*, *81*, 152–162. PMID:7598246

Friedrich, A. (2012). Management of common complications following thoracic surgery. In P. M. Hartigan (Ed.), *Practical Handbook of Thoracic Anesthesia* (pp. 291–310). New York: Springer. doi:10.1007/978-0-387-88493-6_17

Friedrich, I., Simm, A., Kötting, J., Thölen, F., Fischer, B., & Silber, R. E. (2009). Cardiac surgery in the elderly patient. *Deutsches Ärzteblatt International*, *106*, 416–422. PMID:19623310

Fried, T. R., Bradley, E. H., Towle, V. R., & Allore, H. (2002). Understanding the treatment preferences of seriously ill patients. *The New England Journal of Medicine*, *346*(14), 1061–1066. doi:10.1056/NEJMsa012528 PMID:11932474

Fry, D. E. (2008). Surgical site infections and the surgical care improvement project (SCIP): Evolution of national quality measures. *Surgical Infections*, *9*(6), 579–584. doi:10.1089/sur.2008.9951 PMID:19216670

Fry, D. W., Harvey, P. J., Keller, P. R., Elliott, W. L., Meade, M., Trachet, E., & Toogood, P. L. et al. (2004). Specific inhibition of cyclin-dependent kinase 4/6 by PD 0332991 and associated antitumor activity in human tumor xenografts. *Molecular Cancer Therapeutics*, *3*(11), 1427–1438. PMID:15542782

Fujimoto, K., Kubo, K., Yamamoto, H., Yamaguchi, S., & Matsuzawa, Y. (1999). Eosinophilic inflammation in the airway is related to glucocorticoid reversibility in patients with pulmonary emphysema. *Chest. Journal*, *115*(3), 697–702. PMID:10084478

Fujino, Y., Iso, H., Tamakoshi, A., Inaba, Y., Koizumi, A., Kubo, T., & Yoshimura, T. (2006). A prospective cohort study of shift work and risk of ischemic heart disease in Japanese male workers. *American Journal of Epidemiology*, *164*(2), 128–135. doi:10.1093/aje/kwj185 PMID:16707650

Fujita, T., Daiko, H., & Nishimura, M. (2012). Early Enteral Nutrition Reduces the Rate of Life-Threatening Complications after Thoracic Esophagectomy in Patients with Esophageal Cancer. *European Surgical Research*, *48*(2), 79–84. doi:10.1159/000336574 PMID:22377820

Fukuda, K. (2010). Cardiovascular effects of opioids. In Miller's Anesthesia (7th ed.). Elsevier.

Funakoshi, S., Kaji, S., Yamamuro, A., Tani, T., Kinoshita, M., Okada, Y., & Furukawa, Y. (2011). Impact of early surgery in the active phase on long-term outcomes in left-sided native valve infective endocarditis. *The Journal of Thoracic and Cardiovascular Surgery*, *142*(4), 836–842. doi:10.1016/j.jtcvs.2011.01.040 PMID:21397271

Furnary, A. P., Gao, G., Grunkemeier, G. L., Wu, Y., Zerr, K. J., Bookin, S. O., & Starr, A. et al. (2003). Continuous insulin infusion reduces mortality in patients with diabetes undergoing coronary artery bypass grafting. *The Journal of Thoracic and Cardiovascular Surgery*, *125*(5), 1007–1021. doi:10.1067/mtc.2003.181 PMID:12771873

Furnary, A. P., Zerr, K. J., Grunkemeier, G. L., & Starr, A. (1999). Continuous intravenous insulin infusion reduces the incidence of deep sternal wound infection in diabetic patients after cardiac surgical procedures. *The Annals of Thoracic Surgery*, *67*(2), 352–362. doi:10.1016/S0003-4975(99)00014-4 PMID:10197653

Furukawa, N., Kuss, O., Aboud, A., Schonbrodt, M., Renner, A., Hakim Meibodi, K., & Borgermann, J. et al. (2014). Ministernotomy versus conventional sternotomy for aortic valve replacement: Matched propensity score analysis of 808 patients. *European Journal of Cardio-Thoracic Surgery*, *46*(2), 221–226, discussion 226–227. doi:10.1093/ejcts/ezt616 PMID:24446478

Fuster, V. (2013). *Subclinical Athersclerotic Burden: High-Risk Population.* American College of Cardiology Scientific Sessions.

Fuster, V., Rydén, L. E., Cannom, D. S., Crijns, H. J., Curtis, A. B., & Ellenbogen, K. A. et al.. (2006). ACC/AHA/ESC 2006 Guidelines for the Management of Patients With Atrial Fibrillation--Executive Summary. *Circulation*, *114*(7), 700–752. doi:10.1161/CIRCULATIONAHA.106.177031 PMID:16908781

Gaba, D. M. (2004). The future vision of simulation in health care. *Quality and Safety in Health Care, 13*(suppl_1), i2–i10. doi:10.1136/qshc.2004.009878

Gaba, D. M., Howard, S. K., Fish, K. J., Smith, B. E., & Sowb, Y. A. (2001). Simulation-based training in anesthesia crisis resource management (ACRM): A decade of experience. *Simulation & Gaming*, *32*(2), 175–193. doi:10.1177/104687810103200206

Gachet, C., & Aleil, B. (2008). Testing antiplatelet therapy. *European Heart Journal Supplements*, *10*(suppl A), A28–A34. doi:10.1093/eurheartj/sum081

Gage, B., Waterman, A., Shannon, W., Boechler, M., Rich, M., & Radford, M. (2001). Validation of Clinical Classification Schemes for Predicting Stroke. *Journal of the American Medical Association*, *285*(22), 2864–2870. doi:10.1001/jama.285.22.2864 PMID:11401607

Gaillard, R. C., Turnill, D., Sappino, P., & Muller, A. F. (1990). Tumor necrosis factor alpha inhibits the hormonal response of the pituitary gland to hypothalamic releasing factors. *Endocrinology*, *127*(1), 101–106. doi:10.1210/endo-127-1-101 PMID:2163305

Gajic, O., Afessa, B., Hanson, A. C., Krpata, T., Yilmaz, M., Mohamed, S. F., & Wylam, M. E. et al. (2008). Effect of 24-hour mandatory versus on-demand critical care specialist presence on quality of care and family and provider satisfaction in the intensive care unit of a teaching hospital. *Critical Care Medicine*, *36*(1), 36–44. doi:10.1097/01.CCM.0000297887.84347.85 PMID:18007270

Galante, J. M., Bowles, T. L., Khatri, V. P., Schneider, P. D., Goodnight, J. E. Jr, & Bold, R. J. (2005). Experience and attitudes of surgeons toward palliation in cancer. *Archives of Surgery*, *140*(9), 873–878, discussion 878–880. doi:10.1001/archsurg.140.9.873 PMID:16172296

Galiè, N., Beghetti, M., Gatzoulis, M. A., Granton, J., Berger, R. M., & Lauer, A. et al.. (2006). Bosentan therapy in patients with Eisenmenger syndrome: A multicenter, double-blind, randomized, placebo-controlled study. *Circulation*, *114*(1), 48–54. doi:10.1161/CIRCULATIONAHA.106.630715 PMID:16801459

Galiè, N., Hinderliter, A. L., Torbicki, A., Fourme, T., Simonneau, G., Pulido, T., & Rubin, L. et al. (2003). Effects of the oral endothelin-receptorantagonist bosentan on echocardiographic and Doppler measures in patients with pulmonary arterial hypertension. *Journal of the American College of Cardiology*, *41*(8), 1380–1386. doi:10.1016/S0735-1097(03)00121-9 PMID:12706935

Galiè, N., Hoeper, M. M., Humbert, M., Torbicki, A., Vachiery, J. L., Barbera, J. A., & Simonneau, G. et al. (2009). Guidelines for the Diagnosis and Treatment of Pulmonary Hypertension. *The European Respiratory Journal*, *34*(6), 1219–1263. doi:10.1183/09031936.00139009 PMID:19749199

Galiè, N., & Simonneau, G. (2013). Updated Clinical Classification of Pulmonary Hypertension.[_S.]. *Journal of the American College of Cardiology*, *62*, 25. PMID:24355639

Gammie, J. S., Sheng, S., Griffith, B. P., Peterson, E. D., Rankin, J. S., O'Brien, S. M., & Brown, J. M. (2009). Trends in mitral valve surgery in the United States: Results from the Society of Thoracic Surgeons Adult Cardiac Surgery Database. *The Annals of Thoracic Surgery*, *87*(5), 1431–1437, discussion 1437–1439. doi:10.1016/j.athoracsur.2009.01.064 PMID:19379881

Ganière, V., Feihl, F., & Tagan, D. (2006). Dramatic beneficial effects of sildenafil in recurrent massive pulmonary embolism. *Intensive Care Medicine*, *32*(3), 452–454. doi:10.1007/s00134-005-0058-5 PMID:16450094

Gan, T. J., Diemunsch, P., Habib, A. S., Kovac, A., Kranke, P., Meyer, T., & Tramèr, M. R. et al. (2014). Consensus guidelines for the management of postoperative nausea and vomiting. *Anesthesia and Analgesia*, *118*(1), 85–113. doi:10.1213/ANE.0000000000000002 PMID:24356162

Gan, T. J., Meyer, T., Apfel, C. C., Chung, F., Davis, P. J., Eubanks, S., & Watcha, M. et al. (2003). Consensus guidelines for managing postoperative nausea and vomiting. *Anesthesia and Analgesia*, *97*(5), 62–71. doi:10.1213/01.ANE.0000068580.00245.95 PMID:12818945

Gan, T. J., Soppitt, A., Maroof, M., El-Moalem, H., Robertson, K. M., Moretti, E., & Glass, P. S. A. et al. (2002). Goal-directed intraoperative fluid administration reduces length of hospital stay after major surgery. *Anesthesiology*, *97*(4), 820–826. doi:10.1097/00000542-200210000-00012 PMID:12357146

Garg, R., & Yusuf, S. (1995). Overview of randomized trials of angiotensin-converting enzyme inhibitors on mortality and morbidity in patients with heart failure. Collaborative Group on ACE Inhibitor Trials. *Journal of the American Medical Association*, *273*(18), 1450–1456. doi:10.1001/jama.1995.03520420066040 PMID:7654275

Garland, A., & Gershengorn, H. B. (2013). Staffing in ICUs: Physicians and alternative staffing models. *Chest*, *143*(1), 214–221. doi:10.1378/chest.12-1531 PMID:23276844

Garland, A., Roberts, D., & Graff, L. (2012). Twenty-four-hour intensivist presence: A pilot study of effects on intensive care unit patients, families, doctors, and nurses. *American Journal of Respiratory and Critical Care Medicine*, *185*(7), 738–743. doi:10.1164/rccm.201109-1734OC PMID:22246176

Garrett, H. E., Dennies, E. W., & DeBakey, M. E. (1973). Aortocoronary bypass with saphenous vein graft. Seven-year follow-up. *Journal of the American Medical Association*, *223*(7), 792–794. doi:10.1001/jama.1973.03220070046012 PMID:4567689

Garvin, S., Muehlschlegel, J. D., Perry, T. E., Chen, J., Liu, K., Fox, A. A., & Body, S. C. et al. (2010). Postoperative activity, but not preoperative activity, of antithrombin is associated with major adverse cardiac events after coronary artery bypass graft surgery. *Anesthesia and Analgesia*, *111*(4), 862–869. doi:10.1213/ANE.0b013e3181b7908c PMID:19820236

Gasior, M., Zembala, M. O., Tajstra, M., Filipiak, K., Gierlotka, M., Hrapkowicz, T., & Zembala, M. et al. (2014). Hybrid revascularization for multivessel coronary artery disease. *Journal of the American College of Cardiology: Cardiovascular Interventions*, *7*, 1277–1283. PMID:25459040

Gastmeier, P., Geffers, C., Brandt, C., Zuschneid, I., Sohr, D., Schwab, F., & Rüden, H. et al. (2006). Effectiveness of a nationwide nosocomial infection surveillance system for reducing nosocomial infections. *The Journal of Hospital Infection*, *64*(1), 16–22. doi:10.1016/j.jhin.2006.04.017 PMID:16820247

Gatzoulis, M. A., Balaji, S., Webber, S. A., Siu, S. C., Hokanson, J. S., Poile, C., & Redington, A. N. et al. (2000). Risk factors for arrhythmia and sudden cardiac death late after repair of tetralogy of Fallot: A multicentre study. *Lancet*, *356*(9254), 975–981. doi:10.1016/S0140-6736(00)02714-8 PMID:11041398

Gaudreault, P., Guay, J., Thivierge, R. L., & Verdy, I. (1991). Benzodiazepine poisoning: Clinical and pharmacological considerations and treatment. *Drug Safety*, *6*(4), 247–265. doi:10.2165/00002018-199106040-00003 PMID:1888441

Gavaldà, J., Len, O., Miró, J. M., Muñoz, P., Montejo, M., Alarcón, A., & Pahissa, A. et al. (2007). Brief communication: Treatment of Enterococcus faecalis endocarditis with ampicillin plus ceftriaxone. *Annals of Internal Medicine*, *146*(8), 574–579. doi:10.7326/0003-4819-146-8-200704170-00008 PMID:17438316

Gawaz, M. P., Dobos, G., Spath, M., Schollmeyer, P., Gurland, H. J., & Mujais, S. K. (1994). Impaired function of platelet membrane glycoprotein IIb-IIIa in end-stage renal disease. *Journal of the American Society of Nephrology*, *5*(1), 36–46. PMID:7524718

Gaynor, J. W., Nicolson, S. C., Jarvik, G. P., Wernovsky, G., Montenegro, L. M., Burnham, N. B., & Clancy, R. R. et al. (2005). Increasing duration of deep hypothermic circulatory arrest is associated with an increased incidence of postoperative electroencephalographic seizures. *The Journal of Thoracic and Cardiovascular Surgery*, *130*(5), 1278–1286. doi:10.1016/j.jtcvs.2005.02.065 PMID:16256779

Geha, A. S., Krone, R. J., McCormick, J. R., & Baue, A. E. (1975). Selection of coronary bypass. Anatomic, physiological, and angiographic considerations of vein and mammary artery grafts. *The Journal of Thoracic and Cardiovascular Surgery*, *70*(3), 414–431. Retrieved from http://www.ncbi.nlm.nih.gov/pubmed/240984 PMID:240984

Gehi, A. K., Mounsey, J. P., Pursell, I., Landers, M., Boyce, K., Chung, E. H., & Kiser, A. C. et al. (2013). Hybrid epicardial-endocardial ablation using a pericardioscopic technique for the treatment of atrial fibrillation. *Heart Rhythm*, *10*(1), 22–28. doi:10.1016/j.hrthm.2012.08.044 PMID:23064043

Geisen, M., Spray, D., & Nicholas Fletcher, S. (2013). Echocardiography-Based Hemodynamic Management in the Cardiac Surgical Intensive Care Unit. *Journal of Cardiothoracic and Vascular Anesthesia*. Retrieved from http://linkinghub.elsevier.com/retrieve/pii/S1053077013004801

Gelb, A. B., Roth, R. I., Levin, J., London, M. J., Noall, R. A., Hauck, W. W., & Mangano, D. T. et al. (1996). Changes in blood coagulation during and following cardiopulmonary bypass: Lack of correlation with clinical bleeding. *American Journal of Clinical Pathology*, *106*(1), 87–99. PMID:8701939

Gelijns, A. C., Moskowitz, A. J., Acker, M. A., Argenziano, M., Geller, N. L., Puskas, J. D., & Blackstone, E. H. et al. (2014). Management practices and major infections after cardiac surgery. *Journal of the American College of Cardiology*, *64*(4), 372–381. doi:10.1016/j.jacc.2014.04.052 PMID:25060372

Genereux, P., Head, S. J., Hahn, R., Daneault, B., Kodali, S., Williams, M. R., & Leon, M. B. et al. (2013). Paravalvular leak after transcatheter aortic valve replacement: The new Achilles' heel? A comprehensive review of the literature. *Journal of the American College of Cardiology*, *61*(11), 1125–1136. doi:10.1016/j.jacc.2012.08.1039 PMID:23375925

Genereux, P., Head, S. J., Van Mieghem, N. M., Kodali, S., Kirtane, A. J., Xu, K., & Leon, M. B. et al. (2012). Clinical outcomes after transcatheter aortic valve replacement using valve academic research consortium definitions: A weighted meta-analysis of 3,519 patients from 16 studies. *Journal of the American College of Cardiology*, *59*(25), 2317–2326. doi:10.1016/j.jacc.2012.02.022 PMID:22503058

Genereux, P., Kodali, S. K., Green, P., Paradis, J. M., Daneault, B., Rene, G., & Williams, M. R. et al. (2013). Incidence and effect of acute kidney injury after transcatheter aortic valve replacement using the new valve academic research consortium criteria. *The American Journal of Cardiology*, *111*(1), 100–105. doi:10.1016/j.amjcard.2012.08.057 PMID:23040657

George, M. J. (2006). The site of action of epidurally administered opioids and its relevance to postoperative pain management. *Anaesthesia*, *61*(7), 659–664. doi:10.1111/j.1365-2044.2006.04713.x PMID:16792611

George, T. J., Beaty, C. A., Kilic, A., Haggerty, K. A., Frank, S. M., Savage, W. J., & Whitman, G. J. (2012). Hemoglobin drift after cardiac surgery. *The Annals of Thoracic Surgery*, *94*(3), 703–709. doi:10.1016/j.athoracsur.2012.03.038 PMID:22609121

Gerriets, T., Schwarz, N., Sammer, G., Baehr, J., Stolz, E., Kaps, M., & Schonburg, M. et al. (2010). Protecting the brain from gaseous and solid micro-emboli during coronary artery bypass grafting: A randomized controlled trial. *European Heart Journal*, *31*(3), 360–368. doi:10.1093/eurheartj/ehp178 PMID:19541675

Gershengorn, H. B., Johnson, M. P., & Factor, P. (2012). The use of nonphysician providers in adult intensive care units. *American Journal of Respiratory and Critical Care Medicine*, *185*(6), 600–605. doi:10.1164/rccm.201107-1261CP PMID:22135345

Gibbon, J. H. Jr. (1954). Application of a mechanical heart and lung apparatus to cardiac surgery. *Minnesota Medicine*, *37*, 171–180. PMID:13154149

Gibbon, J. H. Jr. (1978). The development of the heart-lung apparatus. *American Journal of Surgery*, *135*(5), 608–619. doi:10.1016/0002-9610(78)90119-8 PMID:347960

Gibbons, R. J., Abrams, J., Chatterjee, K., Daley, J., Deedwania, P. C., Douglas, J. S., & Smith, S. C. Jr et al.. (2003). ACC/AHA 2002 guideline update for the management of patients with chronic stable angina – summary article: A report of the American College of Cardiology/American Heart Association Task Force on Practice Guidelines (Committee on the Management of Patients with Chronic Stable Angina). *Circulation*, *107*(1), 149–158. doi:10.1161/01.CIR.0000047041.66447.29 PMID:12515758

Gibbs, N. M. (2009). Point-of-care assessment of antiplatelet agents in the perioperative period: A review. *Anaesthesia and Intensive Care*, *37*(3), 354–369. PMID:19499855

Gill, R., Herbertson, M., Vuylsteke, A., Olsen, P. S., von Heymann, C., Mythen, M., & Schmidt, T. A. et al. (2009). Safety and Efficacy of Recombinant Activated Factor VII: A Randomized Placebo-Controlled Trial in the Setting of Bleeding After Cardiac Surgery. *Circulation*, *120*(1), 21–27. doi:10.1161/CIRCULATIONAHA.108.834275 PMID:19546387

Gill, S. S., Bronskill, S. E., Normand, S. L., Anderson, G. M., Sykora, K., Lam, K., & Rochon, P. A. et al. (2007). Antipsychotic drug use and mortality in older adults with dementia. *Annals of Internal Medicine*, *146*(11), 775–786. doi:10.7326/0003-4819-146-11-200706050-00006 PMID:17548409

Gilman, S.GILMAN. (1965). Cerebral Disorders after open-heart operations. *The New England Journal of Medicine*, *272*(10), 489–498. doi:10.1056/NEJM196503112721001 PMID:14250198

Gilstrap, D., & MacIntyre, N.Implications for Clinical Management. (2013). Patient-ventilator interactions. Implications for clinical management. *American Journal of Respiratory and Critical Care Medicine*, *188*(9), 1058–1068. doi:10.1164/rccm.201212-2214CI PMID:24070493

Ginsberg, M. D., & Busto, R. (1998). Combating hyperthermia in acute stroke. *Stroke*, *29*(2), 529–534. doi:10.1161/01.STR.29.2.529 PMID:9472901

Giomarelli, P., Scolletta, S., Borrelli, E., & Biagioli, B. (2003). Myocardial and lung injury after cardiopulmonary bypass: Role of interleukin (IL)-10. *The Annals of Thoracic Surgery*, *76*(1), 117–123. doi:10.1016/S0003-4975(03)00194-2 PMID:12842524

Girardi L.N., Shavladze S., Sedrakyan A., Neragi S. (2014). Safety and efficacy of retrograde cerebral perfusion as an adjunct for cerebral protection during surgery on the aortic arch. *The Journal of Thoracic and Cardiovascular Surgery*, Jul 30. pii: S0022-5223(14)00989-1. doi: . [Epub ahead of print].10.1016/j.jtcvs.2014.07.024

Girardi, L. N., Rabotnikov, Y., & Avgerinos, D. V. (2014). Preoperative percutaneous coronary intervention in patients undergoing open thoracoabdominal and descending thoracic aneurysm repair. *The Journal of Thoracic and Cardiovascular Surgery*, *147*(1), 163–168. doi:10.1016/j.jtcvs.2013.09.008 PMID:24176270

Girard, T. D., Kress, J. P., Fuchs, B. D., Thomason, J. W., Schweickert, W. D., Pun, B. T., & Ely, E. W. et al. (2008). Efficacy and safety of a paired sedation and ventilator weaning protocol for mechanically ventilated patients in intensive care (Awakening and Breathing Controlled trial): A randomised controlled trial. *Lancet*, *371*(9607), 126–134. doi:10.1016/S0140-6736(08)60105-1 PMID:18191684

Girard, T. D., Pandharipande, P. P., Carson, S. S., Schmidt, G. A., Wright, P. E., Canonico, A. E., & Ely, E. W. et al. (2010). Feasibility, efficacy, and safety of antipsychotics for intensive care unit delirium: The MIND randomized, placebo-controlled trial. *Critical Care Medicine*, *38*(2), 428–437. doi:10.1097/CCM.0b013e3181c58715 PMID:20095068

Girard, T. D., Shintani, A. K., Jackson, J. C., Gordon, S. M., Pun, B. T., Henderson, M. S., & Ely, E. W. et al. (2007). Risk factors for post-traumatic stress disorder symptoms following critical illness requiring mechanical ventilation: A prospective cohort study. *Critical Care (London, England)*, *11*(1), R28. doi:10.1186/cc5708 PMID:17316452

Girou, E., Loyeau, S., Legrand, P., Oppein, F., & Brun-Buisson, C. (2002). Efficacy of handrubbing with alcohol based solution versus standard handwashing with antiseptic soap: Randomised clinical trial. *British Medical Journal*, *325*(7360), 362. doi:10.1136/bmj.325.7360.362 PMID:12183307

Girou, E., Schortgen, F., Delclaux, C., Brun-Buisson, C., Blot, F., Lefort, Y., & Brochard, L. et al. (2000). Association of noninvasive ventilation with nosocomial infections and survival in critically ill patients. *Journal of the American Medical Association*, *284*(18), 2361–2367. doi:10.1001/jama.284.18.2361 PMID:11066187

Giugliano, R., White, J., Bode, C., Armstrong, P., Montalescot, G., Lewis, B., & Newby, L. et al. (2009). Early versus Delayed, Provisional Eptifibatide in Acute Coronary Syndromes. *The New England Journal of Medicine*, *360*(21), 2176–2190. doi:10.1056/NEJMoa0901316 PMID:19332455

Glenny, R. W., Lamm, W. J., Bernard, S. L., An, D., Chornuk, M., Pool, S. L., . . . Robertson, H. T. (2000). Selected contribution: redistribution of pulmonary perfusion during weightlessness and increased gravity. *Journal of Applied Physiology (1985)*, *89*(3), 1239-1248.

Glower, D. D. (2003). Management of chronic aortic regurgitation. *Current Treatment Options in Cardiovascular Medicine*, *5*(6), 511–520. doi:10.1007/s11936-003-0040-x PMID:14575628

Go, A. S., Mozaffarian, D., Roger, V. L., Benjamin, E. J., Berry, J. D., Borden, W. B., & Turner, M. B. et al.Stroke Statistics, Subcommittee. (2013). Heart disease and stroke statistics--2013 update: A report from the American Heart Association. *Circulation, 127*(1), e6–e245. doi:10.1161/CIR.0b013e31828124ad PMID:23239837

Go, A., Mozaffarian, D., Roger, V., Benjamin, E., Berry, J., Borden, W., & Turner, M. et al. (2013). Heart Disease and Stroke Statistics-2013 Update: A report from the American Heart Association. *Circulation, 127*(1), e6–e245. PMID:23239837

Gödje, O., Gallmeier, U., Schelian, M., Grünewald, M., & Mair, H. (2006). Coagulation factor XIII reduces postoperative bleeding after coronary surgery with extracorporeal circulation. *The Thoracic and Cardiovascular Surgeon, 54*(1), 26–33. doi:10.1055/s-2005-872853 PMID:16485185

Gödje, O., Haushofer, M., Lamm, P., & Reichart, B. (1998). The effect of factor XIII on bleeding in coronary surgery. *The Thoracic and Cardiovascular Surgeon, 46*(5), 263–267. doi:10.1055/s-2007-1010236 PMID:9885116

Goepfert. (2007). Goal-directed fluid management reduces vasopressor and catecholamine use in cardiac surgery patients. *Intensive Care Medicine, 33*, 96–103.

Gokgoz, L., Gunaydin, S., Sinci, V., Unlu, M., & Boratav, C. Babacan, a, ... Ersoz, a. (1997). Psychiatric complications of cardiac surgery postoperative delirium syndrome. *Scandinavian Cardiovascular Journal : SCJ, 31*(4), 217–22. Retrieved from http://www.ncbi.nlm.nih.gov/pubmed/9291540

Gold, J. P., Charlson, M. E., Williams-Russo, P., Szatrowski, T. P., Peterson, J. C., & Pirraglia, P. A. ... Barbut, D. (1995). Improvement of outcomes after coronary artery bypass. A randomized trial comparing intraoperative high versus low mean arterial pressure. *The Journal of Thoracic and Cardiovascular Surgery, 110*(5), 1302–11; discussion 1311–4. Retrieved from http://www.ncbi.nlm.nih.gov/pubmed/7475182

Goldberg, P. A., Siegel, M. D., Sherwin, R. S., Halickman, J. I., Lee, M., Bailey, V. A., & Inzucchi, S. E. et al. (2004). Implementation of a safe and effective insulin infusion protocol in a medical intensive care unit. *Diabetes Care, 27*(2), 461–467. doi:10.2337/diacare.27.2.461 PMID:14747229

Goldhaber, S. Z. (2006). "Bridging" and mechanical heart valves: Perils, promises, and predictions. *Circulation, 113*(4), 470–472. doi:10.1161/CIRCULATIONAHA.105.598268 PMID:16449725

Gold, J. P., Charlson, M. E., & Szatrowski, T. P. (1995). Improvement of outcomes after cardiac surgery. *The Journal of Thoracic and Cardiovascular Surgery, 110*, 1302–1314. doi:10.1016/S0022-5223(95)70053-6 PMID:7475182

Gold, J., Cullinane, S., Chen, J., Oz, M., Olover, J., & Landry, D. (2000). Vasopressin As An Alternative To Norepinephrine In The Treatment Of Milrinone-Induced Hypotension. *Critical Care Medicine, 28*(1), 249–252. doi:10.1097/00003246-200001000-00043 PMID:10667533

Goldman, S., Sutter, F., Ferdinand, F., & Trace, C. (2004). Optimizing intraoperative cerebral oxygen delivery using noninvasive cerebral oximetry decreases the incidence of stroke for cardiac surgical patients. *The Heart Surgery Forum, 7*(5), E376–E381. doi:10.1532/HSF98.20041062 PMID:15799908

Goldstein, D. J., Naftel, D., Holman, W., Bellumkonda, L., Pamboukian, S. V., Pagani, F. D., & Kirklin, J. (2012). Continuous-flow devices and percutaneous site infections: Clinical outcomes. *The Journal of Heart and Lung Transplantation, 31*(11), 1151–1157. doi:10.1016/j.healun.2012.05.004 PMID:22766022

Goldstein, R., O'Neill, J. A. Jr, Holcomb, G. W. III, Morgan, W. M. III, Neblett, W. W. III, Oates, J. A., & Scott, H. W. Jr et al.. (1999). Clinical experience over 48 years with pheochromocytoma. *Annals of Surgery, 229*(6), 755–764. doi:10.1097/00000658-199906000-00001 PMID:10363888

Gologorsky, E., Macedo, F. I. B., Carvalho, E. M., Gologorsky, A., Ricci, M., & Salerno, T. a. (2010). Postoperative cardiac arrest after heart surgery: Does extracorporeal perfusion support a paradigm change in management? *Anesthesiology Research and Practice, 2010*. doi:10.1155/2010/937215 PMID:20798770

Gonzalez-Fernandez, C., Gonzalez-Castro, A., Rodriguez-Borregan, J. C., Lopez-Sanchez, M., Suberviola, B., Francisco Nistal, J., & Martin-Duran, R. (2009). Pulmonary venous obstruction after lung transplantation. Diagnostic advantages of transesophageal echocardiography. *Clinical Transplantation*, *23*(6), 975–980. doi:10.1111/j.1399-0012.2009.01078.x

Goodnick, P. J., Jerry, J., & Parra, F. (2002). Psychotropic drugs and the ECG: Focus on the QTc interval. *Expert Opinion on Pharmacotherapy*, *3*(5), 479–498. doi:10.1517/14656566.3.5.479 PMID:11996627

Goodnough, L. T., & Shander, A. (2012). Patient blood management. *Anesthesiology*, *116*(6), 1367–1376. doi:10.1097/ALN.0b013e318254d1a3 PMID:22487863

Goodnough, L. T., Soegiarso, R. W., Birkmeyer, J. D., & Welch, H. G. (1993). Economic impact of inappropriate blood transfusions in coronary artery bypass graft surgery. *The American Journal of Medicine*, *94*(5), 509–514. doi:10.1016/0002-9343(93)90086-5 PMID:8498396

Gordon, J. (2003). Fostering students' personal and professional development in medicine: A new framework for PPD. *Medical Education*, *37*(4), 341–349. doi:10.1046/j.1365-2923.2003.01470.x PMID:12654119

Gordon, M., Darbyshire, D., & Baker, P. (2012). Non-technical skills training to enhance patient safety: A systematic review. *Medical Education*, *46*(11), 1042–1054. doi:10.1111/j.1365-2923.2012.04343.x PMID:23078681

Gorlinger, K., Dirkmann, D., Hanke, A. A., Kamler, M., Kottenberg, E., Thielmann, M., & Peters, J. et al. (2011). First-line therapy with coagulation factor concentrates combined with point-of-care coagulation testing is associated with decreased allogeneic blood transfusion in cardiovascular surgery: A retrospective, single-center cohort study. *Anesthesiology*, *115*(6), 1179–1191. doi:10.1097/ALN.0b013e31823497dd PMID:21970887

Görlinger, K., Shore-Lesserson, L., Dirkmann, D., Hanke, A. A., Rahe-Meyer, N., & Tanaka, K. A. (2013). Management of hemorrhage in cardiothoracic surgery. *Journal of Cardiothoracic and Vascular Anesthesia*, *27*(4Suppl), S20–S34. doi:10.1053/j.jvca.2013.05.014 PMID:23910533

Gosselin, R. C., Dager, W. E., King, J. H., Janatpour, K., Mahackian, K., Larkin, E. C., & Owings, J. T. (2004). Effect of direct thrombin inhibitors, bivalirudin, lepirudin, and argatroban on prothrombin time and INR values. *American Journal of Clinical Pathology*, *121*(4), 593–599. doi:10.1309/D79K4YG78NTNYY38 PMID:15080313

Gottesman, R. F., & Grega, M. a, Bailey, M. M., Pham, L. D., Zeger, S. L., Baumgartner, W. a, … McKhann, G. M. (2010). Delirium after coronary artery bypass graft surgery and late mortality. *Annals of Neurology*, *67*(3), 338–344. doi:10.1002/ana.21899 PMID:20373345

Gottesman, R. F., Sherman, P. M., Grega, M. A., Yousem, D. M., Borowicz, L. M. Jr, Selnes, O. A., & McKhann, G. M. et al. (2006). Watershed strokes after cardiac surgery: Diagnosis, etiology, and outcome. *Stroke*, *37*(9), 2306–2311. doi:10.1161/01.STR.0000236024.68020.3a PMID:16857947

Gott, V. L. (2005). Lillehei, Lewis, and Wangensteen: The right mix for giant achievements in cardiac surgery. *The Annals of Thoracic Surgery*, *79*(6), S2210–S2213. doi:10.1016/j.athoracsur.2005.02.078 PMID:15919253

Gould, M. K., Garcia, D. A., Wren, S. M., Karnicolas, P. J., Arcelus, J. I., Heit, J. A., & Samama, C. M. (2012). Prevention of VTE in nonorthopedic surgical patients. *Chest*, *141*(2Suppl), e227s–e277s. PMID:22315263

Goulenok, T., Klein, I., Mazighi, M., Messika-Zeitoun, D., Alexandra, J. F., Mourvillier, B., & Duval, X. et al. (2013). Infective endocarditis with symptomatic cerebral complications; Contribution of cerebral magnetic resonance imaging. *Cerebrovascular Diseases (Basel, Switzerland)*, *35*(4), 327–336. doi:10.1159/000348317 PMID:23615478

Gozu, A., Clay, C., & Younus, F. (2011). Hospital-wide reduction in central line-associated bloodstream infections: A tale of two small community hospitals. *Infection Control and Hospital Epidemiology*, *32*(6), 619–622. doi:10.1086/660098 PMID:21558777

Gracey, D., Divertie, M., Howard, F., & Payne, W. (1984). Postoperative respiratory care after transsternal thymectomy in myasthenia gravis. A 3-year experience in 53 patients. *Chest*, *86*(1), 67–71. doi:10.1378/chest.86.1.67 PMID:6734295

Gracias, V. H., Sicoutris, C. P., Stawicki, S. P., Meredith, D. M., Horan, A. D., Gupta, R., & Schwab, C. W. et al. (2008). Critical care nurse practitioners improve compliance with clinical practice guidelines in "semiclosed" surgical intensive care unit. *Journal of Nursing Care Quality*, *23*(4), 338–344. doi:10.1097/01.NCQ.0000323286.56397.8c PMID:18521045

Grady, K. L., Naftel, D., Stevenson, L., Dew, M. A., Weidner, G., Pagani, F. D., & Young, J. et al. (2014). Overall quality of life improves to similar levels after mechanical circulatory support regardless of severity of heart failure before implantation. *The Journal of Heart and Lung Transplantation*, *33*(4), 412–421. doi:10.1016/j.healun.2013.10.017 PMID:24360203

Graham, M. M., Norris, C. M., Galbraith, P. D., Knudtson, M. L., & Ghali, W. A. (2006). Quality of life after coronary revascularization in the elderly. *European Heart Journal*, *27*(14), 1690–1698. doi:10.1093/eurheartj/ehl038 PMID:16717072

Grajales, F. J. III, Sheps, S., Ho, K., Novak-Lauscher, H., & Eysenbach, G. (2014). Social Media: A Review and Tutorial of Applications in Medicine and Health Care. *Journal of Medical Internet Research*, *16*(2), e13. doi:10.2196/jmir.2912 PMID:24518354

Granger, C. B., Alexander, J. H., McMurray, J. J., Lopes, R. D., Hylek, E. M., Hanna, M., & Wallentin, L. et al. (2011). Apixaban versus warfarin in patients with atrial fibrillation. *The New England Journal of Medicine*, *365*(11), 981–992. doi:10.1056/NEJMoa1107039 PMID:21870978

Grantcharov, T. P., & Reznick, R. K. (2008). Teaching procedural skills. *BMJ (Clinical Research Ed.)*, *336*(7653), 1129–1131. doi:10.1136/bmj.39517.686956.47 PMID:18483056

Grant, G. (1979). *On Competence*. San Francisco, USA: Jossey-Bass.

Grant, J., Abdelrahmen, M. Y. H., & Zachariah, A. (2013). Curriculum in Context. In K. Walsh (Ed.), *Oxford Textbook of Medical Education* (1st ed.). Oxford: Oxford University Press.

Grau, T., Bonet, A., Rubio, M., Mateo, D., Farré, M., Acosta, J. A., & Mesejo, A. et al. (2007). Liver dysfunction associated with artificial nutrition in critically ill patients. *Critical Care (London, England)*, *11*(1), R10. doi:10.1186/cc5670 PMID:17254321

Gray, K., & Tobin, J. (2010). Introducing an online community into a clinical education setting: A pilot study of student and staff engagement and outcomes using blended learning. *BMC Medical Education*, *10*(6). doi:10.1186/1472-6920-10-6 PMID:20100354

Greenbaum, A. B., O'Neill, W. W., Paone, G., Guerrero, M. E., Wyman, J. F., Cooper, R. L., & Lederman, R. J. (2014). Caval-aortic access to allow transcatheter aortic valve replacement in otherwise ineligible patients: Initial human experience. *Journal of the American College of Cardiology*, *63*(2525 Pt A), 2795–2804. doi:10.1016/j.jacc.2014.04.015 PMID:24814495

Greenberg, L. W., Goldberg, R. M., & Jewett, L. S. (1984). Teaching in the clinical setting: Factors influencing residents' perceptions, confidence and behaviour. *Medical Education*, *18*(5), 360–365. doi:10.1111/j.1365-2923.1984.tb01283.x PMID:6472144

Greene, M. T., Chang, R., Kuhn, L., Rogers, M. A. M., Chenoweth, C. E., Shuman, E., & Saint, S. (2012). Predictors of hospital-acquired urinary tract-related bloodstream infection. *Infection Control and Hospital Epidemiology*, *33*(10), 1001–1007. doi:10.1086/667731 PMID:22961019

Grgurich, P. E., Hudcova, J., Lei, Y., Sarwar, A., & Craven, D. E. (2013). Diagnosis of ventilator-associated pneumonia: Controversies and working toward a gold standard. *Current Opinion in Infectious Diseases*, *26*(2), 140–150. doi:10.1097/QCO.0b013e32835ebbd0 PMID:23411419

Gries, C. J., Curtis, J. R., Wall, R. J., & Engelberg, R. A. (2008). Family member satisfaction with end-of-life decision making in the ICU. *Chest*, *133*(3), 704-712. doi: chest.07-1773 [pii] 10.1378/chest.07-1773

Griffin, C. E. III, Kaye, A. M., Bueno, F. R., & Kaye, A. D. (2013). Benzodiazepine pharmacology and central nervous system-mediated effects. *Ochsner Journal*, *13*, 214–223. PMID:23789008

Grigore, A. M., Grocott, H. P., Mathew, J. P., Phillips-Bute, B., Stanley, T. O., Butler, A., & Newman, M. F. et al. (2002). The Rewarming Rate and Increased Peak Temperature Alter Neurocognitive Outcome After Cardiac Surgery. *Anesthesia and Analgesia*, *94*(1), 4–10. doi:10.1213/00000539-200201000-00002 PMID:11772792

Grigore, A. M., Murray, C. F., Ramakrishna, H., & Djaiani, G. (2009). A core review of temperature regimens and neuroprotection during cardiopulmonary bypass: Does rewarming rate matter? *Anesthesia and Analgesia*, *109*(6), 1741–1751. doi:10.1213/ANE.0b013e3181c04fea PMID:19923500

Grillo, H., Donahue, D., Mathisen, D., Wain, J., & Wright, C. (1995). Postintubation tracheal stenosis. Treatment and results. *The Journal of Thoracic and Cardiovascular Surgery*, *109*(3), 486–492. doi:10.1016/S0022-5223(95)70279-2 PMID:7877309

Grogan, D. R., Irwin, R. S., Channick, R., Raptopoulos, V., Curley, F. J., Bartter, T., & Corwin, R. W. (1990). Complications associated with thoracentesis. A prospective, randomized study comparing three different methods. *Archives of Internal Medicine*, *150*(4), 873–877. doi:10.1001/archinte.1990.00390160119023 PMID:2183735

Gronseth, G., & Barohn, R. (2000). Practice parameter: thymectomy for autoimmune myasthenia gravis (an evidence-based review): report of the Quality Standards Subcommittee of the American Academy of Neurology. *Neurology*, *55*(1), 7–15. doi:10.1212/WNL.55.1.7 PMID:10891896

Group, I. D. a. C. I. S. (2013). *Awakening and Breathing Coordination*. Retrieved June 5, 2014, from http://www.icu-delirium.org/medicalprofessionals.html

Group, T. h. a. c. s. (2002). Mild therapeutic hypothermia to improve the neurologic outcome after cardiac arrest. *N Engl J Med*, *346*, 549-556.

Grubitzsch, H., Schaefer, A., Melzer, C., Wernecke, K. D., Gabbieri, D., & Konertz, W. (2014). Outcome after surgery for prosthetic valve endocarditis and the impact of preoperative treatment. *The Journal of Thoracic and Cardiovascular Surgery*, *148*(5), 2052–2059. doi:10.1016/j.jtcvs.2014.05.025 PMID:24951022

Gruntzig, A. (1978). Transluminal dilatation of coronary-artery stenosis. *Lancet*, *1*(8058), 263. doi:10.1016/S0140-6736(78)90500-7 PMID:74678

Grüntzig, A. R., Senning, A., & Siegenthaler, W. E. (1979). Nonoperative dilatation of coronary-artery stenosis: Percutaneous transluminal coronary angioplasty. *The New England Journal of Medicine*, *301*(2), 61–68. doi:10.1056/NEJM197907123010201 PMID:449946

Guay, J. (2006). The benefits of adding epidural analgesia to general anesthesia: A metaanalysis. *Journal of Anesthesia*, *20*(4), 335–340. doi:10.1007/s00540-006-0423-8 PMID:17072704

Guazzi, M., & Borlaug, B. (2012). Pulmonary Hypertension Due to Left Heart Disease. *Circulation*, *126*(8), 975–990. doi:10.1161/CIRCULATIONAHA.111.085761 PMID:22908015

Guenther, U., Theuerkauf, N., Frommann, I., Brimmers, K., Malik, R., Stori, S., & Popp, J. et al. (2013). Predisposing and precipitating factors of delirium after cardiac surgery: A prospective observational cohort study. *Annals of Surgery*, *257*(6), 1160–1167. doi:10.1097/SLA.0b013e318281b01c PMID:23426334

Guerin, C., Reignier, J., Richard, J. C., Beuret, P., Gacouin, A., Boulain, T., . . . Group, P. S. (2013). Prone positioning in severe acute respiratory distress syndrome. *N Engl J Med*, *368*(23), 2159-2168.

Guerin, C., Reignier, J., Richard, J. C., Beuret, P., Gacouin, A., Boulain, T., & Ayzac, L. et al. (2013). Prone positioning in severe acute respiratory distress syndrome. *The New England Journal of Medicine*, *368*(23), 2159–2168. doi:10.1056/NEJMoa1214103

Guignard, B., Bossard, A. E., Coste, C., Sessler, D. I., Lebrault, C., Alfonsi, P., & Chauvin, M. et al. (2000). Acute opioid tolerance: Intraoperative remifentanil increases postoperative pain and morphine requirement. *Anesthesiology*, *93*(2), 409–417. doi:10.1097/00000542-200008000-00019 PMID:10910490

Guney, M. R., Ketenci, B., Yapici, F., Sokullu, O., Firat, M. F., Uyarel, H., & Demirtas, M. et al. (2008). Results of treatment methods in cardiac arrest following coronary artery bypass grafting. *Journal of Cardiac Surgery*, *24*(3), 227–233. doi:10.1111/j.1540-8191.2008.00760.x PMID:19040406

Gurbel, P. A., Bliden, K. P., DiChiara, J., Newcomer, J., Weng, W., Neerchal, K., & Etherington, A. et al. (2007). Evaluation of dose related effects of aspirin on platelet function: Results from the aspirin induced platelet effect (ASPECT) study. *Circulation*, *115*(25), 3156–3164. doi:10.1161/CIRCULATIONAHA.106.675587 PMID:17562955

Gurbel, P. A., Bliden, K. P., Hayes, K. M., Yoho, J. A., Herzog, W. R., & Tantry, U. S. (2005). The Relation of Dosing to Clopidogrel Responsiveness and the Incidence of High Post-Treatment Platelet Aggregation in Patients Undergoing Coronary Stenting. *Journal of the American College of Cardiology*, *45*(9), 1392–1396. doi:10.1016/j.jacc.2005.01.030 PMID:15862408

Gurman, G., Samri, M., Sarov, B., Bearman, J. E., & Heilig, I. (1990). The rate of gastrointestinal bleeding in a general ICU population: A retrospective study. *Intensive Care Medicine*, *16*(1), 44–49. doi:10.1007/BF01706324 PMID:2107235

Gürntke, S., Kohler, C., Steinmetz, I., Pfeifer, Y., Eller, C., Gastmeier, P., & Leistner, R. et al. (2014). Molecular epidemiology of extended-spectrum beta-lactamase (ESBL)-positive Klebsiella pneumonia from bloodstream infections and risk factors for mortality. *Journal of Infection and Chemotherapy*, *20*(12), 817–819. doi:10.1016/j.jiac.2014.08.012 PMID:25224765

Gutsche, J. T., Cheung, A. T., McGarvey, M. L., Moser, W. G., Szeto, W., Carpenter, J. P., & Bavaria, J. E. et al. (2007). Risk factors for perioperative stroke after thoracic endovascular aortic repair. *The Annals of Thoracic Surgery*, *84*(4), 1195–1200, discussion 1200. doi:10.1016/j.athoracsur.2007.04.128 PMID:17888969

Guyatt, G. H., Akl, E. A., Crowther, M., Gutterman, D. D., & Schuunemann, H. J. (2012). Executive summary: Antithrombotic therapy and prevention of thrombosis, 9th ed: American College of Chest Physicians Evidence-Based Clinical Practice Guidelines. Chest. 141(2 Suppl), 7S-47S.

Guyton, R. A., Block, P. C., Thourani, V. H., Lerakis, S., & Babaliaros, V. (2013). Carotid artery access for transcatheter aortic valve replacement. *Catheterization and Cardiovascular Interventions*, *82*(4), E583–E586. doi:10.1002/ccd.24596 PMID:22887932

Guzman, F., & Farinde, A. (2014). *First-generation antipsychotics: an introduction.* Retrieved from http://psychopharmacologyinstitute.com/antipsychotics/first-generation-antipsychotics/

Haase, M., Bellomo, R., Devarajan, P., Ma, Q., Bennett, M. R., Möckel, M., & Haase-Fielitz, A. et al. (2009). Novel Biomarkers Early Predict the Severity of Acute Kidney Injury After Cardiac Surgery in Adults. *The Annals of Thoracic Surgery*, *88*(1), 124–130. doi:10.1016/j.athoracsur.2009.04.023 PMID:19559209

Haase, M., Bellomo, R., & Haase-Fielitz, A. (2010). Novel Biomarkers, Oxidative Stress, and the Role of Labile Iron Toxicity in Cardiopulmonary Bypass-Associated Acute Kidney Injury. *Journal of the American College of Cardiology*, *55*(19), 2024–2033. doi:10.1016/j.jacc.2009.12.046 PMID:20447525

Haas, G. S., & Massachusetts, B. (1985). Acute Pancreatitis After Cardiopulrnonary Bypass. *American Journal of Surgery*, *149*(4), 508–515. doi:10.1016/S0002-9610(85)80048-9 PMID:2580453

Habib, G., Badano, L., Tribouilloy, C., Vilacosta, I., Zamorano, J. L., Galderisi, M., & Aakhus, S. et al. (2010). Recommendations for the practice of echocardiography in infective endocarditis. *European Journal of Echocardiography*, *11*(2), 202–219. doi:10.1093/ejechocard/jeq004 PMID:20223755

Habib, G., Hoen, B., Tornos, P., Thuny, F., Prendergast, B., Vilacosta, I., & van Camp, G. et al. (2009). Guidelines on the prevention, diagnosis, and treatment of infective endocarditis (new version 2009): The Task Force on the Prevention, Diagnosis, and Treatment of Infective Endocarditis of the European Society of Cardiology (ESC). *European Heart Journal*, *30*(19), 2369–2413. doi:10.1093/eurheartj/ehp285 PMID:19713420

Hackert, T., Kienle, P., Weitz, J., Werner, J., Szabo, G., Hagl, S., & Schmidt, J. et al. (2003). Accuracy of diagnostic laparoscopy for early diagnosis of abdominal complications after cardiac surgery. *Surgical Endoscopy*, *17*(10), 1671–1674. doi:10.1007/s00464-003-9004-1 PMID:12915977

Haddad, F., Couture, P., Tousignant, C., & Denault, A. Y. (2009). The right ventricle in cardiac surgery, a perioperative perspective: II. Pathophysiology, clinical importance, and management. *Anesthesia and Analgesia*, *108*(2), 422–433. doi:10.1213/ane.0b013e31818d8b92 PMID:19151265

Haglund, N. A., Maltais, S., Bick, J. S., Costello, W., Keebler, M., Davis, M. E., & Wagner, C. E. et al. (2014). Hemodynamic transesophageal echocardiography after left ventricular assist device implantation. *Journal of Cardiothoracic and Vascular Anesthesia*, *28*(5), 1184–1190. doi:10.1053/j.jvca.2014.02.012 PMID:25104081

Hajjar, L. A., Vincent, J.-L., Galas, F. R. B. G., Nakamura, R. E., Silva, C. M. P., Santos, M. H., & Auler, J. O. C. et al. (2010). Transfusion requirements after cardiac surgery: The TRACS randomized controlled trial. *Journal of the American Medical Association*, *304*(14), 1559–1567. doi:10.1001/jama.2010.1446 PMID:20940381

Hakim, T. S., Lisbona, R., & Dean, G. W. (1987). Gravity-independent inequality in pulmonary blood flow in humans. *Journal of Applied Physiology (1985)*, *63*(3), 1114-1121.

Hall, A. H., & Rumack, B. H. (1986). Clinical toxicology of CN. *Annals of Emergency Medicine*, *15*(9), 1067–1074. doi:10.1016/S0196-0644(86)80131-7 PMID:3526995

Hall, N. A., & Fox, A. J. (2006). Renal replacement therapies in critical care. *Continuing Education in Anaesthesia. Critical Care & Pain*, *6*(5), 197–202.

Hall, R. I., Sandham, D., Cardinal, P., Tweeddale, M., Moher, D., Wang, X., & Anis, A. H. (2001). Propofol vs midazolam for ICU sedation: A Canadian multicenter randomized trial. *Chest*, *119*(4), 1151–1159. doi:10.1378/chest.119.4.1151 PMID:11296183

Hall, T. S., Brevetti, G. R., Skoultchi, A. J., Sines, J. C., Gregory, P., & Spotnitz, A. J. (2001). Re-exploration for hemorrhage following open heart surgery differentiation on the causes of bleeding and the impact on patient outcomes. *Annals of Thoracic and Cardiovascular Surgery*, *7*(6), 352–357. PMID:11888475

Halonen, J. H. P., & Jarvinen, O. (2007). Corticosteroids for the prevention of atrial fibrillation after cardiac surgery. *Journal of the American Medical Association*, *297*(14), 1562–1567. doi:10.1001/jama.297.14.1562 PMID:17426275

Halpern, S. D. (2014). Cross-coverage in the intensive care unit: More than meets the "i"? *American Journal of Respiratory and Critical Care Medicine*, *189*(11), 1297–1298. doi:10.1164/rccm.201405-0801ED PMID:24881934

Hamilton, T. T., Huber, L. M., & Jessen, M. E. (2002). PulseCO: A Less-Invasive Method to Monitor Cardiac Output from Arterial Pressure after Cardiac Surgery. *The Annals of Thoracic Surgery*, *74*(4), S1408–S1412. doi:10.1016/S0003-4975(02)04059-6 PMID:12400827

Hamilton, W. F. (1932). Studies on the circulation IV. Further analysis of the injection methods and of changes in hemodynamics under physiological conditions. *The American Journal of Physiology*, *99*, 534–551.

Hamrahian, A. H., Oseni, T. S., & Arafah, B. M. (2004). Measurements of serum free cortisol in critically ill patients. *The New England Journal of Medicine*, *350*(16), 1629–1638. doi:10.1056/NEJMoa020266 PMID:15084695

Handschin, A. E., Weber, M., Renner, E., & Clavien, P.-A. (2005). Abdominal compartment syndrome after liver transplantation. *Liver Transplantation*, *11*(1), 98–100. doi:10.1002/lt.20295 PMID:15690542

Hanlon-Pena, M., & Quaal, S. J. (2011). Intra-Aortic Balloon Pump: Review of evidence supporting current practice. *American Journal of Critical Care*, *10*(4), 323–334. doi:10.4037/ajcc2011542 PMID:21724636

Han, M. K., McLaughlin, V. V., Criner, G. J., & Martinez, F. J. (2007). Pulmonary diseases and the heart. *Circulation*, *116*(25), 2992–3005. doi:10.1161/CIRCULATIONAHA.106.685206 PMID:18086941

Hannan, E. L., Wu, C., Walford, G., Culliford, A. T., Gold, J. P., Smith, C. R., & Jones, R. H. et al. (2008). Drug-eluting stents vs. coronary-artery bypass grafting in multivessel coronary disease. *The New England Journal of Medicine*, *358*(4), 331–341. doi:10.1056/NEJMoa071804 PMID:18216353

Hannan, M. M., Husain, S., Matner, F., Danziger-Isakov, L., Drew, R. J., Corey, G. R., & Mooney, M. L. et al. (2011). Working formulation for the standardization of definitions of infections in patients using ventricular assist devices. *The Journal of Heart and Lung Transplantation*, *30*(4), 375–384. doi:10.1016/j.healun.2011.01.717 PMID:21419995

Hansalia, S., Biswas, M., Dutta, R., Hage, F. G., Hsiung, M. C., Nanda, N. C., & Yin, W. et al. (2009). The value of live/real time three-dimensional transesophageal echocardiography in the assessment of valvular vegetations. *Echocardiography (Mount Kisco, N.Y.)*, *26*(10), 1264–1273. doi:10.1111/j.1540-8175.2009.01042.x PMID:19929872

Hansson, E. C., Rexius, H., Dellborg, M., Albertsson, P., & Jeppsson, A. (2014). Coronary artery bypass grafting-related bleeding complications in real-life acute coronary syndrome patients treated with clopidogrel or ticagrelor. *European Journal of Cardio-Thoracic Surgery*, *46*(4), 699–705. doi:10.1093/ejcts/ezt662 PMID:24482383

Harbarth, S., Fankhauser, C., Schrenzel, J., Christenson, J., Gervaz, P., Bandiera-Clerc, C., & Pittet, D. et al. (2008). Universal screening for methicillin-resistant Staphylococcus aureus at hospital admission and nosocomial infection in surgical patients. *Journal of the American Medical Association*, *299*, 1149–1157. doi:10.1001/jama.299.10.1149 PMID:18334690

Harden, R. M., Crosby, J. R., & Davis, M. H. M. (1999). AMEE Guide No. 14: Outcome-based education: Part 5-From competency to meta-competency: a model for the specification of learning outcomes. *Medical Teacher*, *21*(6), 546–552. doi:10.1080/01421599978951 PMID:21281173

Harenberg, J., Jorg, I., & Fenyvesi, T. (2004). Treatment of heparin-induced thrombocytopenia with fondaparinux. *Haematologica*, *89*(8), 1017–1018. PMID:15339691

Harken, D. E. (1946). Foreign bodies in, and in relation to, thoracic blood vessels and heart, I: Techniques for approaching and removing foreign bodies from chambers of heart. *Surgery, Gynecology & Obstetrics*, *83*, 117–125. PMID:20988045

Harken, D. E., Black, H., Dickson, J. F. III, & Wilson, H. E. III. (1955). De-epicardialization: A simple, effective surgical treatment for angina pectoris. *Circulation*, *12*(6), 955–962. doi:10.1161/01.CIR.12.6.955 PMID:13270351

Harlen, W., & James, M. (1997). Assessment and Learning: Differences and relationships between formative and summative assessment. *Assessment in Education: Principles, Policy & Practice*, *4*(3), 365–379. doi:10.1080/0969594970040304

Harloff, A., Strecker, C., Reinhard, M., Kollum, M., Handke, M., Olschewski, M., & Hetzel, A. et al. (2006). Combined measurement of carotid stiffness and intima-media thickness improves prediction of complex aortic plaques in patients with ischemic stroke. *Stroke*, *37*(11), 2708–2712. doi:10.1161/01.STR.0000244763.19013.dc PMID:17008632

Harpole, D. Jr, Decamp, M. Jr, Daley, J., Hur, K., Oprian, C., Henderson, W., & Khuri, S. (1999). Prognostic models of thirty-day mortality and morbidity after major pulmonary resection. *The Journal of Thoracic and Cardiovascular Surgery*, *117*(5), 969–979. doi:10.1016/S0022-5223(99)70378-8 PMID:10220692

Harrington, R. A., Mc, G. W., Nulty, S., White, H. D., Lincoff, A. M., Gibson, C. M., & Kleiman, N. S. et al. (2009). Platelet inhibition with cangrelor in patients undergoing PCI. *The New England Journal of Medicine*, *361*(24), 2318–2329. doi:10.1056/NEJMoa0908628 PMID:19915221

Harrison, D. C., & Collinsworth, K. A. (1974). Antiarrhythmic actions of lidocaine. *Annual Review of Medicine*, *25*(1), 143–148. doi:10.1146/annurev.me.25.020174.001043 PMID:4596228

Harrison, R. W., Hasselblad, V., Mehta, R. H., Levin, R., Harrington, R. A., & Alexander, J. H. (2013). Effect of levosimendan on survival and adverse events after cardiac surgery: A meta-analysis. *Journal of Cardiovascular and Vascular Anesthesia*, *27*(6), 1224–1232. doi:10.1053/j.jvca.2013.03.027 PMID:24050857

Harskamp, R. E., Lopes, R. D., Baisden, C. E., de Winter, R. J., & Alexander, J. H. (2013). Saphenous vein graft failure after coronary artery bypass surgery: Pathophysiology, management, and future directions. *Annals of Surgery*, *257*(5), 824–833. doi:10.1097/SLA.0b013e318288c38d PMID:23574989

Hartman, G. S., Yao, F. F., & Bruefach, M. (1996). Severity of aortic atheromatous disease diagnosed by transesophageal echocardiography predicts stroke and other outcomes associated with coronary artery surgery: A prospective study. *Anesthesia and Analgesia*, *83*, 701–708. PMID:8831306

Härtter, S., Sennewald, R., Nehmiz, G., & Reilly, P. et al.. (2013). Oral bioavailability of dabigatran etexilate (Pradaxa®) after co-medication with verapamil in healthy subjects. *British Journal of Clinical Pharmacology*, *75*(4), 1053–1062. doi:10.1111/j.1365-2125.2012.04453.x PMID:22946890

Hartwig, M. G., Walczak, R., Lin, S. S., & Davis, R. D. (2012). Improved survival but marginal allograft function in patients treated with extracorporeal membrane oxygenation after lung transplantation. *The Annals of Thoracic Surgery*, *93*(2), 366–371. doi:10.1016/j.athoracsur.2011.05.017

Hartz, R. S. et al.. (1999). Esophageal Doppler ultrasound monitor versus Pulmonary artery catheter in hemodynamic management of critically ill surgical patients. *Journal of Trauma and Acute Care Surgery*, *46*(4), 607–611. doi:10.1097/00005373-199904000-00008 PMID:10217222

Harvey, M. A. (2012). The truth about consequences--post-intensive care syndrome in intensive care unit survivors and their families. *Critical Care Medicine*, *40*(8), 2506–2507. doi:10.1097/CCM.0b013e318258e943 PMID:22809925

Hasan, A. (2010). *Understanding Mechanical Ventilation: A Practical Handbook* (2nd ed.). Dordrecht: Springer. doi:10.1007/978-1-84882-869-8

Hata, M., Yoshitake, I., Wakui, S., Unosawa, S., Kimura, H., Hata, H., & Shiono, M. (2011). Long-term patency rate for radial artery vs. saphenous vein grafts using same-patient materials. *Circulation Journal : Official Journal of the Japanese Circulation Society*, *75*(6), 1373–7. Retrieved from http://www.ncbi.nlm.nih.gov/pubmed/21467657

Hatherill, M., Salie, S., Waggie, Z., Lawrenson, J., Hewitson, J., Reynolds, L., & Argent, A. (2005). Hyperchloraemic metabolic acidosis following open cardiac surgery. *Archives of Disease in Childhood*, *90*(12), 1288–1292. doi:10.1136/adc.2005.078006

Hattler, B., Messenger, J. C., Shroyer, A. L., Collins, J. F., Haugen, S. J., Garcia, J. A., & Grover, F. L. et al. (2012). Off-Pump coronary artery bypass surgery is associated with worse arterial and saphenous vein graft patency and less effective revascularization: Results from the Veterans Affairs Randomized On/Off Bypass (ROOBY) trial. *Circulation*, *125*(23), 2827–2835. doi:10.1161/CIRCULATIONAHA.111.069260 PMID:22592900

Hauck, A. J., Freeman, D. P., Ackermann, D. M., Danielson, G. K., & Edwards, W. D. (1988). Surgical pathology of the tricuspid valve: A study of 363 cases spanning 25 years. *Mayo Clinic Proceedings*, *63*(9), 851–863. doi:10.1016/S0025-6196(12)62687-1 PMID:3045434

Hauer, K. E., Ciccone, A., Henzel, T. R., Katsufrakis, P., Miller, S. H., Norcross, W. A., & Irby, D. M. et al. (2009). Remediation of the deficiencies of physicians across the continuum from medical school to practice: A thematic review of the literature. *Academic Medicine: Journal of the Association of American Medical Colleges*, *84*(12), 1822–1832. doi:10.1097/ACM.0b013e3181bf3170 PMID:19940595

Hawker, G. A., Mian, S., Kendzerska, T., & French, M. (2011). Measures of adult pain. *Arthritis Care and Research*, *63*(S11), S240–S252. doi:10.1002/acr.20543 PMID:22588748

Hawkey, C. J. (2000). Nonsteroidal anti-inflammatory drug gastropathy. *Gastroenterology*, *119*(2), 521–535. doi:10.1053/gast.2000.9561 PMID:10930388

Hawn, M. T., Richman, J. S., Vick, C. C., Deierhoi, R. J., Graham, L. A., Henderson, W. G., & Itani, K. M. (2013). Timing of surgical antibiotic prophylaxis and the risk of surgical site infection. *JAMA Surgery*, *148*(7), 649–657. doi:10.1001/jamasurg.2013.134 PMID:23552769

Hawn, M. T., Vick, C. C., Richman, J., Holman, W., Deierhoi, R. J., Graham, L. A., & Itani, K. M. et al. (2011). Surgical site infection prevention: Time to move beyond the surgical care improvement program. *Annals of Surgery*, *254*(3), 494–499, discussion 499–501. doi:10.1097/SLA.0b013e31822c6929 PMID:21817889

Hawryluck, L. A., Espin, S. L., Garwood, K. C., Evans, C. A., & Lingard, L. A. (2002). Pulling together and pushing apart: Tides of tension in the ICU team. *Academic Medicine*, *77*(10Suppl), S73–S76. doi:10.1097/00001888-200210001-00024 PMID:12377711

Haynes, D., & Baumann, M. H. (2010). Management of pneumothorax. *Seminars in Respiratory and Critical Care Medicine*, *31*(6), 769–780. doi:10.1055/s-0030-1269837 PMID:21213209

Hayward, P., & Buxton, B. F. (2007). Contemporary coronary graft patency: 5-year observational data from a randomized trial of conduits. *The Annals of Thoracic Surgery*, *84*(3), 795–799. doi:10.1016/j.athoracsur.2007.04.028 PMID:17720377

Hayward, P., Gordon, I. R., Hare, D. L., Matalanis, G., Horrigan, M. L., Rosalion, A., & Buxton, B. F. (2010). Comparable patencies of the radial artery and right internal thoracic artery or saphenous vein beyond 5 years: Results from the Radial Artery Patency and Clinical Outcomes trial. *The Journal of Thoracic and Cardiovascular Surgery*, *139*(1), 60–65, discussion 65–67. doi:10.1016/j.jtcvs.2009.09.043 PMID:20106358

Hazinski, M. F., Nolan, J. P., Billi, J. E., Böttiger, B. W., Bossaert, L., de Caen, A. R., & Zideman, D. et al. (2010). Part 1: Executive summary: 2010 International Consensus on Cardiopulmonary Resuscitation and Emergency Cardiovascular Care Science With Treatment Recommendations. *Circulation*, *122*(16Suppl 2), S250–S275. doi:10.1161/CIRCULATIONAHA.110.970897 PMID:20956249

Head, S. J., Kieser, T. M., Falk, V., Huysmans, H. A., & Kappetein, A. P. (2013). Coronary artery bypass grafting: Part 1 – the evolution over the first 50 years. *European Heart Journal*, *34*(37), 2862–2872. doi:10.1093/eurheartj/eht330 PMID:24086085

Healey, S., O'Neill, B., Bilal, H., & Waterworth, P. (2013). Does retraction of the sternum during median sternotomy result in brachial plexus injuries? *Interactive Cardiovascular and Thoracic Surgery*, *17*(1), 151–157. doi:10.1093/icvts/ivs565 PMID:23513004

Hébert, P. C., Wells, G., Blajchman, M. A., Marshall, J., Martin, C., Pagliarello, G., & Yetisir, E. et al. (1999). A multicenter, randomized, controlled clinical trial of transfusion requirements in critical care. Transfusion Requirements in Critical Care Investigators, Canadian Critical Care Trials Group. *The New England Journal of Medicine*, *340*(6), 409–417. doi:10.1056/NEJM199902113400601 PMID:9971864

Hedenstierna, G., Tokics, L., Strandberg, A., Lundquist, H., & Brismar, B. (1986). Correlation of gas exchange impairment to development of atelectasis during anaesthesia and muscle paralysis. *Acta Anaesthesiologica Scandinavica*, *30*(2), 183–191. doi:10.1111/j.1399-6576.1986.tb02393.x PMID:3085429

He, G.-W. (2013). Arterial grafts: Clinical classification and pharmacological management. *Annals of Cardiothoracic Surgery*, *2*(4), 507–518. doi:10.3978/j.issn.2225-319X.2013.07.12 PMID:23977630

Heidegger, C. P., Berger, M. M., Graf, S., Zingg, W., Darmon, P., Costanza, M. C., & Pichard, C. et al. (2013). Optimisation of energy provision with supplemental parenteral nutrition in critically ill patients: A randomised controlled clinical trial. *Lancet*, *381*(9864), 385–393. doi:10.1016/S0140-6736(12)61351-8 PMID:23218813

Heidegger, C. P., Graf, S., Thibault, R., Darmon, P., Berger, M., & Pichard, C. (2011). Supplemental parenteral nutrition (SPN) in intensive care unit (ICU) patients for optimal energy coverage: Improved clinical outcome. *Clinical Nutrition Supplements*, *1*(1), 2–3. doi:10.1016/S1744-1161(11)70006-0

Heilmann, C., Stahl, R., Schneider, C., Sukhodolya, T., Siepe, M., Olschewski, M., & Beyersdorf, F. (2013). Wound complications after median sternotomy: A single-center study. *Interactive Cardiovascular and Thoracic Surgery*, *16*(5), 643–648. doi:10.1093/icvts/ivs554 PMID:23355648

Hein, O. V., Birnbaum, J., Wernecke, K., England, M., Konertz, W., & Spies, C. (2006). Prolonged intensive care unit stay in cardiac surgery: Risk factors and long-term-survival. *The Annals of Thoracic Surgery*, *81*(3), 880–885. doi:10.1016/j.athoracsur.2005.09.077 PMID:16488688

Heller, J., Gabbay, J. S., Ghadjar, K., Jourabchi, M., O'Hara, C., Heller, M., & Bradley, J. P. (2006). Top-10 list of herbal and supplemental medicines used by cosmetic patients: what the plastic surgeon needs to know. *Plast Reconstr Surg*, *117*(2), 436-445; discussion 446-437. doi: 10.1097/01.prs.0000197217.46219.a7

Hemmerling, T. M., Cyr, S., & Terrasini, N. (2013). Epidural catheterization in cardiac surgery: The 2012 risk assessment. *Annals of Cardiac Anaesthesia*, *16*(3), 169–177. doi:10.4103/0971-9784.114237 PMID:23816670

Henderson, W. R., Griesdale, D. E., Walley, K. R., & Sheel, A. W. (2010). Clinical review: Guyton--the role of mean circulatory filling pressure and right atrial pressure in controlling cardiac output. *Critical Care (London, England)*, *14*(6), 243. doi:10.1186/cc9247 PMID:21144008

Henry, D. A. (Ed.). (2011). Anti-fibrinolytic use for minimising perioperative allogeneic blood transfusion. *Cochrane Database of Systematic Reviews*, (1): CD001886. PMID:21249650

Herbert, J. M., Frehel, D., Vallee, E., Kieffer, G., Gouy, D., Berger, Y., & Maffrand, J. P. et al. (1993). Clopidogrel, a novel antiplatelet and antithrombotic agent. *Cardiovascular Drug Reviews*, *11*(2), 180–198. doi:10.1111/j.1527-3466.1993.tb00275.x

Heringlake, M. G. C., & Kabler, J. H. (2011). Preoperative cerebral oxygen saturation and clinical outcomes in cardiac surgery. *Anesthesiology*, *114*(1), 58–69. doi:10.1097/ALN.0b013e3181fef34e PMID:21178669

Hermanides, J., Vriesendorp, T. M., Bosman, R. J., Zandstra, D. F., Hoekstra, J. B., & DeVries, J. H. (2010). Glucose variability is associated with intensive care unit mortality. *Critical Care Medicine*, *38*(3), 838–842. doi:10.1097/CCM.0b013e3181cc4be9 PMID:20035218

Herridge, M. S., Cheung, A. M., Tansey, C. M., Matte-Martyn, A., Diaz-Granados, N., Al-Saidi, F., & Slutsky, A. S. et al. (2003). One-year outcomes in survivors of the acute respiratory distress syndrome. *The New England Journal of Medicine*, *348*(8), 683–693. doi:10.1056/NEJMoa022450 PMID:12594312

Herridge, M. S., Tansey, C. M., Matte, A., Tomlinson, G., Diaz-Granados, N., Cooper, A., & Cheung, A. M. et al. (2011, April07). Cheung, A. M. Functional disability 5 years after acute respiratory distress syndrome. *The New England Journal of Medicine*, *364*(14), 1293–1304. doi:10.1056/NEJMoa1011802 PMID:21470008

Herzig, S. J., Howell, M. D., Ngo, L. H., & Marcantonio, E. R. (2009). Acid-suppressive medication use and the risk for hospital-acquired pneumonia. *Journal of the American Medical Association*, *301*(20), 2120–2128. doi:10.1001/jama.2009.722 PMID:19470989

Herzig, S. J., Rothberg, M. B., Feinbloom, D. B., Howell, M. D., Ho, K. K., Ngo, L. H., & Marcantonio, E. R. (2013). Risk factors for nosocomial gastrointestinal bleeding and use of acid-suppressive medication in non-critically ill patients. *Journal of General Internal Medicine*, *28*(5), 683–690. doi:10.1007/s11606-012-2296-x PMID:23292499

He, S., Chen, B., Li, W., Yan, J., Chen, L., Wang, X., & Xiao, Y. (2014). Ventilator-associated pneumonia after cardiac surgery: A meta-analysis and systematic review. *The Journal of Thoracic and Cardiovascular Surgery*, *148*(6), 3148–3155.e5. doi:10.1016/j.jtcvs.2014.07.107 PMID:25240522

Hess, D. R. (2005). Noninvasive positive-pressure ventilation and ventilator-associated pneumonia. *Respiratory Care*, *50*, 924–929. PMID:15972113

Hess, D. R., & Fessler, H. E. (2007). Respiratory controversies in the critical care setting. Should noninvasive positive-pressure ventilation be used in all forms of acute respiratory failure? *Respiratory Care*, *52*(5), 568–578, discussion 578–581. PMID:17484789

Hess, D. R., & MacIntyre, N. R. (2011). Ventilator discontinuation: Why are we still weaning? *American Journal of Respiratory and Critical Care Medicine*, *184*(4), 392–394. doi:10.1164/rccm.201105-0894ED PMID:21844511

Hessel, E. A. II, & Levy, J. H. (2010). Guidelines for perioperative blood transfusion and conservation in cardiac surgery: Lessons and challenges. *Anesthesia and Analgesia, 111*(6), 1555–1559. doi:10.1213/ANE.0b013e3181fbb386 PMID:21106971

Heyland, D. K., Dodek, P., Muscedere, J., Day, A., & Cook, D.Canadian Critical Care Trials Group. (2008). Randomized trial of combination versus monotherapy for the empiric treatment for suspected ventilator-associated pneumonia. *Critical Care Medicine, 36*(3), 737–744. doi:10.1097/01.CCM.0B013E31816203D6 PMID:18091545

Heyland, D. K., Drover, J. W., Dhaliwal, R., & Greenwood, J. (2002). Optimizing the benefits and minimizing the risks of enteral nutrition in the critically ill: Role of small bowel feeding. *Journal of Parenteral and Enteral Nutrition, 26*(6Suppl), S51–S55. doi:10.1177/014860710202600608 PMID:12405623

Heyland, D., Muscedere, J., Wischmeyer, P. E., Cook, D., Jones, G., Albert, M., & Day, A. G. et al. (2013). A randomized trial of glutamine and antioxidants in critically ill patients. *The New England Journal of Medicine, 368*(16), 1489–1497. doi:10.1056/NEJMoa1212722 PMID:23594003

Hidron, A. I., Edwards, J. R., Patel, J., Horan, T. C., Sievert, D. M., Pollock, D. A., & Fridkin, S. K. (2008). NHSN annual update: Antimicrobial-resistant pathogens associated with healthcare-associated infections: Annual summary of data reported to the National Healthcare Safety Network at the Centers for Disease Control and Prevention, 2006-2007. *Infection Control and Hospital Epidemiology, 29*(11), 996–1011. doi:10.1086/591861 PMID:18947320

Higenbottam, T., Pepke-Zaba, J., Scott, J., Woolman, P., Coutts, C., & Wallwork, J. (1988). Inhaled endothelial derived-relaxing factor (EDRF) in primary pulmonary hypertension (PPH). *The American Review of Respiratory Disease, 137*, A107.

Higgins, T. L., McGee, W. T., Steingrub, J. S., Rapoport, J., Lemeshow, S., & Teres, D. (2003). Early indicators of prolonged intensive care unit stay: Impact of illness severity, physician staffing, and pre-intensive care unit length of stay. *Critical Care Medicine, 31*(1), 45–51. doi:10.1097/00003246-200301000-00007 PMID:12544992

Hill, A. G., Yu, T.-C., Barrow, M., & Hattie, J. (2009). A systematic review of resident-as-teacher programmes. *Medical Education, 43*(12), 1129–1140. doi:10.1111/j.1365-2923.2009.03523.x PMID:19930503

Hillarp, A., Baghhaei, F., Bagerber Blixter, I., Gustafsson, K. M., Stigendal, L., Sten-Linder, M., & Lindahl, T. L. et al. (2011). Effects of oral, direct factor Xa inhibitor rivaroxaban on commonly used coagulation assays. *Journal of Thrombosis and Haemostasis, 9*(1), 133–139. doi:10.1111/j.1538-7836.2010.04098.x PMID:20946166

Hillis, L. D., Smith, P. K., Anderson, J. L., Bittl, J. A., Bridges, C. R., Byrne, J. G., et al. (2011). *2011 ACCF/AHA Guideline for Coronary Artery Bypass Graft Surgery: a report of the American College of Cardiology Foundation/American Heart Association Task Force on Practice Guidelines* (Vol. 124, pp. e652–735). ACCF/AHA.

Hillis, L. D., Smith, P. K., Anderson, J. L., Bittl, J., Bridges, C. R., Byrne, J. G., & Winniford, M. D. et al. (2011). ACCF/AHA Guideline for Coronary Artery Bypass Graft Surgery: executive summary: a report of the American College of Cardiology Foundation/American Heart Association Task Force on Practice Guidelines. *Circulation, 124*(23), 2610–2642. doi:10.1161/CIR.0b013e31823b5fee PMID:22064600

Hillis, L., Smith, P., Anderson, J., Bittl, J., Bridges, C., Byrne, J., & Puskas, J. et al. (2011). 2011 ACCF/AHA guideline for Coronary Artery Bypass Graft Surgery. *Circulation, 124*(23), e652–e735. doi:10.1161/CIR.0b013e31823c074e PMID:22064599

Hill, J. D., O'Brien, T. G., Murray, J. J., Dontigny, L., Bramson, M. L., Osborn, J. J., & Gerbode, F. (1972). Extracorporeal oxygenation for acute post-traumatic respiratory failure (shock-lung syndrome): Use of the Bramson membrane lung. *The New England Journal of Medicine, 286*, 629–634. doi:10.1056/NEJM197203232861204 PMID:5060491

Hill, N. (2013). Noninvasive Positive-Pressure Ventilation. In M. J. Tobin (Ed.), *Principles and practice of mechanical ventilation* (3rd ed.). New York: McGraw-Hill Medical.

Hill, S. A. (2004). Pharmacokinetics of drug infusions. *Continuing Education in Anaesthesia, Critical Care, and Pain, 4*(3), 76–80. doi:10.1093/bjaceaccp/mkh021

Hinson, J. A., Roberts, D. W., & James, L. P. (2010). Mechanisms of acetaminophen-induced liver necrosis. *Handbook of Experimental Pharmacology, 196*, 369–405. doi:10.1007/978-3-642-00663-0_12 PMID:20020268

Hirai, S. (2003). Systemic inflammatory response syndrome after cardiac surgery under cardiopulmonary bypass. *Annals of Thoracic and Cardiovascular Surgery, 9*, 365–370. PMID:15003097

Hiraoka, H., Yamamoto, K., Miyoshi, S., Morita, T., Nakamura, K., Kadoi, Y., & Horiuchi, R. et al. (2005). Kidneys contribute to the extrahepatic clearance of propofol in humans, but not lungs and brain. *British Journal of Clinical Pharmacology, 60*(2), 176–182. doi:10.1111/j.1365-2125.2005.02393.x PMID:16042671

Hirota, K., & Lambert, D. G. (1996). Ketamine: Its mechanism(s) of action and unusual clinical uses. *British Journal of Anaesthesia, 77*(4), 441–444. doi:10.1093/bja/77.4.441 PMID:8942324

Hirsh, J., Bauer, K. A., Donati, M. B., Gould, M., Samama, M. M., & Weitz, J. I. (2008). Parenteral anticoagulants: American College of Chest Physicians Evidence-Based Clinical Practice Guidelines (8th edition). Chest, 133(6 Suppl), 141S-159S.

Hirsh, J., Guyatt, G., Albers, G. W., Harrington, R., Schunemann, H. J., & American College of Chest, P. (2008). Antithrombotic and thrombolytic therapy: American College of Chest Physicians Evidence-Based Clinical Practice Guidelines (8th Edition). *Chest, 133*(6 Suppl), 110S-112S. doi: 10.1378/chest.08-0652

Hirsh, J., & Levine, M. N. (1992). Low molecular weight heparin. *Blood, 79*(1), 1–17. PMID:1309422

Hirst, J., Smithers, B., Gotley, D., Thomas, J., & Barbour, A. (2011). Defining Cure for Esophageal Cancer: Analysis of Actual 5-Year Survivors Following Esophagectomy. *Annals of Surgical Oncology, 18*(6), 1766–1774. doi:10.1245/s10434-010-1508-z PMID:21213056

Hlatky, M. A., Boothroyd, B. D., Bravata, D. M., Boersma, E., Booth, J., Brooks, M. M., & Pocock, S. J. et al. (2009). Coronary artery bypass surgery compared with percutaneous coronary interventions for multivessel disease: A collaborative analysis of individual patients data from ten randomised trials. *Lancet, 373*(9670), 1190–1197. doi:10.1016/S0140-6736(09)60552-3 PMID:19303634

Hochman, J., Sleeper, L., Webb, J., Sanborn, T., White, H., Talley, J., & LeJemtel, T. et al. (1999). Early Revascularization in Acute Myocardial Infarction Complicated by Cardiogenic Shock. *The New England Journal of Medicine, 341*(9), 625–634. doi:10.1056/NEJM199908263410901 PMID:10460813

Hockenhull, J. C., Dwan, K. M., Smith, G. W., Gamble, C. L., Boland, A., Walley, T. J., & Dickson, R. C. (2009). The clinical effectiveness of central venous catheters treated with anti-infective agents in preventing catheter-related bloodstream infections: A systematic review. *Critical Care Medicine, 37*(2), 702–712. doi:10.1097/CCM.0b013e3181958915 PMID:19114884

Hoekstra, H. J., Hawkins, K., de Boer, W. J., Rottier, K., & van der Bij, W. (2001). Gastrointestinal complications in lung transplant survivors that require surgical intervention. *British Journal of Surgery, 88*(3), 433–438. doi:10.1046/j.1365-2168.2001.01693.x

Hoen, B., Alla, F., Selton-Suty, C., Béguinot, I., Bouvet, A., & Briançon, S., … Vandenesch, F., for the Association pour l'Etude et la Prévention de l'Endocardite Infectieuse (AEPEI) Study Group. (. (2002). Changing profile of infective endocarditis. Results of a 1-year survey in France. *Journal of the American Medical Association*, *288*, 75–81. doi:10.1001/jama.288.1.75 PMID:12090865

Hoen, B., & Duval, X. (2013). Infective endocarditis. *The New England Journal of Medicine*, *368*(15), 1425–1433. doi:10.1056/NEJMcp1206782 PMID:23574121

Hoeper, M. M., Bogaard, H. J., Condliffe, R., Frantz, R., Khanna, D., Kurzyna, M., & Badesch, D. B. et al. (2013). Definitions and diagnosis of pulmonary hypertension. *Journal of the American College of Cardiology*, *62*(25Suppl), D42–D50. doi:10.1016/j.jacc.2013.10.032 PMID:24355641

Hoette, S., O'Callaghan, D., Jardim, C., & Souza, R. (2010). Dual receptor blockade by bosentan: Clinical experience in treatment of pulmonary hypertension. *Journal of Receptor. Ligand and Channel Research*, *3*, 113–121.

Hoffman, M., & Monroe, D. M. (2007). Coagulation 2006: A modern view of hemostasis. *Hematology/Oncology Clinics of North America*, *21*(1), 1–11. doi:10.1016/j.hoc.2006.11.004 PMID:17258114

Hoff, T. J., Pohl, H., & Bartfield, J. (2004). Creating a learning environment to produce competent residents: The roles of culture and context. *Academic Medicine*, *79*(6), 532–539. doi:10.1097/00001888-200406000-00007 PMID:15165972

Hofhuis, J. G., Spronk, P. E., van Stel, H. F., Schrijvers, G. J., Rommes, J. H., & Bakker, J. (2008). The impact of critical illness on perceived health-related quality of life during ICU treatment, hospital stay, and after hospital discharge: A long-term follow-up study. *Chest*, *133*(2), 377–385. doi:10.1378/chest.07-1217 PMID:17925419

Hogue, C. W. Jr, Lappas, G. D., Creswell, L. L., Ferguson, T. B. Jr, Sample, M., Pugh, D., & Lappas, D. G. et al. (1995). Swallowing dysfunction after cardiac operations. Associated adverse outcomes and risk factors including intraoperative transesophageal echocardiography. *The Journal of Thoracic and Cardiovascular Surgery*, *110*(2), 517–522. doi:10.1016/S0022-5223(95)70249-0 PMID:7637370

Hogue, C. W. Jr, Talke, P., Stein, P. K., Richardson, C., Domitrovich, P. P., & Sessler, D. I. (2002). Autonomic nervous system responses during sedative infusions of dexmedetomidine. *Anesthesiology*, *97*(3), 592–598. doi:10.1097/00000542-200209000-00012 PMID:12218525

Hohnloser, S., Kuck, K., Dorian, P., Roberts, R., Hampton, J., Hatala, R., & Connoly, S. et al. (2004). Prophylactic use of an implantable cardioverter-defibrillator after acute myocardial infarction. *The New England Journal of Medicine*, *351*(24), 2481–2488. doi:10.1056/NEJMoa041489 PMID:15590950

Ho, J., Reslerova, M., Gali, B., Nickerson, P. W., Rush, D. N., Sood, M. M., & Rigatto, C. et al. (2012). Serum creatinine measurement immediately after cardiac surgery and prediction of acute kidney injury. *American Journal of Kidney Diseases : The Official Journal of the National Kidney Foundation*, *59*(2), 196–201. doi:10.1053/j.ajkd.2011.08.023 PMID:21967775

Ho, K. M., Dobb, G. J., & Webb, S. A. R. (2006). A comparison of early gastric and post-pyloric feeding in critically ill patients: A meta-analysis. *Intensive Care Medicine*, *32*(5), 639–649. doi:10.1007/s00134-006-0128-3 PMID:16570149

Ho, K. M., & Tan, J. A. (2009). Benefits and risks of corticosteroid prophylaxis in adult cardiac surgery: A dose-response meta-analysis. *Circulation*, *119*(14), 1853–1866. doi:10.1161/CIRCULATIONAHA.108.848218 PMID:19332460

Ho, K. M., & Tan, J. A. (2011). Benefits and risks of maintaining normothermia during cardiopulmonary bypass in adult cardiac surgery: A systematic review. *Cardiovascular Therapeutics*, *29*(4), 260–279. doi:10.1111/j.1755-5922.2009.00114.x PMID:20041882

Hollander, J. M., & Mechanick, J. I. (2006). Nutrition support and the chronic critical illness syndrome. *Nutrition in Clinical Practice*, *21*(6), 587–604. doi:10.1177/0115426506021006587 PMID:17119165

Holland, L., Warkentin, T. E., Refaai, M., Crowther, M. A., Johnston, M. A., & Sarode, R. (2009). Suboptimal effect of a three-factor prothrombin complex concentrate (Profilnine-SD) in correcting supratherapeutic international normalized ratio due to warfarin overdose. *Transfusion*, *49*(6), 1171–1177. doi:10.1111/j.1537-2995.2008.02080.x PMID:19210325

Holland, T. L., Arnold, C., & Fowler, V. G. Jr. (2014). Clinical management of Staphylococcus aureus bacteremia. A review. *Journal of the American Medical Association*, *312*(13), 1330–1341. doi:10.1001/jama.2014.9743 PMID:25268440

Hollenberg, S. M. (2011). Vasoactive Drugs in Circulatory Shock. *American Journal of Respiratory and Critical Care Medicine*, *183*(7), 847–855. doi:10.1164/rccm.201006-0972CI PMID:21097695

Holmes, C. L., Patel, B. M., Russell, J. A., & Walley, K. R. (2001). Physiology of vasopressin relevant to management of septic shock. *Chest*, *120*(3), 989–1002. doi:10.1378/chest.120.3.989 PMID:11555538

Holmes, D. R. Jr, Dehmer, G. J., Kaul, S., Leifer, D., O'Gara, P. T., & Stein, M. (2010). ACCF/AHA clopidogrel clinical alert: approaches to the FDA "boxed warning": a report of the American College of Cardiology Foundation Task Force on clinical expert consensus documents and the American Heart Association endorsed by the Society for Cardiovascular Angiography and Interventions and the Society of Thoracic Surgeons. *Journal of the American College of Cardiology*, *65*(4), 321–341. doi:10.1016/j.jacc.2010.05.013 PMID:20633831

Holmes, D. R. Jr, Mack, M. J., Kaul, S., Agnihotri, A., Alexander, K. P., Bailey, S. R., & Thomas, J. D. et al. (2012). 2012 ACCF/AATS/SCAI/STS expert consensus document on transcatheter aortic valve replacement. *Journal of the American College of Cardiology*, *59*(13), 1200–1254. doi:10.1016/j.jacc.2012.01.001 PMID:22300974

Holmes, J. H. IV, Connolly, N. C., Paull, D. L., Hill, M. E., Guyton, S. W., Ziegler, S. F., & Hall, R. A. (2002). Magnitude of the inflammatory response to cardiopulmonary bypass and its relation to adverse clinical outcomes. *Inflammation Research*, *51*(12), 579–586. doi:10.1007/PL00012432 PMID:12558191

Holodinsky, J. K., Roberts, D. J., Ball, C. G., Reintam Blaser, A., Starkopf, J., & Zygun, D. (2013). Risk factors for intra-abdominal hypertension and abdominal compartment syndrome among adult intensive care unit patients: A systematic review and meta-analysis. *Critical Care (London, England)*, *17*(5), R249. doi:10.1186/cc13075 PMID:24144138

Hoogenberg, K., Smit, A. J., & Girbes, A. R. (1998). Effects of low-dose dopamine on renal and systemic hemodynamics during incremental norepinephrine infusion in healthy volunteers. *Critical Care Medicine*, *26*(2), 260–265. doi:10.1097/00003246-199802000-00022 PMID:9468162

Hooton, T. M., Bradley, S. F., Cardenas, D. D., Colgan, R., Geerlings, S. E., Rice, J. C., & Nicolle, L. E. et al. (2010). Diagnosis, prevention, and treatment of catheter-associated urinary tract infection in adults: 2009 international clinical practice guidelines from the Infectious Diseases Society of America. *Clinical Infectious Diseases*, *50*(5), 625–663. doi:10.1086/650482 PMID:20175247

Horan, T. C., Andrus, M., & Dudeck, M. A. (2008). CDC/NHSN surveillance definition of healthcare-associated infection and criteria for specific types of infections in the acute care setting. *American Journal of Infection Control*, *36*(5), 309–332. doi:10.1016/j.ajic.2008.03.002 PMID:18538699

Horstkotte, D., & Burckardt, D. (1995). Prosthetic valve thrombosis. *The Journal of Heart Valve Disease*, *4*(2), 141–153. PMID:8556174

Horstkotte, D., Niehues, R., & Strauer, E. (1991). Pathomorphological aspects, aetiology and natural history of acquired mitral valve stenosis. *European Heart Journal*, *12*(suppl B), 55–60. doi:10.1093/eurheartj/12.suppl_B.55 PMID:1936027

Hortal, J., Giannella, M., Perez, M. J., Barrio, J. M., Desco, M., Bouza, E., & Munoz, P. (2009). Incidence and risk factors for ventilator-associated pneumonia after major heart surgery. *Intensive Care Medicine*, *35*(9), 1518–1525. doi:10.1007/s00134-009-1523-3 PMID:19557389

Hosseinian, L., Chiang, Y., Itagaki, S., Polanco, A., Rhee, A., & Chikwe, J. (2014). Earlier versus later tracheostomy in patients with respiratory failure after cardiac surgery in the United States. *Journal of Cardiothoracic and Vascular Anesthesia*, *28*(3), 488–492. doi:10.1053/j.jvca.2013.07.023 PMID:24295717

Houlind, K., Kjeldsen, B. J., Madsen, S. N., Rasmussen, B. S., Holme, S. J., Nielsen, P. H., & Mortensen, P. E. (2012). On-pump versus off-pump coronary artery bypass surgery in elderly patients: Results from the Danish on-pump versus off-pump randomization study. *Circulation*, *125*(20), 2431–2439. doi:10.1161/CIRCULATIONAHA.111.052571 PMID:22523305

Howell, M. D., Novack, V., Grgurich, P., Soulliard, D., Novack, L., Pencina, M., & Talmor, D. (2010). Iatrogenic gastric acid suppression and the risk of nosocomial Clostridium difficile infection. *Archives of Internal Medicine*, *170*(9), 784–790. doi:10.1001/archinternmed.2010.89 PMID:20458086

Hruska, L. A., Smith, J. M., Hendy, M. P., Fritz, V. L., & McAdams, S. (2005). Continuous insulin infusion reduces infectious complications in diabetics following coronary surgery. *Journal of Cardiac Surgery*, *20*(5), 403–407. doi:10.1111/j.1540-8191.2005.200472.x PMID:16153268

Hsu, P.-S., Chen, J.-L., Hong, G.-J., Tsai, Y.-T., Lin, C.-Y., & Lee, C.-Y. et al.. (2010). Extracorporeal membrane oxygenation for refractory cardiogenic shock after cardiac surgery: Predictors of early mortality and outcome from 51 adult patients. *European Journal of Cardio-Thoracic Surgery: Official Journal of the European Association for Cardio-Thoracic Surgery*, *37*(2), 328–333. doi:10.1016/j.ejcts.2009.07.033 PMID:19748279

Hsu, Y. J., Weeks, K., Yang, T., Sawyer, M. D., & Marsteller, J. A. (2014). Impact of self-reported guideline compliance: Bloodstream infection prevention in a national collaborative. *American Journal of Infection Control*, *42*(10Suppl), S191–S196. doi:10.1016/j.ajic.2014.05.010 PMID:25239709

Hua, M. S., Li, G., Blinderman, C. D., & Wunsch, H. (2014). Estimates of the Need for Palliative Care Consultation across United States Intensive Care Units Using a Trigger-based Model. *American Journal of Respiratory and Critical Care Medicine*, *189*(4), 428–436. doi:10.1164/rccm.201307-1229OC PMID:24261961

Huang, C. T., Tsai, Y. J., Tsai, P. R., & Ko, W. J. (2013). Extracorporeal membrane oxygenation resuscitation in adult patients with refractory septic shock. *The Journal of Thoracic and Cardiovascular Surgery*, *146*(5), 1041–1046. doi:10.1016/j.jtcvs.2012.08.022 PMID:22959322

Huang, D. T., Clermont, G., Kong, L., Weissfeld, L. A., Sexton, J. B., Rowan, K. M., & Angus, D. C. (2010). Intensive care unit safety culture and outcomes: A US multicenter study. *International Journal for Quality in Health Care*, *22*(3), 151–161. doi:10.1093/intqhc/mzq017 PMID:20382662

Huang, J., Cao, Y., Liao, C., Wu, L., & Gao, F. (2010). Effect of histamine-2-receptor antagonists versus sucralfate on stress ulcer prophylaxis in mechanically ventilated patients: A meta-analysis of 10 randomized controlled trials. *Critical Care (London, England)*, *14*(5), R194. doi:10.1186/cc9312 PMID:21034484

Huang, S. J., & McLean, A. S. (2012). Appreciating the Strengths and Weaknesses of Transthoracic Echocardiography in Hemodynamic Assessments. *Cardiology Research and Practice*, *2012*, 1–7. doi:10.1155/2012/894308 PMID:22454777

Huang, S. S., Yokoe, D. S., Hinrichsen, V. L., Spurchise, L. S., Datta, R., Miroshnik, I., & Platt, R. (2006). Impact of routine intensive care unit surveillance cultures and resultant barrier precautions on hospital-wide methicillin-resistant Staphylococcus aureus bacteremia. *Clinical Infectious Diseases*, *43*(8), 971–978. doi:10.1086/507636 PMID:16983607

Huang, S., Datta, R., & Platt, R. (2006). Risk of acquiring antibiotic-resistant bacteria from previous room occupants. *Archives of Internal Medicine*, *166*(18), 1945–1951. doi:10.1001/archinte.166.18.1945 PMID:17030826

Huber, C. H., Goeber, V., Berdat, P., Carrel, T., & Eckstein, F. (2007). Benefits of cardiac surgery in octogenarians--a postoperative quality of life assessment. *European Journal of Cardio-Thoracic Surgery*, *31*(6), 1099–1105. doi:10.1016/j.ejcts.2007.01.055 PMID:17369044

Hudetz, J. A., Iqbal, Z., Gandhi, S. D., Patterson, K. M., Byrne, A. J., & Pagel, P. S. (2011). Postoperative delirium and short-term cognitive dysfunction occur more frequently in patients undergoing valve surgery with or without coronary artery bypass graft surgery compared with coronary artery bypass graft surgery alone: Results of a pilot study. *Journal of Cardiothoracic and Vascular Anesthesia*, *25*(5), 811–816. doi:10.1053/j.jvca.2010.05.003 PMID:20655248

Hudetz, J. A., Patterson, K. M., Iqbal, Z., Gandhi, S. D., Byrne, A. J., Hudetz, A. G., & Pagel, P. S. et al. (2009). Ketamine attenuates delirium after cardiac surgery with cardiopulmonary bypass. *Journal of Cardiothoracic and Vascular Anesthesia*, *23*(5), 651–657. doi:10.1053/j.jvca.2008.12.021 PMID:19231245

Hug, C. C. Jr, Murphy, M. R., Rigel, E. P., & Olson, W. A. (1981). Pharmacokinetics of morphine injected intravenously into the anesthetized dog. *Anesthesiology*, *54*(1), 38–47. doi:10.1097/00000542-198101000-00008 PMID:7457981

Hughes, M. A., Glass, P. S. A., & Jacobs, J. R. (1992). Context-sensitive half-time in multicompartment pharmacokinetic models for intravenous anesthetic drugs. *Anesthesiology*, *76*(3), 334–341. doi:10.1097/00000542-199203000-00003 PMID:1539843

Hugonnet, S., Chevrolet, J., & Pittet, D. (2007). The effect of workload on infection risk in critically ill patients. *Critical Care Medicine*, *35*(1), 76–81. doi:10.1097/01.CCM.0000251125.08629.3F PMID:17095946

Hu, K. K., Lipsky, B. A., Veenstra, D. L., & Saint, S. (2004). Using maximal sterile barriers to prevent central venous catheter-related infection: A systematic evidence-based review. *American Journal of Infection Control*, *32*(3), 142–146. doi:10.1016/j.ajic.2003.10.006 PMID:15153925

Hulscher, J., Sandick, J., Boer, A., Wijnhoven, B., Tijssen, J., Fockens, P., & Lanschot, J. et al. (2002). Extended Transthoracic Resection Compared with Limited Transhiatal Resection for Adenocarcinoma of the Esophagus. *The New England Journal of Medicine*, *347*(21), 1662–1669. doi:10.1056/NEJMoa022343 PMID:12444180

Hulzebos, E. H., Helders, P. J., Favié, N. J., De Bie, R. A., Brutel de la Riviere, A., & Van Meeteren, N. L. (2006). Preoperative intensive inspiratory muscle training to prevent postoperative pulmonary complications in high-risk patients undergoing CABG surgery: A randomized clinical trial. *Journal of the American Medical Association*, *296*(15), 1851–1857. doi:10.1001/jama.296.15.1851 PMID:17047215

Humphrey, H. J. (2010). *Mentoring in Academic Medicine* (1st ed.). Philadelphia: American College of Physicians.

Hundert, E. M., Douglas-Steele, D., & Bickel, J. (1996). Context in medical education: The informal ethics curriculum. *Medical Education*, *30*(5), 353–364. doi:10.1111/j.1365-2923.1996.tb00847.x PMID:8949475

Hunt, S. A., Abraham, W. T., Chin, M. H., Feldman, A. M., Francis, G. S., Ganiats, T. G., . . . Yancy, C. W. (2009). 2009 Focused Update Incorporated Into The Acc/Aha 2005 Guidelines For The Diagnosis And Management Of Heart Failure In Adults: A Report Of The American College Of Cardiology Foundation/American Heart Association Task Force On Practice Guidelines Developed In Collaboration With The International Society For Heart And Lung Transplantation. *Journal Of The American College Of Cardiology, 53*(15), E1-E90. Retrieved from http://www.sciencedirect.com/science/article/pii/s0735109708038023

Hunter, G. R., & Young, G. B. (2011). Seizures after cardiac surgery. *Journal of Cardiothoracic and Vascular Anesthesia*, *25*(2), 299–305. doi:10.1053/j.jvca.2010.08.004 PMID:21036061

Hunziker, S., Tschan, F., Semmer, N. K., Zobrist, R., Spychiger, M., Breuer, M., & Marsch, S. C. et al. (2009). Hands-on time during cardiopulmonary resuscitation is affected by the process of teambuilding: A prospective randomised simulator-based trial. *BMC Emergency Medicine*, *9*(1), 3. doi:10.1186/1471-227X-9-3 PMID:19216796

Husain, F. A., Martin, M. J., Mullenix, P. S., Steele, S. R., & Elliott, D. C. (2003). Serum lactate and base deficit as predictors of mortality and morbidity. *American Journal of Surgery*, *185*(5), 485–491. doi:10.1016/S0002-9610(03)00044-8 PMID:12727572

Hussain, S. I., Gilkeson, R. C., Suarez, J. I., Tarr, R., Schluchter, M., Landis, D. M., & Zaidat, O. O. (2008). Comparing multislice electrocardiogram-gated spiral computerized tomography and transesophageal echocardiography in evaluating aortic atheroma in patients with acute ischemic stroke. *Journal of Stroke and Cerebrovascular Diseases*, *17*(3), 134–140. doi:10.1016/j.jstrokecerebrovasdis.2007.12.008 PMID:18436154

Hylek, E. M., Evans-Molina, C., Shea, C., Henault, L., & Regan, S. (2007). Major hemorrhage and tolerability of warfarin in the first year of therapy among elderly patients with atrial fibrillation. *Circulation*, *115*(21), 2689–2696. doi:10.1161/CIRCULATIONAHA.106.653048 PMID:17515465

Ibanez, B., Macaya, C., Sánchez-Brunete, V., Pizarro, G., Fernández-Friera, L., Mateos, A., & Fuster, V. et al. (2013). Effect of Early Metoprolol on Infarct Size in ST-Segment-Elevation Myocardial Infarction Patients Undergoing Primary Percutaneous Coronary Intervention. *Circulation*, *128*(14), 1495–1503. doi:10.1161/CIRCULATIONAHA.113.003653 PMID:24002794

Ibañez, J., Riera, M., Anezaga, R., Herrero, J., Colomar, A., & Campillo-Artero, C. … Bonnin, O. (2014). Long-term mortality after pneumonia in cardiac surgery patients.: A propensity-matched analysis. *Journal of Intensive Care Medicine*; Advance online publication. doi:10.1177/0885066614523918

Ibrahim, K. S., Vitale, N., Tromsdal, A., Kirkeby-Garstad, I., Fraser, A. G., & Haaverstad, R. (2008). Enhanced intra-operative grading of ascending aorta atheroma by epiaortic ultrasound vs echocardiography. *International Journal of Cardiology*, *128*(2), 218–223. doi:10.1016/j.ijcard.2007.05.035 PMID:17643531

Ichinose, F., Roberts, J. D., & Zapol, W. M. (2004). Inhaled Nitric Oxide: A Selective Pulmonary Vasodilator: Current Uses and Therapeutic Potential. *Circulation*, *109*(25), 3106–3111. doi:10.1161/01.CIR.0000134595.80170.62 PMID:15226227

Immer, F. F., Ackermann, A., Gygax, E., Stalder, M., Englberger, L., Eckstein, F. S., & Carrel, T. P. et al. (2007). Minimal extracorporeal circulation is a promising technique for coronary artery bypass grafting. *The Annals of Thoracic Surgery*, *84*(5), 1515–1520, discussion 1521. doi:10.1016/j.athoracsur.2007.05.069 PMID:17954055

Imrie, C. W., McKay, A. J., Benjamin, I. S., & Blumgart, L. H. (1978). Secondary acute pancreatitis: Aetiology, prevention, diagnosis and management. *British Journal of Surgery*, *65*(6), 399–402. doi:10.1002/bjs.1800650609 PMID:656756

Ingraham, A. M., Cohen, M. E., Bilimoria, K. Y., Dimick, J. B., Richards, K. E., Raval, M. V., & Ko, C. Y. et al. (2010). Association of surgical care improvement project infection-related process measure compliance with risk-adjusted outcomes: Implications for quality measurement. *Journal of the American College of Surgeons*, *211*(6), 705–714. doi:10.1016/j.jamcollsurg.2010.09.006 PMID:21109157

Inhaled Nitric Oxide/INOpulse for Pulmonary Arterial Hypertension. (2015). In *ClinicalTrials.gov*. Retrieved from http://clinicaltrials.gov/ct2/show/record/NCT01457781

Innouye, S., Dyck, C., Alessi, C., & Balkin, S. (1990). Clarifying confusion: the confusion assessment. *Ann Intern Med*. Retrieved from http://scholar.google.com/scholar?hl=en&btnG=Search&q=intitle:Clarifying+confusion:+the+confusion+assessment#1

Inouye, S. K., Bogardus, S. T. Jr, Charpentier, P. A., Leo-Summers, L., Acampora, D., Holford, T. R., & Cooney, L. M. Jr. (1999). A multicomponent intervention to prevent delirium in hospitalized older patients. *The New England Journal of Medicine*, *340*(9), 669–676. doi:10.1056/NEJM199903043400901 PMID:10053175

Iobst, W. F., Sherbino, J., Cate, O. T., Richardson, D. L., Dath, D., Swing, S. R., & Frank, J. R. et al. (2010). Competency-based medical education in postgraduate medical education. *Medical Teacher*, *32*(8), 651–656. doi:10.3109/0142159X.2010.500709 PMID:20662576

Iregui, M., Ward, S., Sherman, G., Fraser, V., & Kollef, M. (2002). Clinical importance of delays in the initiation of appropriate antibiotic treatment for ventilator-associated pneumonia. *Chest*, *122*(1), 262–268. doi:10.1378/chest.122.1.262 PMID:12114368

Irshad, K., Feldman, L., Chu, V., Dorval, J., Baslaim, G., & Morin, J. (2002). Causes of increased length of hospitalization on a general thoracic surgery service: A prospective observational study. *Canadian Journal of Surgery*, *45*(4), 264–268. PMID:12174980

Ishikawa, S., Kugawa, S., Neya, K., Suzuki, Y., Kawasaki, A., Hayama, T., & Ueda, K. (2006). Hemodynamic effects of dexmedetomidine in patients after cardiac surgery. *Minerva Chirurgica*, *61*, 215–219. PMID:16858303

Issenberg, S. B. (2006). The scope of simulation-based healthcare education. *Simulation in Healthcare: the Journal of the Society for Simulation in Healthcare*, *1*(4), 203–208. doi:10.1097/01.SIH.0000246607.36504.5a PMID:19088590

Issenberg, S. B., McGaghie, W. C., Petrusa, E. R., Gordon, D. L., & Scalese, R. J. (2005). Features and uses of high-fidelity medical simulations that lead to effective learning: A BEME systematic review. *Medical Teacher*, *27*(1), 10–28. doi:10.1080/01421590500046924 PMID:16147767

Iung, B., Gohlke-Barwolf, C., Tornos, P., Tribouilloy, C., Hall, R., Butchart, E., & Vahanian, A. (2002). Recommendations on the management of the asymptomatic patient with valvular heart disease. *European Heart Journal*, *23*(16), 1253–1266. doi:10.1053/euhj.2002.3320 PMID:12698958

Iung, B., & Vahanian, A. (2014). Epidemiology of Acquired Valvular Heart Disease. *The Canadian Journal of Cardiology*, *30*(9), 962–970. doi:10.1016/j.cjca.2014.03.022 PMID:24986049

Ivankovich, A. D., Braverman, B., Stephens, T. S., Shulman, M., & Heyman, H. J. (1983). Sodium thiosulfate disposition in humans: Relation to sodium nitroprusside toxicity. *Anesthesiology*, *58*(1), 11–17. doi:10.1097/00000542-198301000-00003 PMID:6600205

Iyer, D., Rastogi, P., Åneman, A., & D'Amours, S. (2014). Early screening to identify patients at risk of developing intra-abdominal hypertension and abdominal compartment syndrome. *Acta Anaesthesiologica Scandinavica*, *58*(10), 1267–1275. doi:10.1111/aas.12409 PMID:25307712

Izuha, H., Hattori, M., Igari, T., Wakamatsu, D., Watanabe, M., & Yokoyama, H. (2005). Changes in platelet aggregation during cardiopulmonary bypass: Comparison of poly-2-methoxyethylacrylate and heparin as a circuit coating material. *Journal of Artificial Organs*, *8*(1), 41–46. doi:10.1007/s10047-004-0280-x PMID:15951979

Jabbari, A. (2013). Serum lactate as a prognostic factor in coronary artery bypass graft operation by on pump method. *Caspian Journal of Internal Medicine*, *4*(2), 662–666. PMID:24009956

Jabbar, U., Leischner, J., Kasper, D., Gerber, R., Sambol, S. P., Parada, J. P., & Gerding, D. N. et al. (2010). Effectiveness of alcohol-based hand rubs for removal of Clostridium difficile spores from hands. *Infection Control and Hospital Epidemiology*, *31*(6), 565–570. doi:10.1086/652772 PMID:20429659

Jackson, A. P. F., Dhadphale, P. R., Callaghan, M. L., & Alseri, S. (1978). Haemodynamic studies during induction of anaesthesia for open-heart surgery using diazepam and ketamine. *British Journal of Anaesthesia*, *50*(4), 375–377. doi:10.1093/bja/50.4.375 PMID:656254

Jacobi, J., Fraser, G. L., Coursin, D. B., Riker, R. R., Fontaine, D., Wittbrodt, E. T., & Lumb, P. D. et al. (2002). … Lumb, P.D. (2002). Clinical practice guidelines for the sustained use of sedatives and analgesics in the critically ill adult: Sedation and Analgesia Task Force of the American College of Critical Care Medicine. *Critical Care Medicine*, *30*(1), 119–141. doi:10.1097/00003246-200201000-00020 PMID:11902253

Jacob, K. A., Nathoe, H. M., Dieleman, J. M., van Osch, D., Kluin, J., & van Dijk, D. (2014). Inflammation in new-onset atrial fibrillation after cardiac surgery. *European Journal of Clinical Investigation*, *44*(4), 402–408. doi:10.1111/eci.12237 PMID:24387767

Jacob, M., Smedira, N., Blackstone, E., Williams, S., & Cho, L. (2011). Effect of timing of chronic preoperative aspirin discontinuation on morbidity and mortality in coronary artery bypass surgery. *Circulation*, *123*(6), 577–583. doi:10.1161/CIRCULATIONAHA.110.957373 PMID:21282503

Jacobsohn, E., Lee, T. W., Amadeo, R. J., Syslak, P. H., Debrouwere, R. G., Bell, D., & Avidan, M. et al. (2005). Low-dose intrathecal morphine does not delay early extubation after cardiac surgery. *Canadian Journal of Anaesthesia*, *52*, 848–857. PMID:16189338

Jaeger, J. M., & Blank, R. S. (2011). Essential Anatomy and Physiology of the Respiratory System and the Pulmonary Circulation. In P. D. Slinger (Ed.), *Principles and Practice of Anesthesia for Thoracic Surgery* (pp. 51–69). New York: Springer. doi:10.1007/978-1-4419-0184-2_4

Jaïs, X., D'Armini, A. M., Jansa, P., Torbicki, A., Delcroix, M., Ghofrani, H. A., & Rubin, L. J. et al. (2008). Bosentan for treatment of inoperable chronic thromboembolic pulmonary hypertension. *Journal of the American College of Cardiology*, *52*(25), 2127–2134. doi:10.1016/j.jacc.2008.08.059 PMID:19095129

Jakob, S. M., Ruokonen, E., Grounds, M., Sarapohja, T., Garratt, C., Pocock, S. J., & Takala, J. et al. (2012). Dexmedetomidine vs. midazolam of propofol for sedation during prolonged mechanical ventilation: Two randomized controlled trials. *Journal of the American Medical Association*, *307*(11), 1151–1160. doi:10.1001/jama.2012.304 PMID:22436955

Jamieson, W. R., Ye, J., Higgins, J., Cheung, A., Fradet, G. J., Skarsgard, P., & Lichtenstein, S. V. et al. (2010). Effect of prosthesis-patient mismatch on long-term survival with aortic valve replacement: Assessment to 15 years. *The Annals of Thoracic Surgery*, *89*(1), 51–58, discussion 59. doi:10.1016/j.athoracsur.2009.08.070 PMID:20103205

Jarvis, W. R. (2003). Benchmarking for prevention: The Centers for Disease Control and Prevention's National Nosocomial Infections Surveillance (NNIS) system experience. *Infection*, *31*(Suppl 2), 44–48. PMID:15018472

Jauch, E. C., Saver, J. L., Adams, H. P. Jr, Bruno, A., Connors, J. J., Demaerschalk, B. M., & Yonas, H. et al. (2013). Guidelines for the early management of patients with acute ischemic stroke: A guideline for healthcare professionals from the American Heart Association/American Stroke Association. *Stroke*, *44*(3), 870–947. doi:10.1161/STR.0b013e318284056a PMID:23370205

Jellish, W. S., Blakeman, B., Warf, P., & Slogoff, S. (1997). Hands-up position during asymmetric sternal retraction for internal mammary artery harvest: A possible method to reduce brachialplexus injury. *Anesthesia and Analgesia*, *84*, 260. PMID:9024012

Jenkins, I. (2007). Linezolid- and vancomycin-resistant Enterococcus faecium endocarditis: Successful treatment with tigecycline and daptomycin. *Journal of Hospital Medicine*, *5*(5), 343–344. doi:10.1002/jhm.236 PMID:17935250

Jennings, D. L., & Thompson, M. L. (2009). Use of combination therapy with a beta-blocker and milrinone in patients with advanced heart failure. *The Annals of Pharmacotherapy*, *43*(11), 1872–1876. doi:10.1345/aph.1M357 PMID:19789358

Jensen, M. B., Sloth, E., Larsen, K. M., & Schmidt, M. B. (2004). Transthoracic echocardiography for cardiopulmonary monitoring in intensive care. *European Journal of Anaesthesiology*, *21*(9), 700–707. doi:10.1097/00003643-200409000-00006 PMID:15595582

Jernigan, J. A., Titus, M. G., Gröschel, D. H., Getchell-White, S., & Farr, B. M. (1996). Effectiveness of contact isolation during a hospital outbreak of methicillin-resistant Staphylococcus aureus. *American Journal of Epidemiology*, *143*(5), 496–504. doi:10.1093/oxfordjournals.aje.a008770 PMID:8610665

Jia, H., Abtahian, F., Aguirre, A., Lee, S., Chia, S., Lowe, H., & Jang, I. et al. (2013). In Vivo Diagnosis of Plaque Erosion and Calcified Nodule in Patients With Acute Coronary Syndrome by Intravascular Optical Coherence Tomography. *Journal of the American College of Cardiology*, *62*(19), 1748–1758. doi:10.1016/j.jacc.2013.05.071 PMID:23810884

Jneid, H., Anderson, J. L., Wright, R. S., Adams, C. D., Bridges, C. R., Casey, D. E. Jr, & Zidar, J. P. et al. (2012). 2012 ACCF/AHA focused update of the guideline for the management of patients with unstable angina/non-ST-elevation myocardial infarction (updating the 2007 guideline and replacing the 2011 focused update): A report of the American College of Cardiology Foundation/American Heart Association Task Force on Practice Guidelines. *Journal of the American College of Cardiology*, *60*(7), 645–681. doi:10.1016/j.jacc.2012.06.004 PMID:22809746

Johnson, J. R., Kuskowski, M. A., & Wilt, T. J. (2006). Systematic review: Antimicrobial urinary catheters to prevent catheter-associated urinary tract infection in hospitalized patients. *Annals of Internal Medicine*, *144*(2), 116–126. doi:10.7326/0003-4819-144-2-200601170-00009 PMID:16418411

Jokinen, J., Smith, A. F., Roewer, N., Eberhart, L. H. J., & Kranke, P. (2012). Management of Postoperative Nausea and Vomiting. How to Deal with Refractory PONV. *Anesthesiology Clinics*, *30*(3), 481–493. doi:10.1016/j.anclin.2012.07.003 PMID:22989590

Jones, C., Griffiths, R. D., Humphris, G., & Skirrow, P. M. (2001). Memory, delusions, and the development of acute posttraumatic stress disorder-related symptoms after intensive care. *Critical Care Medicine*, *29*(3), 573–580. doi:10.1097/00003246-200103000-00019 PMID:11373423

Jongman, R. M., Zijlstra, J. G., Kok, W. F., van Harten, A. E., Mariani, M. A., Moser, J., & van Meurs, M. et al. (2014). Off-pump CABG surgery reduces systemic inflammation compared wth on-pump surgery but does not change systemic endothelial responses: A prospective randomized study. *Shock (Augusta, Ga.)*, *42*, 121–128. doi:10.1097/SHK.0000000000000190 PMID:24727871

Jordan, B., & Devi, L. A. (1998). Molecular mechanisms of opioid receptor signal transduction. *British Journal of Anaesthesia*, *81*(1), 12–19. doi:10.1093/bja/81.1.12 PMID:9771268

Jordan, S., Mitchell, J. A., Quinlan, G. J., Goldstraw, P., & Evans, T. W. (2000). The pathogenesis of lung injury following pulmonary resection. *The European Respiratory Journal*, *15*(4), 790–799. doi:10.1034/j.1399-3003.2000.15d26.x PMID:10780775

Josa, M., Siouffi, S. Y., Silverman, A. B., Barsamian, E. M., Khuri, S. F., & Sharma, G. V. (1993). Pulmonary embolism after cardiac surgery. *Journal of the American College of Cardiology*, *21*(4), 990–996. doi:10.1016/0735-1097(93)90358-8 PMID:8450170

Joshi, G. P., Bonnet, F., Shah, R., Wilkinson, R. C., Camu, F., Fischer, B., & Kehlet, H. et al. (2008). A systemic review of randomized trials evaluating regional techniques for postthoracotomy analgesia. *Anesthesia and Analgesia*, *107*(3), 1026–1040. doi:10.1213/01.ane.0000333274.63501.ff PMID:18713924

Jox, R. J., Schaider, A., Marckmann, G., & Borasio, G. D. (2012). Medical futility at the end of life: The perspectives of intensive care and palliative care clinicians. *Journal of Medical Ethics*, *38*(9), 540–545. doi:10.1136/medethics-2011-100479 PMID:22562948

Judson, M. A., Handy, J. R., & Sahn, S. A. (1996). Pleural effusions following lung transplantation. Time course, characteristics, and clinical implications. *Chest Journal*, *109*(5), 1190–1194. doi:10.1378/chest.109.5.1190 PMID:8625665

Judson, M. A., Handy, J. R., & Sahn, S. A. (1997). Pleural effusion from acute lung rejection. *Chest Journal*, *111*(4), 1128–1130. doi:10.1378/chest.111.4.1128 PMID:9106602

Kahn, J. M., Werner, R. M., David, G., Ten Have, T. R., Benson, N. M., & Asch, D. A. (2013). Effectiveness of long-term acute care hospitalization in elderly patients with chronic critical illness. *Medical Care*, *51*(1), 4–10. doi:10.1097/MLR.0b013e31826528a7 PMID:22874500

Kajdacsy-Balla Amaral, A. C., Barros, B. S., Barros, C. C., Innes, C., Pinto, R., & Rubenfeld, G. D. (2014). Nighttime cross-coverage is associated with decreased intensive care unit mortality. A single-center study. *American Journal of Respiratory and Critical Care Medicine*, *189*(11), 1395–1401. doi:10.1164/rccm.201312-2181OC PMID:24779652

Kaki, R., Elligsen, M., Walker, S., Simor, A., Palmay, L., & Daneman, N. (2011). Impact of antibiotic stewardship in critical care: A systematic review. *The Journal of Antimicrobial Chemotherapy*, *66*(6), 1223–1230. doi:10.1093/jac/dkr137 PMID:21460369

Kalanuria, A. A., Zai, W., & Mirski, M. (2014). Ventilator-associated pneumonia in the ICU. *Critical Care (London, England)*, *18*(2), 208. doi:10.1186/cc13775 PMID:25029020

Kalil, A. C., Van Schooneveld, T. C., Fey, P. D., & Rupp, M. E. (2014). Association between vancomycin minimum inhibitory concentration and mortality among patients with Staphylococcus aureus bloodstream infections. A systematic review and meta-analysis. *Journal of the American Medical Association*, *312*(15), 1552–1564. doi:10.1001/jama.2014.6364 PMID:25321910

Kalina, U., Bickhard, H., & Schulte, S. (2008). Biochemical comparison of seven commercially available prothrombin complex concentrates. *International Journal of Clinical Practice*, *62*(10), 1614–1622. doi:10.1111/j.1742-1241.2008.01859.x PMID:18691229

Kambhampati, S., Park, W., Habtezion, A., Kambhampati, S., Park, W., & Habtezion, A. (2014). Pharmacologic therapy for acute pancreatitis. *World Journal of Gastroenterology*, *20*(45), 16868–16880. doi:10.3748/wjg.v20.i45.16868 PMID:25493000

Kamdar, B. B., King, L. M., Collop, N. A., Sakamuri, S., Colantuoni, E., Neufeld, K. J., & Needham, D. M. et al. (2013). The effect of a quality improvement intervention on perceived sleep quality & cognition in a medical ICU. *Critical Care Medicine*, *41*(3), 800–809. doi:10.1097/CCM.0b013e3182746442 PMID:23314584

Kam, P. C. A., & Cardone, D. (2007). Propofol infusion syndrome. *Anaesthesia*, *62*(7), 690–701. doi:10.1111/j.1365-2044.2007.05055.x PMID:17567345

Kang, C., Chung, D. R., Son, J. S., Ko, K. S., Peck, K. R., & Song, J.Korean Network for Study of Infectious Diseases (KONSID). (2011). Clinical significance of nosocomial acquisition in urinary tract-related bacteremia caused by gram-negative bacilli. *American Journal of Infection Control*, *39*(2), 135–140. doi:10.1016/j.ajic.2010.03.022 PMID:21176996

Kang, D., Kim, Y., Kim, S., Sun, B. J., Kim, D., Yun, S., & Sohn, D. et al. (2012). Early surgery versus conventional treatment for infective endocarditis. *The New England Journal of Medicine*, *366*(26), 2466–2473. doi:10.1056/NEJMoa1112843 PMID:22738096

Kanto, J., & Gepts, E. (1989). Pharmacokinetic implications for the clinical use of propofol. *Clinical Pharmacokinetics*, *17*(5), 308–326. doi:10.2165/00003088-198917050-00002 PMID:2684471

Kantrowitz, A., Tjonneland, S., Freed, P. S., Phillips, S. J., Butner, A. N., & Sherman, J. L. (1968). Initial clinical experience with intraaortic balloon pumping in cardiogenic shock. *Journal of the American Medical Association*, *203*(2), 113–118. doi:10.1001/jama.1968.03140020041011 PMID:5694059

Kaplan, J. A. (2008). *Essentials of Cardiac Anesthesia*. Philadelphia, PA: Saunders.

Kapoor, P. M., Kakani, M., Chowdhury, U., Choudhury, M., Lakshmy, R., & Kiran, U. (2008). Early goal-directed therapy in moderate to high-risk cardiac surgery patients. *Annals of Cardiac Anaesthesia*, *11*(1), 27–34. doi:10.4103/0971-9784.38446 PMID:18182756

Kappetein, A. P., Head, S. J., Genereux, P., Piazza, N., van Mieghem, N. M., Blackstone, E. H., & Leon, M. B. et al. (2012). Updated standardized endpoint definitions for transcatheter aortic valve implantation: The Valve Academic Research Consortium-2 consensus document. *Journal of the American College of Cardiology*, *60*(15), 1438–1454. doi:10.1016/j.jacc.2012.09.001 PMID:23036636

Kapur, A., Hall, R. J., Malik, I. S., Qureshi, A. C., Butts, J., de Belder, M., & Beatt, K. J. et al. (2010). Randomized comparison of percutaneous coronary intervention with coronary artery bypass grafting in diabetic patients. 1-year results of the CARDia (Coronary Artery Revascularization in Diabetes) trial. *Journal of the American College of Cardiology*, *55*(5), 432–440. doi:10.1016/j.jacc.2009.10.014 PMID:20117456

Karkouti, K. (2012). Transfusion and risk of acute kidney injury in cardiac surgery. *British Journal of Anaesthesia*, *109*(suppl 1), i29–i38. doi:10.1093/bja/aes422 PMID:23242748

Karkouti, K., Callum, J., Crowther, M. A., McCluskey, S. A., Pendergrast, J., Tait, G., & Beattie, W. S. et al. (2013). The relationship between fibrinogen levels after cardiopulmonary bypass and large volume red cell transfusion in cardiac surgery: An observational study. *Anesthesia and Analgesia*, *117*(1), 14–22. doi:10.1213/ANE.0b013e318292efa4 PMID:23687229

Karkouti, K., Djaiani, G., Borger, M. A., Beattie, W. S., Fedorko, L., Wijeysundera, D., & Karski, J. et al. (2005). Low hematocrit during cardiopulmonary bypass is associated with increased risk of perioperative stroke in cardiac surgery. *The Annals of Thoracic Surgery*, *80*(4), 1381–1387. doi:10.1016/j.athoracsur.2005.03.137 PMID:16181875

Karkouti, K., von Heymann, C., Jespersen, C. M., Korte, W., Levy, J. H., Ranucci, M., & Song, H. K. et al. (2013). Efficacy and safety of recombinant factor XIII on reducing blood transfusions in cardiac surgery: A randomized, placebo-controlled, multicenter clinical trial. *The Journal of Thoracic and Cardiovascular Surgery*, *146*(4), 927–939. doi:10.1016/j.jtcvs.2013.04.044 PMID:23820174

Karkouti, K., Wijeysundera, D. N., & Beattie, W. S.Reducing Bleeding in Cardiac Surgery (RBC) Investigators. (2008a). Risk associated with preoperative anemia in cardiac surgery: A multicenter cohort study. *Circulation*, *117*(4), 478–484. doi:10.1161/CIRCULATIONAHA.107.718353 PMID:18172032

Karkouti, K., Wijeysundera, D. N., Yau, T. M., Callum, J. L., Cheng, D. C., Crowther, M., & Beattie, W. S. et al. (2009). Acute kidney injury after cardiac surgery: Focus on modifiable risk factors. *Circulation*, *119*(4), 495–502. doi:10.1161/CIRCULATIONAHA.108.786913 PMID:19153273

Karkouti, K., Wijeysundera, D. N., Yau, T. M., McCluskey, S. A., van Rensburg, A., & Beattie, W. S. (2008b). The influence of baseline hemoglobin concentration on tolerance of anemia in cardiac surgery. *Transfusion*, *48*(4), 666–672. doi:10.1111/j.1537-2995.2007.01590.x PMID:18194382

Karlsson, M., Ternstrom, L., Hyllner, M., Baghaei, F., Flinck, A., Skrtic, S., & Jeppsson, A. (2009). Prophylactic fibrinogen infusion reduces bleeding after coronary artery bypass surgery. A prospective randomised pilot study. *Thrombosis and Haemostasis*, *102*(1), 137–144. doi:10.1160/TH08-09-0587 PMID:19572078

Karlsson, M., Ternström, L., Hyllner, M., Baghaei, F., Nilsson, S., & Jeppsson, A. (2008). Plasma fibrinogen level, bleeding, and transfusion after on-pump coronary artery bypass grafting surgery: A prospective observational study. *Transfusion*, *48*(10), 2152–2158. doi:10.1111/j.1537-2995.2008.01827.x PMID:18657083

Karthik, S., Grayson, A. D., McCarron, E. E., Pullan, D. M., & Desmond, M. J. (2004). Reexploration for bleeding after coronary artery bypass surgery: risk factors, outcomes, and the effect of time delay. *The Annals of Thoracic Surgery*, *78*(2), 527–34– discussion 534.

Karthik, S., Grayson, A. D., McCarron, E. E., Pullan, D. M., & Desmond, M. J. (2004). Reexploration for bleeding after coronary artery bypass surgery: Risk factors, outcomes, and the effect of time delay. *The Annals of Thoracic Surgery*, *78*(2), 527–534, discussion 534. doi:10.1016/j.athoracsur.2004.02.088 PMID:15276512

Karvellas, C. J., Farhat, M. R., Sajjad, I., Mogensen, S. S., Leung, A. A., Wald, R., & Bagshaw, S. M. (2011). A comparison of early versus late initiation of renal replacement therapy in critically ill patients with acute kidney injury: A systematic review and meta-analysis. *Critical Care (London, England)*, *15*(1), R72. PMID:21352532

Kastrati, A., Mehilli, J., Pache, J., Kaiser, C., Valgimigli, M., Kelbaek, H., & Schömig, A. et al. (2007). Analysis of 14 trials comparing sirolimus-eluting stents with bare-metal stents. *The New England Journal of Medicine*, *356*(10), 1030–1039. doi:10.1056/NEJMoa067484 PMID:17296823

Kato, R., Sato, J., & Nishino, T. (1998). Milrinone decreases both pulmonary arterial and venous resistances in the hypoxic dog. *British Journal of Anaesthesia*, *81*(6), 920–924. doi:10.1093/bja/81.6.920 PMID:10211020

Kats, S., Schönberger, J. P., Brands, R., Seinen, W., & van Oeveren, W. (2011). Endotoxin release in cardiac surgery with cardiopulmonary bypass: Pathophysiology and possible therapeutic strategies. An update. *European Journal of Cardio-Thoracic Surgery*, *39*(4), 451–458. doi:10.1016/j.ejcts.2010.06.011 PMID:20663682

Katz, A. M. (1996). Calcium channel diversity in the cardiovascular system. *Journal of the American College of Cardiology*, *28*(2), 522–529. doi:10.1016/0735-1097(96)00170-2 PMID:8800134

Katz, J. N., Jensen, B. C., Chang, P. P., Myers, S. L., Pagani, F. D., & Kirklin, J. K. (2015). A multicenter analysis of clinical hemolysis in patients supported with durable, long-term left ventricular assist device therapy. *The Journal of Heart and Lung Transplantation*, *34*(5), 701–709. doi:10.1016/j.healun.2014.10.002 PMID:25582036

Katz, N. M. (2011). The evolution of cardiothoracic critical care. *The Journal of Thoracic and Cardiovascular Surgery*, *141*(1), 3–6. doi:10.1016/j.jtcvs.2010.09.005 PMID:21168010

Katznelson, R., Djaiani, G., Tait, G., Wasowicz, M., Sutherland, A. M., Styra, R., … Beattie, W. S. (2010). Hospital administrative database underestimates delirium rate after cardiac surgery. *Canadian Journal of Anaesthesia = Journal Canadien D'anesthésie*, *57*(10), 898–902. doi:10.1007/s12630-010-9355-8

Kaul, P., Newby, L. K., Fu, Y., Hasselblad, V., Mahaffey, K., Christenson, R., & Armstrong, P. et al. (2003). Troponin T and Quantitative ST-Segment Depression Offer Complementary Prognostic Information in the Risk Stratification of Acute Coronary Syndrome Patients. *Journal of the American College of Cardiology*, *41*(3), 371–380. doi:10.1016/S0735-1097(02)02824-3 PMID:12575962

Kaw, R., Pasupuleti, V., Deshpande, A., Hamieh, T., Walker, E., & Minai, O. A. (2011). Pulmonary hypertension: An important predictor of outcomes in patients undergoing non-cardiac surgery. *Respiratory Medicine*, *105*(4), 619–624. doi:10.1016/j.rmed.2010.12.006 PMID:21195595

Kehara, H., Takano, T., Ohashi, N., Terasaki, T., & Amano, J. (2014). Platelet Function During Cardiopulmonary Bypass Using Multiple Electrode Aggregometry: Comparison of Centrifugal and Roller Pumps. *Artificial Organs*, *38*(11), 924–930. doi:10.1111/aor.12299 PMID:24720284

Kehlet, H., & Holte, K. (2001). Review of postoperative ileus. *American Journal Surgery, 182*(5A Suppl), 3S–10S.

Keith, J. D., Rowe, R. D., & Vlad, P. (1978). *Heart Disease in Infancy and Childhood* (3rd ed.). New York, NY: MacMillan.

Kellermann, K., & Jungwirth, B. (2010). Avoiding stroke during cardiac surgery. *Seminars in Cardiothoracic and Vascular Anesthesia*, *14*(2), 95–101. doi:10.1177/1089253210370902 PMID:20478949

Kelly, A. M., Weldon, D., Tsang, A. Y., & Graham, C. A. (2006). Comparison between two methods for estimating pneumothorax size from chest X-rays. *Respiratory Medicine*, *100*(8), 1356–1359. doi:10.1016/j.rmed.2005.11.022 PMID:16406560

Kelly, A. V. (2009). *The Curriculum* (6th ed.). London: SAGE Publications.

Kelly, D. M., Kutney-Lee, A., McHugh, M. D., Sloane, D. M., & Aiken, L. H. (2014). Impact of critical care nursing on 30-day mortality of mechanically ventilated older adults. *Critical Care Medicine*, *42*(5), 1089–1095. doi:10.1097/CCM.0000000000000127 PMID:24368346

Kelton, J. G. (2002). Heparin induced thrombocytopenia: An overview. *Blood Reviews*, *16*(1), 77–80. doi:10.1054/blre.2001.0189 PMID:11914002

Kenchaiah, S., Evans, J., Levy, D., Wilson, P., Benjamin, E., Larson, M., & Vasan, R. et al. (2002). Obesity and the risk of heart failure. *The New England Journal of Medicine*, *347*(5), 305–313. doi:10.1056/NEJMoa020245 PMID:12151467

Kendall, A., Landers, T., Kirk, J., & Young, E. (2012). Point-of-care hand hygiene: Preventing infection behind the curtain. *American Journal of Infection Control*, *40*(4), S3–S10. doi:10.1016/j.ajic.2012.02.009 PMID:22546271

Kepler, C. K., Huang, R. C., Meredith, D., Kim, J. H., & Sharma, A. K. (2012). Omega-3 and fish oil supplements do not cause increased bleeding during spinal decompression surgery. *Journal of Spinal Disorders & Techniques*, *25*(3), 129–132. doi:10.1097/BSD.0b013e3182120227 PMID:21423055

Keren, H. (2007). Evaluation of a noninvasive continuous cardiac output monitoring system based on thoracic bioreactance. *The American Journal of Physiology*, *293*, H583–H589. PMID:17384132

Kerlin, M. P., Harhay, M. O., Kahn, J. M., & Halpern, S. D. (2014). Nighttime Intensivist Staffing, Mortality, and Limits on Life Support: A Retrospective Cohort Study. *Chest*. doi:10.1378/chest.14-0501 PMID:25321489

Kerlin, M. P., Small, D. S., Cooney, E., Fuchs, B. D., Bellini, L. M., Mikkelsen, M. E., & Halpern, S. D. et al. (2013). A randomized trial of nighttime physician staffing in an intensive care unit. *The New England Journal of Medicine*, *368*(23), 2201–2209. doi:10.1056/NEJMoa1302854 PMID:23688301

Keroack, M. A., Youngberg, B. J., Cerese, J. L., Krsek, C., Prellwitz, L. W., & Trevelyan, E. W. (2007). Organizational factors associated with high performance in quality and safety in academic medical centers. *Academic Medicine*, *82*(12), 1178–1186. doi:10.1097/ACM.0b013e318159e1ff PMID:18046123

Kett, D. H., Azoulay, E., Echeverria, P. M., & Vincent, J.Extended Prevalence of Infection in the ICU Study. (2011). Candida bloodstream infections in intensive care units: Analysis of the extended prevalence of infection in intensive care unit study. *Critical Care Medicine*, *39*(4), 665–670. doi:10.1097/CCM.0b013e318206c1ca PMID:21169817

Kett, D. H., Cano, E., Quartin, A. A., Mangino, J. E., Zervos, M. J., Peyrani, P., & Ramirez, J. A. et al. (2011). Implementation of guidelines for management of possible multidrug-resistant pneumonia in intensive care: An observational, multicentre cohort study. *The Lancet Infectious Diseases*, *11*(3), 181–189. doi:10.1016/S1473-3099(10)70314-5 PMID:21256086

Keusch, G. T. (2003). The history of nutrition: Malnutrition, infection and immunity. *The Journal of Nutrition*, *133*, 336S–340S. PMID:12514322

Key, J. A., Kergin, F. G., Martineau, Y., & Leckey, R. G. (1954). A method of supplementing the coronary circulation by a jejunal pedicle graft. *The Journal of Thoracic Surgery*, *28*, 320–330. PMID:13192879

Khan, N. E. D., & Mister, R. (2004). A randomized comparison of Off-pump and On-pump multivessel coronary-artery bypass surgery. *2004*, *350*, 21-28.

Khan, N. E., De Souza, A., Mister, R., Flather, M., Clague, J., Davies, S., & Pepper, J. et al. (2004). A randomized comparison of off-pump and on-pump multivessel coronary-artery bypass surgery. *The New England Journal of Medicine*, *350*(1), 21–28. doi:10.1056/NEJMoa031282 PMID:14702424

Khatri, P. J., Webb, J. G., Rodes-Cabau, J., Fremes, S. E., Ruel, M., Lau, K., & Ko, D. T. et al. (2013). Adverse effects associated with transcatheter aortic valve implantation: A meta-analysis of contemporary studies. *Annals of Internal Medicine*, *158*(1), 35–46. doi:10.7326/0003-4819-158-1-201301010-00007 PMID:23277899

Khot, U. N., Novaro, G. M., Popović, Z. B., Mills, R. M., Thomas, J. D., Tuzcu, E. M., & Francis, G. S. et al. (2003). Nitroprusside in critically ill patients with left ventricular dysfunction and aortic stenosis. *The New England Journal of Medicine*, *348*(18), 1756–1763. doi:10.1056/NEJMoa022021 PMID:12724481

Khot, U., Jia, G., Moliterno, D., Lincoff, A., Khot, M., Harrington, R., & Topol, E. (2003). Prognostic Importance of Physical Examination for Heart Failure in Non–ST-Elevation Acute Coronary Syndromes. *Journal of the American Medical Association*, *290*(16), 2174–2181. doi:10.1001/jama.290.16.2174 PMID:14570953

Khuri, S. F., Wolfe, J. A., Josa, M., Axford, T. C., Szymanski, I., & Assousa, S. et al.. (1992). Hematologic changes during and after cardiopulmonary bypass and their relationship to the bleeding time and nonsurgical blood loss. *The Journal of Thoracic and Cardiovascular Surgery*, *104*(1), 94–107. PMID:1614220

Kidney Disease; Improving Global Outcomes (KDIGO) Acute Kidney Injury Work Group. (2012). KDIGO Clinical Practice Guideline for Acute Kidney Injury. *Kidney International. Supplement*, *2*(1), 1–138.

Kidney DiseaseImproving Global Outcomes (KDIGO) CKD Work Group. (2012). Notice. *Kidney International. Supplement*, *2*(1), 1–138. doi:10.1038/kisup.2012.1 PMID:25028630

Kiefer, T., Park, L., Tribouilloy, C., Cortes, C., Casillo, R., Chu, V., & ICE-PCS Investigators, et al.. (2011). Association between valvular surgery and mortality among patients with infective endocarditis complicated by heart failure. *Journal of the American Medical Association*, *306*(20), 2239–2247. doi:10.1001/jama.2011.1701 PMID:22110106

Kiely, D. G., Cargill, R. I., & Lipworth, B. J. (1996). Angiotensin II receptor blockade and effects on pulmonary hemodynamics and hypoxic pulmonary vasoconstriction in humans. *Chest Journal*, *110*(3), 698–703. doi:10.1378/chest.110.3.698 PMID:8797414

Kiessling, A., Reyher, C., Philipp, M., Beiras-fernandez, A., & Moritz, A. (2015). Real-Time Measurement of Rectal Mucosal Microcirculation During Cardiopulmonary Bypass. *Journal of Cardiothoracic and Vascular Anesthesia*, *29*(1), 89–94. doi:10.1053/j.jvca.2014.07.003 PMID:25440640

Kihara, S., Kawai, A., Fukuda, T., Yamamoto, N., Aomi, S., Nishida, H., & Koyanagi, H. et al. (2002). Effects of milrinone for right ventricular failure after left ventricular assist device implantation. *Heart and Vessels*, *16*(2), 69–71. doi:10.1007/s380-002-8320-z PMID:11833845

Kilger, E., Weis, F., Briegel, J., Frey, L., Goetz, A. E., Reuter, D., & Peter, K. et al. (2003). Stress doses of hydrocortisone reduce severe systemic inflammatory response syndrome and improve early outcome in a risk group of patients after cardiac surgery. *Critical Care Medicine*, *31*(4), 1068–1074. doi:10.1097/01.CCM.0000059646.89546.98 PMID:12682474

Kilminster, S., Cottrell, D., Grant, J., & Jolly, B. (2007). AMEE Guide No. 27: Effective educational and clinical supervision. *Medical Teacher*, *29*(1), 2–19. doi:10.1080/01421590701210907 PMID:17538823

Kirk, R., Edwards, L. B., Aurora, P., Taylor, D. O., Christie, J. D., Dobbels, F., . . . Hertz, M. I. (2009). Registry Of The International Society For Heart And Lung Transplantation: Twelfth Official Pediatric Heart Transplantation Report–2009. *The Journal Of Heart And Lung Transplantation, 28*(10), 993-1006. Retrieved From http://www.jhltonline.org/article/s1053-2498(09)00634-2/abstract

Kirklin, J. K., Naftel, D. C., Pagani, F. D., Kormos, R. L., Stevenson, L. W., Blume, E. D., & Young, J. B. et al. (2014). Sixth INTERMACS annual report: A 10,000-patient database. *The Journal of Heart and Lung Transplantation*, *33*(6), 555–564. doi:10.1016/j.healun.2014.04.010 PMID:24856259

Kirklin, J. K., Naftel, D. C., Pagani, F. D., Kormos, R. L., Stevenson, L., Miller, M., & Young, J. B. (2012). Long-term mechanical circulatory support (destination therapy): On track to compete with heart transplantation? *The Journal of Thoracic and Cardiovascular Surgery*, *144*(3), 584–603. doi:10.1016/j.jtcvs.2012.05.044 PMID:22795459

Kirklin, J., Naftel, D., Kormos, R., Stevenson, L., Pagani, F., Ph, D., & Young, J. et al. (2013). Fifth INTERMACS annual report: Risk factor analysis from more than 6,000 mechanical circulatory support patients. *The Journal of Heart and Lung Transplantation*, *32*(2), 141–156. doi:10.1016/j.healun.2012.12.004 PMID:23352390

Kirsh, M. M., Magee, K. R., Gago, O., Kahn, D. R., & Sloan, H. (1971). Brachial plexus injury following median sternotomy incision. *The Annals of Thoracic Surgery*, *11*(4), 315–319. doi:10.1016/S0003-4975(10)65455-0 PMID:4927044

Kissin, I., Bright, C. A., & Bradley, E. L. Jr. (2000). The effect of ketamine on opioid-induced acute tolerance: Can it explain reduction of opioid consumption with ketamine-opioid analgesic combinations? *Anesthesia and Analgesia*, *91*(6), 1483–1488. doi:10.1097/00000539-200012000-00035 PMID:11094005

Kitsios, G. D., Mascari, P., Ettunsi, R., & Gray, A. W. (2014). Co-administration of furosemide with albumin for overcoming diuretic resistance in patients with hypoalbuminemia: A meta-analysis. *Journal of Critical Care*, *29*(2), 253–259. doi:10.1016/j.jcrc.2013.10.004 PMID:24268626

Kittleson, M., Hurwitz, S., Shah, M., Nohria, A., Lewis, E., Givertz, M., & Stevenson, L. et al. (2003). Development of circulatory-renal limitations to angiotensin-converting enzyme inhibitors identifies patients with severe heart failure and early mortality. *Journal of the American College of Cardiology*, *41*(11), 2029–2035. doi:10.1016/S0735-1097(03)00417-0 PMID:12798577

Kivikko, M., Antila, S., Eha, J., Lehtonen, L., & Pentikäinen, P. J. (2002). Pharmacodynamics and safety of a new calcium sensitizer, levosimendan, and its metabolites during an extended infusion in patients with severe heart failure. *Journal of Clinical Pharmacology*, *42*(1), 43–51. doi:10.1177/0091270002042001005 PMID:11808823

Klabunde, R. (2012). *Nitric Oxide*. Retrieved from www.cvphysiology.com/bloodflow/BF011.htm

Klabunde, R. (2012). *Nitrodilators*. Retrieved from http://www.cvpharmacology.com/vasodilator/nitro.htm

Klevens, R. M., Edwards, J. R., Richards, C. L. Jr, Horan, T. C., Gaynes, R. P., Pollock, D. A., & Cardo, D. M. (2007). Estimating health care-associated infections and deaths in U.S. hospitals, 2002. *Public Health Reports*, *122*, 160–166. PMID:17357358

Klip, A., Tsakiridis, T., Marrette, A., & Ortiz, P. A. (1994). Regulation of expression of glucose transporters by glucose: A review of studies in vivo and in cell cultures. *The FASEB Journal*, *8*, 43–53. PMID:8299889

Klocke. (1991). Thoracic Electrical Bioimpedance Alternative or Complement in Cardio-pulmonary Exercise Testing? *Computerized Cardiopulmonary Exercise Testing*, 63-70.

Klompas, M. (2007). Does this patient have ventilator-associated pneumonia? *Journal of the American Medical Association*, *297*(14), 1583–1593. doi:10.1001/jama.297.14.1583 PMID:17426278

Klompas, M. (2010). Prevention of ventilator-associated pneumonia. *Expert Review of Anti-Infective Therapy*, *8*(7), 791–800. doi:10.1586/eri.10.59 PMID:20586564

Klompas, M. (2013). Complications of mechanical ventilation – The CDC's new surveillance paradigm. *The New England Journal of Medicine*, *368*(16), 1472–1475. doi:10.1056/NEJMp1300633 PMID:23594002

Klompas, M., Branson, R., Eichenwald, E. C., Greene, L. R., Howell, M. D., Lee, G., & Berenholtz, S. M. et al. (2014). Strategies to prevent ventilator-associated pneumonia in acute care hospitals: 2014 update. *Infection Control and Hospital Epidemiology*, *35*(8), 915–936. doi:10.1086/677144 PMID:25026607

Klompas, M., Speck, K., Howell, M. D., Greene, L. R., & Berenholtz, S. M. (2014). Reappraisal of routine oral care with chlorhexidine gluconate for patients receiving mechanical ventilation: Systematic review and meta-analysis. *JAMA Internal Medicine*, *174*(5), 751–761. doi:10.1001/jamainternmed.2014.359 PMID:24663255

Klovaite, J., Gustafsson, F., Mortensen, S. A., Sander, K., & Nielsen, L. B. (2009). Severely impaired von Willebrand factor-dependent platelet aggregation in patients with a continuous-flow left ventricular assist device (HeartMate II). *Journal of the American College of Cardiology*, *53*(23), 2162–2167. doi:10.1016/j.jacc.2009.02.048 PMID:19497443

Kneebone, R. L., Nestel, D., Vincent, C., & Darzi, A. (2007). Complexity, risk and simulation in learning procedural skills. *Medical Education*, *41*(8), 808–814. doi:10.1111/j.1365-2923.2007.02799.x PMID:17661889

Kneebone, R., Nestel, D., Wetzel, C., Black, S., Jacklin, R., Aggarwal, R., & Darzi, A. et al. (2006). The human face of simulation: Patient-focused simulation training. *Academic Medicine*, *81*(10), 919–924. doi:10.1097/01.ACM.0000238323.73623.c2 PMID:16985358

Knowles, M. S., Holton, E. F. III, & Swanson, R. A. (2011). *The Adult Learner* (7th ed.). Woburn: Butterworth-Heinemann.

Kobal, S. L., Trento, L., Baharami, S., Tolstrup, K., Naqvi, T. Z., Cercek, B., & Siegel, R. J. et al. (2005). Comparison of effectiveness of hand-carried ultrasound to bedside cardiovascular physical examination. *The American Journal of Cardiology*, *96*(7), 1002–1006. doi:10.1016/j.amjcard.2005.05.060 PMID:16188532

Kobashigawa, J. A. (2012). The Future Of Heart Transplantation. *American Journal Of Transplantation, 12*(11), 2875-2891. doi:10.1111/j.1600-6143.2012.04223.x

Kobashigawa, J. A., Miller, L. W., Russell, S. D., Ewald, G. A., Zucker, M. J., Goldberg, L. R., ... First, R. and the study Investigators (2006). Tacrolimus With Mycophenolate Mofetil (Mmf) Or Sirolimus Vs. Cyclosporine With Mmf In Cardiac Transplant Patients: 1-Year Report. *American Journal Of Transplantation, 6*(6), 1377-1386. doi:10.1111/j.1600-6143.2006.01290.x

Kobashigawa, J., Miller, L., Renlund, D., Mentzer, R., Alderman, E., Bourge, R., ... Valentine, H. The Mycophenolate Mofetil Investigators (1998). A Randomized Active-Controlled Trial Of Mycophenolate Mofetil In Heart Transplant Recipients. *Transplantation, 66*(4). Retrieved from http://journals.lww.com/transplantjournal/fulltext/1998/08270/a_randomized_active_controlled_trial_of.16.aspx

Kobayashi, M., Horvath, D. J., Mielke, N., Shiose, A., Kuban, B., Goodin, M., & Golding, L. A. et al. (2012). Progress on the design and development of the continuous-flow total artificial heart. *Artificial Organs*, *36*(8), 705–713. doi:10.1111/j.1525-1594.2012.01489.x PMID:22747979

Koch, C. G., Li, L., Duncan, A. I., Mihaljevic, T., Cosgrove, D. M., Loop, F. D., & Blackstone, E. H. et al. (2006). Morbidity and mortality risk associated with red blood cell and blood-component transfusion in isolated coronary artery bypass grafting. *Critical Care Medicine*, *34*(6), 1608–1616. doi:10.1097/01.CCM.0000217920.48559.D8 PMID:16607235

Koch, C. G., Li, L., Sessler, D. I., Figueroa, P., Hoeltge, G. A., Mihaljevic, T., & Blackstone, E. H. (2008). Duration of red-cell storage and complications after cardiac surgery. *The New England Journal of Medicine*, *358*(12), 1229–1239. doi:10.1056/NEJMoa070403 PMID:18354101

Kodali, S. K., Williams, M. R., Smith, C. R., Svensson, L. G., Webb, J. G., & Makkar, R. R. et al. Investigators, Partner Trial. (2012). Two-year outcomes after transcatheter or surgical aortic-valve replacement. *The New England Journal of Medicine*, *366*(18), 1686–1695. doi:10.1056/NEJMoa1200384 PMID:22443479

Koerber, J. M., Smythe, M. A., Begle, R. L., Mattson, J. C., Kershaw, B. P., & Westley, S. J. (1999). Correlation of activated clotting time and activated partial thromboplastin time to plasma heparin concentration. *Pharmacotherapy*, *19*(8), 922–931. doi:10.1592/phco.19.11.922.31573 PMID:10453963

Kogan, A., Preisman, S., Berkenstadt, H., Segal, E., Kassif, Y., Sternik, L., & Raanani, E. et al. (2013). Evaluation of the impact of a quality improvement program and intensivist-directed ICU team on mortality after cardiac surgery. *Journal of Cardiothoracic and Vascular Anesthesia*, *27*(6), 1194–1200. doi:10.1053/j.jvca.2013.02.028 PMID:24008163

Kohman, L., Meyer, J., Ikins, P., & Oates, R. (1986). Random versus predictable risks of mortality after thoracotomy for lung cancer. *The Journal of Thoracic and Cardiovascular Surgery*, *91*(4). PMID:3959574

Kohn, L. T., Corrigan, J. M., & Donaldson, M. S. (2000). *To err is human: building a safer health system* (p. 287). Washington, D.C.: National Academy Press.

Kolh, P., Lahaye, L., Gerard, P., & Limet, R. (1999). Aortic valve replacement in the octogenarians: Perioperative outcome and clinical follow-up. *European Journal of Cardio-Thoracic Surgery*, *16*(1), 68–73. doi:10.1016/S1010-7940(99)00146-3 PMID:10456406

Kollef, M. H. (1999). Epidemiology and risk factors for nosocomial pneumonia. Emphasis on prevention. *Clinics in Chest Medicine*, *20*(3), 653–670. doi:10.1016/S0272-5231(05)70242-2 PMID:10516910

Kollef, M. H., Afessa, B., Anzueto, A., Veremakis, C., Kerr, K. M., & Margolis, B. D. (2008). Silver-coated endotracheal tubes and incidence of ventilator-associated pneumonia. The NASCENT randomized trial. *Journal of the American Medical Association*, *300*(7), 805–813. doi:10.1001/jama.300.7.805 PMID:18714060

Kollef, M. H., Sharpless, L., Vlasnik, J., Pasque, C., Murphy, D., & Fraser, V. J. (1997). The impact of nosocomial infections on patient outcomes following cardiac surgery. *Chest*, *112*(3), 666–675. doi:10.1378/chest.112.3.666 PMID:9315799

Kononowicz, A. A., & Hege, I. (2014). Virtual patients as a practical realisation of the e-learning idea in medicine. In S. Soomro (Ed.), *E-learning Experiences and Future* (pp. 345–370). Intech; doi:10.5772/8803

Konvalinka, A., Errett, L., & Fong, I. W. (2006). Impact of treating Staphylococcus aureus nasal carriers on wound infections in cardiac surgery. *The Journal of Hospital Infection*, *64*(2), 162–168. doi:10.1016/j.jhin.2006.06.010 PMID:16930768

Kornfeld, D. S., Heller, S. S., & Frank, K. a, & Moskowitz, R. (1974). Personality and psychological factors in post-cardiotomy delirium. *Archives of General Psychiatry*, *31*(2), 249–53. Retrieved from http://www.ncbi.nlm.nih.gov/pubmed/4853590

Kory, P. D., Pellecchia, C. M., Shiloh, A. L., Mayo, P. H., DiBello, C., & Koenig, S. (2011). Accuracy of ultrasonography performed by critical care physicians for the diagnosis of DVT. *Chest*, *139*(3), 538–542. doi:10.1378/chest.10-1479 PMID:21030490

Koster, A., Dyke, C. M., Aldea, G., Smedira, N. G., McCarthy, H. L. II, Aronson, S., & Lincoff, A. M. et al. (2007). Bivalirudin during cardiopulmonary bypass in patients with previous or acute heparin-induced thrombocytopenia and heparin antibodies: Results of the CHOOSE-ON trial. *The Annals of Thoracic Surgery*, *83*(2), 572–577. doi:10.1016/j.athoracsur.2006.09.038 PMID:17257990

Koster, A., & Schirmer, U. (2011). Re-evaluation of the role of antifibrinolytic therapy with lysine analogs during cardiac surgery in the post aprotinin era. *Current Opinion in Anaesthesiology*, *24*(1), 92–97. doi:10.1097/ACO.0b013e32833ff3eb PMID:20881484

Koster, S., Hensens, A. G., Schuurmans, M. J., & van der Palen, J. (2012). Consequences of delirium after cardiac operations. *The Annals of Thoracic Surgery*, *93*(3), 705–711. doi:10.1016/j.athoracsur.2011.07.006 PMID:21992939

Koster, S., Hensens, A. G., Schuurmans, M. J., & van der Palen, J. (2013). Prediction of delirium after cardiac surgery and the use of a risk checklist. *European Journal of Cardiovascular Nursing : Journal of the Working Group on Cardiovascular Nursing of the European Society of Cardiology*, *12*(3), 284–292. doi:10.1177/1474515112450244 PMID:22694810

Koster, S., Hensens, A. G., & van der Palen, J. (2009). The long-term cognitive and functional outcomes of postoperative delirium after cardiac surgery. *The Annals of Thoracic Surgery*, *87*(5), 1469–1474. doi:10.1016/j.athoracsur.2009.02.080 PMID:19379886

Kotloff, R. M., & Thabut, G. (2011). Lung transplantation. *American Journal of Respiratory and Critical Care Medicine*, *184*(2), 159–171. doi:10.1164/rccm.201101-0134CI

Koval, C. E., Thuita, L., Moazami, N., & Blackstone, E. (2014). Evolution and impact of drive-line infection in a large cohort of continuous-flow ventricular assist device recipients. *The Journal of Heart and Lung Transplantation*, *33*(11), 1164–1172. doi:10.1016/j.healun.2014.05.011 PMID:25034793

Kowey, P., Stebbins, D., Igidbashian, L., Goldman, S., Sutter, F., Rials, S., & Marinchak, R. (2001). Clinical Outcome of Patients Who Develop PAF After CABG Surgery. *Pacing and Clinical Electrophysiology*, *24*(2), 191–193. doi:10.1046/j.1460-9592.2001.00191.x PMID:11270698

Kozar, R. A., McQuiggan, M. M., Moore, E. E., Kudsk, K. A., Jurkovich, G. J., & Moore, F. A. (2002). Postinjury enteral tolerance is reliably achieved by a standardized protocol. *The Journal of Surgical Research*, *104*(1), 70–75. doi:10.1006/jsre.2002.6409 PMID:11971680

Kozek-Langenecker, S. A. (2010). Perioperative coagulation monitoring. *Best Practice & Research. Clinical Anaesthesiology*, *24*(1), 27–40. doi:10.1016/j.bpa.2009.09.009 PMID:20402168

Krag, M., Perner, A., Wetterslev, J., Wise, M. P., & Hylander Møller, M. (2014). Stress ulcer prophylaxis versus placebo or no prophylaxis in critically ill patients: A systematic review of randomised clinical trials with meta-analysis and trial sequential analysis. *Intensive Care Medicine*, *40*(1), 11–22. doi:10.1007/s00134-013-3125-3 PMID:24141808

Kramer, D. B., Mitchell, S. L., & Brock, D. W. (2012). Deactivation of Pacemakers and Implantable Cardioverter-Defibrillators. *Progress in Cardiovascular Diseases*, *55*(3), 290–299. doi:10.1016/j.pcad.2012.09.003 PMID:23217433

Kramer, N., Meyer, T. J., Meharg, J., Cece, R. D., & Hill, N. S. (1995). Randomized, prospective trial of noninvasive positive pressure ventilation in acute respiratory failure. *American Journal of Respiratory and Critical Care Medicine*, *151*(6), 1799–1806. doi:10.1164/ajrccm.151.6.7767523 PMID:7767523

Krawczyk, M., Flinta, I., Garncarek, M., Jankowska, E., Banasiak, W., Germany, R., & Ponikowski, P. et al. (2013). Sleep disordered breathing in patients with heart failure. *Cardiology Journal*, *20*(4), 345–355. doi:10.5603/CJ.2013.0092 PMID:23913452

Kress, J. P., Gehlbach, B., Lacy, M., Pliskin, N., Pohlman, A. S., & Hall, J. B. (2003). The long-term psychological effects of daily sedation interruption on critically ill patients. *American Journal of Respiratory and Critical Care Medicine*, *168*(12), 1457–1461. doi:10.1164/rccm.200303-455OC PMID:14525802

Kress, J. P., Pohlman, A. S., O'Connor, M. F., & Hall, J. B. (2000). Daily interruption of sedative infusions in critically ill patients undergoing mechanical ventilation. *The New England Journal of Medicine*, *342*(20), 1471–1477. doi:10.1056/NEJM200005183422002 PMID:10816184

Kreymann, K. G., Berger, M. M., Deutz, N. E. P., Hiesmayr, M., Jolliet, P., Kazandjiev, G., & Spies, C. et al. (2006). ESPEN Guidelines on Enteral Nutrition: Intensive care. *Clinical Nutrition (Edinburgh, Lothian)*, *25*(2), 210–223. doi:10.1016/j.clnu.2006.01.021 PMID:16697087

Krinsley, J. S. (2009). Glycemic variability and mortality in critically ill patients: The impact of diabetes. *Journal of Diabetes Science and Technology*, *3*(6), 1292–1301. doi:10.1177/193229680900300609 PMID:20144383

Krinsley, J. S., Egi, M., Kiss, A., Devendra, A. N., Schuetz, P., Maurer, P. M., & Bellomo, R. et al. (2013). Diabetic status and the relation of the three domains of glycemic control to mortality in critically ill patients: An international multicenter cohort study. *Critical Care (London, England)*, *17*(2), R37. doi:10.1186/cc12547 PMID:23452622

Kroenke, K., Lawrence, V. A., Theroux, J. F., Tuley, M. R., & Hilsenbeck, S. (1993). Postoperative complications after thoracic and major abdominal surgery in patients with and without obstructive lung disease. *Chest Journal*, *104*(5), 1445–1451. doi:10.1378/chest.104.5.1445 PMID:8222804

Kross, E. K., Engelberg, R. A., Downey, L., Cuschieri, J., Hallman, M. R., Longstreth, W. T. Jr, & Curtis, J. R. et al. (2014). Differences in end-of-life care in the ICU across patients cared for by medicine, surgery, neurology, and neurosurgery physicians. *Chest*, *145*(2), 313–321. doi:10.1378/chest.13-1351 PMID:24114410

Kruklitis, R. J., Tracy, J. A., & McCambridge, M. M. (2014). Clinical and financial considerations for implementing an ICU telemedicine program. *Chest*, *145*(6), 1392–1396. doi:10.1378/chest.13-0868 PMID:24889437

Kubitza, D., Becka, M., Roth, A., & Mueck, W. (2008). Dose-escalation study of the pharmacokinetics and pharmacodynamics of rivaroxaban in healthy elderly subjects. *Current Medical Research and Opinion*, *24*(10), 2757–2765. doi:10.1185/03007990802361499 PMID:18715524

Kubo, T., Ozasa, K., Mikami, K., Wakai, K., Fujino, Y., Watanabe, Y., & Tamakoshi, A. et al. (2006). Prospective cohort study of the risk of prostate cancer among rotating-shift workers: Findings from the Japan collaborative cohort study. *American Journal of Epidemiology*, *164*(6), 549–555. doi:10.1093/aje/kwj232 PMID:16829554

Kubota, H., Miyata, H., Motomura, N., Ono, M., Takamoto, S., Harii, K., & Kyo, S. et al. (2013). Deep sternal wound infection after cardiac surgery. *Journal of Cardiothoracic Surgery*, *8*(1), 132. doi:10.1186/1749-8090-8-132 PMID:23688324

Kubota, H., Miyata, H., Motomura, N., Ono, M., Takamoto, S., Harii, K., & Kyo, S. et al. (2013). Deep sternal wound infections after cardiac surgery. *Journal of Cardiothoracic Surgery*, *8*, 132. PMID:23688324

Kuhn, E. W., Liakopoulos, O. J., Stange, S., Deppe, A., Slottosch, I., Choi, Y., & Wahlers, T. (2014). Preoperative statin therapy in cardiac surgery: A meta-analysis of 90000 patients. *European Journal of Cardio-Thoracic Surgery*, *45*(1), 17–26. doi:10.1093/ejcts/ezt181 PMID:23562936

Kulik, A., Le May, M. R., Voisine, P., Tardif, J. C., DeLarochelliere, R., Naidoo, S., & Ruel, M. et al. (2010). Aspirin plus clopidogrel versus aspirin alone after coronary artery bypass grafting. *Circulation*, *122*(25), 2680–2687. doi:10.1161/CIRCULATIONAHA.110.978007 PMID:21135365

Kulik, A., Rubens, F. D., Wells, P. S., Kearon, C., Mesana, T. G., van Berkom, J., & Lam, B. K. (2006). Early postoperative anticoagulation after mechanical valve replacement: A systematic review. *The Annals of Thoracic Surgery*, *81*(2), 770–781. doi:10.1016/j.athoracsur.2005.07.023 PMID:16427905

Kumar, A. (2009). Optimizing antimicrobial therapy in sepsis and septic shock. *Critical Care Clinics*, *25*(4), 733–751. doi:10.1016/j.ccc.2009.08.004 PMID:19892250

Kumar, A. B., Suneja, M., Bayman, E. O., Weide, G. D., & Tarasi, M. (2012). Association Between Postoperative Acute Kidney Injury and Duration of Cardiopulmonary Bypass: A Meta-Analysis. *Journal of Cardiothoracic and Vascular Anesthesia*, *26*(1), 64–69. doi:10.1053/j.jvca.2011.07.007 PMID:21924633

Kumar, A., Roberts, D., Wood, K. E., Light, B., Parillo, J. E., Sharma, S., & Cheang, M. et al. (2006). Duration of hypotension before initiation of effective antimicrobial therapy is the critical determinant of survival in human septic shock. *Critical Care Medicine*, *34*(6), 1589–1596. doi:10.1097/01.CCM.0000217961.75225.E9 PMID:16625125

Kumar, K., Singal, R., Manji, R. A., Zarychanski, R., Bell, D. D., Freed, D. H., & Arora, R. C. (2014). The benefits of 24/7 in-house intensivist coverage for prolonged-stay cardiac surgery patients. *The Journal of Thoracic and Cardiovascular Surgery*, *148*(1), 290–297.e296. doi:10.1016/j.jtcvs.2014.02.074 PMID:24703332

Kumon, K., Tanaka, K., Hirata, T., Naito, Y., & Fujita, T. (1986). Organ failures due to low cardiac output syndrome following open heart surgery. *Japanese Circulation Journal*, *50*(4), 329–335. doi:10.1253/jcj.50.329 PMID:3489109

Kunin, C. M., & McCormack, R. C. (1966). Prevention of catheter-induced urinary-tract infections by sterile closed drainage. *The New England Journal of Medicine*, *274*(21), 1155–1161. doi:10.1056/NEJM196605262742101 PMID:5934951

Kuroda, S., Houkin, K., Abe, H., Hoshi, Y., & Tamura, M. (1996). Near-infrared monitoring of carebral oxygenation state during carotid endarterectomy. *Surgical Neurology*, *45*(5), 450–458. doi:10.1016/0090-3019(95)00463-7 PMID:8629246

Kwak, Y. L., Lee, C. S., Park, Y. H., & Hong, Y. W. (2002). The effect of phenylephrine and norepinephrine in patients with chronic pulmonary hypertension*. *Anaesthesia*, *57*(1), 9–14. doi:10.1046/j.1365-2044.2002.02324.x PMID:11843735

Kwok, H., McCormack, J., Cece, R., Houtchens, J., & Hill, N. S. (2003). Controlled trial of oronasal versus nasal mask ventilation in the treatment of acute respiratory failure. *Critical Care Medicine*, *31*(2), 468–473. doi:10.1097/01.CCM.0000045563.64187.20 PMID:12576953

Kyne, L., Sougioultzis, S., McFarland, L. V., & Kelly, C. P. (2002). Underlying disease severity as a major risk factor for nosocomial Clostridium difficile diarrhea. *Infection Control and Hospital Epidemiology*, *23*(11), 653–659. doi:10.1086/501989 PMID:12452292

Laas, J., Kleine, P., Hasenkam, M. J., & Nygaard, H. (1999). Orientation of tilting disc and bileaflet aortic valve substitutes for optimal hemodynamics. *The Annals of Thoracic Surgery*, *68*(3), 1096–1099. doi:10.1016/S0003-4975(99)00780-8 PMID:10510028

Labovitz, A. J., Noble, V. E., Bierig, M., Goldstein, S. A., Jones, R., Kort, S., & Wei, K. et al. (2010). Focused Cardiac Ultrasound in the Emergent Setting: A Consensus Statement of the American Society of Echocardiography and American College of Emergency Physicians. *Journal of the American Society of Echocardiography*, *23*(12), 1225–1230. doi:10.1016/j.echo.2010.10.005 PMID:21111923

Lacasse, H., Perreault, M. M., & Williamson, D. R. (2006). Systematic review of antipsychotics for the treatment of hospital-associated delirium in medically or surgically ill patients. *The Annals of Pharmacotherapy*, *40*(11), 1966–1973. doi:10.1345/aph.1H241 PMID:17047137

Lachaine, J., & Beauchemin, C. (2012). Economic evaluation of dexmedetomidine relative to midazolam for sedation in the intensive care unit. *The Canadian Journal of Hospital Pharmacy*, *65*(2), 103–110. doi:10.4212/cjhp.v65i2.1116 PMID:22529402

Lacherade, J. C., De Jonghe, B., Guezennec, P., Debbat, K., Hayon, J., Monsel, A., & Bastuji-Garin, S. et al. (2010). Intermittent subglottic secretion drainage and ventilator-associated pneumonia: A multicenter trial. *American Journal of Respiratory and Critical Care Medicine*, *182*(7), 910–917. doi:10.1164/rccm.200906-0838OC PMID:20522796

Ladak, S. S., Katznelson, R., Muscat, M., Sawhney, M., Beattie, W. S., & O'Leary, G. (2009). Incidence of urinary retention in patients with thoracic patient-controlled epidural analgesia (TPCEA) undergoing thoracotomy. *Pain Management Nursing*, *10*(2), 94–98. doi:10.1016/j.pmn.2008.08.001 PMID:19481048

Lador, A., Nasir, H., Mansur, N., Sharoni, E., Biderman, P., Leibovici, L., & Paul, M. (2012). Antibiotic prophylaxis in cardiac surgery: Systematic review and meta-analysis. *The Journal of Antimicrobial Chemotherapy*, *67*(3), 541–550. doi:10.1093/jac/dkr470 PMID:22083832

Laffey, J. G., Boylan, J. F., & Cheng, D. C. (2002). The systemic inflammatory response to cardiac surgery: Implications for the anesthesiologist. *Anesthesiology*, *97*(1), 215–252. doi:10.1097/00000542-200207000-00030 PMID:12131125

Lafuente-Lafuente, C., Longas-Tejero, M. A., Bergman, J. F., & Belmin, J. (2012). Antiarrhythmics for maintaining sinus rhythm after cardioversion of atrial fibrillation. *Cochrane Database of Systematic Reviews*, *5*, CD005049. PMID:22592700

Lahon, B., Mordant, P., Thabut, G., Georger, J. F., Dauriat, G., Mal, H., & Castier, Y. et al. (2011). Early severe digestive complications after lung transplantation. *European Journal of Cardio-Thoracic Surgery*, *40*(6), 1419–1424.

Lai, N. M., Chaiyakunapruk, N., Lai, N. A., O'Riordan, E., Pau, W. S. C., & Saint, S. (2013). Catheter impregnation, coating or bonding for reducing central venous catheter-related infections in adults. *Cochrane Database of Systematic Reviews*, CD007878. PMID:23740696

Lalani, T., Cabell, C. H., Benjamin, D. K., Lasca, O., Naber, C., Fowler, V. G. Jr, & Wang, A. et al. (2010). Analysis of the impact of early surgery on in-hospital mortality of native valve endocarditis: Use of propensity score and instrumental variable methods to adjust for treatment-selection bias. *Circulation*, *121*(8), 1005–1013. doi:10.1161/CIRCULATIONAHA.109.864488 PMID:20159831

Lalonde, S. D., Alba, A. C., Rigobon, A., Ross, H. J., Delgado, D. H., Billia, F., & Rao, V. et al. (2013). Clinical differences between continuous flow ventricular assist devices: A comparison between HeartMate II and HeartWare HVAD. *Journal of Cardiac Surgery*, *28*(5), 604–610. doi:10.1111/jocs.12158 PMID:23844652

Lamarche, Y., Sirounis, D., & Arora, R. C. (2011). A survey of standardized management protocols after coronary artery bypass grafting surgery in Canadian intensive care units. *The Canadian Journal of Cardiology*, *27*(6), 705–710. doi:10.1016/j.cjca.2011.08.123 PMID:22019278

Lam, J. H., Ranganathan, N., Wigle, E. D., & Silver, M. D. (1970). Morphology of the human mitral valve. I. Chordae tendineae: A new classification. *Circulation*, *41*(3), 449–458. doi:10.1161/01.CIR.41.3.449 PMID:5415982

Lampert, R., Hayes, D. L., Annas, G. J., Farley, M. A., Goldstein, N. E., Hamilton, R. M., & Zellner, R. et al. (2010). HRS Expert Consensus Statement on the Management of Cardiovascular Implantable Electronic Devices (CIEDs) in patients nearing end of life or requesting withdrawal of therapy. *Heart Rhythm*, *7*(7), 1008–1026. doi:10.1016/j.hrthm.2010.04.033 PMID:20471915

Lamy, A., Devereaux, P. J., Prabhakaran, D., Taggart, D. P., Hu, S., Paolasso, E., & Yusuf, S. et al. (2013). Effects of off-pump and on-pump coronary-artery bypass grafting at 1 year. *The New England Journal of Medicine*, *368*(13), 1179–1188. doi:10.1056/NEJMoa1301228 PMID:23477676

Lancellotti, P., Tribouilloy, C., Hagendorff, A., Popescu, B. A., Edvardsen, T., Pierard, L. A., Badano, L., & Zamorano, J. L. (2013). Recommendations for the echocardiographic assessment of native valvular regurgitation: An executive summary from the European Association of Cardiovascular Imaging. *European Heart Journal – Cardiovascular Imaging, 14*(7), 611-644.

Landymore, R. W., & Howell, F. (1991). Recurrent atrial arrhythmias following treatment for postoperative atrial fibrillation after coronary bypass operations. *European Journal of Cardio-Thoracic Surgery*, *5*(8), 436–439. doi:10.1016/1010-7940(91)90191-L PMID:1910852

Landzberg, J. S., Pflugfelder, P. W., Cassidy, M. M., Schiller, N. S., Higgins, C. B., & Cheitlin, M. D. (1992). Etiology of the Austin Flint murmur. *Journal of the American College of Cardiology*, *20*(2), 408–413. doi:10.1016/0735-1097(92)90110-9 PMID:1634679

Lang, C., Piergiuseppe, A., & Mancini, D. (2007). Prognostic Significance and Measurement of Exercise-Derived Hemodynamic Variables in Patients With Heart Failure. *Journal of Cardiac Failure*, *13*(8), 672–697. doi:10.1016/j.cardfail.2007.05.004 PMID:17923361

Langewouters, et al.. (1979). Computing the total arterial compliance of the arterial system from its input impedance. *Medical & Biological Engineering & Computing*, *17*(5), 623–628. doi:10.1007/BF02440907 PMID:316077

Langouche, L., & Van den Berghe, G. (2006). Glucose metabolism and insulin therapy. *Critical Care Clinics*, *22*(1), 119–129. doi:10.1016/j.ccc.2005.09.005 PMID:16399023

Langouche, L., Vander Perre, S., Marques, M., Boelen, A., Wouters, P. J., Casaer, M. P., & Van den Berghe, G. (2013). Impact of early nutrient restriction during critical illness on the nonthyroidal illness syndrome and its relation with outcome: A randomized, controlled clinical study. *The Journal of Clinical Endocrinology and Metabolism*, *98*(3), 1006–1013. doi:10.1210/jc.2012-2809 PMID:23348400

Lanier, G., Orlanes, K., Hayashi, Y., Murphy, J., Flannery, M., Te-Frey, R., & Colombo, P. C. et al. (2013). Validity and reliability of a novel slow cuff-deflation system for noninvasive blood pressure monitoring in patients with continuous-flow left ventricular assist device. *Circulation: Heart Failure*, *6*(5), 1005–1012. doi:10.1161/CIRCHEARTFAILURE.112.000186 PMID:23811966

Lanken, P. N., Terry, P. B., Delisser, H. M., Fahy, B. F., Hansen-Flaschen, J., & Heffner, J. E. et al. Force, A. T. S. E.-o.-L. C. T. (2008). An official American Thoracic Society clinical policy statement: Palliative care for patients with respiratory diseases and critical illnesses. *American Journal of Respiratory and Critical Care Medicine*, *177*(8), 912–927. doi:10.1164/rccm.200605-587ST PMID:18390964

Lanning, C. F., & Harmel, M. H. (1975). Ketamine anesthesia. *Annual Review of Medicine*, *26*(1), 137–141. doi:10.1146/annurev.me.26.020175.001033 PMID:1096753

Lanuti, M., Delva, P., Maher, A., Wright, C., Gaissert, H., Wain, J., & Mathisen, D. et al. (2006). Feasibility and Outcomes of an Early Extubation Policy After Esophagectomy. *The Annals of Thoracic Surgery*, *82*(6), 2037–2041. doi:10.1016/j.athoracsur.2006.07.024 PMID:17126107

LaPar, D. J., Crosby, I. K., Ailawadi, G., Ad, N., Choi, E., Spiess, B. D., et al. (2013). Blood product conservation is associated with improved outcomes and reduced costs after cardiac surgery. *The Journal of Thoracic and Cardiovascular Surgery*, *145*(3), 796–803– discussion 803–4.

LaPar, D. J., Isbell, J. M., Kern, J. A., Ailawadi, G., & Kron, I. L. (2014). Surgical Care Improvement Project measure for postoperative glucose control should not be used as a measure of quality after cardiac surgery. *The Journal of Thoracic and Cardiovascular Surgery*, *147*(3), 1041–1048. doi:10.1016/j.jtcvs.2013.11.028 PMID:24418668

Larmann, J., & Theilmeier, G. (2004). Inflammatory response to cardiac surgery: Cardiopulmonary bypass versus non-cardiopulmonary bypass surgery. *Best Practice & Research. Clinical Anaesthesiology*, *18*(3), 425–438. doi:10.1016/j.bpa.2003.12.004 PMID:15212337

Larsen, G. Y., Donaldson, A. E., Parker, H. B., & Grant, M. J. (2007). Preventable harm occurring to critically ill children. *Pediatric Critical Care Medicine*, *8*(4), 331–336. doi:10.1097/01.PCC.0000263042.73539.99 PMID:17417126

Latham, R., Lancaster, A. D., Covington, J. F., Pirolo, J. S., & Thomas, C. S. Jr. (2001). The association of diabetes and glucose control with surgical-site infections among cardiothoracic surgery patients. *Infection Control and Hospital Epidemiology*, *22*(10), 607–612. doi:10.1086/501830 PMID:11776345

Laupland, K. B., Kirkpatrick, A. W., Kortbeek, J. B., & Zuege, D. J. (2006). Long-term mortality outcome associated with prolonged admission to the ICU. *Chest*, *129*(4), 954–959. doi:10.1378/chest.129.4.954 PMID:16608944

Lavoie, J. (2011). Blood transfusion risks and alternative strategies in pediatric patients. *Paediatric Anaesthesia*, *21*(1), 12–24. doi:10.1111/j.1460-9592.2010.03470.x PMID:21155923

Lawrence, V. A., Hilsenbeck, S. G., Mulrow, C. D., Dhanda, R., Sapp, J., & Page, C. P. (1995). Incidence and hospital stay for cardiac and pulmonary complications after abdominal surgery. *Journal of General Internal Medicine*, *10*(12), 671–678. doi:10.1007/BF02602761 PMID:8770719

Lazar, H. L., Chipkin, S. R., Fitzgerald, C. A., Bao, Y., Cabral, H., & Apstein, C. S. (2004). Tight glycemic control in diabetic coronary artery bypass graft patients improves perioperative outcomes and decreases recurrent ischemic events. *Circulation*, *109*(12), 1497–1502. doi:10.1161/01.CIR.0000121747.71054.79 PMID:15006999

Lazar, H. L., McDonnell, M. M., Chipkin, S., Fitzgerald, C., Bliss, C., & Cabral, H. (2011). Effects of aggressive versus moderate glycemic control on clinical outcomes in diabetic coronary artery bypass graft patients. *Annals of Surgery*, *254*(3), 458–464. doi:10.1097/SLA.0b013e31822c5d78 PMID:21865944

Lazar, H. L., McDonnell, M. M., Chipkin, S., Furnary, A. P., Engelman, R. M., Sadhu, A. R., & Shemin, R. J. et al. (2009). The Society for Thoracic Surgeons practice guideline series: Blood glucose management during adult cardiac surgery. *The Annals of Thoracic Surgery*, *87*(2), 663–669. doi:10.1016/j.athoracsur.2008.11.011 PMID:19161815

Le Roith, D. (2004). Molecular mechanisms by which metabolic control may improve outcomes. *Endocrine Practice*, *10*(2Supple), 57–62. doi:10.4158/EP.10.S2.57 PMID:15251642

Leape, L. L., Cullen, D. J., Clapp, M. D., Burdick, E., Demonaco, H. J., Erickson, J. I., & Bates, D. W. (1999). Pharmacist participation on physician rounds and adverse drug events in the intensive care unit. *Journal of the American Medical Association*, *282*(3), 267–270. doi:10.1001/jama.282.3.267 PMID:10422996

LeBlanc, V. R. (2012). Review article: simulation in anesthesia: state of the science and looking forward. *Canadian Journal of Anesthesia/Journal Canadien D'anesthésie, 59*(2), 193–202. doi:10.1007/s12630-011-9638-8

Lee, C. M., Herridge, M. S., Gabor, J. Y., Tansey, C. M., Matte, A., & Hanly, P. J. (2009). Chronic sleep disorders in survivors of the acute respiratory distress syndrome. *Intensive Care Medicine, 35*(2), 314–320. doi:10.1007/s00134-008-1277-3 PMID:18802684

Lee, D. H., Buth, K. J., Martin, B. J., Yip, A. M., & Hirsch, G. M. (2010). Frail patients are at increased risk for mortality and prolonged institutional care after cardiac surgery. *Circulation, 121*(8), 973–978. doi:10.1161/CIRCULATIONAHA.108.841437 PMID:20159833

Lee, G. M., Kleinman, K., Soumerai, S. B., Tse, A., Cole, D., Fridkin, S. K., & Jha, A. K. et al. (2012). Effect of nonpayment for preventable infections in U.S. hospitals. *The New England Journal of Medicine, 367*(15), 1428–1437. doi:10.1056/NEJMsa1202419 PMID:23050526

Lee, J. C., Raman, J., & Song, D. H. (2010). Primary sternal closure with titanium plate fixation: Plastic surgery effecting a paradigm shift. *Plastic and Reconstructive Surgery, 125*(6), 1720–1724. doi:10.1097/PRS.0b013e3181d51292 PMID:20517097

Lenihan, C. R., Montez-Rath, M. E., Mangano, C. T., Chertow, G. M., & Winkelmayer, W. C. (2013). Trends in Acute Kidney Injury, Associated Use of Dialysis, and Mortality After Cardiac Surgery, 1999 to 2008. *The Annals of Thoracic Surgery, 95*(1), 20–28. doi:10.1016/j.athoracsur.2012.05.131 PMID:23272825

Lennon, M. J., Gibbs, N. M., Weightman, W. M., McGuire, D., & Michalopoulos, N. (2004). A comparison of plateletworks and platelet aggregometry for the assessment of aspirin induced platelet dysfunction in cardiac surgical patients. *Journal of Cardiothoracic and Vascular Anesthesia, 18*(2), 136–140. doi:10.1053/j.jvca.2004.01.015 PMID:15073699

Lentschener, C., Gaujoux, S., Tesniere, A., & Dousset, B. (2011). Point of Controversy: Perioperative care of patients undergoing pheochromocytoma removal – time for a reappraisal? *European Journal of Endocrinology, 165*(3), 365–373. doi:10.1530/EJE-11-0162 PMID:21646289

Lentschener, C., Gaujoux, S., Thillois, J. M., Duboc, D., Bertherat, J., Ozier, Y., & Dousset, B. (2009). Increased arterial pressure is not predictive of haemodynamic instability in patients undergoing adrenalectomy for phaeochromocytoma. *Acta Anaesthesiologica Scandinavica, 53*(4), 522–527. doi:10.1111/j.1399-6576.2008.01894.x PMID:19239408

Leon, M. B., Smith, C. R., Mack, M., Miller, D. C., Moses, J. W., Svensson, L. G., & Pocock, S. et al. (2010). Transcatheter aortic-valve implantation for aortic stenosis in patients who cannot undergo surgery. *The New England Journal of Medicine, 363*(17), 1597–1607. doi:10.1056/NEJMoa1008232 PMID:20961243

Le, T., & Bayer, A. S. (2003). Combination antibiotic therapy for infective endocarditis. *Clinical Infectious Diseases, 36*(5), 615–621. doi:10.1086/367661 PMID:12594643

Letheulle, J., Tattevin, P., Saunders, L., Kerjouan, M., Léna, H., Descrues, B., & Jouneau, S. et al. (2013). Iterative thoracentesis as first-line treatment of complicated parapneumonic effusion. *PLoS ONE, 9*(1), e84788. doi:10.1371/journal.pone.0084788 PMID:24400113

Leung, J. M., Sands, L. P., Vaurio, L. E., & Wang, Y. (2006). Nitrous oxide does not change the incidence of postoperative delirium or cognitive decline in elderly surgical patients. *British Journal of Anaesthesia, 96*(6), 754–760. doi:10.1093/bja/ael106 PMID:16670110

Levi, M., Levy, J. H., Andersen, H. F., & Truloff, D. (2010). Safety of recombinant activated factor VII in randomized clinical trials. *The New England Journal of Medicine, 363*(19), 1791–1800. doi:10.1056/NEJMoa1006221 PMID:21047223

Levi, M., Toh, C. H., Thachil, J., & Watson, H. G. (2009). Guidelines for the diagnosis and management of disseminated intravascular coagulation. British Committee for Standards in Haematology. *British Journal of Haematology*, *145*(1), 24–33. doi:10.1111/j.1365-2141.2009.07600.x PMID:19222477

Levine, H. J., & Gaasch, W. H. (1996). Vasoactive drugs in chronic regurgitant lesions of the mitral and aortic valves. *Journal of the American College of Cardiology*, *28*(5), 1083–1091. doi:10.1016/S0735-1097(96)00288-4 PMID:8890799

Levy, B., Bollaert, P. E., Charpentier, C., Nace, L., Audibert, G., Bauer, P., & Larcan, A. et al. (1997). Comparison of norepinephrine and dobutamine to epinephrine for hemodynamics, lactate metabolism, and gastric tonometric variables in septic shock: A prospective, randomized study. *Intensive Care Medicine*, *23*(3), 282–287. doi:10.1007/s001340050329 PMID:9083230

Levy, J. H., & Tanaka, K. A. (2003). Inflammatory response to cardiopulmonary bypass. *The Annals of Thoracic Surgery*, *75*(2), S715–S720. doi:10.1016/S0003-4975(02)04701-X PMID:12607717

Levy, M. M., Rapoport, J., Lemeshow, S., Chalfin, D. B., Phillips, G., & Danis, M. (2008). Association between critical care physician management and patient mortality in the intensive care unit. *Annals of Internal Medicine*, *148*(11), 801–809. doi:10.7326/0003-4819-148-11-200806030-00002 PMID:18519926

Levy, W., Mozaffarian, D., Linker, D., Sutradhar, S., Anker, S., Cropp, A., & Packer, M. et al. (2006). The Seattle Heart Failure Model. Prediction of Survival in Heart Failure. *Heart Failure*, *133*(11), 1424–1433. PMID:16534009

Lewis, G. D., Bloch, K. D., & Semigran, M. J. (2004). Pulmonary thromboembolism superimposed on a congenital ventricular septal defect in a 50-year-old man inhaled nitric oxide and sildenafil to the rescue. *Cardiology in Review*, *12*(4), 188–190. doi:10.1097/01.crd.0000122635.12743.57 PMID:15191635

Leyh, R. G., & Bartels, C. Nötzold, a, & Sievers, H. H. (1999). Management of porcelain aorta during coronary artery bypass grafting. *The Annals of Thoracic Surgery*, *67*(4), 986–8. Retrieved from http://www.ncbi.nlm.nih.gov/pubmed/11603471

Liakopoulos, O. J., Choi, Y.-H., Haldenwang, P. L., Strauch, J., Wittwer, T., Dörge, H., & Wahlers, T. et al. (2008). Impact of preoperative statin therapy on adverse postoperative outcomes in patients undergoing cardiac surgery: A meta-analysis of over 30,000 patients. *European Heart Journal*, *29*(12), 1548–1559. doi:10.1093/eurheartj/ehn198 PMID:18506053

Liakopoulos, O. J., Dörge, H., Schmitto, J. D., Nagorsnik, U., Grabedünkel, J., & Schoendube, F. A. (2006). Effects of preoperative statin therapy on cytokines after cardiac surgery. *The Thoracic and Cardiovascular Surgeon*, *54*(4), 250–254. doi:10.1055/s-2006-923836 PMID:16755446

Liang, X., Liu, S., Chen, Y., Yan, L., Li, H., Xuan, H., & Shi, W. et al. (2010). Combination of urinary kidney injury molecule-1 and interleukin-18 as early biomarker for the diagnosis and progressive assessment of acute kidney injury following cardiopulmonary bypass surgery: A prospective nested case–control study. *Biomarkers*, *15*(4), 332–339. doi:10.3109/13547501003706558 PMID:20233133

Libby, P. (2013). Mechanisms of Acute Coronary Syndromes and Their Implications for Therapy. *The New England Journal of Medicine*, *368*(21), 2004–2013. doi:10.1056/NEJMra1216063 PMID:23697515

Lichtenstein, D. A., & Mezière, G. A. (2008). Relevance of lung ultrasound in the diagnosis of acute respiratory failure: The BLUE protocol. *Chest*, *134*(1), 117–125. doi:10.1378/chest.07-2800 PMID:18403664

Lichtenstein, D. A., Mezière, G., Lascols, N., Biderman, P., Courret, J.-P., Gepner, A., & Tenoudji-Cohen, M. et al. (2005). Ultrasound diagnosis of occult pneumothorax*. *Critical Care Medicine*, *33*(6), 1231–1238. doi:10.1097/01.CCM.0000164542.86954.B4 PMID:15942336

Lichtenstein, D., Mezière, G., Biderman, P., & Gepner, A. (1999). The comet-tail artifact: An ultrasound sign ruling out pneumothorax. *Intensive Care Medicine, 25*(4), 383–388. doi:10.1007/s001340050862 PMID:10342512

Lichtenstein, D., Mézière, G., Biderman, P., Gepner, A., & Barré, O. (1997). The comet-tail artifact. An ultrasound sign of alveolar-interstitial syndrome. *American Journal of Respiratory and Critical Care Medicine, 156*(5), 1640–1646. doi:10.1164/ajrccm.156.5.96-07096 PMID:9372688

Lichtenstein, D., Mezière, G., & Seitz, J. (2009). The dynamic air bronchogram. A lung ultrasound sign of alveolar consolidation ruling out atelectasis. *Chest, 135*(6), 1421–1425. doi:10.1378/chest.08-2281 PMID:19225063

Licker, M., Cikirikcioglu, M., Inan, C., Cartier, V., Kalangos, A., Theologou, T., & Diaper, J. et al. (2010). Preoperative diastolic function predicts the onset of left ventricular dysfunction following aortic valve replacement in high-risk patients with aortic stenosis. *Critical Care (London, England), 14*(3), R101. doi:10.1186/cc9040 PMID:20525242

Licker, M., Diaper, J., Cartier, V., Ellenberger, C., Cikirikcioglu, M., Kalangos, A., & Bendjelid, K. et al. (2012). Clinical review: Management of weaning from cardiopulmonary bypass after cardiac surgery. *Annals of Cardiac Anaesthesia, 15*(3), 206–223. doi:10.4103/0971-9784.97977 PMID:22772515

Licker, M., Spiliopoulos, A., Frey, J., Robert, J., Hohn, L., De Perrot, M., & Tschopp, J. (2002). Risk Factors for Early Mortality and Major Complications Following Pneumonectomy for Non-small Cell Carcinoma of the Lung. *Chest, 121*(6), 1890–1897. doi:10.1378/chest.121.6.1890 PMID:12065354

Light, R. W., Rogers, J. T., Moyers, J. P., Lee, Y. C., Rodriguez, R. M., Alford, W. C. Jr, & Tedder, M. et al. (2002). Prevalence and clinical course of pleural effusions at 30 days after coronary artery and cardiac surgery. *American Journal of Respiratory and Critical Care Medicine, 166*(12 Pt 1), 1567–1571. doi:10.1164/rccm.200203-184OC PMID:12406850

Li, H. T., Long, C. S., Rokosh, D. G., Honbo, N. Y., & Karliner, J. S. (1995). Chronic hypoxia differentially regulates alpha 1-adrenergic receptor subtype mRNAs and inhibits alpha 1-adrenergic receptor-stimulated cardiac hypertrophy and signaling. *Circulation, 92*(4), 918–925. doi:10.1161/01.CIR.92.4.918 PMID:7641375

Li, J. S., Sexton, D. J., Mick, N., Nettles, R., Fowler, V. G., Ryan, T., & Corey, G. R. et al. (2000). Proposed modifications to the Duke criteria for the diagnosis of infective endocarditis. *Clinical Infectious Diseases, 30*(4), 633–638. doi:10.1086/313753 PMID:10770721

Likosky, D. S., FitzGerald, D. C., Groom, R. C., Jones, D. K., Baker, R. A., Shann, K. G., & Body, S. C. et al. (2010). Effect of the perioperative blood transfusion and blood conservation in cardiac surgery clinical practice guidelines of the Society of Thoracic Surgeons and the Society of Cardiovascular Anesthesiologists upon clinical practices. *Anesthesia and Analgesia, 111*(2), 316–323. doi:10.1213/ANE.0b013e3181e329f1 PMID:20488928

Likosky, D. S., Marrin, C. A., Caplan, L. R., Baribeau, Y. R., Morton, J. R., Weintraub, R. M., & O'Connor, G. T. et al. (2003). Determination of etiologic mechanisms of strokes secondary to coronary artery bypass graft surgery. *Stroke, 34*(12), 2830–2834. doi:10.1161/01.STR.0000098650.12386.B3 PMID:14605327

Likosky, D. S., Sorensen, M. J., Dacey, L. J., Baribeau, Y. R., Leavitt, B. J., DiScipio, A. W., & O'Connor, G. T. et al. Northern New England Cardiovascular Disease Study, Group. (2009). Long-term survival of the very elderly undergoing aortic valve surgery. *Circulation, 120*(11Suppl), S127–S133. doi:10.1161/CIRCULATIONAHA.108.842641 PMID:19752357

Lillehei, C. W. (1955). Controlled cross circulation for direct-vision intracardiac surgery: Correction of ventricular septal defects, atrioventricularis cummuis, and tetralogy of Fallot. *Postgraduate Medical Journal, 1*, 388–396.

Lilly, C. M., Zuckerman, I. H., Badawi, O., & Riker, R. R. (2011). Benchmark data from more than 240,000 adults that reflect the current practice of critical care in the United States. *Chest*, *140*(5), 1232–1242. doi:10.1378/chest.11-0718 PMID:21868469

Lim, S. Y., & Hausenloy, D. J. (2012). Remote Ischemic Conditioning: From Bench to Bedside. *Frontiers in Physics*, *3*. doi:10.3389/fphys.2012.00027 PMID:22363297

Lin, D. M., Weeks, K., Bauer, L., Combes, J. R., George, C. T., Goeschel, C. A., & Pham, J. C. et al. (2012). Eradicating central line-associated bloodstream infections statewide: The Hawaii experience. *American Journal of Medical Quality*, *27*(2), 124–129. doi:10.1177/1062860611414299 PMID:21918016

Lindblad, B., Wakefield, T. W., Whitehouse, W. M., & Stanley, J. C. (1988). The effect of protamine sulfate on platelet function. *Scandinavian Journal of Thoracic and Cardiovascular Surgery*, *22*(1), 55–59. doi:10.3109/14017438809106052 PMID:3387950

Linden, A. V., Kempfert, J., Rastan, A. J., Holzhey, D., Blumenstein, J., Schuler, G., & Walther, T. et al. (2011). Risk of acute kidney injury after minimally invasive transapical aortic valve implantation in 270 patients. *European Journal of Cardio-Thoracic Surgery*, *39*(6), 835–843. doi:10.1016/j.ejcts.2010.11.034 PMID:21186126

Lindroos, M., Kupari, M., Heikkila, J., & Tilvis, R. (1993). Prevalence of aortic valve abnormalities in the elderly: an echocardiographic study of a random population sample. *Journal of the American College of Cardiology, 21*(5), 1220-1225. doi: 0735-1097(93)90249-Z [pii]

Lingard, L., Espin, S., Whyte, S., Regehr, G., Baker, G. R., & Reznick, R. et al.. (2004). Communication failures in the operating room: An observational classification of recurrent types and effects. *Quality & Safety in Health Care*, *13*(5), 330–334. doi:10.1136/qshc.2003.008425 PMID:15465935

Linkins, L. A., Dans, A. L., Moores, L. K., Bona, R., Davidson, B. L., Schulman, S., & Crowther, M. (2012). Treatment of prevention of heparin-induced thrombocytopenia: Antithrombotic therapy and prevention of thrombosis, 9th ed: American College of Chest Physicians Evidence-Based Clinical Practice Guidelines. Chest, 141(2 Suppl), e495S-530S.

Linkins, L. A., Dans, A. L., Moores, L. K., Bona, R., Davidson, B., Schulman, S., & Crowther, M. (2012). Treatment and prevention of heparin induced thrombocytopenia. *Chest*, *141*(2), e495s–e530s. PMID:22315270

Liolios, A. (2008). E-learning. In *Controversies in Intensive Care Medicine* (pp. 373–392). Berlin: Medizinisch Wissenschaftliche Verlagsgesellschaft.

Lip, G. Y. H., Lip, P. L., Zafaris, J., Watson, R. D., Bareford, D., Lowe, G. D., & Beevers, D. G. (1996). Fibrin D-dimer and B-thromboglobulin as markers of thrombogenesis and platelet activation in atrial fibrillation. Effects of introducing ultralow-dose warfarin and aspirin. *Circulation*, *94*(3), 425–431. doi:10.1161/01.CIR.94.3.425 PMID:8759084

Lipner, R. S., Hess, B. J., & Phillips, R. L. Jr. (2013). Specialty board certification in the United States: Issues and evidence. *The Journal of Continuing Education in the Health Professions*, *33*(S1Suppl 1), S20–S35. doi:10.1002/chp.21203 PMID:24347150

Lipsett, P. A., Swoboda, S. M., Dickerson, J., Ylitalo, M., Gordon, T., Breslow, M., & Rosenfeld, B. et al. (2000). Survival and functional outcome after prolonged intensive care unit stay. *Annals of Surgery*, *231*(2), 262–268. doi:10.1097/00000658-200002000-00016 PMID:10674619

Liu, S. S., Block, B. M., & Wu, C. L. (2004). Effects of perioperative central neuraxial analgesia on outcome after coronary artery bypass surgery. *Anesthesiology*, *101*(1), 153–161. doi:10.1097/00000542-200407000-00024 PMID:15220785

Livermore, D. M. (2005). Minimising antibiotic resistance. *The Lancet Infectious Diseases*, *5*(7), 450–459. doi:10.1016/S1473-3099(05)70166-3 PMID:15978531

Li, Y., Zheng, Z., & Hu, S. (2009). The Chinese coronary artery bypass grafting registry study: Analysis of the national multicentre database of 9248 patients. *Heart (British Cardiac Society)*, *95*(14), 1140–1144. doi:10.1136/hrt.2008.146563 PMID:18632834

Loach, A., Young, A., Spalding, J., & Smith, A. (1975). Postoperative management after thymectomy. *British Medical Journal*, *1*(5953), 309–312. doi:10.1136/bmj.1.5953.309 PMID:1111793

Lockwood, A., Patka, J., Rabinovich, M., Wyatt, K., & Abraham, P. (2010). Nitroprusside-associated cyanide toxicity in adult patients - fact or fiction? A critical review of the evidence and clinical relevance. *Open Access Journal of Clinical Trials*, *2*(133), 148.

Lodise, T. P., McKinnon, P. S., Swiderski, L., & Rybak, M. J. (2003). Outcomes analysis of delayed antibiotic treatment for hospital-acquired Staphylococcus aureus bacteremia. *Clinical Infectious Diseases*, *36*(11), 1418–1423. doi:10.1086/375057 PMID:12766837

Loef, B. G., Epema, A. H., Smilde, T. D., Henning, R. H., Ebels, T., Navis, G., & Stegeman, C. (2005). Immediate postoperative renal function deterioration in cardiac surgical patients predicts in-hospital mortality and long-term survival. *Journal of the American Society of Nephrology : JASN*, *16*(1), 195–200. doi:10.1681/ASN.2003100875 PMID:15563558

Loforte, A., Stepanenko, A., Potapov, E. V., Musumeci, F., Dranishnikov, N., Schweiger, M., & Hetzer, R. et al. (2013). Temporary right ventricular mechanical support in high-risk left ventricular assist device recipients versus permanent biventricular or total artificial heart support. *Artificial Organs*, *37*(6), 523–530. doi:10.1111/aor.12038 PMID:23550592

Lola, I., Levidiotou, S., Petrou, A., Arnaoutoglou, H., Apostolakis, E., & Papadopoulos, G. S. (2011). Are there independent predisposing factors for postoperative infections following open heart surgery? *Journal of Cardiothoracic Surgery*, *6*(1), 151. doi:10.1186/1749-8090-6-151 PMID:22082355

Loop, F. D., Lytle, B. W., Cosgrove, D. M., Stewart, R. W., Goormastic, M., Williams, G. W., & Sheldon, W. C. et al. (1986). Influence of the internal-mammary-artery graft on 10-year survival and other cardiac events. *The New England Journal of Medicine*, *314*(1), 1–6. doi:10.1056/NEJM198601023140101 PMID:3484393

Loor, G., Li, L., Sabik, J. F. III, Rajeswaran, J., Blackstone, E. H., & Koch, C. G. (2012). Nadir hematocrit during cardiopulmonary bypass: End-organ dysfunction and mortality. *The Journal of Thoracic and Cardiovascular Surgery*, *144*(3), 654–662.e4. doi:10.1016/j.jtcvs.2012.03.058 PMID:22507841

Lopes, R. J., Almeida, J., Dias, P. J., Pinho, P., & Maciel, M. J. (2009). Infectious thoracic aortitis: A literature review. *Clinical Cardiology*, *32*(9), 488–490. doi:10.1002/clc.20578 PMID:19743492

Loponen, P., Luther, M., Wistbacka, J.-O., Nissinen, J., Sintonen, H., Huhtala, H., & Tarkka, M. R. (2008). Postoperative delirium and health related quality of life after coronary artery bypass grafting. *Scandinavian Cardiovascular Journal : SCJ*, *42*(5), 337–344. doi:10.1080/14017430801939217 PMID:18609064

Lorente, L., Lecuona, M., Jimenez, A., Mora, M. L., & Sierra, A. (2007). Influence of an endotracheal tube with polyurethane cuff and subglottic secretion drainage on pneumonia. *American Journal of Respiratory and Critical Care Medicine*, *176*(11), 1079–1083. doi:10.1164/rccm.200705-761OC PMID:17872488

Lorsomradee, S., Lorsomradee, S., Cromheecke, S., & De Hert, S. G. (2007). Uncalibrated arterial pulse contour analysis versus continuous thermodilution technique: Effects of alterations in arterial waveform. *Journal of Cardiothoracic and Vascular Anesthesia*, *21*(5), 636–643. doi:10.1053/j.jvca.2007.02.003 PMID:17905266

Loscalzo, J. (2012). From clinical observation to mechanism--Heyde's syndrome. *The New England Journal of Medicine*, *367*(20), 1954–1956. doi:10.1056/NEJMcibr1205363 PMID:23150964

Lottes, A. E., Rundell, A. E., Geddes, L., Kemeny, A. E., Otlewski, M. P., & Babbs, C. F. (2007). Sustained abdominal compression during CPR raises coronary perfusion pressures as much as vasopressor drugs. *Resuscitation*, *75*(3), 515–524. doi:10.1016/j.resuscitation.2007.05.012 PMID:17630090

Loutzenhiser, R., Griffin, K., Williamson, G., & Bidani, A. (2006). Renal autoregulation: new perspectives regarding the protective and regulatory roles of the underlying mechanisms. *AJP: Regulatory. Integrative and Comparative Physiology*, *290*(5), R1153–R1167. doi:10.1152/ajpregu.00402.2005

Love, J. E., Ferrell, C., & Chandler, W. L. (2007). Monitoring direct thrombin inhibitors with a plasma diluted thrombin time. *Journal of Thrombosis and Haemostasis*, *98*(1), 234–242. PMID:17598018

Lowe, G. D., Rumley, A., & Mackie, I. J. (2004). Plasma fibrinogen. *Annals of Clinical Biochemistry*, *41*(Pt 6), 430–440. doi:10.1258/0004563042466884 PMID:15588432

Lower, R., Stofer, R., & Shumway, N. (1961). Homovital Transplantation Of The Heart. *The Journal of Thoracic and Cardiovascular Surgery*, *41*, 196–204. PMID:13763849

Lubetkin, E. I., Lipson, D. A., Palevsky, H. I., Kotloff, R., Morris, J., Berry, G. T., & Lichtenstein, G. R. et al. (1996). GI complications after orthotopic lung transplantation. *The American Journal of Gastroenterology*, *91*(11), 2382–2390.

Luecke, T., & Pelosi, P. (2005). Clinical review: Positive end-expiratory pressure and cardiac output. *Critical Care (London, England)*, *9*(6), 607–621. doi:10.1186/cc3877 PMID:16356246

Lu, J. C., Grayson, A. D., Jha, P., Srinivasan, A. K., & Fabri, B. M. (2003). Risk factors for sternal wound infection and mid-term survival following coronary artery bypass surgery. *European Journal of Cardio-Thoracic Surgery*, *23*(6), 943–949. doi:10.1016/S1010-7940(03)00137-4 PMID:12829070

Lumb, A. B., & Nunn, J. F. (2005). *Nunn's applied respiratory physiology* (6th ed.). Edinburgh, Philadelphia: Elsevier Butterworth Heinemann.

Luna, C. M., Aruj, P., Niederman, M. S., Garzón, J., Violi, D., & Prignoni, A. (2006). Appropriateness and delay to initiate therapy in ventilator-associated pneumonia. *The European Respiratory Journal*, *27*(1), 158–164. doi:10.1183/09031936.06.00049105 PMID:16387949

Lundquist, H., Hedenstierna, G., Strandberg, A., Tokics, L., & Brismar, B. (1995). CT-assessment of dependent lung densities in man during general anaesthesia. *Acta Radiologica*, *36*(6), 626–632. doi:10.3109/02841859509176761 PMID:8519574

Lupu, D. (2010). Estimate of current hospice and palliative medicine physician workforce shortage. *Journal of Pain and Symptom Management*, *40*(6), 899–911. doi:10.1016/j.jpainsymman.2010.07.004 PMID:21145468

Lurati Buse, G. A., Koller, M. T., Grapow, M., Bolliger, D., Seeberger, M., & Filipovic, M. (2010). The prognostic value of troponin release after adult cardiac surgery - a meta-analysis. *European Journal of Cardio-Thoracic Surgery: Official Journal of the European Association for Cardio-Thoracic Surgery*, *37*(2), 399–406. doi:10.1016/j.ejcts.2009.05.054 PMID:19699102

Luyt, C.-E., Chastre, J., & Fagon, J.-Y. (2004). Value of the clinical pulmonary infection score for the identification and management of ventilator-associated pneumonia. *Intensive Care Medicine*, *30*(5), 844–852. doi:10.1007/s00134-003-2125-0 PMID:15127196

Lytle, B. W., Blackstone, E. H., Sabik, J. F., Houghtaling, P., Loop, F. D., & Cosgrove, D. M. (2004). The effect of bilateral internal thoracic artery grafting on survival during 20 postoperative years. *The Annals of Thoracic Surgery, 78*(6), 2005–12; discussion 2012–4. doi:10.1016/j.athoracsur.2004.05.070

Lytle, B. W., Cosgrove, D. M., Taylor, P. C., Goormastic, M., Stewart, R. W., Golding, L. A., & Loop, F. D. et al. (1989). Primary isolated aortic valve replacement. Early and late results. *The Journal of Thoracic and Cardiovascular Surgery, 97*(5), 675–694. PMID:2709860

MacCallum, N. S., Finney, S. J., Gordon, S. E., Quinlan, G. J., & Evans, T. W. (2014). Modified criteria for the systemic inflammatory response syndrome improves their utility following cardiac surgery. *Chest, 145*(6), 1197–1203. doi:10.1378/chest.13-1023 PMID:24576975

MacDougall, J., & Drummond, M. J. (2005). The development of medical teachers: An enquiry into the learning histories of 10 experienced medical teachers. *Medical Education, 39*(12), 1213–1220. doi:10.1111/j.1365-2929.2005.02335.x PMID:16313580

MacIver, J., & Ross, H. J. (2005). Withdrawal of ventricular assist device support. *Journal of Palliative Care, 21*(3), 151–156. PMID:16334969

Mackay, J. H., Powell, S. J., Osgathorp, J., & Rozario, C. J. (2002). Six-year prospective audit of chest reopening after cardiac arrest. *European Journal of Cardio-Thoracic Surgery : Official Journal of the European Association for Cardio-Thoracic Surgery, 22*(3), 421–425. http://www.ncbi.nlm.nih.gov/pubmed/12204734 doi:10.1016/S1010-7940(02)00294-4 PMID:12204734

Mack, M. J., Pfister, A., Bachand, D., Emery, R., Magee, M. J., Connolly, M., & Subramanian, V. (2004). Comparison of coronary bypass surgery with and without cardiopulmonary bypass in patients with multivessel disease. *The Journal of Thoracic and Cardiovascular Surgery, 127*(1), 167–173. doi:10.1016/j.jtcvs.2003.08.032 PMID:14752427

MacLeod, J. B. A., Lefton, J., Houghton, D., Roland, C., Doherty, J., Cohn, S. M., & Barquist, E. S. (2007). Prospective randomized control trial of intermittent versus continuous gastric feeds for critically ill trauma patients. *The Journal of Trauma, 63*(1), 57–61. doi:10.1097/01.ta.0000249294.58703.11 PMID:17622869

Maddox, R. R., Oglesby, H., Williams, C. K., Fields, M., & Danello, S. (2006). Continuous respiratory monitoring and a "smart" infusion system improve safety of patient-controlled analgesia in the postoperative. *American Journal of Health-System Pharmacy, 63*, 157–164. doi:10.2146/ajhp050194 PMID:16390930

Madsen, B., Hansen, J., Stokholm, K., Brons, J., Husum, D., & Mortensen, L. (1994). Chronic congestive heart failure. Description and survival of 190 consecutive patients with a diagnosis of chronic congestive heart failure based on clinical signs and symptoms. *European Heart Journal, 15*(3), 303–310. PMID:8013501

Madsen, E. H., Saw, J., Kristensen, S. R., Schmidt, E. B., Pittendreigh, C., & Maurer-Spurej, E. (2010). Long term aspirin and clopidogrel response evaluated by light transmission aggregometry, verifynow, and thromboelastography in patients undergoing percutaneous coronary intervention. *Clinical Chemistry, 56*(5), 839–847. doi:10.1373/clinchem.2009.137471 PMID:20224050

Maganti, M. D., Rao, V., Borger, M. A., Ivanov, J., & David, T. E. (2005). Predictors of low cardiac output syndrome after isolated aortic valve surgery. *Circulation, 112*(9Suppl), I448–I452. doi:10.1161/CIRCULATIONAHA.104.526087 PMID:16159861

Maganti, M., Badiwala, M., Sheikh, A., Scully, H., Feindel, C., David, T. E., & Rao, V. (2010). Predictors of low cardiac output syndrome after isolated mitral valve surgery. *The Journal of Thoracic and Cardiovascular Surgery, 140*(4), 790–796. doi:10.1016/j.jtcvs.2009.11.022 PMID:20152992

Magee, K., Campbell, S. G., Moher, D., & Rowe, B. H. (2008). Heparin versus placebo for acute coronary syndromes. *Cochrane Database of Systematic Reviews*, CD003462. PMID:18425889

Maggioni, A., Anand, I., Gottlieb, S., Latini, R., Tognoni, G., & Cohn, J. (2002). Effects of valsartan on morbidity and mortality in patients with heart failure not receiving angiotensin-converting enzyme inhibitors. *Journal of the American College of Cardiology*, *40*(8), 1414–1421. doi:10.1016/S0735-1097(02)02304-5 PMID:12392830

Magill, S. S., Klompas, M., Balk, R., Burns, S. M., Deutschman, C. S., Diekema, D., & Lipsett, P. et al. (2013). Developing a new, national approach to surveillance for ventilator-associated events. *American Journal of Critical Care*, *22*(6), 469–473. doi:10.4037/ajcc2013893 PMID:24186816

Magill, S. S., Klompas, M., Balk, R., Burns, S. M., Deutschman, C. S., Diekema, D., & Lipsett, P. et al. (2013). Developing a new, national approach to surveillance for ventilator-associated events. *Critical Care Medicine*, *41*(11), 2467–2475. doi:10.1097/CCM.0b013e3182a262db PMID:24162674

Magnusson, L., & Spahn, D. R. (2003). New concepts of atelectasis during general anaesthesia. *British Journal of Anaesthesia*, *91*(1), 61–72. doi:10.1093/bja/aeg085 PMID:12821566

Mahaffey, K. W., Wojdyla, D. M., Carroll, K., Becker, R. C., Storey, R. F., Angiolillo, D. J., & Wallentin, L. et al. (2011). Ticagrelor Compared With Clopidogrel by Geographic Region in the Platelet Inhibition and Patient Outcomes (PLATO) Trial. *Circulation*, *124*(5), 544–554. doi:10.1161/CIRCULATIONAHA.111.047498 PMID:21709065

Mahajerin, A., Gurm, H. S., Tsai, T. T., Chan, P. S., & Nallamothu, B. K. (2007). Vasodilator therapy in patients with aortic insufficiency: A systematic review. *American Heart Journal*, *153*(4), 454–461. doi:10.1016/j.ahj.2007.01.006 PMID:17383279

Maharaj, R., & Metaxa, V. (2011). Levosimendan and mortality after coronary revascularisation: A meta-analysis of randomised controlled trials. *Critical Care (London, England)*, *15*(3), R140. doi:10.1186/cc10263 PMID:21651806

Mahidhara, R., Bastani, S., Ross, D. J., Saggar, R., Lynch, J. III, Schnickel, G. T., & Ardehali, A. et al. (2008). Lung transplantation in older patients? *The Journal of Thoracic and Cardiovascular Surgery*, *135*(2), 412–420. doi:10.1016/j.jtcvs.2007.09.030

Mahla, E., Suarez, T. A., Bliden, K. P., Rehak, P., Metzler, H., Sequeira, A. J., & Gurbel, P. A. et al. (2012). Platelet function measurement-based strategy to reduce bleeding and waiting time in clopidogrel-treated patients undergoing coronary artery bypass graft surgery: The timing based on platelet function strategy to reduce clopidogrel-associated bleeding related to CABG (TARGET-CABG) study. *Circulation: Cardiovascular Interventions*, *5*(2), 261–269. doi:10.1161/CIRCINTERVENTIONS.111.967208 PMID:22396581

Mahood, S. C. (2011). Medical education: Beware the hidden curriculum. *Canadian Family Physician Medecin de Famille Canadien*, *57*(9), 983–985. PMID:21918135

Maisel, W. H., Rawn, J. D., & Stevenson, W. G. (2001). Atrial fibrillation after cardiac surgery. *Annals of Internal Medicine*, *135*(12), 1061–1073. doi:10.7326/0003-4819-135-12-200112180-00010 PMID:11747385

Majure, D. T., Greco, T., Greco, M., Ponschab, M., Biondi-Zoccai, G., Zangrillo, A., & Landoni, G. (2013). Meta-analysis of randomized trials of effect of milrinone on mortality in cardiac surgery: An update. *Journal of Cardiothoracic and Vascular Anesthesia*, *27*(2), 220–229. doi:10.1053/j.jvca.2012.08.005 PMID:23063100

Makar, M., Taylor, J., Zhao, M., Farrohi, A., & Trimming, M. (2010). *Perioperative Coagulopathy, Bleeding, and Hemostasis During Cardiac Surgery A Comprehensive Review*. ICU Director.

Makaroun, M. S., Dillaviy, E. D., Wheatley, G. H., & Cambria, R. P. (2008). Five year results of endovascular treatment with the Gore TAG device compared with open repair of thoracic aortic aneurysms. *Journal of Vascular Surgery*, *47*(5), 912–918. doi:10.1016/j.jvs.2007.12.006 PMID:18353605

Makaroun, M. S., Dillavou, E. D., Kee, S. T., Sicard, G., Chaikof, E., Bavaria, J., & Mitchell, R. S. et al. (2005). Endovas.cular treatment of thoracic aortic aneurysms: Results of the phase II multicenter trial of the GORE TAG thoracic endoprosthesis. *Journal of Vascular Surgery*, *41*(1), 1–9. doi:10.1016/j.jvs.2004.10.046 PMID:15696036

Maki, D. G., Kluger, D. M., & Crnich, C. J. (2006). The risk of bloodstream infection in adults with different intravascular devices: A systematic review of 200 published prospective studies. *Mayo Clinic Proceedings*, *81*(9), 1159–1171. doi:10.4065/81.9.1159 PMID:16970212

Makkar, R. R., Fontana, G. P., Jilaihawi, H., Kapadia, S., Pichard, A. D., Douglas, P. S., & Leon, M. B. et al. (2012). Transcatheter aortic-valve replacement for inoperable severe aortic stenosis. *The New England Journal of Medicine*, *366*(18), 1696–1704. doi:10.1056/NEJMoa1202277 PMID:22443478

Malbrain, M. L. N. G., Chiumello, D., Pelosi, P., Bihari, D., Innes, R., Ranieri, V. M., & Gattinoni, L. et al. (2005). Incidence and prognosis of intraabdominal hypertension in a mixed population of critically ill patients: A multiple-center epidemiological study. *Critical Care Medicine*, *33*(2), 315–322. doi:10.1097/01.CCM.0000153408.09806.1B PMID:15699833

Malbrain, M. L. N. G., Chiumello, D., Pelosi, P., Wilmer, A., Brienza, N., Malcangi, V., & Gattinoni, L. et al. (2004). Prevalence of intra-abdominal hypertension in critically ill patients: A multicentre epidemiological study. *Intensive Care Medicine*, *30*(5), 822–829. doi:10.1007/s00134-004-2169-9 PMID:14758472

Maldonado, J. R., Wysong, A., van der Starre, P. J., Block, T., Miller, C., & Reitz, B. A. (2009). Dexmedetomidine and the reduction of postoperative delirium after cardiac surgery. *Psychosomatics*, *50*(3), 206–217. doi:10.1176/appi.psy.50.3.206 PMID:19567759

Malouf, J. F., Alam, S., Gharzeddine, W., & Stefadouros, M. A. (1993). The role of anticoagulation in the development of pericardial effusion and late tamponade after cardiac surgery. *European Heart Journal*, *14*(11), 1451–1457. doi:10.1093/eurheartj/14.11.1451 PMID:8299624

Maltais, S., Costello, W. T., Billings, F. T. IV, Bick, J. S., Byrne, J. G., Ahmad, R. M., & Wagner, C. E. (2013). Episodic Monoplane Transesophageal Echocardiography Impacts Postoperative Management of the Cardiac Surgery Patient. *Journal of Cardiothoracic and Vascular Anesthesia*, *27*(4), 665–669. doi:10.1053/j.jvca.2013.02.012 PMID:23849522

Malvindi, P. G., Jacob, S., Kallikourdis, A., & Vitale, N. (2007). What is the patency of the gastroepiploic artery when used for coronary artery bypass grafting? *Interactive Cardiovascular and Thoracic Surgery*, *6*(3), 397–402. doi:10.1510/icvts.2007.155259 PMID:17669877

Managing Trainees in Difficulty. (2013, October). Managing Trainees in Difficulty. *General Medical COuncil*. London. Retrieved May 12, 2014, from http://www.gmc-uk.org/Final_Appendix_5_Trainees_in_Difficulty.pdf_53816759.pdf

Mangano, C. M., Diamondstone, L. S., Ramsay, J. G., Aggarwal, A., Herskowitz, A., & Mangano, D. T. (1998). Renal dysfunction after myocardial revascularization: Risk factors, adverse outcomes, and hospital resource utilization. The Multicenter Study of Perioperative Ischemia Research Group. *Annals of Internal Medicine*, *128*(3), 194–203. http://www.ncbi.nlm.nih.gov/pubmed/9454527 doi:10.7326/0003-4819-128-3-199802010-00005 PMID:9454527

Mangano, D. T. (2002). Aspirin and mortality from coronary bypass surgery. *The New England Journal of Medicine*, *347*(17), 1309–1317. doi:10.1056/NEJMoa020798 PMID:12397188

Mangano, D. T., Rieves, R. D., & Weiss, K. D. (2006). Judging the safety of aprotinin. *The New England Journal of Medicine*, *355*(21), 2261–2262. doi:10.1056/NEJMc066520 PMID:17124031

Mangano, D. T., Tudor, I. C., & Dietzel, C.Multicenter Study of Perioperative Ischemia Research Group, Ischemia Research and Education Foundation. (2006). The risk associated with aprotinin in cardiac surgery. *The New England Journal of Medicine*, *354*(4), 353–365. doi:10.1056/NEJMoa051379 PMID:16436767

Mangi, A. A., Christison-Lagay, E. R., Torchiana, D. F., Warshaw, A. L., & Berger, D. L. (2005). Gastrointestinal complications in patients undergoing heart operation: An analysis of 8709 consecutive cardiac surgical patients. *Annals of Surgery*, *241*(6), 895–901. doi:10.1097/01.sla.0000164173.05762.32 PMID:15912039

Mangoush, O., Purkayastha, S., Haj-Yahia, S., Kinross, J., Hayward, M., Bartolozzi, F., & Athanasiou, T. et al. (2007). Heparin-bonded circuits versus nonheparin-bonded circuits: An evaluation of their effect on clinical outcomes. *European Journal of Cardio-Thoracic Surgery*, *31*(6), 1058–1069. doi:10.1016/j.ejcts.2007.01.029 PMID:17306555

Manji, R. A., Grocott, H. P., Leake, J., Ariano, R. E., Manji, J. S., Menkis, A. H., & Jacobsohn, E. (2012). Seizures following cardiac surgery: The impact of tranexamic acid and other risk factors. *Canadian Journal of Anaesthesia*, *59*(1), 6–13. doi:10.1007/s12630-011-9618-z PMID:22065333

Mann D. L., Zipes, D. P., Libby, P., Bonow, R. O., & Braunwald, E. (2014). *Braunwald's Heart Disease*. Elsevier.

Manning, W. J., Reis, G. J., & Douglas, P. S. (1992). Use of transoesophageal echocardiography to detect left atrial thrombi before percutaneous balloon dilation of the mitral valve: A prospective study. *British Heart Journal*, *67*(2), 170–173. doi:10.1136/hrt.67.2.170 PMID:1540437

Manno, E., Navarra, M., Faccio, L., Motevallian, M., Bertolaccini, L., Mfochivè, A., & Evangelista, A. et al. (2012). Deep impact of ultrasound in the intensive care unit: The "ICU-sound" protocol. *Anesthesiology*, *117*(4), 801–809. doi:10.1097/ALN.0b013e318264c621 PMID:22990179

Mansfield, D., Gollogly, C., Kaye, D., Richardson, M., Bergin, P., & Naughton, M. (2004). Controlled Trial of Continuous Positive Airway Pressure in Obstructive Sleep Apnea and Heart Failure. *American Journal of Respiratory and Critical Care Medicine*, *169*(3), 361–366. doi:10.1164/rccm.200306-752OC PMID:14597482

Manthous, C. A., & Hollingshead, A. B. (2011). Team science and critical care. *American Journal of Respiratory and Critical Care Medicine*, *184*(1), 17–25. doi:10.1164/rccm.201101-0185CI PMID:21471081

Maquelin, K. N., Berckmans, R. J., Nieuwland, R., Schaap, M. C., ten Have, K., Eijsman, L., & Sturk, A. (1998). Disappearance of glycoprotein Ib from the platelet surface in pericardial blood during cardiopulmonary bypass. *The Journal of Thoracic and Cardiovascular Surgery*, *115*(5), 1160–1165. doi:10.1016/S0022-5223(98)70416-7 PMID:9605086

Marcantonio, E., Goldman, L., Mangione, C., Ludwig, L., Muraca, B., Haslauer, C., & Lee, T. et al. (1994). A Clinical Prediction Rule for Delirium After Elective Noncardiac Surgery. *Journal of the American Medical Association*, *271*(2), 134–139. doi:10.1001/jama.1994.03510260066030 PMID:8264068

Marengo-Rowe, A. J. J. L. (1988). Fibrinolysis: A frequent cause of bleeding (N. Ellison, D.R. Jobes Ed.). Philadelphia: WB Saunders.

Marik, P. E. (2009). Critical illness-related corticosteroid insufficiency. *Chest*, *135*(1), 181–193. doi:10.1378/chest.08-1149 PMID:19136406

Marik, P. E., Baram, M., & Vahid, B. (2008). Does central venous pressure predict fluid responsiveness? A systematic review of the literature and the tale of seven mares. *Chest*, *134*(1), 172–178. doi:10.1378/chest.07-2331 PMID:18628220

Marik, P. E., Cavallazzi, R., Vasu, T., & Hirani, A. (2009). Dynamic changes in arterial waveform derived variables and fluid responsiveness in mechanically ventilated patients: A systematic review of the literature. *Critical Care Medicine*, *37*(9), 2642–2647. doi:10.1097/CCM.0b013e3181a590da PMID:19602972

Marik, P. E., Flemmer, M., & Harrison, W. (2012). The risk of catheter-related bloodstream infection with femoral venous catheters as compared to subclavian and internal jugular venous catheters: A systematic review of the literature and meta-analysis. *Critical Care Medicine*, *40*(8), 2479–2485. doi:10.1097/CCM.0b013e318255d9bc PMID:22809915

Marik, P. E., Levitov, A., Young, A., & Andrews, L. (2013). The use of bioreactance and carotid Doppler to determine volume responsiveness and blood flow redistribution following passive leg raising in hemodynamically unstable patients. *Chest*, *143*(2), 364–370. doi:10.1378/chest.12-1274 PMID:22910834

Marik, P. E., Monnet, X., & Teboul, J.-L. (2011). Hemodynamic parameters to guide fluid therapy. *Annals of Intensive Care*, *1*(1), 1. doi:10.1186/2110-5820-1-1 PMID:21906322

Marik, P. E., Pastores, S. M., Annane, D., Meduri, G. U., Sprung, C. L., Arlt, W., & Vogeser, M. et al.American College of Critical Care Medicine. (2008). Recommendations for the diagnosis and management of corticosteroid insufficiency in critically ill adult patients: Consensus statements from an international task force by the American College of Critical Care Medicine. *Critical Care Medicine*, *36*(6), 1937–1949. doi:10.1097/CCM.0b013e31817603ba PMID:18496365

Marik, P. E., Vasu, T., Hirani, A., & Pachinburavan, M. (2010). Stress ulcer prophylaxis in the new millennium: A systematic review and meta-analysis. *Critical Care Medicine*, *38*(11), 2222–2228. doi:10.1097/CCM.0b013e3181f17adf PMID:20711074

Marik, P. E., & Zaloga, G. P. (2001). Early enteral nutrition in acutely ill patients: A systematic review. *Critical Care Medicine*, *29*(12), 2264–2270. doi:10.1097/00003246-200112000-00005 PMID:11801821

Marik, P. E., & Zaloga, G. P. (2003). Adrenal insufficiency during septic shock. *Critical Care Medicine*, *31*(1), 141–145. doi:10.1097/00003246-200301000-00022 PMID:12545007

Marik, P. E., & Zaloga, G. P. (2003). Gastric versus post-pyloric feeding: A systematic review. *Critical Care (London, England)*, *7*(3), R46–R51. doi:10.1186/cc2190 PMID:12793890

Marik, P. E., & Zaloga, G. P. (2008). Immunonutrition in critically ill patients: A systematic review and analysis of the literature. *Intensive Care Medicine*, *34*(11), 1980–1990. doi:10.1007/s00134-008-1213-6 PMID:18626628

Marin, M., Hollier, L., & Cha, A. (2003). Endovascular stent graft repair of abdominal and thoracic aortic aneurysms. *Annals of Surgery*, *238*(4), 586–595. PMID:14530730

Marino, P. (2007). *The ICU Book* (3rd ed.). Philadelphia: Lippincott Williams and Wilkins.

Mariscalco, G., Lorusso, R., Dominici, C., Renzulli, A., & Sala, A. (2011). Acute kidney injury: A relevant complication after cardiac surgery. *The Annals of Thoracic Surgery*, *92*(4), 1539–1547. doi:10.1016/j.athoracsur.2011.04.123 PMID:21872837

Mariya Joseph, N., Sistla, S., Kumar Dutta, T., Shankar Badhe, A., Rasitha, D., & Chandra Parija, S. (2012). Outcome of ventilator-associated pneumonia: Impact of antibiotic therapy and other factors. *Australasian Medical Journal*, *5*, 135–140. PMID:22905055

Markham, D. (2013). Sympathetic neural and hemodynamic responses to upright tilt in patients with pulsatile and non-pulsatile left ventricular assist devices. *Circulation: Heart Failure*, *6*, 293–299. PMID:23250982

Marques, M. B., & Langouche, L. (2012). Endocrine, Metabolic, and Morphologic Alterations of Adipose Tissue During Critical Illness. *Critical Care Medicine*. PMID:23135416

Marschall, J., Mermel, L. A., Fakih, M., Hadaway, L., Kallen, A., O'Grady, N. P., & Yokoe, D. S. et al. (2014). Strategies to prevent central line-associated infections in acute care hospitals: 2014 update. *Infection Control and Hospital Epidemiology*, *35*(7), 753–771. doi:10.1086/676533 PMID:24915204

Marshall, J. C. (2001). Inflammation, coagulopathy, and the pathogenesis of multiple organ dysfunction syndrome. *Critical Care Medicine*, *29*, S99–S106. doi:10.1097/00003246-200107001-00032 PMID:11445742

Marsh, S. A., & Coombes, J. S. (2006). Vitamin E and alpha-lipoic acid supplementation increase bleeding tendency via an intrinsic coagulation pathway. *Clinical and Applied Thrombosis/Hemostasis*, *12*(2), 169–173. doi:10.1177/107602960601200204 PMID:16708118

Martens, S., Neumann, K., Sodemann, C., Deschka, H., Wimmer-Greinecker, G., & Moritz, A. (2008). Carbon dioxide field flooding reduces neurologic impairment after open heart surgery. *The Annals of Thoracic Surgery*, *85*(2), 543–547. doi:10.1016/j.athoracsur.2007.08.047 PMID:18222261

Martin, B.-J., Buth, K. J., Arora, R. C., & Baskett, R. J. F. (2010). Delirium as a predictor of sepsis in post-coronary artery bypass grafting patients: A retrospective cohort study. *Critical Care (London, England)*, *14*(5), R171. doi:10.1186/cc9273 PMID:20875113

Martin, B.-J., Buth, K. J., Arora, R. C., & Baskett, R. J. F. (2012). Delirium: A cause for concern beyond the immediate postoperative period. *The Annals of Thoracic Surgery*, *93*(4), 1114–1120. doi:10.1016/j.athoracsur.2011.09.011 PMID:22200370

Martin, D. S., & Grocott, M. P. (2013). Oxygen therapy in critical illness: Precise control of arterial oxygenation and permissive hypoxemia. *Critical Care Medicine*, *41*(2), 423–432. doi:10.1097/CCM.0b013e31826a44f6 PMID:23263574

Martindale, R. G., McClave, S. A., Vanek, V. W., McCarthy, M., Roberts, P., Taylor, B., & Cresci, G. et al. (2009). Guidelines for the provision and assessment of nutrition support therapy in the adult critically ill patient: Society of Critical Care Medicine and American Society for Parenteral and Enteral Nutrition: Executive Summary. *Critical Care Medicine*, *37*(5), 1757–1761. doi:10.1097/CCM.0b013e3181a40116 PMID:19373044

Martínez-Comendador, J. M., Alvarez, J. R., Mosquera, I., Sierra, S., Adrio, B., Carro, J. G., & Bengochea, J. et al. (2009). Preoperative statin treatment reduces systemic inflammatory response and myocardial damage in cardiac surgery. *European Journal of Cardio-Thoracic Surgery*, *36*(6), 998–1005. doi:10.1016/j.ejcts.2009.05.022 PMID:19581104

Martinez, E. A., Epstein, A. E., & Bass, E. B. (2005a). Pharmacologic control of ventricular rate: American College of Chest Physicians guidelines for the prevention and management of postoperative atrial fibrillation after cardiac surgery. *Chest*, *128*(2Suppl), 56S–60S. doi:10.1378/chest.128.2_suppl.56S PMID:16167666

Martinez, E.A., Bass, E.B., & Zimetbaum, P., & American College of Chest Physicians. (2005b). Pharmacologic control of rhythm: American College of Chest Physicians guidelines for the prevention and management of postoperative atrial fibrillation after cardiac surgery. *Chest*, *128*(2Suppl), 48S–55S.

Martinez, J. A., Nicolas, J. M., Marco, F., Horcajada, J. P., Garcia-Seggara, G., & Trilla, A. (2006). Comparison of antimicrobial cycling and mixing strategies in two medical intensive care units. *Critical Care Medicine*, *34*, 275–279. PMID:16424711

Martin, K., Wiesner, G., Breuer, T., Lange, R., & Tassani, P. (2008). The risks of aprotinin and tranexamic acid in cardiac surgery: A one-year follow-up of 1188 consecutive patients. *Anesthesia and Analgesia*, *107*(6), 1783–1790. doi:10.1213/ane.0b013e318184bc20 PMID:19020118

Martin, L. M., Halpin, L. S., Barnett, S. D., Speir, A. M., Hunt, S. L., Mukherjee, N., & Ad, N. (2008). The association between early outcome, health-related quality of life, and survival following elective open-heart surgery. *The Journal of Cardiovascular Nursing*, *23*(5), 432–442. doi:10.1097/01.JCN.0000317453.10521.5b PMID:18728516

Marty, J., Nitenberg, A., Blanchet, F., Zouioueche, S., & Desmonts, J. M. (1986). Effects of midazolam on the coronary circulation in patients with coronary artery disease. *Anesthesiology*, *64*(2), 206–210. doi:10.1097/00000542-198602000-00013 PMID:2936281

Mascioli, E. A., Lopes, S. M., Champagne, C., & Driscoll, D. F. (1996). Essential fatty acid deficiency and home total parenteral nutrition patients. *Nutrition (Burbank, Los Angeles County, Calif.)*, *12*(4), 245–249. doi:10.1016/S0899-9007(96)90850-3 PMID:8862529

Masla, M., Gottschalk, A., Durieux, M. E., & Groves, D. S. (2011). HbA1c and diabetes predict perioperative hyperglycemia and glycemic variability in on-pump coronary artery bypass graft patients. *Journal of Cardiothoracic and Vascular Anesthesia*, *25*(5), 799–803. doi:10.1053/j.jvca.2010.09.028 PMID:21111636

Massell, B. F., Chute, C. G., Walker, A. M., & Kurland, G. S. (1988). Penicillin and the marked decrease in morbidity and mortality from rheumatic fever in the United States. *The New England Journal of Medicine*, *318*(5), 280–286. doi:10.1056/NEJM198802043180504 PMID:3336421

Massoudy, P., Wagner, S., Thielmann, M., Herold, U., Kottenberg-Assenmacher, E., Marggraf, G., & Herget-Rosenthal, S. et al. (2008). Coronary artery bypass surgery and acute kidney injury--impact of the off-pump technique. *Nephrology, Dialysis, Transplantation*, *23*(9), 2853–2860. doi:10.1093/ndt/gfn153 PMID:18388121

Mathew, J. P. F. (2004). A multicenter risk index for atrial fibrillation after cardiac surgery. *Journal of the American Medical Association*, *291*(14), 1720–1729. doi:10.1001/jama.291.14.1720 PMID:15082699

Mathias, J., Mathias, E., Jausset, F., Oliver, A., Sellal, C., Laurent, V., & Regent, D. (2012). Aorto-enteric fistulas: A physiopathological approach and computed tomography diagnosis. *Diagnostic and Interventional Imaging*, *93*(11), 840–851. doi:10.1016/j.diii.2012.07.003 PMID:23092721

Mathru, M., Esch, O., Lang, J., Herbert, M. E., Chaljub, G., Goodacre, B., & vanSonnenberg, E. (1996). Magnetic resonance imaging of the upper airway: Effects of propofol anesthesia and nasal continuous positive airway pressure in humans. *Anesthesiology*, *84*(2), 273–279. doi:10.1097/00000542-199602000-00004 PMID:8602656

Matsumura, J. S., Cambria, R. P., Dake, M. D., Moore, R. D., Svensson, L. G., & Snyder, S. (2008). International controlled clinical trial of thoracic endovascular aneurysm repair with the Zenith TX2 endovascular graft: 1-year results. *Journal of Vascular Surgery*, *47*(2), 247–257. doi:10.1016/j.jvs.2007.10.032 PMID:18241743

Mauermann, W. J., Sampathkumar, P., & Thompson, R. L. (2008). Sternal wound infections. *Best Practice & Research. Clinical Anaesthesiology*, *22*(3), 423–436. doi:10.1016/j.bpa.2008.04.003 PMID:18831296

Maung, A., Johnson, D. C., Piper, G. L., Barbosa, R. R., Rowell, S. E., Bokhari, F., & Kerwin, A. J. et al. (2012). Evaluation and management of small-bowel obstruction. *Journal of Trauma and Acute Care Surgery*, *73*(5), S362–S369. doi:10.1097/TA.0b013e31827019de PMID:23114494

Mayberg, T. S., Lam, A. M., Matta, B. F., Domino, K. B., & Winn, H. R. (1995). Ketamine does not increase cerebral blood flow velocity or intracranial pressure during isoflurane/nitrous oxide anesthesia in patients undergoing craniotomy. *Anesthesia and Analgesia*, *81*, 84–89. PMID:7598288

Mayer, J. (1978). Subclavian artery approach for insertion of intraaortic balloon. *The Journal of Thoracic and Cardiovascular Surgery*, *76*, 61–63. PMID:661368

Maynard, N., Bihari, D., Beale, R., Smithies, M., Baldock, G., Mason, R., & McColl, I. (1993). Assessment of splanchnic oxygenation by gastric tonometry in patients with acute circulatory failure. *Journal of the American Medical Association*, *270*(10), 1203–1210. doi:10.1001/jama.1993.03510100053032 PMID:8355382

Mayo, P. H., Beaulieu, Y., Doelken, P., Feller-Kopman, D., Harrod, C., Kaplan, A., & Lichtenstein, D. et al. (2009). American College of Chest Physicians/La Société de Réanimation de Langue Française statement on competence in critical care ultrasonography. *CHEST Journal*, *135*(4), 1050–1060. doi:10.1378/chest.08-2305 PMID:19188546

Mazer, C. D. (2014). Blood conservation in cardiac surgery: Guidelines and controversies. *Transfusion and Apheresis Science*, *50*(1), 20–25. doi:10.1016/j.transci.2013.12.008 PMID:24529682

McAlister, F. A., Man, J., Bistritz, L., Amad, H., & Tandon, P. (2003). Diabetes and coronary artery bypass surgery: An examination of perioperative glycemic control and outcomes. *Diabetes Care*, *26*(5), 1518–1524. doi:10.2337/diacare.26.5.1518 PMID:12716815

McCollough, J. N., Zhang, N., & Reich, D. L. (1999). Cerebral metabolic suppression during hypothermic circulatory arrest in humans. *The Annals of Thoracic Surgery*, *67*(6), 1895–1899. doi:10.1016/S0003-4975(99)00441-5 PMID:10391334

McCrory, D. C., & Brown, C. D. (2002). Anti-cholinergic bronchodilators versus beta2-sympathomimetic agents for acute exacerbations of chronic obstructive pulmonary disease. *Cochrane Database of Systematic Reviews*, (4): CD003900. doi:10.1002/14651858.CD003900 PMID:12519615

McCrory, D. C., Brown, C., Gelfand, S. E., & Bach, P. B. (2001). Management of acute exacerbations of COPD: A summary and appraisal of published evidence. *Chest Journal*, *119*(4), 1190–1209. doi:10.1378/chest.119.4.1190 PMID:11296189

McCrum, M. L., Joynt, K. E., Orav, E. J., Gawande, A. A., & Jha, A. K. (2013). Mortality for publicly reported conditions and overall hospital mortality rates. *JAMA Internal Medicine*, *173*(14), 1351–1357. doi:10.1001/jamainternmed.2013.7049 PMID:23797306

McDaid, C., Maund, E., Rice, S., Wright, K., Jenkins, B., & Woolacott, N. (2010). Paracetamol and selective and non-selective non-steroidal anti-inflammatory drugs (NSAIDs) for the reduction of morphine-related side effects after major surgery: A systematic review. *Health Technology Assessment*, *14*(17), 1–153. doi:10.3310/hta14170 PMID:20346263

McDonagh, D. L., Berger, M., Mathew, J. P., Graffagnino, C., Milano, C., & Newman, M. F. (2014). Neurological complications of cardiac surgery. *Lancet Neurology*, *13*(May), 490–502. doi:10.1016/S1474-4422(14)70004-3 PMID:24703207

McDonnell, M. E., Alexanian, S. M., Junqueira, A., Cabral, H., & Lazar, H. L. (2013). Relevance of the Surgical Care Improvement Project on glycemic control in patients undergoing cardiac surgery who receive continuous insulin infusions. *The Journal of Thoracic and Cardiovascular Surgery*, *145*(2), 590–594, discussion 595–597. doi:10.1016/j.jtcvs.2012.09.031 PMID:23062416

McDonnel, M. E., Alexanian, S. M., White, L., & Lazar, H. L. (2012). A primer for achieving glycemic control in the cardiac surgical patient. *Journal of Cardiac Surgery*, *27*(4), 470–477. doi:10.1111/j.1540-8191.2012.01471.x PMID:22640228

McFarlane, H. J., MacDonald, J., Collins, T. C., Molyneaux, P. J., & Carman, W. F. (2009). Severe pneumonia after cardiac surgery as a result of infection with parainfluenza virus type 4. *Journal of Cardiothoracic and Vascular Anesthesia*, *23*(1), 84–86. doi:10.1053/j.jvca.2008.02.008 PMID:18834791

McGaghie, W. C., Issenberg, S. B., Petrusa, E. R., & Scalese, R. J. (2006). Effect of practice on standardised learning outcomes in simulation-based medical education. *Medical Education*, *40*(8), 792–797. doi:10.1111/j.1365-2929.2006.02528.x PMID:16869926

McGaghie, W. C., Issenberg, S. B., Petrusa, E. R., & Scalese, R. J. (2010). A critical review of simulation-based medical education research: 2003-2009. *Medical Education*, *44*(1), 50–63. doi:10.1111/j.1365-2923.2009.03547.x PMID:20078756

McGeehin, W., Sheikh, F., Donahoo, J. S., Lechman, M. J., & MacVaugh, H. III. (1987). Transthoracic intraaortic balloon pump support: Experience in 39 patients. *The Annals of Thoracic Surgery*, *44*(1), 26–30. doi:10.1016/S0003-4975(10)62350-8 PMID:3606257

McGlynn, E. A., Asch, S. M., Adams, J., Keesey, J., Hicks, J., DeCristofaro, A., & Kerr, E. A. (2003). The quality of health care delivered to adults in the United States. *The New England Journal of Medicine*, *348*(26), 2635–2645. doi:10.1056/NEJMsa022615 PMID:12826639

McGovern, P. G., Jacobs, D. R. Jr, Shahar, E., Arnett, D. K., Folsom, A. R., Blackburn, H., & Luepker, R. (2001). Trends in Acute Coronary Heart Disease Mortality, Morbidity, and Medical Care From 1985 Through 1997. *Circulation*, *104*(1), 19–24. doi:10.1161/01.CIR.104.1.19 PMID:11435332

McGuinness, S., & Sidebotham, D. (2007). Specific Causes of Respiratory Failure. In D. Sidebotham, A. McKee, M. Gillham, & J. H. Levy (Eds.), *Cardiothoracic Critical Care*. Philadelphia: Butterworth Heinemann Elsevier. doi:10.1016/B978-075067572-7.50030-8

Mcilroy, D. R., Wagener, G., & Lee, H. T. (2010). Neutrophil Gelatinase-Associated Lipocalin and Acute Kidney Injury after Cardiac Surgery: The Effect of Baseline Renal Function on Diagnostic Performance. *Clinical Journal of the American Society of Nephrology; CJASN*, *5*(2), 211–219. doi:10.2215/CJN.04240609 PMID:20056755

McKhann, G. M., & Grega, M. A., & BorowiczJr, L. M. (2002). Encephalopathy and stroke after Coronary artery bypass grafting. *JAMA Neurology*, *59*, 1422–1428. PMID:12223028

McKhann, G. M., Grega, M. A., Borowicz, L. M. Jr, Baumgartner, W. A., & Selnes, O. A. (2006). Stroke and encephalopathy after cardiac surgery: An update. *Stroke*, *37*(2), 562–571. doi:10.1161/01.STR.0000199032.78782.6c PMID:16373636

McKhann, G. M., Grega, M., Borowicz, L. M. Jr, Selnes, O., Baumgartner, W., & Royall, R. M. (2004). Encephalopathy and Stroke After Coronary Artery Bypass Grafting. *Current Treatment Options in Cardiovascular Medicine*, *6*(3), 171–178. http://www.ncbi.nlm.nih.gov/pubmed/15096308 doi:10.1007/s11936-996-0011-0 PMID:15096308

McKinley, R. K., Strand, J., Ward, L., Gray, T., Alun-Jones, T., & Miller, H. (2008). Checklists for assessment and certification of clinical procedural skills omit essential competencies: A systematic review. *Medical Education*, *42*(4), 338–349. doi:10.1111/j.1365-2923.2007.02970.x PMID:18338987

McLean, J. (1959). The discovery of heparin. *Circulation*, *19*(1), 75–78. doi:10.1161/01.CIR.19.1.75 PMID:13619023

McLeod, P. J., Steinert, Y., Trudel, J., & Gottesman, R. (2001). Seven principles for teaching procedural and technical skills. *Academic Medicine*, *76*(10), 1080. doi:10.1097/00001888-200110000-00023 PMID:11597855

McMurray, J. J., Adamopoulos, S., Anker, S. D., Auricchio, A., Böhm, M., Dickstein, K., & Ponikowski, P. et al. (2012). ESC guidelines for the diagnosis and treatment of acute and chronic heart failure 2012: The Task Force for the Diagnosis and Treatment of Acute and Chronic Heart Failure 2012 of the European Society of Cardiology. Developed in collaboration with the Heart Failure Association (HFA) of the ESC. *European Heart Journal*, *33*(14), 1787–1847. doi:10.1093/eurheartj/ehs104 PMID:22611136

McMurray, J., Ostergren, J., Swedberg, K., Granger, C., Held, P., Michelson, E., & Pfeffer, M. et al. (2003). Effects of candesartan in patients with chronic heart failure and reduced left-ventricular systolic function taking angiotensin-converting-enzyme inhibitors: The CHARM-Added trial. *Lancet*, *362*(9386), 767–771. doi:10.1016/S0140-6736(03)14283-3 PMID:13678869

McMurray, J., Packer, M., Desai, A., Gong, J., Lefkowitz, M., Rizkala, A., & Zile, M. et al. (2014). Angiotensin-neprilysin inhibition versus enalapril in heart failure. *The New England Journal of Medicine*, *371*(11), 993–1004. doi:10.1056/NEJMoa1409077 PMID:25176015

McPherson, J. A., Wagner, C. E., Boehm, L. M., Hall, J. D., Johnson, D. C., Miller, L. R., & Pandharipande, P. P. et al. (2013). Delirium in the cardiovascular ICU: Exploring modifiable risk factors. *Critical Care Medicine*, *41*(2), 405–413. doi:10.1097/CCM.0b013e31826ab49b PMID:23263581

McSweeney, M. E., Garwood, S., Levin, J., Marino, M. R., Wang, S. X., Kardatzke, D., & Wolman, R. L. et al. (2004). Adverse gastrointestinal complications after cardiopulmonary bypass: Can outcome be predicted from preoperative risk factors? *Anesthesia and Analgesia*, *98*(6), 1610–1617. doi:10.1213/01.ANE.0000113556.40345.2E PMID:15155313

McWilliams, D., Weblin, J., Atkins, G., Bion, J., Williams, J., & Elliott, C. … Snelson, C. (2014). Enhancing rehabilitation of mechanically ventilated patients in the intensive care unit: A quality improvement project. *Journal of Critical Care*; Advance online publication. doi:10.1016/j.jcrc.2014.09.018

Meade, M. O., Granton, J. T., Matte-Martyn, A., McRae, K., Weaver, B., Cripps, P., & Keshavjee, S. H. (2003). A randomized trial of inhaled nitric oxide to prevent ischemia-reperfusion injury after lung transplantation. *American Journal of Respiratory and Critical Care Medicine*, *167*(11), 1483–1489. doi:10.1164/rccm.2203034

Meade, M., Guyatt, G., Cook, D., Griffith, L., Sinuff, T., Kergl, C., & Epstein, S. et al. (2001). Predicting success in weaning from mechanical ventilation. *Chest Journal*, *120*(6Suppl), 400S–424S. doi:10.1378/chest.120.6_suppl.400S PMID:11742961

Meade, M., Jacka, M. J., Cook, D. J., Dodek, P., Griffith, L., & Guyatt, G. H. (2004). Survey of interventions for the prevention and treatment of acute respiratory distress syndrome. *Critical Care Medicine*, *32*(4), 946–954. doi:10.1097/01.CCM.0000120056.76356.AD PMID:15071383

Meadow, W., Pohlman, A., Frain, L., Ren, Y., Kress, J. P., Teuteberg, W., & Hall, J. (2011). Power and limitations of daily prognostications of death in the medical intensive care unit. *Critical Care Medicine*, *39*(3), 474–479. doi:10.1097/CCM.0b013e318205df9b PMID:21150582

Mebazaa, A., Karpati, P., Renaud, E., & Algotsson, L. (2004). Acute right ventricular failure--from pathophysiology to new treatments. *Intensive Care Medicine*, *30*(2), 185–196. doi:10.1007/s00134-003-2025-3 PMID:14618229

Mebazaa, A., Nieminen, M. S., Packer, M., Cohen-Solal, A., Kleber, F. X., Pocock, S. J., & SURVIVE Investigators, et al.. (2007). Levosimendan vs dobutamine for patients with acute decompensated heart failure: The SURVIVE randomized trial. *Journal of the American Medical Association*, *297*(17), 1883–1891. doi:10.1001/jama.297.17.1883 PMID:17473298

Mechanick, J. I. (2006). Metabolic Mechanisms of stress hyperglycemia. *Journal of Parenteral and Enteral Nutrition*, *30*(2), 157–163. doi:10.1177/0148607106030002157 PMID:16517960

Mechanick, J. I., & Brett, E. M. (2002). Endocrine and metabolic issues in the management of the chronically critically ill patient. *Critical Care Clinics*, *18*(3), 619–641. doi:10.1016/S0749-0704(02)00005-2 PMID:12140916

Mechanick, J. I., & Brett, E. M. (2002). Nutrition support of the chronically critically ill patient. *Critical Care Clinics*, *18*(3), 597–618. doi:10.1016/S0749-0704(02)00006-4 PMID:12140915

Meddings, J., Rogers, M. A., Macy, M., & Saint, S. (2010). Systematic review and meta-analysis: Reminder systems to reduce catheter-associated urinary tract infections and urinary catheter use in hospitalized patients. *Clinical Infectious Diseases*, *51*(5), 550–560. doi:10.1086/655133 PMID:20673003

Medicine, S. C. C. (2013). *Guidelines.* Retrieved June 5, 2014, from http://www.iculiberation.org/Guidelines/Pages/default.aspx

Medin, D. L., Brown, D. T., Wesley, R., Cunnion, R. E., & Ognibene, F. F. (1998). Validation of continuous thermodilution cardiac output in critically ill patients with analysis of systematic errors. *Journal of Critical Care, 13*(4), 184–189. doi:10.1016/S0883-9441(98)90004-1 PMID:9869545

Meduri, G. U., & Yates, C. R. (2004). Systemic inflammation-associated glucocorticoid resistance and outcome of ARDS. *Annals of the New York Academy of Sciences, 1024*(1), 24–53. doi:10.1196/annals.1321.004 PMID:15265772

Mega, J. L., Braunwald, E., Wiviott, S. D., Bassand, J.-P., Bhatt, D. L., Bode, C., & Sun, X. et al. (2012). Rivaroxaban in Patients with a Recent Acute Coronary Syndrome. *The New England Journal of Medicine, 366*(1), 9–19. doi:10.1056/NEJMoa1112277 PMID:22077192

Mehlhorn, J., Freytag, A., Schmidt, K., Brunkhorst, F. M., Graf, J., Troitzsch, U., & Gensichen, J. et al. (2014). Rehabilitation Interventions for Postintensive Care Syndrome: A Systematic Review. *Critical Care Medicine, 42*(5), 1263–1271. doi:10.1097/CCM.0000000000000148 PMID:24413580

Mehra, M. R., Kobashigawa, J., Starling, R., Russell, S., Uber, P. A., & Parameshwar, J. … Barr, M. (2006). Listing Criteria For Heart Transplantation: International Society For Heart And Lung Transplantation Guidelines For The Care Of Cardiac Transplant Candidates–2006. *The Journal Of Heart And Lung Transplantation, 25*(9), 1024-1042. Retrieved From http://www.jhltonline.org/article/s1053-2498(06)00460-8/abstract

Mehra, M., Jessup, M., Gronda, E., & Costanzo, M. (2006). Rationale and Process: International Society for Heart and Lung Transplantation Guidelines for the Care of Cardiac Transplant Candidates—2006. *The Journal of Heart and Lung Transplantation, 25*(9), 1001–1002. doi:10.1016/j.healun.2006.06.006 PMID:16962462

Mehta, N. B., Hull, A. L., Young, J. B., & Stoller, J. K. (2013). Just Imagine. *Academic Medicine, 88*(10), 1418–1423. doi:10.1097/ACM.0b013e3182a36a07 PMID:23969368

Mehta, R. L., Kellum, J., Shah, S. V., Molitoris, B. A., Ronco, C., Warnock, D. G., & Levin, A. (2007). Acute Kidney Injury Network: Report of an initiative to improve outcomes in acute kidney injury. *Critical Care (London, England), 11*(2), R31. doi:10.1186/cc5713 PMID:17331245

Mehta, S. R., Yusuf, S., Peters, R. J., Bertrand, M. E., Lewis, B. S., Natarajan, M. K., & Fox, K. A. et al. (2001). Effects of pretreatment with clopidogrel and aspirin followed by long-term therapy in patients undergoing percutaneous coronary intervention: The PCI-CURE study. *Lancet, 358*(9281), 527–533. doi:10.1016/S0140-6736(01)05701-4 PMID:11520521

Mehta, S., Burry, L., Cook, D., Fergusson, D., Steinberg, M., Granton, J., & Meade, M. et al. (2012). Daily sedation interruption in mechanically ventilated critically ill patients cared for with a sedation protocol: A randomized controlled trial. *Journal of the American Medical Association, 308*(19), 1985–1992. doi:10.1001/jama.2012.13872 PMID:23180503

Mehta, S., & Hill, N. S. (2001). Noninvasive ventilation. *American Journal of Respiratory and Critical Care Medicine, 163*(2), 540–577. doi:10.1164/ajrccm.163.2.9906116 PMID:11179136

Mehta, S., McCullagh, I., & Burry, L. (2009). Current sedation practices: Lessons learned from international surveys. *Critical Care Clinics, 25*(3), 471–488. doi:10.1016/j.ccc.2009.04.001 PMID:19576525

Mehta, S., Tanguay, J.-F., Eikelboom, J. W., Jolly, S. S., Joyner, C. D., Granger, C. B., & Yusuf, S. et al. (2010). Double-dose versus standard-dose clopidogrel and high-dose versus low-dose aspirin in individuals undergoing percutaneous coronary intervention for acute coronary syndromes (CURRENT-OASIS 7): A randomised factorial trial. *Lancet, 376*(9748), 1233–1243. doi:10.1016/S0140-6736(10)61088-4 PMID:20817281

Melican, K., Sandoval, R. M., Kader, A., Josefsson, L., Tanner, G. A., Molitoris, B. A., & Richter-Dahlfors, A. (2011). Uropathogenic *Escherichia coli* P and Type 1 Fimbriae Act in Synergy in a Living Host to Facilitate Renal Colonization Leading to Nephron Obstruction. *PLoS Pathogens*, *7*(2), e1001298. doi:10.1371/journal.ppat.1001298 PMID:21383970

Meltzer, E. C., Gallagher, J. J., Suppes, A., & Fins, J. J. (2012). Lip-reading and the ventilated patient. *Critical Care Medicine*, *40*(5), 1529–1531. doi:10.1097/CCM.0b013e318241e56c PMID:22430239

Meltzer, E. C., Ivascu, N. S., Acres, C. A., Stark, M., Kirkpatrick, J. N., Paul, S., & Fins, J. J. et al. (2014). Extracorporeal membrane oxygenation in adults: A grief review and ethical prconsiderations for nonspecialist health providers and hospitalists. *Journal of Hospital Medicine*, *9*(12), 808–813. doi:10.1002/jhm.2262 PMID:25332093

Meltzer, H. Y. (2012). Update on typical and atypical antipsychotic drugs. *Annual Review of Medicine*, *64*(1), 393–406. doi:10.1146/annurev-med-050911-161504 PMID:23020880

Memon, M. A., Joughin, G. R., & Memon, B. (2010). Oral assessment and postgraduate medical examinations: Establishing conditions for validity, reliability and fairness. *Advances in Health Sciences Education: Theory and Practice*, *15*(2), 277–289. doi:10.1007/s10459-008-9111-9 PMID:18386152

Mercaldi, C. J., & Lanes, S. F. (2013). Ultrasound guidance decreases complications and improves the cost of care among patients undergoing thoracentesis and paracentesis. *Chest*, *143*(2), 532–538. doi:10.1378/chest.12-0447 PMID:23381318

Meredith, D. S., Kepler, C. K., Huang, R. C., Hirsch, B., Nguyen, J., Farmer, J. C., & Cammisa, F. P. et al. (2012). The effect of omega-3 fatty-acid supplements on perioperative bleeding following posterior spinal arthrodesis. *European Spine Journal*, *21*(12), 2659–2663. doi:10.1007/s00586-012-2365-1 PMID:22581258

Mermel, L. A., Allon, M., Bouza, E., Craven, D. E., Flynn, P., O'Grady, N. P., & Warren, D. K. et al. (2009). Clinical practice guidelines for the diagnosis and management of intravascular catheter-related infection: 2009 update by the Infectious Disease Society of America. *Clinical Infectious Diseases*, *49*(1), 1–45. doi:10.1086/599376 PMID:19489710

Merriam, S. B., Caffarella, R. S., & Baumgartner, L. M. (2007). *Learning in Adulthood* (3rd ed.). San Francisco: Jossey-Bass.

Messent, M., Sullivan, K., Keogh, B. F., Morgan, C. J., & Evans, T. W. (1992). Adult respiratory distress syndrome following cardiopulmonary bypass: Incidence and prediction. *Anaesthesia*, *47*(3), 267–268. doi:10.1111/j.1365-2044.1992.tb02134.x PMID:1566999

Methangkool, E., Howard-Quijano, K., Ho, J. K., & Mahajan, A. (2014). Infective endocarditis: The importance of intraoperative echocardiography. *Anesthesia and Analgesia*, *119*(1), 35–40. doi:10.1213/ANE.0000000000000195 PMID:24945122

Metzelder, S., Coburn, M., Fries, M., Reinges, M., Reich, S., Rossaint, R., & Rex, S. et al. (2011). Performance of cardiac output measurement derived from arterial pressure waveform analysis in patients requiring high-dose vasopressor therapy. *British Journal of Anaesthesia*, *106*(6), 776–784. doi:10.1093/bja/aer066 PMID:21441548

Meyer, A. L., Malehsa, D., Bara, C., Budde, U., Slaughter, M. S., Haverich, A., & Streuber, M. (2010). Acquired von Willebrand syndrome in patients with an axial flow left ventricular assist device. *Circulation: Heart Failure*, *3*(6), 675–681. doi:10.1161/CIRCHEARTFAILURE.109.877597 PMID:20739614

Meyer, G. S., & Massagli, M. P. (2001). The forgotten component of the quality triad: Can we still learn something from "structure"? *The Joint Commission Journal on Quality Improvement*, *27*(9), 484–493. PMID:11556257

Meyer, T., & Krishnamani, R. (2010). Acute heart failure and pulmonary edema. In A. Jeremias & D. L. Brown (Eds.), *Cardiac Intensive Care* (pp. 291–308). Philadelphia: Saunders. doi:10.1016/B978-1-4160-3773-6.10024-2

Micek, S. T., Ward, S., Fraser, V. J., & Kollef, M. H. (2004). A randomized controlled trial of an antibiotic discontinuation policy for clinically suspected ventilator-associated pneumonia. *Chest Journal*, *125*(5), 1791–1799. doi:10.1378/chest.125.5.1791 PMID:15136392

Michalopoulos, A., Geroulanos, S., Rosmarakis, E. S., & Falagas, M. E. (2006). Frequency, characteristics, and predictors of microbiologically documented nosocomial infections after cardiac surgery. *European Journal of Cardio-Thoracic Surgery*, *29*(4), 456–460. doi:10.1016/j.ejcts.2005.12.035 PMID:16481186

Michard, F. (2005). Changes in arterial pressure during mechanical ventilation. *Anesthesiology*, *103*(2), 419–428. doi:10.1097/00000542-200508000-00026 PMID:16052125

Michard, F., & Teboul, J. L. (2000). Using heart-lung interactions to assess fluid responsiveness during mechanical ventilation. *Critical Care (London, England)*, *4*(5), 282–289. doi:10.1186/cc710 PMID:11094507

Michelena, H. I., Desjardins, V. A., Avierinos, J. F., Russo, A., Nkomo, V. T., Sundt, T. M., & Enriquez-Sarano, M. et al. (2008). Natural history of asymptomatic patients with normally functioning or minimally dysfunctional bicuspid aortic valve in the community. *Circulation*, *117*(21), 2776–2784. doi:10.1161/CIRCULATIONAHA.107.740878 PMID:18506017

Michelson, A. D. (1994). Platelet activation by thrombin can be directly measured in whole blood through the use of the peptide GPRP and flow cytometry: Methods and clinical applications. *Blood Coagulation & Fibrinolysis*, *5*(1), 121–131. doi:10.1097/00001721-199402000-00014 PMID:8180332

Mietto, C., Pinciroli, R., Patel, N., & Berra, L. (2013). Ventilator-associated pneumonia: Evolving definitions and preventive strategies. *Respiratory Care*, *58*(6), 990–1003. doi:10.4187/respcare.02380 PMID:23709196

Milbrandt, E. B., Deppen, S., Harrison, P. L., Shintani, A. K., Speroff, T., Stiles, R. A., & Ely, E. W. et al. (2004). Costs associated with delirium in mechanically ventilated patients. *Critical Care Medicine*, *32*(4), 955–962. doi:10.1097/01.CCM.0000119429.16055.92 PMID:15071384

Milgrom, L. B., Brooks, J. A., Qi, R., Bunnell, K., Wuestfeld, S., & Beckman, D. (2004). Pain levels experienced with activities after cardiac surgery. *American Journal of Critical Care*, *13*(2), 116–125. PMID:15043239

Millar, B. C., & Moore, J. E. (2004). Current trends in the molecular diagnosis of infective endocarditis. *European Journal of Clinical Microbiology & Infectious Diseases*, *23*(5), 353–365. doi:10.1007/s10096-004-1132-6 PMID:15112074

Miller, C. B., Malaisrie, S. C., Patel, J., Garrity, E., Vigneswaran, W. T., & Gamelli, R. L. (2006). Intraabdominal complications after lung transplantation. *Journal of the American College of Surgeons*, *203*(5), 653–660. doi:10.1016/j.jamcollsurg.2006.07.024

Miller, D. C., Blackstone, E. H., Mack, M. J., Svensson, L. G., Kodali, S. K., Kapadia, S., & Smith, C. R. et al. (2012). Transcatheter (TAVR) versus surgical (AVR) aortic valve replacement: Occurrence, hazard, risk factors, and consequences of neurologic events in the PARTNER trial. *The Journal of Thoracic and Cardiovascular Surgery*, *143*(4), 832–843.e13. doi:10.1016/j.jtcvs.2012.01.055 PMID:22424519

Miller, G. E. (1990). The assessment of clinical skills/competence/performance. *Academic Medicine*, *65*(9), S63–S67. doi:10.1097/00001888-199009000-00045 PMID:2400509

Minai, O. A., Yared, J. P., Kaw, R., Subramaniam, K., & Hill, N. S. (2013). Perioperative risk and management in patients with pulmonary hypertension. *Chest Journal*, *144*(1), 329–340. doi:10.1378/chest.12-1752 PMID:23880683

Minneci, P. C., Deans, K. J., Banks, S. M., Eichacker, P. Q., & Natanson, C. (2004). Meta-analysis: The effect of steroids on survival and shock during sepsis depends on the dose. *Annals of Internal Medicine*, *141*(1), 47–56. doi:10.7326/0003-4819-141-1-200407060-00014 PMID:15238370

Minoxidil. (2009). In *Official FDA Information, Side effects and Uses.* Retrieved from http://www.drugs.com/mtm/minoxidil.html

Mirtallo, J. M., Dasta, J. F., Kleinschmidt, K. C., & Varon, J. (2010). State of the art review: intravenous fat emulsions: current applications, safety profile, and clinical implications. *The Annals of Pharmacotherapy*, *44*, 688–700. PMID:20332339

Misfeld, M., Girrbach, F., Etz, C. D., Binner, C., Aspern, K. V., Dohmen, P. M., & Mohr, F. et al. (2014). Surgery for infective endocarditis complicated by cerebral embolism; A consecutive series of 375 patients. *The Journal of Thoracic and Cardiovascular Surgery*, *147*(6), 1837–1846. doi:10.1016/j.jtcvs.2013.10.076 PMID:24837722

Missant, C., Rex, S., & Wouters, P. F. (2008). Accuracy of cardiac output measurements with pulse contour analysis (PulseCO) and Doppler echocardiography during off-pump coronary artery bypass grafting. *European Journal of Anaesthesiology*, *25*(3), 243–24. doi:10.1017/S0265021507002979 PMID:17996125

Mitchell, J. B., Shaw, A. D., Donald, S., & Farrimond, J. G. (2002). Differential lung ventilation after single-lung transplantation *Cardiothorac Vasc Anesth, 16*(4), 459-462.

Mitchell, L. B. C., E.; Heilbron, B. (2004). Atrial fibrillation after cardiac surgery. *The Canadian Journal of Cardiology*, *21*(Suppl B), 45B–50B. PMID:16239988

Mitchell, L. B., Exner, D. V., Wyse, D. G., Connolly, C. J., Prystai, G. D., Bayes, A. J., & Maitland, A. et al. (2005). Prophylactic oral amiodarone for the prevention of arrhythmias that begin early after revascularization, valve replacement or repair: PAPABEAR: a randomized controlled trial. *Journal of the American Medical Association*, *294*(24), 3093–3100. doi:10.1001/jama.294.24.3093 PMID:16380589

Mittnacht, A., Fanshawe, M., & Konstadt, S. (2008). Anesthetic considerations in the patient with valvular heart disease undergoing noncardiac surgery. *Seminars in Cardiothoracic and Vascular Anesthesia*, *12*(1), 33–59. doi:10.1177/1089253208316442 PMID:18397904

Miyahara, K., Matsuura, A., Takemura, H., Mizutani, S., Saito, S., & Toyama, M. (2014). Implementation of bundled interventions greatly decreases deep sternal wound infection following cardiovascular surgery. *The Journal of Thoracic and Cardiovascular Surgery*, *148*(5), 2381–2388. doi:10.1016/j.jtcvs.2014.04.005 PMID:24820192

Miyata, H., Yamasaki, M., Kurokawa, Y., Takiguchi, S., Nakajima, K., Fujiwara, Y., & Doki, Y. et al. (2011). Multimodal treatment for resectable esophageal cancer. *General Thoracic and Cardiovascular Surgery*, *59*(7), 461–466. doi:10.1007/s11748-011-0780-6 PMID:21751104

Moat, N. E., Ludman, P., de Belder, M. A., Bridgewater, B., Cunningham, A. D., Young, C. P., & Mullen, M. J. et al. (2011). Long-term outcomes after transcatheter aortic valve implantation in high-risk patients with severe aortic stenosis: The U.K. TAVI (United Kingdom Transcatheter Aortic Valve Implantation) Registry. *Journal of the American College of Cardiology*, *58*(20), 2130–2138. doi:10.1016/j.jacc.2011.08.050 PMID:22019110

Moat, N. E., Shore, D. F., & Evans, T. W. (1993). Organ dysfunction and cardiopulmonary bypass: The role of complement and complement regulatory proteins. *European Journal of Cardio-Thoracic Surgery*, *7*(11), 563–573. doi:10.1016/1010-7940(93)90241-3 PMID:8297608

Moazami, N., Fukamachi, K., Kobayashi, M., Smedira, N. G., Hoercher, K. J., Massiello, A., & Starling, R. C. et al. (2013). Axial and centrifugal continuous-flow rotary pumps: A translation from pump mechanics to clinical practice. *The Journal of Heart and Lung Transplantation*, *32*(1), 1–11. doi:10.1016/j.healun.2012.10.001 PMID:23260699

Modena, S., Bearelly, D., Swartz, K., & Friedenberg, F. K. (2005). Clostridium difficile among hospitalized patients receiving antibiotics: A case-control study. *Infection Control and Hospital Epidemiology*, *26*(8), 685–690. doi:10.1086/502603 PMID:16156324

Modest, V. E., & Butterworth, J. F. IV. (1995). Effect of pH and lidocaine on beta adrenergic receptor binding: Interaction during resuscitation? *Chest*, *108*(5), 1373–1379. doi:10.1378/chest.108.5.1373 PMID:7587445

Moen, V., Dahlgren, N., & Irestedt, L. (2004). Severe neurological complications after central neuraxial blockades in Sweden, 1990-1999. *Anesthesiology*, *101*(4), 950–959. doi:10.1097/00000542-200410000-00021 PMID:15448529

Moghissi, E. S., Korytkowski, M. T., DiNardo, M., Einhorn, D., Hellman, R., Hirsch, I. B., & Umpierrez, G. E. et al. (2009). American Association of Clinical Endocrinologists and American Diabetes Association consensus statement on inpatient glycemic control. *Diabetes Care*, *32*(6), 1119–1131. doi:10.2337/dc09-9029 PMID:19429873

Mohammed, A., Agnihotri, A. K., van Kimmenade, R. R. J., Martinez-Rumayor, A., Green, S. M., Quiroz, R., & Januzzi, J. L. (2009). Prospective, comprehensive assessment of cardiac troponin T testing after coronary artery bypass graft surgery. *Circulation*, *120*(10), 843–850. doi:10.1161/CIRCULATIONAHA.108.837278 PMID:19704098

Mohr, F. W., Morice, M. C., Kappetein, A. P., Feldman, T. E., Stahle, E., Colombo, A., & Serruys, P. W. et al. (2013). Coronary artery bypass graft surgery versus percutaneous coronary intervention in patients with three-vessel disease and left main coronary disease: 5-year follow-up of the randomised, clinical SYNTAX trial. *Lancet*, *381*(9867), 629–638. doi:10.1016/S0140-6736(13)60141-5 PMID:23439102

Mohr, F. W., Morice, M.-C., Keppetein, A. P., Feldman, T. E., Stahle, E., Colombo, A., & Serruys, P. W. et al. (2013). Coronary artery bypass graft surgery versus percutaneous coronary intevention in patients with three-vessel disease and lef tmain cornoary disease: 5 -year follow-up of the randomised, clinical SYNTAX trial. *Lancet*, *381*(9748), 629–638. PMID:23439102

Moller, C. H., Penninga, L., Wetterslev, J., Steinbruchel, D. A., & Gluud, C. (2008). Clinical outcomes in randomized trials of off- vs. on-pump coronary artery bypass surgery: Systematic review with meta-analyses and trial sequential analyses. *European Heart Journal*, *29*(21), 2601–2616. doi:10.1093/eurheartj/ehn335 PMID:18628261

Moller, J. H., Shumway, S. J., & Gott, V. L. (2009). The first open-heart repairs using extracorporeal circulation by cross-circulation: A 53-year follow-up. *The Annals of Thoracic Surgery*, *88*(3), 1044–1046. doi:10.1016/j.athoracsur.2009.05.077 PMID:19699962

Monnet, X., Anguel, N., Jozwiak, M., Richard, C., & Teboul, J.-L. (2012). Third-generation FloTrac/Vigileo does not reliably track changes in cardiac output induced by norepinephrine in critically ill patients. *British Journal of Anaesthesia*, *108*(4), 615–622. doi:10.1093/bja/aer491 PMID:22265900

Montejo, J. C., Grau, T., Acosta, J., Ruiz-Santana, S., Planas, M., García-De-Lorenzo, A., & López-Martínez, J. et al. (2002). Multicenter, prospective, randomized, single-blind study comparing the efficacy and gastrointestinal complications of early jejunal feeding with early gastric feeding in critically ill patients. *Critical Care Medicine*, *30*(4), 796–800. doi:10.1097/00003246-200204000-00013 PMID:11940748

Montejo, J. C., Miñambres, E., Bordejé, L., Mesejo, A., Acosta, J., Heras, A., & Manzanedo, R. et al. (2010). Gastric residual volume during enteral nutrition in ICU patients: The REGANE study. *Intensive Care Medicine*, *36*(8), 1386–1393. doi:10.1007/s00134-010-1856-y PMID:20232036

Moon, M. R., Pasque, M. K., Munfakh, N. A., Melby, S. J., Lawton, J. S., Moazami, N., & Damiano, R. J. Jr et al.. (2006). Prosthesis-patient mismatch after aortic valve replacement: Impact of age and body size on late survival. *The Annals of Thoracic Surgery*, *81*(2), 481–488, discussion 489. doi:10.1016/j.athoracsur.2005.07.084 PMID:16427836

Moote, M., Krsek, C., Kleinpell, R., & Todd, B. (2011). Physician assistant and nurse practitioner utilization in academic medical centers. *American Journal of Medical Quality*, *26*(6), 452–460. doi:10.1177/1062860611402984 PMID:21555487

Mora, B., Ince, I., Birkenberg, B., Skhirtladze, K., Pernicka, E., Ankersmit, H. J., & Dworschak, M. (2011). Validation of cardiac output measurement with the LiDCO™ pulse contour system in patients with impaired left ventricular function after cardiac surgery. *Anaesthesia*, *66*(8), 675–681. doi:10.1111/j.1365-2044.2011.06754.x PMID:21564044

Morales, D. L., Gregg, D., Helman, D. N., Williams, M. R., Naka, Y., Landry, D. W., & Oz, M. C. (2000). Arginine vasopressin in the treatment of 50 patients with postcardiotomy vasodilatory shock. *The Annals of Thoracic Surgery*, *69*(1), 102–106. doi:10.1016/S0003-4975(99)01197-2 PMID:10654495

Morcos, W. E., & Payne, J. P. (1985). The induction of anaesthesia with propofol compared in normal and renal failure patients. *Postgraduate Medical Journal*, *61*, 62–63. PMID:3877297

Moreillon, P., & Que, Y. (2004). Infective endocarditis. *Lancet*, *363*(9403), 139–149. doi:10.1016/S0140-6736(03)15266-X PMID:14726169

Moreno, P. R. (2010). Vulnerable Plaque: Definition, Diagnosis, and Treatment. *Cardiology Clinics*, *28*(1), 1–30. doi:10.1016/j.ccl.2009.09.008 PMID:19962047

Moreyra, A. E., Wilson, A. C., Deac, R., Suciu, C., Kostis, J. B., Ortan, F., & Mahalingham, B. et al. (1998). Factors associated with atrial fibrillation in patients with mitral stenosis: A cardiac catheterization study. *American Heart Journal*, *135*(1), 138–145. doi:10.1016/S0002-8703(98)70354-0 PMID:9453533

Morgan, I. S., Codispoti, M., Sanger, K., & Mankad, P. S. (1998). Superiority of centrifugal pump over roller pump in paediatric cardiac surgery: Prospective randomised trial. *European Journal of Cardio-Thoracic Surgery*, *13*(5), 526–532. doi:10.1016/S1010-7940(98)00067-0 PMID:9663533

Morice, M.-C., Serruys, P. W., Sousa, J. E., Fajadet, J., Ban Hayashi, E., Perin, M., & Falotico, R. et al. (2002). A randomized comparison of a sirolimus-eluting stent with a standard stent for coronary revascularization. *The New England Journal of Medicine*, *346*(23), 1773–1780. doi:10.1056/NEJMoa012843 PMID:12050336

Moritz, A. R., Hudson, C. L., & Orgain, E. S. (1932). Augmentation of the extracardiac anastomoses of the coronary arteries through pericardial adhesions. *The Journal of Experimental Medicine*, *56*(6), 927–931. doi:10.1084/jem.56.6.927 PMID:19870113

Morris, A. H., Wallace, C. J., Menlove, R. L., Clemmer, T. P., Orme, J. F. Jr, Weaver, L. K., & Rasmusson, B. et al. (1994). Randomized clinical trial of pressure-controlled inverse ratio ventilation and extracorporeal CO2 removal for adult respiratory distress syndrome. *American Journal of Respiratory and Critical Care Medicine*, *149*(2 Pt 1), 295–305. doi:10.1164/ajrccm.149.2.8306022

Morris, D. S., Reilly, P., Rohrbach, J., Telford, G., Kim, P., & Sims, C. A. (2012). The influence of unit-based nurse practitioners on hospital outcomes and readmission rates for patients with trauma. *J Trauma Acute Care Surg*, *73*(2), 474–478. doi:10.1097/TA.0b013e31825882bb PMID:22846959

Morrison, D., Sethi, G., Sacks, J., Henderson, W., Grover, F., Sedlis, S., & Lewis, D. et al. (2001). Percutaneous coronary intervention versus coronary artery bypass graft surgery for patients with medically refractory myocardial ischemia and risk factors for adverse outcomes with bypass: A multicenter, randomized trial. *Journal of the American College of Cardiology*, *38*(1), 143–149. doi:10.1016/S0735-1097(01)01366-3 PMID:11451264

Morrison, E. H., Friedland, J. A., Boker, J., Rucker, L., Hollingshead, J., & Murata, P. (2001). Residents-as-teachers training in US residency programs and offices of graduate medical education. *Academic Medicine: Journal of the Association of American Medical Colleges*, *76*(10Supplement), S1–S4. doi:10.1097/00001888-200110001-00002 PMID:11597856

Morrison, E. H., Shapiro, J. F., & Harthill, M. (2005). Resident doctors' understanding of their roles as clinical teachers. *Medical Education*, *39*(2), 137–144. doi:10.1111/j.1365-2929.2004.02063.x PMID:15679680

Morrison, R. S., Dietrich, J., Ladwig, S., Quill, T., Sacco, J., Tangeman, J., & Meier, D. E. (2011). Palliative care consultation teams cut hospital costs for Medicaid beneficiaries. *Health Affairs*, *30*(3), 454–463. doi:10.1377/hlthaff.2010.0929 PMID:21383364

Morrison, R. S., Magaziner, J., Gilbert, M., Koval, K. J., McLaughlin, M. A., Orosz, G., & Siu, A. L. et al. (2003). Relationship between pain and opioid analgesics on the development of delirium following hip fracture. *The Journals of Gerontology. Series A, Biological Sciences and Medical Sciences*, *58*(1), 76–81. doi:10.1093/gerona/58.1.M76 PMID:12560416

Morrison, R. S., Penrod, J. D., Cassel, J. B., Caust-Ellenbogen, M., Litke, A., & Spragens, L. et al.. (2008). Cost savings associated with US hospital palliative care consultation programs. *Archives of Internal Medicine*, *168*(16), 1783–1790. doi:10.1001/archinte.168.16.1783 PMID:18779466

Morris, P. E., Goad, A., Thompson, C., Taylor, K., Harry, B., Passmore, L., & Haponik, E. et al. (2008). Early intensive care unit mobility therapy in the treatment of acute respiratory failure. *Critical Care Medicine*, *36*(8), 2238–2243. doi:10.1097/CCM.0b013e318180b90e PMID:18596631

Morrone, T. M., Buck, L. A., Catanese, K. A., Goldsmith, R. L., Cahalin, L. P., Oz, M. C., & Levin, H. R. (1996). Early progressive mobilization of patients with left ventricular assist devices is safe and optimizes recovery before heart transplantation. *The Journal of Heart and Lung Transplantation*, *15*(4), 423–429. PMID:8732603

Morrow, D. A., Fang, J. C., Fintel, D. J., Granger, C. B., Katz, J. N., Kushner, F. G., & Winkelman, C. et al. (2012). Evolution of critical care cardiology: Transformation of the cardiovascular intensive care unit and the emerging need for new medical staffing and training models. A scientific statement from the American Heart Association. *Circulation*, *126*(11), 1408–1428. doi:10.1161/CIR.0b013e31826890b0 PMID:22893607

Morrow, D., Cannon, C., Rifai, N., Frey, M., Vicari, N., Lakkis, N., & Braunwald, E. et al. (2001). Ability of minor elevations of troponins I and T to predict benefit from an early invasive strategy in patients with unstable angina and non-ST elevation myocardial infarction: Results from a randomized trial. *Journal of the American Medical Association*, *286*(19), 2405–2412. doi:10.1001/jama.286.19.2405 PMID:11712935

Morrow, L. E. (2009). Probiotics in the intensive care unit. *Current Opinion in Critical Care*, *15*(2), 144–148. doi:10.1097/MCC.0b013e3283252d2d PMID:19300087

Mosenthal, A. C., & Murphy, P. A. (2006). Interdisciplinary model for palliative care in the trauma and surgical intensive care unit: Robert Wood Johnson Foundation Demonstration Project for Improving Palliative Care in the Intensive Care Unit. *Critical Care Medicine*, *34*(11Suppl), S399–S403. doi:10.1097/01.CCM.0000237044.79166.E1 PMID:17057605

Mosenthal, A. C., Weissman, D. E., Curtis, J. R., Hays, R. M., Lustbader, D. R., Mulkerin, C., & Nelson, J. E. et al. (2012). Integrating palliative care in the surgical and trauma intensive care unit: A report from the Improving Palliative Care in the Intensive Care Unit (IPAL-ICU) Project Advisory Board and the Center to Advance Palliative Care. *Critical Care Medicine*, *40*(4), 1199–1206. doi:10.1097/CCM.0b013e31823bc8e7 PMID:22080644

Mosesson, M. W. (2005). Fibrinogen and fibrin structure and functions. *Journal of Thrombosis and Haemostasis*, *3*(8), 1894–1904. doi:10.1111/j.1538-7836.2005.01365.x PMID:16102057

Moskowitz, D. M., McCullough, J. N., Shander, A., Klein, J. J., Bodian, C. A., Goldweit, R. S., & Ergin, M. A. (2010). The impact of blood conservation on outcomes in cardiac surgery: Is it safe and effective? *The Annals of Thoracic Surgery*, *90*(2), 451–458. doi:10.1016/j.athoracsur.2010.04.089 PMID:20667328

Moss, E., & Lamarche, Y. (2012). Acute Kidney Injury Following Cardiac Surgery: Prevention, Diagnosis, and Management. In M. Polenakovic (Ed.), Renal Failure: The Facts (pp. 129–156). Rijeka, Croatia: InTech; Retrieved from http://www.intechopen.com/books/renal-failure-the-facts/acute-kidney-injury-following-cardiac-surgery-prevention-diagnosis-and-treatment, doi:10.5772/37434

Mourvillier, B., Trouillet, J. L., Timsit, J. F., Baudot, J., Chastre, J., Régnier, B., & Wolff, M. et al. (2004). Infective endocarditis in the intensive care unit: Clinical spectrum and prognostic factors in 228 consecutive patients. *Intensive Care Medicine*, *30*(11), 2046–2052. doi:10.1007/s00134-004-2436-9 PMID:15372147

Moussa, I. D., Klein, L. W., Shah, B., Mehran, R., Mack, M. J., Brilakis, E. S., ... (2013). Consideration of a new definition of clinically relevant myocardial infarction after coronary revascularization: an expert consensus document from the Society for Cardiovascular Angiography and Interventions (SCAI). (Vol. 62, pp. 1563–1570). doi:10.1016/j.jacc.2013.08.720

Mudd, J. O., & Gelow, J. M. (2013). Bleeding after heartmate II implantation: A cloud in the silver lining. *Journal of the American College of Cardiology*, *62*(23), 2197–2198. doi:10.1016/j.jacc.2013.08.696 PMID:23994418

Mueller, C., Neumann, F.-J., Perach, W., Perruchoud, A., & Buettner, H. (2004). Prognostic value of the admission electrocardiogram in patients with unstable angina/non–ST-segment elevation myocardial infarction treated with very early revascularization. *The American Journal of Medicine*, *117*(3), 145–150. doi:10.1016/j.amjmed.2004.02.034 PMID:15276591

Mughal, M. M., Gildea, T. R., Murthy, S., Pettersson, G., DeCamp, M., & Mehta, A. C. (2005). Short-term deployment of self-expanding metallic stents facilitates healing of bronchial dehiscence. *American Journal of Respiratory and Critical Care Medicine*, *172*(6), 768–771. doi:10.1164/rccm.200410-1388OC

Muir, K. W., Weir, C. J., Murray, G. D., Povey, C., & Lees, K. R. (1996). Comparison of neurological scales and scoring systems for acute stroke prognosis. *Stroke*, *27*(10), 1817–1820. doi:10.1161/01.STR.27.10.1817 PMID:8841337

Mularski, R. A., Heine, C. E., Osborne, M. L., Ganzini, L., & Curtis, J. R. (2005). Quality of dying in the ICU: Ratings by family members. *Chest*, *128*(1), 280–287. doi:10.1378/chest.128.1.280 PMID:16002947

Muralidhar, K., Bhagyashri, K., Guptha, R., Hegde, N., Ahmed, I., & Vincent, L. (2013). Determinants of renal replacement therapy after adult cardiac surgery. *Asian Cardiovascular & Thoracic Annals*, *21*(5), 533–538. doi:10.1177/0218492312461638 PMID:24570554

Murdoch, D. R., Corey, G. R., Hoen, B., Miró, J. M., Fowler, V. G., Bayer, A. S., & Cabell, C. H. et al. (2009). Clinical presentation, etiology, and outcome of infective endocarditis in the 21st century: The international collaboration on endocarditis-prospective cohort study. *Archives of Internal Medicine*, *169*(5), 463–473. doi:10.1001/archinternmed.2008.603 PMID:19273776

Murkin, J. M. (2013). Is it better to shine a light, or rather to curse the darkness? Cerebral near-infrared spectroscopy and cardiac surgery. *European Journal of Cardio-Thoracic Surgery*, *43*(6), 1081–1083. doi:10.1093/ejcts/ezt186 PMID:23543201

Murkin, J. M., & Arango, M. (2009). Near-infrared spectroscopy as an index of brain and tissue oxygenation. *British Journal of Anaesthesia*, *103*(Suppl), i3–i13. doi:10.1093/bja/aep299 PMID:20007987

Murkin, J. M., Falter, F., Granton, J., Young, B., Burt, C., & Chu, M. (2010). High-dose tranexamic Acid is associated with nonischemic clinical seizures in cardiac surgical patients. *Anesthesia and Analgesia*, *110*(2), 350–353. doi:10.1213/ANE.0b013e3181c92b23 PMID:19996135

Murkin, J. M., Farrar, J. K., Tweed, W. A., McKenzie, F. N., & Guiraudon, G. (1987). Cerebral autoregulation and flow/metabolism coupling during cardiopulmonary bypass: The influence of PaCO2. *Anesthesia and Analgesia*, *66*(9), 825–832. doi:10.1213/00000539-198709000-00003 PMID:3113288

Murphy, M. A., Whitman, I., Campfield, A., Moxey, E., Haddad, M., & Whitman, G. (2010). Intense implementation of a strict insulin infusion protocol does not guarantee postoperative glycemic control. *Journal of the American College of Surgeons, 211*(4), 465-469. doi: 10.1016/j.jamcollsurg.2010.06.003

Murphy, G. J., & Angelini, G. D. (2006). Indications for blood transfusion in cardiac surgery. *The Annals of Thoracic Surgery*, *82*(6), 2323–2334. doi:10.1016/j.athoracsur.2006.06.020 PMID:17126171

Murphy, G. J., Reeves, B. C., Rogers, C. A., Rizvi, S. I. A., Culliford, L., & Angelini, G. D. (2007). Increased mortality, postoperative morbidity, and cost after red blood cell transfusion in patients having cardiac surgery. *Circulation*, *116*(22), 2544–2552. doi:10.1161/CIRCULATIONAHA.107.698977 PMID:17998460

Murphy, G. S., Szokol, J. W., Nitsun, M., Alspach, D. A., Avram, M. J., Vender, J. S., & Hoff, W. J. et al. (2006). Retrograde autologous priming of the cardiopulmonary bypass circuit: Safety and impact on postoperative outcomes. *Journal of Cardiothoracic and Vascular Anesthesia*, *20*(2), 156–161. doi:10.1053/j.jvca.2005.04.003 PMID:16616653

Murphy, G. S., Whitlock, R. P., Gutsche, J. T., & Augoustides, J. G. (2013). Steroids for adult cardiac surgery with cardiopulmonary bypass: Update on dose and key randomized trials. *Journal of Cardiothoracic and Vascular Anesthesia*, *27*(5), 1053–1059. doi:10.1053/j.jvca.2013.04.022 PMID:24054192

Murthy, S. C., Gildea, T. R., & Machuzak, M. S. (2010). Anastomotic airway complications after lung transplantation. *Current Opinion in Organ Transplantation*, *15*(5), 582–587. doi:10.1097/MOT.0b013e32833e3e6e

Muscedere, J., Dodek, P., Keenan, S., Fowler, R., Cook, D., & Heyland, D. (2008). Comprehensive evidence-based clinical practice guidelines for ventilator-associated pneumonia: Prevention. *Journal of Critical Care*, *23*(1), 126–137. doi:10.1016/j.jcrc.2007.11.014 PMID:18359430

Muscedere, J., Rewa, O., Mckechnie, K., Jiang, X., Laporta, D., & Heyland, D. K. (2011). Subglottic secretion drainage for the prevention of ventilator-associated pneumonia: A systematic review and meta-analysis. *Critical Care Medicine*, *39*(8), 1985–1991. doi:10.1097/CCM.0b013e318218a4d9 PMID:21478738

Musci, M., Weng, Y., Hübler, M., Amiri, A., Pasic, M., Kosky, S., & Hetzer, R. et al. (2010). Homograft aortic root replacement in native or prosthetic active infective endocarditis: Twenty-year single-center experience. *The Journal of Thoracic and Cardiovascular Surgery*, *139*(3), 665–673. doi:10.1016/j.jtcvs.2009.07.026 PMID:19767017

Mutlu, G. M., Mutlu, E. A., & Factor, P. (2001). GI complications in patients receiving mechanical ventilation. *Chest*, *119*(4), 1222–1241. doi:10.1378/chest.119.4.1222 PMID:11296191

Myers, M. G., & Fremes, S. E. (2003). Prevention of radial artery graft spasm: A survey of Canadian surgical centres. *The Canadian Journal of Cardiology*, *19*(6), 677–681. Retrieved from http://www.ncbi.nlm.nih.gov/pubmed/12772018 PMID:12772018

Myles, P. S., & McIlroy, D. (2005). Fast-track cardiac anesthesia: Choice of anesthetic agents and techniques. *Seminars in Cardiothoracic and Vascular Anesthesia*, *9*(1), 5–16. doi:10.1177/108925320500900102 PMID:15735840

Mylonakis, E., & Calderwood, S. B. (2001). Infective Endocarditis in Adults. *The New England Journal of Medicine*, *345*(18), 1318–1330. doi:10.1056/NEJMra010082 PMID:11794152

Myslobodsky, M. S., Golovchinsky, V., & Mintz, M. (1981). Ketamine: Convulsant or anti-convulsant? *Pharmacology, Biochemistry, and Behavior*, *14*(1), 27–33. doi:10.1016/0091-3057(81)90099-X PMID:7465607

Mythen, M. (1995). Perioperative plasma volume expansion reduces the incidence of gut mucosal hypoperfusion during cardiac surgery. *Archives of Surgery*, *130*(4), 423–429. doi:10.1001/archsurg.1995.01430040085019 PMID:7535996

Nagayasu, T., Yamayoshi, T., Matsumoto, K., Ide, N., Hashizume, S., Nomura, M., & Oka, T. et al. (2005). Beneficial effects of plasmapheresis before thymectomy on the outcome in myasthenia gravis. *Japanese Journal of Thoracic and Cardiovascular Surgery*, *53*(1), 2–7. doi:10.1007/s11748-005-1001-y PMID:15724495

Nagendran, J., Norris, C. M., Graham, M. M., Ross, D. B., MacArthur, R. G., Kieser, T. M., & Meyer, S. R. et al. (2013). Coronary Revascularization for Patients With Severe Left Ventricular Dysfunction. *The Annals of Thoracic Surgery*, *96*(6), 2038–2044. doi:10.1016/j.athoracsur.2013.06.052 PMID:23968761

Nagler, A., Andolsek, K., Rudd, M., Sloane, R., Musick, D., & Basnight, L. (2014). The professionalism disconnect: Do entering residents identify yet participate in unprofessional behaviors? *BMC Medical Education*, *14*(1), 60. doi:10.1186/1472-6920-14-60 PMID:24674275

Nakahara, K., Ohno, K., Hashimoto, J., Miyoshi, S., Maeda, H., Matsumura, A., & Kawashima, Y. et al. (1988). Prediction of postoperative respiratory failure in patients undergoing lung resection for lung cancer. *The Annals of Thoracic Surgery*, *46*(5), 549–552. doi:10.1016/S0003-4975(10)64694-2 PMID:3190329

Nalla, B. P., Freedman, J., Hare, G. M. T., & Mazer, C. D. (2012). Update on blood conservation for cardiac surgery. *Journal of Cardiothoracic and Vascular Anesthesia*, *26*(1), 117–133. doi:10.1053/j.jvca.2011.07.024 PMID:22000983

Nalysnyk, L., Fahrbach, K., Reynolds, M. W., Zhao, S. Z., & Ross, S. (2003). Adverse events in coronary artery bypass graft (CABG) trials: A systematic review and analysis. *Heart (British Cardiac Society)*, *89*(7), 767–772. http://www.pubmedcentral.nih.gov/articlerender.fcgi?artid=1767742&tool=pmcentrez&rendertype=abstract doi:10.1136/heart.89.7.767 PMID:12807853

Nasca, T. J., Day, S. H., & Amis, E. S. Jr. (2010). The New Recommendations on Duty Hours from the ACGME Task Force. *The New England Journal of Medicine*, *363*(2), e3. doi:10.1056/NEJMsb1005800 PMID:20573917

Nashef, S. A., Roques, F., Sharples, L. D., Nilsson, J., Smith, C., Goldstone, A. R., & Lockowandt, U. (2012). EuroSCORE II. *European Journal of Cardio-Thoracic Surgery, 41*(4), 734-744; discussion 744-735. doi: 10.1093/ejcts/ezs043

Nassimiha, D., Aronow, W. S., Ahn, C., & Goldman, M. E. (2001). Rate of progression of valvular aortic stenosis in patients > or = 60 years of age. *American Journal of Cardiology, 87*(6), 807-809, A809.

Nasso, G., Coppola, R., Bonifazi, R., Piancone, F., Bozzetti, G., & Speziale, G. (2009). Arterial revascularization in primary coronary artery bypass grafting: Direct comparison of 4 strategies--results of the Stand-in-Y Mammary Study. *The Journal of Thoracic and Cardiovascular Surgery*, *137*(5), 1093–1100. doi:10.1016/j.jtcvs.2008.10.029 PMID:19379973

Nath, J., Forster, E., & Heidenreich, P. A. (2004). Impact of tricuspid regurgitation on long-term survival. *Journal of the American College of Cardiology*, *43*(3), 405–409. doi:10.1016/j.jacc.2003.09.036 PMID:15013122

Nathoe, H. M., van Dijk, D., Jansen, E. W. L., Suyker, W. J. L., Diephuis, J. C., van Boven, W.-J., & de Jaegere, P. P. T. et al. (2003). A comparison of On-pump and Off-pump coronary bypass surgery in low-risk patients. *The New England Journal of Medicine*, *348*(5), 394–402. doi:10.1056/NEJMoa021775 PMID:12556542

National Committee of Quality Assurance. (2006). *Guidelines for Medical Documentation.* Retrieved May 2014, from http://www.ncqa.org/Portals/0/PolicyUpdates/Supplemental/Guidelines_Medical_Record_Review.pdf

National Heart, Lung, and Blood Institute Coronary Artery Surgery Study (CASS). (1981). A multi-center comparison of the effects of randomized medical and surgical treatment of mildly symptomatic patients with coronary artery disease, and a registry of consecutive patients undergoing coronary angiography. *Circulation, 63*, I1-I81.

National Heart. (2006). Comparison of two fluid-management strategies in acute lung injury. *The New England Journal of Medicine*, *354*(24), 2564–2575. doi:10.1056/NEJMoa062200 PMID:16714767

National Kidney Foundation. (2014). *Frequently asked questions about GFR estimates*. Retrieved from http://www.kidney.org/professionals

Navia, D., Vrancic, M., Piccinini, F., Camporrotondo, M., Thierer, J., Gil, C., & Benzadon, M. (2014). Is the second internal thoracic artery better than the radial artery in total arterial off-pump coronary artery bypass grafting? A propensity score-matched follow-up study. *The Journal of Thoracic and Cardiovascular Surgery*, *147*(2), 632–638. doi:10.1016/j.jtcvs.2013.02.012 PMID:23566513

Needham, D. M., Dinglas, V. D., Morris, P. E., Jackson, J. C., Hough, C. L., Mendez-Tellez, P. A., & Hopkins, R. O. et al. (2013). Physical and cognitive performance of patients with acute lung injury 1 year after initial trophic versus full enteral feeding EDEN Trial follow-up. *American Journal of Respiratory and Critical Care Medicine*, *188*(5), 567–576. doi:10.1164/rccm.201304-0651OC PMID:23805899

Nelson, J. E., Meier, D. E., Litke, A., Natale, D. A., Siegel, R. E., & Morrison, R. S. (2004). The symptom burden of chronic critical illness. *Crit Care Med, 32*(7), 1527-1534. doi: 00003246-200407000-00010 [pii]

Nelson, J. E. (2006a). Identifying and overcoming the barriers to high-quality palliative care in the intensive care unit. *Critical Care Medicine*, *34*(11Suppl), S324–S331. doi:10.1097/01.CCM.0000237249.39179.B1 PMID:17057594

Nelson, J. E., Angus, D. C., Weissfeld, L. A., Puntillo, K. A., Danis, M., & Deal, D. et al. Critical Care Peer Workgroup of the Promoting Excellence in End-of-Life Care, P. (2006b). End-of-life care for the critically ill: A national intensive care unit survey. *Critical Care Medicine*, *34*(10), 2547–2553. doi:10.1097/01.CCM.0000239233.63425.1D PMID:16932230

Nelson, J. E., Curtis, J. R., Mulkerin, C., Campbell, M., Lustbader, D. R., Mosenthal, A. C., & Weissman, D. E. et al. (2013). Choosing and using screening criteria for palliative care consultation in the ICU: A report from the Improving Palliative Care in the ICU (IPAL-ICU) Advisory Board. *Critical Care Medicine*, *41*(10), 2318–2327. doi:10.1097/CCM.0b013e31828cf12c PMID:23939349

Nelson, J. E., Meier, D. E., Litke, A., Natale, D. A., Siegel, R. E., & Morrison, R. S. (2004). The symptoms burden of chronic critical illness. *Critical Care Medicine*, *32*(7), 1527–1534. doi:10.1097/01.CCM.0000129485.08835.5A PMID:15241097

Nelson, J. E., Meier, D. E., Oei, E. J., Nierman, D. M., Senzel, R. S., Manfredi, P. L., & Morrison, R. S. et al. (2001). Self-reported symptom experience of critically ill cancer patients receiving intensive care. *Critical Care Medicine*, *29*(2), 277–282. doi:10.1097/00003246-200102000-00010 PMID:11246306

Nelson, J. E., Puntillo, K. A., Pronovost, P. J., Walker, A. S., McAdam, J. L., Ilaoa, D., & Penrod, J. (2010). In their own words: Patients and families define high-quality palliative care in the intensive care unit. *Critical Care Medicine*, *38*(3), 808–818. doi:10.1097/CCM.0b013e3181c5887c PMID:20198726

Network, T. A. R. D. S. (2000). Ventilation with lower tidal volumes as compared with traditional tidal volumes for acute lung injury and the acute respiratory distress syndrome. The Acute Respiratory Distress Syndrome Network. *The New England Journal of Medicine*, *342*(18), 1301–1308. doi:10.1056/NEJM200005043421801 PMID:10793162

Neumar, R. W., Otto, C. W., Link, M. S., Kronick, S. L., Shuster, M., Callaway, C. W., & Morrison, L. J. et al. (2010). Part 8: adult advanced cardiovascular life support: 2010 American Heart Association Guidelines for Cardiopulmonary Resuscitation and Emergency Cardiovascular Care. *Circulation*, *122*(18Suppl 3), S729–S767. doi:10.1161/CIRCULATIONAHA.110.970988 PMID:20956224

Newman, M. F., Mathew, J. P., Grocott, H. P., Mackensen, G. B., Monk, T., Welsh-Bohmer, K. A., & Mark, D. B. et al. (2006). Central nervous system injury associated with cardiac surgery. *Lancet*, *368*(9536), 694–703. doi:10.1016/S0140-6736(06)69254-4 PMID:16920475

Ngaage, D. L., & Bland, J. M. (2010). Lessons from aprotinin: Is the routine use and inconsistent dosing of tranexamic acid prudent? Meta-analysis of randomised and large matched observational studies. *European Journal of Cardio-Thoracic Surgery*, *37*(6), 1375–1383. doi:10.1016/j.ejcts.2009.11.055 PMID:20117944

Nguyen, D. T., Delahaye, F., Obadia, J., Duval, X., Selton-Suty, C., Carteaux, J., & Alla, F. et al. (2010). Aortic valve replacement for active infective endocarditis: 5-year survival comparison of bioprostheses, homografts and mechanical prostheses. *European Journal of Cardio-Thoracic Surgery*, *37*(5), 1025–1032. doi:10.1016/j.ejcts.2009.11.035 PMID:20036573

Nguyen, K., & Marks, J. G. Jr. (2003). Pseudoacromegaly induced by the long-term use of minoxidil. *Journal of the American Academy of Dermatology*, *48*(6), 962–965. doi:10.1067/mjd.2003.325 PMID:12789195

Nguyen, T. C., Babaliaros, V. C., Razavi, S. A., Kilgo, P. D., Guyton, R. A., Devireddy, C. M., & Thourani, V. H. et al. (2013). Impact of varying degrees of renal dysfunction on transcatheter and surgical aortic valve replacement. *The Journal of Thoracic and Cardiovascular Surgery*, *146*(6), 1399–1407. doi:10.1016/j.jtcvs.2013.07.065 PMID:24075566

NICE-SUGAR Study Investigators. (2009). Intensive Versus Conventional Glucose Control In Critically Ill Patients. *The New England Journal of Medicine*, *360*(13), 1283–1297. doi:10.1056/NEJMoa0810625 PMID:19318384

NICE-SUGAR Study Investigators. (2012). Hypoglycemia and risk of death in critically ill patients. *The New England Journal of Medicine*, *367*(12), 1108–1118. doi:10.1056/NEJMoa1204942 PMID:22992074

Niedner, M. F., Muething, S. E., & Sutcliffe, K. M. (2013). The high-reliability pediatric intensive care unit. *Pediatric Clinics of North America*, *60*(3), 563–580. doi:10.1016/j.pcl.2013.02.005 PMID:23639655

Nielsen, D. V., Hansen, M. K., Johnsen, S. P., Hansen, M., Hindsholm, K., & Jakobsen, C. J. (2014). Health outcomes with and without use of inotropic therapy in cardiac surgery: Results of a propensity score-matched analysis. *Anesthesiology*, *120*(5), 1098–1108. doi:10.1097/ALN.0000000000000224 PMID:24614322

Nieminen, M. S., Akkila, J., Hasenfuss, G., Kleber, F. X., Lehtonen, L. A., Mitrovic, V., & Remme, W. J. et al. (2000). Hemodynamic and neurohumoral effects of continuous infusion of levosimendan in patients with congestive heart failure. *Journal of the American College of Cardiology*, *36*(6), 1903–1912. doi:10.1016/S0735-1097(00)00961-X PMID:11092663

Nienaber, C. A., Kische, S., Rosseau, H., Eggebrecht, H., Rehders, T. C., Kundt, G., & Ince, H. et al. (2013). Endovascular repair of type B aortic dissection: Long-term results of the randomized investigation of stent grafts in aortic dissection trial. *Circulation: Cardiovascular Interventions*, *6*(4), 407–416. doi:10.1161/CIRCINTERVENTIONS.113.000463 PMID:23922146

Nienaber, J. J. C., Kusne, S., Riaz, T., Walker, R. C., Baddour, L. M., Wright, A. J., & Sohail, M. R. et al. (2013). Clinical manifestations and management of left ventricular assist device-associated infections. *Clinical Infectious Diseases*, *57*(10), 1438–1448. doi:10.1093/cid/cit536 PMID:23943820

Nietlispach, F., Johnson, M., Moss, R. R., Wijesinghe, N., Gurvitch, R., Tay, E. L., & Webb, J. G. et al. (2010). Transcatheter closure of paravalvular defects using a purpose-specific occluder. *JACC: Cardiovascular Interventions*, *3*(7), 759–765. doi:10.1016/j.jcin.2010.04.013 PMID:20650438

Nijjer, S., Watson, G., Athanasiou, T., & Malik, I. (2011). Safety of clopidogrel being continued until the time of coronary artery bypass grafting in patients with acute coronary sundrome: A meta-analysis of 34 studies. *European Heart Journal*, *32*(23), 2970–2988. doi:10.1093/eurheartj/ehr151 PMID:21609973

Nilsson, J., Algotsson, L., Hoglund, P., Luhrs, C., & Brandt, J. (2004). Early mortality in coronary bypass surgery: The EuroSCORE versus The Society of Thoracic Surgeons risk algorithm. *The Annals of Thoracic Surgery*, *77*(4), 1235–1239. doi:10.1016/j.athoracsur.2003.08.034 PMID:15063242

Nishimura, R. A., Otto, C. M., Bonow, R. O., Carabello, B. A., Erwin, J. P. III, Guyton, R. A., & Thomas, J. D. et al. (2014). 2014 AHA/ACC guideline for the management of patients with valvular heart disease. *Journal of the American College of Cardiology*, *63*(22), e57–e185. doi:10.1016/j.jacc.2014.02.536 PMID:24603191

Nishimura, R. A., Otto, C. M., Bonow, R. O., Carabello, B. A., Erwin, J. P. III, Guyton, R. A., & Thomas, J. D. et al. (2014). 2014 AHA/ACC guideline for the management of patients with valvular heart disease: Executive summary: A report of the American College of Cardiology/American Heart Association task force on practice guidelines. *Journal of the American College of Cardiology*, *63*(22), 2438–2488. doi:10.1016/j.jacc.2014.02.537 PMID:24603192

Nkomo, V. T., Gardin, J. M., Skelton, T. N., Gottdiener, J. S., Scott, C. G., & Enriques-Sarano, M. (2006). Burden of valvular heart disease: A population-based study. *Lancet*, *368*(9540), 1005–1011. doi:10.1016/S0140-6736(06)69208-8 PMID:16980116

Nolan, T., & Berwick, D. M. (2006). All-or-none measurement raises the bar on performance. *Journal of the American Medical Association*, *295*(10), 1168–1170. doi:10.1001/jama.295.10.1168 PMID:16522838

Nombela-Franco, L., Webb, J. G., de Jaegere, P. P., Toggweiler, S., Nuis, R. J., Dager, A. E., & Rodes-Cabau, J. et al. (2012). Timing, predictive factors, and prognostic value of cerebrovascular events in a large cohort of patients undergoing transcatheter aortic valve implantation. *Circulation*, *126*(25), 3041–3053. doi:10.1161/CIRCULATIONAHA.112.110981 PMID:23149669

Noppen, M., & De Keukeleire, T. (2008). Pneumothorax. *Respiration*, *76*(2), 121–127. doi:10.1159/000135932 PMID:18708734

Norman, G. R., Van der Vleuten, C. P., & De Graaff, E. (1991). Pitfalls in the pursuit of objectivity: Issues of validity, efficiency and acceptability. *Medical Education*, *25*(2), 119–126. doi:10.1111/j.1365-2923.1991.tb00037.x PMID:2023553

Norton, S. A., Hogan, L. A., Holloway, R. G., Temkin-Greener, H., Buckley, M. J., & Quill, T. E. (2007). Proactive palliative care in the medical intensive care unit: Effects on length of stay for selected high-risk patients. *Critical Care Medicine*, *35*(6), 1530–1535. doi:10.1097/01.CCM.0000266533.06543.0C PMID:17452930

Nothnagle, M., Anandarajah, G., Goldman, R. E., & Reis, S. (2011). Struggling to Be Self-Directed: Residents - Paradoxical Beliefs About Learning. *Academic Medicine*, *86*(12), 1539–1544. doi:10.1097/ACM.0b013e3182359476 PMID:22030764

Nourdine, K., Combes, P., Carton, M. J., Beuret, P., Cannamela, A., & Ducreux, J. C. (1999). Does noninvasive ventilation reduce the ICU nosocomial infection risk? A prospective clinical survey. *Intensive Care Medicine*, *25*(6), 567–573. doi:10.1007/s001340050904 PMID:10416907

Novak, F., Heyland, D. K., Avenell, A., Drover, J. W., & Su, X. (2002). Glutamine supplementation in serious illness: A systematic review of the evidence. *Critical Care Medicine*, *30*(9), 2022–2029. doi:10.1097/00003246-200209000-00011 PMID:12352035

Novy, E., Sonneville, R., Mazighi, M., Klein, I. F., Mariotte, E., Mourvillier, B., & Wolff, M. et al. (2013). Neurological complications of infective endocarditis: New breakthroughs in diagnosis and management. *Medecine et Maladies Infectieuses*, *43*(11-12), 443–450. doi:10.1016/j.medmal.2013.09.010 PMID:24215865

Nussmeier, N. A., Whelton, A. A., Brown, M. T., Langford, R. M., Hoeft, A., Parlow, J. L., & Verburg, K. M. et al. (2005). Complications of the COX-2 inhibitors parecoxib and valdecoxib after cardiac surgery. *The New England Journal of Medicine*, *352*(11), 1081–1091. doi:10.1056/NEJMoa050330 PMID:15713945

O'Connor, C. J. (2010). Glycemic control during cardiac surgery: A moving target? *Current Opinion in Anaesthesiology*, *23*, 47–48. doi:10.1097/ACO.0b013e328333c115 PMID:19858716

O'Grady, N. P., Alexander, M., Burns, L. A., Dellinger, E. P., Garland, J., Heard, S. O., & Saint, S. et al. (2011). Guidelines for the prevention of intravascular catheter-related infections. *Clinical Infectious Diseases*, *52*(9), e162–e193. doi:10.1093/cid/cir257 PMID:21460264

O'Horo, J. C., Maki, D. G., Krupp, A. E., & Safdar, N. (2014). Arterial catheters as a source of bloodstream infection: A systematic review and meta-analysis. *Critical Care Medicine*, *42*(6), 1334–1339. doi:10.1097/CCM.0000000000000166 PMID:24413576

O'Shaughnessy, L. (1936). An experimental method of providing collateral circulation to the heart. *British Journal of Surgery*, *23*(91), 665–670. doi:10.1002/bjs.1800239122

O'Brien, S. M., Shahian, D. M., Filardo, G., Ferraris, V. A., Haan, C. K., Rich, J. B., . . . Anderson, R. P. (2009). The Society of Thoracic Surgeons 2008 cardiac surgery risk models: part 2--isolated valve surgery. *Annals of Thoracic Surgery, 88*(1 Suppl), S23-42. doi: S0003-4975(09)01059-5 [pii] 10.1016/j.athoracsur.2009.05.056

O'Croinin, D., Ni Chonghaile, M., Higgins, B., & Laffey, J. G. (2005). Bench-to-bedside review: Permissive hypercapnia. *Critical Care (London, England)*, *9*(1), 51–59. doi:10.1186/cc2918 PMID:15693984

Oderda, G. M., Said, Q., Evans, R. S., Stoddard, G. J., Lloyd, J., Jackson, K., & Samore, M. H. et al. (2007). Opioid-related adverse drug events in surgical hospitalizations: Impact on costs and length of stay. *The Annals of Pharmacotherapy*, *41*(3), 400–406. doi:10.1345/aph.1H386 PMID:17341537

Oelkers, W. (1996). Adrenal insufficiency. *The New England Journal of Medicine*, *335*(16), 1206–1212. doi:10.1056/NEJM199610173351607 PMID:8815944

Ofori-Krakye, S. K., Tyberg, T. I., Geha, A. S., Hammond, G. L., Cohen, L. S., & Langou, R. A. (1981). Late cardiac tamponade after open heart surgery: Incidence, role of anticoagulants in its pathogenesis and its relationship to the post-cardiotomy syndrome. *Circulation*, *63*(6), 1323–1328. doi:10.1161/01.CIR.63.6.1323 PMID:7226478

O'Gara, P., Kushner, F. G., Ascheim, D. D., Casey, D. E., Chung, M. K., Lemos, J. A., & Zhao, D. et al. (2013). 2013 ACCF/AHA Guideline for the Management of ST-Elevation Myocardial Infarction. *Journal of the American College of Cardiology*, *61*(4), e78–e140. doi:10.1016/j.jacc.2012.11.019 PMID:23256914

O'Grady, N. P., Alexander, M., Dellinger, E. P., Gerberding, J. L., Heard, S. O., Maki, D. G., & Weinstein, R. A. et al. (2002). Guidelines for the prevention of intravascular catheter-related infections. Centers for Disease Control and Prevention. *MMWR. Recommendations and Reports*, *51*(RR-10), 1–29. PMID:12233868

Ohman, E. M., George, B. S., White, C. J., Kern, M. J., Gurbel, P. A., Freedman, R. J., & Frey, M. J. et al.The Randomized IABP Study Group. (1994). Use of Aortic Counterpulsation to Improve Sustained Coronary Artery Patency During Acute Myocardial Infarction. *Circulation*, *90*(2), 792–799. doi:10.1161/01.CIR.90.2.792 PMID:8044950

Ohri, S. K., & Velissaris, T. (2006). Gastrointestinal dysfunction following cardiac surgery. *Perfusion*, *21*(4), 215–223. doi:10.1191/0267659106pf871oa PMID:16939115

Olaison, L., & Schadewitz, K. (2002). Enterococcal endocarditis in Sweden, 1995-1999: Can shorter therapy with aminoglycosides be used? *Clinical Infectious Diseases*, *34*(2), 159–166. doi:10.1086/338233 PMID:11740702

Oldgren, J., Budaj, A., Granger, C. B., Khder, Y., Roberts, J., Siegbahn, A., & Frans Van de Werf, L. W. et al. (2011). Dabigatran vs. placebo in patietns with acute coronary syndromes on dual antiplatelet therapy: A randomized, double-blind, phase II trial. *European Heart Journal*, *32*(22), 2781–2789. doi:10.1093/eurheartj/ehr113 PMID:21551462

Olearchyk, A.S., & Vasilii, I., & Kolesov. (1988). A pioneer of coronary revascularization by internal mammary-coronary artery grafting. *Journal of Cardiovascular and Thoracic Surgery*, *96*, 13–18. PMID:2898559

Olkkola, K. T., & Ahonen, J. (2008). Midazolam and other benzodiazepines. *Handbook of Experimental Pharmacology*, *182*, 335–360. doi:10.1007/978-3-540-74806-9_16 PMID:18175099

Olsen, R. W. (1981). GABA-benzodiazepine-barbiturate receptor interactions. *Journal of Neurochemistry*, *37*(1), 1–13. doi:10.1111/j.1471-4159.1981.tb05284.x PMID:6265597

Olson, L. J., Subramanian, R., Ackermann, D. M., Orszulak, T. A., & Edwards, W. D. (1987). Surgical pathology of the mitral valve: A study of 712 cases spanning 21 years. *Mayo Clinic Proceedings*, *62*(1), 22–34. doi:10.1016/S0025-6196(12)61522-5 PMID:3796056

O'Mahony, S., McHenry, J., Blank, A. E., Snow, D., Eti Karakas, S., Santoro, G., & Kvetan, V. et al. (2010). Preliminary report of the integration of a palliative care team into an intensive care unit. *Palliative Medicine*, *24*(2), 154–165. doi:10.1177/0269216309346540 PMID:19825893

Ong, A., Dysert, K., Herbert, C., Laux, L., Granato, J., Crawford, J., & Cortes, V. et al. (2011). Trends in central line-associated bloodstream infections in a trauma-surgical intensive care unit. *Archives of Surgery*, *146*(3), 302–307. doi:10.1001/archsurg.2011.9 PMID:21422361

Oostdijk, E. A. N., Kesecioglu, J., Schultz, M. J., Visser, C. E., de Jonge, E., van Essen, E. H. R., & Bonten, M. J. M. et al. (2014). Effects of decontamination of the oropharynx and digestive tract on antibiotic resistance in ICUs. A randomized clinical trial. *Journal of the American Medical Association*, *312*, 1429–1437. doi:10.1001/jama.2014.7247 PMID:25271544

Orme, R. M. L., Oram, M. P., & McKinstry, C. E. (2009). Impact of echocardiography on patient management in the intensive care unit: An audit of district general hospital practice. *British Journal of Anaesthesia*, *102*(3), 340–344. doi:10.1093/bja/aen378 PMID:19151420

Ormrod, J. E. (2011). *Human Learning*. Boston: Pearson.

Ornstein, E. (1998). Systolic pressure variation predicts the response to acute blood loss. *Journal of Clinical Anesthesia*, *10*, 137–140. doi:10.1016/S0952-8180(97)00257-2 PMID:9524899

Osler, W. (1885). The Gulstonian lectures, on malignant endocarditis. *British Medical Journal*, *1*(1263), 522–526. doi:10.1136/bmj.1.1263.522 PMID:20751196

Oto, T., Rosenfeldt, F., Rowland, M., Pick, A., Rabinov, M., Preovolos, A., & Esmore, D. et al. (2004). Extracorporeal membrane oxygenation after lung transplantation: Evolving technique improves outcomes. *The Annals of Thoracic Surgery*, *78*(4), 1230–1235. doi:10.1016/j.athoracsur.2004.03.095

Ottens, T. H. D., Dieleman, J. M., Sauër, A.-M. C., Peelen, L. M., Nierich, A. P., de Groot, W. J., & van Dijk, D. et al. (2014). Effects of dexamethasone on cognitive decline after cardiac surgery. *Anesthesiology*, *121*(3), 492–500. doi:10.1097/ALN.0000000000000336 PMID:25225745

Otto, C. M., Burwash, I. G., Legget, M. E., Munt, B. I., Fujioka, M., Healy, N. L., & Schwaegler, R. G. et al. (1997). Prospective study of asymptomatic valvular aortic stenosis. Clinical, echocardiographic, and exercise predictors of outcome. *Circulation*, *95*(9), 2262–2270. doi:10.1161/01.CIR.95.9.2262 PMID:9142003

Otto, C. M., Pearlman, A. S., & Gardner, C. L. (1989). Hemodynamic progression of aortic stenosis in adults assessed by Doppler echocardiography. *Journal of the American College of Cardiology*, *13*(3), 545–550. doi:10.1016/0735-1097(89)90590-1 PMID:2918158

Overgaard, C. B., & Dzavik, V. (2008). Inotropes and Vasopressors. *Circulation, 118*(10), 1047–1056. doi:10.1161/CIRCULATIONAHA.107.728840 PMID:18765387

Oxorn, D., & Pearlman, A. (2012). CON: physician-performed ultrasound: the time has come for routine use in acute care medicine. *Anesthesia and Analgesia, 115*(5), 1004–1006. doi:10.1213/ANE.0b013e31826a118a PMID:23093582

Ozkaynak, B., Kayalar, N., Gümüs, F., Yücel, C., Mert, B., Boyacioğlu, K., & Erentuğ, V. (2014). *Time from cardiac catheterization to cardiac surgery: a risk factor for acute kidney injury? Interactive Cardiovascular and Thoracic Surgery*. Retrieved from; doi:10.1093/icvts/ivu023

Packer, M., Bristow, M., Cohn, J., Colucci, W., Fowler, M., Gilbert, E., & Shusterman, N. (1996). The effect of carvedilol on morbidity and mortality in patients with chronic heart failure. US carvedilol heart failure study group. *The New England Journal of Medicine, 334*(21), 1349–1355. doi:10.1056/NEJM199605233342101 PMID:8614419

Packer, M., Colucci, W., Fisher, L., Massie, B. M., Teerlink, J. R., Young, J., & Sarapohja, T. et al. (2013). Effect of levosimendan on the short-term clinical course of patients with acutel decompensated heart failure. *Journal of American College Cardiology Heart Failure, 1*(2), 103–111. doi:10.1016/j.jchf.2012.12.004 PMID:24621834

Packer, M., Poole-Wilson, P., Armstrong, P., Cleland, J., Horowitz, J., Massie, B., & Uretsky, B. et al. (1999). Comparative effects of low and high doses of the angiotensin-converting enzyme inhibitor, lisinopril, on morbidity and mortality in chronic heart failure. ATLAS Study Group. *Circulation, 100*(23), 2312–2318. doi:10.1161/01.CIR.100.23.2312 PMID:10587334

Padial, L. R., Abascal, V. M., Moreno, P. R., Weyman, A. E., Levine, R. A., & Palacios, I. F. (1999). Echocardiography can predict the development of severe mitral regurgitation after percutaneous mitral valvuloplasty by the Inoue technique. *The American Journal of Cardiology, 83*(8), 1210–1213. doi:10.1016/S0002-9149(99)00061-2 PMID:10215286

Page, V. J., Ely, E. W., Gates, S., Zhao, X. B., Alce, T., Shintani, A., & McAuley, D. F. et al. (2013). Effect of intravenous haloperidol on the duration of delirium and coma in critically ill patients (Hope-ICU): A randomised, double-blind, placebo-controlled trial. *Lancet Respiratory Medicine, 1*(7), 515–523. doi:10.1016/S2213-2600(13)70166-8 PMID:24461612

Pagni, S., Ganzel, B. L., Williams, M., Slater, A. D., & Trivedi, J. R. (2012). Inflammatory aneurysms of the ascending aorta: Diagnosis and surgical treatment. *Journal of Cardiac Surgery, 27*(1), 70–74. doi:10.1111/j.1540-8191.2011.01335.x PMID:22103645

Paice, E., & Orton, V. (2004). Early signs of the trainee in difficulty. *Hospital Medicine (London, England), 65*(4), 238–240. doi:10.12968/hosp.2004.65.4.12739 PMID:15127680

Palanzo, D. A., El-Banayosy, A., Stephenson, E., Brehm, C., Kunselman, A., & Pae, W. E. (2013). Comparison of hemolysis between CentriMag and RotaFlow rotary blood pumps during extracorporeal membrane oxygenation. *Artificial Organs, 37*(9), E162–E166. PMID:23981131

Palmbergen, W., van Sonderen, A., Keyhan-Falsafi, A. M., Keunen, R. W. M., & Wolterbeek, R. (2012). Improved perioperative neurological monitoring of coronary artery bypass graft patients reduces the incidence of postoperative delirium: The Haga Brain Care Strategy. *Interactive Cardiovascular and Thoracic Surgery, 15*(4), 671–677. doi:10.1093/icvts/ivs317 PMID:22778141

Palmer, L. B., & Smaldone, G. C. (2014). Reduction of bacterial resistance with inhaled antibiotics in the intensive care unit. *American Journal of Respiratory and Critical Care Medicine, 189*(10), 1225–1233. doi:10.1164/rccm.201312-2161OC PMID:24646034

Palter, V. N., & Grantcharov, T. P. (2010). Simulation in surgical education. *CMAJ: Canadian Medical Association Journal = Journal De l'Association Medicale Canadienne, 182*(11), 1191–1196. doi:10.1503/cmaj.091743

Pandharipande, P. P., Girard, T. D., Jackson, J. C., Morandi, A., Thompson, J. L., Pun, B. T., & Ely, E. W. et al. (2013). Long-term cognitive impairment after critical illness. *The New England Journal of Medicine*, *369*(14), 1306–1316. doi:10.1056/NEJMoa1301372 PMID:24088092

Pandharipande, P., Pun, B. T., Herr, D. L., Maze, M., Girard, T. D., Miller, R. R., & Ely, E. W. et al. (2007). Effect of sedation with dexmedetomidine vs. lorazepam on acute brain dysfunction in mechanically ventilated patients: The MENDS randomized controlled trial. *Journal of the American Medical Association*, *298*(22), 2644–2653. doi:10.1001/jama.298.22.2644 PMID:18073360

Pandharipande, P., Shintani, A., Peterson, J., Pun, B. T., Wilkinson, G. R., Dittus, R. S., & Ely, E. W. et al. (2006). Lorazepam is an independent risk factor for transitioning to delirium in intensive care unit patients. *Anesthesiology*, *104*(1), 21–26. doi:10.1097/00000542-200601000-00005 PMID:16394685

Pandharipande, PP, J. J., Ely EW. (2005). Delirium: Acute cognitive dysfunction in the critically ill. *Current Opinion in Critical Care*, *11*, 360–368. PMID:16015117

Pang, P. Y., Sin, Y. K., Lim, C. H., Tan, T. E., Lim, S. L., Chao, V. T., & Chua, Y. L. (2014). Surgical management of infective endocarditis: An analysis of early and late outcomes. *European Journal of Cardio-Thoracic Surgery*; Advance online publication. doi:10.1093/ejcts/ezu281 PMID:25027271

Paparella, D., Brister, S. J., & Buchanan, M. R. (2004). Coagulation disorders of cardiopulmonary bypass: A review. *Intensive Care Medicine*, *30*(10), 1873–1881. doi:10.1007/s00134-004-2388-0 PMID:15278267

Paparella, D., Yau, T. M., & Young, E. (2002). Cardiopulmonary bypass induced inflammation: Pathophysiology and treatment. An update. *European Journal of Cardio-Thoracic Surgery*, *21*(2), 232–244. doi:10.1016/S1010-7940(01)01099-5 PMID:11825729

Papazian, L., Forel, J. M., Gacouin, A., Penot-Ragon, C., Perrin, G., Loundou, A., & Investigators, A. S. et al. (2010). Neuromuscular blockers in early acute respiratory distress syndrome. *The New England Journal of Medicine*, *363*(12), 1107–1116. doi:10.1056/NEJMoa1005372 PMID:20843245

Papazian, L., Thomas, P., Garbe, L., Guignon, I., Thirion, X., Charrel, J., & Gouin, F. et al. (1995). Bronchoscopic or blind sampling techniques for the diagnosis of ventilator-associated pneumonia. *American Journal of Respiratory and Critical Care Medicine*, *152*(6 Pt 1), 1982–1991. doi:10.1164/ajrccm.152.6.8520766 PMID:8520766

Park, C. M., Chun, H. K., Lee, D. S., Jeon, K., Suh, G. Y., & Jeong, J. C. (2014). Impact of a surgical intensivist on the clinical outcomes of patients admitted to a surgical intensive care unit. *Annals of Surgical Treatment and Research*, *86*(6), 319–324. doi:10.4174/astr.2014.86.6.319 PMID:24949324

Park, S. J., Liao, K. K., Segurola, R., Madhu, K. P., & Miller, L. W. (2004). Management of aortic insufficiency in patients with left ventricular assist devices: A simple coaptation stitch method (Park's stitch). *The Journal of Thoracic and Cardiovascular Surgery*, *127*(1), 264–266. doi:10.1016/S0022-5223(03)01301-1 PMID:14752440

Parks, N. A., Magnotti, L. J., Weinberg, J. A., Zarzaur, B. L., Schroeppel, T. J., Swanson, J. M., & Croce, M. A. et al. (2012). Use of the clinical pulmonary infection score to guide therapy for ventilator-associated pneumonia risks antibiotic overexposure in patients with trauma. *Journal of Trauma and Acute Care Surgery*, *73*(1), 52–58. doi:10.1097/TA.0b013e31825ac37b PMID:22743372

Parolari, A., Loardi, C., Mussoni, L., Cavallotti, L., Camera, M., Biglioli, P., & Alamanni, F. et al. (2009). Nonrheumatic calcific aortic stenosis: An overview from basic science to pharmacological prevention. *European Journal of Cardio-Thoracic Surgery*, *35*(3), 493–504. doi:10.1016/j.ejcts.2008.11.033 PMID:19162497

Parr. (1975). Cardiac performance and early mortality after cardiac surgery in infants and young children. *Circulation, 51*, 867.

Parry, M. F., Grant, B., & Sestovic, M. (2013). Successful reduction in catheter-associated urinary tract infections: Focus on nurse-directed catheter removal. *American Journal of Infection Control, 41*(12), 1178–1181. doi:10.1016/j.ajic.2013.03.296 PMID:23768439

Pasala, K. K., Gujja, K., Prabhu, H., Vasavada, B., & Konka, S. et al.. (2012). Short-term Minoxidil Use Associated With Pericardial Effusion and Cardiac Tamponade: An Uncommon Presentation. *American Journal of Therapeutics, 19*(6), e186–e188. doi:10.1097/MJT.0b013e3181f5371c PMID:21519225

Pasin, L., Greco, T., Feltracco, P., Vittorio, A., Neto, C. N., Cabrini, L., & Zangrillo, A. et al. (2013). Dexmedetomidine as a sedative agent in critically ill patients: A meta-analysis of randomized controlled trials. *PLoS ONE, 8*(12), e82913. doi:10.1371/journal.pone.0082913 PMID:24391726

Pasquina, P., Tramèr, M. R., & Walder, B. (2003). Prophylactic respiratory physiotherapy after cardiac surgery: Systematic review. *British Medical Journal, 327*(7428), 1379. doi:10.1136/bmj.327.7428.1379 PMID:14670881

Patel, V., Lim, M., Massin, E., Jonsyn, G., Ates, P., Abou-Awdi, N., . . . Frazier, O. H. (1996). Sudden Cardiac Death In Cardiac Transplant Recipients. *Circulation, 94*(9 Suppl) i273-Ii277. Retrieved From http://www.ncbi.nlm.nih.gov/pubmed/8901759

Patel, M. R., Mahaffey, K. W., Garg, J., Pan, G., Singer, D. E., Werner, H., & Califf, R. M. et al. (2011). Rivaroxaban versus warfarin in nonvalvular atrial fibrillation. *The New England Journal of Medicine, 365*(10), 883–891. doi:10.1056/NEJMoa1009638 PMID:21830957

Patel, N. N., Lin, H., Toth, T., Jones, C., Ray, P., Welsh, G. I., & Murphy, G. J. et al. (2011). Phosphodiesterase-5 Inhibition Prevents Postcardiopulmonary Bypass Acute Kidney Injury in Swine. *The Annals of Thoracic Surgery, 92*(6), 2168–2176. doi:10.1016/j.athoracsur.2011.07.002 PMID:21983073

Patel, P. A., Ernst, F. R., & Gunnarsson, C. L. (2012). Ultrasonography guidance reduces complications and costs associated with thoracentesis procedures. *Journal of Clinical Ultrasound: JCU, 40*(3), 135–141. doi:10.1002/jcu.20884 PMID:21994047

Patel, R., & Gallagher, J. C. (2014). Vancomycin-resistant enterococcal bacteremia pharmacotherapy. *The Annals of Pharmacotherapy*; Advance online publication. doi:10.1177/1060028014556879 PMID:25352037

Patel, R., Rouse, M. S., Piper, K. E., & Steckelberg, J. M. (2001). Linezolid therapy of vancomycin-resistant Enterococcus faecium experimental endocarditis. *Antimicrobial Agents and Chemotherapy, 45*(2), 621–623. doi:10.1128/AAC.45.2.621-623.2001 PMID:11158767

Pate, P., Tenholder, M., Griffin, J., Eastridge, C., & Weiman, D. (1996). Preoperative assessment of the high-risk patient for lung resection. *The Annals of Thoracic Surgery, 61*(5), 1494–1500. doi:10.1016/0003-4975(96)00087-2 PMID:8633965

Patey, R., Flin, R., Fletcher, G., Maran, N., & Glavin, R. (2005). Developing a Taxonomy of Anesthetists' Nontechnical Skills (ANTS). (K. Henricksen, J. B. Battles, & E. S. Marks, Eds.). Rockville: Advances in Patient Safety: From Research to Implementation (Volume 4: Programs, Tools, and Products).

Patterson, G. A., Cooper, J. D., Dark, J. H., & Jones, M. T. (1988). Experimental and clinical double lung transplantation. *The Journal of Thoracic and Cardiovascular Surgery, 95*(1), 70–74.

Patterson, G. A., Cooper, J. D., Goldman, B., Weisel, R. D., Pearson, F. G., Waters, P. F., & Ginsberg, R. J. et al. (1988). Technique of successful clinical double-lung transplantation. *The Annals of Thoracic Surgery*, *45*(6), 626–633. doi:10.1016/S0003-4975(10)64763-7

Paul Olson, T. J., Brasel, K. J., Redmann, A. J., Alexander, G. C., & Schwarze, M. L. (2013). Surgeon-reported conflict with intensivists about postoperative goals of care. *JAMA Surgery*, *148*(1), 29–35. doi:10.1001/jamasurgery.2013.403 PMID:23324837

Paul, S., Escareno, C. E., Clancy, K., Jaklitsch, M. T., Bueno, R., & Lautz, D. B. (2009). Gastrointestinal complications after lung transplantation. *The Journal of Heart and Lung Transplantation*, *28*(5), 475–479. doi:10.1016/j.healun.2009.02.011

Pavese, P., Saurel, N., Labarère, J., Decouchon, C., Vittoz, J., Foroni, L., & François, P. et al. (2009). Does an educational session with an infectious diseases physician reduce the use of inappropriate antibiotic therapy for inpatients with positive urine culture results? A controlled before-and-after study. *Infection Control and Hospital Epidemiology*, *30*(6), 596–599. doi:10.1086/597514 PMID:19419329

Pawlik, A. J., & Kress, J. P. (2013). Issues affecting the delivery of physical therapy services for individuals with critical illness. *Physical Therapy*, *93*(2), 256–265. doi:10.2522/ptj.20110445 PMID:23162041

Payen, J. F., Bru, O., Bosson, J. L., Lagrasta, A., Novel, E., Deschaux, I., & Jacquot, C. et al. (2001). Assessing pain in critically ill sedated patients by using a behavioral pain scale. *Critical Care Medicine*, *29*(12), 2258–2263. doi:10.1097/00003246-200112000-00004 PMID:11801819

Pearse, R. M., Harrison, D. A., MacDonald, N., Gillies, M. A., Blunt, M., Ackland, G., & Rowan, K. et al. (2014). Effect of a perioperative, cardiac output-guided hemodynamic therapy algorithm on outcomes following major gastrointestinal surgery: A randomized clinical trial and systematic review. *Journal of the American Medical Association*, *311*(21), 2181–2190. doi:10.1001/jama.2014.5305 PMID:24842135

Pearse, R., Dawson, D., Fawcett, J., Rhodes, A., Grounds, R. M., & Bennett, E. D. (2005). Early goal-directed therapy after major surgery reduces complications and duration of hospital stay. A randomised, controlled trial. *Critical Care (London, England)*, *9*(6), R687–R693. doi:10.1186/cc3887 PMID:16356219

Pecanac, K. E., Kehler, J. M., Brasel, K. J., Cooper, Z., Steffens, N. M., McKneally, M. F., & Schwarze, M. L. (2014). It's big surgery: Preoperative expressions of risk, responsibility, and commitment to treatment after high-risk operations. *Annals of Surgery*, *259*(3), 458–463. doi:10.1097/SLA.0000000000000314 PMID:24253139

Peek, G. J., Mugford, M., Tiruvoipati, R., Wilson, A., Allen, E., Thalanany, M. M., & Elbourne, D. et al. (2009). Efficacy and economic assessment of conventional ventilatory support versus extracorporeal membrane oxygenation for severe adult respiratory failure (CESAR): A multicentre randomised controlled trial. *Lancet*, *374*(9698), 1351–1363. doi:10.1016/S0140-6736(09)61069-2

Pellegrino, E. D. (2005). Futility in medical decisions: The word and the concept. *HEC Forum*, *17*(4), 308–318. doi:10.1007/s10730-005-5156-9 PMID:16637443

Pellikka, P. A., Sarano, M. E., Nishimura, R. A., Malouf, J. F., Bailey, K. R., Scott, C. G., & Tajik, A. J. et al. (2005). Outcome of 622 adults with asymptomatic, hemodynamically significant aortic stenosis during prolonged follow-up. *Circulation*, *111*(24), 3290–3295. doi:10.1161/CIRCULATIONAHA.104.495903 PMID:15956131

Pelosi, P., Quintel, M., & Malbrain, M. L. N. G. (2007). Effect of intra-abdominal pressure on respiratory mechanics. *Acta Clinica Belgica*, *62*(Suppl 1), 78–88. doi:10.1179/acb.2007.62.s1.011 PMID:24881704

Peña, A. (2010). The Dreyfus model of clinical problem-solving skills acquisition: A critical perspective. *Medical Education Online*, *15*(0). doi:10.3402/meo.v15i0.4846 PMID:20563279

Penderson, A. K., & Fitzgerald, G. A. (1984). Dose related kinetics of aspirin: Presystemic acetylation of platelet cyclooxygenase. *The New England Journal of Medicine*, *311*(19), 1206–1211. doi:10.1056/NEJM198411083111902 PMID:6436696

Pendleton, D. (1984). *The Consultation*. Oxford: Oxford University Press.

Pennefather, S., & Russell, G. (2004). Postthoracotomy analgesia: Recent advances and future directions. In *Progress in Thoracic Anesthesia* (pp. 163–185). Baltimore: Lippincott Williams & Wilkins.

Penrod, J. D., Deb, P., Dellenbaugh, C., Burgess, J. F. Jr, Zhu, C. W., Christiansen, C. L., & Morrison, R. S. et al. (2010). Hospital-based palliative care consultation: Effects on hospital cost. *Journal of Palliative Medicine*, *13*(8), 973–979. doi:10.1089/jpm.2010.0038 PMID:20642361

Peredo, R., Sabatier, C., Villagrá, A., González, J., Hernández, C., Pérez, F., & Vallés, J. et al. (2010). Reduction in catheter-related bloodstream infections in critically ill patients through a multiple system intervention. *European Journal of Clinical Microbiology & Infectious Diseases*, *29*(9), 1173–1177. doi:10.1007/s10096-010-0971-6 PMID:20533071

Perencevich, E. N., Fisman, D. N., Lipsitch, M., Harris, A. D., Morris, J. G. Jr, & Smith, D. L. (2004). Projected benefits of active surveillance for vancomycin-resistant enterococci in intensive care units. *Clinical Infectious Diseases*, *38*(8), 1108–1115. doi:10.1086/382886 PMID:15095215

Perera, P., Mailhot, T., Riley, D., & Mandavia, D. (2010). The RUSH exam: Rapid Ultrasound in SHock in the evaluation of the critically Ill.[vii.]. *Emergency Medicine Clinics of North America*, *28*(1), 29–56. doi:10.1016/j.emc.2009.09.010 PMID:19945597

Peretto, G., Durante, A., Limite, L. R., & Cianflone, D. (2014). Postoperative arrhythmias after cardiac surgery: Incidence, risk factors, and therapeutic management. *Cardiology Research and Practice*, (3): 615987–15. doi:10.1155/2014/615987 PMID:24511410

Perez-Gomez, F., Salvador, A., Zumalde, J., Iriarte, J. A., Berjon, J., Alegria, E., & Fernandez, C. et al. (2006). Effect of antithrombotic therapy in patients with mitral stenosis and atrial fibrillation: A sub-analysis of NASPEAF randomized trial. *European Heart Journal*, *27*(8), 960–967. doi:10.1093/eurheartj/ehi667 PMID:16330464

Perl, T. M., & Golub, J. E. (1998). New approaches to reduce Staphylococcus aureus nosocomial infection rates: Treating S. aureus nasal carriage. *The Annals of Pharmacotherapy*, *32*(1), S7–S16. doi:10.1177/106002809803200104 PMID:9475834

Perme, C. S., Southard, R. E., Joyce, D. L., Noon, G. P., & Loebe, M. (2006). Early mobilization of LVAD recipients who require prolonged mechanical ventilation. *Texas Heart Institute Journal*, *33*(2), 130–133. PMID:16878612

Perneby, C., Wallen, N. H., Rooney, C., Fitzgerald, D., & Hjemdahi, P. (2006). Dose and time-dependent antiplatelet effects of aspirin. *Journal of Thrombosis and Haemostasis*, *95*(4), 652–658. PMID:16601836

Petäjä, L., Salmenperä, M., Pulkki, K., & Pettilä, V. (2009). Biochemical injury markers and mortality after coronary artery bypass grafting: A systematic review. *The Annals of Thoracic Surgery*, *87*(6), 1981–1992. doi:10.1016/j.athoracsur.2008.12.063 PMID:19463650

Peter, J. V., Moran, J. L., & Phillips-Hughes, J. (2005). A meta-analysis of treatment outcomes of early enteral versus early parenteral nutrition in hospitalized patients. *Critical Care Medicine*, *33*(1), 213–220. doi:10.1097/01.CCM.0000150960.36228.C0 PMID:15644672

Petersen, P., Kastrup, J., Wilhelmsen, R., & Schutten, H. J. (1988). Atrial natriuretic peptide in atrial fibrillation before and after electrical cardioversion therapy. *European Heart Journal*, *9*, 639–641. PMID:2970387

Peterson, L. R., & Smith, B. A. (2014). Non-utility of catheter tip cultures for the diagnosis of central line-associated blood stream infection (CLABSI). *Clinical Infectious Diseases*; Advance online publication. doi:10.1093/cid/ciu845 PMID:25355902

Petroni, T., Harrois, A., Amour, J., Lebreton, G., Brechot, N., Tanaka, S., & Combes, A. et al. (2014). Intra-aortic balloon pump effects on macrocirculation and microcirculation in cardiogenic shock patients supported by venoarterial extracorporeal membrane oxygenation. *Critical Care Medicine*, *42*(9), 2075–2082. doi:10.1097/CCM.0000000000000410 PMID:24810530

Petterson, G. B., Hussain, S. T., Shrestha, S. K., Gordon, S., Fraser, T. G., Ibrahim, K. S., & Blackstone, E. H. (2014). Infective endocarditis: An atlas of disease progression for describing, staging, coding, and understanding the pathology. *The Journal of Thoracic and Cardiovascular Surgery*, *147*(4), 1142–1149. doi:10.1016/j.jtcvs.2013.11.031 PMID:24507402

Peura, D. A. (1986). Stress-related mucosal damage. *Clinical Therapeutics*, *8*(Suppl A), 14–23. PMID:2878727

Pfuntner, A., Wier, L. M., & Stocks, C. (2013). Most Frequent Conditions in U.S. Hospitals, 2011. *HCUP Statistical Brief #162. Agency for Healthcare Research and Quality*, Retrieved May 25, 2015, from http://www.hcup-us.ahrq.gov/reports/statbriefs/sb162.pdf

Phan, K., Xie, A., Di Eusanio, M., & Yan, T. D. (2014). A Meta-Analysis of Minimally Invasive Versus Conventional Sternotomy for Aortic Valve Replacement. *The Annals of Thoracic Surgery*, *98*(4), 1499–1511. doi:10.1016/j.athoracsur.2014.05.060 PMID:25064516

Phan, T. D. (2011). A comparison of three minimally invasive cardiac output devices with thermodilution in elective cardiac surgery. *Anaesthesia and Intensive Care Journal*, *39*, 1014–1021. PMID:22165352

Phillips, J. O., Metzler, M. H., Palmieri, M. T., Huckfeldt, R. E., & Dahl, N. G. (1996). A prospective study of simplified omeprazole suspension for the prophylaxis of stress-related mucosal damage. *Critical Care Medicine*, *24*(11), 1793–1800. doi:10.1097/00003246-199611000-00006 PMID:8917027

Phurrough, S., Farrell, J., Ulrich, M., & Long, K. (2003). *Decision Memo for Ventricular Assist Devices as Destination Therapy (CAG-00119N).* Retrieved May 25, 2015, from http://www.cms.gov/medicare-coverage-database/details/nca-decision-memo.aspx?ncaid=79&ncaname=ventricular+assist+devices+as+destination+therapy&ncdid=246&ispopup=y&bc=aaaaaaaaeaaa&

Pibarot, P., & Dumesnil, J. G. (2000). Hemodynamic and clinical impact of prosthesis-patient mismatch in the aortic valve position and its prevention. *Journal of the American College of Cardiology*, *36*(4), 1131–1141. doi:10.1016/S0735-1097(00)00859-7 PMID:11028462

Pierpont, L., Cohn, J., & Franciosa, J. (1978). Combined oral hydralazine-nitrate therapy in left ventricular failure: Hemodynamic equivalency to sodium nitroprusside. *American College of Chest Physicians*, *73*(1), 8–13. PMID:620563

Pierri, M. D., Capestro, F., Zingaro, C., & Torracca, L. (2010). The changing face of cardiac surgery patients: An insight into a Mediterranean region. *European Journal of Cardio-Thoracic Surgery*, *38*(4), 407–413. doi:10.1016/j.ejcts.2010.02.040 PMID:20399675

Pilcher, D. V., Scheinkestel, C. D., Snell, G. I., Davey-Quinn, A., Bailey, M. J., & Williams, T. J. (2005). High central venous pressure is associated with prolonged mechanical ventilation and increased mortality after lung transplantation. *The Journal of Thoracic and Cardiovascular Surgery*, *129*(4), 912–918. doi:10.1016/j.jtcvs.2004.07.006

Pincock, T., Bernstein, P., Warthman, S., & Holst, E. (2012). Bundling hand hygiene interventions and measurement to decrease health care-associated infections. *American Journal of Infection Control*, *40*(4), S18–S27. doi:10.1016/j.ajic.2012.02.008 PMID:22546269

Pinhu, L., Whitehead, T., Evans, T., & Griffiths, M. (2003). Ventilator-associated lung injury. *Lancet*, *361*(9354), 332–340. doi:10.1016/S0140-6736(03)12329-X PMID:12559881

Piquette, D., Fowler, R. A., & Slutsky, A. S. (2010). Impact of intensivist staffing on patient care and trainee education: A Canadian perspective. *American Journal of Respiratory and Critical Care Medicine*, *182*(4), 442–444. doi:10.1164/rccm.201006-0973ED PMID:20713639

Pisani, M. (2003). Underrecognition of Preexisting Cognitive Impairment by Physicians in Older ICU Patients<xref rid="AFF1">*</xref>. *CHEST Journal*, *124*(6), 2267. doi:10.1378/chest.124.6.2267

Pitt, B., Remme, W., Zannad, F., Neaton, J., Martinez, F., Roniker, B., & Gatlin, M. et al. (2003). Eplerenone, a Selective Aldosterone Blocker, in Patients with Left Ventricle Dysfunction after Myocardial Infarction. *The New England Journal of Medicine*, *348*(14), 1309–1321. doi:10.1056/NEJMoa030207 PMID:12668699

Pitt, B., Zannad, F., Remme, W., Cody, R., Castaigne, A., Perez, A., & Wittes, J. et al. (1999). The effect of spironolactone on morbidity and mortality in patients with severe heart failure. *The New England Journal of Medicine*, *341*(10), 709–717. doi:10.1056/NEJM199909023411001 PMID:10471456

Pittet, D., Allegranzi, B., & Boyce, J.World Health Organization World Alliance for Patient Safety Challenge Core Group of Experts. (2009). The World Health Organization guidelines on hand hygiene in health care and their consensus recommendations. *Infection Control and Hospital Epidemiology*, *30*(7), 611–622. doi:10.1086/600379 PMID:19508124

Plummer, M. P., Blaser, A. R., & Deane, A. M. (2014). Stress ulceration: prevalence, pathology and association with adverse outcomes. *Critical Care, 18*(2), 213.

Poch, D. S., & Ost, D. E. (2009). What are the important risk factors for healthcare-associated pneumonia? *Seminars in Respiratory and Critical Care Medicine*, *30*(01), 26–35. doi:10.1055/s-0028-1119806 PMID:19199184

Podcast. (n.d.). Podcast. *Merriam-Webster.com*. Retrieved May 11, 2014, from http://www.merriam-webster.com/dictionary/Podcast

Poelaert, J., Depuydt, P., De Wolf, A., Van de Velde, S., Herck, I., & Blot, S. (2008). Polyurethane cuffed endotracheal tubes to prevent early postoperative pneumonia after cardiac surgery: A pilot study. *The Journal of Thoracic and Cardiovascular Surgery*, *135*(4), 771–776. doi:10.1016/j.jtcvs.2007.08.052 PMID:18374755

Poelaert, J., Haentjens, P., & Blot, S. (2014). Association among duration of mechanical ventilation, cuff material of endotracheal tube, and postoperative nosocomial pneumonia in cardiac surgical patients: A prospective study. *The Journal of Thoracic and Cardiovascular Surgery*, *148*(4), 1622–1627. doi:10.1016/j.jtcvs.2014.05.085 PMID:25127550

Pogorzelska, M., Stone, P. W., Furuya, E. Y., Perencevich, E. N., Larson, E. L., Goldmann, D., & Dick, A. (2011). Impact of the ventilator bundle on ventilator-associated pneumonia in intensive care unit. *International Journal for Quality in Health Care*, *23*(5), 538–544. doi:10.1093/intqhc/mzr049 PMID:21821603

Polderman, K. H., & Girbes, A. R. (2002). Central venous catheter use. Part 2: Infectious complications. *Intensive Care Medicine*, *28*(1), 18–28. doi:10.1007/s00134-001-1156-7 PMID:11818995

Polderman, K. H., van Zanten, A., & Girbes, A. R. J. (2004). Free cortisol and critically ill patients. *The New England Journal of Medicine*, *351*(4), 395–397. doi:10.1056/NEJM200407223510419 PMID:15278953

Pollack, L. A., & Srinivasan, A. (2014). Core elements of hospital antibiotic stewardship programs from the Centers for Disease Control and Prevention. *Clinical Infectious Diseases*, *59*(Suppl 3), S97–S100. doi:10.1093/cid/ciu542 PMID:25261548

Polomsky, M., & Puskas, J. D. (2012). Off-pump coronary artery bypass grafting--the current state. *Circulation Journal : Official Journal of the Japanese Circulation Society, 76*(4), 784–90. Retrieved from http://www.ncbi.nlm.nih.gov/pubmed/22451446

Polson, J., & Lee, W. M. (2005). AASLD position paper: The management of acute liver failure. *Hepatology (Baltimore, Md.), 41*(5), 1179–1197. doi:10.1002/hep.20703 PMID:15841455

Pomianowski, P., & Elefteriades, J. A. (2013). The genetics and genomics of thoracic aortic disease. *Annals of Cardiothoracic Surgery, 2*(3), 271–279. PMID:23977594

Popma, J. J., Adams, D. H., Reardon, M. J., Yakubov, S. J., Kleiman, N. S., & Heimansohn, D. et al.. CoreValve United States Clinical, Investigators. (2014). Transcatheter Aortic Valve Replacement Using A Self-Expanding Bioprosthesis in Patients With Severe Aortic Stenosis at Extreme Risk for Surgery. *Journal of the American College of Cardiology*. doi:10.1016/j.jacc.2014.02.556

Popov, A. F., Schmitto, J. D., Jebran, A. F., Bireta, C., Friedrich, M., Rajaruthnam, D., & Schoendube, F. A. et al. (2011). Treatment of gram-positive deep sternal wound infections in cardiac surgery – Experiences with daptomycin. *Journal of Cardiothoracic Surgery, 6*(1), 112. doi:10.1186/1749-8090-6-112 PMID:21929771

Popping, D. M., Elia, N., Marret, E., Remy, C., & Tramer, M. R. (2008). Protective effects of epidural analgesia on pulmonary complications after abdominal and thoracic surgery: A meta-analysis. *Archives of Surgery, 143*(10), 990–999. doi:10.1001/archsurg.143.10.990 PMID:18936379

Preeshagul, I., Gharbaran, R., Jeong, K. H., Abdel-Razek, A., Lee, L. Y., Elman, E., & Suh, K. S. (2013). Potential biomarkers for predicting outcomes in CABG cardiothoracic surgeries. *Journal of Cardiothoracic Surgery, 8*(1), 176. doi:10.1186/1749-8090-8-176 PMID:23866777

Preslaski, C. R., Lat, I., MacLaren, R., & Poston, J. (2013). Pharmacist contributions as members of the multidisciplinary ICU team. *Chest, 144*(5), 1687–1695. doi:10.1378/chest.12-1615 PMID:24189862

Price, L. C., Wort, S. J., Finney, S. J., Marino, P. S., & Brett, S. J. (2010). Pulmonary vascular and right ventricular dysfunction in adult critical care: current and emerging options for management: a systematic literature review. *Critical Care (London, England), 14*(5), R169. doi:10.1186/cc9264 PMID:20858239

Price, S., Prout, J., Jaggar, S. I., Gibson, D. G., & Pepper, J. R. (2004). "Tamponade" following cardiac surgery: Terminology and echocardiography may both mislead. *European Journal of Cardio-Thoracic Surgery: Official Journal of the European Association for Cardio-Thoracic Surgery, 26*(6), 1156–1160. doi:10.1016/j.ejcts.2004.08.020 PMID:15541977

Prondzinsky, R., Lemm, H., Swyter, M., Wegener, N., Unverzagt, S., Carter, J., & Buerke, M. et al. (2010). Intra-aortic balloon counterpulsation in patients with acute myocardial infarction complicated by cardiogenic shock: The prospective, randomized IABP SHOCK Trial for attenuation of multiorgan dysfunction syndrome. *Critical Care Medicine, 38*(1), 152–160. doi:10.1097/CCM.0b013e3181b78671 PMID:19770739

Pronovost, P. J., Angus, D. C., Dorman, T., Robinson, K. A., Dremsizov, T. T., & Young, T. L. (2002). Physician staffing patterns and clinical outcomes in critically ill patients: A systematic review. *Journal of the American Medical Association, 288*(17), 2151–2162. doi:10.1001/jama.288.17.2151 PMID:12413375

Pronovost, P. J., Goeschel, C. A., Colantuoni, E., Watson, S., Lubomski, L. H., Berenholtz, S. M., & Needham, D. et al. (2010). Sustaining reductions in catheter related bloodstream infections in Michigan intensive care units; Observational study. *British Medical Journal, 340*(feb04 1), c309. doi:10.1136/bmj.c309 PMID:20133365

Pronovost, P. J., Jenckes, M. W., Dorman, T., Garrett, E., Breslow, M. J., Rosenfeld, B. A., & Bass, E. et al. (1999). Organizational characteristics of intensive care units related to outcomes of abdominal aortic surgery. *Journal of the American Medical Association*, *281*(14), 1310–1317. doi:10.1001/jama.281.14.1310 PMID:10208147

Pronovost, P. J., King, J., Holzmueller, C. G., Sawyer, M., Bivens, S., Michael, M., & Miller, M. et al. (2006). A web-based tool for the Comprehensive Unit-based Safety Program (CUSP). *Joint Commission Journal on Quality and Patient Safety*, *32*(3), 119–129. PMID:16617943

Pronovost, P. J., Weast, B., Holzmueller, C. G., Rosenstein, B. J., Kidwell, R. P., Haller, K. B., & Rubin, H. R. et al. (2003). Evaluation of the culture of safety: Survey of clinicians and managers in an academic medical center. *Quality & Safety in Health Care*, *12*(6), 405–410. doi:10.1136/qhc.12.6.405 PMID:14645754

Pronovost, P., Needham, D., Berenholtz, S., Sinopoli, D., Chu, H., Cosgrove, S., & Goeschel, C. et al. (2006). An intervention to decrease catheter-related bloodstream infections in the ICU. *The New England Journal of Medicine*, *355*(26), 2725–2732. doi:10.1056/NEJMoa061115 PMID:17192537

Pronovost, P., Weast, B., Schwarz, M., Wyskiel, R. M., Prow, D., Milanovich, S. N., & Lipsett, P. et al. (2003). Medication reconciliation: A practical tool to reduce the risk of medication errors. *Journal of Critical Care*, *18*(4), 201–205. doi:10.1016/j.jcrc.2003.10.001 PMID:14691892

Pugin, J., Auckenthaler, R., Mili, N., Janssens, J. P., Lew, P. D., & Suter, P. M. (1991). Diagnosis of ventilator-associated pneumonia by bacteriologic analysis of bronchoscopic and nonbronchoscopic "blind" bronchoalveolar lavage fluid. *The American Review of Respiratory Disease*, *143*(5 Pt 1), 1121–1129. doi:10.1164/ajrccm/143.5_Pt_1.1121 PMID:2024824

Pulikottil-Jacob, R., Suri, G., Connock, M., Kandala, N. B., Sutcliffe, P., Maheswaran, H., & Clarke, A. et al. (2014). Comparative cost-effectiveness of the HeartWare versus HeartMate II left ventricular assist devices used in the United Kingdom National Health Service bridge-to-transplant program for patients with heart failure. *The Journal of Heart and Lung Transplantation*, *33*(4), 350–358. doi:10.1016/j.healun.2014.01.003 PMID:24582838

Puskas, J. D., Sadiq, A., Vassiliades, T. A., Kilgo, P. D., & Lattouf, O. M. (2012). Bilateral internal thoracic artery grafting is associated with significantly improved long-term survival, even among diabetic patients. *The Annals of Thoracic Surgery*, *94*(3), 710–716. doi:10.1016/j.athoracsur.2012.03.082 PMID:22677228

Puskas, J. D., Williams, W. H., Mahoney, E. M., Huber, P. R., Block, P. C., Duke, P. G., & Guyton, R. A. et al. (2004). Off-pump vs conventional coronary artery bypass grafting: early and 1-year graft patency, cost, and quality-of-life outcomes: a randomized trial. *Journal of the American Medical Association*, *291*(15), 1841–1849. doi:10.1001/jama.291.15.1841 PMID:15100202

Qaseem, A., Humphrey, L. L., Chou, R., Snow, V., & Shekelle, P.Clinical Guidelines Committee of the American College of Physicians. (2011). Use of intensive insulin therapy for the management of glycemic control in hospitalized patients: A clinical practice guideline from the American College of Physicians. *Annals of Internal Medicine*, *154*(4), 260–267. doi:10.7326/0003-4819-154-4-201102150-00007 PMID:21320941

Qayyum, R., Becker, D. M., Yanek, L. R., Moy, T. F., Becker, L. C., Faraday, N., & Vaidya, D. (2008). Platelet inhibition by 81 and 325 mg aspirin daily in men vs women without clinically apparent cardiovascular disease. *The American Journal of Cardiology*, *101*(9), 1359–1363. doi:10.1016/j.amjcard.2007.12.038 PMID:18435972

Quill, T. E., & Abernethy, A. P. (2013). Generalist plus Specialist Palliative Care - Creating a More Sustainable Model. *The New England Journal of Medicine*, *368*(13), 1173–1175. doi:10.1056/NEJMp1215620 PMID:23465068

Raad, I., Hanna, H., & Maki, D. (2007). Intravascular catheter-related infections: Advances, in diagnosis, prevention, and management. *The Lancet Infectious Diseases*, *7*(10), 645–657. doi:10.1016/S1473-3099(07)70235-9 PMID:17897607

Racz, M. J., Hannan, E. L., Isom, O. W., Subramanian, V., Jones, R. H., Gold, J. P., & Rose, E. A. et al. (2004). A comparison of short- and long-term outcomes after off-pump and on-pump coronary artery bypass graft surgery with sternotomy. *Journal of the American College of Cardiology*, *43*(4), 557–564. doi:10.1016/j.jacc.2003.09.045 PMID:14975463

Radrizzani, D., Bertolini, G., Facchini, R., Simini, B., Bruzzone, P., Zanforlin, G., & Iapichino, G. et al. (2006). Early enteral immunonutrition vs. parenteral nutrition in critically ill patients without severe sepsis: A randomized clinical trial. *Intensive Care Medicine*, *32*(8), 1191–1198. doi:10.1007/s00134-006-0238-y PMID:16788808

Rafiq, S., Steinbrüchel, D. A., Wanscher, M. J., Andersen, L. W., Navne, A., Lilleoer, N. B., & Olsen, P. S. (2014). Multimodal analgesia versus traditional opiate based analgesia after cardiac surgery, a randomized controlled trial. *Journal of Cardiothoracic Surgery*, *9*(1), 52. doi:10.1186/1749-8090-9-52 PMID:24650125

Raghunathan, K., Shaw, A., Nathanson, B., Sturmer, T., Brookhart, A., Stefan, M. S., & Lindenauer, P. K. et al. (2014). Association between the choice of IV crystalloid and in-hospital mortality among critically ill adults with sepsis. *Critical Care Medicine*, *42*(7), 1585–1591. doi:10.1097/CCM.0000000000000305

Rahe-Meyer, N., Pichlmaier, M., Haverich, A., Solomon, C., Winterhalter, M., Piepenbrock, S., & Tanaka, K. A. (2009). Bleeding management with fibrinogen concentrate targeting a high-normal plasma fibrinogen level: A pilot study. *British Journal of Anaesthesia*, *102*(6), 785–792. doi:10.1093/bja/aep089 PMID:19411671

Rahe-Meyer, N., Solomon, C., Hanke, A., Schmidt, D. S., Knoerzer, D., Hochleitner, G., & Pichlmaier, M. et al. (2013). Effects of fibrinogen concentrate as first-line therapy during major aortic replacement surgery: A randomized, placebo-controlled trial. *Anesthesiology*, *118*(1), 40–50. doi:10.1097/ALN.0b013e3182715d4d PMID:23249928

Rahe-Meyer, N., Solomon, C., Winterhalter, M., Piepenbrock, S., Tanaka, K., Haverich, A., & Pichlmaier, M. (2009). Thromboelastometry-guided administration of fibrinogen concentrate for the treatment of excessive intraoperative bleeding in thoracoabdominal aortic aneurysm surgery. *The Journal of Thoracic and Cardiovascular Surgery*, *138*(3), 694–702. doi:10.1016/j.jtcvs.2008.11.065 PMID:19698858

Rahe-Meyer, N., & Sørensen, B. (2011). For: Fibrinogen concentrate for management of bleeding. *Journal of Thrombosis and Haemostasis*, *9*(1), 1–5. doi:10.1111/j.1538-7836.2010.04099.x PMID:20946151

Raja, S. G., & Berg, G. A. (2007). Impact of off-pump coronary artery bypass surgery on systemic inflammation: Current best available evidence. *Journal of Cardiac Surgery*, *22*(5), 445–455. doi:10.1111/j.1540-8191.2007.00447.x PMID:17803591

Rajek, A., Pernerstorfer, T., Kastner, J., Mares, P., Grabenwöger, M., Sessler, D. I., . . . Hiesmayr, M. (2000). Inhaled Nitric Oxide Reduces Pulmonary Vascular Resistance More Than Prostaglandin E1 During Heart Transplantation. *Anesthesia & Analgesia, 90*(3). Retrieved From http://journals.lww.com/anesthesia-analgesia/fulltext/2000/03000/inhaled_nitric_oxide_reduces_pulmonary_vascular.5.aspx

Ramakrishnan, N., Hanauer, D., & Keller, B. (2010). Mining electronic health records. *Computer*, *43*(10), 77–81. doi:10.1109/MC.2010.292

Raman, J. S., Kochi, K., Morimatsu, H., Buxton, B., & Bellomo, R. (2002). Severe ischemic early liver injury after cardiac surgery. *The Annals of Thoracic Surgery*, *74*(5), 1601–1606. doi:10.1016/S0003-4975(02)03877-8 PMID:12440615

Ramsay, J. G., Ralley, F. E., Whalley, D. G., DelliColli, P., & Wynands, J. E. (1985). Site of temperature monitoring and prediction of afterdrop after open heart surgery. *Canadian Anaesthetists' Society Journal*, *32*(6), 607–612. doi:10.1007/BF03011406 PMID:3878219

Ramsay, J., & Finley, A. (2011). Postoperative Respiratory Failure and Treatment. In P. D. Slinger (Ed.), *Principles and Practice of Anesthesia for Thoracic Surgery* (pp. 609–633). New York: Springer. doi:10.1007/978-1-4419-0184-2_42

Ranganathan, N., Lam, J. H., Wigle, E. D., & Silver, M. D. (1970). Morphology of the human mitral valve. II. The value leaflets. *Circulation*, *41*(3), 459–467. doi:10.1161/01.CIR.41.3.459 PMID:5415983

Ranucci, M. B. B. (2006). Lowest hematocrit on cardiopulmonary bypass impairs the outcome in coronary surgery. *Texas Heart Institute Journal*, *33*, 300–305. PMID:17041685

Ranucci, M., Aronson, S., Dietrich, W., Dyke, C. M., Hofmann, A., Karkouti, K., & von Heymann, C. et al. (2011a). Patient blood management during cardiac surgery: Do we have enough evidence for clinical practice? *The Journal of Thoracic and Cardiovascular Surgery*, *142*(2), 249.e1–249.e32. doi:10.1016/j.jtcvs.2011.04.007 PMID:21605874

Ranucci, M., Baryshnikova, E., Castelvecchio, S., & Pelissero, G.Surgical and Clinical Outcome Research (SCORE) Group. (2013). Major bleeding, transfusions, and anemia: The deadly triad of cardiac surgery. *The Annals of Thoracic Surgery*, *96*(2), 478–485. doi:10.1016/j.athoracsur.2013.03.015 PMID:23673069

Ranucci, M., La Rovere, M. T., Castelvecchio, S., Maestri, R., Menicanti, L., Frigiola, A., & Febo, O. et al. (2011b). Postoperative anemia and exercise tolerance after cardiac operations in patients without transfusion: What hemoglobin level is acceptable? *The Annals of Thoracic Surgery*, *92*(1), 25–31. doi:10.1016/j.athoracsur.2011.02.058 PMID:21592458

Ranucci, M., Pazzaglia, A., Bianchini, C., Bozzetti, G., & Isgrò, G. (2008). Body size, gender, and transfusions as determinants of outcome after coronary operations. *The Annals of Thoracic Surgery*, *85*(2), 481–486. doi:10.1016/j.athoracsur.2007.10.014 PMID:18222248

Raoof, S., Baumann, M. H., & Collaborative, C. C. S. (2014). An official multi-society statement: ventilator-associated events: the new definition. *Critical Care Medicine*, *42*(1), 228–229. doi:10.1097/CCM.0000000000000191 PMID:24346542

Rapp-Kesek, D., Ståhle, E., & Karlsson, T. (2004). Body mass index and albumin in the preoperative evaluation of cardiac surgery patients. *Clinical Nutrition (Edinburgh, Lothian)*, *23*(6), 1398–1404. doi:10.1016/j.clnu.2004.06.006 PMID:15556262

Raschke, R. A., Reilly, B. M., Guidry, J. R., Fontana, J. R., & Srinivas, S. (1993). The weight-based heparin dosing nomogram compared with a "standard care" nomogram. A randomized controlled trial. *Annals of Internal Medicine*, *119*(9), 874–881. doi:10.7326/0003-4819-119-9-199311010-00002 PMID:8214998

Rasmussen, C., Thiis, J. J., Clemmensen, P., Efsen, F., Arendrup, H. C., & Saunamäki, K. et al.. (1997). Significance and management of early graft failure after coronary artery bypass grafting: Feasibility and results of acute angiography and re-re-vascularization. *European Journal of Cardio-Thoracic Surgery: Official Journal of the European Association for Cardio-Thoracic Surgery*, *12*(6), 847–852. doi:10.1016/S1010-7940(97)00268-6 PMID:9489868

Rathore, S., Wang, Y., & Krumholz, M. (2002). Sex-based differences in the effect of digoxin for the treatment of heart failure. *The New England Journal of Medicine*, *347*(18), 1403–1411. doi:10.1056/NEJMoa021266 PMID:12409542

Raynaud-Simon, A., Revel-Delhom, C., & Hébuterne, X. (2011). Clinical practice guidelines from the French health high authority: Nutritional support strategy in protein-energy malnutrition in the elderly. *Clinical Nutrition (Edinburgh, Lothian)*, *30*(3), 312–319. doi:10.1016/j.clnu.2010.12.003 PMID:21251732

Reader, T. (2006). Non-technical skills in the intensive care unit. *British Journal of Anaesthesia*, *96*(5), 551–559. doi:10.1093/bja/ael067 PMID:16567346

Rea-Neto, A., Youssef, N. C. M., Tuche, F., Brunkhorst, F., Ranieri, V. M., Reinhart, K., & Sakr, Y. (2008). Diagnosis of ventilator-associated pneumonia; A systematic review of the literature. *Critical Care (London, England)*, *12*(2), R56. doi:10.1186/cc6877 PMID:18426596

Recommendations for Clinical Skills Curricula for Undergraduate Medical Education. (2005, May 12). Recommendations for Clinical Skills Curricula for Undergraduate Medical Education. *Association of American Medical Colleges*. Retrieved May 12, 2014, from https://members.aamc.org/eweb/upload/Recommendations%20for%20Clinical%20Skills%20Curricula%202005.pdf

Reed, C. R., Fogel, S. L., Collier, B. R., Bradburn, E. H., Baker, C. C., & Hamill, M. E. (2014). Higher surgical critical care staffing levels are associated with improved National Surgical Quality Improvement Program quality measures. *J Trauma Acute Care Surg, 77*(1), 83-88; discussion 88. doi: 10.1097/TA.0000000000000279

Reed, D. A., & Wright, S. M. (2010). Role Models in Medicine. In H. J. Humphrey (Ed.), *Mentoring in Academic Medicine*. Philadelphia: American College of Physicians.

Rehman, S. M., Yi, G., & Taggart, D. P. (2013). The radial artery: Current concepts on its use in coronary artery revascularization. *The Annals of Thoracic Surgery*, *96*(5), 1900–1909. doi:10.1016/j.athoracsur.2013.06.083 PMID:24090580

Reich, D. L., Bodian, C. A., Krol, M., Kuroda, M., Osinski, T., & Thys, D. M. (1999). Intraoperative hemodynamic predictors of mortality, stroke, and myocardial infarction after coronary artery bypass surgery. *Anesthesia and Analgesia*, *89*(4), 814–822. PMID:10512249

Reichenberger, F., Kohstall, M. G., Seeger, T., Olschewski, H., Grimminger, F., Seeger, W., & Ghofrani, H. A. (2007). Effect of sildenafil on hypoxia-induced changes in pulmonary circulation and right ventricular function. *Respiratory Physiology & Neurobiology*, *159*(2), 196–201. doi:10.1016/j.resp.2007.07.005 PMID:17851140

Reid, C. L., Anton-Culver, H., Yunis, C., & Gardin, J. M. (2007). Prevalence and clinical correlates of isolated mitral, isolated aortic regurgitation, and both in adults aged 21 to 35 years (from the CARDIA study). *The American Journal of Cardiology*, *99*(6), 830–834. doi:10.1016/j.amjcard.2006.10.048 PMID:17350376

Reid, C. W., Slinger, P. D., & Lenis, S. (1996). A comparison of the effects of propofol-alfentanil versus isoflurane anesthesia on arterial oxygenation during one-lung ventilation. *Journal of Cardiothoracic and Vascular Anesthesia*, *10*(7), 860–863. doi:10.1016/S1053-0770(96)80046-2 PMID:8969391

Reignier, J., Mercier, E., Le Gouge, A., Boulain, T., Desachy, A., Bellec, F., & Lascarrou, J.-B. et al. (2013). Effect of not monitoring residual gastric volume on risk of ventilator-associated pneumonia in adults receiving mechanical ventilation and early enteral feeding: A randomized controlled trial. *Journal of the American Medical Association*, *309*(3), 249–256. doi:10.1001/jama.2012.196377 PMID:23321763

Reineck, L. A., Wallace, D. J., Barnato, A. E., & Kahn, J. M. (2013). Nighttime intensivist staffing and the timing of death among ICU decedents: A retrospective cohort study. *Critical Care (London, England)*, *17*(5), R216. doi:10.1186/cc13033 PMID:24090194

Rekha, G., Gorlin, R., Smith, T., & Yusuf, S. (1997). The effect of digoxin on mortality and morbidity in patients with heart failure. *The New England Journal of Medicine*, *336*(8), 525–533. doi:10.1056/NEJM199702203360801 PMID:9036306

Rello, J., Ochagavia, A., Sabanes, E., Roque, M., Mariscal, D., Reynaga, E., & Valles, J. (2000). Evaluation of outcome of intravenous catheter-related infections in critically ill patients. *American Journal of Respiratory and Critical Care Medicine*, *162*(3 Pt 1), 1027–1030. doi:10.1164/ajrccm.162.3.9911093 PMID:10988125

Resar, R., Pronovost, P., Haraden, C., Simmonds, T., Rainey, T., & Nolan, T. (2005). Using a bundle approach to improve ventilator care processes and reduce ventilator-associated pneumonia. *Joint Commission Journal on Quality and Patient Safety*, *31*(5), 243–248. PMID:15960014

Reston, J. T., Tregear, S. J., & Turkelson, C. M. (2003). Meta-analysis of short-term and mid-term outcomes following off-pump coronary artery bypass grafting. *The Annals of Thoracic Surgery*, *76*(5), 1510–1515. doi:10.1016/S0003-4975(03)01195-0 PMID:14602277

Restrepo, R. D. (2009). A stepwise approach to management of stable COPD with inhaled pharmacotherapy: A review. *Respiratory Care*, *54*(8), 1058–1081. PMID:19650947

Reuler, J. B., & Nardone, D. A. (1994). Role modeling in medical education. *The Western Journal of Medicine*, *160*(4), 335–337. PMID:8023482

Reznick, R. K., & MacRae, H. (2006). Teaching surgical skills--changes in the wind. *The New England Journal of Medicine*, *355*(25), 2664–2669. doi:10.1056/NEJMra054785 PMID:17182991

Ribeiro, H. B., Webb, J. G., Makkar, R. R., Cohen, M. G., Kapadia, S. R., Kodali, S., & Rodes-Cabau, J. et al. (2013). Predictive factors, management, and clinical outcomes of coronary obstruction following transcatheter aortic valve implantation: Insights from a large multicenter registry. *Journal of the American College of Cardiology*, *62*(17), 1552–1562. doi:10.1016/j.jacc.2013.07.040 PMID:23954337

Rice, T. W., Wheeler, A. P., Thompson, B. T., DeBoisblanc, B. P., Steingrub, J., & Rock, P. (2011). Enteral omega-3 fatty acid, gamma-linolenic acid, and antioxidant supplementation in acute lung injury. *Journal of the American Medical Association*, *306*(14), 1574–1581. doi:10.1001/jama.2011.1435 PMID:21976613

Rice, T. W., Wheeler, A. P., Thompson, B. T., Steingrub, J., Hite, R. D., Moss, M., & Rock, P. et al. (2012). Initial trophic vs full enteral feeding in patients with acute lung injury. *Journal of the American Medical Association*, *307*(8), 795–803. doi:10.1001/jama.2012.137 PMID:22307571

Richardson, J., Lonnqvist, P. A., & Naja, Z. (2011). Bilateral thoracic paravertebral block: Potential and practice. *British Journal of Anaesthesia*, *106*(2), 164–171. doi:10.1093/bja/aeq378 PMID:21233114

Richey, R., Wray, D., & Stokes, T.Guideline Development Group. (2008). Prophylaxis against infective endocarditis: Summary of NICE guidance. *British Medical Journal*, *336*(7647), 770–771. doi:10.1136/bmj.39510.423148.AD PMID:18390528

Riddington, D. W., Venkatesh, B., Bolvin, C. M., Bonser, R. S., Elliott, T. S., Marshall, T., & Bion, J. F. et al. (1996). Intestinal permeability, gastric intramucosal pH, and systemic endotoxemia in patients undergoing cardiopulmonary bypass. *Journal of the American Medical Association*, *275*(13), 1007–1012. doi:10.1001/jama.1996.03530370045029 PMID:8596232

Riker, R. R., & Fraser, G. L. (2001). Monitoring sedation, agitation, analgesia, neuromuscular blockade, and delirium in adult ICU patients. *Seminars in Respiratory and Critical Care Medicine*, *22*(02), 189–198. doi:10.1055/s-2001-13832 PMID:16088673

Riker, R. R., Shehabi, Y., Bokesch, P. M., Ceraso, D., Wisemandle, W., Koura, F., & Rocha, M. G. et al. (2009). Dexmedetomidine vs. midazolam for sedation of critically ill patients: A randomized trial. *Journal of the American Medical Association*, *301*, 489–499. doi:10.1001/jama.2009.56 PMID:19188334

Rinaldi, P., Mecocci, P., Benedetti, C., Ercolani, S., Bregnocchi, M., Menculini, G., & Cherubini, A. et al. (2003). Validation of the Five-Item Geriatric Depression Scale in Elderly Subjects in Three Different Settings. *Journal of the American Geriatrics Society*, *51*(5), 694–698. doi:10.1034/j.1600-0579.2003.00216.x PMID:12752847

Rinder, C. S., Bohnert, J., Rinder, H. M., Mitchell, J., Ault, K., & Hillman, R. (1991). Platelet activation and aggregation during cardiopulmonary bypass. *Anesthesiology*, *75*(3), 388–393. doi:10.1097/00000542-199109000-00002 PMID:1716077

RISC Group. (1990). Risk of myocardial infarction and death during treatment with low dose aspirin and intravenous heparin in men with unstable coronary artery disease. *Lancet*, *336*(8719), 827–830. doi:10.1016/0140-6736(90)92336-G PMID:1976875

Risnes, I., Abdelnoor, M., Almdahl, S. M., & Svennevig, J. L. (2010). Mediastinitis after coronary artery bypass grafting risk factors and long-term survival. *The Annals of Thoracic Surgery*, *89*(5), 1502–1510. doi:10.1016/j.athoracsur.2010.02.038 PMID:20417768

Roach, G. W., Kanchuger, M., & Mora-Mangano, C. T. (1996). Adverse cerebral outcomes after coronary artery bypass surgery. *The New England Journal of Medicine*, *335*(25), 1857–1863. doi:10.1056/NEJM199612193352501 PMID:8948560

Roberts, F. L., Dixon, J., Lewis, G. T., Tackley, R. M., & Prys-Roberts, C. (1988). Induction and maintenance of propofol anaesthesia. *Anaesthesia*, *43*(s1), 14–17. doi:10.1111/j.1365-2044.1988.tb09061.x PMID:3259089

Roberts, W. C., & Ko, J. M. (2005). Frequency by decades of unicuspid, bicuspid, and tricuspid aortic valves in adults having isolated aortic valve replacement for aortic stenosis, with or without associated aortic regurgitation. *Circulation*, *111*(7), 920–925. doi:10.1161/01.CIR.0000155623.48408.C5 PMID:15710758

Robiscek, A., Beaumont, J. L., Paule, S. M., Hacek, D. M., Thomson, R. B. Jr, Kaul, K. L., & Peterson, L. R. et al. (2008). Universal surveillance for methicillin-resistant Staphylococcus aureus in 3 affiliated hospitals. *Annals of Internal Medicine*, *148*(6), 409–418. doi:10.7326/0003-4819-148-6-200803180-00003 PMID:18347349

Rockwood, K., Song, X., MacKnight, C., Bergman, H., Hogan, D. B., McDowell, I., & Mitnitski, A. (2005). A global clinical measure of fitness and frailty in elderly people. *CMAJ : Canadian Medical Association Journal*, *173*(5), 489–95. doi:10.1503/cmaj.050051

Rodes-Cabau, J., Dumont, E., Boone, R. H., Larose, E., Bagur, R., Gurvitch, R., & Webb, J. G. et al. (2011). Cerebral embolism following transcatheter aortic valve implantation: Comparison of transfemoral and transapical approaches. *Journal of the American College of Cardiology*, *57*(1), 18–28. doi:10.1016/j.jacc.2010.07.036 PMID:21185496

Rodriguez, A., Bernardi, V., Navia, J., Baldi, J., Grinfeld, L., Martinez, J., … O'Neill, W. (2001). Argentine Randomized Study: Coronary Angioplasty with Stenting versus Coronary Bypass Surgery in patients with Multiple-Vessel Disease (ERACI II): 30-day and one-year follow-up results. ERACI II Investigators. *Journal of the American College of Cardiology, 37*(1), 51–8. Retrieved from http://www.ncbi.nlm.nih.gov/pubmed/11153772

Rodriguez, R., Robich, M. P., Plate, J. F., Trooskin, S. Z., & Sellke, F. W. (2010). Gastrointestinal complications following cardiac surgery: A comprehensive review. *Journal of Cardiac Surgery*, *25*(2), 188–197. doi:10.1111/j.1540-8191.2009.00985.x PMID:20149010

Rogers, J.G., Boyle, A.J., O'Connell, J.B., Horstmanshof, D.A., Haas, D.C., Slaughter, M.S., … Starling, R.C. (2014). Risk Assessment and Comparative Effectiveness of Left Ventricular Assist Device and Medical Management in Ambulatory Heart Failure Patients: Design and Rationale of the ROADMAP Clinical Trial. *American Heart Journal*. DOI:10.1016/j.ahj.2014.11.004

Rogers, C. A., Pike, K., Angelini, G. D., Reeves, B. C., Glauber, M., Ferrarini, M., & Murphy, G. J. (2013). An open randomized controlled trial of median sternotomy versus anterolateral left thoracotomy on morbidity and health care resource use in patients having off-pump coronary artery bypass surgery : The Sternotomy Versus Thoracotomy (STET) trial. *The Journal of Thoracic and Cardiovascular Surgery*, *146*(2), 306–316.e9. doi:10.1016/j.jtcvs.2012.04.020 PMID:22944093

Rogers, J. G., Bostic, R. R., Tong, K. B., Adamson, R., Russo, M., & Slaughter, M. S. (2012). Cost-effectiveness analysis of continuous-flow left ventricular assist devices as destination therapy. *Circulation: Heart Failure*, *5*(1), 10–16. doi:10.1161/CIRCHEARTFAILURE.111.962951 PMID:22052901

Rogers, J. H., & Bolling, S. F. (2009). The tricuspid valve: Current perspective and evolving management of tricuspid regurgitation. *Circulation*, *119*(20), 2718–2725. doi:10.1161/CIRCULATIONAHA.108.842773 PMID:19470900

Roguin, A., Rinkevich, D., Milo, S., Markiewicz, W., & Reisner, S. A. (1998). Long-term follow-up of patients with severe rheumatic tricuspid stenosis. *American Heart Journal*, *136*(1), 103–108. doi:10.1016/S0002-8703(98)70189-9 PMID:9665226

Rohde, J. M., Dimcheff, D. E., Blumberg, N., Saint, S., Langa, K. M., Kuhn, L., & Rogers, M. A. M. et al. (2014). Health care-associated infection after red blood cell transfusion. A systematic review and meta-analysis. *Journal of the American Medical Association*, *311*(13), 1317–1326. doi:10.1001/jama.2014.2726 PMID:24691607

Rohrer, M. J., & Natale, A. M. (1992). Effect of hypothermia on the coagulation cascade. *Critical Care Medicine*, *20*(10), 1402–1405. doi:10.1097/00003246-199210000-00007 PMID:1395660

Ronco, C., Haapio, M., House, A., Anavekar, N., & Bellomo, R. (2008). Cardiorenal Syndrome. *Journal of the American College of Cardiology*, *52*(19), 1527–1539. doi:10.1016/j.jacc.2008.07.051 PMID:19007588

Roques, F., Nashef, S. A., Michel, P., Gauducheau, E., de Vincentiis, C., Baudet, E., . . . Thulin, L. (1999). Risk factors and outcome in European cardiac surgery: analysis of the EuroSCORE multinational database of 19030 patients. *European Journal of Cardiothoracic Surgery, 15*(6), 816-822; discussion 822-813.

Rosa, G., Conti, G., Orsi, P., D'Alessandro, F., La Rosa, I., DiGiugno, G., & Gasparetto, A. (1992). Effects of low-dose propofol administration on central respiratory drive, gas exchanges and respiratory pattern. *Acta Anaesthesiologica Scandinavica*, *36*(2), 128–131. doi:10.1111/j.1399-6576.1992.tb03438.x PMID:1549931

Rose, E. A., Gelijns, A. C., Moskowitz, A. J., Heitjan, D. F., Stevenson, L. W., Dembitsky, W., & Poirier, V. L. et al. (2001). Long-term use of a left ventricular assist device for end-stage heart failure. *The New England Journal of Medicine*, *345*, 1435–1443. PMID:11794191

Rose, E., Gelijns, A., Moskowitz, A., Heitjan, D., Stevenson, L., Dembitsky, W., & Meier, P. et al. (2001). Long-Term Use of a Left Ventricular Assist Device for End-Stage Heart Failure. *The New England Journal of Medicine*, *345*(20), 1435–1443. doi:10.1056/NEJMoa012175 PMID:11794191

Roselli, E., Murthy, S., Rice, T., Houghtaling, P., Pierce, C., Karchmer, D., & Blackstone, E. (2005). Atrial fibrillation complicating lung cancer resection. *The Journal of Thoracic and Cardiovascular Surgery*, *130*(2), 438.e1–438.e9. doi:10.1016/j.jtcvs.2005.02.010 PMID:16077410

Rosenberger, P., Shernan, S. K., Loffler, M., Shekar, P. S., Fox, J. A., Tuli, J. K., & Eltzschig, H. K. et al. (2008). The influence of epiaortic ultrasonography on intraoperative surgical management in 6051 cardiac surgical patients. *The Annals of Thoracic Surgery*, *85*(2), 548–553. doi:10.1016/j.athoracsur.2007.08.061 PMID:18222262

Rosenhek, R., Rader, F., Klaar, U., Gabriel, H., Krejc, M., Kalbeck, D., & Baumgartner, H. et al. (2006). Outcome of watchful waiting in asymptomatic severe mitral regurgitation. *Circulation*, *113*(18), 2238–2244. doi:10.1161/CIRCULATIONAHA.105.599175 PMID:16651470

Rossaint, R., Falke, K. J., López, F., Slama, K., Pison, U., & Zapol, W. M. (1993). Inhaled nitric oxide for the adult respiratory distress syndrome. *The New England Journal of Medicine*, *328*(6), 399–405. doi:10.1056/NEJM199302113280605 PMID:8357359

Rossebø, A. B., Pedersen, T. R., Boman, K., Brudi, P., Chambers, J. B., Egstrup, K., & Willenheimer, R. et al. (2008). Intensive lipid lowering with simvastatin and ezetimibe in aortic stenosis. *The New England Journal of Medicine*, *359*(13), 1343–1356. doi:10.1056/NEJMoa0804602 PMID:18765433

Ross, J. Jr, & Braunwald, E. (1968). Aortic stenosis. *Circulation*, *38*(1Suppl), 61–67. PMID:4894151

Rouby, J. J., Eurin, B., Glaser, P., Guillosson, J. J., Nafziger, J., Guesde, R., & Viars, P. (1981). Hemodynamic and metabolic effects of morphine in the critically ill. *Circulation*, *64*(1), 53–59. doi:10.1161/01.CIR.64.1.53 PMID:7237725

Roudaut, R., Serri, K., & Lafitte, S. (2007). Thrombosis of prosthetic heart valves: Diagnosis and therapeutic considerations. *Heart (British Cardiac Society)*, *93*(1), 137–142. doi:10.1136/hrt.2005.071183 PMID:17170355

Rousou, J. A., Tighe, D. A., Garb, J. L., Krasner, H., Engelman, R. M., Flack, J. E. III, & Deaton, D. W. (2000). Risk of dysphagia after transesophageal echocardiography during cardiac operations. *The Annals of Thoracic Surgery*, *69*(2), 486–489. doi:10.1016/S0003-4975(99)01086-3 PMID:10735685

Roy, D., Talajic, M., Dorian, P., Connolly, S., Eisenberg, M. J., Green, M., & Thibault, B. et al. (2000). Amiodarone to prevent recurrence of atrial fibrillation. Canadian Trial of Atrial Fibrillation Investigators. *The New England Journal of Medicine*, *342*(13), 913–920. doi:10.1056/NEJM200003303421302 PMID:10738049

Royse, C., Royse, A., & Blake, D. (1998). Screening the thoracic aorta for atheroma: A comparison of manual palpation, Transesophageal and epiaortic ultrasonography. *Annals of Thoracic and Cardiovascular Surgery*, *4*, 347–350. PMID:9914464

Royston, D., & von Kier, S. (2001). Reduced haemostatic factor transfusion using heparinase-modified thrombelastography during cardiopulmonary bypass. *British Journal of Anaesthesia*, *86*(4), 575–578. doi:10.1093/bja/86.4.575 PMID:11573637

Rozental, T., & Shore-Lesserson, L. (2012). Pharmacologic management of coagulopathy in cardiac surgery: An update. *Journal of Cardiothoracic and Vascular Anesthesia*, *26*(4), 669–679. doi:10.1053/j.jvca.2012.03.030 PMID:22608465

Rubenfeld, G. D., & Angus, D. C. (2008). Are intensivists safe? *Annals of Internal Medicine*, *148*(11), 877–879. doi:10.7326/0003-4819-148-11-200806030-00010 PMID:18519933

Rubin, L. J., Badesch, D. B., Barst, R. J., Galie, N., Black, C. M., Keogh, A., & Simonneau, G. et al. (2002). Bosentan therapy for pulmonary arterial hypertension. *The New England Journal of Medicine*, *346*(12), 896–903. doi:10.1056/NEJMoa012212 PMID:11907289

Rubino, A. S., Onorati, F., Serraino, F., & Renzulli, A. (2009). Safety and efficacy of transbrachial intra-aortic balloon pumping with the use of 7-Fr catheters in patients undergoing coronary bypass surgery. *Interactive Cardiovascular and Thoracic Surgery*, *9*(1), 135–137. doi:10.1510/icvts.2009.205823 PMID:19383637

Rudis, M. I., & Brandl, K. M. (2000). Position paper on critical care pharmacy services. Society of Critical Care Medicine and American College of Clinical Pharmacy Task Force on Critical Care Pharmacy Services. *Critical Care Medicine*, *28*(11), 3746–3750. doi:10.1097/00003246-200011000-00037 PMID:11098984

Rudolph, J. L., Inouye, S. K., Jones, R. N., Yang, F. M., Fong, T. G., Levkoff, S. E., & Marcantonio, E. R. (2010). Delirium: An independent predictor of functional decline after cardiac surgery. *Journal of the American Geriatrics Society*, *58*(4), 643–649. doi:10.1111/j.1532-5415.2010.02762.x PMID:20345866

Rudolph, J. L., Jones, R. N., Grande, L. J., Milberg, W. P., King, E. G., Lipsitz, L. A., & Marcantonio, E. R. et al. (2006). Impaired executive function is associated with delirium after coronary artery bypass graft surgery. *Journal of the American Geriatrics Society*, *54*(6), 937–941. doi:10.1111/j.1532-5415.2006.00735.x PMID:16776789

Rudolph, J. L., Jones, R. N., Levkoff, S. E., Rockett, C., Inouye, S. K., Sellke, F. W., & Marcantonio, E. R. et al. (2009). Derivation and validation of a preoperative prediction rule for delirium after cardiac surgery. *Circulation*, *119*(2), 229–236. doi:10.1161/CIRCULATIONAHA.108.795260 PMID:19118253

Ruel, M., Shariff, M., Lapierre, H., Goyal, N., Dennie, C., Sadel, S. M., & McGinn, J. T. Jr et al.. (2014). Results of the Minimally Invasive Coronary Artery Bypass Grafting Angiographic Patency Study. *The Journal of Thoracic and Cardiovascular Surgery*, *147*(1), 203–208. doi:10.1016/j.jtcvs.2013.09.016 PMID:24183338

Ruffolo, R. R. Jr. (1987). The pharmacology of dobutamine. *The American Journal of the Medical Sciences*, *294*(4), 244–248. doi:10.1097/00000441-198710000-00005 PMID:3310640

Ruggeri, L., Landoni, G., Guarrancino, F., Scolletta, S., Bignami, E., & Zangrillo, A. (2011). Remifentanil in critically ill cardiac patients. *Annals of Cardiac Anaesthesia*, *14*, 6–12. PMID:21196668

Rugolotto, M., Chang, C.-P., Hu, B., Schnittger, I., & Liang, D. H. (2002). Clinical use of cardiac ultrasound performed with a hand-carried device in patients admitted for acute cardiac care. *The American Journal of Cardiology*, *90*(9), 1040–1042. doi:10.1016/S0002-9149(02)02700-5 PMID:12398985

Ruiz, J. G., Mintzer, M. J., & Leipzig, R. M. (2006). The impact of E-learning in medical education. *Academic Medicine*, *81*(3), 207–212. doi:10.1097/00001888-200603000-00002 PMID:16501260

Rushton, A. (2005). Formative assessment: A key to deep learning? *Medical Teacher*, *27*(6), 509–513. doi:10.1080/01421590500129159 PMID:16199357

Russell, J. A., Walley, K. R., Singer, J., Gordon, A. C., Hébert, P. C., Cooper, D. J., & Ayers, D. et al. (2008). Vasopressin versus norepinephrine infusion in patients with septic shock. *The New England Journal of Medicine*, *358*(9), 877–887. doi:10.1056/NEJMoa067373 PMID:18305265

Russo, M. J., Iribarne, A., Hong, K. N., Ramlawi, B., Chen, J. M., Takayama, H., . . . Naka, Y. (2010). Factors Associated With Primary Graft Failure After Heart Transplantation. *Transplantation, 90*(4). Retrieved From http://journals.lww.com/transplantjournal/fulltext/2010/08270/factors_associated_with_primary_graft_failure.19.aspx

Ruttmann, E., Willeit, J., Ulmer, H., Chevtchik, O., Höfer, D., Poewe, W., & Müller, L. C. et al. (2006). Neurological outcome of septic cardioembolic stroke after infective endocarditis. *Stroke*, *37*(8), 2094–2099. doi:10.1161/01.STR.0000229894.28591.3f PMID:16794213

Sabashnikov, A., Popov, A. F., Bowles, C. T., Mohite, P. N., Weymann, A., Hards, R., & Simon, A. R. et al. (2014). Outcomes after implantation of partial-support left ventricular assist devices in inotropic-dependent patients: Do we still need full-support assist devices? *The Journal of Thoracic and Cardiovascular Surgery*, *148*(3), 1115–1121, discussion 1021–1022. doi:10.1016/j.jtcvs.2014.05.063 PMID:25129605

Sabik, J. F., Lytle, B. W., McCarthy, P. M., & Cosgrove, D. M. (1995). Axillary artery: An alternative site of arterial cannulation for patients with extensive aortic and peripheral vascular disease. *The Journal of Thoracic and Cardiovascular Surgery*, *109*(5), 885–890, discussion 890–891. http://www.ncbi.nlm.nih.gov/pubmed/7739248 doi:10.1016/S0022-5223(95)70312-8 PMID:7739248

Sacar, M., Sacar, S., Kaleli, I., Cevahir, N., Teke, Z., Kavas, S. T., & Turgut, H. et al. (2008). Efficacy of linezolid in the treatment of mediastinitis due to methicillin-resistant Staphylococcus aureus: An experimental study. *International Journal of Infectious Diseases*, *12*, 396–401. PMID:18162429

Saczkowski, R., Maklin, M., Mesana, T., Boodhwani, M., & Ruel, M. (2012). Centrifugal pump and roller pump in adult cardiac surgery: A meta-analysis of randomized controlled trials. *Artificial Organs*, *36*(8), 668–676. doi:10.1111/j.1525-1594.2012.01497.x PMID:22804106

Saczynski, J. S., Marcantonio, E. R., Quach, L., Fong, T. G., Gross, A., Inouye, S. K., & Jones, R. N. (2012). Cognitive trajectories after postoperative delirium. *The New England Journal of Medicine, 367*(1), 30–39. doi:10.1056/NEJMoa1112923 PMID:22762316

Safdar, N., Dezfoulian, C., Collard, H. R., & Saint, S. (2005). Clinical and economic consequences of ventilator-associated pneumonia: A systematic review. *Critical Care Medicine, 33*(10), 2184–2193. doi:10.1097/01.CCM.0000181731.53912.D9 PMID:16215368

Safdar, N., Kluger, D. M., & Maki, D. G. (2002). A review of risk factors for catheter-related bloodstream infection caused by percutaneously inserted, noncuffed central venous catheters: Implications for preventive strategies. *Medicine; Analytical Reviews of General Medicine, Neurology, Psychiatry, Dermatology, and Pediatries, 81*(6), 466–479. doi:10.1097/00005792-200211000-00007 PMID:12441903

Safdar, N., & Maki, D. G. (2004). The pathogenesis of catheter-related bloodstream infection with noncuffed short-term central venous catheters. *Intensive Care Medicine, 30*(1), 62–67. doi:10.1007/s00134-003-2045-z PMID:14647886

Safdar, N., O'Horo, J. C., Ghufran, A., Bearden, A., Didier, M. E., Chateau, D., & Maki, D. G. (2014). Chlorhexidine-impregnated dressing for prevention of catheter-related bloodstream infection: A meta-analysis. *Critical Care Medicine, 42*(7), 1703–1713. doi:10.1097/CCM.0000000000000319 PMID:24674924

Sagawa, K. (1990). "Translation of Otto Frank's Paper" Otto Frank. (1899). "Die Grundform des Arteriellen Pulses" Zeitschriftfür Biologie, 37, 483-526. *Journal of Molecular and Cellular Cardiology, 22*(3), 253–254. doi:10.1016/0022-2828(90)91459-K PMID:2192068

Sagie, A., Freitas, N., Padial, L. R., Leavitt, M., Weyman, A. E., & Levine, R. A. (1996). Doppler echocardiographic assessment of long-term progression of mitral stenosis in 103 patients: Valve area and right heart disease. *Journal of the American College of Cardiology, 28*(2), 472–479. doi:10.1016/0735-1097(96)00153-2 PMID:8800128

Sahu, B., Chauhan, S., Kiran, U., Bisoi, A., Lakshmy, R., Selvaraj, T., & Nehra, A. (2009). Neurocognitive function in patients undergoing coronary artery bypass graft surgery with cardiopulmonary bypass: The effect of two different rewarming strategies. *Journal of Cardiothoracic and Vascular Anesthesia, 23*(1), 14–21. doi:10.1053/j.jvca.2008.07.010 PMID:18834816

Saint, S., & Chenoweth, C. E. (2003). Biofilms in catheter-associated urinary tract infections. *Infectious Disease Clinics of North America, 17*(2), 411–432. doi:10.1016/S0891-5520(03)00011-4 PMID:12848477

Saint, S., Greene, M. T., Kowalski, C. P., Watson, S. R., Hofer, T. P., & Krein, S. L. (2013). Preventing catheter-associated urinary tract infection in the United States. A national comparative study. *JAMA Internal Medicine, 173*(10), 874–879. doi:10.1001/jamainternmed.2013.101 PMID:23529579

Saint, S., Meddings, J. A., Calfee, D., Kowalski, C. P., & Krein, S. L. (2009). Catheter-associated urinary tract infection and the Medicare rule changes. *Annals of Internal Medicine, 150*(12), 877–884. doi:10.7326/0003-4819-150-12-200906160-00013 PMID:19528567

Saint, S., Olmsted, R. N., Fakih, M. G., Kowalski, C. P., Watson, S. R., Sales, A. E., & Krein, S. L. (2009). Translating health care-associated urinary tract infection prevention research into practice via the bladder bundle. *Joint Commission Journal on Quality and Patient Safety, 35*, 449–455. PMID:19769204

Saint, S., Wiese, J., Amory, J. K., Bernstein, M. L., Patel, U. D., Zemencuk, J. K., & Hofer, T. P. et al. (2000). Are physicians aware of which of their patients have indwelling urinary catheters? *The American Journal of Medicine, 109*(6), 476–480. doi:10.1016/S0002-9343(00)00531-3 PMID:11042237

Sainz, I. M., Pixley, R. A., & Colman, R. W. (2007). Fifty years of research on the plasma kallikrein-kinin system: From protein structure and function to cell biology and in-vivo pathophysiology. *Thrombosis and Haemostasis*, *98*, 77–83. PMID:17597995

Sakka, S. G., Kozieras, J., Thuemer, O., & van Hout, N. (2007). Measurement of cardiac output: A comparison between transpulmonary thermodilution and uncalibrated pulse contour analysis. *British Journal of Anaesthesia*, *99*(3), 337–342. doi:10.1093/bja/aem177 PMID:17611251

Salas, E., Wilson, K. A., Burke, C. S., & Priest, H. A. (2005). Using simulation-based training to improve patient safety: what does it take? *Joint Commission Journal on Quality and Patient Safety / Joint Commission Resources*, *31*(7), 363–371.

Salis, S., Mazzanti, V. V., Merli, G., Salvi, L., Tedesco, C. C., Veglia, F., & Sisillo, E. (2008). Cardiopulmonary Bypass Duration Is an Independent Predictor of Morbidity and Mortality After Cardiac Surgery. *Journal of Cardiothoracic and Vascular Anesthesia*, *22*(6), 814–822. doi:10.1053/j.jvca.2008.08.004 PMID:18948034

Samama, M. M., Martinoli, J. L., LeFlem, L., Guinet, C., Plu-Bureau, G., Depasse, F., & Perzborn, E. (2010). Assessment of laboratory assays to measure rivaroxaban-an oral, direct factor Xa inhibitor. *Journal of Thrombosis and Haemostasis*, *103*(4), 815–825. doi:10.1160/TH09-03-0176 PMID:20135059

Sambunjak, D., Straus, S. E., & Marusić, A. (2006). Mentoring in academic medicine: A systematic review. *Journal of the American Medical Association*, *296*(9), 1103–1115. doi:10.1001/jama.296.9.1103 PMID:16954490

Sampat, U., Varadarajan, P., Turk, R., Kamath, A., Khandhar, S., & Pai, R. G. (2009). Effect of beta-blocker therapy on survival in patients with severe aortic regurgitation. *Journal of the American College of Cardiology*, *54*(5), 452–457. doi:10.1016/j.jacc.2009.02.077 PMID:19628121

Sander, M., Spies, C. D., Grubitzsch, H., Foer, A., Müller, M., & von Heymann, C. (2006). Comparison of uncalibrated arterial waveform analysis in cardiac surgery patients with thermodilution cardiac output measurements. *Critical Care (London, England)*, *10*(6), R164. doi:10.1186/cc5103 PMID:17118186

Sandham. (2003). Randomized, Controlled Trial of the Use of Pulmonary-Artery Catheters in High-Risk Surgical Patients. *The New England Journal of Medicine, 348*, 5-14.

Sandiumenge, A., Diaz, E., Bodi, M., & Rello, J. (2003). Therapy of ventilator-associated pneumonia. A patient-based approach based on the ten rules of "The Tarragona Strategy". *Intensive Care Medicine*, *29*, 876–883. PMID:12677369

Sandner, S. E., Zimpfer, D., Zrunek, P., Rajek, A., Schima, H., Dunkler, D., & Wieselthaler, G. M. et al. (2009). Renal function and outcome after continuous flow left ventricular assist device implantation. *The Annals of Thoracic Surgery*, *87*(4), 1072–1078. doi:10.1016/j.athoracsur.2009.01.022 PMID:19324130

Sanford, T. J. Jr, Smith, N. T., Dec-Silver, H., & Harrison, W. K. (1986). A comparison of morphine, fentanyl, and sufentanil anesthesia for cardiac surgery: Induction, emergence, and extubation. *Anesthesia and Analgesia*, *65*(3), 259–266. doi:10.1213/00000539-198603000-00007 PMID:2937352

Sarr, M. G., Gott, V. L., & Townsend, T. R. (1984). Mediastinal infection after cardiac surgery. *The Annals of Thoracic Surgery*, *38*(4), 415–423. doi:10.1016/S0003-4975(10)62300-4 PMID:6385892

Sarvotham, S. S. (1987). Nitroprusside therapy in post-open heart hypertensives: A ritual tryst with CN death? *Chest*, *91*(5), 796. doi:10.1378/chest.91.5.796b PMID:3568793

Sastry, B. K., Narasimhan, C., Reddy, N. K., & Raju, B. S. (2004). Clinical Efficacy of Sildenafil in Primary Pulmonary Hypertension. *Journal of the American College of Cardiology*, *43*(7), 1149–1153. doi:10.1016/j.jacc.2003.10.056 PMID:15063421

Sauër, A. C., Slooter, A. J. C., Veldhuijzen, D. S., van Eijk, M. M. J., Devlin, J. W., & van Dijk, D. (2014). Intraoperative dexamethasone and delirium after cardiac surgery: A randomized clinical trial. *Anesthesia and Analgesia*, *119*(5), 1046–1052. doi:10.1213/ANE.0000000000000248 PMID:24810262

Savage, E. B., Grab, J. D., O'Brien, S. M., Ali, A., Okum, E. J., Perez-Tamayo, A., & Higgins, R. S. D. et al. (2007). Use of both internal thoracic arteries in diabetic patients increases deep sternal wound infections. *The Annals of Thoracic Surgery*, *83*(3), 1002–1007. doi:10.1016/j.athoracsur.2006.09.094 PMID:17307448

Savage, E. B., Saha-Chaudhuri, P., Asher, C. R., Brennan, J. M., & Gammie, J. S. (2014). Outcomes and prosthesis choice for active aortic valve infective endocarditis: Analysis of the Society of Thoracic Surgeons Adult Cardiac Surgery Database. *The Annals of Thoracic Surgery*, *98*(3), 806–814. doi:10.1016/j.athoracsur.2014.05.010 PMID:25085561

Savonitto, S., D'Urbano, M., Caracciolo, M., Barlocco, F., Mariani, G., Nichelatti, M., & De Servi, S. et al. (2010). Urgent surgery in patients with a recently implanted coronary drug-eluting stent: A phase II study of "bridging" antiplatelet therapy with tirofiban during temporary withdrawal of clopidogrel. *British Journal of Anaesthesia*, *104*(3), 285–291. doi:10.1093/bja/aep373 PMID:20047898

Sayer, G., Baker, J., & Parks, K. (2012). Heart rescue: The role of mechanical circulatory support in the management of severe refractory cardiogenic shock. *Current Opinion in Critical Care*, *18*(5), 409–416. doi:10.1097/MCC.0b013e328357f1e6 PMID:22895213

Sayer, G., & Bhat, G. (2014). The renin-angiotensin-aldosterone system and heart failure. *Cardiology Clinics*, *32*(1), 21–32. doi:10.1016/j.ccl.2013.09.002 PMID:24286576

Scalea, T. M., Rodriguez, A., Chiu, W. C., Brenneman, F. D., Fallon, W. F. Jr, Kato, K., & Yoshii, H. et al. (1999). Focused Assessment with Sonography for Trauma (FAST): Results from an international consensus conference. *The Journal of Trauma*, *46*(3), 466–472. doi:10.1097/00005373-199903000-00022 PMID:10088853

Schelling, G., Stoll, C., Kapfhammer, H. P., Rothenhäusler, H. B., Krauseneck, T., Durst, K., & Briegel, J. et al. (1999). The effect of stress doses of hydrocortisone during septic shock on posttraumatic stress disorder and health-related quality of life in survivors. *Critical Care Medicine*, *27*(12), 2678–2683. doi:10.1097/00003246-199912000-00012 PMID:10628609

Schepens, M. A., Heijmen, R. H., Ranschaert, W., Sonker, U., & Morshuis, W. J. (2009). Thoracoabdominal aortic aneurysm repair: Results of conventional open surgery. *European Journal of Vascular and Endovascular Surgery*, *37*(6), 640–645. doi:10.1016/j.ejvs.2009.03.011 PMID:19362499

Scheunemann, L. P., McDevitt, M., Carson, S. S., & Hanson, L. C. (2011). Randomized, controlled trials of interventions to improve communication in intensive care: A systematic review. *Chest*, *139*(3), 543–554. doi:10.1378/chest.10-0595 PMID:21106660

Schmidt, E. B., Varming, K., Ernst, E., Madsen, P., & Dyerberg, J. (1990). Dose-response studies on the effect of n-3 polyunsaturated fatty acids on lipids and haemostasis. *Thrombosis and Haemostasis*, *63*(1), 1–5. PMID:2339345

Schmidt, M., Bailey, M., Sheldrake, J., Hodgson, C., Aubron, C., Rycus, P. T., & Pilcher, D. et al. (2014). Predicting Survival after Extracorporeal Membrane Oxygenation for Severe Acute Respiratory Failure. The Respiratory Extracorporeal Membrane Oxygenation Survival Prediction (RESP) Score. *American Journal of Respiratory and Critical Care Medicine*, *189*(11), 1374–1382. doi:10.1164/rccm.201311-2023OC PMID:24693864

Schneiderman, L. J. (2011). Defining medical futility and improving medical care. *Journal of Bioethical Inquiry*, *8*(2), 123–131. doi:10.1007/s11673-011-9293-3 PMID:21765643

Schneiderman, L. J., Gilmer, T., Teetzel, H. D., Dugan, D. O., Blustein, J., Cranford, R., & Young, E. W. et al. (2003). Effect of ethics consultations on nonbeneficial life-sustaining treatments in the intensive care setting: A randomized controlled trial. *Journal of the American Medical Association*, *290*(9), 1166–1172. doi:10.1001/jama.290.9.1166 PMID:12952998

Schnoor, M., Schäfer, T., Lühmann, D., & Sievers, H. H. (2007). Bicaval Versus Standard Technique In Orthotopic Heart Transplantation: A Systematic Review And Meta-Analysis. *The Journal Of Thoracic And Cardiovascular Surgery*, *134*(5), 1322-1331. Retrieved From http://www.jtcvsonline.org/article/s0022-5223(07)00935-x/abstract

Schulman, P. M., Stecker, E. C., & Rozner, M. A. (2012). R-on-T and cardiac arrest from dual-chamber pacing without an atrial lead. *Heart Rhythm: the Official Journal of the Heart Rhythm Society*, *9*(6), 970–973. doi:10.1016/j.hrthm.2012.01.023 PMID:22300663

Schulman, R. C., & Mechanick, J. I. (2012). Metabolic and nutrition support in the chronic critical illness syndrome. *Respiratory Care*, *57*(6), 958–977. doi:10.4187/respcare.01620 PMID:22663970

Schulman, R. C., & Mechanick, J. I. (2013). Can Nutrition Support Interfere with Recovery from Acute Critical Illness? *World Review of Nutrition and Dietetics*, *105*, 69–81. doi:10.1159/000341272 PMID:23075588

Schulman, R. C., Moshier, E. L., Rho, L., Casey, M. F., Godbold, J. H., & Mechanick, J. I. (2014). Association of Glycemic Control Parameters with Clinical Outcomes in Chronic Critical Illness.[Epub ahead of print]. *Endocrine Practice*, *20*(9), 884–893. doi:10.4158/EP13324.OR PMID:24641919

Schultz, J. E., Hsu, A. K., & Gross, G. J. (1996). Morphine mimics the cardioprotective effect of ischemic preconditioning via a glibenclamide-sensitive mechanism in the rat heart. *Circulation Research*, *78*(6), 1100–1104. doi:10.1161/01.RES.78.6.1100 PMID:8635241

Schulze, C., Kitada, S., Clerkin, K., Jin, Z., & Mancini, D. (2014). Regional Differences in Recipient Waitlist Time and Pre- and Post-Transplant Mortality After the 2006 United Network for Organ Sharing Policy Changes in the Donor Heart Allocation Algorithm. *Journal of the American College of Cardiology: Heart Failure*, *2*(2), 166–177. PMID:24720925

Schulz, S., Kastrati, A., Ferenc, M., Massberg, S., Birkmeier, K., Laugwitz, K., & Neumann, F. et al. (2013). One-year outcomes with abciximab and unfractionated heparin versus bivalirudin during percutaneous coronary interventions in patients with non-ST-segment elevation myocardial infarction: Updated results from the ISAR-REACT 4 trial. *EuroIntervention*, *9*(4), 430–436. doi:10.4244/EIJV9I4A71 PMID:23455033

Schurink, C. A., Van Nieuwenhoven, C. A., Jacobs, J. A., Rozenberg-Arska, M., Joore, H. C., Buskens, E., & Bonten, M. J. et al. (2004). Clinical pulmonary infection score for ventilator-associated pneumonia: Accuracy and inter-observer variability. *Intensive Care Medicine*, *30*(2), 217–224. doi:10.1007/s00134-003-2018-2 PMID:14566455

Schussler, O., Dermine, H., Alifano, M., Casetta, A., Coignard, S., Roche, N., & Regnard, J. F. et al. (2008). Should we change antibiotic prophylaxis for lung surgery? Postoperative pneumonia is the critical issue. *The Annals of Thoracic Surgery*, *86*(6), 1727–1734. doi:10.1016/j.athoracsur.2008.08.005 PMID:19021965

Schuurmans, M., Diacon, A., & Bolliger, C. (2002). Functional evaluation before lung resection. *Clinics in Chest Medicine*, *23*(1), 159–172. doi:10.1016/S0272-5231(03)00066-2 PMID:11901909

Schuwirth, L. W. T., & Van Der Vleuten, C. P. M. (2004). Changing education, changing assessment, changing research? *Medical Education*, *38*(8), 805–812. doi:10.1111/j.1365-2929.2004.01851.x PMID:15271040

Schuwirth, L. W. T., & Vleuten, C. (2011). How to Design a Useful Test. In T. Swanwick (Ed.), *Understanding Medical Education* (p. 24). Oxford: Wiley-Blackwell.

Schwann, T. A., Kistler, L., Engoren, M. C., & Habib, R. H. (2010). Incidence and predictors of postoperative deep vein thrombosis in cardiac surgery in the era of aggressive thromboprophylaxis. *The Annals of Thoracic Surgery*, *90*(3), 760–766. doi:10.1016/j.athoracsur.2010.03.117 PMID:20732491

Schwartz, D. A., & Horwitz, L. D. (n.d.). Effects of ketamine on left ventricular performance. *The Journal of Pharmacology and Experimental Therapeutics*, *194*, 410–414. PMID:1151766

Schwarze, M. L., Bradley, C. T., & Brasel, K. J. (2010). Surgical "buy-in": The contractual relationship between surgeons and patients that influences decisions regarding life-supporting therapy. *Critical Care Medicine*, *38*(3), 843–848. doi:10.1097/CCM.0b013e3181cc466b PMID:20048678

Schwarze, M. L., Redmann, A. J., Brasel, K. J., & Alexander, G. C. (2012). The role of surgeon error in withdrawal of postoperative life support. *Annals of Surgery*, *256*(1), 10–15. doi:10.1097/SLA.0b013e3182580de5 PMID:22584696

Schweickert, W. D., Pohlman, M. C., Pohlman, A. S., Nigos, C., Pawlik, A. J., Esbrook, C. L., & Kress, J. P. et al. (2009). Early physical and occupational therapy in mechanically ventilated, critically ill patients: A randomised controlled trial. *Lancet*, *373*(9678), 1874–1882. doi:10.1016/S0140-6736(09)60658-9 PMID:19446324

Schweigert, M., Solymosi, N., Dubecz, A., Fernández, M. J., Stadlhuber, R., Ofner, D., & Stein, H. J. (2014). Surgery for parapneumonic pleural empyema – What influence does the rising prevalence of multimorbidity and advanced age has on the current outcome? *The Surgeon*. doi:10.1016/j.surge.2014.05.002 PMID:24930000

Scognamiglio, R., Rahimtoola, S. H., Fasoli, G., Nistri, S., & Volta, S. D. (1994). Nifedipine in asymptomatic patients with severe aortic regurgitation and normal left ventricular function. *The New England Journal of Medicine*, *331*(1), 689–694. doi:10.1056/NEJM199409153311101 PMID:8058074

Scurlock, C. S., Raikhelkar, J., & Mechanick, J. (2010). Parenteral nutrition in the critically ill patient[letter]. *The New England Journal of Medicine*, *362*(1), 81–84, author reply 83–84. doi:10.1056/NEJMc0909589 PMID:20054053

Searle, N. R., & Sahab, P. (1993). Propofol in patients with cardiac disease. *Canadian Journal of Anesthesiology*, *40*(8), 730–747. doi:10.1007/BF03009770 PMID:8403158

Sedgwick, J. F., & Burstow, D. J. (2012). Update on echocardiography in the management of infective endocarditis. *Current Infectious Disease Reports*, *14*(2), 373–380. doi:10.1007/s11908-012-0262-8 PMID:22544484

Sedrakyan, A., Wu, A. W., Parashar, A., Bass, E. B., & Treasure, T. (2006). Off-pump surgery is associated with reduced occurrence of stroke and other morbidity as compared with traditional coronary artery bypass grafting: A meta-analysis of systematically reviewed trials. *Stroke*, *37*(11), 2759–2769. doi:10.1161/01.STR.0000245081.52877.f2 PMID:17008617

Segers, P., Speekenbrink, R. G. H., Ubbink, D. T., van Ogtrop, M. L., & de Mol, B. A. (2006). Prevention of nosocomial infection in cardiac surgery by decontamination of the nasopharynx and oropharynx with chlorhexidine gluconate. *Journal of the American Medical Association*, *296*(20), 2460–2466. doi:10.1001/jama.296.20.2460 PMID:17119142

Selnes, O. A. G. R., & Grega, M. A. (2012). Cognitive and neurologic outcomes after Coronary artery bypass grafting. *The New England Journal of Medicine*, *366*(3), 250–257. doi:10.1056/NEJMra1100109 PMID:22256807

Selton-Suty, C., Célard, M., Le Moing, V., Doco-Lecompte, T., Chirouze, C., Iung, B., & Hoen, B. et al. (2012). Preeminence of Staphylococcus aureus in infective endocarditis: A 1-year population-based survey. *Clinical Infectious Diseases*, *54*(9), 1230–1239. doi:10.1093/cid/cis199 PMID:22492317

Sendelbach, S. E., Halm, M. A., Doran, K. A., Miller, E. H., & Gaillard, P. (2006). Effects of music therapy on physiological and psychological outcomes for patients undergoing cardiac surgery. *The Journal of Cardiovascular Nursing*, *21*(3), 194–200. doi:10.1097/00005082-200605000-00007 PMID:16699359

Senge, P. M. (2010). *The Fifth Discipline: The Art and Practice of the Learning Organization* (2nd ed.). London: Random House.

Senn, A., Button, D., Zollinger, A., & Hofer, C. K. (2007). Assessment of the cardiac output changes using a modified FloTrac/Vigileo Algorithm in cardiac surgery patients. *Critical Care (London, England)*, *13*(2), R32. doi:10.1186/cc7739 PMID:19261180

Senturk, M., Ozcan, P. E., Talu, G. K., Kiyan, E., Camci, E., Ozyalcin, S., & Pembeci, K. et al. (2002). The effects of three different analgesia techniques on long-term postthoracotomy pain. *Anesthesia and Analgesia*, *94*(1), 11–15. doi:10.1213/00000539-200201000-00003 PMID:11772793

Serebruany, V. L. (2010). Mortality in the TRITON trial: Update from the FDA prasugrel action package. *The American Journal of Cardiology*, *105*(9), 1356–1357. doi:10.1016/j.amjcard.2009.12.052 PMID:20403493

Serruys, P. W., Kutryk, M. J. B., & Ong, A. T. L. (2006). Coronary-artery stents. *The New England Journal of Medicine*, *354*(5), 483–495. doi:10.1056/NEJMra051091 PMID:16452560

Serruys, P. W., Morice, M.-C., Keppetein, A. P., Colombo, A., Holmes, D. R., Mack, M. J., & Mohr, F. et al. (2009). Percutaneous Coronary Intervention versus Coronary-Artery Bypass Grafting for Severe Coronary Artery Disease. *The New England Journal of Medicine*, *360*(10), 961–972. doi:10.1056/NEJMoa0804626 PMID:19228612

Serruys, P. W., Ong, A. T. L., & van Herwerden, L. a, Sousa, J. E., Jatene, A., Bonnier, J. J. R. M., … Unger, F. (2005). Five-year outcomes after coronary stenting versus bypass surgery for the treatment of multivessel disease: The final analysis of the Arterial Revascularization Therapies Study (ARTS) randomized trial. *Journal of the American College of Cardiology*, *46*(4), 575–581. doi:10.1016/j.jacc.2004.12.082 PMID:16098418

Sessler, C. N., Gosnell, M. S., Grap, M. J., Brophy, G. M., O'Neal, P. V., Keane, K. A., & Elswick, R. K. et al. (2002). The Richmond agitation-sedation scale: Validity and reliability in adult intensive care unit patients. *American Journal of Respiratory and Critical Care Medicine*, *166*(10), 1338–1344. doi:10.1164/rccm.2107138 PMID:12421743

Sessler, C. N., Grap, M. J., & Ramsay, M. A. E. (2009). Evaluating and monitoring analgesia and sedation in the intensive care unit. *Critical Care (London, England)*, *12*, 1–13. doi:10.1186/cc6147 PMID:18495053

Sessums, L. L., Zembruzuska, H., & Jackson, J. L. (2011). Does this patient have decision-making capacity? *Journal of the American Medical Association*, *306*(4), 420–427. doi:10.1001/jama.2011.1023 PMID:21791691

Setoguchi, S., Stevenson, L., & Schneeweiss, S. (2007). Repeated hospitalizations predict mortality in the community population with heart failure. *American Heart Journal*, *154*(2), 260–266. doi:10.1016/j.ahj.2007.01.041 PMID:17643574

Sexton, D. J., Tenenbaum, M. J., Wilson, W. R., Steckelberg, J. M., Tice, A. D., Gilbert, D., & Durack, D. T. et al.Endocarditis Treatment Consortium Group. (1998). Ceftriaxone once daily for four weeks compared with ceftriaxone plus gentamycin once daily for two weeks for treatment of endocarditis due to penicillin-susceptible streptococci. *Clinical Infectious Diseases*, *27*(6), 1470–1474. doi:10.1086/515038 PMID:9868662

Seyfer, A. E., Grammer, N. Y., Bogumill, G. P., Provost, J. M., & Chandry, U. (1985). Upper extremity neuropathies after cardiac surgery. *The Journal of Hand Surgery*, *10*(1), 16–19. doi:10.1016/S0363-5023(85)80241-0 PMID:2981914

Seymour, N. E., Gallagher, A. G., Roman, S. A., O'Brien, M. K., Bansal, V. K., Andersen, D. K., & Satava, R. M. (2002). Virtual reality training improves operating room performance: results of a randomized, double-blinded study. *Annals of Surgery*, *236*(4), 458–63– discussion 463–4. doi:10.1097/01.SLA.0000028969.51489.B4

Shadvar, K., Baastani, F., Mahmoodpoor, A., & Bilehjani, E. (2013). Evaluation of the prevalence and risk factors of delirium in cardiac surgery ICU. *J Cardiovasc Thorac Res*, *5*(4), 157–161. doi:10.5681/jcvtr.2013.034 PMID:24404347

Shafii, A. E., Chamogeorgakis, T., Mountis, M., & Gonzalez-Stawinski, G. (2012). Fate of retained right ventricular assist device outflow grafts after right ventricular recovery. *The Journal of Heart and Lung Transplantation*, *31*(6), 672–673. doi:10.1016/j.healun.2012.02.028 PMID:22483411

Shahian, D. M., Edwards, F. H., Jacobs, J. P., Prager, R. L., Normand, S. L., Shewan, C. M., & Grover, F. L. et al. (2011). Public reporting of cardiac surgery performance: Part 2--implementation. *The Annals of Thoracic Surgery*, *92*(3Suppl), S12–S23. doi:10.1016/j.athoracsur.2011.06.101 PMID:21867788

Shahian, D. M., O'Brien, S. M., Sheng, S., Grover, F. L., Mayer, J. E., Jacobs, J. P., & Edwards, F. H. et al. (2012). Predictors of long-term survival after coronary artery bypass grafting surgery: Results from the Society of Thoracic Surgeons Adult Cardiac Surgery Database (the ASCERT study). *Circulation*, *125*(12), 1491–1500. doi:10.1161/CIRCULATIONAHA.111.066902 PMID:22361330

Shah, K. B., Levenson, J. L., & Mehra, M. R. (2014). Emergent use of mechanical circulatory support devices: Ethical dilemmas. *Current Opinion in Cardiology*, *29*(3), 281–284. doi:10.1097/HCO.0000000000000058 PMID:24686401

Shah, P. J., Gordon, I., Fuller, J., Seevanayagam, S., Rosalion, A., Tatoulis, J., & Buxton, B. F. et al. (2003). Factors affecting saphenous vein graft patency: Clinical and angiographic study in 1402 symptomatic patients operated on between 1977 and 1999. *The Journal of Thoracic and Cardiovascular Surgery*, *126*(6), 1972–1977. doi:10.1016/S0022-5223(03)01276-5 PMID:14688715

Shah, R. M., Singh, M., Bhuriya, R., Molnar, J., Arora, R. R., & Khosla, S. (2012). Favorable effects of vasodilators on left ventricular remodeling in asymptomatic patients with chronic moderate-severe aortic regurgitation and normal ejection fraction: A meta-analysis of clinical trials. *Clinical Cardiology*, *35*(10), 619–625. doi:10.1002/clc.22019 PMID:22707241

Shahzad, A., & Stables, R. (2014). *HEAT PPCI: How Effective are Antithrombotic Therapies in PPCI*. American College of Cardiology Scientific Sessions.

Shander, A., Van Aken, H., Colomina, M. J., Gombotz, H., Hofmann, A., Krauspe, R., & Spahn, D. R. et al. (2012). Patient blood management in Europe. *British Journal of Anaesthesia*, *109*(1), 55–68. doi:10.1093/bja/aes139 PMID:22628393

Shanmugam, G. (2005). Vasoplegic syndrome--the role of methylene blue. *European Journal of Cardio-Thoracic Surgery: Official Journal of the European Association for Cardio-Thoracic Surgery*, *28*(5), 705–710. doi:10.1016/j.ejcts.2005.07.011 PMID:16143539

Shao, X., Tian, L., Xu, W., Zhang, Z., Wang, C., Qi, C., & Mou, S. et al. (2014). Diagnostic Value of Urinary Kidney Injury Molecule 1 for Acute Kidney Injury: A Meta-Analysis. *PLoS ONE*, *9*(1), e84131. doi:10.1371/journal.pone.0084131 PMID:24404151

Shapiro, A., Zohar, E., Zaslansky, R., Hoppenstein, D., Shabat, S., & Fredman, B. (2005). The frequency and timing of respiratory depression in 1524 postoperative patients treated with systemic or neuraxial morphine. *Journal of Clinical Anesthesia*, *17*(7), 536–542. doi:10.1016/j.jclinane.2005.01.006 PMID:16297754

Shapiro, I. (2001). Doctor means teacher. *Academic Medicine*, *76*(7), 711–711. doi:10.1097/00001888-200107000-00013 PMID:11448826

Shapiro, M. J., & Melendez, M. M. (2010). Billing for Bedside Procedures. In H. L. Frankel & B. P. deBoisblanc (Eds.), *Bedside Procedures for the Intensivist*. New York: Springer Science & Business. doi:10.1007/978-0-387-79830-1_17

Shargall, Y., Guenther, G., Ahya, V. N., Ardehali, A., Singhal, A., & Keshavjee, S. (2005). Report of the ISHLT Working Group on Primary Lung Graft Dysfunction part VI: Treatment. *The Journal of Heart and Lung Transplantation*, *24*(10), 1489–1500. doi:10.1016/j.healun.2005.03.011

Sharma, V., Deo, S. V., Stulak, J. M., Durham, L. A. III, Daly, R. C., Park, S. J., & Joyce, L. D. et al. (2012). Driveline infections in left ventricular assist devices: Implications for destination therapy. *The Annals of Thoracic Surgery*, *94*(5), 1381–1386. doi:10.1016/j.athoracsur.2012.05.074 PMID:22818961

Sharrock, N. E. (1998). Anesthesia. In The Adult Hip. Philadelphia: Lippincott - Raven Publishers.

Sharshar, T., Gray, F., Lorin de la Grandmaison, G., Hopkinson, N. S., Ross, E., Dorandeu, A., & Annane, D. et al. (2003). Apoptosis of neurons in cardiovascular autonomic centres triggered by inducible nitric oxide synthase after death from septic shock. *Lancet*, *362*(9398), 1799–1805. doi:10.1016/S0140-6736(03)14899-4 PMID:14654318

Shear, W., & Rosner, M. H. (2006). Acute kidney dysfunction secondary to the abdominal compartment syndrome. *Journal of Nephrology*, *19*(5), 556–565. PMID:17136682

Shehabi, Y., Botha, J. A., Ernest, D., Freebairn, R. C., Reade, M., Roberts, B. L., & Seppelt, I. (2010). Clinical application, the use of dexmedetomidine in intensive care sedation, *13*(2), 40–50.

Shehabi, Y., Grant, P., Wolfenden, H., Hammond, N., Bass, F., Campbell, M., & Chen, J. (2009). Prevalence of delirium with dexmedetomidine compared with morphine based therapy after cardiac surgery: A randomized controlled trial (DEXmedetomidine COmpared to Morphine-DEXCOM Study). *Anesthesiology*, *111*(5), 1075–1084. doi:10.1097/ALN.0b013e3181b6a783 PMID:19786862

Sheng, W., Xing, Q., Hou, W., Sun, L., Niu, Z., Lin, M., & Chi, Y. (2014). Independent risk factors for ventilator-associated pneumonia after cardiac surgery. *Journal of Investigative Surgery*, *27*(5), 256–261. doi:10.3109/08941939.2014.892652 PMID:24660655

Shigemura, N., Bhama, J., Gries, C. J., Kawamura, T., Crespo, M., Johnson, B., & Bermudez, C. et al. (2012). Lung transplantation in patients with prior cardiothoracic surgical procedures. *American Journal of Transplantation*, *12*(5), 1249–1255. doi:10.1111/j.1600-6143.2011.03946.x

Shigemura, N., Orhan, Y., Bhama, J. K., D'Cunha, J., Zaldonis, D., Pilewski, J. M., & Bermudez, C. A. et al. (2014). Delayed chest closure after lung transplantation: Techniques, outcomes, and strategies. *The Journal of Heart and Lung Transplantation*, *33*(7), 741–748. doi:10.1016/j.healun.2014.03.003

Shin, J.-S., & Abah, U. (2012). Is routine stress ulcer prophylaxis of benefit for patients undergoing cardiac surgery? *Interactive Cardiovascular and Thoracic Surgery*, *14*(5), 622–628. doi:10.1093/icvts/ivs019 PMID:22345061

Shi, Z., Xie, H., Wang, P., Zhang, Q., Wu, Y., Chen, E., & Furness, S. et al. (2013). Oral hygiene for critically ill patients to prevent ventilator-associated pneumonia. *Cochrane Database of Systematic Reviews*, CD008367. PMID:23939759

Shore-Lesserson, L., Manspeizer, H. E., DePerio, M., Francis, S., Vela-Cantos, F., & Ergin, M. A. (1999). Thromboelastography-guided transfusion algorithm reduces transfusions in complex cardiac surgery. *Anesthesia and Analgesia*, *88*(2), 312–319. PMID:9972747

Shostak, E., Brylka, D., Krepp, J., Pua, B., & Sanders, A. (2013). Bedside sonography for detection of postprocedure pneumothorax. *Journal of Ultrasound in Medicine: Official Journal of the American Institute of Ultrasound in Medicine*, *32*(6), 1003–1009. doi:10.7863/ultra.32.6.1003 PMID:23716522

Shroyer, A. L., Coombs, L. P., Peterson, E. D., Eiken, M. C., DeLong, E. R., Chen, A., . . . Edwards, F. H. (2003). The Society of Thoracic Surgeons: 30-day operative mortality and morbidity risk models. *Annals of Thoracic Surgery, 75*(6), 1856-1864; discussion 1864-1855.

Shroyer, A. L., Grover, F. L., Hattler, B., Collins, J. F., McDonald, G. O., Kozora, E., & Novitzky, D. et al. (2009). On-pump versus off-pump coronary-artery bypass surgery. *The New England Journal of Medicine*, *361*(19), 1827–1837. doi:10.1056/NEJMoa0902905 PMID:19890125

Shumway, N., Lower, R., & Stofer, R. (1966). Transplantation Of The Heart. *Advances in Surgery*, *2*, 265–284. PMID:5333297

Sidebotham, McKee, Gillham, & Levy. (2007). *Cardiothoracic Critical Care*. Elsevier Health Sciences.

Sievers, H. H., Weyand, M., Kraatz, G., & Bernhard, A. (1991). An Alternative Technique For Orthotopic Cardiac Transplantation, With Preservation Of The Normal Anatomy Of The Right Atrium. *The Thoracic and Cardiovascular Surgeon*, *39*(02), 70–72. doi:10.1055/s-2007-1013934 PMID:1877054

Sievert, D. M., Ricks, P., Edwards, J. R., Schneider, A., Patel, J., Srinivasan, A., & Fridkin, S. et al. (2013). Antimicrobial-resistant pathogens associated with healthcare-associated infections: Summary of data reported to the National Healthcare Safety Network at the Centers for Disease Control and Prevention, 2009-2010. *Infection Control and Hospital Epidemiology*, *34*(1), 1–14. doi:10.1086/668770 PMID:23221186

Silvain, J., Bellemain-Appaix, A., Barthelemy, O., Beygui, F., Collet, J. P., & Montalescot, G. (2011). Optimal use of thienopyridines in non-ST-elevation acute coronary syndrome following CURRENT-OASIS 7. *Circulation: Cardiovascular Interventions*, *4*(1), 95–103. doi:10.1161/CIRCINTERVENTIONS.109.910406 PMID:21325198

Silverman, J. D., Draper, J., & Kurtz, S. M. (1997). The Calgary-Cambridge approach to communications skills teaching 2: The Set-Go method of descriptive feedback. *Education for General Practice*, (8), 16–23.

Silverman, J. D., Kurtz, S. M., & Draper, J. (1996). The Calgary-Cambridge approach to communication skills teaching. 1. Agenda-led, outcome-based analysis of the consultation. *Education for General Practice*, (7), 288–299.

Silvestri, L., van Saene, H. K., Casarin, A., Berlot, G., & Gullo, A. (2008). Impact of selective decontamination of the digestive tract on carriage and infection due to Gram-negative and Gram-positive bacteria: A systematic review of randomised controlled trials. *Anaesthesia and Intensive Care*, *36*, 324–338. PMID:18564793

Simonneau, G., Gatzoulis, M. A., Adatia, I., Celermajer, D., Denton, C., Ghofrani, A., & Souza, R. et al. (2013). Updated clinical classification of pulmonary hypertension. *Journal of the American College of Cardiology*, *62*(25Suppl), D34–D41. doi:10.1016/j.jacc.2013.10.029 PMID:24355639

Simpson, E. J. (1972). *The classification of educational objectives in the psychomotor domain*. Washington, D. C.: Gryphon House.

Sinclair. (1997). Intraoperative intravascular volume optimization and length of hospital stay after repair of proximal femoral fracture: randomized controlled trial. *The BMJ, 315*, 909–12.

Singer, D. E., Albers, G. W., Dalen, J. E., Fang, M. C., & Go, A. Ss, Halperin J.L., Lip G.Y. & Manning WJ. (2008). Antithrombotic therapy in atrial fibrillation: American College of Chest Physicians Evidence-Based Clinical Practice Guidelines (8th Edition). Chest, 133(6 suppl), 546S-592S.

Singer, M., De Santis, V., Vitale, D., & Jeffcoate, W. (2004). Multiorgan failure is an adaptive, endocrine-mediated, metabolic response to overwhelming systemic inflammation. *Lancet*, *364*(9433), 545–548. doi:10.1016/S0140-6736(04)16815-3 PMID:15302200

Singer, P., Anbar, R., Cohen, J., Shapiro, H., Shalita-Chesner, M., Lev, S., & Madar, Z. et al. (2011). The tight calorie control study (TICACOS): A prospective, randomized, controlled pilot study of nutritional support in critically ill patients. *Intensive Care Medicine*, *37*(4), 601–609. doi:10.1007/s00134-011-2146-z PMID:21340655

Singer, P., Berger, M. M., Van den Berghe, G., Biolo, G., Calder, P., Forbes, A., & Pichard, C. et al. (2009). ESPEN Guidelines on Parenteral Nutrition: Intensive care. *Clinical Nutrition (Edinburgh, Lothian)*, *28*(4), 387–400. doi:10.1016/j.clnu.2009.04.024 PMID:19505748

Singh, B. N., Singh, S. N., Reda, D. J., Tang, X. C., Lopez, B., Harris, C. L., & Ezekowitz, M. D. et al. (2005). Amiodarone versus sotalol for atrial fibrillation. *The New England Journal of Medicine*, *352*(18), 1861–1872. doi:10.1056/NEJMoa041705 PMID:15872201

Singh, D., Gupta, K., & Vacek, J. L. (2014). Anticoagulation and antiplatelet therapy in acute coronary syndromes. *Cleveland Clinic Journal of Medicine*, *81*(2), 103–114. doi:10.3949/ccjm.81a.13016 PMID:24493493

Singh, J. P., Evans, J. C., Levy, D., Larson, M. G., Freed, L. A., Fuller, D. L., & Benjamin, E. J. et al. (1999). Prevalence and clinical determinants of mitral, tricuspid, and aortic regurgitation (the Framingham Heart Study). *The American Journal of Cardiology*, *83*(6), 897–902. doi:10.1016/S0002-9149(98)01064-9 PMID:10190406

Singh, M., Gersh, B. J., Li, S., Rumsfeld, J. S., Spertus, J., O'Brien, S. M., & Peterson, E. D. et al. (2008). Mayo Clinic Risk Score for percutaneous coronary intervention predicts in-hospital mortality in patients undergoing coronary artery bypass graft surgery. *Circulation*, *117*(3), 356–362. doi:10.1161/CIRCULATIONAHA.107.711523 PMID:18172033

Sinning, J. M., Hammerstingl, C., Vasa-Nicotera, M., Adenauer, V., Lema Cachiguango, S. J., Scheer, A. C., & Werner, N. et al. (2012). Aortic regurgitation index defines severity of peri-prosthetic regurgitation and predicts outcome in patients after transcatheter aortic valve implantation. *Journal of the American College of Cardiology*, *59*(13), 1134–1141. doi:10.1016/j.jacc.2011.11.048 PMID:22440213

Siontis, G. C., Juni, P., Pilgrim, T., Stortecky, S., Bullesfeld, L., Meier, B., & Windecker, S. et al. (2014). Predictors of permanent pacemaker implantation in patients with severe aortic stenosis undergoing TAVR: A meta-analysis. *Journal of the American College of Cardiology*, *64*(2), 129–140. doi:10.1016/j.jacc.2014.04.033 PMID:25011716

Siraux, V., De Backer, D., Yalavatti, G., Melot, C., Gervy, C., Mockel, J., & Vincent, J. L. (2005). Relative adrenal insufficiency in patients with septic shock: Comparison of low-dose and conventional corticotropin tests. *Critical Care Medicine*, *33*, 2479–2486. doi:10.1097/01.CCM.0000185641.87051.7C PMID:16276169

Sirbu, H., Busch, T., Aleksic, I., Lotfi, S., Ruschewski, W., & Dalichau, H. (1999). Chest re-exploration for complications after lung surgery. *The Thoracic and Cardiovascular Surgeon*, *47*(2), 73–76. doi:10.1055/s-2007-1013114 PMID:10363604

Sitbon, O., Gressin, V., Speich, R., Macdonald, P. S., Opravil, M., Cooper, D. A., & Simonneau, G. et al. (2004). Bosentan for the treatment of human immunodeficiency virus-associated pulmonary arterial hypertension. *American Journal of Respiratory and Critical Care Medicine*, *170*(11), 1212–1217. doi:10.1164/rccm.200404-445OC PMID:15317666

Sitbon, O., McLaughlin, V., Badesch, D., Barst, R., Black, C., & Galie, N. et al.. (2005). Survival in patients with class III idiopathic pulmonary arterial hypertension treated with first line oral bosentan compared with an historical cohort of patients startedon intravenous epoprostenol. *Thorax*, *60*(12), 1025–1030. doi:10.1136/thx.2005.040618 PMID:16055621

Sjögren, J., Malmsjö, M., Gustafsson, R., & Ingemansson, R. (2006). Poststernotomy mediastinitis: A review of conventional surgical treatments, vacuum-associated closure therapy and presentation of the Lund University Hospital mediastinitis algorithm. *European Journal of Cardio-Thoracic Surgery*, *30*(6), 898–905. doi:10.1016/j.ejcts.2006.09.020 PMID:17056269

Skipper, A. (2012). Refeeding syndrome or refeeding hypophosphatemia: A systematic review of cases. *Nutrition in Clinical Practice*, *27*(1), 34–40. doi:10.1177/0884533611427916 PMID:22307490

Skrupky, L. P., McConnell, K., Dallas, J., & Kollef, M. H. (2012). A comparison of ventilator-associated pneumonia rates as identified according to the National Healthcare Safety Network and American College of Chest Physicians criteria. *Critical Care Medicine*, *40*(1), 281–284. doi:10.1097/CCM.0b013e31822d7913 PMID:21926609

Slater, J. P., Guarino, T., Stack, J., Vinod, K., Bustami, R. T., Brown, J. M., 3rd, . . . Parr, G. V. (2009). Cerebral oxygen desaturation predicts cognitive decline and longer hospital stay after cardiac surgery. *Ann Thorac Surg, 87*(1), 36-44; discussion 44-35. doi: 10.1016/j.athoracsur.2008.08.070

Slaughter, M. S., Rogers, J. G., Milano, C. A., Russell, S. D., Conte, J. V., Feldman, D., & Frazier, O. H. et al. (2009). Advanced heart failure treated with continuous-flow left ventricular assist device. *The New England Journal of Medicine*, *361*(23), 2241–2251. doi:10.1056/NEJMoa0909938 PMID:19920051

Slottosch, I., Liakopoulos, O., Kuhn, E., Deppe, A. C., Scherner, M., Madershahian, N., & Wahlers, T. et al. (2013). Outcomes after peripheral extracorporeal membrane oxygenation therapy for postcardiotomy cardiogenic shock: A single-center experience. *The Journal of Surgical Research*, *181*(2), e47–e55. doi:10.1016/j.jss.2012.07.030 PMID:22878151

Slutsky, A. S., & Ranieri, V. M. (2013). Ventilator-induced lung injury. *The New England Journal of Medicine*, *369*(22), 2126–2136. doi:10.1056/NEJMra1208707 PMID:24283226

Smedira, N., Moazami, N., Golding, C., McCarthy, P., Apperson-Hansen, C., Blackstone, E., & Cosgrove, D. (2001). Clinical experience with 202 adults receiving extracorporeal membrane oxygenation for cardiac failure: Survival at five years. *The Journal of Thoracic and Cardiovascular Surgery*, *122*(1), 92–102. doi:10.1067/mtc.2001.114351 PMID:11436041

Smiley, R. M., Navedo, A. T., Kirby, T., & Schulman, L. L. (1991). Postoperative independent lung ventilation in a single-lung transplant recipient. *Anesthesiology*, *74*(6), 1144–1148. doi:10.1097/00000542-199106000-00026

Smith, A. M., Elliot, C. M., Kiely, D. G., & Channer, K. S. (2006). The role of vasopressin in cardiorespiratory arrest and pulmonary hypertension. *Open Journal of Medicine*, *99*(3), 127–133. doi:10.1093/qjmed/hcl009 PMID:16467356

Smith, C. R., Leon, M. B., Mack, M. J., Miller, D. C., Moses, J. W., Svensson, L. G., & Pocock, S. J. et al. (2011). Transcatheter versus surgical aortic-valve replacement in high-risk patients. *The New England Journal of Medicine*, *364*(23), 2187–2198. doi:10.1056/NEJMoa1103510 PMID:21639811

Smith, P. C., Slaughter, M. S., Petty, M. G., Shumway, S. J., Kshettry, V. R., & Bolman, R. M. III. (1995). Abdominal complications after lung transplantation. *The Journal of Heart and Lung Transplantation*, *14*(1 Pt 1), 44–51.

Smith, P. K., Goodnough, L. T., Levy, J. H., Poston, R. S., Short, M. A., Weerakkody, G. J., & LeNarz, L. A. (2012). Mortality Benefit With Prasugrel in the TRITON-TIMI 38 Coronary Artery Bypass Grafting Cohort: Risk-Adjusted Retrospective Data Analysis. *Journal of the American College of Cardiology*, *60*(5), 388–396. doi:10.1016/j.jacc.2012.03.030 PMID:22633653

Snadden, D., & Thomas, M. (1998). The use of portfolio learning in medical education. *Medical Teacher*, *20*(3), 192–199. doi:10.1080/01421599880904

Snell-Bergeon, J. K., & Wadwa, R. P. (2012). Hypoglycemia, diabetes, and cardiovascular disease. *Diabetes Technology & Therapeutics*, *14*(S1Supple 1), S51–S58. doi:10.1089/dia.2012.0031 PMID:22650225

Snellen, H. A., Hartman, H., Buis-Liem, T. N., Kole, E. H., & Rohmer, J. (1968). Pulmonic Stenosis. *Circulation*, *38*(1S5suppl V), V93–V101. doi:10.1161/01.CIR.38.1S5.V-93 PMID:4889601

Snow, C. E., Varela, B. R., Pardi, D. A., Adelman, R. D., Said, S., & Reid, M. C. (2009). Identifying factors affecting utilization of an inpatient palliative care service: A physician survey. *Journal of Palliative Medicine*, *12*(3), 231–237. doi:10.1089/jpm.2008.0235 PMID:19254200

Snyder, C. W., Graham, L. A., Byers, R. E., & Holman, W. L. (2009). Primary sternal plating to prevent sternal wound complications after cardiac surgery: Early experience and patterns of failure. *Interactive Cardiovascular and Thoracic Surgery*, *9*(5), 763–766. doi:10.1510/icvts.2009.214023 PMID:19710069

Snyder-Ramos, S. A., Mohnle, P., Weng, Y. S., Bottiger, B. W., Kulier, A., Levin, J., & Mangano, D. T. (2008). The ongoing variability in blood transfusion practices in cardiac surgery. *Transfusion*, *48*(7), 1284–1299. doi:10.1111/j.1537-2995.2008.01666.x PMID:18422857

Soar, J., Deakin, C. D., Nolan, J. P., Abbas, G., Alfonzo, A., Handley, A. J., & Thies, K. et al. (2005). European Resuscitation Council guidelines for resuscitation 2005. Section 7. Cardiac arrest in special circumstances. *Resuscitation*, *67*(Suppl 1), S135–S170. doi:10.1016/j.resuscitation.2005.10.004 PMID:16321711

Society of Thoracic Surgeons Blood Conservation Guideline Task Force, Ferraris, V. A., Ferraris, S. P., Saha, S. P., Hessel, E. A., Haan, C. K., et al. (2007, May). Perioperative blood transfusion and blood conservation in cardiac surgery: The Society of Thoracic Surgeons and The Society of Cardiovascular Anesthesiologists clinical practice guideline. *The Annals of Thoracic Surgery*. doi:10.1016/j.athoracsur.2007.02.099

Soja, S. L., Pandharipande, P. P., Fleming, S. B., Cotton, B. A., Miller, L. R., Weaver, S. G., & Ely, E. W. et al. (2008). Implementation, reliability testing, and compliance monitoring of the Confusion Assessment Method for the Intensive Care Unit in trauma patients. *Intensive Care Medicine*, *34*(7), 1263–1268. doi:10.1007/s00134-008-1031-x PMID:18297270

Soldati, G., Testa, A., Sher, S., Pignataro, G., La Sala, M., & Silveri, N. G. (2008). Occult traumatic pneumothorax: Diagnostic accuracy of lung ultrasonography in the emergency department. *Chest*, *133*(1), 204–211. doi:10.1378/chest.07-1595 PMID:17925411

Soliman, M. G., Brinale, G. F., & Kuster, G. (1975). Response to hypercapnia under ketamine anaesthesia. *Canadian Anaesthetists' Society Journal*, *22*(4), 486–494. doi:10.1007/BF03004864 PMID:1139389

Song, D. H., Lohman, R. F., Renucci, J. D., Jeevanandam, V., & Raman, J. (2004). Primary sternal plating in high-risk patients prevents mediastinitis. *European Journal of Cardio-Thoracic Surgery*, *26*(2), 367–372. doi:10.1016/j.ejcts.2004.04.038 PMID:15296898

Song, H. K., Tibayan, F. A., Kahl, E. A., Sera, V. A., Slater, M. S., Deloughery, T. G., & Scanlan, M. M. (2014). Safety and efficacy of prothrombin complex concentrates for the treatment of coagulopathy after cardiac surgery. *The Journal of Thoracic and Cardiovascular Surgery*, *147*(3), 1036–1040. doi:10.1016/j.jtcvs.2013.11.020 PMID:24365268

Song, J. W., Shim, J. K., Yoo, K. J., Oh, S. Y., & Kwak, Y. L. (2013). Impact of intraoperative hyperglycaemia on renal dysfunction after off-pump coronary artery bypass. *Interactive Cardiovascular and Thoracic Surgery*, *17*(3), 473–478. doi:10.1093/icvts/ivt209 PMID:23690431

Sonnenblick, E. H., Frishman, W. H., & LeJemtel, T. H. (1979). Dobutamine: A new synthetic cardioactive sympathetic amine. *The New England Journal of Medicine*, *300*(1), 17–22. doi:10.1056/NEJM197901043000105 PMID:362214

Søraas, C. L., Friis, C., Engebretsen, K. V. T., Sandvik, L., Kjeldsen, S. E., & Tønnessen, T. (2012). Troponin T is a better predictor than creatine kinase-MB of long-term mortality after coronary artery bypass graft surgery. *American Heart Journal*, *164*(5), 779–785. doi:10.1016/j.ahj.2012.05.027 PMID:23137510

Sørensen, B., Spahn, D. R., Innerhofer, P., Spannagl, M., & Rossaint, R. (2011). Clinical review: Prothrombin complex concentrates -evaluation of safety and thrombogenicity. *Critical Care (London, England)*, *15*(1), 201. doi:10.1186/cc9311 PMID:21345266

Sousa-Uva, M., Storey, R., Huber, K., Falk, V., Leite-Moreira, A. F., Amour, J., & Collet, J.-P. et al. (2014). Expert position paper on the management of antiplatelet therapy in patients undergoing coronary artery bypass graft surgery. *European Heart Journal*, *35*(23), 1510–1514. doi:10.1093/eurheartj/ehu158 PMID:24748565

Souza, R., Jardim, C., Martins, B., Cortopassi, F., Yaksic, M., Rabelo, R., & Bogossian, H. (2005). Effect of bosentan treatment on surrogate markers in pulmonary arterial hypertension. *Current Medical Research and Opinion*, *21*(6), 907–911. doi:10.1185/030079905X46232 PMID:15969891

Spady, W. G. (1994). *Outcome-based Education*. Arlington, USA: Amer Assn School Administrator.

Spaulding, C., Daemen, J., Boersma, E., Cutlip, D. E., & Serruys, P. W. (2007). A pooled analysis of data comparing sirolimus-eluting stents with bare-metal stents. *The New England Journal of Medicine*, *356*(10), 989–997. doi:10.1056/NEJMoa066633 PMID:17296825

Speiss, B. D. (2002). Transfusion and outcome in heart surgery. *The Annals of Thoracic Surgery*, *74*(4), 986–987. doi:10.1016/S0003-4975(02)03906-1 PMID:12400732

Spencer, K. T., Kimura, B. J., Korcarz, C. E., Pellikka, P. A., Rahko, P. S., & Siegel, R. J. (2013). Focused Cardiac Ultrasound: Recommendations from the American Society of Echocardiography. *Journal of the American Society of Echocardiography*, *26*(6), 567–581. doi:10.1016/j.echo.2013.04.001 PMID:23711341

Sperry, J., & Cohen, M. J. (2014). Acute Obstruction. *The Surgical Clinics of North America*, *94*(1), 77–96. doi:10.1016/j.suc.2013.10.001 PMID:24267500

Spertus, J. a, Winder, J. a, Dewhurst, T. a, Deyo, R. a, & Fihn, S. D. (1994). Monitoring the quality of life in patients with coronary artery disease. *The American Journal of Cardiology, 74*(12), 1240–4. Retrieved from http://www.ncbi.nlm.nih.gov/pubmed/7977097

Spertus, J. a, Winder, J. a, Dewhurst, T. a, Deyo, R. a, Prodzinski, J., McDonell, M., & Fihn, S. D. (1995). Development and evaluation of the Seattle Angina Questionnaire: a new functional status measure for coronary artery disease. *Journal of the American College of Cardiology, 25*(2), 333–41. Retrieved from http://www.ncbi.nlm.nih.gov/pubmed/7829785

Spiess, B. D., Horrow, J., & Kaplan, J. A. (2011). Kaplan's Cardiac Anesthesia (D. L. R. Joel A. Kaplan, Joseph S. Savino Ed. 6th edition ed.). St. Louis, MO: Elsevier Saunders.

Spiess, B. D., Tuman, K. J., McCarthy, R. J., DeLaria, G. A., Schillo, R., & Ivankovich, A. D. (1987). Thromboelastography as an indicator of post-cardiopulmonary bypass coagulopathies. *Journal of Clinical Monitoring*, *3*(1), 25–30. doi:10.1007/BF00770880 PMID:3819793

Springer, T. A. (1994). Traffic signals for lymphocyte recirculation leukocyte emigration: The multistep paradigm. *Cell*, *76*(2), 301–314. doi:10.1016/0092-8674(94)90337-9 PMID:7507411

Sprung, C. L., Annane, D., Keh, D., Moreno, R., Singer, M., Freivogel, K., & Briegel, J. et al. (2008). Hydrocortisone therapy for patients with septic shock. *The New England Journal of Medicine*, *358*(2), 111–124. doi:10.1056/NEJMoa071366 PMID:18184957

Squara, P., Denjean, D., Estagnasie, P., Brusset, A., Dib, J. C., & Dubois, C. (2007). Noninvasive cardiac output monitoring (NICOM): A clinical validation. *Intensive Care Medicine*, *33*(7), 1191–1194. doi:10.1007/s00134-007-0640-0 PMID:17458538

Srinivasan, A., Song, X., Ross, T., Merz, W., Brower, R., & Perl, T. M. (2002). A prospective study to determine whether cover gowns in addition to gloves decrease nosocomial transmission of vancomycin-resistant enterococci in an intensive care unit. *Infection Control and Hospital Epidemiology*, *23*(8), 424–428. doi:10.1086/502079 PMID:12186206

Srivastava, V., D'silva, C., Tang, A., Sogliani, F., & Ngaage, D. L. (2012). The impact of major perioperative renal insult on long-term renal function and survival after cardiac surgery. *Interactive Cardiovascular and Thoracic Surgery*, *15*(1), 14–17. doi:10.1093/icvts/ivs106 PMID:22473666

St André, A. C., & DelRossi, A. (2005). Hemodynamic management of patients in the first 24 hours after cardiac surgery. *Critical Care Medicine*, *33*(9), 2082–2093. doi:10.1097/01.CCM.0000178355.96817.81 PMID:16148484

Stafford-Smith, M., Shaw, A., & Swaminathan, M. (2009). Cardiac surgery and acute kidney injury: Emerging concepts. *Current Opinion in Critical Care*, *15*(6), 498–502. doi:10.1097/MCC.0b013e328332f753 PMID:19812485

Stamou, S. C., Hill, P. C., Dangas, G., Pfister, J., Boyce, S. W., Dullum, M. K. C., & Silver, B. et al. (2001). Stroke after coronary artery bypass: Incidence, predictors, and clinical outcome. *Stroke*, *32*(7), 1508–1513. doi:10.1161/01.STR.32.7.1508 PMID:11441193

Stapleton, R. D., Jones, N., & Heyland, D. K. (2007). Feeding critically ill patients: What is the optimal amount of energy? *Critical Care Medicine*, *5*(9Suppl), 535–540. doi:10.1097/01.CCM.0000279204.24648.44 PMID:17713405

Starling, R. C., Moazami, N., Silvestry, S. C., Ewald, G., Rogers, J. G., Milano, C. A., & Smedira, N. G. et al. (2014). Unexpected abrupt increase in left ventricular assist device thrombosis. *The New England Journal of Medicine*, *370*(1), 33–40. doi:10.1056/NEJMoa1313385 PMID:24283197

Staub, N. C., Nagano, H., & Pearce, M. L. (1967). Pulmonary edema in dogs, especially the sequence of fluid accumulation in lungs. *Journal of Applied Physiology*, *22*(2), 227–240. PMID:6017888

Stecker, M. M., Cheung, A. T., Pochettino, A., Kent, G. P., Patterson, T., Weiss, S. J., & Bavaria, J. E. (2001). Deep hypothermic circulatory arrest: 1. Effects of cooling on electroencephalogram and evoked potentials. *The Annals of Thoracic Surgery*, *71*(1), 14–21. doi:10.1016/S0003-4975(00)01592-7 PMID:11216734

Stefanidis, D., Korndorffer, J. R. Jr, Black, F. W., Dunne, J. B., Sierra, R., Touchard, C. L., & Scott, D. J. et al. (2006). Psychomotor testing predicts rate of skill acquisition for proficiency-based laparoscopic skills training. *Surgery*, *140*(2), 252–262. doi:10.1016/j.surg.2006.04.002 PMID:16904977

Steg, P., van'tHof, A., Hamm, C., Clemmensen, P., Lapostelle, F., Coste, P., & Goldstein, P. et al. (2013). Bivalirudin Started during Emergency Transport for Primary PCI. *The New England Journal of Medicine*, *369*(23), 2207–2217. doi:10.1056/NEJMoa1311096 PMID:24171490

Stehlik, J., Edwards, L. B., Kucheryavaya, A. Y., Benden, C., Christie, J. D., Dipchand, A. I., . . . Hertz, M. I. (2012). The Registry Of The International Society For Heart And Lung Transplantation: 29th Official Adult Heart Transplant Report−2012. *The Journal Of Heart And Lung Transplantation*, *31*(10), 1052-1064. Retrieved From http://www.jhltonline.org/article/s1053-2498(12)01210-7/abstract

Stehlik, J., Edwards, L. B., Kucheryavaya, A. Y., Benden, C., Christie, J. D., Dipchand, A. I., & Hertz, M. I. et al. (2012). The Registry of the International Society for Heart and Lung Transplantation: 29th official adult heart transplant report – 2012. *The Journal of Heart and Lung Transplantation*, *31*(10), 1052–1064. doi:10.1016/j.healun.2012.08.002 PMID:22975095

Steinbeck, G., Andrensen, D., Seidl, K., Brachmann, J., Hoffman, E., Wojciechowski, D., & Senges, J. et al. (2009). Defibrillator Implantation Early after Myocardial Infarction. *The New England Journal of Medicine*, *361*(15), 1427–1436. doi:10.1056/NEJMoa0901889 PMID:19812399

Steinberg, A. (2003). *Encyclopedia of Jewish medical ethics: a compilation of Jewish medical law on all topics of medical interest*. Jerusalem, New York: Feldheim Publishers.

Steiner, M. E., Ness, P. M., Assman, S. F., Triulzi, D. J., Sloan, S. R., & Delaney, M. et al.. (2015). Effects of red-cell storage duration on patients undergoing cardiac surgery. *The New England Journal of Medicine*, *372*(15), 1419–1429. doi:10.1056/NEJMoa1414219 PMID:25853746

Steinert, Y. (2004). Student perceptions of effective small group teaching. *Medical Education*, *38*(3), 286–293. doi:10.1046/j.1365-2923.2004.01772.x PMID:14996338

Steinkraus, G., White, R., & Friedrich, L. (2007). Vancomycin MIC creep in non-vancomycin-intermediate Staphylococcus aureus (VISA), vancomycin-susceptible clinical methicillin-resistant S. aureus (MRSA) blood isolates from 2001-05. *The Journal of Antimicrobial Chemotherapy*, *60*(4), 788–794. doi:10.1093/jac/dkm258 PMID:17623693

Steinlechner, B., Zeidler, P., Base, E., Birkenberg, B., Ankersmit, H. J., Spannagl, M., & Jilma, B. et al. (2011). Patients with severe aortic valve stenosis and impaired platelet function benefit from preoperative desmopressin infusion. *The Annals of Thoracic Surgery*, *91*(5), 1420–1426. doi:10.1016/j.athoracsur.2011.01.052 PMID:21439546

Steinthorsdottir, K. J., Kandler, K., Agerlin Windeløv, N. A., & Steinbrüchel, D. A. (2013). Renal replacement therapy after cardiac surgery; renal function recovers. *Scandinavian Cardiovascular Journal*, *47*(5), 303–306. doi:10.3109/14017431.2013.821625 PMID:23915029

Stephan, H., Sonntag, H., Schenk, H. D., Kettler, D., & Khambatta, H. J. (1986). Effects of propofol on cardiovascular dynamics, myocardial blood flow and myocardial metabolism in patients with coronary artery disease. *British Journal of Anaesthesia*, *58*(9), 969–975. doi:10.1093/bja/58.9.969 PMID:3489478

Stevenson, L. (2003). Clinical use of inotropic therapy for heart failure: looking backward or forward? Part II: chronic inotropic therapy. *Circulation*, *108*(4), 492–497. doi:10.1161/01.CIR.0000078349.43742.8A PMID:12885733

Stewart, B. F., Siscovick, D., Lind, B. K., Gardin, J. M., Gottdiener, J. S., Smith, V. E., & Otto, C. M. et al. (1997). Clinical factors associated with calcific aortic valve disease. Cardiovascular Health Study. *Journal of the American College of Cardiology*, *29*(3), 630–634. doi:10.1016/S0735-1097(96)00563-3 PMID:9060903

Stewart, N. I., Jagelman, T. A., & Webster, N. R. (2011). Emerging modes of ventilation in the intensive care unit. *British Journal of Anaesthesia*, *107*(1), 74–82. doi:10.1093/bja/aer114 PMID:21613281

Stinson, E. B., Caves, P. K., Griepp, R. B., Oyer, P. E., Rider, A. K., & Shumway, N. E. (1975). Hemodynamic observations in the early period after human heart transplantation. *The Journal of Thoracic and Cardiovascular Surgery*, *69*(2), 264–270. PMID:1089847

Stinson, L., Pearson, D., & Lucas, B. (2006). Developing a learning culture: Twelve tips for individuals, teams and organizations. *Medical Teacher*, *28*(4), 309–312. doi:10.1080/01421590600726433 PMID:16807167

Stoelting, R. K. (1981). Hemodynamic effects of barbiturates and benzodiazepines. *Cleveland Clinic Journal of Medicine*, *48*(1), 9–13. doi:10.3949/ccjm.48.1.9 PMID:7261393

Stollerman, G. H. (2001). Rheumatic fever in the 21st century. *Clinical Infectious Diseases*, *33*(6), 806–814. doi:10.1086/322665 PMID:11512086

Stone, P. W., Braccia, D., & Larson, E. (2005). Systematic review of economic analyses of health care-associated infections. *American Journal of Infection Control*, *33*(9), 501–509. doi:10.1016/j.ajic.2005.04.246 PMID:16260325

Stone, P. W., Pogorzelska-Maziarz, M., Herzig, C. T. A., Weiner, L. M., Furuya, E. Y., Dick, A., & Larson, E. (2014). State of infection prevention in US hospitals enrolled in the National Health and Safety Network. *American Journal of Infection Control*, *42*(2), 94–99. doi:10.1016/j.ajic.2013.10.003 PMID:24485365

Strange, C. (1999). Pleural complications in the intensive care unit. *Clinics in Chest Medicine*, *20*(2), 317–327. doi:10.1016/S0272-5231(05)70144-1 PMID:10386259

Stransky, M., Schmidt, C., Ganslmeier, P., Grossmann, E., Haneya, A., Moritz, S., & Trabold, B. et al. (2011). Hypoactive delirium after cardiac surgery as an independent risk factor for prolonged mechanical ventilation. *Journal of Cardiothoracic and Vascular Anesthesia*, *25*(6), 968–974. doi:10.1053/j.jvca.2011.05.004 PMID:21741272

Strassburg, C. P. (2003). Shock liver. *Best Practice & Research. Clinical Gastroenterology*, *17*(3), 369–381. doi:10.1016/S1521-6918(03)00025-8 PMID:12763502

Strøm, T., Martinussen, T., & Toft, P. (2010). A protocol of no sedation for critically ill patients receiving mechanical ventilation: A randomised trial. *Lancet*, *375*(9713), 475–480. doi:10.1016/S0140-6736(09)62072-9 PMID:20116842

Strueber, M., O'Driscoll, G., Jansz, P., Khaghani, A., Levy, W. C., & Wieselthaler, G. M. (2011). Multicenter evaluation of an intrapericardial left ventricular assist system. *Journal of the American College of Cardiology*, *57*(12), 1375–1382. doi:10.1016/j.jacc.2010.10.040 PMID:21414534

Stuklis, R. G., O'Shaughnessy, D. F., & Ohri, S. K. (2001). Novel approach to bleeding in patients undergoing cardiac surgery with liver dysfunction. *European Journal of Cardio-Thoracic Surgery: Official Journal of the European Association for Cardio-Thoracic Surgery*, *19*(2), 219–220. doi:10.1016/S1010-7940(00)00641-2 PMID:11167117

Stulberg, J. J., Delaney, C. P., Neuhauser, D. V., Aron, D. C., Fu, P., & Koroukian, S. M. (2010). Adherence to surgical care improvement project measures and the association with postoperative infections. *Journal of the American Medical Association*, *303*(24), 2479–2485. doi:10.1001/jama.2010.841 PMID:20571014

Sturm, L. P., Windsor, J. A., Cosman, P. H., Cregan, P., Hewett, P. J., & Maddern, G. J. (2008). A systematic review of skills transfer after surgical simulation training. *Annals of Surgery*, *248*(2), 166–179. doi:10.1097/SLA.0b013e318176bf24 PMID:18650625

Subramanian, V. A., Mccabe, J. C., Geller, C. M., Hospital, L. H., & York, N. (1997). Grafting : Two-Year Clinical Experience, *4975*(97).

Sullivan, M. E., Yates, K. A., Inaba, K., Lam, L., & Clark, R. E. (2014). The Use of Cognitive Task Analysis to Reveal the Instructional Limitations of Experts in the Teaching of Procedural Skills. *Academic Medicine*, *89*(5), 811–816. doi:10.1097/ACM.0000000000000224 PMID:24667500

Suma, H., Tanabe, H., Takahashi, A., Horii, T., Isomura, T., Hirose, H., & Amano, A. (2007). Twenty years experience with the gastroepiploic artery graft for CABG. *Circulation*, *116*(11Suppl), I188–I191. doi:10.1161/CIRCULATIONAHA.106.678813 PMID:17846302

Suman, A. B., Barnes, D. S., Zein, N. N., Levinthal, G. N., Connor, J. T., & Carey, W. D. (2004). Predicting outcomes after cardiac surgery in patients with cirrhosis: A comparison of Child-Pugh and MELD scores. *Clinical Gastroenterology and Hepatology*, *2*(8), 719–723. doi:10.1016/S1542-3565(04)00296-4 PMID:15290666

Sun, J., Whitlock, R., Cheng, J., Eikelboom, J., Thabane, L., Crowther, M., & Teoh, K. (2008). The effect of pre-operative aspirin on bleeding, transfusion, myocardial infarction, and mortality in coronary artery bypass surgery: A systematic review of randomized and observational studies. *European Heart Journal*, *29*(8), 1057–1071. doi:10.1093/eurheartj/ehn104 PMID:18346962

Surawicz, C. M., Brandt, L. J., Binion, D. G., Ananthakrishnan, A. N., Curry, S. R., Gilligan, P. H., & Zuckerbraun, B. S. et al. (2013). Guidelines for diagnosis, treatment, and prevention of Clostridum difficile infections. *The American Journal of Gastroenterology*, *108*(4), 478–498. doi:10.1038/ajg.2013.4 PMID:23439232

Surgical Care Improvement Project, version 4.3 (2014). *Specifications Manual for National Hospital Inpatient Quality Measures*. QualityNet.org.

Sutcliffe, K. M., Lewton, E., & Rosenthal, M. M. (2004). Communication failures: An insidious contributor to medical mishaps. *Academic Medicine*, *79*(2), 186–194. doi:10.1097/00001888-200402000-00019 PMID:14744724

Sutherland, E. R., & Martin, R. J. (2003). Airway inflammation in chronic obstructive pulmonary disease: Comparisons with asthma. *The Journal of Allergy and Clinical Immunology*, *112*(5), 819–827, quiz 828. doi:10.1016/S0091-6749(03)02011-6 PMID:14610463

Suttner, S., Piper, S. N., Kumle, B., Lang, K., Röhm, K. D., Isgro, F., & Boldt, J. (2004). The influence of allogeneic red blood cell transfusion compared with 100% oxygen ventilation on systemic oxygen transport and skeletal muscle oxygen tension after cardiac surgery. *Anesthesia and Analgesia*, *99*(1), 2–11. doi:10.1213/01.ANE.0000120163.44315.47 PMID:15281492

Sutton, M., Plappert, T., Hilpisch, K., Abraham, W., Hayes, D., & Chinchoy, E. (2006). Sustained reverse left ventricular structural remodeling with cardiac resynchronization at one year is a function of etiology: Quantitative Doppler echocardiographic evidence from the Multicenter InSync Randomized Clinical Evaluation (MIRACLE). *Circulation*, *113*(2), 266–272. doi:10.1161/CIRCULATIONAHA.104.520817 PMID:16401777

Sutton, T. A., Fisher, C. J., & Molitoris, B. A. (2002). Microvascular endothelial injury and dysfunction during ischemic acute renal failure. *Kidney International*, *62*(5), 1539–1549. doi:10.1046/j.1523-1755.2002.00631.x PMID:12371954

Suvarna, S., Smith, A., Stygall, J., Kolvecar, S., Walesby, R., Harrison, M., & Newman, S. (2007). An intraoperative assessment of the ascending aorta: A comparison of digital palpation, transesophageal echocardiography, and epiaortic ultrasonography. *Journal of Cardiothoracic and Vascular Anesthesia*, *21*(6), 805–809. doi:10.1053/j.jvca.2007.05.014 PMID:18068056

Svensson, L. G., Adams, D. H., Bonow, R. O., Kouchoukos, N. T., Miller, D. C., O'Gara, P. T., & Williams, M. R. et al. (2013). Aortic valve and ascending aorta guidelines for management and quality measures. *The Annals of Thoracic Surgery*, *95*(6Suppl), S1–S66. doi:10.1016/j.athoracsur.2013.01.083 PMID:23688839

Svensson, L. G., Hess, K. R., Coselli, J. S., Safi, H. J., & Crawford, S. (1991). A prospective study of respiratory failure after high-risk surgery on the thoracoabdominal aorta. *Journal of Vascular Surgery*, *14*(3), 271–282. doi:10.1016/0741-5214(91)90077-8 PMID:1880835

Svensson, L. G., Tuzcu, M., Kapadia, S., Blackstone, E. H., Roselli, E. E., Gillinov, A. M., & Lytle, B. W. et al. (2013). A comprehensive review of the PARTNER trial. *The Journal of Thoracic and Cardiovascular Surgery*, *145*(3Suppl), S11–S16. doi:10.1016/j.jtcvs.2012.11.051 PMID:23410766

Svircevic, V., Nierich, A. P., Moons, K. G. M., Diephuis, J. C., Ennema, J. J., Brandon Bravo Bruinsma, G. J., & van Dijk, D. et al. (2011). Thoracic epidural anesthesia for cardiac surgery: A randomized trial. *Anesthesiology*, *114*(2), 262–270. doi:10.1097/ALN.0b013e318201d2de PMID:21239976

Svircevic, V., Passier, M. M., Nierich, A. P., van Dijk, D., Kalkman, C. J., & van der Heijden, G. J. (2013). Epidural analgesia for cardiac surgery. *Cochrane Database of Systematic Reviews*, *6*, CD006715. PMID:23740694

Sweet, S. C. (2013). Induction therapy in lung transplantation. *Transplant International*, *26*(7), 696–703. doi:10.1111/tri.12115

Swetz, K. M., & Mansel, J. K. (2013). Ethical Issues and Palliative Care in the Cardiovascular Intensive Care Unit. *Cardiology Clinics*, *31*(4), 657–668. doi:10.1016/j.ccl.2013.07.013 PMID:24188227

Swetz, K. M., Ottenberg, A. L., Freeman, M. R., & Mueller, P. S. (2011). Palliative care and end-of-life issues in patients treated with left ventricular assist devices as destination therapy. *Current Heart Failure Reports*, *8*(3), 212–218. doi:10.1007/s11897-011-0060-x PMID:21538039

Swidler, R. N. (2010). The Family Health Care Decisions Act: A Summary of Key Provisions. *Health Law Journal*, *15*(1), 32–35.

Swing, S. R. S., Clyman, S. G. S., Holmboe, E. S. E., & Williams, R. G. R. (2009). Advancing resident assessment in graduate medical education. *Journal of Graduate Medical Education*, *1*(2), 278–286. doi:10.4300/JGME-D-09-00010.1 PMID:21975993

Szabo, Z., Hakanson, E., & Svedjeholm, R. (2002). Early postoperative outcome and medium-term survival in 540 diabetic and 2239 nondiabetic patients undergoing coronary artery bypass grafting. *The Annals of Thoracic Surgery*, *74*(3), 712–719. doi:10.1016/S0003-4975(02)03778-5 PMID:12238829

Szeto, W. Y., Kreisel, D., Karakousis, G. C., Pochettino, A., Sterman, D. H., Kotloff, R. M., & Rosengard, B. R. et al. (2002). Cardiopulmonary bypass for bilateral sequential lung transplantation in patients with chronic obstructive pulmonary disease without adverse effect on lung function or clinical outcome. *The Journal of Thoracic and Cardiovascular Surgery*, *124*(2), 241–249. doi:10.1067/mtc.2002.121303

Taggart, D. P. (2006). Thomas B. Ferguson Lecture. Coronary artery bypass grafting is still the best treatment for multivessel and left main disease, but patients need to know. *The Annals of Thoracic Surgery*, *82*(6), 1966–1975. doi:10.1016/j.athoracsur.2006.06.035 PMID:17126093

Taggart, D. P. (2013). The FREEDOM trial: A definitive answer to coronary artery bypass grafting or stents in patients with diabetes and multivessel coronary artery disease. *European Journal of Cardio-Thoracic Surgery : Official Journal of the European Association for Cardio-Thoracic Surgery*, *44*(6), 978–979. doi:10.1093/ejcts/ezt450 PMID:24047712

Taggart, D. P., D'Amico, R., & Altman, D. G. (2001). Effect of arterial revascularisation on survival: A systematic review of studies comparing bilateral and single internal mammary arteries. *Lancet*, *358*(9285), 870–875. doi:10.1016/S0140-6736(01)06069-X PMID:11567701

Taghavi, S., Zuckermann, A., Ankersmit, J., Wieselthaler, G., Rajek, A., Laufer, G., . . . Grimm, M. (2004). Extracorporeal Membrane Oxygenation Is Superior To Right Ventricular Assist Device For Acute Right Ventricular Failure After Heart Transplantation. *The Annals Of Thoracic Surgery, 78*(5), 1644-1649. Retrieved From http://www.annalsthoracicsurgery.org/article/S0003-4975(04)00997-X/abstract

Taira, K., Suzuki, A., Fujino, A., Watanabe, T., Ogyu, A., & Ashikawa, K. (2006). Tricuspid valve stenosis related to subvalvular adhesion of pacemaker lead: A case report. *Journal of Cardiology*, *47*(6), 301–306. PMID:16800373

Takagi, H., Goto, S.-N., Watanabe, T., Mizuno, Y., Kawai, N., & Umemoto, T. (2014). A meta-analysis of adjusted hazard ratios from 20 observational studies of bilateral versus single internal thoracic artery coronary artery bypass grafting. *The Journal of Thoracic and Cardiovascular Surgery*, 1–10. doi:10.1016/j.jtcvs.2014.01.010 PMID:24521973

Takagi, H., Niwa, M., Mizuno, Y., Goto, S. N., & Umemoto, T. (2013). Incidence, predictors, and prognosis of acute kidney injury after transcatheter aortic valve implantation: A summary of contemporary studies using Valve Academic Research Consortium definitions. *International Journal of Cardiology*, *168*(2), 1631–1635. doi:10.1016/j.ijcard.2013.01.273 PMID:23453450

Takagi, H., Tanabashi, T., Kawai, N., & Umemoto, T. (2007). Off-pump surgery does not reduce stroke, compared with results of on-pump coronary artery bypass grafting: A meta-analysis of randomized clinical trials. *The Journal of Thoracic and Cardiovascular Surgery*, *134*(4), 1059–1060. doi:10.1016/j.jtcvs.2007.07.006 PMID:17903537

Takahashi, M. (2014). NLRP3 Inflammasome as a Novel Player in Myocardial Infarction. *International Heart Journal*, *55*(2), 101–105. doi:10.1536/ihj.13-388 PMID:24632952

Takayama, H., Leone, R. J., & Aldea, G. S. (2006). *Open-chest management after heart transplantation*. Texas Heart Institute.

Talmor, D., Sarge, T., Malhotra, A., O'Donnell, C. R., Ritz, R., Lisbon, A., & Loring, S. H. et al. (2008). Mechanical ventilation guided by esophageal pressure in acute lung injury. *The New England Journal of Medicine*, *359*(20), 2095–2104. doi:10.1056/NEJMoa0708638 PMID:19001507

Tamburino, C., Capodanno, D., Ramondo, A., Petronio, A. S., Ettori, F., Santoro, G., & Ussia, G. P. et al. (2011). Incidence and predictors of early and late mortality after transcatheter aortic valve implantation in 663 patients with severe aortic stenosis. *Circulation*, *123*(3), 299–308. doi:10.1161/CIRCULATIONAHA.110.946533 PMID:21220731

Tambyah, P. A., Halvorson, K. T., & Maki, D. G. (1999). A prospective study of pathogenesis of catheter-associated urinary tract infections. *Mayo Clinic Proceedings*, *74*(2), 131–136. doi:10.4065/74.2.131 PMID:10069349

Tambyah, P. A., & Maki, D. G. (2000). Catheter-associated urinary tract infection is rarely symptomatic. A prospective study of 1497 catheterized patients. *Archives of Internal Medicine*, *160*(5), 678–682. doi:10.1001/archinte.160.5.678 PMID:10724054

Tanaka, K. A., Key, N. S., & Levy, J. H. (2009). Blood coagulation: Hemostasis and thrombin regulation. *Anesthesia and Analgesia*, *108*(5), 1433–1446. doi:10.1213/ane.0b013e31819bcc9c PMID:19372317

Tang, A., Wells, G., Taljic, M., Arnold, M., Sheldon, R., Connolly, S., & Rouleau, J. et al. (2010). Cardiac resynchronization therapy for mild-to-moderate heart failure. *The New England Journal of Medicine*, *363*(25), 2385–2395. doi:10.1056/NEJMoa1009540 PMID:21073365

Tang, H., Lin, H., Lin, Y., Leung, P., Chuang, Y., & Lai, C. (2014). The impact of central line insertion bundle on central line-associated bloodstream infection. *BMC Infectious Diseases*, *14*(1), 356. doi:10.1186/1471-2334-14-356 PMID:24985729

Tarakji, K. G. S. (2011). Temporal Onset, risk factors and outcomes associated with stroke after coronary artery nypass grafting. *Journal of the American Medical Association*, *305*(4), 381–390. doi:10.1001/jama.2011.37 PMID:21266685

Taramasso, M., Maisano, F., Latib, A., Denti, P., Guidotti, A., Sticchi, A., & Alfieri, O. (2014). *Conventional surgery and transcatheter closure via surgical transapical approach for paravalvular leak repair in high-risk patients: results from a single-centre experience*. European Heart Journal Cardiovascular Imaging; doi:10.1093/ehjci/jeu105

Tarhan, S., Moffitt, E. A., Sessler, A. D., Douglas, W. W., & Taylor, W. F. (1973). Risk of anesthesia and surgery in patients with chronic bronchitis and chronic obstructive pulmonary disease. *Surgery*, *74*(5), 720–726. PMID:4742756

Tasanarong, A., Duangchana, S., Sumransurp, S., Homvises, B., & Satdhabudha, O. (2013). Prophylaxis with Erythropoietin versus Placebo Reduces Acute Kidney Injury and Neutrophil Gelatinase-Associated Lipocalin in Patients Undergoing Cardiac Surgery: A Randomized, Double-Blind Controlled Trial. *BMC Nephrology*, *14*(1), 136. doi:10.1186/1471-2369-14-136 PMID:23829828

Tasca, G., Mhagna, Z., Perotti, S., Centurini, P. B., Sabatini, T., Amaducci, A., & Pibarot, P. et al. (2006). Impact of prosthesis-patient mismatch on cardiac events and midterm mortality after aortic valve replacement in patients with pure aortic stenosis. *Circulation*, *113*(4), 570–576. doi:10.1161/CIRCULATIONAHA.105.587022 PMID:16401767

Tatoulis, J., Buxton, B. F., & Fuller, J. (2004). Patencies of 2127 arterial to coronary conduits over 15 years. *The Annals of Thoracic Surgery*, *77*(1), 93–101. doi:10.1016/S0003-4975(03)01331-6 PMID:14726042

Tatoulis, J., Buxton, B. F., & Fuller, J. (2011). The right internal thoracic artery: The forgotten conduit--5,766 patients and 991 angiograms. *The Annals of Thoracic Surgery*, *92*(1), 9–15, discussion 15–17. doi:10.1016/j.athoracsur.2011.03.099 PMID:21718825

Tattevin, P., Donal, E., & Revest, M. (2010). Can we really achieve a 1-year mortality rate lower than 10% in patients with infective endocarditis? *Archives of Internal Medicine*, *170*(2), 211–212. PMID:20101020

Tayama, E., Ueda, T., Shojima, T., Akasu, K., Oda, T., Fukunaga, S., & Aoyagi, S. et al. (2007). Arginine vasopressin is an ideal drug after cardiac surgery for the management of low systemic vascular resistant hypotension concomitant with pulmonary hypertension. *Interactive Cardiovascular and Thoracic Surgery*, *6*(6), 715–719. doi:10.1510/icvts.2007.159624 PMID:17704123

Taylor, D. O., Edwards, L. B., Aurora, P., Christie, J. D., Dobbels, F., Kirk, R., . . . Hertz, M. I. (2008). Registry Of The International Society For Heart And Lung Transplantation: Twenty-Fifth Official Adult Heart Transplant Report-2008. *The Journal Of Heart And Lung Transplantation, 27*(9), 943-956. Retrieved From http://www.jhltonline.org/article/s1053-2498(08)00501-9/abstract

Taylor, A., Ziesche, S., Yancy, C., Carson, P., D'Agostino, R. Jr, Ferdinand, K., & Cohn, J. et al. (2004). Combination of isosorbide dinitrate and hydralazine in blacks with heart failure. *The New England Journal of Medicine*, *351*(20), 2049–2057. doi:10.1056/NEJMoa042934 PMID:15533851

Taylor, R. W., Zimmerman, J. L., Dellinger, R. P., Straube, R. C., Criner, G. J., & Davis, K. et al.. (2004). Low-dose inhaled nitric oxide in patients with acute lung injury: A randomized controlled trial. *Journal of the American Medical Association*, *291*, 1603–1609. doi:10.1001/jama.291.13.1603 PMID:15069048

Tenofsky, P. L., Beamer, L., & Smith, R. S. (2000). Ogilvie syndrome as a postoperative complication. *Archives of Surgery*, *135*(6), 682–687. doi:10.1001/archsurg.135.6.682 PMID:10843364

Terragni, P. P., Antonelli, M., Fumagalli, R., Faggiano, C., Berardino, M., Pallavicini, F. B., & Ranieri, V. M. et al. (2010). Early vs late tracheotomy for prevention of pneumonia in mechanically ventilated adult ICU patients: A randomized controlled trial. *Journal of the American Medical Association*, *303*(15), 1483–1489. doi:10.1001/jama.2010.447 PMID:20407057

Tessitore, E., Rundek, T., Jin, Z., Homma, S., Sacco, R. L., & Di Tullio, M. R. (2010). Association between carotid intima-media thickness and aortic arch plaques. *Journal of the American Society of Echocardiography*, *23*(7), 772–777. doi:10.1016/j.echo.2010.04.012 PMID:20510582

Teunissen, P. W., Scheele, F., Scherpbier, A. J. J. A., van der Vleuten, C. P. M., Boor, K., van Luijk, S. J., & van Diemen-Steenvoorde, J. A. A. M. (2007). How residents learn: Qualitative evidence for the pivotal role of clinical activities. *Medical Education*, *41*(8), 763–770. doi:10.1111/j.1365-2923.2007.02778.x PMID:17661884

Thakar, C. V., Arrigain, S., Worley, S., Yared, J.-P., & Paganini, E. P. (2005). A clinical score to predict acute renal failure after cardiac surgery. *Journal of the American Society of Nephrology : JASN*, *16*(1), 162–168. doi:10.1681/ASN.2004040331 PMID:15563569

Thanassoulis, G., Campbell, C. Y., Owens, D. S., Smith, J. G., Smith, A. V., Peloso, G. M., & Post, W. S. et al. (2013). Genetic associations with valvular calcification and aortic stenosis. *The New England Journal of Medicine*, *368*(6), 503–512. doi:10.1056/NEJMoa1109034 PMID:23388002

Thanavaro, K. L., & Nixon, J. V. (2014). Endocarditis 2014: An update. *Heart & Lung*, *43*(4), 334–337. doi:10.1016/j.hrtlng.2014.03.009 PMID:24780242

The Acute Respiratory Distress Syndrome Network. (2000). Ventilation with lower tidal volumes as compared with traditional tidal volumes for acute lung injury and the acute respiratory distress syndrome. *New England Journal of Medicine, 342*(18), 1301-1308.

The Anesthesiology Milestone Project. (2013, December 13). The Anesthesiology Milestone Project. *Acgme*. Retrieved May 2014, from https://www.acgme.org/acgmeweb/Portals/0/PDFs/Milestones/AnesthesiologyMilestones.pdf

The BARI Investigators. (2007). The final 10-year follow-up results from the BARI randomized trial. *Journal of the American College of Cardiology, 49*(15), 1600–1606. doi:10.1016/j.jacc.2006.11.048 PMID:17433949

The Clopidogrel in Unstable Angina to Prevent Recurrent Events Trial Investigators. (2001). Effects of Clopidogrel in Addition to Aspirin in Patients with Acute Coronary Syndromes without ST-Segment Elevation. *The New England Journal of Medicine, 345*(7), 494–502. doi:10.1056/NEJMoa010746 PMID:11519503

The Criteria Committee of the New York Heart Association. (1994). *Nomenclature and criteria for diagnosis of diseases of the heart and great vessels* (9th ed.). Boston, MA.

The EINSTEIN investigators. (2010). Oral rivaroxaban for symptomatic venous thromboembolism. *The New England Journal of Medicine, 363*(26), 2499–2510. doi:10.1056/NEJMoa1007903 PMID:21128814

The EINSTEIN-PE Investigators. (2012). Oral rivaroxaban for the treatment of symptomatic pulmonary embolism. *The New England Journal of Medicine, 366*(14), 1287–1297. doi:10.1056/NEJMoa1113572 PMID:22449293

The Syntax Score. (n.d.).

The Trainee Doctor. (2011). *The Trainee Doctor*. Manchester: General Medical Council.

Theodorakopoulou, M., Perros, E., Giamarellos-Bourboulis, E. J., & Dimopoulos, G. (2013). Controversies in the management of the critically ill: The role of probiotics. *International Journal of Antimicrobial Agents, 42*(Suppl), S41–S44. doi:10.1016/j.ijantimicag.2013.04.010 PMID:23664676

Thiagarajan, R. R., Brogan, T. V., Scheurer, M. A., Laussen, P. C., Rycus, P. T., & Bratton, S. L. (2009). Extracorporeal membrane oxygenation to support cardiopulmonary resuscitation in adults. *The Annals of Thoracic Surgery, 87*(3), 778–785. doi:10.1016/j.athoracsur.2008.12.079 PMID:19231388

Thiele, H., Zeymer, U., Neumann, F.-J., Ferenc, M., Olbrich, H.-G., Hausleiter, J., & Schuler, G. et al. (2013). Intra-aortic balloon counterpulsation in acute myocardial infarction complicated by cardiogenic shock (IABP-SHOCK II): Final 12 month results of a randomised, open-label trial. *Lancet, 382*(9905), 1638–1645. doi:10.1016/S0140-6736(13)61783-3 PMID:24011548

Thiele, H., Zeymer, U., Neumann, F.-J., Ferenc, M., Olbrich, H.-G., Hausleiter, J., & Werdan, K. et al. (2012). Intraaortic Balloon Support for Myocardial Infarction with Cardiogenic Shock. *The New England Journal of Medicine, 367*(14), 1287–1296. doi:10.1056/NEJMoa1208410 PMID:22920912

Thiele, R. H., & Raphael, J. (2014). A 2014 Update on Coagulation Management for Cardiopulmonary Bypass. *Seminars in Cardiothoracic and Vascular Anesthesia, 18*(2), 177–189. doi:10.1177/1089253214534782 PMID:24876232

Thomas, M., Schymik, G., Walther, T., Himbert, D., Lefevre, T., Treede, H., & Wendler, O. et al. (2010). Thirty-day results of the SAPIEN aortic Bioprosthesis European Outcome (SOURCE) Registry: A European registry of transcatheter aortic valve implantation using the Edwards SAPIEN valve. *Circulation, 122*(1), 62–69. doi:10.1161/CIRCULATIONAHA.109.907402 PMID:20566953

Thompson, M. L., Flynn, J. D., & Clifford, T. M. (2013). Pharmacotherapy of lung transplantation: An overview. *Journal of Pharmacy Practice, 26*(1), 5–13. doi:10.1177/0897190012466048

Thomson, I. R., Harding, G., & Hudson, R. J. (2000). A comparison of fentanyl and sufentanil in patients undergoing coronary artery bypass surgery. *Journal of Cardiothoracic and Vascular Anesthesia*, *14*(6), 652–656. doi:10.1053/jcan.2000.18307 PMID:11139103

Thorel, C. H. (1903). Pathologie der Kreislauforgane. *Ergebnisse der Allgemeinen Pathologie und Pathologischen Anatomie*, *9*, 559.

Thourani, V. H., Ailawadi, G., Szeto, W. Y., Dewey, T. M., Guyton, R. A., Mack, M. J., . . . Bavaria, J. E. (2011). Outcomes of surgical aortic valve replacement in high-risk patients: a multiinstitutional study. *Annals of Thoracic Surgery*, *91*(1), 49-55; discussion 55-46. doi: 10.1016/j.athoracsur.2010.09.040

Thourani, V. H., Razavi, S. A., Nguyen, T. C., Kilgo, P. D., Puskas, J. D., Guyton, R. A., & Halkos, M. E. et al. (2014). Incidence of postoperative stroke using the Heartstring device in 1,380 coronary artery bypass graft patients with mild to severe atherosclerosis of the ascending aorta. *The Annals of Thoracic Surgery*, *97*(6), 2066–2072, discussion 2072. doi:10.1016/j.athoracsur.2014.02.044 PMID:24726605

Thuny, F., Avierinos, J., Tribouilloy, C., Giorgi, R., Casalta, J., Milandre, L., & Habib, G. et al. (2007). Impact of cerebrovascular complications on mortality and neurologic outcome during infective endocarditis: A prospective multicentre study. *European Heart Journal*, *28*(9), 1155–1161. doi:10.1093/eurheartj/ehm005 PMID:17363448

Thuny, F., Beurtheret, S., Mancini, J., Gariboldi, V., Casalta, J., Riberi, A., & Habib, G. et al. (2011). The timing of surgery influences mortality and morbidity in adults with severe complicated infective endocarditis: A propensity analysis. *European Heart Journal*, *32*(16), 2027–2033. doi:10.1093/eurheartj/ehp089 PMID:19329497

Thuny, F., Grisoli, D., Collart, F., Habib, G., & Raoult, D. (2012). Management of infective endocarditis: Challenges and perspectives. *Lancet*, *379*(9819), 965–975. doi:10.1016/S0140-6736(11)60755-1 PMID:22317840

Thygesen, K., Alpert, J. S., Jaffe, A. S., Simoons, M. L., Chaitman, B. R., White, H. D., ... (2012). Third universal definition of myocardial infarction. (Vol. 126, pp. 2020–2035). doi:10.1161/CIR.0b013e31826e1058

Thygesen, K., Alpert, J. S., Jaffe, A. S., Simoons, M. L., Chaitman, B. R., White, H. D., & Mendis, S. et al. (2012). Third universal definition of myocardial infarction. *European Heart Journal*, *33*(20), 2551–2567. doi:10.1093/eurheartj/ehs184 PMID:22922414

Tiberius, R. G. (1999). *Small Group Teaching*. London: Kogan Page Publishers.

Tilden, L. B., Williams, B. R., Tucker, R. O., MacLennan, P. A., & Ritchie, C. S. (2009). Surgeons' attitudes and practices in the utilization of palliative and supportive care services for patients with a sudden advanced illness. *Journal of Palliative Medicine*, *12*(11), 1037–1042. doi:10.1089/jpm.2009.0120 PMID:19663713

Timmermans, P., Willems, J. L., Piessens, J., & De Geest, H. (1988). Angina pectoris and coronary artery disease in severe aortic regurgitation. *The American Journal of Cardiology*, *61*(10), 826–829. doi:10.1016/0002-9149(88)91074-0 PMID:3354447

Timrott, K., Vondran, F. W., Kleine, M., Warnecke, G., Haverich, A., Lehner, F., & Klempnauer, J. (2014). The impact of abdominal complications on the outcome after thoracic transplantation-a single center experience. *Langenbeck's Archives of Surgery*, *399*(6), 789–793. doi:10.1007/s00423-014-1193-7

Timsit, J., Mimoz, O., Mourvillier, B., Souweine, B., Garrouste-Orgeas, M., Alfandari, S., & Lucet, J. et al. (2012). Randomized controlled trial of chlorhexidine dressing and highly adhesive dressing for preventing catheter-related infections in critically ill adults. *American Journal of Respiratory and Critical Care Medicine*, *186*(12), 1272–1278. doi:10.1164/rccm.201206-1038OC PMID:23043083

Timsit, J., Schwebel, C., Bouadma, L., Geffroy, A., Garrouste-Orgeas, M., Pease, S., & Dressing Study Group, et al.. (2009). Chlorhexidine-impregnated sponges and less frequent dressing changes for prevention of catheter-related infections in critically ill adults: A randomized controlled trial. *Journal of the American Medical Association, 301*(12), 1231–1241. doi:10.1001/jama.2009.376 PMID:19318651

Tjia, M. W., & Gitlin, D. F. (2010). Use of antipsychotics in medically ill patients. In A. J. Rothschild (Ed.), *The evidence-based guide to antipsychotic medications* (pp. 215–243). Arlington, VA: American Psychiatric Publishing.

Tleyjeh, I. M., Abdel-Latif, A., Rahbi, H., Scott, C. G., Bailey, K. R., Steckelbert, J. M., & Baddour, L. M. et al. (2007). A systematic review of population-based studies of infective endocarditis. *Chest, 132*(3), 1025–1035. doi:10.1378/chest.06-2048 PMID:17873196

Tobin, M. J. (2001). Advances in mechanical ventilation. *The New England Journal of Medicine, 344*(26), 1986–1996. doi:10.1056/NEJM200106283442606 PMID:11430329

Tocco, M. P., Constantino, A., Ballardini, M., D'Andrea, C., Masala, M., Merico, E., & Sordini, P. et al. (2009). Improved results of the vacuum-assisted closure and Nitinol clips sternal closure after postoperative deep sternal wound infection. *European Journal of Cardio-Thoracic Surgery, 35*(5), 833–838. doi:10.1016/j.ejcts.2008.12.036 PMID:19216084

Tochel, C., Haig, A., Hesketh, A., Cadzow, A., Beggs, K., Colthart, I., & Peacock, H. (2009). The effectiveness of portfolios for post-graduate assessment and education: BEME Guide No 12. *Medical Teacher, 31*(4), 299–318. doi:10.1080/01421590902883056 PMID:19404890

Toff, N. J. (2010). Human factors in anaesthesia: Lessons from aviation. *British Journal of Anaesthesia, 105*(1), 21–25. doi:10.1093/bja/aeq127 PMID:20507856

Toktas, F., Yavuz, S., Eris, C., & Surer, S. (2014). Transaortic intra-aortic balloon pump catheter insertion through a separate saphenous vein graft in patients with severe aortoiliac disease. *TheScientificWorldJournal, 247803*. doi:10.1155/2014/247803 PMID:24516360

Tomasi, R., & von Dossow-Hanfstingl, V. (2014). Critical care strategies to improve neurocognitive outcome in thoracic surgery. *Current Opinion in Anaesthesiology, 27*(1), 44–48. doi:10.1097/ACO.0000000000000026 PMID:24263687

Tomorrow's Doctors. (1993). *Tomorrow's Doctors*. London: General Medical Council.

Topkara, V. K., O'Neill, J. K., Carlisle, A., Novak, E., Silvestry, S. C., & Ewald, G. A. (2014). HeartWare and HeartMate II left ventricular assist devices as bridge to transplantation: A comparative analysis. *The Annals of Thoracic Surgery, 97*(2), 506–512. doi:10.1016/j.athoracsur.2013.08.048 PMID:24140211

Torbeck, L., & Canal, D. F. (2009). Remediation practices for surgery residents. *American Journal of Surgery, 197*(3), 397–402. doi:10.1016/j.amjsurg.2008.10.008 PMID:19245922

Toronto Lung Transplant Group. (1986). Unilateral lung transplantation for pulmonary fibrosis. *New England Journal of Medicine, 314*(18), 1140-1145.

Toumpoulis, I. K., Anagnostopoulos, C. E., DeRose, J. J., & Swistel, D. G. (2005). The impact of deep sternal wound infection on long-term survival after coronary artery bypass grafting. *Chest, 127*(2), 464–471. doi:10.1378/chest.127.2.464 PMID:15705983

Tousoulis, D., Psarros, C., Demosthenous, M., Patel, R., Antoniades, C., & Stefanadis, C. (2014). Innate and adaptive inflammation as a therapeutic target in vascular disease. *Journal of the American College of Cardiology, 63*(23), 2491–2502. doi:10.1016/j.jacc.2014.01.054 PMID:24613322

Tranbaugh, R. F., Dimitrova, K. R., Lucido, D. J., Hoffman, D. M., Dincheva, G. R., Geller, C. M., & Swistel, D. G. et al. (2014). The second best arterial graft: A propensity analysis of the radial artery versus the free right internal thoracic artery to bypass the circumflex coronary artery. *The Journal of Thoracic and Cardiovascular Surgery*, *147*(1), 133–140. doi:10.1016/j.jtcvs.2013.08.040 PMID:24100104

Trento, A., Hardesty, R., Griffith, B., Zerbe, T., Kormos, R., & Bahnson, H. (1988). Role Of The Antibody To Vascular Endothelial Cells In Hyperacute Rejection In Patients Undergoing Cardiac Transplantation. *The Journal of Thoracic and Cardiovascular Surgery*, *95*(1), 37–41. PMID:2447445

Trettin, A., Böhmer, A., Suchy, M. T., Probst, I., Staerk, U., & Stichtenoth, D. O. ... Tsikas, D. (2014). Effects of paracetamol on NOS, COX, and CYP activity and on oxidative stress in healthy male subjects, rat hepatocytes, and recombinant NOS. *Oxidative Medicine and Cellular Longevity*. doi:10.1155/2014/212576 PMID:24799980

Triantafillou, A. N., Pasque, M. K., Huddleston, C. B., Pond, C. G., Cerza, R. F., Forstot, R. M., & Lappas, D. G. et al. (1994). Predictors, frequency, and indications for cardiopulmonary bypass during lung transplantation in adults. *The Annals of Thoracic Surgery*, *57*(5), 1248–1251. doi:10.1016/0003-4975(94)91367-6

Tribouilloy, C. M., Enriquez-Sarano, M., Schaff, H. V., Orszulak, T. A., Bailey, K. R., Tajik, A. J., & Frye, R. L. (1999). Impact of preoperative symptoms on survival after surgical correction of organic mitral regurgitation: Rationale for optimizing surgical indications. *Circulation*, *99*(3), 400–405. doi:10.1161/01.CIR.99.3.400 PMID:9918527

Troianos, C. A., Hartman, G. S., Glas, K. E., Skubas, N. J., Eberhardt, R. T., Walker, J. D., & Reeves, S. T. (2011). Guidelines for Performing Ultrasound Guided Vascular Cannulation: Recommendations of the American Society of Echocardiography and the Society of Cardiovascular Anesthesiologists. *Journal of the American Society of Echocardiography*, *24*(12), 1291–1318. doi:10.1016/j.echo.2011.09.021 PMID:22115322

Truog, R. D., Campbell, M. L., Curtis, J. R., Haas, C. E., Luce, J. M., Rubenfeld, G. D., & Kaufman, D. C. et al. (2008). Recommendations for end-of-life care in the intensive care unit: A consensus statement by the American College [corrected] of Critical Care Medicine. *Critical Care Medicine*, *36*(3), 953–963. doi:10.1097/CCM.0B013E3181659096 PMID:18431285

Tsai, B., Turrentine, M. W., Sheridan, B. C., Wang, M., Fiore, A. C., Brown, J. W., & Meldrum, D. R. (2006). Differential Effects of Phosphodiesterase-5 Inhibitors on Hypoxic Pulmonary Vasoconstriction and Pulmonary Artery Cytokine Expression. *The Annals of Thoracic Surgery*, *81*(1), 272–278. doi:10.1016/j.athoracsur.2005.06.040 PMID:16368379

Tsai, T. C., Joynt, K. E., Orav, E. J., Gawande, A. A., & Jha, A. K. (2013). Variation in surgical-readmission rates and quality of hospital care. *The New England Journal of Medicine*, *369*(12), 1134–1142. doi:10.1056/NEJMsa1303118 PMID:24047062

Tsiotos, G. G., Mullany, C. J., Zietlow, S., & van Heerden, J. (1994). Abdominal complications following cardiac surgery. *American Journal of Surgery*, *167*(6), 553–557. doi:10.1016/0002-9610(94)90096-5 PMID:8209926

Tu, C. P., Tsai, C. H., Tsai, C. C., Huang, T. S., Cheng, S. P., & Liu, T. P. (2014). Postoperative ileus in the elderly. *International Journal of Gerontology*, *8*(1), 1–5. doi:10.1016/j.ijge.2013.08.002

Tufo, H. M., Ostfeld, A. M., & Shekelle, R. (1970). Central nervous system dysfunction following open-heart surgery. *Journal of the American Medical Association*, *212*(8), 1333–1340. doi:10.1001/jama.1970.03170210039006 PMID:5467674

Turina, J., Hess, O., Sepulcri, F., & Krayenbuehl, H. P. (1987). Spontaneous course of aortic valve disease. *European Heart Journal*, *8*(5), 471–483. PMID:3609042

Tweed, W. A., Minuck, M., & Mymin, D. (1972). Circulatory responses to ketamine anesthesia. *Anesthesiology*, *37*(6), 613–619. doi:10.1097/00000542-197212000-00008 PMID:4652778

Twele, L., Moyen, E., Zhang, K., Dalton, B., Church, D., & Conly, J. (2010). Methicillin-resistant Staphylococcus aureus endocarditis and de novo development of daptomycin resistance during therapy. *The Canadian Journal of Infectious Diseases & Medical Microbiology = Journal Canadien des Maladies Infectieuses et de la Microbiologie Medicale / AMMI Canada*, *21*, 89–93. PMID:21629617

Tyler, R. W. (2013). *Basic Principles of Curriculum and Instruction*. University of Chicago Press. doi:10.7208/chicago/9780226086644.001.0001

Ucer, E., Gungor, B., Erdinler, I. C., Akyol, A., Alper, A. T., Eksik, A., & Ulufer, T. et al. (2008). High sensitivity CRP levels predict atrial tachyarrhythmias in rheumatic mitral stenosis. *Annals of Noninvasive Electrocardiology*, *13*(1), 31–38. doi:10.1111/j.1542-474X.2007.00198.x PMID:18234004

Uchino S, et al., (2006). Pulmonary artery catheter versus pulse contour analysis: a prospective epidemiological study. *Critical Care, 10*(6), R 174.

Udy, A. A., Roberts, J. A., & Lipman, J. (2013). Clinical implications of antibiotic pharmacokinetic principles in the critically ill. *Intensive Care Medicine*, *39*(12), 2070–2082. doi:10.1007/s00134-013-3088-4 PMID:24045886

Uhlig, C., Silva, P. L., Deckert, S., Schmitt, J., & de Abreu, M. G. (2014). Albumin versus crystalloid solutions in patients with the acute respiratory distress syndrome: A systematic review and meta-analysis. *Critical Care (London, England)*, *18*(2), R10. doi:10.1186/cc13187

Ullman, A. J., Cooke, M. L., Gillies, D., Marsh, N. M., Daud, A., McGrail, M. R., & Rickard, C. M. et al. (2013). Optimal timing for intravascular administration set replacement. *Cochrane Database of Systematic Reviews*, CD003588. PMID:24037784

Umpierrez, G. E., Hellman, R., Korytkowski, M. T., Kosiborod, M., Maynard, G. A., Montori, V. M., & Van den Berghe, G. et al. (2012). Management of hyperglycemia in hospitalized patients in non-critical care setting: An Endocrine Society clinical practice guideline. *The Journal of Clinical Endocrinology and Metabolism*, *97*(1), 16–38. doi:10.1210/jc.2011-2098 PMID:22223765

Unahalekhaka, A., Jamulitrat, S., Chongsuvivatwong, V., & Ovretveit, J. (2007). Using a collaborative to reduce ventilator-associated pneumonia in Thailand. *Joint Commission Journal on Quality and Patient Safety*, *33*(7), 387–394. PMID:17711140

Unlu, Y., Velioglu, Y., Kocak, H., Becit, N., & Ceviz, M. (2007). Brachial plexus injury following median sternotomy. *Interactive Cardiovascular and Thoracic Surgery*, *6*(2), 235–237. doi:10.1510/icvts.2006.137380 PMID:17669822

Unverferth, D. A., Blanford, M., Kates, R. E., & Leier, C. V. (1980). Tolerance to dobutamine after a 72 hour continuous infusion. *The American Journal of Medicine*, *69*(2), 262–266. doi:10.1016/0002-9343(80)90387-3 PMID:7405947

Vahanian, A., Alfieri, O., Andreotti, F., Antunes, M. J., Baron-Esquivias, G., Baumgartner, H., & Zembala, M. et al. (2012). Guidelines on the management of valvular heart disease (version 2012). *European Heart Journal*, *33*(19), 2451–2496. doi:10.1093/eurheartj/ehs109 PMID:22922415

Vahanian, A., Alfieri, O., Andreotti, F., Antunes, M. J., Barón-Esquivias, G., Baumgartner, H., & Zembala, M. et al. (2012). Guidelines on the management of valvular heart disease (version 2012): The Joint Task Force on the Management of Valvular Heart Disease of the European Society of Cardiology (ESC) and the European Association for Cardio-Thoracic Surgery (EACTS). *European Journal of Cardio-Thoracic Surgery*, *42*(4), S1–S44. doi:10.1093/ejcts/ezs455 PMID:22922698

Vahl, C. F., Carl, I., Muller-Vahl, H., & Struck, E. (1991). Brachial plexus injury after cardiac surgery. The role of internal mammary artery preparation: A prospective study on 1000 consecutive patients. *The Journal of Thoracic and Cardiovascular Surgery*, *102*(5), 724–729. PMID:1682532

Valeri, C. R., Cassidy, G., Pivacek, L. E., Ragno, G., Lieberthal, W., Crowley, J. P., & Loscalzo, J. et al. (2001). Anemia-induced increase in the bleeding time: Implications for treatment of nonsurgical blood loss. *Transfusion*, *41*(8), 977–983. doi:10.1046/j.1537-2995.2001.41080977.x

Valeri, C. R., Feingold, H., Cassidy, G., Ragno, G., Khuri, S., & Altschule, M. D. (1987). Hypothermia-induced reversible platelet dysfunction. *Annals of Surgery*, *205*(2), 175–181. doi:10.1097/00000658-198702000-00012 PMID:3813688

Vallés, J., Fernández, I., Alcaraz, D., Chacón, E., Cazorla, A., Canals, M., & Morón, A. et al. (2008). Prospective randomized trial of 3 antiseptic solutions for prevention of catheter colonization in an intensive care unit for adult patients. *Infection Control and Hospital Epidemiology*, *29*(9), 847–853. doi:10.1086/590259 PMID:18665819

Van den Berghe, G. (2002). Neuroendocrine pathobiology of chronic critical illness. *Critical Care Clinics*, *18*(3), 509–528. doi:10.1016/S0749-0704(02)00007-6 PMID:12140911

Van den Berghe, G., Baxter, R. C., Weekers, F., Wouters, P., Bowers, C. Y., Iranmanesh, A., & Bouillon, R. et al. (2002). The combined administration of GH-releasing peptide-2 (GHRP-2), TRH and GnRH to men with prolonged critical illness evokes superior endocrine and metabolic effects compared to treatment with GHRP-2 alone. *Horumon To Rinsho*, *56*, 655–669. PMID:12030918

Van den Berghe, G., Wilmer, A., Hermans, G., Meersseman, W., Wouters, P. J., Milants, I., & Bouillon, R. et al. (2006). Intensive insulin therapy in the medical ICU. *The New England Journal of Medicine*, *354*(5), 449–461. doi:10.1056/NEJMoa052521 PMID:16452557

Van den Berghe, G., Wilmer, A., Milants, I., Wouters, P. J., Bouckaert, B., Bruyninckx, F., & Schetz, M. et al. (2006). Intensive insulin therapy in mixed medical/surgical intensive care units. *Diabetes*, *55*(11), 3151–3159. doi:10.2337/db06-0855 PMID:17065355

Van den Berghe, G., Wouters, P., Weekers, F., Verwaest, C., Bruyninckx, F., Schetz, M., & Bouillon, R. et al. (2001). Intensive insulin therapy in critically ill patients. *The New England Journal of Medicine*, *345*(19), 1359–1367. doi:10.1056/NEJMoa011300 PMID:11794168

Van der linden, J., Hadjinikolaou, L., & Bergman, P. (2001). Postoperative stroke in cardiac surgery is related to the location and extent of atherosclerotic disease inthe ascending aorta. *J Am Coll Cardiol, 38*(1), 131-135.

Van der Mast, R. C., & Roest, F. H. (1996). Delirium after cardiac surgery: A critical review. *Journal of Psychosomatic Research*, *41*(1), 13–30. http://www.ncbi.nlm.nih.gov/pubmed/8887815 doi:10.1016/0022-3999(96)00005-0 PMID:8887815

Van Der Vleuten, C. (1996). The assessment of professional competence: Developments, research and practical implications. *Advances in Health Sciences Education: Theory and Practice*, *1*(1), 41–67. doi:10.1007/BF00596229 PMID:24178994

Van der Vleuten, C. P., Norman, G. R., & De Graaff, E. (1991). Pitfalls in the pursuit of objectivity: Issues of reliability. *Medical Education*, *25*(2), 110–118. doi:10.1111/j.1365-2923.1991.tb00036.x PMID:2023552

van der Wilden, G. M., Schmidt, U., Chang, Y., Bittner, E. A., Cobb, J. P., Velmahos, G. C., & King, D. R. et al. (2013). Implementation of 24/7 intensivist presence in the SICU: Effect on processes of care. *Journal of Trauma and Acute Care Surgery*, *74*(2), 563–567. doi:10.1097/TA.0b013e31827880a8 PMID:23354251

Van Dijk, D., Keizer, A. M. A., Diephuis, J. C., Durand, C., Vos, L. J., & Hijman, R. (2000). Neurocognitive dysfunction after coronary artery bypass surgery: A systematic review. *The Journal of Thoracic and Cardiovascular Surgery*, *120*(4), 632–639. doi:10.1067/mtc.2000.108901 PMID:11003741

Van Gulik, L., Ahlers, S. J., Brkic, Z., Belitser, S. V., van Boven, W. J., van Dongen, E. P., & Bruins, P. et al. (2010). Improved analgesia after the realisation of a pain management programme in ICU patients after cardiac surgery. *European Journal of Anaesthesiology*, *27*(10), 900–905. doi:10.1097/EJA.0b013e32833d91c3 PMID:20848698

Van Hagen, P., Hulshof, M., Van Lanschot, J., Steyerberg, E., Van Berge Henegouwen, M., Wijnhoven, B., & Van der Gaast, A. (2012). Preoperative chemoradiotherapy for esophageal or junctional cancer. *The New England Journal of Medicine*, *366*(22), 2074–2084. doi:10.1056/NEJMoa1112088 PMID:22646630

Van Reit, J., Hill, E. E., Gheysens, O., Dymarkowski, S., Herregods, M., Herijgers, P., & Mortelmans, L. et al. (2010). ^{18}F-FDG PET/CT for early detection of embolism and metastatic infection in patients with infective endocarditis. *European Journal of Nuclear Medicine and Molecular Imaging*, *37*(6), 1189–1197. doi:10.1007/s00259-010-1380-x PMID:20204357

Van Sickle, K. R., Ritter, E. M., & Smith, C. D. (2006). The pretrained novice: Using simulation-based training to improve learning in the operating room. *Surgical Innovation*, *13*(3), 198–204. doi:10.1177/1553350606293370 PMID:17056786

van Straten, A. H. M., Hamad, M. A. S., van Zundert, A. J., Martens, E. J., Schönberger, J. P. A. M., & de Wolf, A. M. (2009). Preoperative hemoglobin level as a predictor of survival after coronary artery bypass grafting: A comparison with the matched general population. *Circulation*, *120*(2), 118–125. doi:10.1161/CIRCULATIONAHA.109.854216 PMID:19564556

Van Zanten, A. R. H., Sztark, F., Kaisers, U. X., Zielmann, S., Felbinger, T. W., Sablotzki, A. R., & Hofman, Z. et al. (2014). High-protein enteral nutrition enriched with immune-modulating nutrients vs standard high-protein enteral nutrition and nosocomial infections in the ICU: A randomized clinical trial. *Journal of the American Medical Association*, *312*(5), 514–524. doi:10.1001/jama.2014.7698 PMID:25096691

Vanden Hoek, T. L., Morrison, L. J., Shuster, M., Donnino, M., Sinz, E., Lavonas, E. J., & Gabrielli, A. et al. (2010). Part 12: cardiac arrest in special situations: 2010 American Heart Association Guidelines for Cardiopulmonary Resuscitation and Emergency Cardiovascular Care. *Circulation*, *122*(18Suppl 3), S829–S861. doi:10.1161/CIRCULATIONAHA.110.971069 PMID:20956228

Vander Salm, T. J., Cereda, J. M., & Cutler, B. S. (1980). Brachial plexus injury following median sternotomy. *The Journal of Thoracic and Cardiovascular Surgery*, *80*(3), 447–452. PMID:7412350

Vane, J. R., Bakhle, Y. S., & Botting, R. M. (1998). Cyclooxygenases 1 and 2. *Annual Review of Pharmacology and Toxicology*, *38*(1), 97–120. doi:10.1146/annurev.pharmtox.38.1.97 PMID:9597150

Vanhorebeek, I., Gunst, J., Derde, S., Derese, I., Boussemaere, M., Guiza, F., & Van den Berghe, G. et al. (2011). Insufficient activation of autophagy allows cellular damage to accumulate in critically ill patients. *The Journal of Clinical Endocrinology and Metabolism*, *96*(4), E633–E645. doi:10.1210/jc.2010-2563 PMID:21270330

vanWerkum, J., Kleibeuker, M., Postma, S., Bouman, H. J., Elsenberg, E. H., ten Berg, J. M., & Hackeng, C. M. (2010). A comparison between plateletworks assay and light transmittance aggregometry for monitoring the inhibitory effects of clopidogrel. *International Journal of Cardiology*, *140*(1), 123–126. doi:10.1016/j.ijcard.2008.10.046 PMID:19091430

Vanwijngaerden, Y. M., Wauters, J., Langouche, L., Vander Perre, S., Liddle, C., Coulter, S., & Mesotten, D. et al. (2011). Critical illness evokes elevated circulating bile acids related to altered hepatic transporter and nuclear receptor expression. *Hepatology (Baltimore, Md.)*, *54*(5), 1741–1752. doi:10.1002/hep.24582 PMID:21800341

Varenhorst, C., Alstrom, U., Scirica, B., Hogue, C., Asenblad, N., Storey, R., & Held, C. et al. (2012). Factors Contributing to the Lower Mortality With Ticagrelor Compared with Clopidogrel in Patients Undergoing Coronary Artery Bypass Surgery. *Journal of the American College of Cardiology*, *60*(17), 1623–20. PMID:23021325

Varghese, R., & Adams, D.H. (2014). Techniques in repairing posterior leaflet prolapse. *Operative Techniques in Thoracic and Cardiovascular Surgery* (pp. 293-308). Academic Press.

Varghese, R., Akujuo, A., & Adams, D. H. (2010). Right coronary artery injury after tricuspid valve repair. *Seminars in Thoracic and Cardiovascular Surgery*, *22*(2), 189–190. doi:10.1053/j.semtcvs.2010.09.004 PMID:21092900

Varghese, R., Anyanwu, A. C., Itagaki, S., Milla, F., Castillo, J., & Adams, D. H. (2012). Management of systolic anterior motion after mitral valve repair: An algorithm. *The Journal of Thoracic and Cardiovascular Surgery*, *143*(4Suppl), S2–S7. doi:10.1016/j.jtcvs.2012.01.063 PMID:22423603

Varghese, R., Itagaki, S., Anyanwu, A. C., Milla, F., & Adams, D. H. (2014). Predicting early left ventricular dysfunction after mitral valve reconstruction: The effect of atrial fibrillation and pulmonary hypertension. *The Journal of Thoracic and Cardiovascular Surgery*, *148*(2), 422–427. doi:10.1016/j.jtcvs.2013.08.073 PMID:24176266

Varghese, R., Itagaki, S., Anyanwu, A. C., Trigo, P., Fischer, G., & Adams, D. H. (2014). Predicting systolic anterior motion after mitral valve reconstruction: Using intraoperative transoesophageal echocardiography to identify those at greatest risk. *European Journal of Cardio-Thoracic Surgery*, *45*(1), 132–137, discussion 137–138. doi:10.1093/ejcts/ezt234 PMID:23657548

Vassiliadi, D. A., Ilias, I., Tzanela, M., Nikitas, N., Theodorakopoulou, M., Kopteridea, P., & Dimopoulou, I. et al. (2013). Interstitial cortisol obtained by microdialysis in mechanically ventilated septic patients: Correlations with total and free serum cortisol. *Journal of Critical Care*, *28*, 158–165. PMID:22981531

Velazquez, E. J., Lee, K. L., Deja, M. A., Jain, A., Sopko, G., Marchenko, A., & Rouleau, J. et al. (2011). Coronary-Artery Bypass Surgery in Patients with Left Ventricular Dysfunction. *The New England Journal of Medicine*, *364*(17), 1607–1616. doi:10.1056/NEJMoa1100356 PMID:21463150

Velik-Salchner, C., Maier, S., Innerhofer, P., Kolbitsch, C., Streif, W., Mittermayr, M., & Fries, D. et al. (2009). An assessment of cardiopulmonary bypass-induced changes in platelet function using whole blood and classical light transmission aggregometry: The results of a pilot study. *Anesthesia and Analgesia*, *108*(6), 1747–1754. doi:10.1213/ane.0b013e3181a198ac PMID:19448196

Velissaris, T., Tang, A., Murray, M., El-Minshawy, A., Hett, D., & Ohri, S. (2003). A prospective randomized study to evaluate splanchnic hypoxia during beating-heart and conventional coronary revascularization. *European Journal of Cardio-Thoracic Surgery*, *23*(6), 917–924. doi:10.1016/S1010-7940(03)00167-2 PMID:12829067

Venn, R. (2002). Randomized controlled trial to investigate influence of the fluid challenge on duration of hospital stay and perioperative morbidity in patients with hip fractures. *British Journal of Anaesthesia*, *88*(1), 65–67. doi:10.1093/bja/88.1.65 PMID:11881887

Venn, R. M., Hell, J., & Grounds, R. M. (2000). Respiratory effects of dexmedetomidine in the surgical patient requiring intensive care. *Critical Care (London, England)*, *4*(5), 302–308. doi:10.1186/cc712 PMID:11056756

Verapamil. (2013). In *Official FDA Information, Side effects and Uses*. Retrieved from http://www.drugs.com/verapamil.html

Verma, S., Fedak, P. W., Weisel, R. D., Butany, J., Rao, V., Maitland, A., & Yau, T. M. et al. (2002). Fundamentals of reperfusion injury for the clinical cardiologist. *Circulation*, *105*(20), 2332–2336. doi:10.1161/01.CIR.0000016602.96363.36 PMID:12021216

Verma, S., & Siu, S. C. (2014). Aortic dilatation in patients with bicuspid aortic valve. *The New England Journal of Medicine*, *370*(20), 1920–1929. doi:10.1056/NEJMra1207059 PMID:24827036

Vermes, I., Beishuizen, A., Hampsink, R. M., & Haanen, C. (1995). Dissociation of plasma adrenocorticotropin and cortisol levels in critically ill patients: Possible role of endothelin and atrial natriuretic hormone. *The Journal of Clinical Endocrinology and Metabolism*, *80*(4), 1238–1242. PMID:7714094

Veroli, P., O'Kelly, B., Bertrand, F., Trouvin, J. H., Farinotti, R., & Ecoffey, C. (1992). Extrahepatic metabolism of propofol in man during the anhepatic phase of orthotopic liver transplantation. *British Journal of Anaesthesia*, *68*(2), 183–186. doi:10.1093/bja/68.2.183 PMID:1540462

Verrier, E. D., Shernan, S. K., Taylor, K. M., Van de Werf, F., Newman, M. F., Chen, J. C., & Levy, J. H. et al.for the PRIMO-CABG Investigators. (2004). Terminal complement blockade with pexelizumab during coronary artery bypass graft surgery requiring cardiopulmonary bypass: A randomized trial. *Journal of the American Medical Association*, *291*(19), 2319–2327. doi:10.1001/jama.291.19.2319 PMID:15150203

Via, M. A., Scurlock, C., Adams, D. H., Weiss, A. J., & Mechanick, J. I. (2010). Impaired postoperative hyperglycemic stress response associated with increased mortality in patients in the cardiothoracic surgery intensive care unit. *Endocrine Practice*, *16*(5), 798–804. doi:10.4158/EP10017.OR PMID:20350912

Viana, F. F., Chen, Y., Almeida, A., Baxter, H. D., Cochrane, A. D., & Smith, J. (2013). Gastrointestinal complications after cardiac surgery: 10-year experience of a single australian centre. *ANZ Journal of Surgery*, *83*(9), 651–656. doi:10.1111/ans.12134 PMID:23530720

Vicchio, M., Della Corte, A., De Santo, L. S., De Feo, M., Caianiello, G., Scardone, M., & Cotrufo, M. (2008). Tissue versus mechanical prostheses: Quality of life in octogenarians. *The Annals of Thoracic Surgery*, *85*(4), 1290–1295. doi:10.1016/j.athoracsur.2007.12.039 PMID:18355512

Vidal, M. G., Ruiz Weisser, J., Gonzalez, F., Toro, M. A., Loudet, C., Balasini, C., & Estenssoro, E. et al. (2008). Incidence and clinical effects of intra-abdominal hypertension in critically ill patients. *Critical Care Medicine*, *36*(6), 1823–1831. doi:10.1097/CCM.0b013e31817c7a4d PMID:18520642

Vida, V. L., Mack, R., & Castaneda, A. R. (2005). The role of vasopressin in treating systemic inflammatory syndrome complicated by right ventricular failure. *Cardiology in the Young*, *15*(1), 88–90. doi:10.1017/S1047951105000193 PMID:15831170

Vieillard-Baron, A., Slama, M., Mayo, P., Charron, C., Amiel, J.-B., Esterez, C., & Vignon, P. et al. (2013). A pilot study on safety and clinical utility of a single-use 72-hour indwelling transesophageal echocardiography probe. *Intensive Care Medicine*, *39*(4), 629–635. doi:10.1007/s00134-012-2797-4 PMID:23287876

Vignon, P. (2012). PRO: physician-performed ultrasound: the time has come for routine use in acute care medicine. *Anesthesia and Analgesia*, *115*(5), 999–1003. doi:10.1213/ANE.0b013e31826bfa7d PMID:23093581

Vignon, P., Mücke, F., Bellec, F., Marin, B., Croce, J., Brouqui, T., & Amiel, J.-B. et al. (2011). Basic critical care echocardiography: Validation of a curriculum dedicated to noncardiologist residents*. *Critical Care Medicine*, *39*(4), 636–642. doi:10.1097/CCM.0b013e318206c1e4 PMID:21221001

Villanueva, C., Colomo, A., Bosch, A., Concepción, M., Hernandez-Gea, V., Aracil, C., & Guarner, C. et al. (2013). Transfusion strategies for acute upper gastrointestinal bleeding. *The New England Journal of Medicine*, *368*(1), 11–21. doi:10.1056/NEJMoa1211801 PMID:23281973

Vind, S. H., & Hess, S. (2010). Possible role of PET/CT in infective endocarditis. *Journal of Nuclear Cardiology*, *17*(3), 516–519. doi:10.1007/s12350-009-9174-x PMID:19953353

Vital signs: central line-associated blood stream infections--United States, 2001, 2008, and 2009. (2011). *MMWR Morbidity and Mortality Weekly Report, 60*(8), 243-248.

Vivacqua, A., Koch, C. G., Yousuf, A. M., Nowicki, E. R., Houghtaling, P. L., Blackstone, E. H., & Sabik, J. F. III. (2011). Morbidity of bleeding after cardiac surgery: Is it blood transfusion, reoperation for bleeding, or both? *The Annals of Thoracic Surgery, 91*(6), 1780–1790. doi:10.1016/j.athoracsur.2011.03.105 PMID:21619974

Vives, M., Wijeysundera, D., & Rao, V. (2014). Cardiac surgery-associated acute kidney injury. *Interactive Cardiovascular and Thoracic Surgery*, 1–9. doi:10.1093/icvts/ivu014 PMID:24535092

Vlahakes, G. J. (2012). Right Ventricular Failure After Cardiac Surgery. *Cardiology Clinics, 30*(2), 283-289. Retrieved From http://www.sciencedirect.com/science/article/pii/s073386511200029x

Vuylsteke, A., Pagel, C., Gerrard, C., Reddy, B., Nashef, S., Aldam, P., & Utley, M. (2011). The Papworth Bleeding Risk Score: A stratification scheme for identifying cardiac surgery patients at risk of excessive early postoperative bleeding. *European Journal of Cardio-Thoracic Surgery : Official Journal of the European Association for Cardio-Thoracic Surgery, 39*(6), 924–930. doi:10.1016/j.ejcts.2010.10.003 PMID:21094051

Wademan, B. H., & Galvin, S. D. (2014). Desmopressin for reducing postoperative blood loss and transfusion requirements following cardiac surgery in adults. *Interactive Cardiovascular and Thoracic Surgery, 18*(3), 360–370. doi:10.1093/icvts/ivt491 PMID:24263581

Wagner, F. M. (2011a). Donor Heart Preservation And Perfusion. *Applied Cardiopulmonary Pathophysiology, 15*, 198–206.

Wagner, F. M. (2011b). Monitoring And Management Of Right Ventricular Function Following Cardiac Transplantation. *Applied Cardiopulmonary Pathophysiology, 15*, 220–229.

Wagnetz, D., & de Perrot, M. (2011). Postthoracotomy surgical management and complications. In P. D. Slinger (Ed.), *Principles and Practice of Anesthesia for Thoracic Surgery* (pp. 661–673). New York: Springer. doi:10.1007/978-1-4419-0184-2_45

Wahr, J. A., Parks, R., Boisvert, D., Comunale, M., Fabian, J., Ramsay, J., & Mangano, D. T. (1999). Preoperative serum potassium levels and perioperative outcomes in cardiac surgery patients. Multicenter Study of Perioperative Ischemia Research Group. *Journal of the American Medical Association, 281*(23), 2203–2210. doi:10.1001/jama.281.23.2203 PMID:10376573

Wakeling, H. G., Barclay, G. R., & Fleming, S. C. (2005). Intraoperative Oesophageal Doppler guided fluid management shortens postoperative hospital stay after major bowel surgery. *British Journal of Anaesthesia, 95*(5), 634–642. doi:10.1093/bja/aei223 PMID:16155038

Wald, H. L., Ma, A., Bratzler, D. W., & Kramer, A. M. (2008). Indwelling urinary catheter use in the postoperative period: Analysis of the National Surgical Infection Prevention Project data. *Archives of Surgery, 143*(6), 551–557. doi:10.1001/archsurg.143.6.551 PMID:18559747

Wald, R., Liangos, O., Perianayagam, M. C., Kolyada, A., Herget-Rosenthal, S., Mazer, C. D., & Jaber, B. L. (2010). Plasma Cystatin C and Acute Kidney Injury after Cardiopulmonary Bypass. *Clinical Journal of the American Society of Nephrology; CJASN, 5*(8), 1373–1379. doi:10.2215/CJN.06350909 PMID:20522534

Waldron, N. (2012). *A Prospective Comparison of Outcomes in NICOM- Versus EDM-Guided Goal Directed Fluid Therapy*. Duke Anesthesia Celebration of Research.

Walkden, G. J., Verheyden, V., Goudie, R., & Murphy, G. J. (2013). Increased perioperative mortality following aprotinin withdrawal: A real-world analysis of blood management strategies in adult cardiac surgery. *Intensive Care Medicine, 39*(10), 1808–1817. doi:10.1007/s00134-013-3020-y PMID:23863975

Walker, T. G., Kalva, S. P., Yeddula, K., Wicky, S., Kundu, S., Drescher, P., & Cardella, J. F. et al. (2010). Clinical practice guideline for endovascular abdominal aortic aneurysm repair. *Journal of Vascular and Interventional Radiology, 21*(11), 1632–1655. doi:10.1016/j.jvir.2010.07.008 PMID:20884242

Walkey, A. J., O'Donnell, M. R., & Wiener, R. S. (2011). Linezolid vs glycopeptide antibiotics for the treatment of suspected methicillin-resistant Staphylococcus aureus nosocomial pneumonia: A meta-analysis of randomized controlled trials. *Chest, 139*(5), 1148–1155. doi:10.1378/chest.10-1556 PMID:20864609

Wallace, D. J., Angus, D. C., Barnato, A. E., Kramer, A. A., & Kahn, J. M. (2012). Nighttime intensivist staffing and mortality among critically ill patients. *The New England Journal of Medicine, 366*(22), 2093–2101. doi:10.1056/NEJMsa1201918 PMID:22612639

Wallentin, L., Becker, R. C., Budaj, A., Cannon, C. P., Emanuelsson, H., Held, C., & Harrington, R. A. et al. (2009). Ticagrelor versus Clopidogrel in Patients with Acute Coronary Syndromes. *The New England Journal of Medicine, 361*(11), 1045–1057. doi:10.1056/NEJMoa0904327 PMID:19717846

Waller, B. F. (1987). Etiology of pure tricuspid regurgitation. *Cardiovascular Clinics, 17*(2), 53–95. PMID:3536106

Wallis, D., Workman, D., Lewis, B., Steen, L., Pifarre, R., & Moran, J. (1999). Failure of early heparin cessation as treatment for heparin-induced thrombocytopenia. *The American Journal of Medicine, 106*(6), 629–635. doi:10.1016/S0002-9343(99)00124-2 PMID:10378620

Walshe, C., & Kevin, L. (2010). *Pulmonary Hypertension in ARDS: Is It Important and Should We Treat It? Evidence Based Practice of Critical Care.* Philadelphia: Saunders Elsevier. doi:10.1016/B978-1-4160-5476-4.00049-3

Walsh, K. (2005). The Rules. *BMJ: British Medical Journal, 331*(7516), 574. doi:10.1136/bmj.331.7516.574

Walton, H. (1997). Small group methods in medical teaching. *Medical Education, 31*(6), 459–464. doi:10.1046/j.1365-2923.1997.00703.x PMID:9463650

Wang, A., Athan, E., Pappas, P. A., Fowler, V. G., Olaison, L., Paré, C., & Cabell, C. H. et al. (2007). Contemporary clinical profile and outcome of prosthetic valve endocarditis. *Journal of the American Medical Association, 297*(12), 1354–1361. doi:10.1001/jama.297.12.1354 PMID:17392239

Wang, F., Pan, W., Wang, H., Wang, S., Pan, S., & Ge, J. (2012). Relationship between thyroid function and ICU mortality: A prospective observation study. *Critical Care (London, England), 16*(1), R11. doi:10.1186/cc11151 PMID:22257427

Wang, H., Gong, M., Zhou, B., & Dai, A. (2009). Comparison of inhaled and intravenous milrinone in patients with pulmonary hypertension undergoing mitral valve surgery. *Advances in Therapy, 26*(4), 462–468. doi:10.1007/s12325-009-0019-4 PMID:19381522

Wang, W., Li, H., Wang, D., Zhu, X., Li, S., Yao, G., & Zhu, S. et al. (2012). Haloperidol prophylaxis decreases delirium incidence in elderly patients after noncardiac surgery: A randomized controlled trial. *Critical Care Medicine, 40*(3), 731–739. doi:10.1097/CCM.0b013e3182376e4f PMID:22067628

Wan, S., Leclerc, J. L., & Vincent, J. L. (1997). Inflammatory response to cardiopulmonary bypass: Mechanisms involved and possible therapeutic strategies. *Chest, 112*(3), 676–692. doi:10.1378/chest.112.3.676 PMID:9315800

Ward, N. S., Afessa, B., Kleinpell, R., Tisherman, S., Ries, M., Howell, M., & Kahn, J. et al. (2013). Intensivist/patient ratios in closed ICUs: A statement from the Society of Critical Care Medicine Taskforce on ICU Staffing. *Critical Care Medicine*, *41*(2), 638–645. doi:10.1097/CCM.0b013e3182741478 PMID:23263586

Wareing, T. H., Davila-Roman, V. G., Barzilai, B., Murphy, S. F., & Kouchoukos, N. T. (1992). Management of the severely atherosclerotic ascending aorta during cardiac operations. A strategy for detection and treatment. *The Journal of Thoracic and Cardiovascular Surgery*, *103*(3), 453–462. Retrieved from http://www.ncbi.nlm.nih.gov/pubmed/1545544 PMID:1545544

Ware, L. B., Golden, J. A., Finkbeiner, W. E., & Matthay, M. A. (1999). Alveolar epithelial fluid transport capacity in reperfusion lung injury after lung transplantation. *American Journal of Respiratory and Critical Care Medicine*, *159*(3), 980–988. doi:10.1164/ajrccm.159.3.9802105

Warkentin, T. E., & Kelton, J. G. (1996). A 14 year study of heparin induced thrombocytopenia. *The American Journal of Medicine*, *101*(5), 502–507. doi:10.1016/S0002-9343(96)00258-6 PMID:8948273

Warnes, C. A., Williams, R. G., Bashore, T. M., Child, J. S., Connolly, H. M., Dearani, J. A., & Webb, G. D. et al. (2008). ACC/AHA 2008 guidelines for the management of adults with congenital heart disease: Executive summary. *Journal of the American College of Cardiology*, *52*(23), e143–e263. doi:10.1016/j.jacc.2008.10.001 PMID:19038677

Warren, D. K., Zack, J. E., Mayfield, J. L., Chen, A., Prentice, D., Fraser, V. J., & Kollef, M. H. (2004). The effect of an education program on the incidence of central venous catheter-associated bloodstream infection in a medical ICU. *Chest*, *126*(5), 1612–1618. doi:10.1378/chest.126.5.1612 PMID:15539735

Watanabe, A., Watanabe, T., Obama, T., Mawatari, T., Ohsawa, H., Ichimiya, Y., & Abe, T. et al. (2004). Prognostic factors for myasthenic crisis after transsternal thymectomy in patients with myasthenia gravis. *The Journal of Thoracic and Cardiovascular Surgery*, *127*(3), 868–876. doi:10.1016/j.jtcvs.2003.07.036 PMID:15001919

Weber, A., Noureddine, H., Englberger, L., Dick, F., Gahl, B., Aymard, T., & Carrel, T. P. et al. (2012). Ten-year comparison of pericardial tissue valves versus mechanical prostheses for aortic valve replacement in patients younger than 60 years of age. *The Journal of Thoracic and Cardiovascular Surgery*, *144*(5), 1075–1083. doi:10.1016/j.jtcvs.2012.01.024 PMID:22341653

Weber, D. J., Sickbert-Bennett, E. E., Gould, C. V., Brown, V. M., Huslage, K., & Rutala, W. A. (2011). Incidence of catheter-associated and non-catheter-associated urinary tract infections in a healthcare system. *Infection Control and Hospital Epidemiology*, *32*(8), 822–823. doi:10.1086/661107 PMID:21768769

Webster, J., & Osborne, S. (2007). Preoperative bathing or showering with skin antiseptics to prevent surgical site infections. *Cochrane Database of Systematic Reviews*, CD004985. PMID:17443562

Weeks, K. R., Hsu, Y. J., Yang, T., Sawyer, M., & Marsteller, J. A. (2014). Influence of a multifaceted intervention on central line days in intensive care units: Results of a national multisite study. *American Journal of Infection Control*, *42*(10Suppl), S197–S202. doi:10.1016/j.ajic.2014.06.003 PMID:25239710

Weerasinghe, A., Athanasiou, T., Philippidis, P., Day, J., Mandal, K., Warren, O., & Taylor, K. et al. (2006). Platelet-monocyte pro-coagulant interactions in on-pump coronary surgery. *European Journal of Cardio-Thoracic Surgery*, *29*(3), 312–318. doi:10.1016/j.ejcts.2005.11.036 PMID:16423536

Weigert, A. L., & Schafer, A. I. (1998). Uremic bleeding: Pathogenesis and therapy. *The American Journal of the Medical Sciences*, *316*(2), 94–104. doi:10.1097/00000441-199808000-00005 PMID:9704663

Weijs, P. J., Stapel, S. N., de Groot, S. D., Driessen, R. H., de Jong, E., Girbes, A. R., & Beishuizen, A. et al. (2012). Optimal protein and energy nutrition decreases mortality in mechanically ventilated, critically ill patients: A prospective observational cohort study. *Journal of Parenteral and Enteral Nutrition*, *36*(1), 60–68. doi:10.1177/0148607111415109 PMID:22167076

Weimar, C., Konig, I. R., Kraywinkel, K., Ziegler, A., & Diener, H. C. (2004). Age and National Institutes of Health Stroke Scale Score within 6 hours after onset are accurate predictors of outcome after cerebral ischemia: Development and external validation of prognostic models. *Stroke*, *35*(1), 158–162. doi:10.1161/01.STR.0000106761.94985.8B PMID:14684776

Weinberger, B., Laskin, D. L., Heck, D. E., & Laskin, J. D. (2001). The Toxicology of Inhaled Nitric Oxide. *Toxicological Sciences*, *59*(1), 5–16. doi:10.1093/toxsci/59.1.5 PMID:11134540

Weintraub, W. S., Grau-Sepulveda, M. V., Weiss, J. M., O'Brien, S. M., Peterson, E. D., Kolm, P., & Edwards, F. H. et al. (2012). Comparative effectiveness of revascularization strategies. *The New England Journal of Medicine*, *366*(16), 1467–1476. doi:10.1056/NEJMoa1110717 PMID:22452338

Weisenack, C. et al.. (2001). Assessment of intrathoracic blood volume as an indicator of cardiac preload: Single transpulmonary thermodilution technique vs assessment of pressure preloadparameters derived from a pulmonary artery catheter. *Journal of Cardiothoracic and Vascular Anesthesia*, *15*(5), 584–588. doi:10.1053/jcan.2001.26536 PMID:11687999

Weiskopf, R. B., & Silverman, T. A. (2013). Balancing potential risks and benefits of hemoglobin-based oxygen carriers. *Transfusion*, *53*(10), 2327–2333. PMID:23869543

Weiss, A. J., & Mechanick, J. M. (2011). Glycemic control: How tight in the intensive care unit? *Seminars in Thoracic and Cardiovascular Surgery*, *23*(1), 1–4. doi:10.1053/j.semtcvs.2011.04.006 PMID:21807288

Weiss, A. J., Zhao, S., Tian, D. H., Taggart, D. P., & Yan, T. D. (2013). A meta-analysis comparing bilateral internal mammary artery with left internal mammary artery for coronary artery bypass grafting. *Annals of Cardiothoracic Surgery*, *2*(4), 390–400. doi:10.3978/j.issn.2225-319X.2013.07.16 PMID:23977614

Weissman, D. E., & Meier, D. E. (2011). Identifying patients in need of a palliative care assessment in the hospital setting: A consensus report from the Center to Advance Palliative Care. *Journal of Palliative Medicine*, *14*(1), 17–23. doi:10.1089/jpm.2010.0347 PMID:21133809

Weissmann, N., Gerigk, B., Kocer, O., Nollen, M., Hackemack, S., Ghofrani, H. A., & Grimminger, F. et al. (2007). Hypoxia-induced pulmonary hypertension: Different impact of iloprost, sildenafil, and nitric oxide. *Respiratory Medicine*, *101*(10), 2125–2132. doi:10.1016/j.rmed.2007.05.025 PMID:17643279

Westaby, S., Anastasiadis, K., & Wieselthaler, G. (2012). Cardiogenic shock in ACS. Part 2: Role of mechanical circulatory support. *Nature Reviews. Cardiology*, *9*(4), 195–208. doi:10.1038/nrcardio.2011.205 PMID:22231716

Westenbrink, B. D., Kleijn, L., de Boer, R. A., Tijssen, J. G., Warnica, W. J., Baillot, R., & van Gilst, W. H. et al. (2011). Sustained postoperative anaemia is associated with an impaired outcome after coronary artery bypass graft surgery: Insights from the IMAGINE trial. *Heart (British Cardiac Society)*, *97*(19), 1590–1596. doi:10.1136/heartjnl-2011-300118 PMID:21757458

West, J. B. (2012). *Respiratory physiology: the essentials* (9th ed.). Philadelphia: Wolters Kluwer Health/Lippincott Williams & Wilkins.

Westley, J. (1973). Rhodanese. *Advances in Enzymology and Related Areas of Molecular Biology*, *39*, 327–368. PMID:4583640

Westley, J., Adler, H., Westley, L., & Nishida, C. (1983). The sulfur transferases. *Fundamental and Applied Toxicology*, *3*(5), 377–382. doi:10.1016/S0272-0590(83)80008-6 PMID:6357923

Whelan, K., Judd, P. A., Preedy, V. R., & Taylor, M. A. (2004). Enteral feeding: The effect on faecal output, the faecal microflora and SCFA concentrations. *The Proceedings of the Nutrition Society*, *63*(1), 105–113. doi:10.1079/PNS2003317 PMID:15099408

Whelton, A., & Hamilton, C. W. (1991). Nonsteroidal anti-inflammatory drugs: Effects on kidney function. *Journal of Clinical Pharmacology*, *31*(7), 588–598. doi:10.1002/j.1552-4604.1991.tb03743.x PMID:1894754

White, H., Assmann, S. F., Sanborn, T. A., Jacobs, A. K., Webb, J. G., Sleeper, L. A., & Hochman, J. S. et al. (2005). Comparison of Percutaneous Coronary Intervention and Coronary Artery Bypass Graft After Acute Myocardial Infarction Complicated by Cardiogenic Shock. *Circulation*, *112*(13), 1992–2001. doi:10.1161/CIRCULATIONAHA.105.540948 PMID:16186436

White, P. F., Way, W. L., & Trevor, A. J. (1982). Ketamine- its pharmacology and therapeutic uses. *Anesthesiology*, *56*(2), 119–136. doi:10.1097/00000542-198202000-00007 PMID:6892475

White, R. A., Miller, D. C., Criado, F. J., Dake, M. D., Diethrich, E. B., Greenberg, R. K., & Siami, F. S. et al. (2011). Report on the results of thoracic endovascular aortic repair for acute, complicated, type B aortic dissection at 30 days and 1 year from a multidisciplinary subcommittee of the Society for Vascular Surgery Outcomes Committee. *Journal of Vascular Surgery*, *53*(4), 1082–1090. doi:10.1016/j.jvs.2010.11.124 PMID:21334174

Whiting, D., & DiNardo, J. A. (2014). TEG and ROTEM: Technology and clinical applications. *American Journal of Hematology*, *89*(2), 228–232. doi:10.1002/ajh.23599 PMID:24123050

Whitlock, R. P., Sun, J. C., Fremes, S. E., Rubens, F. D., Teoh, K. H., & American College of Chest, P. (2012). Antithrombotic and thrombolytic therapy for valvular disease: Antithrombotic Therapy and Prevention of Thrombosis, 9th ed: American College of Chest Physicians Evidence-Based Clinical Practice Guidelines. *Chest, 141*(2 Suppl), e576S-600S. doi: 10.1378/chest.11-2305

Whitlock, E. L., Torres, B. A., Lin, N., Helsten, D. L., Nadelson, M. R., Mashour, G. A., & Avidan, M. S. (2014). Postoperative delirium in a substudy of cardiothoracic surgical patients in the BAG-RECALL clinical trial. *Anesthesia and Analgesia*, *118*(4), 809–817. doi:10.1213/ANE.0000000000000028 PMID:24413548

Whitlock, R. P., Chan, S., Devereaux, J. P., Sun, J., Rubens, F. D., Thorlund, K., & Teoh, K. H. T. (2008). Clinical benefit of steroid use in patients undergoing cardiopulmonary bypass: A meta-analysis of randomized trials. *European Heart Journal*, *29*(21), 2592–2600. doi:10.1093/eurheartj/ehn333 PMID:18664462

Whitlock, R. P., Sun, J. C., Fremes, S. E., Rubens, F. D., & Teoh, K. H. (2012). Antithrombotic and thrombolytic therapy for valvular disease. *Chest*, *141*(2), e576s–e600s. PMID:22315272

Whitlock, R., Crowther, M. A., & Ng, H. J. (2005). Bleeding in cardiac surgery: Its prevention and treatment--an evidence-based review. *Critical Care Clinics*, *21*(3), 589–610. doi:10.1016/j.ccc.2005.04.003 PMID:15992674

Whitman, G. J., Haddad, M., Hirose, H., Allen, J. G., Lusardi, M., & Murphy, M. A. (2011). Cardiothoracic surgeon management of postoperative cardiac critical care. *Archives of Surgery*, *146*(11), 1253–1260. doi:10.1001/archsurg.2011.298 PMID:22106316

Widmer, A. F. (2000). Replace hand washing with use of a waterless alcohol hand rub? *Clinical Infectious Diseases*, *31*(1), 136–143. doi:10.1086/313888 PMID:10913411

Wiesenack, C. L. A., & Philipp, A. (2004). Four years' experience with a miniaturized extracorporeal circulation system and its influence on clinical outcomes. *Artificial Organs*, *28*(12), 1082–1088. doi:10.1111/j.1525-1594.2004.00030.x PMID:15554936

Wiesen, P., Van Gossum, A., & Preiser, J.-C. (2006). Diarrhoea in the critically ill. *Current Opinion in Critical Care*, *12*(2), 149–154. doi:10.1097/01.ccx.0000216583.64804.46 PMID:16543792

Wigfield, C. H., Lindsey, J. D., Steffens, T. G., Edwards, N. M., & Love, R. B. (2007). Early institution of extracorporeal membrane oxygenation for primary graft dysfunction after lung transplantation improves outcome. *The Journal of Heart and Lung Transplantation*, *26*(4), 331–338. doi:10.1016/j.healun.2006.12.010

Wiki. (n.d.). Wiki. *Merriam-Webster.com*. Retrieved May 11, 2014, from http://www.merriam-webster.com/dictionary/wiki

Wikkelsø, A. (Ed.). (2013). Fibrinogen concentrate in bleeding patients. *Cochrane Database of Systematic Reviews*, *8*, CD008864. PMID:23986527

Wikkelsoe, A. J., Afshari, A., Wetterslev, J., Brok, J., & Moeller, A. M. (2011). Monitoring patients at risk of massive transfusion with Thrombelastography or Thromboelastometry: A systematic review. *Acta Anaesthesiologica Scandinavica*, *55*(10), 1174–1189. doi:10.1111/j.1399-6576.2011.02534.x PMID:22092122

Wilcox, B. R. (2004). *Surgical Anatomy of the Heart*. Cambridge, UK: Cambridge University Press.

Wilcox, M. E., Chong, C. A., Niven, D. J., Rubenfeld, G. D., Rowan, K. M., Wunsch, H., & Fan, E. (2013). Do intensivist staffing patterns influence hospital mortality following ICU admission? A systematic review and meta-analyses. *Critical Care Medicine*, *421*(10), 2253–2274. doi:10.1097/CCM.0b013e318292313a PMID:23921275

Wilcox, M. E., Harrison, D. A., Short, A., Jonas, M., & Rowan, K. M. (2014). Comparing mortality among adult, general intensive care units in England with varying intensivist cover patterns: A retrospective cohort study. *Critical Care (London, England)*, *18*(4), 491. doi:10.1186/s13054-014-0491-3 PMID:25123141

Wilkins, G. T., Weyman, A. E., Abascal, V. M., Block, P. C., & Palacios, I. F. (1988). Percutaneous balloon dilatation of the mitral valve: An analysis of echocardiographic variables related to outcome and the mechanism of dilatation. *British Heart Journal*, *60*(4), 299–308. doi:10.1136/hrt.60.4.299 PMID:3190958

Wilkins, M. R., Paul, G. A., Strange, J. W., Tunariu, N., Gin-Sing, W., Banya, W. A., & Gibbs, J. S. R. et al. (2005). Sildenafil versus endothelin receptor antagonist for pulmonary hypertension (SERAPH) study. *American Journal of Respiratory and Critical Care Medicine*, *171*(11), 1292–1297. doi:10.1164/rccm.200410-1411OC PMID:15750042

Williams, B. a, Kentor, M. L., Skledar, S. J., Orebaugh, S. L., & Vallejo, M. C. (. (2007). Eliminating postoperative nausea and vomiting in outpatient surgery with multimodal strategies including low doses of nonsedating, off-patent antiemetics: Is "zero tolerance" achievable? *TheScientificWorldJournal*, *7*, 978–986. doi:10.1100/tsw.2007.132 PMID:17619779

Williams, J. B., Alexander, K. P., Morin, J. F., Langlois, Y., Noiseux, N., Perrault, L. P., & Afilalo, J. et al. (2013). Preoperative anxiety as a predictor of mortality and major morbidity in patients aged > 70 years undergoing cardiac surgery. *The American Journal of Cardiology*, *111*(1), 137–142. doi:10.1016/j.amjcard.2012.08.060 PMID:23245838

Williams, J. B., Hernandez, A. F., Li, S., Dokholyan, R. S., O'Brien, S. M., Smith, P. K., & Peterson, E. D. et al. (2011). Postoperative inotrope and vasopressor use following CABG: Outcome data from the CAPS-care study. *Journal of Cardiac Surgery*, *26*(6), 572–578. doi:10.1111/j.1540-8191.2011.01301.x PMID:21951076

Wilson, R. M., De Silva, D. S., Sato, K., Izumiya, Y., & Sam, F. (2009). Effects of fixed-dose Isosorbide Dinitrate/Hydralazine on diastolic function and exercise capacity in hypertension-induced diastolic heart failure. *Hypertension*, *54*(3), 583–590. doi:10.1161/HYPERTENSIONAHA.109.134932 PMID:19620510

Wilson, W. R., Thompson, R. L., Wilkowske, C. J., Washington, J. A. II, Giuliani, E. R., & Geraci, J. E. (1981). Short-term therapy for streptococcal infective endocarditis: Combined intramuscular administration of penicillin and streptomycin. *Clinical Infectious Diseases*, *245*(4), 360–363. PMID:7452862

Wilson, W., Taubert, K. A., Gewitz, M., Lockhart, P. B., Baddour, L. M., Levison, M., & Durack, D. T. et al. (2007). Prevention of infective endocarditis: Guidelines from the American Heart Association: A guideline from the American Heart Association Rheumatic Fever, Endocarditis, and Kawasaki Disease Committee, Council on Cardiovascular Disease in the Young, and the Council on Clinical Cardiology, Council on Cardiovascular Surgery and Anesthesia, and the Quality of Care and Outcomes Research Interdisciplinary Working Group. *Circulation*, *116*(15), 1736–1754. doi:10.1161/CIRCULATIONAHA.106.183095 PMID:17446442

Win, T., Jackson, A., Sharples, L., Groves, A., Wells, F., Ritchie, A., & Laroche, C. (2005). Relationship between pulmonary function and lung cancer surgical outcome. *The European Respiratory Journal*, *25*(4), 594–599. doi:10.1183/09031936.05.00077504 PMID:15802330

Wip, C., & Napolitano, L. (2009). Bundles to prevent ventilator-associated pneumonia: How valuable are they? *Current Opinion in Infectious Diseases*, *22*(2), 159–166. doi:10.1097/QCO.0b013e3283295e7b PMID:19276975

Wirz, S., Wartenberg, H. C., & Nadstawek, J. (2008). Less nausea, emesis, and constipation comparing hydromorphone and morphine? A prospective open-labeled investigation on cancer pain. *Supportive Care in Cancer*, *16*(9), 999–1009. doi:10.1007/s00520-007-0368-y PMID:18095008

Wise, K. R., Akopov, V. A., Williams, B. R. Jr, Ido, M. S., Leeper, K. V. Jr, & Dressler, D. D. (2012). Hospitalists and intensivists in the medical ICU: A prospective observational study comparing mortality and length of stay between two staffing models. *Journal of Hospital Medicine*, *7*(3), 183–189. doi:10.1002/jhm.972 PMID:22069304

Wiviott, S., Braunwald, E., McCabe, C., Montalescot, G., Ruzyllo, W., Gottlieb, S., & Antman, E. et al. (2007). Prasugrel versus clopidogrel in patients with acute coronary syndromes. *The New England Journal of Medicine*, *357*(20), 2001–2015. doi:10.1056/NEJMoa0706482 PMID:17982182

Wolf, A., Weir, P., Segar, P., Stone, J., & Shield, J. (2001). Impaired fatty acid oxidation in propofol infusion syndrome. *Lancet*, *357*(9256), 306–307. doi:10.1016/S0140-6736(00)04064-2 PMID:11558490

Wong, W. W., Gabriel, A., Maxwell, G. P., & Gupta, S. C. (2012). Bleeding risks of herbal, homeopathic, and dietary supplements: A hidden nightmare for plastic surgeons? *Aesthetic Surgery Journal*, *32*(3), 332–346. doi:10.1177/1090820X12438913 PMID:22395325

Wood, D. F. (2011). Formative Assessment. In T. Swanwick (Ed.), *Understanding Medical Education* (pp. 259–270). Oxford: Wiley-Blackwell.

Wood, P. (1954). An appreciation of mitral stenosis. *British Medical Journal*, *1*(4879), 1051–1063. doi:10.1136/bmj.1.4870.1051 PMID:13149899

Wood, P. (1956). *Disease of the heart and circulation*. Philadelphia, PA: Lippincott.

Woods, J. A., Wheeler, J. S., Finch, C. K., & Pinner, N. A. (2014). Corticosteroids in the treatment of acute exacerbations of chronic obstructive pulmonary disease. *International Journal of Chronic Obstructive Pulmonary Disease*, *9*, 421–430. doi:10.2147/COPD.S51012 PMID:24833897

Woolsey, C. A., & Coopersmith, C. M. (2006). Vasoactive drugs and the gut: Is there anything new? *Current Opinion in Critical Care*, *12*(2), 155–159. doi:10.1097/01.ccx.0000216584.72427.e4 PMID:16543793

Wormuth, J., & Heitmiller, R. (2006). Esophageal Conduit Necrosis. *Thoracic Surgery Clinics*, *16*(1), 11–22. doi:10.1016/j.thorsurg.2006.01.003 PMID:16696279

Wozniak, G., Noll, T., Akintürk, H., Thul, J., & Müller, M. (2001). Factor XIII prevents development of myocardial edema in children undergoing surgery for congenital heart disease. *Annals of the New York Academy of Sciences*, *936*(1), 617–620. doi:10.1111/j.1749-6632.2001.tb03549.x PMID:11460520

Wright, A. A., Keating, N. L., Balboni, T. A., Matulonis, U. A., Block, S. D., & Prigerson, H. G. (2010). Place of death: Correlations with quality of life of patients with cancer and predictors of bereaved caregivers' mental health. *Journal of Clinical Oncology*, *28*(29), 4457–4464. doi:10.1200/JCO.2009.26.3863 PMID:20837950

Wright, R. J., & Frier, B. M. (2008). Vascular disease and diabetes: Is hypoglycaemia an aggravating factor? *Diabetes/Metabolism Research and Reviews*, *24*(5), 353–363. doi:10.1002/dmrr.865 PMID:18461635

Wright, R. S., Anderson, J. L., Adams, C. D., Bridges, C. R., Casey, D. E. Jr, Ettinger, S. M., & Zidar, J. P. et al. (2011). ACCF/AHA Focused Update of the Guidelines for the Management of Patients With Unstable Angina/Non–ST-Elevation Myocardial Infarction (Updating the 2007 Guideline). *Journal of the American College of Cardiology*, *57*(19), 1920–1959. doi:10.1016/j.jacc.2011.02.009 PMID:21450428

Wright, S. (1996). Examining what residents look for in their role models. *Academic Medicine*, *71*(3), 290–292. doi:10.1097/00001888-199603000-00024 PMID:8607931

Wu, I., Liang, P., Huang, S., Chi, N., Lin, F., & Wang, S. (2009). The Significance of Endograft Geometry on the Incidence of Intraprosthetic Thrombus Deposits after Abdominal Endovascular Grafting. *European Journal of Vascular and Endovascular Surgery*, *38*(6), 741–747. doi:10.1016/j.ejvs.2009.09.004 PMID:19836272

Wu, J. S., Siewert, B., & Boiselle, P. M. (2010). Resident evaluation and remediation: A comprehensive approach. *Journal of Graduate Medical Education*, *2*(2), 242–245. doi:10.4300/JGME-D-10-00031.1 PMID:21975628

Wunderink, R. G., Niederman, M. S., Kollef, M. H., Shorr, A. F., Kunkel, M. J., Baruch, A., & Chastre, J. et al. (2012). Linezolid in methicillin-resistant Staphylococcus aureus nosocomial pneumonia: A randomized, controlled study. *Clinical Infectious Diseases*, *54*(5), 621–629. doi:10.1093/cid/cir895 PMID:22247123

Wunsch, H., Christiansen, C. F., Johansen, M. B., Olsen, M., Ali, N., Angus, D. C., & Sorensen, H. T. (2014). Psychiatric diagnoses and psychoactive medication use among nonsurgical critically ill patients receiving mechanical ventilation. *Journal of the American Medical Association*, *311*(11), 1133–1142. doi:10.1001/jama.2014.2137 PMID:24643603

Wunsch, H., Guerra, C., Barnato, A. E., Angus, D. C., Li, G., & Linde-Zwirble, W. T. (2010). Three-year outcomes for Medicare beneficiaries who survive intensive care. *Journal of the American Medical Association*, *303*(9), 849–856. doi:10.1001/jama.2010.216 PMID:20197531

Wyckoff, T., & Augoustides, J. G. (2012). Advances in Acute Kidney Injury Associated with Cardiac Surgery: The Unfolding Revolution in Early Detection. *Journal of Cardiothoracic and Vascular Anesthesia*, *26*(2), 340–345. doi:10.1053/j.jvca.2012.01.001 PMID:22405191

Wynia, M. K., Papadakis, M. A., Sullivan, W. M., & Hafferty, F. W. (2014). More Than a List of Values and Desired Behaviors. *Academic Medicine*, *89*(5), 712–714. doi:10.1097/ACM.0000000000000212 PMID:24667515

Wyse, D. G., Waldo, A. L., DiMarco, J. P., Domanski, M. J., Rosenberg, Y., & Schron, E. B. (2002). A Comparison of Rate Control and Rhythm Control in Patients with Atrial Fibrillation. *The New England Journal of Medicine*, *347*(23), 1825–1833. doi:10.1056/NEJMoa021328 PMID:12466506

Xiaobo, Y. (2014). Does pulse pressure variation predict fluid responsiveness in critically ill patients? A systematic review and meta-analysis. *Critical Care (London, England)*, *18*(6), 650. doi:10.1186/s13054-014-0650-6 PMID:25427970

Yacoub, M., Mankad, P., & Ledingham, S. (1990). Donor Procurement And Surgical Techniques For Cardiac Transplantation. *Seminars in Thoracic and Cardiovascular Surgery*, *2*(2), 153–161. PMID:2081225

Yager, P. H., Cummings, B. M., Whalen, M. J., & Noviski, N. (2012). Nighttime telecommunication between remote staff intensivists and bedside personnel in a pediatric intensive care unit: A retrospective study. *Critical Care Medicine*, *40*(9), 2700–2703. doi:10.1097/CCM.0b013e3182591dab PMID:22732287

Yancy, C., Jessup, M., Bozkurt, B., Butler, J., Casey, D., Drazner, M. H., & Wilkoff, B. L. et al. (2013). ACCF/AHA Guideline for the Management of Heart Failure: Executive Summary: A Report of the American College of Cardiology Foundation/American Heart Association Task Force on Practice Guidelines. *Circulation*, *128*(16), 1810–1852. doi:10.1161/CIR.0b013e31829e8807 PMID:23741057

Yancy, C.W., Jessup, M., Bozkurt, B., Butler, J., Casey, D.E. Jr, & Drazner, M.H., … American College of Cardiology Foundation; American Heart Association Task Force on Practice Guidelines. (2013). ACCF/AHA guideline for the management of heart failure: A report of the American College of Cardiology Foundation/American Heart Association Task Force on Practice Guidelines. *Journal of the American College of Cardiology*, *62*(16), e147–e239. doi:10.1016/j.jacc.2013.05.019 PMID:23747642

Yang, G., Wu, X.-T., Zhou, Y., & Wang, Y.-L. (2005). Application of dietary fiber in clinical enteral nutrition: A meta-analysis of randomized controlled trials. *World Journal of Gastroenterology*, *11*(25), 3935–3938. PMID:15991297

Yang, K. L., & Tobin, M. J. (1991). A prospective study of indexes predicting the outcome of trials of weaning from mechanical ventilation. *The New England Journal of Medicine*, *324*(21), 1445–1450. doi:10.1056/NEJM199105233242101 PMID:2023603

Yao, D. C., & Wright, S. M. (2001). The challenge of problem residents. *Journal of General Internal Medicine*, *16*(7), 486–492. doi:10.1046/j.1525-1497.2001.016007486.x PMID:11520388

Yap, F., Chan, A., & Joynt, G. (2000). Timing of extubation after esophagectomy. *Critical Care (London, England)*, *4*(Suppl 1), 101–101. doi:10.1186/cc821

Yarmus, L., & Feller-Kopman, D. (2012). Pneumothorax in the critically ill patient. *Chest Journal*, *141*(4), 1098–1105. doi:10.1378/chest.11-1691 PMID:22474153

Yavagal, D. R., Karnad, D. R., & Oak, J. L. (2000). Metoclopramide for preventing pneumonia in critically ill patients receiving enteral tube feeding: A randomized controlled trial. *Critical Care Medicine*, *28*(5), 1408–1411. doi:10.1097/00003246-200005000-00025 PMID:10834687

Yedidia, M. J., Schwartz, M. D., Hirschkorn, C., & Lipkin, M. Jr. (1995). Learners as teachers. *Journal of General Internal Medicine*, *10*(11), 615–623. doi:10.1007/BF02602745 PMID:8583264

Yeter, R., Hübler, M., Pasic, M., & Hetzer, R. (2011). Organ Preservation With The Organ Care System. *Applied Cardiopulmonary Pathophysiology*, *15*, 207–212.

Yıldızeli, B., Özyurtkan, M., Batırel, H., Kuşcu, K., Bekiroğlu, N., & Yüksel, M. (2005). Factors Associated With Postoperative Delirium After Thoracic Surgery. *The Annals of Thoracic Surgery*, *79*(3), 1004–1009. doi:10.1016/j.athoracsur.2004.06.022 PMID:15734423

Yilmaz, T., Arslan, M., Demirkilç, U., Ozal, E., Kuralay, E., Bingöl, H., … Oztürk, O. Y. (1996). Gastrointestinal complications after cardiac surgery. *European Journal of Cardiothoracic Surgery, 10*(9), 763–7.

Yip, C., Loeb, M., Salama, S., Moss, L., & Olde, J. (2001). Quinolone use as a risk factor for nosocomial Clostridium difficile-associated diarrhea. *Infection Control and Hospital Epidemiology*, *22*(9), 572–575. doi:10.1086/501954 PMID:11732787

Yiu, S., Enriquez-Sarano, M., Tribouilloy, C., & Tajik, A. J. (2000). Determinants of the degree of functional mitral regurgitation in patients with systolic left ventricular dysfunction: A quantitative clinical study. *Circulation*, *102*(12), 1400–1406. doi:10.1161/01.CIR.102.12.1400 PMID:10993859

Yoder, J., & Hochevar, C. (2005). Encouraging Active Learning Can Improve Students' Performance on Examinations. *Teaching of Psychology*, *32*(2), 91–95. doi:10.1207/s15328023top3202_2

Yokoyama, Y., Chaitman, B. R., Hardison, R. M., Guo, P., Krone, R., & Stocke, K. … Detre, K. M. (2000). Association between new electrocardiographic abnormalities after coronary revascularization and five-year cardiac mortality in BARI randomized and registry patients. *The American Journal of Cardiology*, *86*(8), 819–24. Retrieved from http://www.ncbi.nlm.nih.gov/pubmed/11024394

Yonan, N. A., el-Gamel, A., Egan, J., Kakadellis, J., Rahman, A., & Deiraniya, A. K. (1998). Single lung transplantation for emphysema: Predictors for native lung hyperinflation. *The Journal of Heart and Lung Transplantation*, *17*(2), 192–201.

Yoo, Y.-C., Shim, J.-K., Kim, J.-C., Jo, Y.-Y., Lee, J.-H., & Kwak, Y.-L. (2011). Effect of single recombinant human erythropoietin injection on transfusion requirements in preoperatively anemic patients undergoing valvular heart surgery. *Anesthesiology*, *115*(5), 929–937. doi:10.1097/ALN.0b013e318232004b PMID:22027622

Yoo, Y., Shim, J., Song, Y., Yang, S., & Kwak, Y. (2014). Anesthetics influence the incidence of acute kidney injury following valvular heart surgery. *Kidney International*, *86*(2), 414–422. doi:10.1038/ki.2013.532 PMID:24429400

Yorke, J., Wallis, M., & McLean, B. (2004). Patients' perceptions of pain management after cardiac surgery in an Australian critical care unit. *Heart and Lung: The Journal of Acute and Critical Care*, *33*(1), 33–41. doi:10.1016/j.hrtlng.2003.09.002 PMID:14983137

Yoshioka, M., Mori, T., Kobayashi, H., Iwatani, K., Yoshimoto, K., Terasaki, H., & Nomori, H. (2006). The efficacy of epidural analgesia after video-assisted thoracoscopic surgery: A randomized control study. *Annals of Thoracic and Cardiovascular Surgery*, *12*, 313–318. PMID:17095972

You, J. J., Singer, D. E., Howard, P. A., Lane, D. A., Eckman, M. H., Fang, M. C., ... American College of Chest, P. (2012). Antithrombotic therapy for atrial fibrillation: Antithrombotic Therapy and Prevention of Thrombosis, 9th ed: American College of Chest Physicians Evidence-Based Clinical Practice Guidelines. Chest, 141(2 Suppl), e531S-575S. doi:10.1378/chest.11-2304

Young, D., Harrison, D. A., Cuthbertson, B. H., Rowan, K., & TracMan Collaborators, . (2013). Effect of early vs late tracheostomy placement on survival in patients receiving mechanical ventilation: The TracMan randomized trial. *Journal of the American Medical Association*, *309*(20), 2121–2129. doi:10.1001/jama.2013.5154 PMID:23695482

Younger, D., Braun, N., Jaretzki, A., Penn, A., & Lovelace, R. (1984). Myasthenia gravis: Determinants for independent ventilation after transsternal thymectomy. *Neurology*, *34*(3), 336–336. doi:10.1212/WNL.34.3.336 PMID:6538272

Young, J. Q., van Merriënboer, J., Durning, S., & Ten Cate, O. (2014). Cognitive Load Theory: Implications for medical education: AMEE Guide No. 86. *Medical Teacher*, *36*(5), 371–384. doi:10.3109/0142159X.2014.889290 PMID:24593808

Young, L. B., Chan, P. S., Lu, X., Nallamothu, B. K., Sasson, C., & Cram, P. M. (2011). Impact of telemedicine intensive care unit coverage on patient outcomes: A systematic review and meta-analysis. *Archives of Internal Medicine*, *171*(6), 498–506. doi:10.1001/archinternmed.2011.61 PMID:21444842

Young, M. P., & Birkmeyer, J. D. (2000). Potential reduction in mortality rates using an intensivist model to manage intensive care units. *Effective Clinical Practice*, *3*, 284–289. PMID:11151525

Youngquist, P., Carroll, M., Farber, M., Macy, D., Madrid, P., Ronning, J., & Susag, A. (2007). Implementing a ventilator bundle in a community hospital. *Joint Commission Journal on Quality and Patient Safety*, *33*(4), 219–225. PMID:17441560

Yu, A. W., Rippel, R. A., Smock, E., & Jarral, O. A. (2013). In patients with post-sternotomy mediastinitis is vacuum-assisted closure superior to conventional therapy? *Interactive Cardiovascular and Thoracic Surgery*, *17*(5), 861–866. doi:10.1093/icvts/ivt326 PMID:23912622

Yusen, R. D., Christie, J. D., Edwards, L. B., Kucheryavaya, A. Y., Benden, C., Dipchand, A. I., & Stehlik, J. et al. (2013). The Registry of the International Society for Heart and Lung Transplantation: Thirtieth Adult Lung and Heart-Lung Transplant Report--2013; focus theme: age. *The Journal of Heart and Lung Transplantation*, *32*(10), 965–978. doi:10.1016/j.healun.2013.08.007

Zaas, A., Andolsek, K., Weinerth, J. L., Nagler, A., Fortune, R., Tuck, T., & McNeil, D. B. (2013, October). Constructive Corrective Action: Assessing and Developing Comprehensive Learning Plans for the Core Competencies. *Insight*. Retrieved May 12, 2014, from http://www.im.org/Publications/Insight/Archives/2011/V9I2/Pages/corrective.aspx

Zacharias, A., Schwann, T., Riordan, C. J., Durham, S. J., Shah, A. S., & Habib, R. H. (2009). Late results of conventional versus all-arterial revascularization based on internal thoracic and radial artery grafting. *The Annals of Thoracic Surgery*, *87*(1), 19–26.e2. doi:10.1016/j.athoracsur.2008.09.050 PMID:19101262

Zack, J. E., Garrison, T., Trovillion, E., Clinkscale, D., Coopersmith, C. M., Fraser, V. J., & Kollef, M. H. (2002). Effect of an education program aimed at reducing the occurrence of ventilator-associated pneumonia. *Critical Care Medicine*, *30*(11), 2407–2412. doi:10.1097/00003246-200211000-00001 PMID:12441746

Zaloga, G. P., Roberts, P. R., & Marik, P. (2003). Feeding the hemodynamically unstable patient: A critical evaluation of the evidence. *Nutrition in Clinical Practice*, *18*(4), 285–293. doi:10.1177/0115426503018004285 PMID:16215052

Zandstra, D. F., & Stoutenbeek, C. P. (1994). The virtual absence of stress-ulceration related bleeding in ICU patients receiving prolonged mechanical ventilation without any prophylaxis. A prospective cohort study. *Intensive Care Medicine*, *20*(5), 335–340. doi:10.1007/BF01720905 PMID:7930027

Zangrillo, A., Biondi-Zoccai, G. G., Frati, E., Covello, R. D., Cabrini, L., Guarracino, F., & Landoni, G. et al. (2012). Fenoldopam and Acute Renal Failure in Cardiac Surgery: A Meta-Analysis of Randomized Placebo-Controlled Trials. *Journal of Cardiothoracic and Vascular Anesthesia*, *26*(3), 407–413. doi:10.1053/j.jvca.2012.01.038 PMID:22459931

Zannad, F., McMurray, J., Krum, H., Van Veldhuisen, D., Sweedberg, K., Shi, H., & Pitt, B. et al. (2011). Eplerenone in patients with systolic heart failure and mild symptoms. *The New England Journal of Medicine*, *364*(1), 11–21. doi:10.1056/NEJMoa1009492 PMID:21073363

Zaouter, C., Kaneva, P., & Carli, F. (2009). Less urinary tract infection by earlier removal of bladder catheter in surgical patients receiving thoracic epidural analgesia. *Regional Anesthesia and Pain Medicine*, *34*(6), 542–548. doi:10.1097/AAP.0b013e3181ae9fac PMID:19916208

Zaouter, C., & Ouattara, A. (2014). How long is a transurethral catheter necessary in patients undergoing thoracotomy and receiving thoracic epidural analgesia? Literature review. *Journal of Cardiothoracic and Vascular Anesthesia*; Advance online publication. doi:10.1053/j.jcva.2014.05.022 PMID:25287748

Zarbock, A., & Ley, K. (2008). Mechanisms and consequences of neutrophil interaction with the endothelium. *American Journal of Pathology*, *172*(1), 1–7. doi:10.2353/ajpath.2008.070502 PMID:18079440

Zarbock, A., Mueller, E., Netzer, S., Gabriel, A., Feindt, P., & Kindgen-Milles, D. (2009). Prophylactic nasal continuous positive airway pressure following cardiac surgery protects from postoperative pulmonary complications. *Chest, 135*(5), 1252–1259. doi:10.1378/chest.08-1602 PMID:19017864

Zaroff, J. G., Rosengard, B. R., Armstrong, W. F., Babcock, W. D., D'alessandro, A., Dec, G. W., . . . Young, J. B. (2002). Consensus Conference Report: Maximizing use of organs recovered from the cadaver donor: Cardiac recommendations: March 28–29, 2001, Crystal City, Va. *Circulation, 106*(7), 836-841. Retrieved From http://circ.ahajournals.org/content/106/7/836

Zegdi, R., Debièche, M., Latrémouille, C., Lebied, D., Chardigny, C., Grinda, J., & Fabiani, J. et al. (2005). Long-term results of mitral valve repair in active endocarditis. *Circulation, 111*(19), 2532–2536. doi:10.1161/01.CIR.0000165122.08660.1A PMID:15867185

Zeitani, J., Buccisano, F., Nardella, S., Flaminio, M., Prati, P., Chiariello, G., & Chiariello, L. et al. (2013). Mini-extracorporeal circulation minimizes coagulation abnormalities and ameliorates pulmonary outcome in coronary artery bypass grafting surgery. *Perfusion, 28*(4), 298–305. doi:10.1177/0267659113478322 PMID:23411504

Zerr, K. J., Furnary, A. P., Grunkemeier, G. L., Bookin, S., Kanhere, V., & Starr, A. (1997). Glucose control lowers the risk of wound infection in diabetics after open heart operations. *The Annals of Thoracic Surgery, 63*, 356–361. doi:10.1016/S0003-4975(96)01044-2 PMID:9033300

Zhang, Z., Spertus, J., Mahoney, E. M., Booth, J., Nugara, F., Stables, R. H., & Weintraub, W. S. (2005). The impact of acute coronary syndrome on clinical, economic, and cardiac-specific health status after coronary artery bypass surgery versus stent-assisted percutaneous coronary intervention: 1-year results from the stent or surgery (SoS) trial. *American Heart Journal, 150*(1), 175–181. doi:10.1016/j.ahj.2005.01.019 PMID:16084166

Zhao, S., Qi, G., Tian, W., Chen, L., & Sun, Y. (2014). Effect of Intracoronary Nitroprusside in Preventing No Reflow Phenomenon during Primary Percutaneous Coronary Intervention: A Meta-Analysis. *Journal of Interventional Cardiology, 27*(4), 356–364. doi:10.1111/joic.12133 PMID:25041036

Zhu, F. L., A.; Chee, Y.E. (2012). Fast-track cardiac care for adult cardiac surgical patients. *The Cochrane Collaboration,* (10).

Zhu, F., Lee, A., & Chee, Y.E. (2012). Fast-track cardiac care for adult cardiac surgical patients. *Cochrane Database of Systematic Reviews, Oct 17*, 10:CD003587.

Zhu, F., Lee, A., & Chee, Y. E. (2012). Fast-track cardiac care for adult cardiac surgical patients. *Cochrane Database of Systematic Reviews, 10*, Cd003587. doi:10.1002/14651858.CD003587.pub2 PMID:23076899

Zier, L. S., Sottile, P. D., Hong, S. Y., Weissfield, L. A., & White, D. B. (2012). Surrogate decision makers' interpretation of prognostic information: A mixed-methods study. *Annals of Internal Medicine, 156*(5), 360–366. doi:10.7326/0003-4819-156-5-201203060-00008 PMID:22393131

Zilberberg, M. D., & Shorr, A. F. (2013). Preventing Clostridium Difficile Infection in the Intensive Care Unit. *Critical Care Clinics, 29*(1), 11–18. doi:10.1016/j.ccc.2012.10.006 PMID:23182524

Zilberberg, M. D., Shorr, A. F., & Kollef, M. H. (2009). Implementing quality improvements in the intensive care unit: Ventilator bundle as an example. *Critical Care Medicine, 37*(1), 305–309. doi:10.1097/CCM.0b013e3181926623 PMID:19050626

Zimetbaum, P. (2007). Amiodarone for atrial fibrillation. *The New England Journal of Medicine, 356*(9), 935–941. doi:10.1056/NEJMct065916 PMID:17329700

Zishiri, E., William, S., Cronin, E., Blackstone, E., Ellis, S., Roselli, E., & Chung, M. et al. (2013). Early Risk of Mortaliy After Coronary Artery Revascularization in Patients with Left Ventricular Dysfunction and Potential Role of the Wearable Cardioverter Defibrillator. *Circulation: Arrhythmia and Electrophysiology*, *6*(1), 117–128. doi:10.1161/CIRCEP.112.973552 PMID:23275233

Ziv, A., Wolpe, P. R., Small, S. D., & Glick, S. (2003). Simulation-based medical education: An ethical imperative. *Academic Medicine*, *78*(8), 783–788. doi:10.1097/00001888-200308000-00006 PMID:12915366

Zoghbi, W. A., Enriquez-Sarano, M., Foster, E., Grayburn, P. A., Kraft, C. D., Levine, R. A., & Weissman, N. J. et al. (2003). Recommendations for evaluation of the severity of native valvular regurgitation with two-dimensional and Doppler echocardiography. *Journal of the American Society of Echocardiography*, *16*(7), 777–802. doi:10.1016/S0894-7317(03)00335-3 PMID:12835667

About the Contributors

Adam S. Evans is currently an assistant professor on the faculty of the Icahn School of Medicine at Mount Sinai where he actively practices cardiac anesthesia and is an intensivist in the cardiothoracic intensive care unit. He completed his anesthesiology residency at Weill Cornell Medical College in 2010 followed by a fellowship in critical care at Columbia Presbyterian and a fellowship in cardiac anesthesia at the Johns Hopkins Hospital. He received his medical degree from Jefferson Medical College as part of the joint five year MD-MBA program with Widener University in Delaware. Dr. Evans is an active member of the Society for Critical Care Medicine, Society for Cardiac Anesthesia, and New York State Society of Anesthesiologists. He has presented locally, nationally, and internationally on issues pertinent to the management of critically ill patients in the cardiothoracic intensive care unit.

Gregory Kerr is an Associate Professor of Anesthesiology at Weill Medical College of Cornell University. His clinical areas of expertise include cardiac anesthesiology and critical care medicine. Leadership roles at New York Presbyterian Hospital include being the Medical Director of the Cardiothoracic ICU and Medical Director of Critical Care Services for NYPH. Dr. Kerr is actively engaged in the American Society of Anesthesiologists, the Society of Critical Care Medicine, the Commission to End Health Care Disparities, and is a fellow of the American College of Critical Care Medicine. Dr. Kerr has worked with New York Presbyterian Hospital and the other intensive care units in the institution to create a strong culture of patient safety and a culture where the best patient care is expected. The creation of the Housestaff Quality Council was a result of some of this work.

Insung Chung grew up in southern California but left for the East Coast to attend Brown University where he graduated with a BA in Economics. He worked in the Chodobski lab doing traumatic brain injury research on mice looking at the expression of VEGF and V1 receptors in the choroid plexus and synaptic proteins. After Providence, he moved to Philadelphia where he attended Drexel University College of Medicine and then trained in anesthesiology at the Hospital of the University of Pennsylvania. He then completed fellowships in Critical Care Medicine and Adult CardioThoracic Anesthesia at New York Presbyterian Columbia University. He then joined the faculty at Mount Sinai School of Medicine where he attends in the divisions of critical care and cardiac anesthesia. His clinical interests are in critical care ultrasonography and the use of real time echocardiography for guiding resuscitation.

Robin Varghese is an Attending Cardiovascular Surgeon and Assistant Professor of Surgery at the Icahn School of Medicine at Mount Sinai and the Mount Sinai Hospital in New York. He is the Surgical Director of the Cardiothoracic Intensive Care Unit.

* * *

Zarah Antongiorgi, MD, is an Assistant Clinical Professor in the Department of Anesthesiology and Perioperative Medicine at the UCLA David Geffen School of Medicine. Following graduation from UCSF School of Medicine she completed her Anesthesia Residency and Critical Care Medicine Fellowship at UCLA and joined the UCLA faculty in 2013.

Anelechi C. Anyanwu, MD, is a Professor and Vice Chairman of Department of Cardiovascular Surgery in the Icahn School of Medicine, Mount Sinai Medical Center.

Rakesh Arora is the first Canadian cardiac surgeon to undergo the formal Royal College of Physicians and Surgeons of Canada Critical Care Medicine Training Program. He is currently the Medical Co-Director of the Intensive Care Cardiac Sciences at the St. Boniface Hospital in Winnipeg, Manitoba. He is also the Co-Founder and Chair of the Canadian Cardiovascular Critical Care (CANCARE) Society (www.cancaresociety.com).

Keki R. Balsara MD obtained his degree at the University of Pennsylvania. He completed his post graduate training in general surgery, critical care and cardiac surgery at Duke and Johns Hopkins. He is currently an Assistant Professor of Surgery with a focus on mechanical circulatory support and thoracic organ transplantation. He is also co-director of the cardiothoracic surgery intensive care unit at Barnes-Jewish Hospital.

Raymond Bietry is an Assistant Professor of Cardiology at the Icahn School of Medicine at Mount Sinai. He attended the University of Maryland where he received his medical degree. He completed residency training at The Mount Sinai Medical Center, a fellowship in cardiology at New York University, and a fellowship in advanced heart failure & transplantation at Mount Sinai.

Eva Boyd, MD, graduated from UC Irvine School of Medicine and completed a residency in Anesthesiology at the University of New Mexico. After finishing residency, she worked as an Assistant Professor in the Department of Anesthesiology and Critical Care Medicine at the University of New Mexico. She is currently an Assistant Professor in the University of California Los Angeles Department of Anesthesiology and Perioperative Medicine. While she does practice in many areas of anesthesiology including obstetric anesthesia, pediatric anesthesia, adult general anesthesia, and trauma anesthesia, Dr. Boyd's main focus is on regional anesthesia and the management of acute post-operative pain. She is involved in resident and medical student education through the resident lecture series, simulator training, and hands-on teaching in the operating room and perioperative setting.

Jordan Brand, a native New Yorker, completed his residency in Anesthesiology at New York Presbyterian Hospital-Weill Cornell Center, and then moved to NYPH-Columbia University for his Critical Care fellowship. He currently practices anesthesiology and critical care medicine at the San Francisco VA Medical Center, where he is also Medical Director of Respiratory Therapy. In addition, he holds an appointment as Assistant Professor at the University of California, San Francisco. Jordan's interests include regional and thoracic anesthesia, prevention and management of lung injury, and the application of alternative and complementary therapies in the ICU. Outside work, Jordan enjoys cycling, spending time with his family, and (as you would expect from a former Jeopardy! champion) playing trivia games.

Peter S. Burrage, MD, PhD, is a clinical fellow at Brigham and Women's Hospital at Harvard Medical School. He did his medical and doctoral training in molecular and cellular biology at the Geisel School of Medicine at Dartmouth in Hanover, NH and then completed a residency and chief residency in anesthesiology at Brigham and Women's Hospital. Dr. Burrage then did a fellowship in adult cardio-thoracic anesthesia at Brigham and Women's Hospital prior to pursuing his current fellowship training in Critical Care Medicine.

Brandon W. Calenda is a fellow in cardiovascular disease at the Icahn School of Medicine at Mount Sinai. He completed his residency in internal medicine at Mount Sinai, and medical school at Tufts University.

June M. Chan is an anesthesiology resident at Weill Cornell Medical College. Originally from Sydney, Australia, she attended the University of New South Wales where she received her bachelor's degrees in Science, Medicine and Surgery in 2002. She spent her requisite clinical years prior to specialist training in internal medicine, general surgery and critical care before starting her residency in anesthesiology in 2006. She completed her fellowship with an emphasis on regional anesthesia, airway management and medical education in 2011 and was subsequently awarded her Fellowship of the Australian and New Zealand College of Anaesthetists (FANZCA) with a dissertation on diagnostic methods in peri-operative anaphylaxis. Her interest in medical education stems from her post-graduate experience at Concord Repatriation General Hospital, which, as a teaching hospital of the University of Sydney, has an especially strong tradition of teaching and mentoring. She continues to further this interest within the Department of Anesthesiology at Cornell, where a she is a member of the Residency Support Council and the Education Curriculum Committee, and a forthcoming Fellow in cardiothoracic anesthesiology.

Aaron M. Cheng is an Assistant Professor of Surgery at the University of Washington and the surgical co-director of the University of Washington Medical Center cardiothoracic critical care unit. His clinical and research interests include general thoracic surgery, lung transplantation, and critical care outcomes in cardiothoracic surgery.

Sheela Pai Cole, Clinical Associate Professor Division of Cardiac Anesthesiology and Critical Care Medicine Department of Anesthesiology, Pain and Perioperative Medicine Stanford University.

Ahmed El-Eshmawi is an Assistant Professor in the Icahn School of Medicine at Mount Sinai, attending surgeon, as well as the Clinical Director of the Mitral Valve Repair Reference Center at Mount Sinai.

Alexander C. P. Fort is originally from Miami, Florida. He attended Brown University where he majored in Latin American studies and completed pre-medical coursework. He went on to obtain his medical degree from the University of Miami Miller School of Medicine. Currently, he is a resident in anesthesiology and critical care medicine at New York Presbyterian/Weill Cornell. Brown University '04 University of Miami Miller School of Medicine '11 NYP/Weill Cornell Anesthesiology '15.

Nishant A. Gandhi is a staff anesthesiologist at the James J. Peters Bronx VA Medical Center in Bronx, NY (affiliated with the Icahn School of Medicine at Mount Sinai). He completed his internship in general surgery at Union Memorial Hospital in Baltimore, MD, followed by a residency in anesthesiology at Johns Hopkins Hospital in Baltimore, MD and a surgical critical care fellowship at New York Presbyterian/Columbia University Medical Center. He worked as an anesthesiologist and critical care physician at Mount Sinai Hospital, and then completed a fellowship in simulation medicine before taking a position at the VA Medical Center. He also helps run anesthesia simulation courses for anesthesia residents, as well as anesthesia attendings undergoing maintenance of certification, at the ASA endorsed simulation center at Mount Sinai. Dr. Gandhi lives in New York City with his wife, Shelley; they enjoy the arts, Broadway shows and fine dining.

Umesh K. Gidwani is the Chief of Cardiac Critical Care at the Zena and Michael A. Wiener Cardiovascular Institute at the Mount Sinai Hospital and Director of the Cardiac Intensive Care Unit at Icahn School of Medicine at Mount Sinai. The mission of the CCU has rapidly evolved. Until the recent past the typical patient would be admitted for post-myocardial infarction monitoring for complications, or for the management of heart failure. The contemporary Cardiac ICU patient has more severe illness and is more likely to have complex multiorgan involvement and require more sophisticated technology. At Mount Sinai Dr. Gidwani had lead this transition of the CCU into a Cardiac Intensive Care Unit equipped to serve precisely such high acuity patients.

Leonard N. Girardi is a Professor of Cardiothoracic Surgery in the Department of Cardiothoracic Surgery at New York Presbyterian-Weill Cornell Medical Center. He is also an Associate Attending Surgeon at the Memorial-Sloan Kettering Cancer Center. Dr. Girardi completed his undergraduate studies at Harvard University in 1985, obtaining a degree in biochemistry. He pursued his medical education at Cornell University Medical College and completed his residency in general surgery at Cornell Medical College, where he remained as a resident in Cardiothoracic Surgery. Dr. Girardi graduated from the program in 1996 under Dr. O. Wayne Isom, his Chairman at present. After completion of a fellowship in aortic surgery at Baylor, Dr. Girardi assumed his present position at New York Presbyterian-Weill Cornell Medical Center. Dr. Girardi is committed to training the next generation of cardiothoracic surgeons and teaches medical students and residents on all levels. He is a member of numerous surgical societies, including the American Association of Thoracic Surgery, Society of Thoracic Surgery, The DeBakey International Surgical Society and the American College of Surgeons. He has published extensively on multiple topics in cardiovascular and aneurysm surgery and has given many lectures at regional and national surgical meetings.

Vadim Gudzenko obtained his medical degree from Odessa Medical University in Ukraine. After moving to the USA he has worked in the laboratory of Dr. Riccardo Olcese studying L-type calcium and BK – channels. Dr. Gudzenko continued his postgraduate medical training in anesthesiology residency at UCLA medical center. After successful completion of anesthesiology residency, he entered critical care fellowship at Massachusetts General Hospital. Upon completion of the fellowship, he has returned to UCLA and joined the newly established division of critical care of anesthesiology department. At present Dr. Gudzenko attends Cardiothoracic Surgical ICU and works in the thoracic and vascular operating room as attending anesthesiologist. Dr. Gudzenko is associate program director of Surgical Critical Care fellowship.

Shawn Hansberry is a native of Boston, Massachusetts. Dr. Hansberry attended his undergraduate and medical school training at Tufts University. He went on to complete his surgical internship at Brown University/Rhode Island Hospital and anesthesiology residency at New York Presbyterian Hospital/Weill Cornell Medical Center where he served as co-chief resident. In 2015 he will start his cardiothoracic anesthesiology fellowship at Duke University Medical Center.

Carrie E. Harvey was born and raised in metro Detroit, will only drive GM, and somehow manages to remain an optimistic Lions fan. Dr. Harvey received a BS from Michigan State University, MS from Boston University, MD from Wayne State University, and completed her residency in Emergency Medicine at the University of Wisconsin. Dr. Harvey is currently a Critical Care fellow at the University of Michigan. Her interests include ethics, end-of-life care, and the ED and ICU interface.

Nadia Hensley is an Assistant Professor at Johns Hopkins University School of Medicine Department of Anesthesiology and Critical Care Medicine.

May Hua is an Assistant Professor of Anesthesiology and Critical Care at Columbia University Medical Center. Her research focuses on the intersection between palliative care and critical care, and on methods for improving the delivery of palliative care to critically ill patients. She is currently supported by a Mentored Training Research Grant from the Foundation for Anesthesia Education and Research.

Natalia S. Ivascu is an Associate Professor of Clinical Anesthesiolgy and Associate Professor of Medical Ethics in Clinical Medicine. She is the Medical Director of the New York Presbyterian Hospital- Weill Cornell, Cardiothoracic Surgical Intensive Care Unit. Dr. Ivascu completed her undergraduate studies in Cellular and Molecular Biology at the University of Michigan, in Ann Arbor. She went on to earn her medical degree from Wayne State University School of Medicine in Detroit, Michigan. She began her career at New York-Presbyterian Hospital/Weill Medical College as a resident in Anesthesiology. Dr. Ivascu completed an additional year of fellowship training at Cornell, in Cardiovascular Anesthesiology. She then spent a year at the Columbia University campus of NYP as a fellow in Critical Care Medicine. Dr. Ivascu is board certified in Anesthesiology and Critical Care Medicine. She is also a Diplomate of the American Board of Echocardiography, with certification in Advanced Perioperative Transesophageal Echocardiography. She is an expert in pulmonary hypertension and is the Director of the Pulmonary Hypertension Anesthesiology team. Dr. Ivascu is also the Director of Liver Transplant Anesthesiology, Pre-Anesthesia testing and the Post-Anesthesia Care Unit.

Jason Katz is an Assistant Professor of Medicine, dually appointed in the Divisions of Cardiology and Pulmonary/Critical Care Medicine at the University of North Carolina. He is Medical Director of the Cardiac Intensive Care Unit, the Cardiothoracic Intensive Care Unit, and the Mechanical Heart Program there, and also Director of the Cardiovascular Clinical Trials Program. His research interests lie at the intersection of cardiovascular disease and critical care, and includes a particular focus on optimal care delivery for patients supported with durable ventricular assist devices.

Wolf Benjamin Kratzert was born in Luebeck and grew up in Hamburg, Germany. After graduating from Hamburg University Medical School in Germany, he completed his medical internship at St. Raphael's hospital in New Haven Connecticut, and anesthesiology residency at UC San Diego. He then went on to subspecialize in critical care medicine at Columbia University, followed by a cardiothoracic fellowship at Stanford University. After conclusion of his training, he worked as an assistant Professor in the Department of Anesthesiology and Critical Medicine at the University of New Mexico. There he held the position as director of the cardiothoracic intensive care unit and perioperative echocardiography. After relocating to UCLA in 2014, Dr. Kratzert works as a critical care and cardiothoracic anesthesiologist at Ronald Reagan UCLA Medical Center. He is board certified in anesthesiology, critical care medicine, and echocardiography.

Shreyajit R. Kumar is an assistant professor in Anesthesiology at Weill Cornell Medical College, board certified in Anesthesiology and in Critical Care Medicine. He received his undergraduate degree in Biology and Biomedical Engineering from the Massachusetts Institute of Technology, and his Doctor of Medicine from the Boston University School of Medicine. He subsequently completed Anesthesiology residency at New York University Langone Medical Center and a fellowship in Critical Care Medicine from Columbia University. He has been honored with numerous teaching awards, and maintains clinical and research interests in mechanical circulatory support, pulmonary hypertension, telemedicine and residency education.

Dong-Seok Daniel Lee is an Assistant Professor in the Department of Thoracic Surgery at the Icahn School of Medicine at Mount Sinai. He obtained his medical degree at Rutgers – Robert Wood Johnson Medical School and completed a residency in General Surgery at Mount Sinai Hospital. He went on to complete a fellowship in Thoracic Surgery at Mount Sinai Hospital. Dr. Lee is certified by both the American Board of Surgery and the American Board of Thoracic Surgery. He is a member of the Society of Thoracic Surgeons. Dr. Lee's practice encompasses all aspects of Thoracic Surgery with extensive expertise in advanced minimally invasive surgical approaches, such as thoracoscopy (VATS) and laparoscopy. He has particular clinical interests in the treatment of lung cancer, esophageal cancer, and benign esophageal diseases with minimally invasive surgery. In addition, Dr. Lee is involved in a clinical trial involving a diaphragmatic pacing system for ventilator-dependent spinal cord injury patients and for patients with ALS/Lou Gehrig's disease.

Christine M. Lennon completed her undergraduate studies at Dartmouth College, and attended medical school at Rutgers New Jersey Medical School. She did her anesthesiology training at Cedars Sinai Medical Center, where she served as co-chief resident. She went on to complete a fellowship in critical care medicine at Northwestern Memorial Hospital. She currently serves as an Assistant Professor of Anesthesiology at New York Presbyterian Hospital/Weill Cornell Medical Center.

Ashleigh Lowery is a clinical pharmacy specialist in the Cardiac Surgery ICU at the University of Maryland Medical Center and a clinical assistant professor for the University of Maryland School of Pharmacy.

Michael D. Maile studied biochemistry at Michigan State University prior to earning his M.D. at Penn State University. Subsequently, he trained in Anesthesiology and Critical Care Medicine at the University of Michigan and accepted a faculty position at this institution upon completion of his residency and fellowship. During his first two years as faculty, he completed a M.S. in Clinical Research

Design & Statistical Analysis from the School of Public Health at the University of Michigan. Dr. Maile is currently the Program Director of the Anesthesiology Critical Care Medicine Fellowship Program and his clinical work involves the cares of adult patients both in the operating room and in the Surgical and Cardiovascular Intensive Care Units. He is engaged in outcomes and translation research with a focus on the etiology and impact of perioperative cardiovascular dysfunction.

Michael Angelo Mazzeffi is a cardio-thoracic anesthesiologist who also practices critical care medicine in the cardiac surgery intensive care unit. HIs research interests include hemostasis and coagulation, outcomes after cardiac surgery, and epidemiology. He currently works as an anesthesiologist and intensivist at the University of Maryland Medical center.

Jeffrey I. Mechanick, Clinical Professor of Medicine and Director, Metabolic Support, Division of Endocrinology, Diabetes and Bone Disease Icahn School of Medicine at Mount Sinai, Past President, American Association of Clinical Endocrinologists; President-Elect, American College of Endocrinology; Editor-in-Chief, President's Council on Fitness, Sports and Nutrition "Elevate Health"; Past President, American Board of Physician Nutrition Specialists; Chancellor, American College of Endocrinology; BS University of Maryland at College Park; MD Mount Sinai School of Medicine Internal Med - Baylor College of Medicine Endocrinology; Fellow - Mount Sinai School of Medicine; 1990-present private practice in endocrinology and metabolic support; >225 publications 6 books research on metabolic support, thyroid cancer, metabolic bone disease, and biomathematics.

Ellen C. Meltzer is an Assistant Attending Physician and an Assistant Professor of Medicine at Weill Cornell Medical College. She is a Fellow of the American College of Physicians. In addition to maintaining an active internal medicine practice at New York Presbyterian Weill Cornell Medical Center, Dr. Meltzer is an Associate Clinical Ethicist. She provides clinical ethics consultation and teaches medical ethics at Weill Cornell Medical College. She is an Assistant Professor of Healthcare Policy and Research and conducts research in novel life-sustaining therapies and their ethical implications. She is a member of the New York Presbyterian Medical Ethics Committee and serves on the Ethics Committee for the New York State Chapter of the American College of Physicians.

Joseph Samuel Meltzer, Associate Professor of Anesthesiology and Critical Care Medicine UCLA.

Michael S. Mulligan is Professor of Surgery at the University of Washington and Director of Lung Transplantation at the University Washington Medical Center. He established and directs a lung transplant research laboratory that has been continuously funded since his arrival to Seattle and has trained more than a dozen research fellows, many of them who have gone on to successful academic careers. Renowned for his teaching abilities, Dr. Mulligan has received the John K. Stevenson Award for Outstanding Teacher in the University Washington Department of Surgery and the prestigious McGoon Award for Outstanding Mentorship in Cardiothoracic Surgery. He has over 200 peer reviewed publications. He has served on the Board of Directors at UNOS and is the current Chair of the Pulmonary Council of the International Society for Heart and Lung Transplantation and the President of the Western Thoracic Surgical Association.

Dave Nagpal, born in Toronto, Ontario, completed his BSc in Physiotherapy at Queen's University in Kingston in 1998, and went on to complete his MD at the University of Western Ontario in 2004. With an interest in healthcare delivery, he completed a Masters of International Health Management, Economics, and Policy at Bocconi University in Milan, Italy in 2007, and interned at the Cardiac Care Network of Ontario in 2007. Following completion of the University of Western Ontario / London Health Sciences Centre cardiac surgery training program in 2010, and the critical care medicine fellowship in 2011, he completed a surgical heart failure fellowship in 2012 at the Cleveland Clinic. He is a fellow of the Royal College of Physicians and Surgeons of Canada with certifications in Cardiac Surgery and Critical Care Medicine, and is currently Assistant Professor in the Divisions of Cardiac Surgery and Critical Care Medicine at the University of Western Ontario / London Health Sciences Centre in London, Ontario.

Michael Nurok, MBChB, PhD, is the Director of the Cardiac-Surgical Intensive Care Unit within the Division of Cardiothoracic Surgery in the Cedars-Sinai Heart Institute – the home of the largest heart transplant program in the world. Dr. Nurok earned his medical degree from the University of Cape Town in South Africa. He completed internships in pediatrics and surgery at Somerset Hospital of the University of Cape Town. At Brigham and Women's Hospital in Boston, Dr. Nurok completed his residency in anesthesia and separate fellowships in critical care medicine, cardiac and thoracic anesthesia. He earned his PhD from the Ecole des Hautes Etudes en Sciences Sociales in Paris with highest honors and completed certificates in clinical effectiveness and value-based healthcare delivery at Harvard University. Prior to joining Cedars-Sinai, he was instrumental in creating the first Intensive Care Unit at the Hospital for Special Surgery in New York, and served as the Unit's first Director.

James Osorio is a faculty member of the department of Anesthesiology at the New York Presbyterian Hospital Weill Cornell Medical College. His clinical practice is a combined practice of Critical Care Medicine in the Cardiothoracic Intensive Care Unit and he practices Cardiac Anesthesiology. During his tenure, he has dedicated much of his time towards student, resident and fellow education. He is currently is the Program Director for the Anesthesiology Critical Care Medicine Fellowship Program, department of Anesthesiology at Weill Cornell. Dr. Osorio is an active member of the Anesthesiology and Critical Care Societies on the regional and national level. He made a number of contributions to the field of Anesthesiology and Critical Care as a society editor, speaker at national conferences as well as faculty member and workshop director at national workshops. He is actively involved in clinical research and is an author of a number of written articles and chapters.

Alexander Papolos is a resident in Internal Medicine at Mount Sinai.

Madhuri Rao is originally from Bangalore, India where she was born, raised and completed her medical education at Kempegowda Institute of Medical Science. She then spent 2 years in England as a Senior House Officer in the National Health Service and completed her Basic Surgical Training through the Mersey Deanery. Dr. Rao passed her membership exams for the Royal College of Surgeons and obtained her M.R.C.S. in 2008. Following that, she decided to pursue further surgical training in the United States. She completed her general surgical residency at SUNY Downstate Medical Center, Brooklyn, NY in 2014 and obtained her board certification in March of 2015. Dr. Rao is currently a fellow in Cardiothoracic Surgery at Mount Sinai Hospital (Icahn School of Medicine at Mount Sinai) in Manhattan, NY.

Bryan Romito, M.D. is an Assistant Professor in the Division of Critical Care Medicine of the Department of Anesthesiology and Pain Management at UT Southwestern Medical Center.

Daniel Rubin, Assistant Professor Department of Anesthesia and Critical Care University of Chicago.

Jennifer Sandadi is an Anesthesiologist who is Board-Certified in Anesthesiology and Critical Care Medicine. Originally from eastern Pennsylvania, she attended the University of Maryland, where she earned two bachelor's degrees – a B.S. in Biology/Neurophysiology and a B.S. in Kinesiology. At Maryland, she was also a full scholarship Division I athlete, and was named an Atlantic Coast Conference Academic Honor Roll student-athlete for four years running. She earned her M.D. at the University of Miami, Miller School of Medicine in 2006. Dr. Sandadi completed her Internship and Residency at Case Medical Center in Cleveland, Ohio. In 2010-11, she was a Fellow at New York-Presbyterian/Columbia University Medical Center, and then joined Weill Cornell Medical College as a faculty member. While focused on providing quality patient care, Dr. Sandadi also engages in clinical research, and has several peer-reviewed publications to her credit. She is a committed and devoted teacher, and in 2013 won the Marjorie Topkins Award, the Weill Cornell Department of Anesthesiology's Teacher of the Year award.

Eric Leo Sarin, Assistant Professor of Surgery Division of Cardiothoracic Surgery Emory University School of Medicine.

Edward Sawey is a senior resident in the Internal Medicine training program at the University of North Carolina. He will be a cardiology fellow at Virginia Commonwealth University and has an interest in cardiac intensive care.

Rifka C. Schulman is an endocrinologist with the Division of Endocrinology, Metabolism and Diabetes of the North Shore LIJ Health System. She is the Director of Inpatient Diabetes at Long Island Jewish Medical Center in New Hyde Park, NY and an assistant professor of the Hofstra North Shore LIJ School of Medicine.

Pranav R. Shah, Fellow, Critical Care Medicine and Adult Cardiothoracic Anesthesiology, Department of Anesthesiology, Vanderbilt University Medical Center.

Andrew Shaw is Professor of Anesthesiology and Chief, Division of Cardiothoracic Anesthesiology at Vanderbilt University Medical Center in Nashville, TN.

Rohit Singal is a cardiac surgeon and intensivist at the University of Manitoba. He is the Surgical Head of the Heart Failure Program with a growing program that ranges in activity from short term mechanical circulatory assistance to implantable left ventricular assist devices. He also manages surgical aspects of arrhythmia management and off-pump coronary artery bypass surgery.

Sheida Tabaie attended the University of Pennsylvania School of Medicine, following which she completed her Anesthesiology Residency at New York Presbyterian-Weill Cornell. She will complete an Adult Anesthesiology Critical Care Fellowship in July, 2015. Her interests include medical ethics and global health.

Christopher Tam is currently an anesthesiology critical care medicine fellow at Weill Cornell medical college. He is a native New Yorker who completed his bachelor degree at the Sophie Davis School of biomedical education; a 7 year combined BS/MD program. He earned his medical degree at the State University of Downstate prior to completing his internship and anesthesiology residency at Stony Brook University Hospital. He has had several publications to his credit including peer reviewed articles and conference presentations. Dr. Tam will begin his fellowship training in cardiothoracic anesthesia at Weill Cornell Medical College starting in July 2015.

Bethany R. Tellor, PharmD, obtained her degree at St. Louis College of Pharmacy. She subsequently completed a two year critical care pharmacy residency at Barnes-Jewish Hospital/Washington University Medical Center. She is currently lead clinical pharmacist for the cardiothoracic surgery intensive care unit at Barnes-Jewish Hospital. She is also an adjunct clinical instructor at St. Louis College of Pharmacy and Goldfarb School of Nursing.

Elrond Teo, MBBS, completed his medical degree at St Bartholomews and the Royal London School of Medicine, University of London. He pursued Anesthesiology training at the University of Vermont and subsequently completed fellowships in Critical Care Medicine and Cardiothoracic Anesthesiology at Columbia University, New York. He is a Fellow of the American Society of Echocardiography and Associated Medical Director of the Cardiothoracic Intensive Care Unit at Emory University Hospital. He manages advanced heart and lung failure in his unit which includes 2nd and 3rd generation continuous flow ventricular assist devices and extracorporeal membrane oxygenation. His interests include the teaching of critical care ultrasound, advanced physiology and anesthesiology to residents, fellows and allied health professionals.

Vinod H. Thourani, MD, received his medical degree from Emory University in Atlanta, Georgia in 1994. He performed his 11 years of postgraduate training at Emory University including general and cardiothoracic clinical surgery training and 3 years of basic science cardiac surgery research. Dr. Thourani joined the faculty of Emory University in 2005 and is currently a Professor of Surgery (Cardiothoracic Surgery) in the Joseph B. Whitehead Department of Surgery. He is also the Chief of Cardiothoracic Surgery at Emory University Hospital Midtown, Co-Director of the Structural Heart and Valve Center, and the Chair of the Executive Committee of CT Surgery Clinical Research Center. He has an active open clinical practice in adult cardiac surgery at Emory University with a concentration in minimally invasive and transcatheter aortic and mitral valve repair and replacement. Dr. Thourani is very active in the cardiac surgical and cardiology societies with a leadership positions in the AATS, ACC, AHA, ISMICS, STS, and the Heart Valve Society. He serves on the editorial boards of *The Annals of Thoracic Surgery, The Journal of Heart Valve Disease, Aging Health, Innovations, and Circulation: Quality and Outcomes*. He has or is in the process of authoring or co-authoring 2 textbooks, 40 book chapters, and has over 200 papers published in peer-reviewed professional journals.

Kei Togashi, from 2005-2008 Dr. Togashi served in the Attending Anesthesiologist Department of Anesthesiology Teikyo University Hospital, Tokyo City, Japan. From 2010-2013 Dr. Togashi was the Acting Instructor Cardiothoracic Anesthesia Division Cardiothoracic Critical Care Division Department of Anesthesiology and Pain Medicine University of Washington, Seattle, WA. Since 2013, Dr. Togashi has been the Assistant Professor Cardiothoracic Anesthesia Division Cardiothoracic Critical Care Division Department of Anesthesiology and Pain Medicine University of Washington, Seattle, WA.

Avery Tung, Professor Department of Anesthesia and Critical Care University of Chicago.

Peter von Homeyer, MD, FASE, completed medical school in Berlin/Germany and did his residency in anesthesiology and fellowship training in cardiothoracic anesthesia and critical care medicine in Münster/Germany. Dr. von Homeyer has been a faculty at the University of Washington since 2008. Dr. von Homeyer is a practicing cardiothoracic anesthesiologist and critical care physician and is co-director of the cardiothoracic ICU at the University of Washington Medical Center.

Zinaida Wadhwani, MD, is a board-certified anesthesiologist. Dr. Wadhwani studied medicine at the New York University School of Medicine, in New York. She completed her Anesthesiology residency followed by Cardiothoracic anesthesia fellowship at the Brigham and Women's Hospital at Harvard Medical School in Boston MA. She is an active member of the Society of Cardiovascular Anesthesiologists. Dr. Wadhwani is a cardiothoracic anesthesiologis at Kaiser Permanente, in San Diego, CA.

Chad Wagner, after receiving his medical degree from the University of Texas Health Science Center in 1998, Dr. Wagner completed an internship in internal medicine in 1999, followed by an anesthesiology residency program at the University of Texas School of Medicine. During his residency, he received the Outstanding Junior Resident award and was a chief resident in his final year. In 2003 he achieved board certification in Anesthesiology. In 2003, he completed a fellowship in Critical Care Anesthesia and subsequently achieved board certification. In addition, he received specialized training in Cardiothoracic Anesthesiology in 2006 and is currently boarded in perioperative echocardiography. Dr. Wagner's focus on Hemodynamic Echocardiography has gained substantial regional and national recognition. In 2011, he was invited to give a presentation at the Tennessee Perfusion Society Annual Meeting. In 2012, he was invited to speak at Vanderbilt University Hospital Respiratory Therapy Spring Seminar to present the Hemodynamic Effects of Mechanical Ventilation. On a national level, Dr. Wagner has given grand rounds at Columbia University Critical Care and Baylor Dallas Anesthesiology Grand Rounds on the topic of Hemodynamic TEE monitoring.

Michael H. Wall, MD, FCCM is currently Professor and Chairman of the Department of Anesthesiology at the University of Minnesota. Dr. Wall is Board Certified in Anesthesiology and Critical Care Medicine, and has practiced in Trauma, Neurosurgical, and Cardiothoracic Intensive Care Units in Military, Veterans Affairs, and University Hospitals. Dr. Wall has held several departmental and hospital leadership positions including Fellowship Director, Chief of Cardiothoracic Anesthesiology, Vice Chairman of Clinical Affairs, and Clinical Chief of Anesthesiology prior to his current position. Dr. Wall has served on the council of the Society of Critical Care Medicine and is currently Chair of the Committee on Critical Care for the American Society of Anesthesiology.

Berhane Worku is an Attending Cardiothoracic Surgeon at New York Methodist Hospital and an Assistant Professor of Cardiothoracic Surgery in the Department of Cardiothoracic Surgery at New York Presbyterian-Weill Cornell Medical Center. Dr. Worku completed his undergraduate studies at Brown University in 1998, obtaining a degree in neuroscience. He pursued his medical education at Harvard Medical School and completed his residency in general surgery at New York University Medical Center. He completed his Cardiothoracic Surgery residency at Weill Cornell Medical Center in 2012 and assumed his present position afterwards. He is a member of several surgical societies, including the Society of Thoracic Surgery. He has published on multiple topics in cardiovascular surgery and presented research at regional and national surgical meetings.

Index

A

B

C

I

J

K

L

M

N

O

P

R

S

T

U

V

W

CPSIA information can be obtained at www.ICGtesting.com
Printed in the USA
BVOW07*0322051015

420620BV00001B/1/P